AF660906

IAP Specialty Series on

PEDIATRIC CARDIOLOGY

IAP Specialty Series on
PEDIATRIC CARDIOLOGY

3rd Edition

Editors

R Krishna Kumar MD DM (Cardio) FAHA
Professor and Head
Department of Pediatric Cardiology
Amrita Institute of Medical Sciences and Research Centre
Amrita Vishwa Vidyapeetham
Kochi, Kerala, India

Shakuntala S Prabhu MD FRCPCH (UK)
Medical Director and Professor
Division of Pediatric Cardiology
Department of Pediatrics
Bai Jerbai Wadia Hospital for Children
Mumbai, Maharashtra, India

Sumitra Venkatesh DNB (Ped) DCH
Head, Division of Pediatric Cardiology
Associate Professor in Pediatric Medicine
Bai Jerbai Wadia Hospital for Children
Mumbai, Maharashtra, India

Shreepal Jain MD FNB (Ped Cardio)
Consultant Pediatric Interventional and
Fetal Cardiologist
Bai Jerbai Wadia Hospital for Children
Mumbai, Maharashtra, India

M Zulfikar Ahamed MD DM
Senior Consultant in Pediatric Cardiology
KIMS Health, Anayara, Thiruvananthapuram
Former Professor and Head, Pediatric Cardiology
Government Medical College
Thiruvananthapuram, Kerala, India

Foreword
Nitin K Shah

JAYPEE

JAYPEE BROTHERS MEDICAL PUBLISHERS
The Health Sciences Publisher
New Delhi | London

Jaypee Brothers Medical Publishers (P) Ltd

Headquarters
Jaypee Brothers Medical Publishers (P) Ltd
EMCA House, 23/23-B
Ansari Road, Daryaganj
New Delhi 110 002, India
Landline: +91-11-23272143, +91-11-23272703
+91-11-23282021, +91-11-23245672
Email: jaypee@jaypeebrothers.com

Corporate Office
Jaypee Brothers Medical Publishers (P) Ltd
4838/24, Ansari Road, Daryaganj
New Delhi 110 002, India
Phone: +91-11-43574357
Fax: +91-11-43574314
Email: jaypee@jaypeebrothers.com

Overseas Office
JP Medical Ltd
83 Victoria Street, London
SW1H 0HW (UK)
Phone: +44 20 3170 8910
Fax: +44 (0)20 3008 6180
Email: info@jpmedpub.com

Website: www.jaypeebrothers.com
Website: www.jaypeedigital.com

IAP Specialty Series on Pediatric Cardiology

Third Edition: **2022**

Second Edition: 2013

First Edition: 2008

ISBN: 978-93-90595-14-3

Printed at: Sterling Graphics Pvt. Ltd.

Dedication

This book is dedicated to our patients,
who with their tender ailing hearts,
have taught us everything.

Contributors

Alice Neetha MPharm
Tutor and Clinical Pharmacist
Department of Pediatric Cardiology
Amrita Institute of Medical Sciences and Research Centre
Amrita Vishwa Vidyapeetham
Kochi, Kerala, India

Alpana Ohri MD DNB FISPN
Associate Professor
Department of Pediatrics
In-Charge, Division of Pediatric Nephrology
Bai Jerbai Wadia Hospital for Children
Consultant, Pediatric Nephrology
Jaslok Hospital
Mumbai, Maharashtra, India

Anand Subramanian DM
Associate Professor
Department of Pediatric Cardiology
Sri Jayadeva Institute of Cardiovascular Sciences and Research
Bengaluru, Karnataka, India

Anil Kumar Singhi
MD (Ped) FNB (Ped Card) Fellow Cardiology CHW (Sydney)
Senior Consultant and Interventional Cardiologist
Specialist in Pediatric Congenital and Structural Heart Disease
Medica Superspecialty Hospital
Kolkata, West Bengal, India

Anita Saxena MD DM
Dean (Academics)
Chief, Cardio-thoracic Center
Head, Department of Cardiology
All India Institute of Medical Sciences
New Delhi, India

Annu Jose MD DM (Ped Card)
Associate Consultant
Pediatric Cardiology
Lisie Hospital
Kochi, Kerala, India

Arun Gopalakrishnan
MD (Ped) DM (Cardio)
Associate Professor
Department of Cardiology
Division of Pediatric Cardiology
Sree Chitra Tirunal Institute for Medical Sciences and Technology
Thiruvananthapuram, Kerala India

Balaganesh Karmegaraj MD (Ped) DM (Ped Cardio)
Clinical Assistant Professor
Department of Pediatric Cardiology
Amrita Institute of Medical Sciences and Research Centre
Amrita Vishwa Vidyapeetham
Kochi, Kerala, India

Balaji Srimurugan MS MCh (CVTS) FPCS
Assistant Professor
Department of Pediatric Cardiac Surgery
Amrita Institute of Medical Sciences and Research Centre
Amrita Vishwa Vidyapeetham
Kochi, Kerala, India

Balu Vaidyanathan
MD DNB (Ped) DM (Cardio)
Clinical Professor
Department of Pediatric Cardiology
Head, Fetal Cardiology Division
Amrita Institute of Medical Sciences and Research Centre
Amrita Vishwa Vidyapeetham
Kochi, Kerala, India

Bharat Dalvi MD DM FACC FPICS
Consultant Cardiologist
Glenmark Cardiac Centre
Mumbai, Maharashtra, India

Biswa Panda
MCh (Cardiothoracic Surgery) Fellowship (Pediatric Cardiac Surgery)
Head
Department of Pediatric Cardiac Surgery
Bai Jerbai Wadia Hospital for Children
Mumbai, Maharashtra, India

Dhanya Yesodharan MD (Ped)
Associate Professor
Department of Pediatric Genetics
Amrita Institute of Medical Sciences and Research Centre
Amrita Vishwa Vidyapeetham
Kochi, Kerala, India

Diane E Spicer PA (ASCP) CM
Pathologist's Assistant
Heart Institute
Johns Hopkins All Children's Hospital
St Petersburg, Florida, USA

Edwin Francis MD DM
Chief Pediatric Cardiologist
Department of Pediatric Cardiology
Lisie Hospital
Kochi, Kerala, India

Harikrishnan KN MD (Ped) DM (Cardio)
Assistant Professor
Department of Cardiology
Sree Chitra Tirunal Institute for Medical Sciences and Technology
Thiruvananthapuram, Kerala, India

Jayashree Mishra
MD (Peds) FNB Pediatric Cardiology
Consultant Pediatric Cardiologist
Bai Jerbai Wadia Hospital for Children
Mumbai, Maharashtra, India

John Valliattu MS FRCS
Chief of Cardiothoracic Surgery and Senior Consultant Pediatric Cardiac Surgeon
Believers International Heart Centre
Believers Church Medical College Hospital
Thiruvalla, Kerala, India

K Sivakumar MD DCH DNB (Ped) DM (Cardio) DNB (Cardio)
Head
Department of Pediatric Cardiology
Senior Consultant, Institute of Cardiovascular Diseases
The Madras Medical Mission
Chennai, Tamil Nadu, India

KS Remadevi MD (Ped) FNB (Ped Cardio)
Senior Consultant
Department of Pediatric Cardiology
Aster Malabar Institute of Medical Sciences (MIMS)
Calicut, Kerala, India

M Jayranganath DM
Professor and Head
Department of Pediatric Cardiology
Sri Jayadeva Institute of Cardiovascular Sciences and Research
Bengaluru, Karnataka, India

M Zulfikar Ahamed MD DM
Senior Consultant in Pediatric Cardiology
KIMS Health, Anayara, Thiruvananthapuram
Former Professor and Head
Pediatric Cardiology
Government Medical College
Thiruvananthapuram, Kerala, India

Mahesh Kappanayil
DCH DNB (Ped) FNB (Ped Cardio)
Professor
Department of Pediatric Cardiology
Amrita Institute of Medical Sciences and Research Centre
Amrita Vishwa Vidyapeetham
Kochi, Kerala, India

Mani Ram Krishna
DNB (Ped) FNB (Ped Cardio)
Consultant Pediatric and Fetal Cardiologist
Tiny Hearts Fetal and Pediatric Cardiac Clinic
RK Hospital for Women and Children
Thanjavur, Tamil Nadu, India

Manu Raj
DCH DNB (Ped) MSc (Health Research Methodology)
Professor and Senior Consultant
Divisions of Pediatrics
Pediatric Cardiology and Health Sciences Research
Amrita Institute of Medical Sciences and Research Centre
Amrita Vishwa Vidyapeetham
Kochi, Kerala, India

MK Usha MD FPC
Associate Professor
Department of Pediatric Cardiology
Sri Jayadeva Institute of Cardiovascular Sciences and Research
Bengaluru, Karnataka, India

Munesh Tomar MD FNB FACC
Consultant Pediatric Cardiologist
Department of Pediatrics
LLRM Medical College
Meerut, Uttar Pradesh, India

Nageswara Rao Koneti MD DM
Chief Pediatric Cardiologist
Rainbow Children's Heart Institute
Hyderabad, Telangana, India

Navaneetha Sasikumar
MD (Ped) DM (Cardio) FACC
Consultant
Department of Pediatric Cardiology
Meditrina Hospital
Kollam, Kerala, India

Nikhil Thatte MBBS
Senior Fellow in Interventional Cardiology
Children's Hospital and Harvard Medical School
Boston, Massachusetts, USA

Nitin Rao MD DNB (Ped) DM DNB (Cardio)
Consultant Pediatric Cardiologist
Department of Pediatric Cardiology
Star Hospitals
Hyderabad, Telangana, India

Prashant Bobhate
MD (Ped) FNB (Ped Cardio)
Consultant
Children's Heart Centre
Kokilaben Dhirubhai Ambani Hospital
Mumbai, Maharashtra, India

Praveen Kumar K
Echocardiography (Cert) (Dip) MBA
Chief Cardiac Sonographer
Hands on Heart (Pediatric Cardiology Group)
RxDx and Teleradiology Solutions
Bengaluru, Karnataka, India

Preeti Ramachandran MD FACC FSCCT
Assistant Professor
Division of Pediatric Cardiology
Department of Pediatrics
University of Kentucky - Kentucky Children's Hospital
Lexington, Kentucky, USA

Priyankar Pal MD
Professor and Head
Department of Pediatric Rheumatology
Institute of Child Health, Kolkata
Past President, Paediatric Rheumatology Society
Hony Secretary of Kawasaki Disease Society

R Krishna Kumar MD DM (Cardio) FAHA
Professor and Head
Department of Pediatric Cardiology
Amrita Institute of Medical Sciences and Research Centre
Amrita Vishwa Vidyapeetham
Kochi, Kerala, India

R Suresh Kumar MD DM FSCAI
Senior Consultant
Department of Pediatric Cardiology and Adult Congenital Heart Disease
Believers International Heart Centre
Believers Church Medical College Hospital
Thiruvalla, Kerala, India

Raghavan Subramanyan
MD DM FRCPI FSCAI FCSI
Honorary Senior Consultant
Former Head
Department of Cardiology
Frontier Lifeline Hospital
Chennai, Tamil Nadu, India

Renu P Kurup
MBBS DCH DNB (Ped) FNB (Ped Cardio)
Senior Consultant and Head
Department of Pediatric Cardiology
Malabar Institute of Medical Sciences (MIMS)
Calicut, Kerala, India

Ritchie Sharon Solomon MD DCH DM
Assistant Professor
Department of Pediatric Cardiology
Institute of Child Health and Hospital for Children
Chennai, Tamil Nadu, India

Robert Anderson MD
Professor
Newcastle University
Newcastle upon Tyne, UK

Rohit S Loomba MD
Assistant Professor
Advocate Children's Hospital
Chicago Medical School
Chicago, Illinois, USA

Saileela Rajan
MD (Ped) DNB (Ped) FNB (Ped Cardio)
Consultant
Pediatric Cardiologist
MIOT Centre for Children's Cardiac Care
MIOT Hospitals
Chennai, Tamil Nadu, India

Saji Philip
MBBS DCH (CMC), F.CARD (Ped) PhD (Cardio) FAAP FAHA
Fetal and Pediatric Cardiologist
Founder President
KD Foundation and Indian Society of Kawasaki Disease
Tiruvalla Medical Mission
Thiruvalla, Kerala, India

Sakshi Sachdeva MD DNB FNB DM
Senior Resident
Department of Cardiology
All India Institute of Medical Sciences
New Delhi, India

Sangeetha Viswanathan
MRCPCH (UK) CCST UK (Ped Cardio)
Consultant Interventional Pediatric and Congenital Cardiologist
Department of Pediatrics
Medcare Hospital
Dubai, UAE

Sanjeev H Naganur MD DM
Associate Professor
Department of Cardiology
Postgraduate Institute of Medical Education and Research
Chandigarh, India

Saurabh Kumar Gupta MD DM
Additional Professor
Department of Cardiology
All India Institute of Medical Sciences
New Delhi, India

Sejal Shah
MD (Ped) Fellowship in Pediatric Cardiology
Senior Pediatric and Fetal Cardiologist
Hands on Heart (Pediatric Cardiology Group)
RxDx and Teleradiology Solutions
Bengaluru, Karnataka, India

Shakuntala S Prabhu MD FRCPCH (UK)
Medical Director and Professor
Division of Pediatric Cardiology
Department of Pediatrics
Bai Jerbai Wadia Hospital for Children
Mumbai, Maharashtra, India

Sheela Nampoothiri
DCH DNB (Ped) MSc Medical Genetics (Glasgow)
Clinical Professor
Department of Pediatric Genetics
Amrita Institute of Medical Sciences and Research Centre
Amrita Vishwa Vidyapeetham
Kochi, Kerala, India

Shilpa Kulkarni
MD DCH DNB MNAMS Fellowship in Pediatric Neurology
Additional Professor
In-Charge, Division of Neurosciences
Bai Jerbai Wadia Hospital For Children
Mumbai, Maharashtra, India

Shine Kumar KH
DCH DNB (Ped) FNB (Ped Cardio)
Associate Professor
Department of Pediatric Cardiology
Amrita Institute of Medical Sciences and Research Centre
Amrita Vishwa Vidyapeetham
Kochi, Kerala, India

Shreepal Jain MD FNB (Ped Cardio)
Consultant Pediatric Interventional and Fetal Cardiologist
Bai Jerbai Wadia Hospital for Children
Mumbai, Maharashtra, India

Shweta Bakhru DNB (Ped) FNB (Ped Cardio)
Pediatric Cardiologist
Rainbow Children Heart Institute
Hyderabad, Telangana, India

Snehal Kulkarni MD DNB (Cardio) FACC
Chief Cardiologist
Sri Satya Sai Sanjeevani Hospitals
Navi Mumbai
Chief of Cardiovascular Sciences
Bai Jerbai Wadia Hospital for Children
Mumbai, Maharashtra, India

Sonam Kothari
MD PhD (Pediatric Neurology)
Consultant in Pediatric Neurology
Bai Jerbai Wadia Hospital for Children
Mumbai, Maharashtra, India

Sudeep Verma MD (Ped) FNB (Ped Cardio)
Consultant Pediatric Cardiologist
Krishna Institute of Medical Sciences (KIMS) Hospital
Secunderabad, Telangana, India

Suman Vyas MD DNB (Cardio)
Consultant Pediatric Cardiologist
Department of Pediatric Cardiology
Star Hospitals
Hyderabad, Telangana, India

Sumitra Venkatesh DNB (Ped) DCH
Head, Division of Pediatric Cardiology
Associate Professor in Pediatric Medicine
Bai Jerbai Wadia Hospital for Children
Mumbai, Maharashtra, India

Sunita Maheshwari ABP ABPC
Senior Pediatric Cardiologist
Hands on Heart (Pediatric Cardiology Group)
RxDx and Teleradiology Solutions
Bengaluru, Karnataka, India

Surjit Singh
MD DCH (Lon) FRCP (Lon) FRCPCH (Lon) FAMS; Fellowship in Pediatric Immunology (Lon) FIAP FICAAI
Head
Department of Pediatrics
Chief
Allergy Immunology Unit
Advanced Pediatrics Centre
Principal Investigator, ICMR Centre for Advanced Research in Primary Immunodeficiency Diseases
Postgraduate Institute of Medical Education and Research
Chandigarh, India

Sushil Azad MD FNB (Ped Cardio)
Principal Consultant
Department of Pediatric Cardiology
Fortis Escorts Heart Institute
New Delhi, India

Swati Garekar
American Board Certified (Ped Cardio)
Consultant, Pediatric Cardiology
Division of Pediatric Cardiology
Fortis Hospital
Mumbai, Maharashtra, India

Tanuja Karande
MBBS DNB (Ped) FNB (Ped Cardio)
Consultant
Pediatric Cardiologist
Kokilaben Dhirubhai Ambani Hospital
Mumbai, Maharashtra, India

Vasu Gooty MD
Assistant Professor
Division of Pediatric Cardiology
LeBonheur Children's Hospital
University of Tennessee Health Sciences
Memphis, Tennessee, USA

Vejendla Gouthami MD (Med) DM (Cardio)
Consultant Pediatric Cardiologist
Krishna Institute of Medical Sciences (KIMS) Hospital
Secunderabad, Telangana, India

Vishal Singh
DCH MD DNB (Ped) Fellowship in Pediatric Cardiac Critical Care
Senior Consultant Pediatric Cardiac Critical Care
Indraprastha Apollo Hospital
New Delhi, India

Foreword

Dramatic advancements have transformed the outlook of children with heart disease world over. Until the late 70s, most neonates and many infants with congenital heart defects would die prematurely or live an extremely restricted life constrained by their poor physical condition. Today, a newborn with transposition can have a near normal life expectancy after a neonatal arterial switch operation.

Though the speciality of pediatric cardiology was initially slow to develop in India, the outlook of children with heart disease progressively improved with the establishment of several new comprehensive pediatric cardiac programs in the country over the past 3 decades. The quality of care and outcomes have also improved significantly and Indian centers are now able to deliver outcomes at par with international centers, with few centers being well-established destinations for children from other countries too.

However, there are several unmet challenges of children with heart disease in India and other low- and middle-income countries (LMICs). Rheumatic heart disease may have declined in selected regions of the country but the overall burden is substantial and many children in poorly served regions are affected with devastating consequences. Congenital heart defects have begun to surface as a significant health problem among infants and newborns in several regions of the country that are now witnessing a rapid and substantial declining trend in infant mortality rates (owing to reduction in mortality by communicable diseases). Myocarditis, cardiomyopathy and Kawasaki diseases are all increasingly being recognized. In the current pandemic, COVID-19 can present in children with MIS-C that can present as Kawasaki like illness in small children and with myocarditis in older children. Childhood obesity and hypertension are assuming epidemic proportions, particularly in urban settings and will contribute to the growing burden of adult cardiovascular disease.

It is very essential for postgraduate students and practicing pediatricians to familiarize themselves with the nuances of modern pediatric cardiac care. Hence, there is a strong need for a textbook that is specifically written for the LMIC context. This book from India will serve as an accessible reference book for postgraduate students in pediatrics and practicing pediatricians looking after children with heart disease. It is also well suited for prospective candidates seeking to specialize in pediatric cardiology.

There have been two previous editions of this book in 2008 and 2013. This third edition is greatly expanded and has been rewritten completely to keep pace with the rapid and dramatic advancements in the field. The collaboration and contribution by a number of expert pediatric cardiologists, pediatric cardiac surgeons and intensivists from India and overseas has ensured the highest possible quality. The book is reorganized into convenient sections and every facet of pediatric cardiac care has been covered. Despite being comprehensive, the book is written in an easily readable style, keeping in mind the diversity of readers. Several illustrations, flowcharts, tables and boxes allow for easy understanding and assimilation of information. There are important new chapters on screening for congenital heart disease, counseling of families, fetal cardiology and intensive care. Individual congenital heart defects are dealt with in greater detail and 20 chapters have been exclusively assigned to them.

I am quite certain that like with the previous two editions, this edition too will be abundantly useful as a reference book for postgraduates and practicing pediatricians, and a comprehensive textbook for all those who are aspiring to become pediatric cardiologists.

Nitin K Shah
Section Head, Pediatrics, PD Hinduja Hospital, Mumbai
Hon Hematologist Oncologist, BJ Wadia Hospital for Children, Mumbai
Fellow and Past President, Indian Academy of Pediatrics
Founder Editor, IAP Specialty Series Books 2006

Preface to the Third Edition

The Indian Academy of Pediatrics (IAP) specialty series in Pediatric Cardiology seeks to provide a comprehensive working knowledge of pediatric cardiac care to a broad audience that includes postgraduate students, practicing pediatricians and pediatric cardiac professionals. The first edition was published in 2008 and the second in 2013. The advancement of Pediatric Cardiology in India has been impressive, particularly in the past decade. We now have several new centers, offering comprehensive pediatric cardiac care and the outlook of children with heart disease have improved dramatically in many parts of the country. There are now dedicated government sponsored programs that seek to provide assistance to children with heart disease. Notable among these is the Hridyam program in the state of Kerala. Hridyam has contributed to marked reductions in deaths due to pediatric heart disease as a result of which there has been a significant decline in the infant mortality rate to single digit levels in the state.

Recognizing the need for a thoroughly revised content, the 3rd edition of this textbook has been entirely re-written from scratch. The book harnesses the collective expertise of a number of pediatric cardiac experts in the country, many of whom are experienced teachers in leading academic institutions. The content has been completely re-organized and greatly expanded. There are 55 chapters in total. Several new chapters have been added to this edition. These include chapters on screening, counseling of parents, pediatric cardiac intensive care and common problems in office practice.

The first section is devoted to foundations that includes chapters on epidemiology and disease burden, anatomy, embryology and physiology. This is followed by sections on diagnostic tools, which include chapters on clinical evaluation, ECG, chest X-ray, echocardiography and advanced imaging modalities such as CT and MRI. A new chapter on screening of congenital heart disease has also been added here. The section on therapeutic tools has chapters on pharmacology, intensive care, catheter interventions, cardiac surgery, and counseling of parents.

The section on cardiovascular disease begins with common medical issues such as heart failure, pulmonary hypertension and syncope, followed by a detailed section on congenital heart disease. An elaborate introduction seeks to unravel essential concepts, that is followed by 20 chapters devoted to individual conditions. The section on acquired heart disease has been substantially expanded with chapters on infective endocarditis, myocarditis, rheumatic fever and rheumatic heart disease, Kawasaki disease and cardiomyopathy. A number of important issues that include fetal cardiology, neonatal heart disease, lifestyle related conditions and rhythm disorders are devoted to the final section.

It is our fervent hope that this endeavor will serve the needs of all pediatricians who care for children with heart disease as well as the postgraduate students seeking to strengthen their knowledge base in this exciting and challenging specialty.

R Krishna Kumar
Shakuntala S Prabhu
Shreepal Jain
Sumitra Venkatesh
M Zulfikar Ahamed

Preface to the First Edition

Impressive advances have occurred in Pediatric cardiac care in India over the last decade. Several new programs have been established and the quality of care has progressively improved. Infant heart surgery is now becoming increasingly available in many Indian centers. Pediatric cardiology is now recognized as a distinct subspecialty and dedicated fellowship training programs have been initiated in selected centers in India. However, several challenges continue to exist. The number of centers is not enough to take care of the number of affected children and cost of care continues to be prohibitive for the average Indian family. Large parts of India still do not have access to pediatric heart care because there are no centers even in many larger states. Most postgraduate training programs in India are in centers which do not offer specialized pediatric cardiac services. As a result the average Indian pediatric postgraduate trainee receives very little systematic exposure in pediatric cardiology.

While it is absolutely clear that early recognition and timely intervention is the key to successful outcome of children with heart disease, the average pediatrician in India has limited opportunities to improve his/her understanding in diagnosis of pediatric heart disease. This book attempts to bridge this gap and aims to provide basic information required for a practising pediatrician and a postgraduate student in pediatrics. The entire text throws light on clinical approach and seeks to examine relatively common problems encountered by practising pediatricians. The text begins with the diagnostic tools required to identify heart disease and the chapters include clinical examination, X-ray, ECG, echocardiography and diagnostic catheterization. Common clinical problems such as chest pain, syncope and arrhythmias are dealt with in the next set of chapters. Congenital heart diseases are described under conventional categories. Specific congenital heart conditions are not dealt with in great detail and readers will need to refer to comprehensive textbooks for details on individual conditions. Acquired conditions such as rheumatic fever, Kawasaki disease, myocardial and pericardial diseases and endocarditis are all described in separate chapters. The final set of chapters includes a variety of special issues relating to pediatric heart care. A chapter on Follow-up of children following Cardiac Surgery and Percutaneous Interventions is specifically included.

We thank all contributors who made this book possible and the Indian Academy of Pediatrics for giving us the opportunity to write this textbook. We also wish to specially acknowledge the editorial assistance of Dr Sumitra Venkatesh and Dr BRJ Kannan. Given the fact that this is the first edition, we recognize that there will be considerable scope for improvement. We sincerely solicit feedback from our readers. We would use them to improve the quality of next edition.

R Krishna Kumar
Shakuntala S Prabhu
M Zulfikar Ahamed

Acknowledgments

We wish to thank the Indian Academy of Pediatrics for the opportunity to contribute significantly to educating of the current and the next generation of caregivers of children with heart disease.

We wish to acknowledge the assistance from all the members of the Pediatric Cardiac Program at Amrita Institute of Medical Sciences and Research Centre who have helped write many chapters. Additionally, many of the resident staff have proof read several chapters at various stages.

We acknowledge Dr Minnie Bodhanwala, Chief Executive Officer, BJ Wadia Hospital for Children for her constant support and encouragement.

We acknowledge the strong support of our family members who have stood by us through the thick and thin of our professional life and withstood the challenges that resulted from precious family-time being devoted to this book. We must also express our deep and heartfelt gratitude to our patients and their families for giving us the opportunity to trust us with their health and the opportunity to serve and learn from them.

We are extremely thankful to Shri Jitendar P Vij (Group Chairman), Mr Ankit Vij (Managing Director), Mr MS Mani (Group President), Ms Chetna Malhotra Vohra (Associate Director—Content Strategy), Ms Pooja Bhandari (Production Head), and Dr Rajul Jain (Senior Development Editor) of M/s Jaypee Brothers Medical Publishers (P) Ltd, New Delhi, India, for giving the go-ahead at the very beginning and helping us in every way possible to bring out this book.

Contents

PART 1
PEDIATRIC CARDIOLOGY FOUNDATIONS

SECTION 1 INTRODUCTION TO THE SPECIALTY OF PEDIATRIC CARDIOLOGY

SECTION 2 FUNDAMENTALS OF PEDIATRIC CARDIOLOGY

SECTION 3 DIAGNOSTIC TOOLS

SECTION 4 THERAPEUTIC TOOLS

SECTION 8 OTHERS

SECTION 9 MISCELLANEOUS

SECTION 10 CARDIOVASCULAR INVOLVEMENT IN OTHER SYSTEM DISORDERS

1

PART

Pediatric Cardiology Foundations

1 CHAPTER

Epidemiology and Burden of Pediatric Heart Disease in India

Anita Saxena, Sakshi Sachdeva

INTRODUCTION

Congenital heart diseases (CHDs) are the most common birth defects. Given the high birth rate in India, the number of children born with CHDs is also very high, approximating to a quarter million every year. Many of these children need early treatment (usually within initial days to months of life), but there is an inadequate reach, both for diagnosis and treatment. Additionally, at least 21% of the deliveries in India still happen at home and many neonates die even before they are diagnosed to have CHD. The institutional infrastructure, human, and material resources required to deliver quality pediatric cardiac diagnosis and care require substantial investments. The patients with simple or mild CHDs survive without any significant worsening in quality of life. Rarely, the natural survivors of critical CHDs also survive till late childhood but at the cost of worsened quality of life. Neonatal and infantile cardiac surgeries are among the most resource-intensive endeavors in medicine. The ability to carry out successful neonatal surgeries defines the quality of a pediatric cardiac care program. It requires a team of dedicated specialists along with huge infrastructure investments.

Added to the burden of CHD is rheumatic heart disease (RHD), which remains a global health problem in many low-income and middle-income countries including India. A large number of children suffer from RHD in the very same regions where facilities for diagnosis and treatment are sparse or unavailable. An important road-block in the field is the unequal regional distribution of centers. The centers are clustered around the metropolitan cities in the country. There are very few centers in the most densely populated Eastern states which have the highest need due to their high birth rates. Although the government is taking multiple steps to improve pediatric cardiac care in the country, it is imperative to increase aware-ness among pediatricians and primary care physicians, who are the first point-of-contact for newborns and children to facilitate appropriate assessment and timely referral for better outcome. This chapter focuses on the unique challenges faced by our country in delivering pediatric cardiac care, the solutions to overcome them, and also the progress that we have made in the country.

EPIDEMIOLOGY OF CONGENITAL HEART DISEASE

Congenital heart diseases are the most common birth defects, accounting for almost 28% of all congenital defects.[1] At birth, the prevalence of CHD is 8–12/1,000 live births, although in a recent study, the prevalence was noted to be 16.8/1,000 live births in South-East Asia.[2-4] Considering a rate of 9/1,000, almost 1.35 million babies are born with CHD globally each year.[5] Extrapolating these figures to India, the estimated number of children born with CHD is approximately 200,000 to 240,000 annually.[6] Even this may be an underestimation as nearly 21% births in our country are home deliveries.[7] This poses a tremendous challenge for families, society, and the health care system.

Critical CHDs are those which require intervention within the first year of life. The birth prevalence of severe CHDs has been reported as 1.5–1.7/1,000 live births.[8,9] In low- and middle-income countries such as India, where a substantial proportion of births occur at home, hospital-based data is invariably subject to sampling bias and unlikely to be representative of community settings.[10-15] Critical CHD, especially duct-dependent lesions, may go undiagnosed in such settings. Profile of patients reaching health care facility is determined by the natural history of individual lesions.

The prevalence or true incidence of CHDs has been reported from a few studies which only included the in-hospital births and varies depending upon the screening modality used. If only clinical examination is used for screening, the prevalence is minimum (3.9/1,000 live births) compared to when echocardiography is used in association with pulse oximetry (8.1/1,000 live births).[6,16-18] Beyond neonatal age, the reported prevalence of CHD during childhood varies from 1.3 to 9.2/1,000 population, again depending upon the screening modality used.[19-27] CHD caused 26,000 deaths globally in 2017, a 34.5% decline from 1990, with 180,000

TABLE 1: Birth prevalence of congenital heart disease (CHD) in India.

Author	*Number screened*	*Method*	*Prevalence per 1,000 live births*
Khalil et al.[16]	10,964	Clinical examination	3.9
Vaidyanathan et al.[17]	5,487	Clinical examination, pulse oximetry, echocardiography in all cases	Minor CHD 74.4 at birth 21.7 at 6 weeks; Major CHD 3.1
Sawant et al.[18]	2,636	Clinical examination, echocardiography in suspected	13.3
Saxena et al.[6]	20,307	Clinical examination, pulse oximetry, echocardiography in all cases	Significant CHD: 8.1

TABLE 2: Prevalence of congenital heart disease in India beyond neonatal age.

Author and study setting	*Age group (y)*	*N*	*Screening method*	*Prevalence per 1,000*
Gupta et al., 1992, community[19]	6–16	10,263	Clinical	0.8
Vashishtha et al., 1993, School[20]	5–15	8,449	Clinical	5.2
Thakur et al., 1995, School[21]	5–16	15,080	Clinical	2.2
Chadha et al., 2001, Community[22]	<15	11,833	Clinical	4.2
Misra et al., 2009, School[23]	4–18	118,212	Clinical, echo for suspected cases	1.3
Kumari et al., 2013, School[24]	5–16	4,213	Clinical and echo in all	9.2
Saxena et al., 2013, School[25]	5–15	14,716	Clinical and echo in all	2.3
Bhardwaj et al., 2016, Community[26]	Up to 19.5	1,882	Clinical, echo for suspected cases	6.3
Nisale et al., 2016, School[27]	1st to 10th class	353,761	Clinical, echo for suspected cases	0.4

deaths in infancy.[4] **Table 1** describes the birth prevalence of CHD in India and **Table 2** lists similar information beyond the neonatal period, mostly in school-age children.

EPIDEMIOLOGY OF RHEUMATIC FEVER AND RHEUMATIC HEART DISEASE

Rheumatic heart disease results from valvular damage caused by acute rheumatic fever (RF) which is an autoimmune response to group A beta hemolytic streptococci (GAS). RF commonly occurs among children and adolescents between the ages of 5 and 15 years, due to the higher incidence of streptococcal pharyngitis in school-aged children.[28] Peak incidence is around 8–9 years of age. According to the studies from last decade, global incidence of RF as measured in school-going children aged 5–14 years varies from as low as 1.25 per 100,000 (in most high-income countries) to as high as 194 per 100,000 annually.[29] Kumar et al. have reported the incidence of RF as 8.7/100,000 in 5–14-year school-aged children in a prospective surveillance in a specific region of North India.[30] Rheumatic fever occurs at a relatively younger age in India, affecting children even as young as 3 years. The incidence of carditis in the children from Indian subcontinent is also higher during an episode of RF. Further, the disease progresses very rapidly with a malignant course and may produce severe mitral stenosis at a very young age.[31] The reason for this accelerated course of the disease is not very clear and may be either due to a genetic predisposition or due to recurrent attacks of RF as secondary prophylaxis is generally inadequate. In general, the aggressive forms of RF and RHD involving young children is largely limited to regions with a high disease prevalence. There is a great deal of variability within India and there are parts of India that are no different from high-income countries and there are also regions that quite mimic the poorest nations of the world.

The prevalence of RHD has ranged from 1.8 to 11/1,000 children (average 6/1,000) in 1970s and 1980s.[32] Studies conducted in the 1990s showed a relatively lower prevalence of 1–3.9/1,000 children.[33,34] Prevalence of 0.5/1,000 children was reported from Gorakhpur (UP) in 2007 and 0.67/1,000 from Vellore and Bikaner.[35-37] The ability to detect murmurs and differentiating functional from pathological murmurs depends on clinical skills of the examining physician and the settings of auscultation. Hence, auscultation-based methods of screening have limited sensitivity and specificity.[38] Echocardiographic studies have shown a 10 times higher prevalence of RHD as compared to prevalence on clinical evaluation alone.[39] The echocardiographic data from a single center study of children aged 5–15 years, showed a prevalence of 20.4/1,000 as compared to 0.8/1,000 by clinical evaluation.[40] However, a multicentric study from India, published at a later date, used standardized World Heart Federation Criteria of 1992 and showed a prevalence of 7.7/1,000 as compared to 0.36/1,000 by clinical evaluation.[41]

There is a declining interest of physicians and cardiologists toward RHD as they believe its incidence is reducing. The number of research publications related to RF or RHD had also greatly reduced over the past 40 years. Last decade however has seen increasing number of publications, mainly related to echocardiographic diagnosis. Some data from India does suggest a declining prevalence; however, the incidence continues to remain high in a number of states with lower levels of human development. According to a study published from Shimla region in Himachal Pradesh, there has been reduction in the prevalence of RHD in school-aged children (5–15 years) from 4.8/1,000 in 1993 to 0.59/1,000 in 2008.[42,43]

A significant proportion of RHD patients in India present at an advanced stage of the disease contributing to high mortality. In 2015, there was 8% global reduction in mortality due to RHD, compared to 1990 statistics. However, in the same year, the maximal mortality world-over, occurred in India with 119,000 deaths.[44] Short-term results from a tertiary hospital-based registry data on children <18 years with RF/RHD showed 3% mortality in just 11 months of follow-up.[45] The cause of death included progressive congestive heart failure in unoperated patients and mechanical valve thrombosis in those with mechanical heart valves.

CURRENT STATUS OF PEDIATRIC CARDIAC CARE IN INDIA

There is a great disparity that exists as far as care for children with CHD is concerned, when we compare the high-income countries with low- and middle-income countries. There is one cardiac center catering to a population of 120,000 in North America, whereas 16 million population is served by one cardiac center in Asia.[46,47] Cardiac surgeons form the backbone of any pediatric cardiac care program. There is one cardiac surgeon per 3.5 million population in North America and Europe, as compared to one per 25 million in Asia,[3] emphasizing that there is a huge deficit of infrastructure, medical professionals, and paramedical staff in our part of the world.

A number of cardiac centers have been established in India over the past two decades. Approximately one-sixth of these are high volume centers, carrying out at least 500 cardiac surgeries a year.[46] In the year 2016-2017, approximately 27,000 CHD surgeries were carried out in the country. Of these, 9,700 were infant cardiac surgeries and 1,700 were neonatal cardiac surgeries. Considering the birth prevalence of serious CHD requiring intervention in first year of life to be 1.6/1,000 live births, approximately 43,000 babies are born with serious CHD in India each year, of which only one-fourth seem to be receiving optimal cardiac care. This proportion is much better compared to what it was a decade ago,[48,49] suggesting that the pediatric cardiac care in the country is steadily improving.

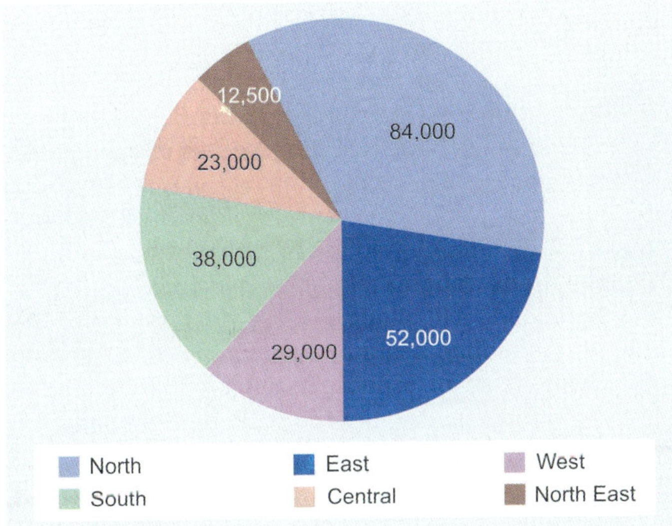

Fig. 1: Regional distribution of infants born with congenital heart disease (CHD) in India.[46]
(*Adapted from*: Saxena A. Congenital heart disease in India: a status report. Indian Pediatr. 2018;55(12):1075-82.)

There is marked regional variation in the population density and birth rates in various parts of country. On comparing the six regions of the country, the total number of births are much higher in Northern and Eastern states (Delhi, Jammu and Kashmir, Punjab, Haryana, Himachal Pradesh, Rajasthan, Uttar Pradesh, Uttarakhand, Bihar, Jharkhand, Orissa, West Bengal) as compared to the other four regions (Southern, Western, Central, and North-East). Consequently, the total number of babies born with CHD is likely to be much more in regions with high birth rates (**Fig. 1**).

Intuitively, the cardiac centers should be located in the areas of need according to the principles of demand and supply. But the reality is completely paradoxical as most centers are located in regions with lower burden of CHD. Children born with serious heart disease in southern India have over 70% chance of receiving good quality cardiac care when compared to those born in Eastern and Central part of the country (**Fig. 2**).

UNIQUE CHALLENGES

Lack of Awareness and Delay in Diagnosis

Twenty one percent of births in India are home deliveries and an infant with a critical, ductus-dependent CHD is more likely to die even before diagnosis.[7] Recently, the number of hospital deliveries have risen significantly, attributable to several incentive-based schemes by the Government of India. Despite this, ductus-dependent CHD may still escape detection as babies are often discharged in 24 hours after

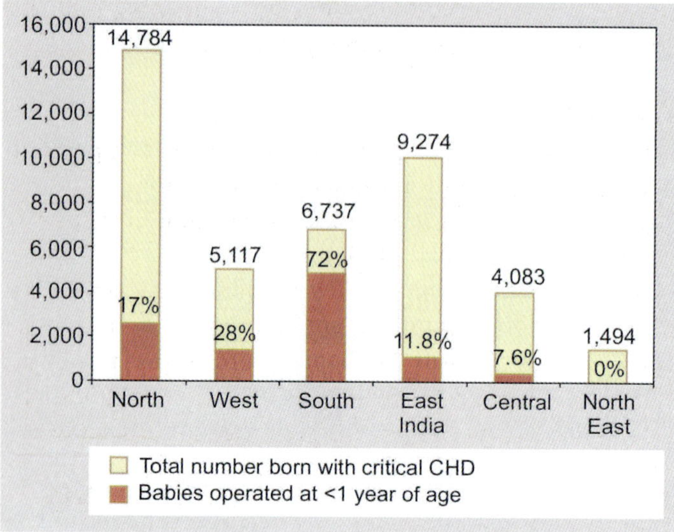

Fig. 2: Regional distribution of infants with critical heart disease accessing surgery as compared to total number born with critical heart disease.[46]
(*Adapted from*: Saxena A. Congenital heart disease in India: a status report. Indian Pediatr. 2018;55(12):1075-82)
(CHD: congenital heart disease)

a normal delivery. Predischarge screening of newborns by pulse oximetry, which may raise suspicion of these CHDs, is often not practiced, especially in rural and semi-urban centers. Even if the CHD is detected, frontline health workers and primary caregivers are not sensitized to the problem of CHD and the need for early intervention. Hence, delayed referrals result in complications and poor outcomes as comorbidities (such as undernutrition and infection) may have already set in. Late presentations also make some diseases inoperable (e.g., large VSD that have developed irreversible pulmonary vascular disease) and for others the risk associated with intervention is increased. At the level of primary care physicians, sometimes there is lower sensitivity towards a serious CHD or oversensitivity towards a trivial CHD. For example, sometimes a patient with small atrial septal defect (ASD) is labeled as hole in the heart and the distressed family flocks to a tertiary center with a 2-day old neonate without the mother, thus depriving the baby of the much needed attention. And on other occasions, a patient with large VSD is referred to tertiary center at 5 years of age when it is inoperable due to irreversible pulmonary vascular disease. Such families are often falsely reassured about the natural closure of the defect. Thus, optimal knowledge regarding the need and timing of intervention for various cardiac lesions is required for primary care physicians to facilitate proper and timely referrals.

Similarly, a large number of physicians are not sensitized to the link between a simple, bacterial sore throat in children and RF. Majority of sore throats are either not treated or treated with home remedies. In contrast, some of the viral sore throats are treated with high end antibiotics, especially in metropolitan cities when concerned parents seek medical attention. This occurs due to the inability to clinically differentiate between viral and bacterial pharyngitis and the under use of throat swab cultures.

Maldistribution of Resources

Along with inadequate number of facilities, their distribution is also uneven. Most of the states in the eastern parts of India which are most poverty stricken have higher birth rates and have little or no pediatric cardiac care facility. Organized transport of newborns with critical CHD is lacking and sick babies reach the tertiary care facility in dismal metabolic states due to long unsupervised transport. This adds to the already compromised circulation and results in suboptimal outcomes despite best available treatment.[50] Children undergoing surgery are often in advanced stages of disease with associated malnutrition, infections, anemia, and other comorbid conditions.[51] The results of intervention in such settings are expected to be less than ideal. Limited resources and inefficient governance further compromise a fair distribution of resources.

Financial Constraints

Management of CHD is very resource intensive and relatively expensive. In sharp contrast to western world, medical insurance is practically nonexistent in India, especially for congenital defects. So, families are expected to meet the treatment expenses by themselves, thus increasing the financial burden. Families lose wages due to long duration of treatments and multiple follow-up visits. The number of public hospitals in the country providing low cost care is very limited. Most recent pediatric cardiac centers are in the private sector and treatment at these centers may not be affordable for the vast majority. Public hospitals are faced with large number of patients and have long waiting lists ranging from months to years. Some government and nongovernment schemes and charitable and philanthropic organizations exist for benefit of economically weaker sections, but awareness about their existence is often lacking in community. Most of these schemes provide one-time funding and do not assist for follow-up care and related medical expenses.

Health-seeking Behavior of the Community

Parents often seek medical care only when the child is significantly symptomatic, even in the absence of financial constraints. This is due to local religious and sociocultural beliefs and practices, coupled with unawareness and illiteracy. Gender bias also plays a role in certain societies, putting girls at a disadvantage compared to boys. In a study from a referral tertiary care center, girls were less likely to undergo cardiac surgery for CHD than boys.[52] In some cases, the parents choose to postpone cardiac intervention or surgery until the child is older, thus wasting precious time.

Lack of Follow-up Care

Most children with CHD, including those who have undergone an intervention or surgery, require long-term care for a good outcome. But a large number of children, specifically from middle and lower socioeconomic strata are lost to follow-up due to various personal reasons. Our healthcare network is not very robust, well connected or interlinked, thus making the follow-up of the child a total responsibility of the family/parents.

Nonavailability of Drugs

Drugs for pediatric age groups are generally a low priority for pharmaceutical companies. Long-acting benzathine penicillin injections are crucial for patients suffering from RHD. Three weekly injections are used as secondary prophylaxis to prevent recurrence of acute RF and hence worsening of valvular damage. Oral penicillin V (phenoxymethylpenicillin) is the drug of choice for the treatment of bacterial sore throat. The pharmaceutical companies are reluctant to manufacturing penicillin due to low profit margins. At times, patients miss the dose due to nonavailability, which puts them at the risk of ARF, thus worsening their cardiac status. Families often have to travel long distances to get the injection, thereby losing their wages and adding to the financial burden. Pediatric preparations of many cardiac medications are often unavailable, forcing the patients to use dose adjusted adult preparations putting them at a risk of critical overdosing or underdosing.

OTHER FACTORS

The other preventable factors associated with CHD are maternal infections (Rubella); exposure to drugs (retinoids) and environmental toxins (lead paints and insecticides); lack of periconceptional folate supplementation and maternal malnutrition (undernutrition or obesity). Rapidly increasing population, inefficient and inadequately equipped infrastructure, and a deficit of trained staff at all levels of healthcare are major roadblocks to optimal cardiac care. Also, investment on public healthcare is one of the lowest in India compared to several other countries.

WAY FORWARD

Although there has been a lot of improvement in pediatric cardiac care in last 20 years, much is left to be done. Strategies to improve should focus on the newborn and infant cardiac care for CHDs and prevention and control of RHD in school children. Health is a state level issue and the various states in India are vastly different with regards to economy, literacy level, population, cultural beliefs, social practices, and human development indices. These factors make the task accomplishment more difficult, given the limited resources.[53]

Increasing Awareness among Community, Primary Care Physicians, and Policy Makers (Table 3)

General pediatricians are often trained in institutions with no dedicated pediatric cardiac care. This translates into poor awareness. This can change through dedicated CME programs targeted to improve awareness. These CME programs and other similar initiatives should especially emphasize the need for early diagnosis and the possible treatment options available on referral. Additionally, there is need for community education regarding the existence of CHDs and their potential for creating specific problems in neonates, infants, and children. This should be thoughtfully accomplished through means of print media, social media, radio, and television as is being done by ministry of maternal and child health. The general public and policy makers should be made aware that a number of CHDs (about 80%) can be treated with very good outcome with timely referral. Similarly, lay people should be educated about the link between sore-throat, joint pain, and serious heart disease in school going children. This will encourage parents to seek early attention for sore throat and RF. It is also essential to formulate and revise treatment guidelines suited for the Indian context.

TABLE 3: Summary of major challenges faced by healthcare system for delivering pediatric cardiac care in India and suggested solutions to overcome them.

Unique challenges	*Solutions*
Lack of awareness and delayed diagnosis	Increasing awareness by continuing education targeting primary care providers
Maldistribution of resources	Geographic distribution of tertiary treatment centers, advocacy with state and central governments to establish newer pediatric heart programs
Financial constraints	Financial support for treatment, engagement of philanthropic organizations, and government sponsored public insurance
Health-seeking behavior of community	Community education and awareness, preventive measures, and screening
Lack of follow-up care	Prioritization of care; integration of pediatric heart care with primary care networks
Nonavailability of drugs	Indigenization and optimization of resources, advocacy for promotion of low cost medication such as penicillin
Others: maternal rubella, lack of folate supplementation	Advocacy to improve primary care services, strengthening health systems

Preventive Measures and Screening

Prevention of CHD has so far received little specific attention perhaps because of the belief that much of CHD is not preventable. However, certain specific strategies need countrywide implementation because they have the potential to prevent specific heart defects in a number of patients. They include mass rubella vaccination and periconceptional folate supplementation. Additionally, improvements in women health and nutrition have the potential of mitigating the problem of low birth weight that have a positive impact on care of babies with CHD. Fetal echocardiography can help in early diagnosis of complex CHDs. A detailed description of prevention of CHD is included in the chapter on Congenital Heart Disease. The programs specific for CHD or RHD are not financially sustainable on their own, hence they should incorporate comprehensive child health care. One such program is Rashtriya Bal Swasthya Karyakram (RBSK), which was started by Government of India in 2013 for screening of children between 0 and 18 years of age, followed by early detection and management of congenital and acquired diseases. Newborn screening with pulse oximetry should become a part of routine newborn care.[54]

Adequate and prompt treatment of streptococcal sore throats with antibiotics will prevent the occurrence of RF; and appropriate penicillin prophylaxis would prevent its recurrence in patients with RHD, thus avoiding further valvular damage. Secondary prophylaxis has been proven to be of benefit in control of RHD. The rates of secondary prophylaxis must improve to control progressive damage to cardiac valves. The primary health centers must have facilities for injecting long-acting penicillin to the patients. This may be best done by incorporating with the existing facilities for maternal and childcare at the health center. Good quality penicillin must be made available consistently all across the country. It should be either free or priced at a subsidized cost. Physicians and others involved in providing injection of penicillin must be educated about the allergic reactions and the importance of skin testing before each injection.

Geographic Distribution of Tertiary Treatment Centers

Establishing new centers is not only challenging due to the huge infrastructure required, but also needs a motivational team of health professionals. Pediatric cardiac care delivery demands a team approach. A dedicated and well-knit team of pediatric cardiologists, pediatric cardiac surgeons, cardiac anesthetists, nursing staff and intensive care specialists is necessary to run a successful program. Each state should have at least one center running such comprehensive program, so that the travel distances for seeking cardiac care is reduced. These centers should be supported by the government so that the financially incapable are also able to obtain benefits. An important initiative by the Government of India is establishment of new AIIMS (All India Institute of Medical Sciences) in many parts of the country, where the departments are being set-up.

Optimal Resource Utilization

The adult cardiology programs are relatively less resource intensive, so initiating a pediatric cardiac program on a successfully ongoing adult program is useful for resource optimization. The entire infrastructure comprising of cardiac catheterization laboratory, operating room, staff, and other services are shared. Hence, by piggybacking, the running costs of the pediatric program are reduced. Also, outcome data collection to assess the quality of program is very important for sustainability.

In-country Training of Staff

The current number of pediatric cardiologists, pediatric cardiac surgeons, and pediatric cardiac intensivists in the country is grossly inadequate. As these specialties are much more demanding and have low monetary returns, fewer number of specialists choose them. Also, the learning curve in these specialties is very long, it requires training for a number of years under the supervision of experts in the fields before a practitioner can independently perform surgeries or interventions. Such kind of long and intensive training and mentoring is best done within the country since training abroad may not be very applicable in Indian settings. Structured training programs for these specialties are being established gradually at the high volume centers in India. Incorporating research in these programs is also very important for sustainability. Other supporting staff such as nurses, perfusionists, and operation room technicians are indispensable part of the team and their training should also be emphasized upon.

Indigenization and Innovation

Local design and manufacturing of healthcare related technology can have many advantages. Apart from cost reduction, there can be inclusion of features as suited for local needs. It also creates jobs in industries in the country. It can be a more efficient process and the technical support and troubleshooting would be easily available as and when required. Cost containment is necessary for the surgery and interventions to be affordable. Hence, encouraging homegrown technology with local manufacture of good quality products is necessary.

Financial Support for Treatment

Many financial models exist for supporting healthcare in India and a number of them cater to children with CHDs. Many schemes including nongovernmental organizations (NGOs); Corporate Social Responsibilities of multinational companies (MNCs); private donations; and State micro finance schemes such as Arogyasri, Yeshaswini scheme; and Employee State Insurance (ESI) are working to financially help the families of CHD patients. Recent initiative by central Government, the Ayushman Bharat Scheme provides free treatment for CHDs included in its ambit. School health schemes and Rashtriya Bal Swasthya Karyakram (RBSK) provide free surgery for CHD and there is also a provision of follow-up care under RBSK. Also, there are special schemes for infants such as JSSK (Janani Shishu Suraksha Karyakaram), which cover all the expenses of investigations and medical as well as surgical treatment. The policy makers are proactively taking note of the pediatric health and in the future, more schemes for the benefit of children with CHD might be seen. But the increasing demand for care must match the available infrastructure thus avoiding long waiting periods at the treating facilities.

CONCLUSION

Pediatric cardiac care in India has advanced impressively in terms of quality of care in selected institutions and the number of new centers that have the capability for the infant and newborn heart surgery. However, the collective capacity for pediatric heart care in the country falls woefully short of the overall national requirements, and the existing centers are not distributed in accordance with regional needs. Improvement from current situations and groundbreaking results will not appear overnight. Each effort takes time to yield results. Not only the government, but other social leaders and seniors in field of pediatrics, in symbiosis with the government can help to define priorities. The efforts from the government and stakeholders need to be continued and consistent.

REFERENCES

1. Dolk H, Loane M, EUROCAT Steering Committee. Congenital Heart Defect in Europe: 2000-2005. Newtownabbey, Northern Ireland: University of Ulster; March 2009. [online] Available from: http://eurocat.bio medical.co.uk/content/Special Report.pdf. [Last accessed September, 2020].
2. Bernier PL, Stefanescu A, Samoukovic G, Tchervenkov CI. The challenge of congenital heart disease worldwide: epidemiologic and demographic facts. Semin Thorac Cardiovasc Surg Pediatr Card Surg Annu. 2010;13(1):26-34.
3. Hoffman JIE. The global burden of congenital heart disease. Cardiovascular J Africa. 2013; 24(4):141-5.
4. GBD 2017 Congenital Heart Disease Collaborators. Global, regional, and national burden of congenital heart disease, 1990–2017: a systematic analysis for the Global Burden of Disease Study 2017. Lancet Child Adolesc Health. 2020;4(3):185-200.
5. Linde DVD, Konings EEM, Slager MA, Witsenburg M, Helbing WA, Takkenberg JJM, et al. Birth prevalence of congenital heart disease worldwide. J Am Coll Cardiol. 2011;58(21):2241-7.
6. Saxena A, Mehta A, Sharma M, Salhan S, Kalaivani M, Ramakrishnan S, et al. Birth prevalence of congenital heart disease: A cross sectional observational study from North India. Ann Pediatr Cardiol. 2016;9(3):205-9.
7. Ministry of Health and Family Welfare. (2017). National Family Health Survey 4. [online] Available from: http://rchiips.org/NFHS/NFHS-4Reports/India.pdf. [Last accessed September, 2020].
8. Hoffman JI, Kaplan S. The incidence of congenital heart disease. J Am Coll Cardiol. 2002;39(12):1890-900.
9. Kothari SS, Gupta SK. Prevalence of congenital heart disease. Indian J Pediatr. 2013;80(4):337-9.
10. Kapoor R, Gupta S. Prevalence of congenital heart disease, Kanpur, India. Indian Pediatr. 2008;45(4):309-11.
11. Bhat NK, Dhar M, Kumar R, Patel A, Rawat A, Kalra BP. Prevalence and pattern of congenital heart disease in Uttarakhand, India. Indian J Pediatr. 2013;80(4):281-5.
12. Wanni KA, Shahzad N, Ashraf M, Ahmed K, Jan M, Rasool S. Prevalence and spectrum of congenital heart diseases in children. Heart India. 2014;2(3):76-9.
13. Kiran B, Chintan S, Reddy C, Savitha S, Medhar SS, Keerthana TN. Study of prevalence of congenital heart diseases in children in a rural tertiary care hospital. J Pediatr Res. 2016; 3(12):887-90.
14. Abqari S, Gupta A, Shahab T, Rabbani MU, Ali SM, Firdaus U. Profile and risk factors for congenital heart defects: a study in a tertiary care hospital. Ann Pediatr Cardiol. 2016; 9(3):216-21.
15. Mahapatra A, Sarangi R, Mahapatra PP. Spectrum of congenital heart disease in a tertiary care centre of Eastern India. Int J Contemp Pediatr. 2017;4(2):314-6.
16. Khalil A, Aggarwal R, Thirupuram S, Arora R. Incidence of congenital heart disease among hospital live births in India. Indian Pediatr. 1994;31(5):519-27.
17. Vaidyanathan B, Sathish G, Mohanan ST, Sundaram KR, Warrier KK, Kumar RK. Clinical screening for congenital heart disease at birth: a prospective study in a community hospital in Kerala. Indian Pediatr. 2011;48(1):25-30.
18. Sawant SP, Amin AS, Bhat M. Prevalence, pattern and outcome of congenital heart disease in Bhabha atomic research centre hospital. Indian J Pediatr. 2013;80(4):286-91.
19. Gupta I, Gupta ML, Parihar A, Gupta CD. Epidemiology of rheumatic and congenital heart disease in rural children. J Indian Med Assoc. 1992;90(3):57-9.
20. Vashishtha VM, Kalra A, Kalra K, Jain VK. Prevalence of congenital heart disease in school children. Indian Pediatr. 1993;30(11):1337-40.
21. Thakur JS, Negi PC, Ahluwalia SK, Sharma R, Bhardwaj R. Congenital heart disease among school children in Shimla hills. Indian Heart J. 1995;47(3):232-5.
22. Chadha SL, Singh N, Shukla DK. Epidemiological study of congenital heart disease. Indian J Pediatr. 2001;68(6):507-10.
23. Misra M, Mittal M, Verma AM, Rai R, Chandra G, Singh DP, et al. Prevalence and pattern of congenital heart disease in school children of eastern Uttar Pradesh. Indian Heart J. 2009;61(1):58-60.
24. Rama Kumari N, Bhaskara Raju I, Patnaik AN, Barik R, Singh A, Pushpanjali A, et al. Prevalence of rheumatic and congenital heart disease in school children of Andhra Pradesh, South India. J Cardiovasc Dis Res. 2013;4(1):11-4.
25. Saxena A. Echocardiographic prevalence of congenital cardiac malformations among 14,716 asymptomatic school children in India. Presented at EuroEcho Imaging 2013.
26. Bhardwaj R, Kandoria A, Marwah R, Vaidya P, Singh B, Dhiman P, et al. Prevalence of congenital heart disease in rural population of Himachal—A population-based study. Indian Heart J. 2016; 68(1):48-51.
27. Nisale SH, Maske GM. A study of prevalence and pattern of congenital heart disease and rheumatic heart disease among school children. Int J Adv Med. 2016;3(4):947-51.
28. World Health Organization. The Current Evidence for the Burden of Group A Streptococcal Diseases. Geneva, Switzerland: World Health Organization, 2005. WHO/FCH/CAH/05.07. [online] Available from: ttps://www.who.int/maternal_child_adolescent/documents/fch_cah_05_07/en/. [Last accessed September, 2020].

29. Karthikeyan G, Guilherme L. Acute rheumatic fever. Lancet. 2018;392(10142):161-74.
30. Kumar R, Sharma YP, Thakur JS. Streptococcal pharyngitis, rheumatic fever and rheumatic heart disease: eight-year prospective surveillance in Rupnagar district of Punjab, India. Natl Med J India. 2014;27(2):70-5.
31. Sanyal SK, Berry AM, Duggal S, Hooja V, Ghosh S. Sequelae of the initial attack of acute rheumatic fever in children from North India. Circulation. 1982;65(2):375-9.
32. Saxena A. Epidemiology of rheumatic heart disease in India and challenges to its prevention and control. J Preventive Cardiol. 2012;2:256-61.
33. Community control of rheumatic fever and rheumatic heart disease. Report of ICMR task force study. New Delhi: Indian Council of Medical Research; 1994.
34. Shrivastava S. Rheumatic heart disease: Is it declining in India? Indian Heart J 2007;59(1):9-10.
35. Misra M, Mittal M, Singh R, Verma A, Rai R, Chandra G, et al. Prevalence of rheumatic heart disease in school-going children of eastern Uttar Pradesh. Indian Heart J. 2007;59(1):42-3.
36. Jose VJ, Gomathi M. Declining prevalence of rheumatic heart disease in rural school-children in India: 2001–2002. Indian Heart J. 2003;55(2):158-60.
37. Periwal KL, Gupta BK, Panwar RB, Khatri PC, Raja S, Gupta R. Prevalence of rheumatic heart disease in school children in Bikaner: an echocardiographic study. J Assoc Physicians India. 2006;54:279-82.
38. Gewitz MH, Baltimore RS, Tani LY, Sable CA, Shulman ST, Carapetis J, et al. Revision of the Jones Criteria for the diagnosis of acute rheumatic fever in the era of Doppler echocardiography: a scientific statement from the American Heart Association. Circulation. 2015; 131(20):1806-18.
39. Marijon E, Ou P, Celermajer DS, Ferreira B, Mocumbi AO, Jani D, et al. Prevalence of rheumatic heart disease detected by echocardiographic screening. N Engl J Med. 2007; 357(5):470-6.
40. Saxena A, Ramakrishnan S, Roy A. Prevalence and outcome of subclinical rheumatic heart disease in India: the rheumatic study. Heart. 2011;97(24):2018-22.
41. Saxena A, Desai A, Narvencar K. Echocardiographic prevalence of rheumatic heart disease in Indian school children using World Heart Federation criteria - a multisite extension of rheumatic study (the e-rheumatic study). Int J Cardiol. 2017;249:438-42.
42. Thakur JS, Negi PC, Ahluwalia SK, Vaidya NK. Epidemiological survey of rheumatic heart disease among school children in the Shimla hills of Northern India: prevalence and risk factors. J Epidemiological Community Health. 1996;50(1):62-7.
43. Negi PC, Kanwar A, Chauhan R, Asotra S, Thakur J, Bhardwaj AK. Epidemiological trends in RF/RHD in school children of Shimla in north India. Indian J Med Res. 2013;137(6):1121-7.
44. Watkins DA, Johnson CO, Colquhoun SM, Karthikeyan G, Beaton A, Bukhman G, et al. Global, regional, and national burden of rheumatic heart disease, 1990–2015. N Eng J Med. 2017; 377(8):713-22.
45. Mehta A, Saxena A, Juneja R, Ramakrishnan S, Gupta S, Kothari SS. Characteristics and outcomes of Indian children enrolled in a rheumatic heart disease registry. Int J Cardiol. 2016;222:1136-40.
46. Saxena A. Congenital heart disease in India: a status report. Indian Pediatr. 2018;55(12):1075-82.
47. Pezzella T. Worldwide maldistribution of access to cardiac surgery. J Thorac Cardiovasc Surg. 2002;123(5):1016-7.
48. Saxena A. Congenital heart disease in India: a status report. Indian J Pediatr. 2005;72(7):595-8.
49. Kumar RK, Shrivastava S. Pediatric heart care in India. Heart. 2008;94(8):984-90.
50. Kumar RK. Congenital heart disease profile: four perspectives. Ann Pediatr Cardiol. 2016; 9(3):203-4.
51. Liu J. Challenges and progress of the pediatric cardiac surgery in Shanghai Children's Medical Center: a 25-year solid collaboration with Project HOPE. Semin Thorac Cardiovasc Surg Pediatr Card Surg Annu. 2009;12:12-8.
52. Ramakrishnan S, Khera R, Jain S, Saxena A, Kailash S, Karthikeyan G, et al. Gender differences in the utilisation of surgery for congenital heart disease in India. Heart. 2011; 97(23): 1920-5.
53. Saxena A. Pediatric cardiac care in India: current status and the way forward. Future Cardiol. 2018;14(1):1-4.
54. Saxena A, Mehta A, Ramakrishnan S, Sharma M, Salhan S, Kalaivani M, et al. Pulse oximetry as a screening tool for detecting major congenital heart defects in Indian newborns. Arch Dis Child Fetal Neonatal Ed. 2015;100(5):F416-21.

2
CHAPTER

Anatomy of the Heart: An Overview

Sanjeev H Naganur, Balaji Srimurugan, Saurabh Kumar Gupta

INTRODUCTION

"Form follows function", the saying by Louis Sullivan with regards to the buildings and architecture, underscores the importance of understanding anatomy of the cardiovascular system. No assessment of cardiac function is possible without a detailed analysis of cardiac anatomy. The cardiac anatomy assumes even greater significance while managing a patient with congenital heart disease. A detailed and accurate depiction of cardiac malformation is the single most important factor determining the clinical outcome of these patients. This chapter provides an overview of clinically relevant cardiac anatomy.

GENERAL FEATURES OF CARDIOVASCULAR ANATOMY

The heart is a complex three-dimensional organ positioned in the chest cavity between 2nd and 5th intercostal space. In most healthy individuals, the heart lies obliquely in the left hemithorax with two-third of the bulk located to the left of midline with its long axis in the direction of right shoulder to left costophrenic angle. An axis different from rest of the body organs mandates a special approach while analyzing anatomy of the heart (**Figs. 1 and 2**).

Anteriorly, the heart is covered by the sternum and costal cartilages while posterior surface of the heart is in relation to esophagus (**Fig. 2**). The cardiac silhouette in anteroposterior projection is like a trapezoid with an inverted right triangle and an equilateral triangle overlying atrial and ventricular chambers, respectively (**Fig. 1**). Being oriented in tilted manner, the ventricular triangle has its base on the right side and apex pointing downward and to the left. Although the true base of the heart is the posterior aspect of the atrial chambers, the term base is usually applied to the base of the ventricular triangle which corresponds to the cardiac crux, a plane where all cardiac valves are located (see further). The obliquity also exists in anteroposterior plane with the right side of the heart lying somewhat anterior compared to rest of the heart.

The size of the heart varies with age, gender, and body habitus. Conventionally, the heart size is measured as cardiothoracic ratio, a ratio of the heart and thoracic cavity

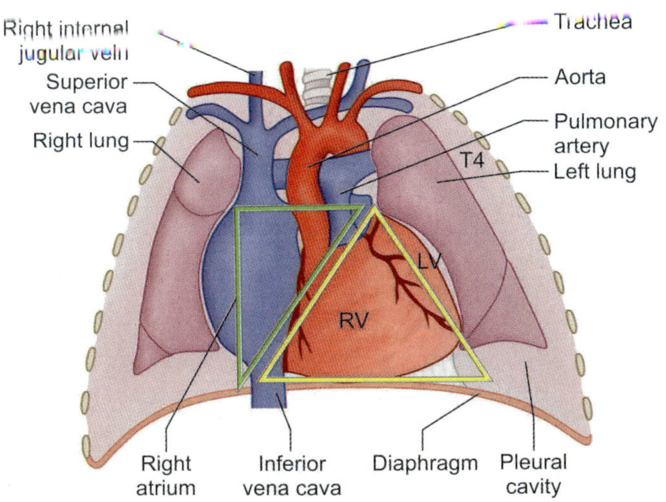

Fig. 1: Relationship of the heart with adjacent structures in anteroposterior view. The green and yellow triangle overlies the atrial and ventricular chambers, respectively.
(LV: left ventricle; RV: right ventricle)

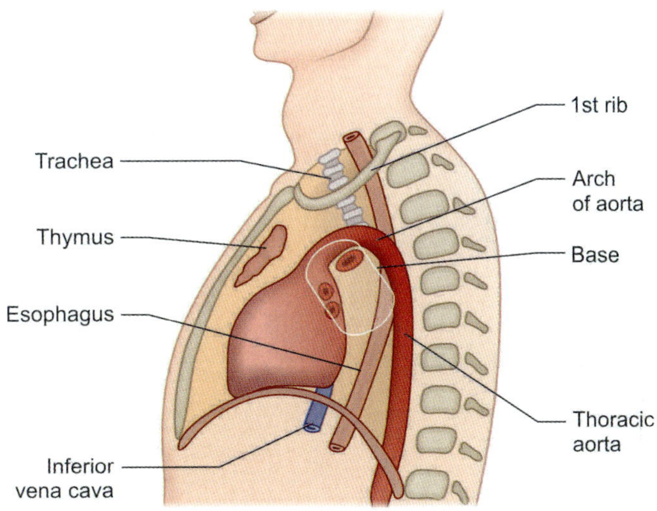

Fig. 2: Relationship of the heart and adjacent structures and bony cage in lateral view.

in transverse diameter, in a chest radiograph obtained in posteroanterior projection in deep inspiration. In health, the cardiothoracic ratio is 60% or less in a newborn and 50% or less in children and adults. Cardiac size correlates better with body surface area and weight than with height.

PERICARDIUM

The pericardium covers the heart all around except the posterior aspect of the left atrium. The pericardial reflection also extends to the proximal part of superior caval vein and great arteries (**Fig. 3**). The pericardium is composed of two layers—an outer fibrous parietal pericardium and an inner serous visceral pericardium. The parietal pericardium is firmly attached to the central tendon of the diaphragm, mediastinal pleura, and the sternum holding the heart in its position. Unique compliance characteristics of the pericardium helps in optimal interaction between the right and left ventricle. A small amount of serous fluid present in between these two layers serves as a lubricant and allows a relatively friction-free movement of the heart within the chest.

GENERAL EXTERNAL FEATURES OF CARDIAC ANATOMY

The external surface of the heart is characterized by atrioventricular and interventricular grooves (**Fig. 4**). As the name suggests, the atrioventricular groove defines the position of ventricular inlet, while the interventricular groove locates the ventricular septum. A cross section at the level of atrioventricular groove exposes all the four valves of the heart (**Fig. 5**). The interventricular groove is oblique and lies between the ventricles. On its inferior surface, the interventricular groove joins the atrioventricular groove and this point of the heart is called "cardiac crux." Externally, right and left coronary artery (LCA) runs in the right and left atrioventricular groove respectively, while left anterior and inferior interventricular arteries run along anterior and inferior interventricular groove, respectively. We draw attention of the readers to the use of attitudinally appropriate term "inferior" in place of "posterior" to describe the diaphragmatic surface of the heart within the chest cavity. This preference of terminology is to deemphasize erroneous description of anatomy of extracted heart in upside down (Valentine heart) orientation.

CARDIAC CHAMBERS

The human heart is a four-chambered organ with complete separation of pulmonary and systemic circulation with a set of thin-walled atrium and thick-walled ventricle on each side. Though commonly labeled as right- and left-sided, the chambers are not strictly left and right. Instead, the so-called

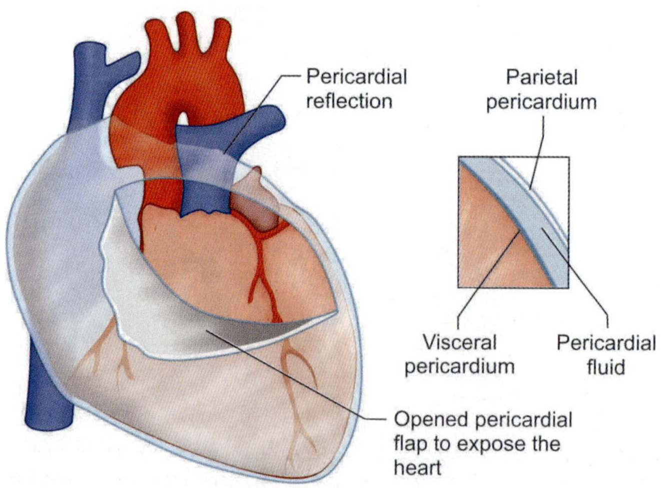

Fig. 3: Reflection of the pericardium around the heart. The image in the inset shows the layers of the pericardium.

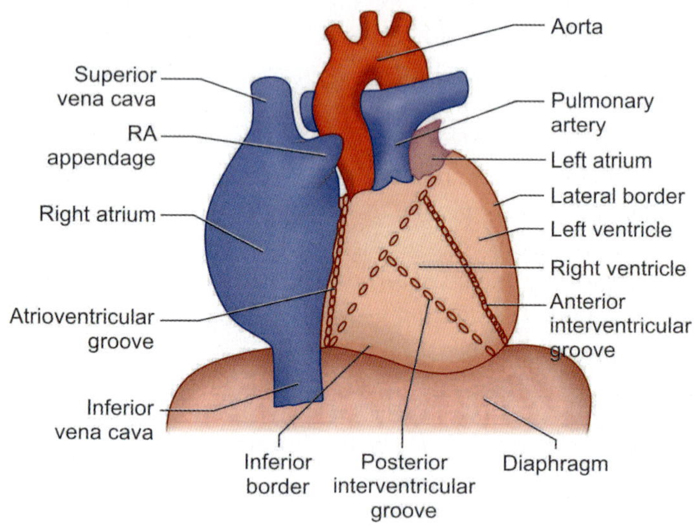

Fig. 4: Various borders and boundaries of the heart. Note the so-called posterior border of the left ventricle is in reality the inferior border which lies in relation with the diaphragm.
(RA: right atrium)

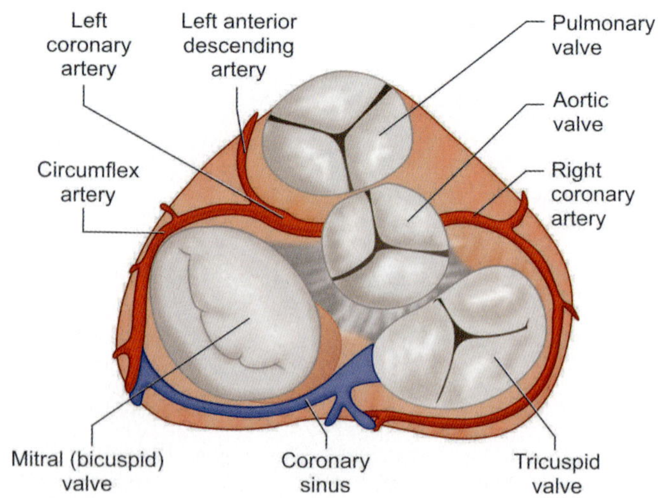

Fig. 5: The heart as seen from the head end after removing the atrial chambers. This shows the relative position of all the four cardiac valves, coronary arteries and coronary sinus. Also, note close relationship of mitral, tricuspid, and aortic valve supported by the fibrous trigone.

right-sided chambers of the heart are located anteriorly with the ventricle situated to the left and inferior relative to the atrium. Nevertheless, for ease of communication, in this chapter, we will continue to use these prevalent terminologies.

Further, the morphological features of a chamber are more important than its relative position. This approach to cardiac anatomy, better known as morphological method, is particularly important while dealing with malformed hearts wherein aberrancy of location and connections is common. Besides, variation in the proximal and distal connections of any chamber in patients with congenital heart disease is well known, it is essential to identify each chamber on its own morphological characteristics and not on the basis of its connections. For example, although pulmonary veins almost always connects to the left atrium, this feature cannot be the defining feature for the left atrium. If it is used then how will one identify the left atrium in a patient with totally anomalous pulmonary venous connection wherein the pulmonary veins are connected to systemic veins or the right atrium in place of the left atrium.

Sequential segmental approach is yet another important concept. As the name suggests, this approach mandates a composite analysis of cardiac anatomy after a detailed independent morphological assessment of all the cardiac chambers and connections. A detailed description of sequential segmental approach is beyond the scope of this chapter. Instead, in this chapter, we will briefly discuss morphological characteristics of all the cardiac chambers.

Right Atrium

The right atrium forms the right lateral border of the heart along with the venae cavae in the chest radiograph. It receives blood from the superior and inferior caval veins, coronary sinus, and thebesian veins and expels blood across the tricuspid valve and into the right ventricle. Structurally right atrium consists of a venous component receiving blood from caval veins, vestibule connecting it to the ventricle and an appendage. Right atrial appendage is the most distinctive and constant feature of the right atrium. It is broad triangular shape with wide orifice with pectinate muscles extending well beyond the appendage and reaching up to the vestibule of the atrium.

The free wall of the right atrium has a smooth posterior and a muscular anterior part. The smooth posterior portion receives superior and inferior caval veins and has a vein-like appearance. C-shaped ridge of muscle, called "crista terminalis" separates these two. Many pectinate muscles arise from the terminal crest and travel as parallel ridges along the anterior aspect of the free wall (**Fig. 6**). The atrial septum on the right side is relatively smooth. As the tricuspid valve is apically displaced relative to the mitral valve (see further), the right atrial aspect of the septum has two components—one between the right and left atrium and the other between the right atrium and left ventricle, better known as atrioventricular septum.

Left Atrium

In reality, the so-called left atrium lies posterior to the right atrium and not to the left as its name suggests. In fact, it is

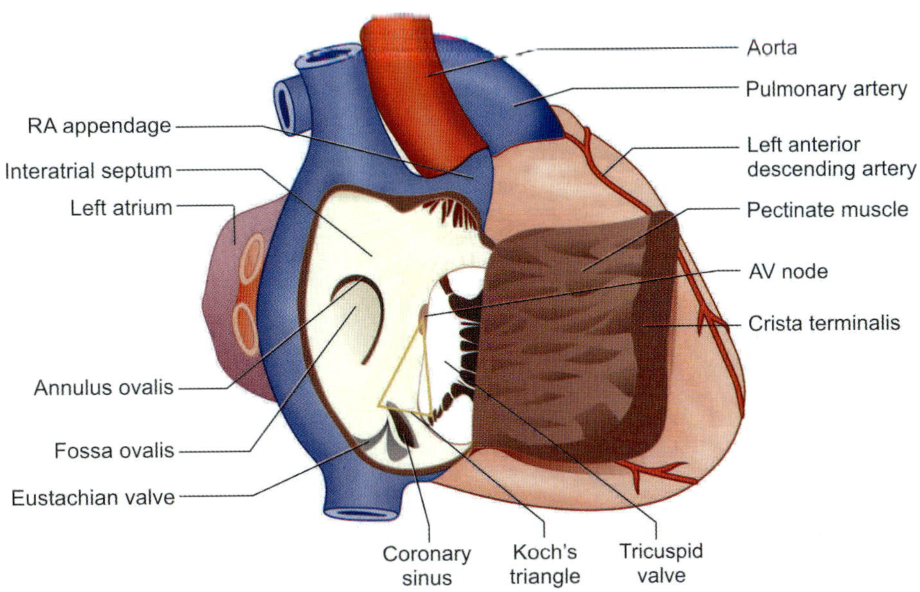

Fig. 6: The heart after removing the anterior wall of the right atrium showing its morphological aspects and right atrial aspect of the atrial septum. The yellow triangle denotes the triangle of Koch with its apex having the atrioventricular node. Note the extension of the pectinate muscles on the anterior wall of the right atrium. In contrast, the pectinate muscles of the left atrium are confined to the left atrial appendage.
(AV: atrioventricular; RA: right atrium)

only a part of the left atrial appendage that forms a small part of the left heart border. The left atrium, like the right atrium, possesses a venous component, an appendage, and a vestibule. Just like the right atrium, the most distinctive and constant component of the left atrium is the left atrial appendage. However, unlike the right atrial appendage, it is a long tubular structure with a narrow orifice and pectinate muscles restricted within it. The internal structure of the appendage is variable with regards to its shape and number of lobes. The left atrial cavity is devoid of crista terminalis. The corners of the posterior smooth portion receives blood from pulmonary veins and direct it to the left ventricle through the mitral valve. When viewed from the left, the atrial septum is entirely interatrial. Neither the limbus of the fossa ovalis nor the atrioventricular septum is visible from this side. Instead, the septal surface represents the flap valve of the oval fossa overlapping the infolded embryonic secondary atrial septum commonly labeled as the superior rim of the oval fossa (**Fig. 7**).

Right Ventricle

Anatomically, right ventricle is divided into three parts namely inlet, trabecular, and outlet regions. The inlet is guarded by the tricuspid valve having three leaflets—septal, inferior or mural, and anterosuperior. The anterosuperior leaflet is the largest of the three. The septal leaflet has multiple chordal attachments to the ventricular septum, which is one of the features to identify the tricuspid valve and in turn, the right ventricle (**Fig. 8**).

The apical trabecular portion of the right ventricle has coarse trabeculations. A relatively trabeculated septal surface is the morphologic hallmark to identify the right ventricle. One of the trabeculations on the septal surface, the septomarginal trabeculation or septal band, is particularly prominent. The septal band divides into two limbs toward the base of the heart to clasp the supraventricular crest. Moderator band is yet another distinctive trabeculation that connects the papillary muscle to the parietal wall of the right ventricle and is used to identify the right ventricle during echocardiographic or angiographic evaluation. Multiple trabeculations also connect anterior surface of septomarginal band to the anterior wall of the right ventricle are known as septoparietal trabeculations.

The outlet component of the right ventricle is relatively free of trabeculations and extends up to the pulmonary valve. A sleeve of tissue, commonly known as supraventricular crest lying between the two limbs of septomarginal trabeculation, separates pulmonary valve from the tricuspid valve. This is unlike the relationship of the mitral and aortic valve on the left side of the heart wherein both the valves are in fibrous continuity. The segment between the inflow and the outflow of the right ventricle is also known as the infundibulum.

Left Ventricle

The left ventricle is the left posterior chamber of the heart and forms major part of the left border of the heart. Like the right ventricle, the left ventricle also has inlet, apical trabecular and apical component. The inlet is guarded by a bileaflet mitral valve. The mitral valve has two leaflets—a larger posterior or mural leaflet and a smaller anterior or aortic leaflet. The morphological features of the valves are better seen in closed position during ventricular systole. Once again, although traditionally claimed to have two commissures—posteromedial and anterolateral, the mitral valve has only a

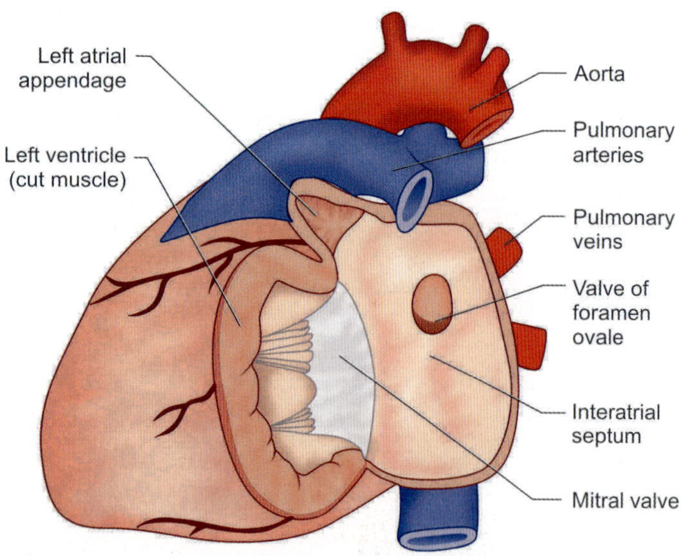

Fig. 7: Left atrial aspect of the atrial septum and mitral valve. The left atrial surface of the atrial septum is relatively smooth and contains valve of the foramen ovale. Unlike the right atrium, the pectinate muscles in the left atrium are confined to the appendage.

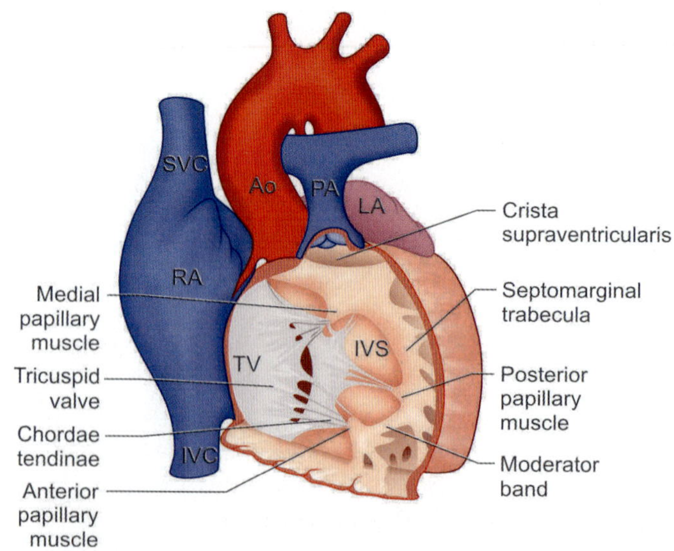

Fig. 8: The heart with anterior wall of the right ventricle removed to show the internal anatomy. The right ventricle is heavily trabeculated with a prominent moderator band connecting septomarginal trabecula with the anterior wall. Also, septal attachment of the atrioventricular valve identifies the tricuspid valve.
(Ao: aorta; IVC: inferior vena cava; IVS: interventricular septum; LA: left atrium; PA: pulmonary artery; RA: right atrium; SVC: superior vena cava; TV: tricuspid valve)

single line of opposition. The leaflets are supported by two papillary muscles and a series of tendinous chords. Unlike the tricuspid valve, there is no septal attachment of the mitral valve. Instead, the anterior leaflet of the mitral valve is separated from the ventricular septum by the left ventricular outflow tract.

The trabecular portion of the left ventricle lies between the papillary muscles of the mitral valve and the apex. The trabeculations are not as coarse as the right ventricle with the septal surface free of trabeculations.

The outlet of the left ventricle is much abbreviated in comparison to the right ventricular outflow tract. The posterior two leaflets of the aortic valve are in fibrous continuity with the anterior mitral leaflet. This is again in contrast to the tricuspid valve which is separated from the pulmonary valve by a free standing infundibulum. The outflow of the left ventricle is guarded by trisinusate aortic valve. Owing to complex looping of various cardiac segments during embryonic life, the left ventricular outflow lies to the right of the right ventricular outflow. This crossing of the ventricular outflows results in typical "circle and sausage" appearance to the arterial trunks (see further).

ARTERIAL TRUNKS

Each of the ventricular outflow supports an arterial trunk connecting the ventricle to its respective circulation. Twisting at the level of the outflow tracts results in the aorta occupying right and posterior position relative to the pulmonary valve. This when viewed in cross section gives rise to typical "circle and sausage" appearance. Any arrangement other than this arrangement, often labeled as normally related great arteries, is known as malposition (*see* **Fig. 5**). These terms, however, are limited to the spatial orientation of the arterial trunks and has no relation with the ventriculoarterial connection. Although mostly associated with abnormality of ventriculoarterial connection, malposition of arterial trunks can be rarely seen in the setting of normal ventriculoarterial connection. It is therefore important to describe both the ventriculoarterial connection and the spatial relationship of the arterial trunks.

Each of the arterial trunks has a semilunar valve at its origin. Unlike atrioventricular valves, the valves guarding the arterial trunks does not have tensor apparatus. The root of the arterial trunks have well-formed bulge, better known as sinus, in number equivalent to the number of leaflets of the underlying valve. The junction of the sinus and the distal part of the root is called sinotubular junction.

The pulmonary artery divides into right and left branches after a short distance from its origin. The aorta, on the other hand, does not divide or branch before giving rise to neck vessels after ascending up in the neck. These features help in identification of aorta and pulmonary artery during echocardiography in cases with complex congenital heart disease. With the exception of anomalous origin of coronary artery from pulmonary artery and coronary atresia, the origin of coronary artery identifies an arterial trunk as aorta.

Aorta and Systemic Arterial Tree

The aorta is the major elastic artery of the systemic circulation. It arises at the level of the aortic valve and terminates at its bifurcation into the common iliac arteries, at the level of the umbilicus and the fourth lumbar vertebra. The aorta may be divided into four regions: ascending aorta, aortic arch, descending thoracic aorta, and abdominal aorta. Ascending aorta consists of sinus and tubular portions, demarcated by the sinotubular junction. During childhood and adolescence, the dimensions of the ascending aorta are related to age and body size. The aortic arch normally travels over the left bronchus, defining a left aortic arch, and overlies the right pulmonary artery. From the top of the arch, the brachiocephalic (or innominate), left common carotid, and left subclavian arteries arise, in that order (**Fig. 9**). The aortic arch contributes to the left superior border of the radiographic frontal cardiac silhouette and forms the aortic knob in adults. The descending thoracic aorta lies posterior in relation to the left atrium, esophagus, and vertebral column.

The arterial tree is the result of a complex series of remodeling during embryonic life with each component of the arterial tree getting contribution from different embryonic aortic arches. This explains frequent occurrence of aortic arch anomalies.

Pulmonary Arteries

As mentioned earlier, the pulmonary arterial trunk lies to the left of aortic root and ascending aorta (*see* **Figs. 1, 4, and 8**). As it bifurcates, left pulmonary artery continues as a smooth arch and courses over the left bronchus, whereas the right pulmonary artery takes off at a right angle and travels beneath the aortic arch and behind the superior vena cava. Within the lung, pulmonary arteries travel with their corresponding airways. As the pulmonary circulation is a low-pressure and low-resistance system, its arteries and veins are thin walled compared to their systemic counterparts. In addition to

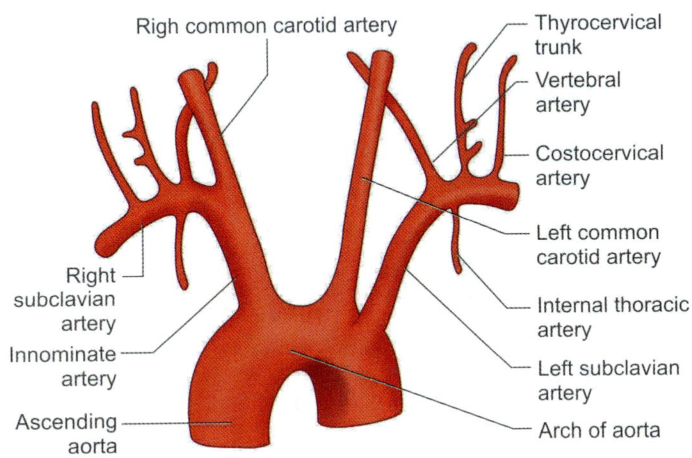

Fig. 9: The aorta and its branches.

pulmonary arteries, the lungs also get their blood supply through bronchial arteries arising from descending aorta. These bronchial arteries provide nutrition to bronchial and pulmonary vascular wall. They are insignificant in health but assumes significance in variety of diseases such as congenital heart diseases with reduced pulmonary blood flow, Eisenmenger syndrome, by providing alternate source of blood supply to lungs. These enlarged bronchial arteries are the major source of hemoptysis in these patients.

CORONARY CIRCULATION

Coronary Arteries

The right and left coronary arteries arise from their corresponding aortic sinuses. The major epicardial arteries include the left main, left anterior descending, left circumflex, and right coronary arteries. Branches of the left anterior descending artery are called diagonals, whereas branches of the right and circumflex arteries are called marginals. Septal perforators represent long intramural branches of the anterior and posterior descending arteries that supply the ventricular septum and hence are not epicardial (**Fig. 10**).

Right Coronary Artery

In about 60% of subjects, the first branch is the conus coronary artery, which supplies the right ventricular outflow tract; in the other 40%, this artery arises independently from the right aortic sinus. Many marginal branches arise with a prominent acute marginal artery. In 70% of human hearts, the right coronary artery is dominant and gives rise to the posterior descending branch and also the posterolateral branches nourishing right ventricular free wall, inferoseptal wall of the left ventricle, posteromedial mitral papillary muscle, and atrioventricular nodal artery.

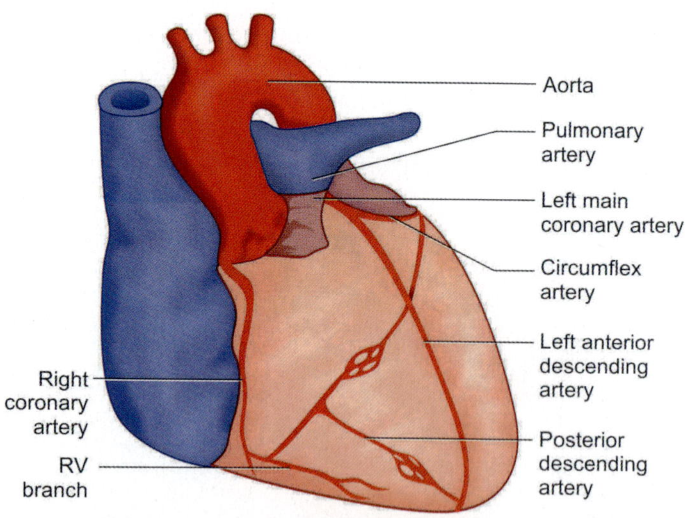

Fig. 10: The heart showing arrangement of coronary arteries and its relationship with the cardiac chambers. The right and left circumflex coronary arteries run in the right and left atrioventricular groove, respectively. The left anterior descending artery runs in the anterior interventricular groove.
(RV: right ventricle)

Left Coronary Artery

Left coronary artery bifurcates into left anterior descending and left circumflex branches in most, but trifurcates in few. Most of the coronary perfusion occurs during ventricular diastole. Left anterior descending artery travels in the anterior interventricular groove, wraps around the apex and extends for a variable distance in the posterior interventricular groove. This vessel also supplies anteroseptal and anterolateral walls, part of the anterolateral mitral papillary muscle, and entire apex of the left ventricle through its diagonal and septal perforating branches.

Left Circumflex Coronary Artery

This vessel travels in the left atrioventricular groove, usually terminating just beyond its obtuse marginal branches and nourishes the lateral wall of the left ventricle and part of the anterolateral mitral papillary muscle. In 10% of subjects, this artery also supplies the posterior descending branch, constituting left dominance and inferoseptal wall of the left ventricle, posteromedial mitral papillary muscle, and atrioventricular nodal artery. About 20% of human hearts exhibit shared coronary dominance, such that both the right coronary artery and left circumflex arteries provide posterior descending branches. The sinus nodal artery arises from right coronary artery in about 60% of hearts and from left circumflex coronary artery in 40%, irrespective of coronary dominance. In contrast, the atrioventricular nodal artery arises from the dominant coronary artery with its origin from right coronary artery in 90% of human hearts.

Coronary Veins

Venous system of the heart consists of a coronary sinus system, anterior cardiac venous system, and thebesian venous system. The great cardiac vein travels beside left anterior descending and left circumflex arteries to merge with the coronary sinus (**Fig. 11**). The coronary sinus also receives left-posterior, middle, and small cardiac veins before draining into the right atrium. Along the anterobasal aspect of the right ventricular free wall, three or four anterior cardiac veins drain into the right atrium or first join either directly or via a common collecting vein. There are numerous small thebesian veins that drain directly into right atrium or right ventricle.

CARDIAC CONDUCTION SYSTEM

General Features

Cardiac conduction system consists of the sinus node, internodal tracts, and atrioventricular conduction tissues. Its function is influenced by sympathetic and parasympathetic innervation, circulating catecholamines, patency of its nutrient blood supply, regional acid-base or electrolyte disturbances, mechanical trauma (such as sutures, synthetic patches, and ablation procedures), etc. Sinus and atrioventricular nodes are both right atrial structures with similar microscopic features, conduction velocities, and action

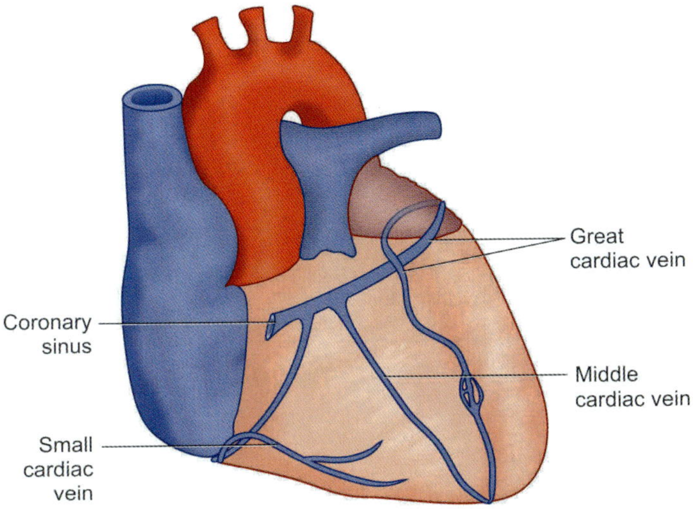

Fig. 11: The arrangement of coronary veins and their relationship with various cardiac chambers.

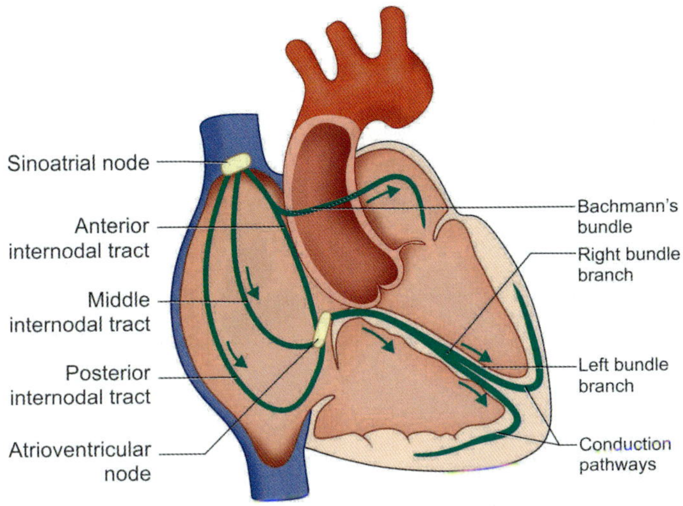

Fig. 12: The cardiac conduction system. Note that the atrioventricular node lies at the apex of the triangle of Koch (also see Figure 6).

potentials. Similarities also exist in the structure, conduction velocities, and action potentials of the atrioventricular (His) bundle, right and left bundle branches, and working cardiac myocytes. All components of the cardiac conduction system are specialized cardiac myocytes (not nerves) whose major function is conduction rather than contraction (**Fig. 12**).

Sinus Node

Being the primary pacemaker of the heart, sinus node represents a right atrial structure that is located subepicardially along the terminal groove near the superior cavoatrial junction. Numerous autonomic nerves approach the sinus node.

Internodal Tracts

The existence of these specialized pathways between sinus and atrioventricular nodes is a subject controversy. Electrophysiologic studies support the concept of preferential pathways, but morphologic studies do not. Recent investigations suggest that both views may be correct.

Atrioventricular Node

Atrioventricular node is also a right atrial structure, richly innervated by parasympathetic and sympathetic fibers. This node is located subendocardially within the triangle of Koch and adjacent to the central fibrous body. The triangle of Koch corresponds to the atrioventricular septum, bordered by septal tricuspid annulus, coronary sinus ostium, and tendon of Todaro (*see* **Fig. 6**).

Atrioventricular (His) Bundle

Atrioventricular (His) bundle arises from the distal portion of the atrioventricular node, travels through the central fibrous body and along the basal ventricular septum, adjacent to the membranous septum, representing the normal route for the electrical conduction between atrial and ventricular myocardium. Atrioventricular bundle is related closely to the annuli of the aortic, mitral, and tricuspid valves. Microscopically, atrioventricular bundle is divided into two regions: penetrating portion, which courses through the central fibrous body and the branching portion, which gives rise to right and left bundle branches.

Bundle Branches

The right bundle branch originates from the distal portion of the atrioventricular bundle and forms a cord-like structure, traveling along the septal and moderator bands toward the anterior tricuspid papillary muscle. The left bundle branch is a broad fenestrated sheet of subendocardial conduction fibers spreading along the septal surface of the left ventricle. It courses toward the ventricular apex and both mitral papillary muscles and may separate into two or three indistinct fascicles.

CONCLUSION

For any reasonable understanding of cardiac physiology and pathology, it is imperative to understand the cardiac anatomy. A sequential segmental analysis based on morphological assessment of individual cardiac chamber and its connections is the key to any meaningful analysis of cardiac anatomy.

SUGGESTED READING

1. Agur AMR, Dalley AF, Moore KL, (Eds). The thorax. In: Clinically Oriented Anatomy, 5th edition. Philadelphia: Lippincott Williams & Wilkins; 2005. pp. 72-181.
2. Anderson RH, Spicer DE, Mori S. Anatomy. In: Wernovsky G, Anderson R, Kumar K, Mussato K, Redington A, Tweddell J, Tretter J, (Eds). Anderson's Textbook of Paediatric Cardiology, 4th edition. Philadelphia: Elsevier; 2019. pp. 17-32.
3. Loukas M. Heart. In: Standring S, (Ed). Gray's Anatomy: The Anatomical Basis of Clinical Practice, 41st edition. Canada: Elsevier; 2016. pp. 994-1033.
4. Sinnatam C. Middle mediastinum and heart. Last's Anatomy, 12th edition. London: Churchill Livingstone; 2011. pp. 106-211.
5. Wikipedia. Form follows function. [online] Available from: https://en.wikipedia.org/wiki/Form_follows_function. [Last accessed September 2020].

3
CHAPTER

Embryology

Sanjeev H Naganur, Balaji Srimurugan, Saurabh Kumar Gupta

INTRODUCTION

A basic knowledge of the development of the cardiovascular system is essential for understanding morphologic and physiologic alterations seen in various congenital heart diseases. This chapter briefly describes cardiac development and seeks to provide foundations that are perhaps essential to understand the wide variety of congenital heart diseases. The chapter has incorporated newer concepts but the overall narrative is kept simple enough for the postgraduate students to understand.

PRIMITIVE HEART TUBE FORMATION

The human heart starts developing from the mesoderm during the third week of gestation with the first sign on days 18–19 of gestation. The heart begins to develop near the head of the embryo in a region known as the cardiogenic area (**Fig. 1A**). The cardiogenic area begins to form two strands called the cardiogenic cords under the influence of certain chemical factors. Before the embryonic folding, angiogenic cell clusters on either side of the neural crest, fuse to form capillaries in the mesoderm of the germ disk. This subsequently forms a pair of blood vessels on either side. These vessels run along the long axis of the germ disk, with one pair of blood vessels at the lateral edge of the embryo (one on each edge) and other pair more medially on either side of the neural tube. When the embryo loops laterally, lateral edges of the germ disk approach each other, giving embryo a tubular form. The two outer endocardial tubes come close to each other in the median, ventral to the primitive gut and start fusing cranial to caudal to form a single median, primitive heart tube (**Figs. 1B to D**).

Primitive Heart Tube

Although the primitive heart starts beating on day 22, the fetal circulation starts around days 27–29 of gestation. The primitive heart tube develops multiple constrictions demarcating the location of future segments of the heart. These structures, cranial to caudal, are bulbus cordis, which extends cranially into truncus arteriosus, primitive ventricle, and primitive atrium. The primitive atrium connects to the sinus venosus, which receives vitelline veins from yolk sac, common cardinal vein from the embryo, and umbilical veins from the placenta (**Fig. 1D**).

> Abnormal development during the formation of primitive heart tube almost always results in embryonic death due to the lack of fetal circulation at an early stage.

LOOPING

Around day 23 of gestation, primitive heart tube loops in a way that its cephalic end curves in counter-clockwise direction. This brings the cephalic portion ventrally, caudally, and slightly to the right. The looping of the primitive heart tube is the result of differential growth—posterior leftward slow growth and anterior rightward fast growth (**Figs. 2A and B**). In most instances, more so in the setting of future situs solitus, it is dextro or right-handed looping that brings the future right ventricle to the right and anterior to the future left ventricle. At this time, the atrial portion starts moving in a cephalic and leftward direction. The primitive ventricle eventually develops into the left ventricle. The proximal portion of the bulbus cordis forms the right ventricle while the distal part of the bulbus cordis forms the outflow tract of both ventricles. The truncus arteriosus forms the roots of both great vessels. The junction between the ventricle and the arterial bulb will be called the primary intraventricular hole. At this time of the development, no septum is present in the heart (**Fig. 2C**).

> The abnormalities of cardiac looping result in abnormalities of atrio-ventricular connection. An isolated discordance at atrioventricular junction result in isolated ventricular inversion. Simultaneous discordance at atrioventricular as well as ventriculoarterial junction leads to congenitally corrected transposition of great arteries (ccTGA).

HEART FIELDS

In recent years, it has become obvious that different parts of the heart and cardiovascular system develops from cells of different lineages. It is now well established that while the majority of the heart, including both the atriums and the

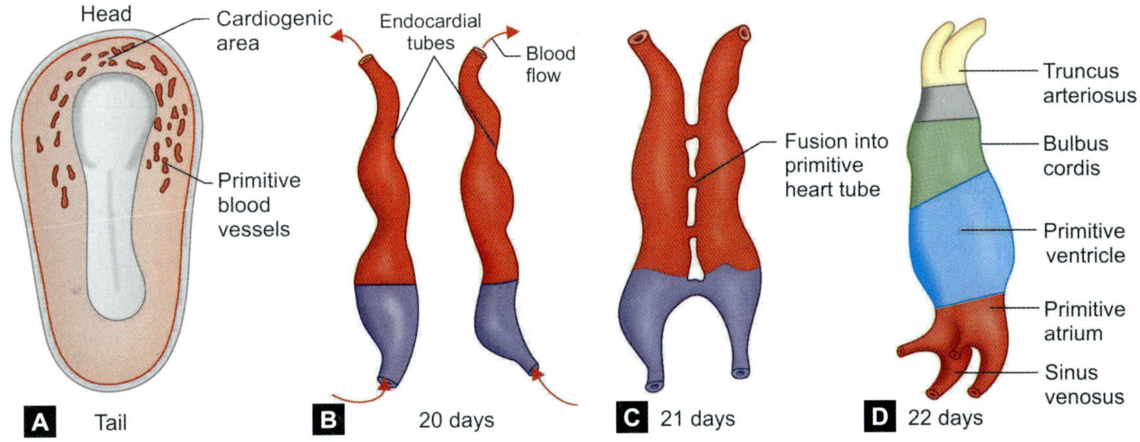

Figs. 1A to D: Early stages of cardiac development showing the cardiogenic area near the head of the embryo (A). Subsequently formed two endocardial tubes (B) fuse cranial to caudal (C) to form a single primitive heart tube (D).

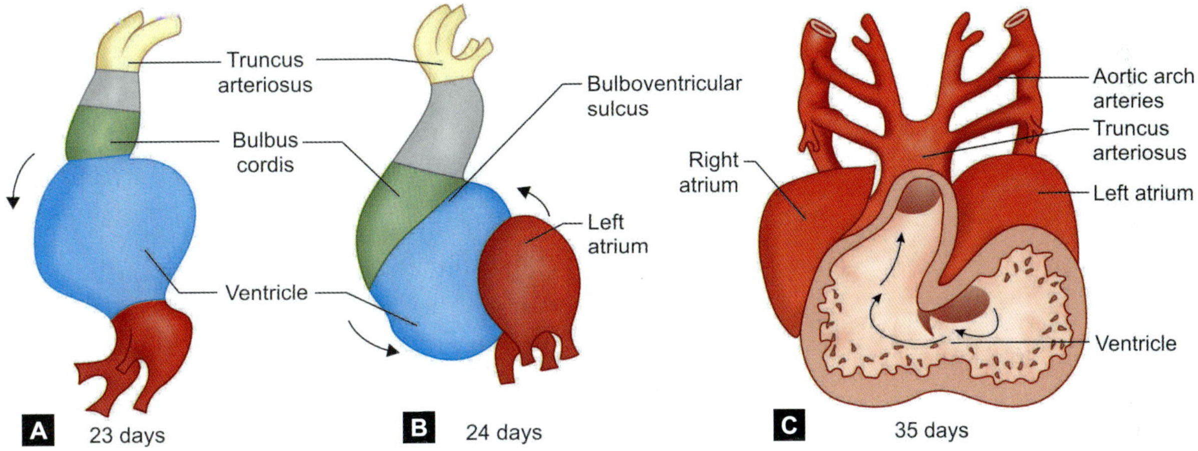

Figs. 2A to C: Looping of the primitive heart tube (A and B) and early differentiation of future cardiac chambers (C). Note that even at day 35 of gestation, the primitive ventricle forms the left ventricle and there is single common outflow.

left ventricle, develops from the first heart field, the right ventricle and outflow tract develop from the second heart field. The second heart field develops late during cardiac development and is believed to be a late addition during the process of evolution. In addition to the first and second heart fields, the heart also receives a contribution from neural crest cells, which contributes to the development of outflow tracts and aortic arches.

The absence of the first heart field is incompatible with life. The abnormalities of the second heart field result in cardiac malformations with maldevelopment of the right ventricle and outflow tract. An abnormal integration of neural crest cells with the developing heart is typically seen in DiGeorge syndrome and manifests as conotruncal and arch anomalies.

DEVELOPMENT OF ATRIOVENTRICULAR VALVES

The atrioventricular valves form during the 5–8th week. Initially, endocardial cushion tissue forms a bulge at the atrioventricular junction, guarded by superior and inferior endocardial cushions. These two masses meet in the middle, dividing the atrioventricular junction into right and left atrioventricular orifices. Endocardial cushions act as a target for the atrial and ventricular septum, as they grow toward the cushions. It is for this reason, the abnormalities of the endocardial cushions are commonly associated with the atrial and ventricular septal defect (**Fig. 3**).

Atrioventricular canal defect, commonly seen in children with Down syndrome, is the result of maldevelopment of endocardial cushions. The malformation includes a primum atrial septal defect, inlet ventricular septal defect as well as abnormalities of atrioventricular valves.

DEVELOPMENT OF ATRIUMS AND ATRIAL SEPTUM

The trabeculated portions of the right and left atriums develop from the primitive atrium. The posterior aspect of the left atrium and right atrium are formed by the pulmonary veins and sinus venosus, respectively. The veins draining into the left sinus venosus (left common cardinal, umbilical, and vitelline veins) degenerate, and the left sinus venosus becomes smaller to form coronary sinus.

Unlike ventricular septum (see further), which develops within the course of gestation, the development of atrial septum concludes only after birth. In the developing heart, the primary atrial septum arises from the posterosuperior region of the primitive common atrium between the left venous valve and orifice of the developing pulmonary veins. The primary septum with a mesenchymal cap on its leading-edge grows toward endocardial cushions. Even before the primary interatrial foramen is closed, the cranial part to the primary septum, near the atrial roof, breaks down to create secondary interatrial foramen (**Figs. 4A to D**).

With further remodeling, the fold between the systemic venous valve and pulmonary vein, located to the right of the primary atrial septum, deepens to form secondary atrial septum. The inferior edge of the secondary atrial septum extends caudally to form the limbus of the oval fossa and covers the flap of the primary septum. The space between the limbus and the flap valve is the definitive foramen ovale. This sequential development of primary and secondary septum is to maintain secondary interatrial foramen through which oxygenated placental blood from inferior vena cava reaches the left side of the developing heart (**Figs. 4A to D**).

> The failure of fusion of primary atrial septum with the endocardial cushion results in primum atrial septal defect. The secundum atrial septal defect, on the other hand, results from deficiency of the superior portion of the primary atrial septum. A complete absence of atrial septum results in common atrium. Restricted foramen ovale during fetal life results in reduced blood flow from inferior vena cava to the left heart and has been shown to cause hypoplastic left heart syndrome.

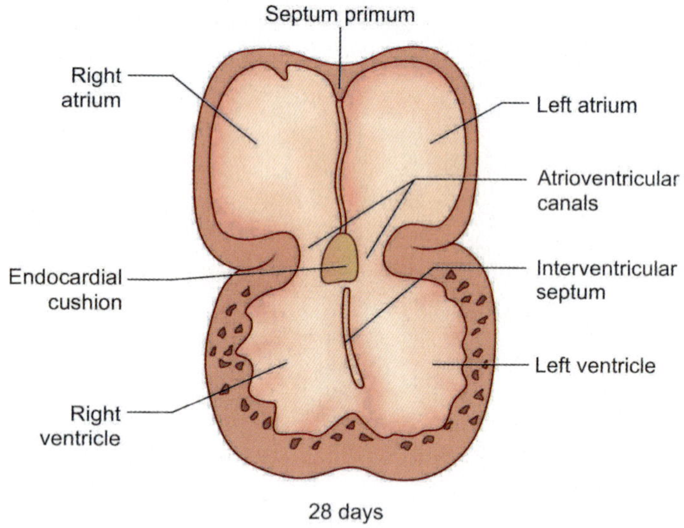

Fig. 3: Development of endocardial cushions dividing the atrioventricular connection into the left and right. Being at the crux of the developing heart, the endocardial cushions form the target for the atrial and ventricular septum.

VENTRICULAR AND OUTFLOW SEPTATION

On day 30, a muscular fold extends from the anterior wall of primitive ventricles, at the apex, and grows toward atrioventricular valves. Most of the initial growth is achieved by the growth of ventricles on the sides (*see* **Figs. 2A to C**). Simultaneously, trabeculations from the inlet region coalesce to form inlet septum in the same plane of the atrial septum. The fusion of these two septa, inlet and trabecular, forms the bulk of the muscular interventricular septum, which then comes in contact with outflow septum to complete the process of ventricular septation (**Fig. 5**). The joining point of these three contributors to the ventricular septum localizes the perimembranous area.

The aortopulmonary septum is formed by ridges separating fourth (future aortic arch) and sixth (future pulmonary arteries) aortic arches. The truncus ridges formed

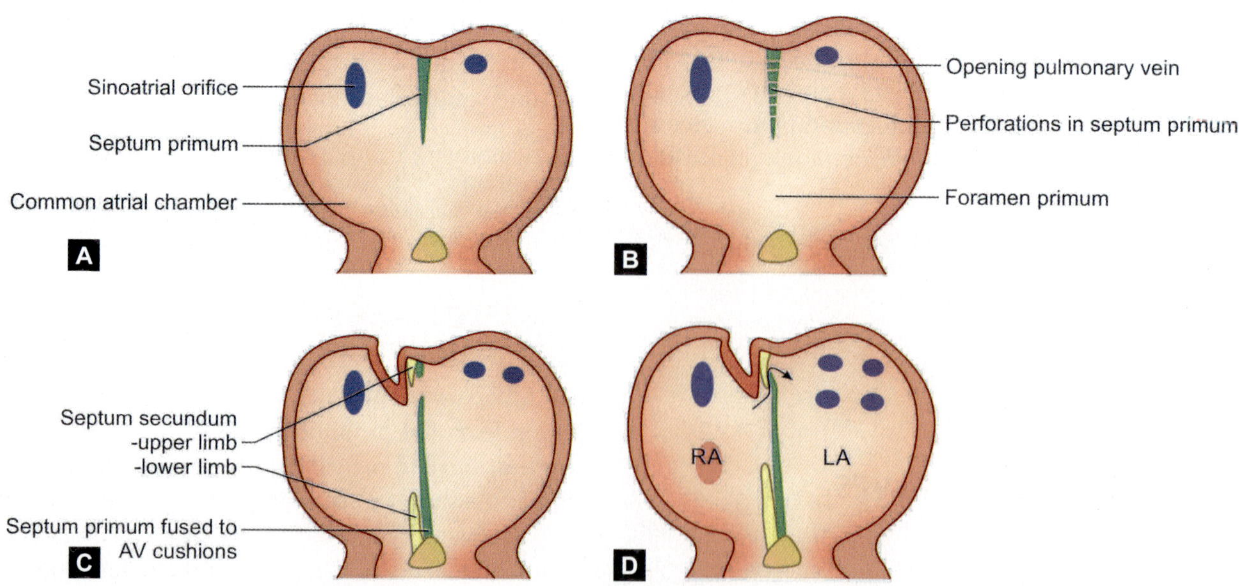

Figs. 4A to D: Various stages of the development of the atrial septum showing sequential formation of the primary atrial septum (A) followed by the development of secondary interatrial foramen (B), secondary atrial septum (C) and foramen ovale (D). The arrangement of atrial septal structures at foramen ovale permits preferential flow of oxygenated blood from inferior vena cava to reach to the left atrium.

in the area of future semilunar valves form the septum between ascending aorta and the main pulmonary artery. The conal ridges form just below the semilunar valves and complete the septation between right and left ventricular outflow tracts (**Fig. 5**). The development of the outflow tract is highly influenced by the integration of neural crest cells.

> Perimembranous area of the ventricular septum, being the junction of all three parts of the ventricular septum, is the most common site of hemodynamically significant ventricular septal defects. A close relation of the development of the ventricular septum with the development of the outflow tract explains common association of ventricular septal defects, particularly in the outflow region, with anomalies of ventricular outflow and ventriculoarterial junction.
>
> A complete absence of aortopulmonary septum results in common arterial trunk. Abnormalities of neural crest integration, as seen in DiGeorge syndrome, is commonly associated with anomalies of outflow tract such as double outlet right ventricle.

PROXIMAL PULMONARY ARTERIES

The proximal main pulmonary artery develops from the truncus arteriosus, whereas the distal main pulmonary artery and proximal right pulmonary artery develop from the ventral sixth aortic arch (see further). The distal right pulmonary artery and left pulmonary arteries are derived from postbranchial arteries, which develop from the lung buds and surrounding mesoderm. The ductus arteriosus develops from the distal left sixth aortic arch.

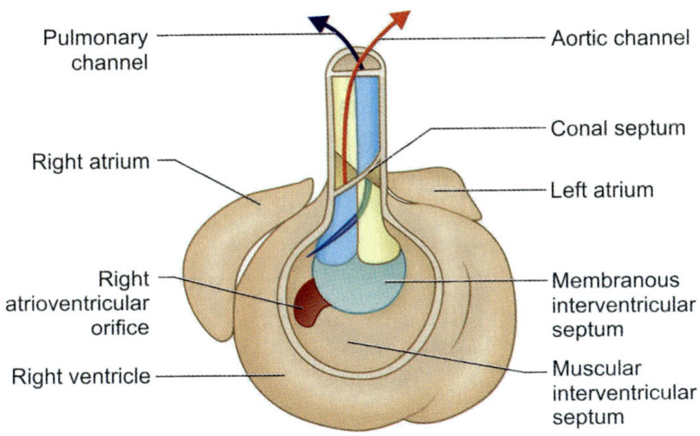

Fig. 5: Ventricular and aortopulmonary septation during development.

GREAT VESSELS AND LARGE ARTERIES

Truncus arteriosus is divided by the aortopulmonary septum to form the pulmonary trunk and the aorta (**Fig. 5**). Aortic arches develop from distal parts of the truncus arteriosus. For long, the human embryo is believed to have six pairs of aortic arches, including a transient fifth arch. The evidence from the developmental biologists to the contrary with no proof, whatsoever, of the existence of the fifth arch in the human embryo (**Fig. 6**). These aortic arches undergo extensive remodeling to form different parts of the future arterial tree.

> Maldevelopment and erroneous remodeling of various segments of aortic arches result in aortic arch anomalies. An understanding of the contribution of various arches in different parts of the atrial tree helps in understanding the morphogenesis of aortic arch anomalies.

SYSTEMIC VENOUS SYSTEM

On day 21, the common atrium is formed due to the fusion of two endocardial tubes, which communicates with two sinus horns (left and right) representing the unfused ends of the endocardial tubes. These two horns subsequently form the dorsally located sinus venosus. The veins draining into the sinus venosus on each side are common cardinal vein (receiving anterior and posterior cardinal vein receiving blood from cranial and caudal part of the embryo,

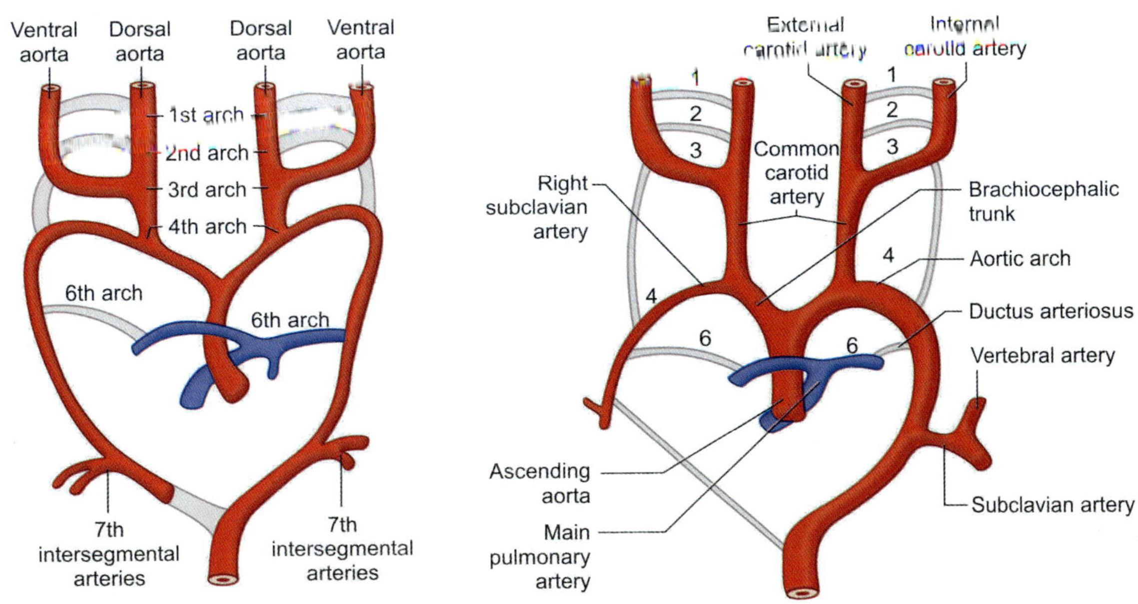

Fig. 6: Development of arterial system based on the Edward's double arch model. Note that unlike the earlier claims by multiple investigators, there is no proof that the fifth arch exists in human embryo.

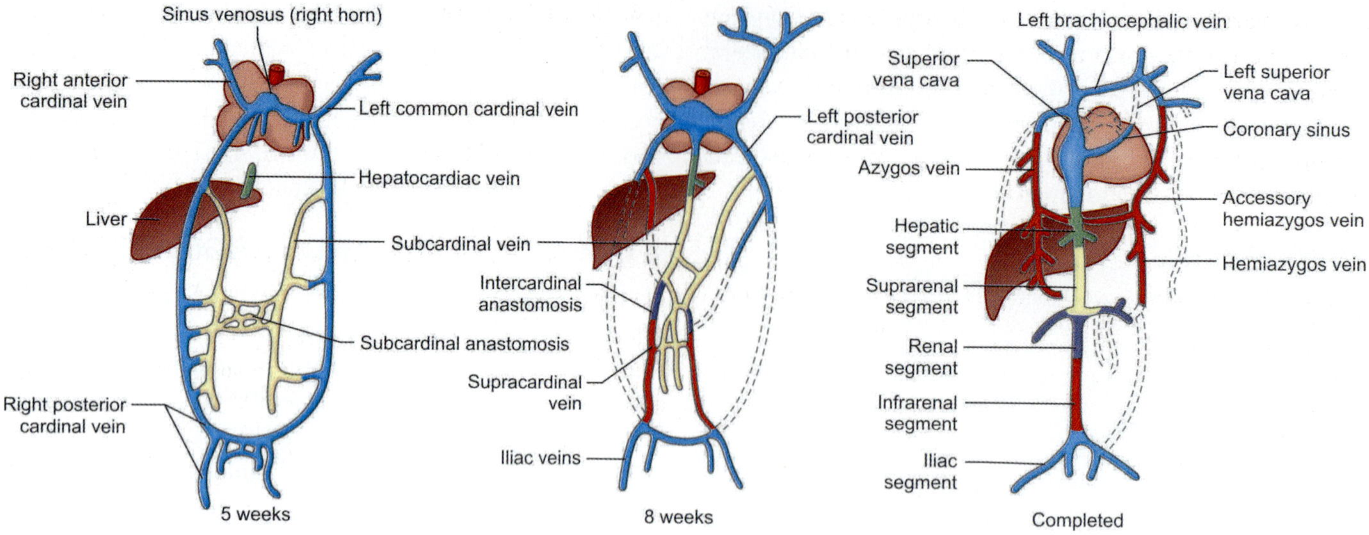

Fig. 7: Development of the venosus system. Note that the inferior vena cava develops from multiple embryonic venous segment.

respectively); umbilical vein (connecting placenta); and vitelline vein (draining yolk sac, gastrointestinal system, and portal circulation) (**Fig. 7**). At 8 weeks, the distal end of the left cardinal vein degenerates, and the proximal portion connects through the anastomosing vein (left brachiocephalic vein) to the right anterior cardinal vein (right brachiocephalic vein) to form superior vena cava. The left posterior cardinal vein degenerates, and the left sinus horn becomes coronary sinus. The right vitelline vein becomes inferior vena cava with the right posterior cardinal vein forming azygos vein. The left umbilical vein degenerates and the right umbilical vein connects to the vitelline system through the ductus venosus.

PULMONARY VENOUS SYSTEM

A primitive vein sprouts out of the left atrium, bifurcating twice to give four pulmonary veins that grow toward the developing lungs. A plexus of veins formed in the mesoderm enveloping the bronchial buds; meet the developing pulmonary veins during week 5. These pulmonary veins form the smooth posterior wall of the left atrium.

CONDUCTION SYSTEM

Primary myocardium, found in the early heart tube, gives rise to the contracting myocardium and the conducting myocardium (nodal and ventricular conducting tissue). The ventricular conduction system starts with the formation of an encircling ring of conducting myocardial tissue around the bulboventricular foramen. The dorsal portion of the ring forms the bundle of His. The portion of the ring covering the septum becomes left and right bundle branches.

DEVELOPMENT OF PERICARDIAL SAC

The right and left intracoelomic cavities extend toward the midline as the median heart tube is formed (day 21), eventually surrounding the heart tube. The ventral mesoderm is immediately absorbed and the two cavities communicate forming the pericardial sac.

TABLE 1: Timeline of cardiac development.

Days after fertilization	*Milestone in cardiac development*
Days 18–19	Heart begins to form
Day 21	Formation of primitive heart tube
Day 22	Heart starts to beat and development of pericardium starts
Day 23	Cardiac looping begins
Days 25–26	Sinus venosus formed and start receiving blood from fetal poles
Days 27–28	Looping completed, shape of the heart is almost complete, septum primum starts to form, two atrioventricular endocardial cushions appear, commencement of circulation
Days 28–35	Venous system formation, development of conduction system, atrial septation is complete, commencement of ventricular septum development, development of aortic arches, pulmonary bud, and pulmonary arteries development starts
Days 28–37	Cardiac "walls" formation
Weeks 5–7	Complete formation of AV valves, complete development of ventricles, and outflow tracts

SUMMARY

The timeline of cardiac development is given in **Table 1**.

CONCLUSION

Knowledge of the basic embryology of cardiovascular system helps in better understanding of the development of congenital heart diseases and their implications on circulation physiology. This forms the basis for advanced knowledge on fetal echocardiography and prenatal counseling. The timing of exposure to teratogenic agents may have various abnormalities from simple septal defects to embryonic deaths depending on the stage of cardiac development at the time of exposure. An understanding of the genetic influences and teratogenic effects at various developmental stages is expected to improve management of various cardiac malformations.

SUGGESTED READING

1. Graham A, Poopalasundaram S, Shone V, Kiecker C. A reappraisal and revision of the numbering of the pharyngeal arches. J Anat. 2019;235(6):1019-23.
2. Gupta SK, Bamforth SD, Anderson RH. How frequent is the fifth arch artery? Cardiol Young. 2015;25(4):628-46.
3. Hosseini HS, Garcia KE, Taber LA. A new hypothesis for foregut and heart tube formation based on differential growth and actomyo-sin contraction. Development. 2017;144(13): 2381-91.
4. Moore K, Persaud TVN, Torchia M (Eds). The Developing Human, 10th edition. St Louis: Saunders; 2015. pp. 245-63.
5. Patton K, Thibodeau G, Hutton A. Development of heart. In: Anatomy and Physiology, 1st edition. Houston: OpenStax; 2013. pp. 787-846.
6. Sadler TW, (Ed). Cardiovascular system. In: Longman's Medical Embryology, 14th edition. Philadelphia: Wolters Kluwer; 2019. pp. 179-222.
7. Schoenwolf G, Bleyl S, Brauer P, Francis-West P, (Eds). Development of heart. In: Larsen's Human Embryology, 5th edition. London: Churchill Livingstone; 2014. pp. 97-122.

4 CHAPTER

Physiology: Essential Hemodynamics and Basic Electrophysiology

Raghavan Subramanyan

HEART AND BLOOD VESSELS: BASIC CONCEPTS AND PROPERTIES

The heart is essentially a pump. It propels blood through two serial circuits, the systemic and the pulmonary circulation. The output of the heart is regulated by a complex interplay of cardiac, neural, and humoral mechanisms that help to maintain adequate perfusion to all tissues.[1] When the metabolic need increases, the heart can increase its output to the necessary level. In addition, the heart helps in balancing the pulmonary and systemic circulations, and in the regulation of blood pressure (BP) and blood volume.

Functionally, the myocardium contains two types of tissues—the contractile tissue and the conducting tissue. The former is a syncytium made up long, branched nucleated cells which contain myofibrils inside a sarcolemma membrane. The myofibrils, in turn, are made of myofilaments of actin and myosin, arranged as a contractile unit called sarcomere. Electrical depolarization of the sarcomere allows influx of sodium ions, in turn leading to influx of calcium ions. Coupling of excitation and contraction then causes sliding of actin over myosin filaments, and shortening of the myofibril. Cessation of contraction and relaxation of myofibrils are brought about by the clearance of calcium ions. A number of factors influence the tension or force developed by the myocardial cell. Increase in initial length (Starling law), catecholamines, sympathetic stimulation, and increased calcium lead to a greater tension being generated during contraction. The myocardium in the left ventricle is thick and arranged in three layers. By a combination of thickening, shortening, and torsion, the left ventricular (LV) myocardium can generate high pressures. In contrast, the right ventricular (RV) wall is a thin layer of muscle wrapped around the LV (**Fig. 1**). The RV functions like a bellow and pumps large volumes at low pressures, mainly by shortening.

Normal circulation is characterized by two distinct vascular beds arranged in a serial fashion with little or no mixing between the two. The systemic vascular bed is a very long circuit made up of arteries, arterioles, capillaries, and veins. The precapillary systemic vasculature is characterized by high resistance and high pressure. Flow in the larger arteries is pulsatile in nature due to the force generated by cardiac contraction during systole. The larger arteries expand to accommodate the excess volume in systole, and recoil during diastole. The kinetic energy imparted by cardiac systole along with arterial recoil helps to propel blood in a more continuous manner (both systole and diastole) through the arterioles, capillaries, and veins. The vast area of the capillary bed allows exchange of oxygen and carbon dioxide in the tissues. The systemic arterioles exhibit active tone which responds to many stimuli. Hypoxia, hypercapnia, and acidosis cause vasodilatation. The autonomic nervous system and circulating catecholamines also exercise important regulatory effects on the systemic arterioles. In contrast to the systemic circulation, the pressure and resistance in pulmonary arterial circulation[2] are quite low. Unlike the systemic arterioles, the pulmonary vessels respond by vasoconstriction to hypoxia, hypercapnia, and acidosis. Conversely, hyperoxia, hypocapnia, and alkalosis result in pulmonary vasodilatation and reduction in pulmonary vascular resistance.

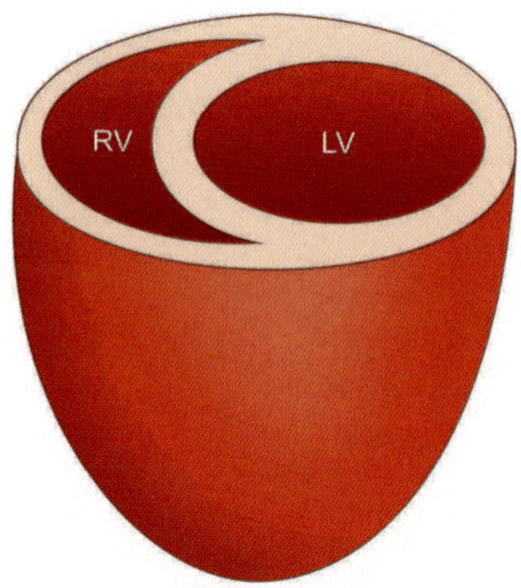

Fig. 1: Diagrammatic representation of the heart showing the right ventricle (RV) wrapped around the left ventricle (LV).

REGULATION OF CARDIAC OUTPUT

The healthy adult heart pumps 3–6 L/min of blood at rest. This is known as the cardiac output (CO). During exercise, the heart can increase its output by four to five times. Other physiological states with increased CO are emotional disturbances, postprandial period, and pregnancy. The factors which determine CO are:

- Diastolic ventricular volume (ventricular preload)
- Strength of myocardial contraction (contractility)
- Resistance to ejection (ventricular afterload)
- Heart rate.

The Frank–Starling law states that within physiological limits the force of myocardial contraction is directly proportional to the initial length of the muscle fiber. In the intact heart, increased diastolic filling volume will accentuate the force of ejection, while decreased filling will have the opposite effect. The venous return, an important determinant of ventricular filling, is influenced by blood volume, venous capacitance, gravity, skeletal muscle contraction, and respiratory changes in intrathoracic pressure. The myocardium also influences ventricular filling by its pumping action and by its diastolic stiffness. Myocardial contractility on the other hand is independent of the filling volume or the resistance. It is enhanced by sympathetic stimulation, circulating catecholamines and calcium, while parasympathetic stimulation, potassium ions, hypoxia, hypercapnia, and acidosis suppress myocardial contractility. Vascular resistance is determined by the net cross-sectional area of all the blood vessels, compliance of the vessel walls, and to a lesser extent, the blood viscosity. Increase in heart rate helps to increase the CO up to a physiological limit. Further increase in rate results in fall in CO due to diminished ventricular filling. Thus, cardiac function is regulated by a complex interplay of multiple mechanisms (**Fig. 2**). Enhancement of contractility by inotropes causes a greater force of contraction at any given end-diastolic volume (shift to left). Myocardial depressants reduce the force of contraction at any given end-diastolic volume (shift to right).

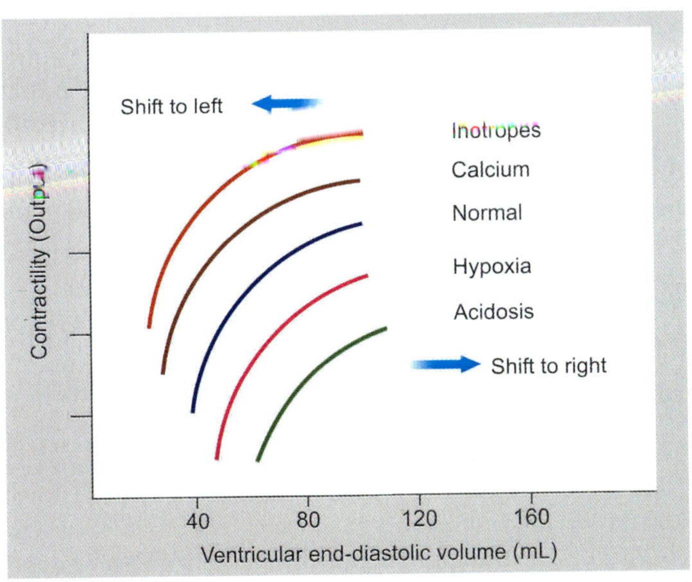

Fig. 2: Relationship between ventricular end-diastolic volume and contractility.

REGULATION OF BLOOD CIRCULATION

The circulation is regulated by the interplay of systemic and local mechanisms. Local regulatory factors include oxygen, acid–base ions, endothelial factors, metabolites, mediators, and local hormones. They mainly act upon the smaller arterioles and the precapillary sphincters, and keep tissue perfusion at a constant level despite wide fluctuations in perfusion pressures. Such short-term autoregulation of perfusion is seen in many organs including heart, brain, kidneys, skin, and muscles. Long-term local modulation of tissue perfusion is mediated by growth of new blood vessels as seen in ischemic tissues and rapidly growing organs. Systemic regulation is mediated by the autonomic nervous system and circulating humoral factors. Neural and chemical mediators alter the CO by changes in the rate and contractility. In addition, they can influence vascular resistance and venous capacity. Epinephrine, norepinephrine, angiotensin II, and vasopressin are examples of circulating vasoconstrictors, while atrial natriuretic peptide, vasoactive intestinal peptide, and bradykinin are vasodilators. Neural control of the circulation by sympathetic and parasympathetic systems is in turn modulated by inputs from medullary, hypothalamic, and cortical cardiovascular centers.

In addition to local and systemic regulation, several cardiovascular reflexes help to adjust CO and BP. The afferent stimuli for these reflexes are conducted by glossopharyngeal or vagus nerves to the medullary cardiovascular and vasomotor centers. The efferent impulses are mediated by the sympathetic ganglia and vagus nerve. Cardiovascular reflexes include the following:

- *Baroreceptor reflexes*: Receptors sensitive to stretch are located in the carotid sinus of internal carotid arteries, aortic arch, pulmonary arteries, pulmonary veins, atrial walls, and LV. Stretch due to rise in aortic pressure leads to a decrease in heart rate, reduction in contractility, and reduced vasomotor tone.
- *Chemoreceptor reflexes*: Chemoreceptors are present in the carotid and aortic bodies. They respond to hypoxia, hypercapnia, and acidosis by stimulating the vasomotor center to raise BP.
- *Atrial baroreceptor reflex*: Stretching of the atrial wall by increased pressure and volume causes an increase in the heart rate (Bainbridge reflex). The effect on BP is less marked. A volume reflex is also initiated with renal vasodilatation, inhibition of antidiuretic hormone secretion, and release of atrial natriuretic peptide. This results in diuresis which contributes to volume and pressure regulation.

- Central chemoreceptors can sense hypoxia and hypercapnia, to produce a reflex rise in arterial pressure and bradycardia (Cushing reflex).
- Chemoreceptors in the lungs respond to hypoxia, hypercapnia, and acidosis by pulmonary vasoconstriction.

Reflex changes in CO, vascular resistance, and pressures are useful in immediate response to acute hemodynamic challenges. Long-term adaptation to unusual demand or disease includes myocardial hypertrophy, chamber enlargement, vascular remodeling, neovascularization, intimal-medial changes, resetting of receptors, volume changes, and neurohormonal activation.

MEASUREMENT OF BLOOD FLOW AND CARDIAC OUTPUT

Measurement of CO in humans is done by indirect or noninvasive methods. The follow-ing techniques are commonly employed: (1) application of Fick principle, (2) indicator dilution method, (3) ultrasonic Doppler method, and (4) echocardiography.

Fick Principle

The blood flow through an organ is equal to the amount of a substance taken up by the organ in unit time divided by the difference in arteriovenous concentration of the substance (**Fig. 3**). Oxygen is commonly used as the marker substance.

$$\text{Blood flow} = \frac{\text{Amount of marker uptake}}{\text{Arteriovenous content difference}}$$

The amount of oxygen taken up by the lungs in a minute can be measured by asking the subject to breathe into a reservoir (Douglas bag). The oxygen consumption is then derived by analysis of the difference in oxygen content in inspired and expired air, and the minute respiratory volume. To obtain the arteriovenous oxygen content difference

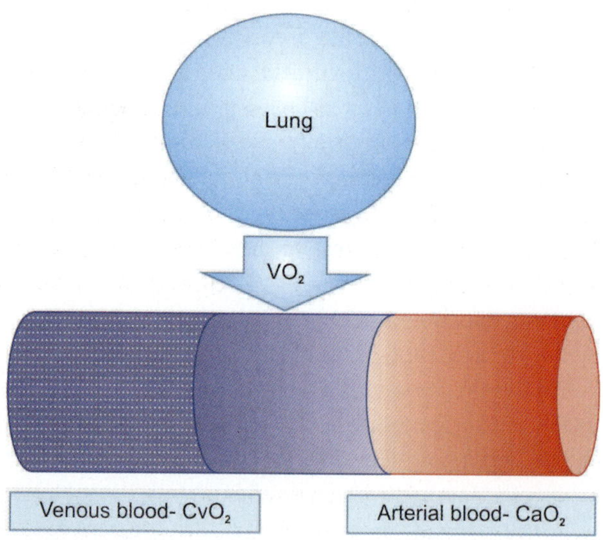

Fig. 3: Measurement of cardiac output (CO) by Fick principle using O_2 as the marker.
(CaO_2: arterial oxygen content; CvO_2: venous oxygen content; VO_2: oxygen uptake or consumption)

for the lung one needs to measure the oxygen contents of pulmonary artery and pulmonary venous blood. A caval blood sample can substitute for pulmonary artery sample, while a systemic arterial sample can be used instead of pulmonary vein sample. Oxygen is transported in two forms in the blood. The major part of the oxygen is combined with hemoglobin (1.36 mL/g). It is calculated as Hb (g%) × 1.36 × (Saturation/100) and expressed as volumes/100 mL of blood (vol%). A smaller portion of the oxygen is dissolved in plasma (0.003 mL O_2/100 mL/mm Hg PO_2). Thus, at normal PO_2 (around 100 mm Hg), 100 mL of plasma will contain 0.3 mL of dissolved O_2 (expressed as 0.3 vol%). The dissolved component increases significantly if oxygen is being administered. The oxygen content of blood is the sum of these two components.

$$\text{CO (mL/min)} = \frac{O_2 \text{ consumption (mL/min)}}{\text{Pulm vein } O_2 \text{ content - Pulm artery } O_2 \text{ content}}$$

A wide arteriovenous oxygen content difference indicates increased oxygen extraction due to reduced tissue flow. If ventilation and inspired oxygen (and thereby arterial oxygen content) remain constant, a rise or fall in venous saturation is a good guide to increase or decrease in CO, respectively. Central venous saturation is therefore often used as a continuous indicator of CO or tissue perfusion in ICU patients. The CO is reported as cardiac index (CI) by dividing it by the subject's body surface area. This normalization allows better interpretation in relation to metabolic needs. Measurement of CO by Fick principle has the advantage of being simple and avoiding use of any extraneous indicators. However, accurate measurement of O_2 consumption is difficult. In practice, therefore, it is common to assume oxygen consumption from population-derived tables. Such assumptions are not useful during exercise or other maneuvers.

Application of the Fick principle is also used to measure regional blood flows. In shunt lesions, the pulmonary blood flow (Qp) can be calculated by measuring the difference in O_2 contents of pulmonary venous blood and pulmonary arterial blood. For calculating systemic blood flow (Qs), the arteriovenous O_2 content difference is measured between the aortic blood and systemic venous blood. Normally Qp and Qs are nearly equal. In left-to-right shunt, Qp is greater than Qs. The ratio (Qp/Qs) is used as a measure of the magnitude of shunt.

Indicator Dilution Method

A number of indicators have been used: dyes (Evans blue or indocyanine green), radioisotopes, or cold sterile saline (thermodilution). The indicator should be measurable, nontoxic, and have no effect on the circulation. A known quantity of the indicator is injected at a proximal point in the circulation. At a given point, downstream measurements are made of the serial changes in concentration or isotope activity or temperature change. The flow or CO is equal to the amount of indicator injected divided by the average concentration of the indicator after a single circulation.

Ultrasound Doppler Method

This method can be employed for serial measurement of CO in the setting of ICU. The CO is calculated as the product of aortic velocity time integral, aortic cross-sectional area and heart rate.

Echocardiography

The volume of the left ventricle can be accurately measured by 2D or 3D echocardiography. The difference in the end-diastolic volume and the end-systolic volume is the stroke volume per beat. CO is equal to the product of stroke volume and heart rate.

CARDIAC CYCLE

The repetitive sequence of cardiac events with each beat of the heart is known as the cardiac cycle. Cardiac systole and diastole refer to the periods of ventricular contraction and ventricular relaxation, respectively. Diastole lasts approximately two times the duration of systole. Atrial systole occurs in ventricular diastole while atrial diastole overlaps both systole and diastole. Physiologists use a diagrammatic depiction of the cardiac events related to excitation, electrocardiogram (ECG), contraction, ejection, valve function, filling volume, pressure, heart sounds, etc., to understand the cardiac cycle. Named after its developer, Carl Wiggers, this diagram charts time on the x-axis and cardiac events on the y-axis (**Fig. 4**).

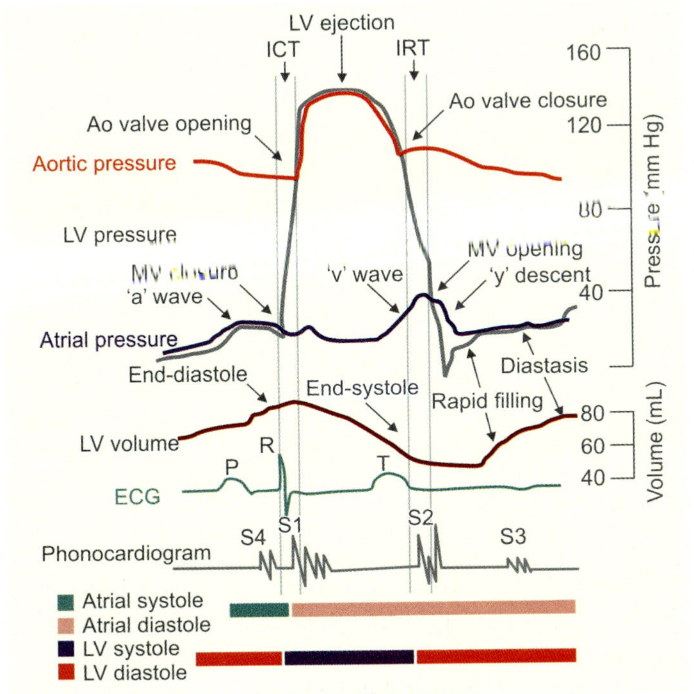

Fig. 4: Wigger diagram showing events during the cardiac cycle. (Ao valve: aortic valve; ICT: isovolumic contraction time; IRT: isovolumic relaxation time; LV: left ventricle; MV: mitral valve; S1: first heart sound, S2: second heart sound; S3: third heart sound; S4: fourth heart sound).

Electrical depolarization of the ventricular myocardium initiates contraction after a 20–30 ms electromechanical delay. This occurs near the peak of the R wave in ECG. The rise in LV pressure closes the MV. With both mitral and aortic valves in closed state, the LV pressure builds up sharply without any change in LV volume (isovolumic contraction). The first heart sound is the clinical indicator of this phase. When the LV pressure rises to above the aortic diastolic pressure, the aortic valve opens to allow flow into the aorta. During the ejection phase (duration about 100 ms), the LV and aortic pressures are similar, but the LV volume decreases rapidly. The end of systole occurs roughly around the peak of T wave in ECG and is indicated by the second heart sound. At this point, the LV pressure falls below the aortic pressure leading to the closure of aortic valve, which coincides with a notch in the aortic pressure tracing (incisura). LV volume is lowest at this point (end-systolic volume). The ensuing isovolumic phase (about 50–60 ms) is characterized by steep fall in LV pressure with no change in LV volume. It is produced by continuing LV relaxation with closed mitral and aortic valves. When the LV pressure falls below the left atrial (LA) pressure, the mitral valve opens leading to rapid ventricular filling. The rapid increase in LV volume and stretching of the wall is audible as the third heart sound. About 60–70% of filling occurs in the initial rapid filling phase, while 5–10% filling occurs in the slow filling phase. The last part of the ventricular filling is due to atrial contraction and coincides with fourth heart sound. The atrial contribution to ventricular filling varies from 20 to 30%. The LV pressure rises rapidly early in diastole, and more slowly in mid-diastole. With atrial contraction, the LV diastolic pressure as well as the LV diastolic volume rises to their maximum levels. It indicates the end of diastole. The end-diastolic volume and end-diastolic pressure are important determinants of ventricular function and output. It is also at this point that the next systole starts. Atrial systole produces an "a" wave followed by the "x" descent caused by atrial diastole. LV contraction also contributes to the fall in atrial pressure during early systole due to downward traction on the closed mitral valve. During this phase, atrial filling leads to increased left atrial volume. Atrial filling continues throughout systole and the resultant rise in pressure produces the atrial "v" wave, approximately at the end of systole. When the LV filling starts in diastole, the atrial pressure falls to produce the "y" descent.

The right heart chambers and pulmonary circulation show similar sequence of events as the left heart with a few differences. RV systole begins earlier due to earlier activation. However, ejection of blood into the pulmonary artery continues and the pulmonary valve remains open for a longer period than on the left side. This is related to the larger capacitance and lower resistance in the pulmonary vascular bed. Ventricular relaxation in early diastole is much more rapid and occurs earlier in the LV.

DYNAMICS OF BLOOD FLOW

Hemodynamics refers to the physics of blood flow in the cardiovascular system.[3] The two main determinants of flow in a channel are pressure difference and resistance in muscular arteries–arterioles. The resistance is predominantly determined by the radius of the smaller arteries and arterioles under physiological conditions. Some factors such as viscosity and blood velocity become important in the abnormal state. The blood flow (Q) is directly proportional to the pressure difference (P1–P2) and inversely proportional to the resistance (R).

$$Q = \frac{P1-P2}{R}$$

R is measured as resistance units (mm Hg/mL/s). It can also be expressed as absolute units, one resistance unit being equal to 80 dynes.sec/cm^5. Pulmonary vascular resistance (PVR) is calculated by dividing Qp by the difference in mean pulmonary artery and mean left atrial pressures. For calculating systemic vascular resistance, Qs is divided by the difference in mean aortic pressure and mean right atrial pressure.

Since the heart ejects blood rhythmically, the flow in aorta and big arteries is pulsatile. However, forward flow is maintained in diastole by the momentum of the blood column. In addition, the aortic distends in systole and recoils back in diastole. This generates the propagating pulse wave. The pulsatile nature of flow gradually decreases toward the smaller vessels due to peripheral resistance and blood viscosity. As a result, circulation in the arterioles, capillaries, and veins is characterized by continuous flow at low velocity and low pressure.

HEMODYNAMIC STUDY

Cardiovascular hemodynamics can be studied by recording the pressures and flows in the cardiac chambers and blood vessels. The ideal method to obtain high fidelity recording is to introduce catheters with micromanometers at their tips into the area of interest. In practice, it is commonly done by connecting the cardiac catheter to external manometers by a fluid-filled tube. Characteristic waveforms are generated by different parts of the circulation. These are useful in understanding and diagnosing normal and abnormal circulation.

The LV pressure (**Fig. 5**) rises sharply with the onset of systole and continues to rise after the aortic valve opening as rapid ejection occurs. Ejection starts slowing down in the second half of systole. The LV pressure and aortic pressure curves together form a parabolic top. In the fluid-filled pressure recording systems used in most catheterization laboratories, it is common to see a notch in the LV pressure tracing in mid-systole. Active myocardial contraction ceases in late systole leading to a smooth descent in pressure curves. The end of systole is indicated by the incisura, a sharp notch in the aortic pressure. It is produced by closure of the aortic valve as the LV pressure falls below aortic diastolic pressure. From this point, the two pressures diverge. The LV diastole deceases sharply to a very low level. This early diastolic dip is particularly marked in the fluid-filled recording systems. Thus, the LV has a high systolic pressure and a low diastolic pressure. This is in contrast to the arteries which have a higher diastolic pressure although the systolic pressure is similar (**Fig. 5**). The ventricular diastolic pressure rises continuously throughout diastole due to filling. Different phases can be sequentially identified in the ventricular filling: rapid filling, slow filling, diastasis or transient equalization, and finally atrial contraction. The aortic pressure on the other hand shows a gradual but continuous fall to its lowest level (diastolic arterial pressure) at end diastole. The atrial and venous pressure tracing can be identified by the presence of "a" and "v" waves in each cardiac cycle (**Fig. 6**).

The normal range of pressures in the different chambers is given in **Table 1**. Pressures and flows are not constant. Beat-to-beat variation as well as phasic changes are normal. Change in intrathoracic pressure with respiration influences

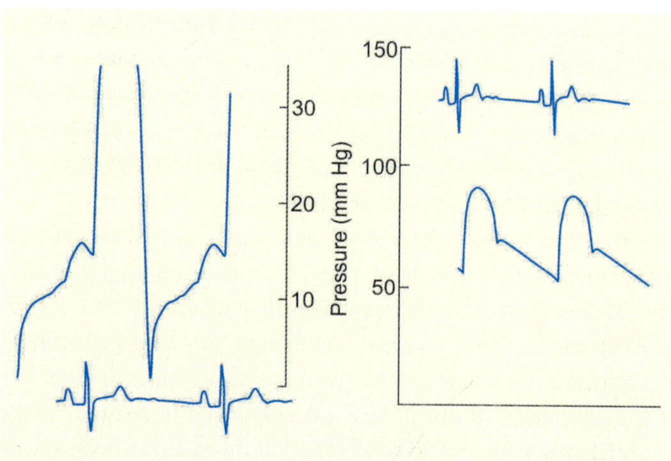

Fig. 5: Pressure recordings from left ventricle (LV) (left) and aorta (right) showing the characteristic waveforms.

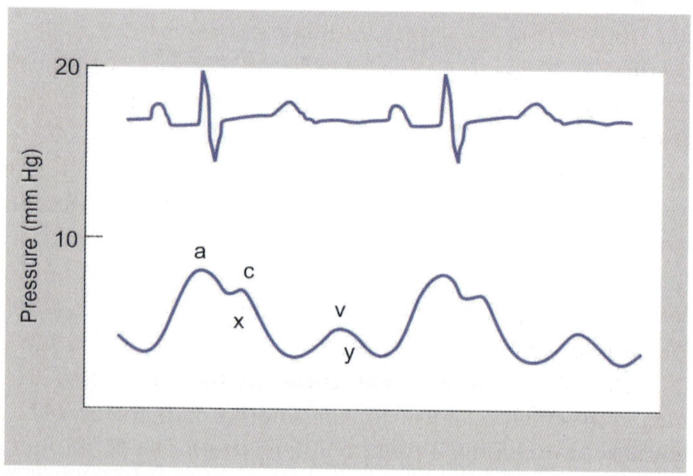

Fig. 6: Atrial pressure recording showing the characteristic waveforms.

TABLE 1: Normal hemodynamic values.

Chamber	*Pressure (mm Hg)*
Right atrium	a = 4–6, v = 2–5, mean 4–6
Right ventricle	Systolic = 20–30, end-diastolic = 3–6
Pulmonary artery	Systolic = 20–30, diastolic = 8–12, mean = 15–18
Left atrium	a = 6–12, v = 7–10, mean 6–12
Left ventricle	Systolic = 100–130, end-diastolic = 6–12
Aorta	Systolic = 100–130, diastolic = 60–80, mean = 65–85
Flow	
Cardiac output	4–6 L/min
Cardiac index	2.5–3.5 L/min/m^2
Resistance	
Pulmonary vascular resistance	0.5–2.0 units or 40–160 dynes.sec/cm^5
Systemic vascular resistance	12–20 units or 1,000–1,600 dynes.sec/cm^5

cardiac filling and transmural pressures, with pressures being higher in expiration than in inspiration. It is customary to report the intracardiac pressures at end-expiration. While the right atrial pressure can be recorded directly, the left atrial pressure is often obtained indirectly by wedging an end-hole catheter in the distal pulmonary artery. The pulmonary artery wedge pressure reflects the left atrial pressure accurately, although there is a delay in transmission of the waves and descents. For atrial pressures, the peak value of the two waves and the mean pressure are reported. In case of ventricles, the peak systolic pressure and the end-diastolic pressure are reported, while in case of arteries, the systolic, end-diastolic, and mean pressures are recorded. The mean or average pressure is best obtained from the area under the pressure curve over a period of time. For practical purposes, the mean arterial pressure can be approximately calculated as the sum of diastolic arterial pressure and one-third of the pulse pressure.

Unusually tall "a" wave in the RA indicates impaired filling of the RV due to hypertrophy, altered myocardium, or TV obstruction. Prominent "v" wave in RA results from tricuspid incompetence. Rise in RA pressure is an early sign of cardiac failure. The LA pressure rises in conditions with mitral inflow obstruction, mitral regurgitation, volume overload of LA, and LV impairment. Mitral regurgitation is associated with prominent "v" waves in LA. In the normal state, the LA pressure is higher than RA pressure. Equalization of LA and RA pressure can occur in the presence of a large atrial septal defect. The systolic pressure in the ventricle is determined by the pressure in the respective arteries. In the presence of outflow tract stenosis in either RV or LV, the ventricular systolic pressure will rise to a higher level than the arterial systolic pressure. The difference in systolic pressures in ventricle and artery (known as pressure gradient) is an indicator of the severity of obstruction. The ventricular diastolic pressure is influenced by the diastolic volume load, myocardial compliance, and myocardial systolic and diastolic functions. Elevation of the end-diastolic pressure is a very early sign of ventricular dysfunction. Impaired ventricular filling due to compression by pericardial tamponade or constrictive pericarditis also increases the ventricular diastolic pressure. Aortic pressure shows characteristic patterns in certain conditions. A low systolic and pulse pressure indicates low CO. A slow upstroke occurs in valvar aortic stenosis. Aortic regurgitation and other causes of aortic run-off are associated with wide pulse pressure and low diastolic pressure.

Hemodynamic parameters obtained by cardiac catheterization is the most direct method of diagnosing normal and abnormal cardiac function. This is the gold standard to study CO, pressures, pressure wave-forms, flows in pulmonary and systemic circulations, vascular resistance, and cardiac function. With the development of echocardiography with Doppler, computerized tomography imaging, and cardiac magnetic resonance imaging, the need for invasive hemodynamic study has diminished in recent years. Currently diagnostic cardiac catheterization is used as a complimentary procedure to obtain essential flow, pressure, and resistance data that are not reliably obtained by the noninvasive techniques.[3] Evaluation of shunt lesions with pulmonary hypertension requires measurement of Qp, Qs, PVR, and SVR. Reactivity to pulmonary vasodilators is important in shunt lesions as well as in patients with idiopathic pulmonary hypertension. When there is a discordance between clinical data and noninvasive test findings, cardiac catheterization data becomes necessary. It can be combined with maneuvers such as exercise, drug administration, or pacing to assess the hemodynamics under stress.

BLOOD PRESSURE: REGULATION AND MEASUREMENT

The lateral pressure on the arterial walls exerted by the blood column is called BP. BP helps to maintain flow of blood and tissue perfusion. The two main determinants of BP are CO and vascular resistance, and factors affecting them would alter the BP. Under normal circumstances, the BP is maintained within a range by a complex interaction of multiple regulatory mechanisms. These can be broadly classified as follows:

- *Short-term mechanisms*: Cardiovascular reflexes, autonomic nervous system, catecholamines, and central vasomotor centers
- *Long-term mechanisms*: Renin–angiotensin system, aldosterone, blood volume, antidiuretic hormone, natriuretic hormones, endothelial nitric oxide, growth factors, vascular remodeling, and resetting of receptors

Blood pressure varies within limits in the normal individual. Factors which rise the BP from the basal level include day-time, physical activity, emotions, and increasing age. The normal range of resting BP at different ages has been studied extensively. Persistent elevation of either systolic or diastolic BP is called hypertension. In general, for adults, a systolic BP of >140 mm Hg or diastolic BP >90 mm Hg, if persistent, is considered abnormal. Hypertension does not cause many symptoms but causes extensive vascular and organ damage. Similarly, hypotension (systolic <90 mm Hg or diastolic BP <50 mm Hg), if prolonged, can cause hypoperfusion and permanent damage. These values are not absolute, and the critical level at which harm occurs, is modulated by other factors such as age, temperature, pre-existing disease, and infection.

The arterial BP can be measured directly by catheterization or by arterial cannulation. The indirect method (Sphygmomanometer) is much more extensively used in clinical practice. A pressure cuff is wrapped around the arm. It should approximately cover two-thirds of the arm circumference and the middle two-thirds of the arm length. The pressure in the cuff is increased by a pumping mechanism, and, measured by either mercury or aneroid meter. The cuff pressure is first raised to above the expected systolic BP. Then the cuff is deflated slowly with continuous palpation of the radial pulse. The pressure at which the obliterated pulse reappears indicates the systolic BP. The palpatory method is a quick way of estimating the systolic BP and is useful in emergency situations. However, it tends to underestimate systolic BP. Korotkoff auscultatory method involves auscultation over the brachial artery as the cuff is deflated. The flow in the artery produces the Korotkoff sounds in five distinct phases: tapping sounds, prolonged sounds of flow turbulence, loud intermittent sounds, muffled sounds, and cessation of sound. Appearance of tapping sound (phase I) indicates systolic BP, while cessation of sound (phase V) indicates diastolic BP. When there is an aortic run-off situation such as severe aortic regurgitation, the sounds may be audible till nearly zero level. In such cases, phase IV or muffling is used to measure diastolic BP.

Special care must be taken to obtain a correct BP reading. Proper sized cuff and method are necessary. The subject must be relaxed, comfortable, and breathing normally. The arm with the cuff should be at the approximate level of the heart. Both palpatory and auscultatory methods must be used. If the initial reading is abnormal, one must take more measurements on the same visit, as well as plan for more readings to be taken. Only persistently elevated BP should be labeled as hypertension. If needed, ambulatory BP record can be done over several hours or more. Automatic sphygmomanometers are also available for recording BP at home. Both these types of BP measurements sense vibrations in the arterial wall with flow (oscillometer).

BASIC ELECTROPHYSIOLOGY

Cardiac Conduction System: Anatomy and Properties

The sequential contraction of atria and ventricles during each cycle is produced by the production of impulses from a controlling pacemaker (sinoatrial or SA node), and their propagation through a specialized conduction system. The SA node is a strip of specialized atrial muscle at the junction of superior vena cava and RA. Pacemaker cells exhibit spontaneous diastolic depolarization. This results in a wave of electrical activation spreading sequentially through the RA and LA myocardium. In addition, three internodal tracts facilitate conduction from the SA node to the atrioventricular (AV) node. The latter is situated at the AV junction in the anteroinferior part of interatrial septum. The AV node ensures unidirectional conduction from atria to ventricles. The physiological delay in conduction through AV node allows adequate time for ventricular filling from atrial systole. The AV node leads to the Bundle of His, which represents the only area of electrical continuity between atria and ventricles in the healthy heart. This is an important factor in preventing re-entrant arrhythmia. At the crest of the muscular septum on the right side, the bundle divides into a smaller right bundle and a larger left bundle which pierces the septum. On reaching the LV side, the left bundle divides into the anterior and posterior fascicles. Both these fascicles then ramify into a broad network of Purkinje fibers in the subendocardial layer. The more compact right bundle travels to the base of the anterior papillary muscle in RV, and then branches into the subendocardial Purkinje network. The His–Purkinje system conducts impulses much more rapidly than the ventricular myocardium.

While any part of the conduction system can produce rhythm, the SA node dominates because of its higher rate (70–80/min). AV nodal rhythm (40–60/min) and ventricular rhythm (20–40/min) are much slower. In pathological states, one of the latter can function as a secondary pacemaker. After traversing the AV node and Bundle of His, the impulse stimulates the ventricular myocardium. Beginning at the midportion of ventricular septum on the LV side, it spreads across the septum toward the right side. Then both ventricles are activated toward the apex, with the LV lagging slightly behind the RV. From the apical area, the wave of excitation travels to the basal regions of the ventricles. The last areas of ventricular activation are the outflow tracts and posterior-basal LV wall. In each region, depolarization occurs from endocardium to epicardium. Recovery of the excitable tissues from depolarized state is called repolarization. This spreads in a reverse direction through the ventricular myocardium.

Surface Electrocardiogram

Every myocardial cell is electrically active. These potentials require special methods to study and record. It is easier to record the summated electrical activity of the heart during each cycle by placing electrodes directly on the heart tissue (electrogram) or on the surface of the body (electrocardiogram or ECG). The potentials are small in magnitude and need to be amplified. Appropriate filters are used to avoid interference from other electric potentials. The record obtained represents the algebraic sum of all electric potentials from the heart occurring at any given moment. The ECG wave represents the net magnitude and direction of the electrical wave (depolarization or repolarization) in the heart. Depending upon the location of electrodes, each lead predominantly reflects one aspect of the heart. Bipolar leads have a negative and a positive electrode, while unipolar leads have an exploring electrode and an indifferent electrode. The ECG is usually recorded on a millimeter graph paper at a speed of 25 mm/s (1 mm on the "X" axis = 0.04 s). The calibration is usually set to produce a 10-mm deflection for 1 mV on the "Y" axis.

Each cardiac cycle produces a set of waves named sequentially as P, Q, R, S, and T waves. The P wave represents atrial activation, while QRS complex is due to ventricular excitation. Atrial repolarization is inconspicuous and occurs during the P-R segment. Ventricular repolarization is represented by the ST segment and T wave. Studies in healthy people have given information on normal patterns, amplitudes, and duration of the ECG complexes. A knowledge of normal and abnormal patterns is necessary to identify physiological variations and pathological abnormalities. The ECG is an extremely valuable tool to the clinician and aids in diagnosing arrhythmia, ischemia, myocardial infarction, electrolyte imbalance, cardiac inflammation, cardiac hypertrophy, and conduction defects. A more extended recording of the ECG over 24–72 hours (Holter ECG monitor) helps to pick up transient abnormalities which occur during wakefulness, sleep, normal activity, or exercise.

Cardiac Electrophysiology Study

Cardiac electrophysiology study (EPS) involves placing multiple electrode catheters in the heart under fluoroscopic guidance. A typical EPS will record electrograms at the following locations: high RA, low RA, TV annulus (close to His bundle), RV apex, and coronary sinus. A multichannel monitor-recorder is necessary to record the above leads along with 3–6 surface leads. In more complex studies, additional electrodes would be necessary in the LA, LV, aorta, epicardium, etc. EPS recorders use appropriate combinations of high-pass and low-pass filters to allow selective recording of intracardiac electrograms at specific sites and surface ECG waves. Since electrical conduction in the heart is fast, EPS recordings are obtained at speeds of 100–250 mm/s. Extraneous electrical stimuli can be introduced at specific times in the cardiac cycle to see the effect on excitation, conduction, and arrhythmia genesis (programmed electrical stimuli). Electrical pacing of the heart is also used to stress the SA node, AV node, and conduction system. These methods have allowed insight into the mechanisms of clinical arrhythmia, and development of effective treatment methods by ablation at critical locations.

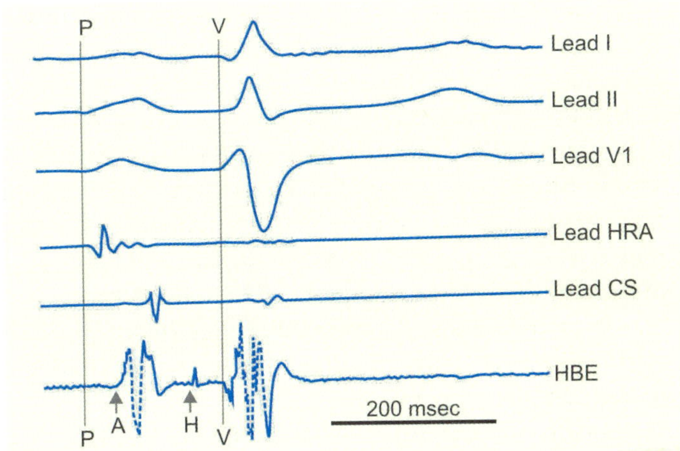

Fig. 7: Multichannel recording during a cardiac electrophysiology study showing normal His bundle electrogram (HBE).
(A: low atrial electrogram; CS: coronary sinus; H: His deflection; HRA: high right atrium, P: atrial activation in surface ECG; V: earliest ventricular activation).

A typical His bundle electrogram (HBE) is shown in **Figure 7**. It records electrograms from the low RA (A), His bundle (H), and ventricle (V). The PA interval, measured from the onset of P wave in ECG to the beginning of the A, represents intra-atrial conduction. AH interval is measured in HBE from the beginning of A to the start of the H spike, reflecting the time taken by the impulse to traverse from low RA to the His bundle. The major component of the AH interval is due to AV nodal conduction. The normal range of AH interval is 50–110 ms. A longer AV interval indicates AV nodal (supra-Hisian) conduction delay, while a shorter AV interval may be due to pre-excitation. Conduction from the His bundle to the ventricles (HV interval) normally takes 35–55 ms. This is measured from the beginning of the H spike to the start of the earliest ventricular activation in any lead. Unusual prolongation of the HV interval reflects infra-Hisian conduction problem. Atrial pacing at incremental rates causes prolongation of AH interval with little change in HV intervals. High atrial pacing rates (>220/min) is associated with increasing degrees of AV block even in the normal heart. A lower threshold for developing AV block is a clue to AV conduction disease. Atrial pacing is also useful to evaluate SA nodal function by measuring its recovery time. This is obtained by measuring the time taken for the first sinus P wave to appear after sudden cessation of pacing.

Mechanisms of Cardiac Arrhythmia

Slow cardiac rhythm (bradyarrhythmia) can occur due to dysfunction of the SA nodal pacemaker or the conduction system.[4] Sick sinus syndrome refers to the clinical picture caused by bradycardia or a combination of intermittent tachycardia and bradycardia. Factors associated with sick sinus syndrome are increasing age, ischemic heart disease, thyroid dysfunction, and diabetes mellitus. AV conduction block can occur due to ischemia, infarction, inflammation, cardiomyopathy, infiltration, or degeneration. Heart block in infants and children can be the result of developmental defect (labeled as idiopathic heart block at present) or damage by maternal antibodies in systemic lupus erythematosus.

Tachyarrhythmia refers to an abnormal intermittent or persistent increase in the heart rate. Three mechanisms have been identified as follows:

- *Increased automaticity*: There is increased repetitive discharge of impulses from a focus due to irritability or stimulation. When the rate of such discharge is higher than that of the SA node tachycardia occurs. It is more commonly seen in disease states such as ischemia, myocarditis, cardiomyopathy, heart failure, pneumonia, and chronic lung diseases. It is aggravated by high sympathetic tone or sympathomimetic substances.
- *Re-entry circuit*: This is the most common form of intermittent or paroxysmal tachyarrhythmia. It is often associated with an otherwise normal heart. The substrate for re-entry is a closed loop of conducting tissue anywhere in the heart. Some potential sites of re-entry exist in the normal heart such as: AV node, SA node, bundle branches, and His-Purkinje system. In addition, presence of accessory conduction bundles, especially if straddling the AV junction, is an important cause of tachyarrhythmia. Homogenous conduction in all parts of the conduction system helps to prevent re-entry by ensuring uniform depolarization and repolarization. This ensures that each impulse gets extinguished at the end of the cardiac cycle. A defect or heterogeneity in conduction or excitability permits a continuous cycle of excitation and recovery which perpetuates the tachycardia. The two most common clinical conditions caused by re-entry mechanisms are AV nodal re-entrant tachycardia and AV re-entrant tachycardia. The latter is also known as pre-excitation or accessory path tachycardia or Wolff–Parkinson–White syndrome.
- *Triggered activation*: A preceding depolarization can cause oscillations in the membrane potential. This is also known as after potential or after depolarization. If it happens to reach threshold level, a wave of depolarization is created leading to an ectopic beat or sustained tachycardia. Triggered activation can be enhanced by many factors: hypoxia, acidosis, stretch, hypokalemia, catecholamines, and drugs.

CONCLUSION

A clear understanding of cardiac physiology is essential to understand pathological changes in the circulation. All diagnostic methods in cardiology including physical examination, rhythm analysis, hemodynamic study, imaging and flow studies, require proper timing and correlation with the events in the cardiac cycle.

REFERENCES

1. Klabunde RE. Cardiovascular Physiology Concepts, 2nd edition. Philadelphia: Wolters Kluwer (Health)/Lippincott, Williams and Wilkins; 2012. pp. 9-140.
2. Naeiji R. Physiology of the pulmonary circu-lation and the right heart. Curr Hypertension Rep. 2013;15(6):623-31.
3. Tharakan JA. Hemodynamic foundations. In: Prabhakaran D, Krishna Kumar R, Naik N, Kaul U (Eds). Tandon's Textbook of Cardiology, 1st edition, Volume 1. New Delhi: Wolters Kluwer (India); 2019. pp. 73-95.
4. Abhilash SP, Namboodri N. Basics of cardiac electrophysiology. In: Prabhakaran D, Krishna Kumar R, Naik N, Kaul U, (Eds). Tandon's Textbook of Cardiology, 1st edition, Volume 1. New Delhi: Wolters Kluwer (India); 2019. pp. 96-111.

5 CHAPTER

Cardiovascular System: History and Physical Examination

M Zulfikar Ahamed, R Krishna Kumar

HISTORY

"The Past is Prologue"

–**William Shakespeare**[1]

Clinical history in suspected heart disease in infants and children differ from that of an adult, both in content and accent. History taking has to be tailored to the age of the child, birth-related matters, and the need for a provisional diagnosis. It should also consider the various clinical presentations of congenital heart disease (CHD) and various acquired heart diseases. Symptom analysis should be undertaken considering the age-specific presentation.[2-4]

History in Newborn and Infant

Both history and physical examination are used to detect and evaluate cardiac problems in the infant. Nearly half of significant CHDs present within 1 month and 90% by 1 year. Hence, queries are to be age specific.[5]

In the newborn and infant, CHD can present in various ways. The common presentations can be as follows:

- Heart failure (HF)
- Hypoxemia
- Both HF and hypoxemia
- Shock
- Arrhythmia
- Asymptomatic murmur
- Failure to thrive (FTT)
- Recurrent respiratory infections
- Stroke
- Hypertension.

History taking must begin with assess-ment of pregnancy details.

Pregnancy

Age of the mother at the time of conception, birth order, and gestational age should be inquired into. History of possible maternal diseases such as diabetes, systemic lupus erythematosus (SLE), phenylketonuria (PKU), and epilepsy should be sought. The other issues are history of maternal infections such as rubella, exposure to teratogenic drugs and agents, smoking, alcohol and exposure to X-rays.

Family History

Family history of CHD is important. History of CHD both in siblings and parents is useful. There could be syndromes with associated CHD which may be familial certain. Acquired heart conditions, specific arrhythmia substrates, and sudden cardiac deaths could be familial and genetically mediated. In certain situations, family screening may also be indicated or initiated.

Perinatal History

Pregnancy-related problems such as hypertension, antepartum bleeding, and intrauterine growth retardation (IUGR) should be asked for. Birth weight and maturity are crucial. IUGR is a feature of congenital rubella syndrome. Prematurity can increase the chance of patent ductus arteriosus (PDA) and perinatal hypoxia can lead to persistent pulmonary hypertension in the newborn (PPHN).

Neonatal History

History of postnatal hypoxemia, feeding difficulties, sweating, breathing difficulty, and poor circulation should be asked for. Nearly half of critical CHD present in the newborn and they have a certain chronological order in presentation.

Infancy

Developmental and growth history can be integrally associated with CHD, especially in a syndromic baby. In a cyanotic CHD, there could be predominant motor delay and in large left-to-right shunts, growth can be affected.

Feeding history, episodes of irritability, lower respiratory infections, history of excessive sweating, and other systemic symptoms have to be sought.

Past Medical History

Medical history relates to specific illnesses which can lead to specific heart diseases, e.g., possible viral myocarditis and cancer chemotherapy leading to dilated cardiomyopathy (DCM). History of cardiac drugs being taken will give a diagnostic clue also. A large post-tricuspid shunt may be receiving diuretics and digoxin.

Immunization History

Widespread use of measles, mumps, and rubella (MMR) vaccine has significantly reduced rubella syndrome-related CHD and possibly endocardial fibroelastosis (EFE). Infants with CHD should be receiving all vaccinations including those against *Haemophilus influenzae* and *Pneumococcus*. It is important to ascertain the specifics of the vaccinations received till the date of evaluation to enable planning of subsequent immunizations.

Diet History

Poor diet intake can be linked to symptomatic CHD. Iron deficiency can precipitate HF. Though rare, Thiamine or vitamin B_1 deficiency can cause high-output HF and pulmonary hypertension (PH). Thiamine deficiency happens in the very specific circumstance of exclusive breastfed infants whose mothers are consuming a thiamine-deficient diet of polished rice.

History in Children and Adolescents

In history taking in children and adolescents, there can be more than one historian and yet the primary one must be the child. Many children and adolescents may present with "adult" like symptoms such as chest pain, palpitation, and exercise intolerance.

Majority of the medical history will go along like a routine history-taking in a growing child. Past medical history is very crucial as these may highlight the impact of cardiac condition on the child's overall health. Additional information should be sought regarding schooling, sports activity, and psychosocial elements and also in specific cardiovascular disease (CVD) risk factors in an adolescent (*see* Chapter 50). Family history is not only relevant to CHD, but also to acquired heart disease.

Clinical presentations can either be due to CHD or acquired heart disease. These acquired illnesses can range from valvar diseases, myocardial diseases, and pericardial diseases to vascular disorders, arrhythmias, and inflammatory condition.

The common presentations in this age group are as follows:

- Overt or covert HF with exercise intolerance with fatigue or dyspnea on effort
- Hypoxemia manifesting as cyanosis
- Arrhythmia manifesting as palpitations
- Asymptomatic murmur identified incidentally
- Stroke, syncope, and sudden cardiac death
- Systemic hypertension.

Shock, FTT, and recurrent respiratory infections are less common presentations.

SYMPTOM ANALYSIS

The symptoms in CVDs in childhood include four cardinal cardiac symptoms—dyspnea, palpitation, chest pain, fatigue, and other symptoms such as respiratory, neurological, hypoxemia related, and various others.

Dyspnea

An uncomfortable awareness of one's own breathing is called dyspnea. Hence, the symptom could be interpreted as an "adult" symptom. But in small children and infants, there are certain measurable symptoms and signs that correlate to exercise intolerance [dyspnea (Greek): Difficult breathing].

- Exertional dyspnea in a child can be caused by both CHD and acquired heart disease. The three major reasons for breathlessness on exertion are:
  1. Pulmonary venous congestion, examples include large ventricular septal defect (VSD)/PDA, mitral valve disease, and cardiomyopathies
  2. Hypoxemia, examples include tetralogy of Fallot (TOF), and Eisenmenger syndrome (ES)
  3. Low fixed cardiac output, examples include idiopathic pulmonary hypertension and severe aortic or pulmonary stenosis (PS).

Note: In admixture lesions like in single ventricle with pulmonary arterial hypertension (PAH), a combination of both pulmonary congestion and mild hypoxemia may be at play.

Additional factors for dyspnea may be compression of bronchi by dilated pulmo-nary arteries and subsequent atelectasis, coincidental respiratory infection, and even less of skeletal muscle content (including respiratory muscles) in CHD.

Orthopnea

Breathlessness on lying down, relieved by sitting up is called orthopnea. Children and adolescents can experience this. Infants who have significant heart disease seem to become comfortable on putting them to mother's shoulders. This could be a variant of orthopnea.

Orthopnea is usually manifest in those with pulmonary venous congestion and subsequent poor lung compliance. It has a good correlation to left-sided filling pressures.

When a child lies down, venous return is more and more of blood reaches the right heart which increases further the pulmonary flow and more of congestion. Lung compliance further declines and work of breathing is more, leading to orthopnea. Unfavorable position of diaphragm can also contribute here.

Paroxysmal Nocturnal Dyspnea

This is an extreme form paroxysmal dyspnea. Characteristically, the patient with left heart disease goes to sleep, sleeps for 2–3 hours, and wakes up with dyspnea which is associated with cough, bringing out pink frothy sputum. He/she stands up for some time and is often relieved.

In the setting of left heart disease such as mitral stenosis (MS), DCM, or other causes of left ventricular (LV) dysfunction, pulmonary venous congestion is quite significant. When a person sleeps for 2–3 hours, there is a redistribution of fluid from extravascular space into intravascular compartment. Venous return further increases on lying down leading to aggravation of pulmonary congestion. In addition, sleep takes away some of the sympathetic drive, which further lead to reduction in contractility and heart rate.

Paroxysmal nocturnal dyspnea as a symptom clearly marks the patient as having left heart disease. In children, we encounter PND in severe MS, mitral regurgitation (MR) with LV dysfunction, severe carditis, DCM with acute decompensation, and viral myocarditis.

Acute Pulmonary Edema

It is the extreme form of dyspnea due to cardiac causes and precipitates abruptly. There is alveolar pulmonary edema and can be lethal unless treated properly. Acute pulmonary edema can occur when left atrial pressure or pulmonary venous pressure is acutely elevated beyond 25 mm Hg. Gradual increase in pulmonary venous pressure does not result in frank pulmonary edema despite significant elevations to levels >25 mm Hg.

Table 1 summarizes the clinical correlates of elevated pulmonary venous pressure.

Miscellaneous

There are certain terminologies which are related to dyspnea. *Cheyne-Stokes* breathing can occur in adults in advanced HF. *Platypnea* refers to a situation where the person is comfortable on supine position, but dyspneic on sitting up. The *trepopnea* refers to a situation where assuming a particular position brings out breathlessness, found in LA myxoma. *Hyperpnea* refers to increase in both rate and depth of breathing, found in acidosis and cyanotic spell. *Tachypnea* is rapid and shallow breathing, which can be in response to elevated pulmonary venous pressure of >10–12 mm Hg in infants and >20 mm Hg in adolescents.

Special Circumstances in Infants

Physical stress in infants includes crying, feeding, passing stools, and playing. These will result in breathing difficulty in various forms.

TABLE 1: Clinical correlates of pulmonary venous hypertension.

Symptom	*Pulmonary venous pressure*
Dyspnea	≥15 mm Hg
Paroxysmal nocturnal dyspnea	≥18 mm Hg
Acute pulmonary edema	≥25 mm Hg

The infant may feed for a short period, stops and rests and again feeds—*suck-rest-suck cycle* due to HF and subsequent pulmonary congestion. Some babies take a long time (normal feeding time is 20 minutes). Babies who are younger than 3 months can typically consume 3–4 Oz in 20 minutes, while those who are ≥3 months take in 6–8 Oz in 20 minutes. Infant with HF may require 30–45 minutes to complete a feed.

Excessive sweating on feeding is another sign that occurs due to the increased sympathetic drive. Babies with cardiac tachypnea seldom grunt. This has been called "happy tachypnea". Retractions involving intercostal (IC), suprasternal, and subcostal regions occur in HF.

Palpitation

Uncomfortable awareness of one's own heart beating is often described as palpitation, which is perceived and vocalized by older child and adolescent (≥4 years). Palpitation can be paroxysmal or exertional and can be brief or prolonged.

Paroxysmal palpitation is often due to paroxysmal arrhythmias. Supraventricular tachycardia (SVT) is the most common cause, followed by ventricular tachycardia and atrial flutter. Atrial fibrillation is uncommon in young children but may happen in advanced rheumatic heart disease in adolescents. Ectopic activity causes palpi-tation. Exertional palpitation is often due to volume overloaded heart conditions, the examples being large atrial septal defect (ASD), PDA, severe MR and aortic regurgitation (AR), and hyperdynamic heart.

Chest Pain

Chest pain is often a common symptom in children and adolescents, though most are noncardiac in origin. Cardiac causes (≤10%) are either anginal or nonanginal. Exertional anginal pain can occur due to aortic stenosis, anomalous coronary artery from pulmonary artery, hypertrophic cardiomyopathy, coronary arterial fistula, Kawasaki disease, SLE, and premature atherosclerotic coronary artery disease in the adolescent. Mitral valve prolapse (MVP)and pericarditis can lead to chest pain. Viral myocarditis is another important cause of chest pain as is pulmonary embolism. Various reasons for chest pain in MS are well known. Severe PH can also cause chest pain due to right ventricular (RV) ischemia. The cardiac causes of chest pain are listed in **Table 2**.

Fatigue

Fatigue is less well defined in young children and there may be an overlap between fatigue and exercise intolerance. Some children avoid symptoms by avoiding exercise and appear to be "normal." Generally, fatigue due to cardiac causes is due to low fixed cardiac output such as DCM, restrictive cardiomyopathy (RCM), severe PAH, severe PS, and

TABLE 2: Cardiac causes of chest pain in children.

Condition	*Description and possible basis*
Anomalous left coronary artery from pulmonary artery	Manifests with episodic sweating, irritability, and lassitude during feeding myocardial ischemia resulting from hypoperfusion and/or coronary steal
Coronary artery fistula	Anginal chest pain on exertion; myocardial ischemia resulting from coronary steal
Severe aortic stenosis	Anginal chest pain on exertion; myocardial ischemia resulting from increased myocardial oxygen demand as a result of ventricular hypertrophy
Hypertrophic cardiomyopathy	Anginal chest pain on exertion; myocardial ischemia resulting from increased myocardial oxygen demand as a result of ventricular hypertrophy
Severe aortic regurgitation	Anginal chest pain at rest and during exertion; myocardial ischemia resulting from coronary hypoperfusion from low diastolic pressure
Mitral stenosis	No specific pattern; reasons not clear; pulmonary hypertension
Pericarditis	Sharp pain with postural variation in pain; pain may be relieved by sitting up; pericardial inflammation
Tachyarrhythmia	Palpitations can be reported erroneously as chest pain (especially young children), ischemia from extreme tachycardia
Pulmonary embolism	Acute right ventricular ischemia; chest pain seldom reported as an isolated complaint; dyspnea and extreme fatigue are far commoner
Aortic dissection	Acute chest pain that characteristically radiates to the back
Mitral valve prolapse	Atypical sharp chest pain with no consistent relation with activity
Post-KD coronary artery disease	Remote history of KD in the past; previous history of giant aneurysm, pain is anginal and severe
Premature atherosclerosis	Familial hypercholesterolemia; pain is anginal; homozygous condition is associated with feature of aortic stenosis

(KD: Kawasaki disease)

TABLE 3: The relationship between visible cyanosis, hemoglobin levels, and oxygen saturation.

Cyanosis	*Reduced hemoglobin (g/dL)*	*Saturation*
±	3	90%
+	4	85%
++	5	80%

tricuspid stenosis. MS can also lead to fatigue, but dyspnea dominates. Fatigue may be a late feature in aortic valve disease. Severe MR causes fatigue due to reduced forward flow.

Hypoxemia-related Symptoms

This section will discuss three specific manifestations of hypoxia. They include cyanosis, cyanotic spell, and squatting.

Cyanosis

Kaunosis (Greek): Blueness

Cyanosis is defined as bluish discoloration of skin and mucous membrane due to elevated amount of reduced hemoglobin (Hb) within capillaries, of >4 g/dL.[2] Other pigments capable of causing cyanosis are methemoglobin (1.5 g/dL) or sulfhemoglobin (>0.5 g/dL). Cyanosis is generally picked up at an arterial saturation of 85% in a child or adolescent (**Table 3**).

Cyanosis can be central or peripheral. Peripheral cyanosis is often due to circulatory compromise as in low cardiac output, shock, and pulmonary edema. Central cyanosis is always pathological and is due to cardiorespiratory conditions. **Table 4** lists the differences between central and peripheral cyanosis.

TABLE 4: Central versus peripheral cyanosis.

	Peripheral	*Central*
Basis	Vasoconstriction and diminished peripheral blood flow	Systemic desaturation
Hands and feet	Present	Present
Lips, tongue, and sublingual	No	Present
Warmth	Abolishes	Remains

Central cyanosis can be physiologic up to 30 minutes of life. Acrocyanosis may persist up to 12 hours of life. *Persistent central cyanosis is pathological.*

In the newborn, two primary reasons for central cyanosis are cardiac and respiratory. Clinical pointers may help in differentiating between them (**Table 5**).

Cyanosis can be *uniform or nonuniform*. Nonuniform cyanosis can be of two types:

1. *Differential cyanosis* refers to a situation when the upper limb is pink and lower limb is blue and this generally requires a >10% difference to be visibly apparent. Measuring saturations in the right upper limb and either lower limbs enables identification of differential saturation. A >3% difference is considered as significant in neonatal screening. This is a valuable component

of neonatal screening of heart disease. The basis of differential saturations or differential cyanosis is right-to-left shunting via the PDA. The causes in neonates include persistent PPHN with a PDA where the elevated pulmonary vascular resistance results in R-L shunting across the duct. Additionally, critical coarctation or arch interruption results in an obligatory R-L shunt across the duct. When arch interruption is proximal to the left subclavian artery (Type B arch interruption), the left upper limb is postductal and would have similar saturations as either lower limb (hence it is prudent to check saturation in the right upper limb and either of the lower limbs). Older patients with PDA and Eisenmenger physiology would also have differential saturation or cyanosis.

2. *Reversed differential cyanosis or saturations* results when lower limb (postductal) saturations are higher than upper limb saturations. This finding is quite specific for transposition of the great arteries with severe PH and a large PDA (with or without coarctation or arch interruption).

TABLE 5: Making a distinction between cardiac and respiratory cause of cyanosis.

Clinical features	*Cardiac*	*Respiratory*
Cyanosis	Deeper	Present
Respiratory rate	↑	↑↑
Grunt	±	+
Retractions	±	+
Response to oxygen inhalation	Poor	Good
Hyperoxia test	Fails	Passes

Additional Noteworthy Points on Cyanosis

- Deep cyanosis in an infant usually indicates a saturation of less than 70%; mild cyanosis, around 85%.
- For a saturation of 85%, an infant will need PO_2 of 32–42 mm Hg; while for an adolescent, the value is 42–52 mm Hg.
- Dark skin, poor ambient light, low Hb can all mask cyanosis. Polycythemia in a newborn may give an impression of mild cyanosis.

The onset and severity of cyanosis are roughly dictated by the specific type of cyanotic CHD (**Table 6**). However, the severity of specific lesions (such as degree of pulmonic stenosis) has an important influence on the age at onset and severity of cyanosis.

Cyanotic Spell

Cyanotic spell, variously called as "Tet" spell, hypoxic spell, anoxic spell, and hypercyanotic spell occurs as a major complication in an infant cyanotic CHD with reduced blood flow. The anatomical substrate is VSD and RV outflow tract obstruction. The classical prototype is TOF. Other lesions which can manifest with cyanotic spells include TOF with pulmonary atresia, other conditions with tetralogy (VSD-PS) physiology that include double-outlet right ventricle with VSD and PS, single ventricle with PS, transposition with VSD and PS, etc.

TABLE 6: Temporal patterns and severity of cyanosis in common cyanotic congenital heart diseases.

Condition	*Onset*	*Severity*
Transposition with intact septum	Early, immediately after birth	Severe (<70%) in most instances
Transposition with VSD	Early after birth	Moderate to severe (70–85%)
Duct-dependent pulmonary atresia	Whenever the ductus arteriosus start to close, typically within 48–72 hours after birth, sometimes later	Mild at first, progresses rapidly as the duct starts to close
Unobstructed total anomalous pulmonary venous communication (TAPVC)	Desaturation is usually manifest soon after birth; however, cyanosis may not be visible until a few months	Mild >85%
Tetralogy of Fallot	Onset dictated by severity of PS; tends to be variable, Severe PS tends to have early onset of cyanosis mild PS may result in cyanosis at a much older age	Severity is also dictated by severity of PS. Mild PS may be pink altogether
Obstructed TAPVC	Early often within a few days after birth	Often severe, depending on the degree of obstruction
Single ventricle with PS	Onset dictated by severity of PS; severe PS: early onset of cyanosis	Severity of cyanosis proportional to severity of PS
Single ventricle with no PS	Cyanosis often not noticeable	Mild cyanosis until there is significant elevation of pulmonary vascular resistance
Persistent truncus arteriosus	Cyanosis often not noticeable until PVR becomes elevated	Mild, saturation typically in the 90s
Ebstein anomaly	Variable (bimodal), a subset of neonates with severe Ebstein's presents early; mild Ebstein's present later in life with cyanosis	Severe in those with severe valve affliction

(PS: pulmonary stenosis; PVR: pulmonary vascular resistance; VSD: ventricular septal defect)

Spells typically present after 2 months of age and may spontaneously improve by 24 months. The occurrence of a spell should be viewed as a medical emergency indicates that the lesion is severe and merits early correction.

The classic triad of spell is:

- Progressive increase in cyanosis
- Hyperpnea
- Extreme irritability.

There is audible and visible respiratory distress. It can last for 5–30 minutes. If prolonged, it can lead to drowsiness, lethargy, and seizures. Stroke can be precipitated by a prolonged spell. It does not occur in sleep.[3]

The spell has to be differentiated from breath-holding spell, seizure, colic, and even an acute asthma.

The mechanism of spell is multifactorial and described in some detail in Chapter 34. When the baby cries, feeds, or is bathed, the ensuing increased physical activity causes systemic vasodilatation. The systemic vascular resistance is reduced and because of the fixed impedance to pulmonary flow, blood reaching right ventricle goes to aorta more and causes further hypoxemia. Hypoxemia initiates a vicious cycle—it stimulates the respiratory center, causes metabolic acidosis; both causing hyperpnea. Infundibular spasm has also been touted as a mechanism by causing an abrupt reduction of pulmonary blood flow. RV mechanoreceptors have also been implicated in the genesis of spell.

Clinically baby is often visibly very blue, irritable, and the outflow murmur diminishes or disappears. ABG shows metabolic acidosis and low saturations.

Squatting

Older children with TOF like conditions may squat while playing or after exertion. A small child who has not started walking will pull up his or her knees to chest wall when tired.

Squatting improves systemic saturation by causing acute increase in systemic vascular resistance (SVR) and facilitating more pulmonary blood flow. It can also limit lower limb venous blood which is significantly desaturated from reaching RV and then to aorta. Squatting goes away in early adolescence presumably due to social pressure. Still, some of them may adopt squatting equivalent postures.

Note: Any child beyond 3 years, who is blue, had a spell in infancy, and has had squatting in childhood is most likely to have TOF or equivalent physiology.

Respiratory Symptoms

Cough and Wheeze

Cough and wheeze in heart disease can be due to pulmonary congestion. Wheeze can predominate in some infants with HF. Both PND and acute pulmonary edema can result in cough or wheeze. Wheeze may also result from small airway compression in patients with TOF and absent pulmonary valve.

Stridor

The most common cause of stridor in patients with CHD is the presence of an associated lesion of the upper respiratory tract such as laryngomalacia. Stridor is particularly common in syndromic babies (Catch 22 and Down syndrome). Stridor has important implications in postoperative recovery and should be formally evaluated by the otorhinolaryngologist. Other leading causes of stridor due to CHD include vascular ring and severe PAH with aneurismal pulmonary artery as in Eisenmenger syndrome. Severe mitral valve disease, aortic aneurism, and idiopathic pulmonary arterial hypertension (IPAH) could cause compression of trachea bronchial tree and stridor in older children.

Hemoptysis

Coughing out blood- or blood-stained sputum can occur in many CHD. Cyanotic CHD like TOF, pulmonary arteriovenous fistula (PAVF) and ES are examples. Hemoptysis occurs in MS, pulmonary embolism, IPAH, and as part of acute pulmonary edema. Massive hemoptysis (pulmonary apoplexy) happens to be a leading cause of death in ES and IPAH. Administration of anticoagulants in the presence of heart disease could precipitate hemoptysis.

Recurrent Respiratory Tract Infection

Recurring RTI occur commonly in post-tricuspid L→R shunts as in VSD or PDA. However, its specificity is limited especially in polluted urban settings where many normal children suffer from recurrent RTI. It can also occur in cyanotic CHD with increased pulmonary blood flow. Various mechanisms can operate to lead to recurrent RTI (≥2 LRTI within 6 months).

- Increased pulmonary flow with lung congestion invites infection.
- Compression of bronchi by dilated PA and branches can cause atelectasis and air trapping, which act as a nidus for infection.
- In a congested lung as in large L→R shunt, mucociliary clearing mechanisms of bronchial tree is compromised.
- Nearly 10–15% of L→R shunts will have gastroesophageal reflux (GERD) which favors infection.
- Large L→R shunts will lead to malnutrition which can increase susceptibility to infections.
- Some syndromes with CHD (Down) have abnormal upper airways and hypotonia which favor recurring infections.
- Some syndromes with CHD will have impaired immune competence, will cause repeated infections, e.g., DiGeorge.

Neurological Presentations

Headache

Headache in an adolescent can be due to systemic hypertension, which could be due to coarctation. Polycythemia in cyanotic CHD often cause severe headache and this is made worse by dehydration.

Syncope

Syncope is an alarming symptom and often quite dramatic. It is a common reason for a school-going child to be brought for a formal cardiac evaluation and is often a source of anxiety for the family. The most important investigation for a child with syncope is a detailed history. A thorough description on the causes of syncope and its diagnostic approach is given in Chapter 19.

Stroke and Transient Ischemic Attack (See Chapter 51)

The occurrence of a stroke may bring to attention the underlying heart disease for the first time in a child.[4] Chapter 51 outlines a comprehensive approach for strokes occurring in younger populations.

Other Symptoms

Failure to Thrive

When an infant has significant growth failure, the term, FTT (**Box 1**) is used. While this symptom is often thought of as a leading clinical problem in many CHD, especially left-to-right shunts, it is important to recognize that this symptom is not very specific for underlying heart disease. FTT in infancy has multiple following contributing factors:

- HF leading to reduced nutrient intake.
- *Reduced growth potential*: In a large cross-sectional study, it has been demonstrated that FTT occurs in all forms of CHD not necessarily left-to-right shunts. Additionally, most syndromic babies with CHD have reduced growth potential.
- IUGR with CHD, e.g., rubella with reduced growth potential.
- Presence of associated GERD.
- Repeated hospitalizations disrupting feeding frequently.

Sweating

Excessive sweating in a CHD occurs in large left-to-right shunt leading to HF, due to excessive sympathetic discharge. Sweating is typically noticed over the forehead and often persists for a few months after correction of the shunt.

BOX 1: Measuring failure to thrive (FTT).

- Normal weight gain in infancy
  - *0–3 months*:
    30 g/day. Approximately, 2.5 kg
  - *3–6 months*:
    20 g/day. Approximately, 1.8 kg
  - *6–12 months*:
    15 g/day. Approximately, 2.7 kg
    Total gain since birth ~ 7 kg
- Weight gain <15 g/day at any period in infancy, especially below 6 months would be considered FTT.

Edema

It is less conspicuous in infants as a manifestation of right HF. In older children, facial puffiness and pedal or presacral pitting edema may be noticeable in those with gross right HF. A recent excess weight gain can also indicate water retention due to HF. Turner syndrome and Noonan syndrome may be associated with CHD and can have bilateral pedal edema that is related to lymphatic fluid accumulation.

Functional Classification

The four major cardinal cardiac symptoms are incorporated into a functional classification known as [New York Heart Association (NYHA)] classification which was originally introduced in 1964.[5] Later many other functional classifications were introduced, mostly applicable to adults.[6] The first exclusive pediatric functional classification came about in 1992—the Ross classification.[7]

The NYHA classification (**Table 7**) was originally introduced to assess functional status in HF in adults and was modified in 1994. It affords a rapid assessment, is quite simple, predicts functional ability, and can predict prognosis. There is poor interobserver agreement and is less reproducible. Still NYHA has had a tremendous staying power and is widely used by both clinicians and clinical researchers.

New York Heart Association classification can be used in older children. There are two other functional classifications which grades only angina. They are Canadian Cardiovascular Society Classification (1976) and Goldman's Specific Activity Scale (1981). In 1998, World Health Organization (WHO) introduced a specific classification for functional assessment in PAH.

Ross Pediatric Functional Classification (**Table 8**) was introduced in 1992 and modified in 2002.

Ross classification is currently used in the assessment of history in CHD and CHF by pediatricians and is eminently reproducible.

For PAH in adults and older children, WHO functional classification is used. Here, palpitation is replaced by presyncope as one of the four major symptoms. There has been a recent functional classification for children with PAH by PVRI Task Force, 2011.

TABLE 7: New York Heart Association (NYHA) classification.

Symptom class	*Functional status*
Class I	No limitations. Ordinary physical activity does not cause dyspnea, chest pain, palpitation, or fatigue
Class II	Slight limitation. Ordinary physical activity results in symptoms
Class III	Marked limitation of physical activity. Less than ordinary activity leads to symptoms
Class IV	Unable to carry out any activity without discomfort. Symptoms often present at rest

TABLE 8: Ross Pediatric Functional Classification.

Symptom class	*Functional status*
Class I	No symptom
Class II	Mild tachypnea or sweating on feeding in infants. Dyspnea on exertion in children
Class III	Marked tachypnea or sweating on feeding. Growth failure in infants. Marked dyspnea on exertion in children
Class IV	Tachypnea/retractions/diaphoresis/grunting at rest in infants. Dyspnea at rest or minimal effort in children

Key standard definitions relating to vital signs are listed in **Box 2**. These definitions should be adhered to while using terms such as tachypnea, tachycardia, and hypotension.

BOX 2: Thresholds for tachypnea, tachycardia, and hypotension.

Tachypnea (rate/minute)		
Newborn/up to 2 months	–	≥60
Infant	–	>50
Child	–	>40
Adolescent	–	≥20
Tachycardia (rate/minute)		
Newborn	–	≥160
Infant	–	>120
Child up to 5 years	–	>100
Hypotension SBP (mm Hg)		
Newborn	–	<60
Infant	–	<70
Child	–	<80
Adolescent	–	<90

(SBP: systolic blood pressure)

PHYSICAL EXAMINATION

General Examination

Physical examination of the cardiovascular examination needs to be systematic and thorough. Several clues to etiology of the underlying CVD emerge from facial appearance (dysmorphisms), skin (e.g., tuberous sclerosis and neurofibromatosis), and skeletal system including digits, limbs and spine (**Table 9**). The chapter on genetics (Chapter 54) provides a comprehensive account of genetic syndromes and their external manifestations. Assessment of growth (anthropometry) and development is crucial in assessing cardiovascular system (CVS) in a growing child. The major measures of growth are weight for age, height for age, head circumference, and degree of wasting. Body mass index (BMI) can also be measured from 2 years onward. In a young child (<5 years), developmental assessment is done on four templates—gross motor, fine motor, adaptive, social, and language. This chapter will focus on general physical examination with special reference to the cardiovascular system and cardiac examination.

An assessment of appearance and state of distress serve to guide the urgency of further investigations and management. Sick infants often appear anxious, fretful, diaphoretic, pale, or breathless and are seldom consolable. Evidence of cyanosis, pallor, clubbing, pattern of respiration, and sweating indicates the clinical condition of the child.

Clubbing is due to soft tissue proliferation at tips of fingers and toes. This usually accompanies cyanotic CHD in cardiology. It can occur without cyanosis in infective endocarditis.[8]

Clubbing is traditionally graded as:

First degree: Increased fluctuation of finger tips
Second degree: Obliteration of angle of nailbed
Third degree: Increased anteroposterior of finger tips
Fourth degree: Extreme clubbing which may resemble a drumstick or parrot beak clubbing can be associated with many lung disease, gastrointestinal and liver diseases, and rarely endocrine problem. It can be occupational or familial.

Edema of feet is rather uncommon as feature of HF in infants and children. The edema in HF is pitting and indicates right HF. Anemia can co-exist with many cardiac problems and is often a major precipitating factor of HF in children with heart disease. Jaundice in a newborn with associated CHD could exist in Rubella syndrome, Down syndrome, and Alagille syndrome. Chronic cardiac illness with cirrhosis can cause icterus. Rashes can occur in many cardiac situations. Rubella syndrome, Kawasaki disease, infective endocarditis, rheumatic fever, Lyme disease, and rhabdomyoma are some such situations. Limb anomalies can coexist with CHD in at least 10%. Some of them may be with associated with syndromes. Nonpitting or lymphedema is a feature of specific conditions that include Turner syndrome and Noonan syndrome. These conditions have a high likelihood of serious CVD and the presence of lymphedema may indicate underlying congenital lymphatic abnormalities that could impact postoperative recovery.

CARDIOVASCULAR EXAMINATION

Arterial Pulse

Arterial pulse wave is a peripheral window to look at heart and the starting point for cardiovascular examination.[9] It is hemodynamically related to:

- LV stroke volume
- Ejection velocity of blood from left ventricle
- Capacity and compliance of arterial system.

Pulse can be *central*—carotid or *peripheral*—radial. The other peripheral pulses are brachial, femoral, popliteal, dorsalis pedis, and posterior tibial.

A central pulse has:

- An early systolic component—*percussion wave*
- Later peak in systole—*tidal wave*

TABLE 9: Cutaneous markers of underlying heart disease in children.

Cutaneous marker	*Description*	*Underlying heart disease*
	Congenital	
Shagreen spots (tuberous sclerosis)	Roughened, raised lesion with orange-peel consistency located primarily in the lumbosacral region	Cardiac rhabdomyoma
Ash-leaf macules (tuberous sclerosis)	Hypomelanotic macules	Cardiac rhabdomyoma
Multiple nevoid basal cell carcinomas (Gorlin syndrome)	Crops of tumors not restricted to sun-exposed areas. Sites of predilection are periorbital skin, nose, malar areas, and upper lip	Fibromas
Lentigines (LAMB syndrome—lentigines, atrial myxomas, myxoid neurofibroma, and blue nevi)	Lentigines are small round dark brown macules that can appear anywhere on the body	Atrial myxoma
Lentigines (Leopard syndrome—lentigines, ECG abnormalities, ocular, pulmonary stenosis, abnormal genitalia, retardation of growth, and deafness)	Lentigines are small round dark brown macules that can appear anywhere on the body	Atrial myxoma
Ephelides (NAME syndrome—nevi, atrial myxoma, myxoid neurofibroma, and ephelides)	Ephelides are well-demarcated macules—light or dark brown, round, oval or irregularly shaped—that occur in sun-exposed areas	Atrial myxoma
Congenital cutaneous hemangioma (PHACES syndrome—posterior fossa brain malformation, hemangioma, arterial lesion, cardiac, eye abnormalities, and sterna cleft)	Facial hemangioma typically ipsilateral to the aortic arch	Coarctation of aorta, aberrant right subclavian artery
Hereditary hemorrhagic telangiectasia	Mucocutaneous lesions which usually develop at puberty are 1–4 mm sharply demarcated red-to-purple macules, papules, or spider-like projections, each composed of a tightly woven mat of tortuous telangiectatic vessels	Pulmonary AVMs
Linear nevus sebaceous syndrome	Large facial nevus usually located on the forehead and nose and tend to be midline in its distribution	Coarctation of aorta
	Acquired	
Erythema multiforme, erythema and cracking of lips, and strawberry tongue (Kawasaki disease)	Erythema multiforme is a cutaneous and mucous hypersensitivity reaction with characteristic lesions in target triggered by antigenic stimuli	Coronary artery aneurysms, myocarditis, pericarditis, and valvar regurgitation
Erythema marginatum	Bright pink macule or papule that spread with serpiginous borders and central clearing	Acute rheumatic fever
Subcutaneous nodules	Discrete nontender nodules on extensor surfaces	Acute rheumatic fever
Janeway lesions	Small, nontender, flat erythematous lesions on the palms or soles	Infective endocarditis
Osler nodes	Small, tender, raised lesions on the pads of the fingers and toes	Infective endocarditis
Malar rash, discoid rash (SLE)	• Malar rash—erythematous flat or raised rash across the bridge of the nose and cheeks, which spares nasolabial folds • Discoid rash—red inflamed patch with a scaling and crusty appearance	Pericarditis, myocarditis, coronary artery aneurysms, and congenital heart block
Erythematous rash (juvenile idiopathic arthritis)	Evanescent and erythematous rash	Pericarditis and myocarditis
Atrophy skin (systemic sclerosis)	Tightened indurated skin	Pulmonary artery hypertension

(AVM: arteriovenous malformation; ECG: electrocardiogram; SLE: systemic lupus erythematosus)

- *A diastolic component*:
  Abrupt negative wave—diastole begins with a *Dicrotic notch*
- Late diastolic component—*dicrotic wave.*

Radial, femoral, and other pulsations are *peripheral* in nature and the pulse changes its character as it becomes peripheral. It assumes greater amplitude, greater velocity—has a steep rise and has a lower dicrotic notch.

Carotid pulse: It is the major central pulse and is the largest palpable proximal vessel closest to aortic valve; hence, the contour resembles that of central aorta. The carotid pulse is best for evaluation of volume and contour of the pulse.

Radial pulse: It is the archetypal peripheral pulse which is traditionally palpated in CVS examination. It is either palpated by thumb or first two fingers with finger pads. It is assessed for rate, rhythm, and is especially useful for assessing pulsus alternans and paradoxus. Traditionally, pulse rate, rhythm, volume, character, and condition of vessel wall is looked for, followed by radiofemoral delay and other peripheral pulses. Pulse wave arrives at radial artery and femoral artery almost simultaneously about 75–80 ms after ascending aorta and radiofemoral palpation is ideal for pulse discrepancy.

Pulse Rate

Unlike adults, pulse rate varies with age, and hence the arbitrary cut-off points for tachycardia and bradycardia vary in infants and children (**Table 10**).

Rhythm

Pulse can be regular or irregular. Minor irregularity in relation to respiratory cycle is common in children, especially when heart rate is slow—sinus arrhythmia. Abnormal irregularity in children can be either regularly irregular or irregularly irregular.

Regularly irregular pulse can be found in ectopics with bigeminy or trigeminy. It can also be caused by sinoatrial exit block or in some instances of atrioventricular block with Wenckebach rhythm. *Irregularly irregular pulse* is associated with atrial fibrillation, atrial flutter with varying block, multifocal atrial tachycardia, frequent atrial or ventricular ectopics, and most instances of atrioventricular block with Wenckebach rhythm.

Pulse Volume

Pulse volume is assessed by feeling both the carotids and radials. This is somewhat subjective. A forceful or "*high volume pulse*" results from increased force of LV ejection, increased stroke volume, and elevated arterial pressures. The most consistent hemodynamic correlate for high volume pulse is a wide pulse pressure that can result from a variety of causes that include anemia, thyrotoxicosis, AR, PDA, and systemic arteriovenous fistula. In these conditions, there is a fall in diastolic pressure because of "steal" from aorta or excessive systemic vasodilation. When the steal is severe, the pulse may be collapsing as a result of very low diastolic pressures. This pulse is also called *Corrigan's pulse* or water hammer pulse. Additionally, systemic hypertension, MR, and hypertrophic cardiomyopathy can have a relatively rapid upstroke that is perceived as a high pulse volume. Here, the diastolic pressures are not lowered.

TABLE 10: Commonly accepted limits of normal heart rates.

Age	*Tachycardia*	*Bradycardia*
Newborn	>150/min	<90/min
Infant and young child	>120/min	<80/min
Older child	>100/min	<60/min

Low volume pulse results from low cardiac output as in severe HF, ventricular dysfunction, aortic stenosis, and severe MS. In aortic stenosis, the pulse has a slow upstroke, low amplitude, and the dicrotic notch occurs later—pulsus *parvus et tardus*. This is best appreciated in carotid artery.

Abnormalities in Character of Pulse

When two palpable pulses per cardiac cycle are felt, it is called *twice beating pulse*. In most instances, both pulses are in systole (bisferiens/bifid) or rarely one is systole and other in diastole (dicrotic). The common causes of bisferiens are AR with or without associated mild aortic stenosis and hypertrophic obstructive cardiomyopathy. *Dicrotic pulse* results from low output states such as impaired ventricular function, cardiac tamponade, and hypovolemic shock. *Pulsus alternans* is best appreciated in radial artery. Alternate strong and weak pulses are felt *regularly*. It is also detected by blood pressure (BP) difference of ≥20 mm Hg. It is classically found in significantly impaired LV function. The possible mechanisms include recruitment of more myocardial fibers that alter a weak contraction with an improved subsequent contraction as a result of the Frank–Starling law.

Pulsus Paradoxus

Pulsus paradoxus is defined as a marked and exaggerated fall in systolic BP in inspiration by >10 mm Hg. It can be appreciated by palpation of a peripheral pulse like radial pulse and has to be elicited during quiet respiration. Pulsus paradoxus generally indicates a high likelihood of cardiac tamponade from pericardial effusion. Severe airway obstruction from asthma or emphysema and constrictive pericarditis can also result in pulsus paradoxus. Occasionally, significant pericardial collection may not be associated with pulsus paradoxus when there are co-existent conditions such as a large ASD, hypovolemia, and AR.

Discrepant Pulses

Unequal pulses between right and left radials (also referred to as anisosphygmia). It can occur in the following circumstances:

- Coarctation which is proximal to left subclavian artery
- Takayasu arteritis
- Supravalvar aortic stenosis (right radial is more prominent here)
- Following a classical Blalock–Taussig operation or after a subclavian flap coarctation repair
- Aortic dissection.

Both radials and femorals can be weak with strong carotids bilaterally can be found in presubclavian coarctation with aberrant right subclavian origin, distal to coarctation and Takayasu arteritis with stenosis of both origins of subclavian with descending aortic narrowing.

Weak femoral with bounding radials are found classically in coarctation of aorta, usually of thoracic descending aorta. Takayasu arteritis, distal thoracic, or abdominal aortic narrowing in association with neurofibromatosis can and cause weak femoral pulses. *Coarctation with well palpable femorals is found in* co-existing AR (due to bicuspid aortic valve), and extensive collaterals to lower limb. A difference in volume between radial and femoral may be more important than radiofemoral delay in an infant with resting heart rate of 120–140/minute. In an infant, it may be difficult to palpate the femoral, and dorsalis pedis examination is a useful way to exclude a significant coarctation.

Blood Pressure

The specifics of measuring BP are presented in the chapter on systemic hypertension (*see* Chapter 49). Indirect methods of BP recording are preferred in routine clinical setting either at hospital or office practice. They are:

- Palpatory method
- Flush method (in newborn)
- Sphygmomanometry
- Oscillometry
- Doppler probe.

The most popular method is sphygmomanometry. This principle is also used in flush method. BP is recorded when child is lying down or sitting up with arm well supported at level of heart. Auscultation is done by bell (ideal) or diaphragm over brachial artery at antecubital fossa, auscultating for Korotkoff sounds. Korotkoff sounds are low-pitched sounds and hence bell is ideal; however, it may be difficult to place the bell beneath the cuff in the antecubital fossa properly and hence diaphragm is used; gently applying over the brachial artery.

- K_1: Initial, soft, increases in intensity—systolic blood pressure (SBP)
- K_2: Murmur-like sounds
- K_3: Crisp and tapping sounds
- K_4: Abrupt muffling
- K_5: Disappearance of sounds—diastolic blood pressure (DBP).

K_1 corresponds to SBP and K_4 is 5–10 mm Hg higher than true DBP and K_5 is 2–5 mm lower than true DBP.

Note: Palpatory SBP is 5 mm Hg lower than auscultatory SBP. BP is ideally taken in the beginning of the CVS examination and end of examination. BP cuff has to be inflated to 20 mm Hg higher than estimated SBP by palpatory method and brought down 2–3 mm per cardiac beat. *Currently, in children as well as adults K_1 corresponds to SBP and K_5 to DBP with a few exceptions.*

- *In atrial fibrillation (AF)*: Multiple readings are done and average taken
- *In obstetric patient*: K_4 is taken as DBP
- *In aortic run off*: K_4 is taken as DBP.

TABLE 11: Recommended cuff diameters for blood pressure measurements in children.

Age group	*Bladder width (cm)*
Newborn	5
Infant	5
Young child	8
Older child	12–13
Adult	12–13
Thigh	18

Note: In children if disappearance of Korotkoff sounds does not occur; i.e., K sounds heard till 0 mm Hg, BP recording is read as $K_1/K_4/K_5$ as in chronic AR.

The 1987 Report of the Second Task Force on BP control in childhood and The National High Blood Pressure Education Program 1996 update recommends that all children 3 years of age or older should have their BP recorded on all consultations and preferably yearly thereafter. This is the only effective way of diagnosing hypertension in children, in the early stages (**Table 11**). BP should be measured with a standard clinical sphygmomanometer, using the stethoscope placed over the brachial artery pulse, proximal, and medial to the cubital fossa and below the bottom edge of the cuff approximately 2 cm above cubital fossa, right upper arm is routinely chosen. BP in both arms should be measured at least once. BP should be measured in a "controlled environment" after 3–5 minutes of rest in the seated position with the cubital fossa supported at heart level. Supine position is recommended for infants and toddlers, as it is easier. Bladder width that is approximately 40% of the child's arm circumference, measured midway between the olecranon and acromion is ideal. The cuff bladder should cover 80–100% of the circumference of the arm. If two cuffs are close in size to the measured width of the arm, the larger cuff should be used. Use of smaller cuff will lead to false high reading and hypertension can be overdiagnosed. The cuff should be inflated to a pressure of 20–30 mm Hg above SBP. Recommended cuff deflation rate is 2–3 mm Hg/second. SBP is taken as the onset of tapping Korotkoff sounds (phase I). Measurement of DBP was more controversial, till recently. Now disappearance of Korotkoff sounds (phase V) is accepted as DBP.

Doppler ultrasound measurement of BP is reliable in children and is especially useful in newborns and infants in whom auscultation is difficult. It is also very useful in the intensive care setting where frequent BP monitoring is required. But the utility of this has not been documented in epidemiological studies.

Ambulatory blood pressure monitoring (ABPM) has become a very useful tool in hypertensive adult especially for diagnosing "white coat hypertension" and "paroxysmal hypertension". The prognostic value of ABPM for end-organ damage exceeds that of casual BP values in adults. But reliable data is lacking on the role of ABPM in childhood hypertension.

Points to Remember

- Auscultatory gap occurs in high BP and can be avoided by initially assessing SBP by palpatory method.
- Larger cuff is likely to cause less error than smaller cuff if suitable cuff width is not available.
- SBP in lower limb can be higher than upper limb by 10–20 mm Hg.

Factors that influence blood pressure measurements:

- *Diurnal variation*: BP is lowest during sleep, between 2 and 5 AM. It has a steep rise from 6 to 8 AM and highest BP recordings are in the afternoon (2–4 PM).
- *Upper limb–lower limb difference*: Normally, in SBP, there is a difference of 10–20 mm Hg, higher in lower limb. If SBP, in lower limb is >20 mm Hg, it suggests aortic run-off (Hill sign) as in AR. A difference of >60 mm Hg or more suggests severe AR and 30–60 mm Hg suggests moderate AR. A false negative Hill sign is found in AR in associated aortic stenosis or with HF.
- *Posture*: On standing, SBP falls by ≤10 mm in adults and 5 mm in children. DBP remains the same or becomes mildly elevated on standing. Postural hypotension as defined as a fall of SBP by >15 mm Hg in adult and 10 mm Hg in children.
- *Difference between upper limbs*: Because LV jet preferentially is directed to innominate artery and subsequently to right subclavian artery, right upper limb BP is marginally higher than left upper limb BP.
- *Pulse pressure*: Normally, it is between 30 and 50 mm of Hg. Wide pulse pressure is defined as >60 mm Hg in adults and >50 mm Hg in children. Narrow pulse pressure occurs when PP is <30 mm Hg. It can occur with reduced stroke volume as in HF and aortic stenosis. Wide pulse pressure is found in fever, anemia, thyrotoxicosis, pregnancy, systemic arteriovenous fistula, patent arterial duct, AR, and cyanotic CHD with collaterals.

Flush Method

Measures mean BP in neonates. The cuff is applied in the arm—forearm or upper arm, palm is squeezed with examiner's hand keeping the limb raised and blanched. BP cuff is inflated to a higher value and slowly decompressed while deflating flushing of palm is observed.

Normal Blood Pressures and Definitions of Hypertension

Normal BP in children is <90th centile for age, sex, and height centiles for SBP, DBP, or both. Between 90th and 95th centile BP is considered high normal and above 95th centile BP is abnormal—hypertensive (**Table 12**). Value above 99th centile is severe hypertension.

TABLE 12: Blood pressure (BP) in children.

Normal	<90th centile
Elevated	90–95th centile
Hypertension	>95th centile
Severe hypertension	>99th centile

A rule of thumb for normal BP in a child for systolic BP is: 90 + (Age × 5/3) mm Hg; diastolic pressures are in the range of 60 ± 10 mm Hg

For example: In a 7-year-old BP is expected to be
SBP: 90 + (7 × 5/3) = 102 mm Hg
DBP: 60 ± 10 mm Hg

Rule of thumb for high BP would be >110/70 between ages 0 and 5; >120/80 between 5 and 10 years and >130/80 for those >10 years of age.

For SBP, boys will have BP readings 1–2 mm more than girls up to 8 years, will have same BP up to 12 years and again will have slightly higher BP (1–2 mm) up to 18 years. Boys will have DBP slightly higher—1 mm up to 12 years compared to girls. So the difference according to sex is negligible in childhood.

Jugular Venous Pressure

Systemic veins are a low pressure, high compliance system where pressure is between 4 and 11 cm of H_2O (3–7 mm Hg). Jugular venous pressure (JVP) offers a *window* to right heart—both right atrium and right ventricle. Normal JVP is assessed by visualizing either external jugular vein (EJV) or internal jugular vein (IJV). The latter, IJV, is preferred as it has direct continuity with SVC, and hence RA, it has no valves (unlike EJV) and it is closer to RA. It is traditionally examined with patient at 45° inclination; but the inclination can range from 30–90°.[10] Two aspects of JVP need to be looked at and they include: height of JVP wave and type of wave pattern.[11,12]

The JVP has 3 positive waves and 2 descents in every cardiac cycle. The "a" wave is due to right atrial contraction and occurs when the tricuspid valve (TV) is open. It follows the P wave in ECG and is almost simultaneous with first heart sound. The "c" wave is due to bulging of TV into the floor of RA during RV isovolumic contraction. This occurs when the TV is closed and is not easily seen, but can be recorded. The "v" wave is due to right atrial filling later in systole while the TV is closed. It ends in early diastole and is almost simultaneous with carotid pulsation (**Fig. 1**).

The "x" descent is due to atrial relaxation and downward displacement of TV during early RV systole as TV is pulled caudally during RV contraction. The TV is closed here. The "y" descent occurs with the opening of the TV and emptying of right atrium in early diastole as TV opens (**Fig. 2**).

Assessment of JVP is most conveniently done in sitting up position and is generally difficult in infants and young children. If venous pulsations are seen above medial end of clavicle, it is elevated. One can measure the height from sternal angle and express in centimeters. Venous pulsations can be seen in supine position even when they are not elevated and the pattern of waveforms can be identified. It is important to distinguish neck venous pulsations from carotid pulses and the differences are listed in **Table 13**.

The JVP is considered elevated, whenever venous pulsations are seen in the upright position. For pulsations to be visible in the root of the neck the JVP should be 4 cm or more from the sternal angle in adults and 3 cm or more in children. To convert JVP height in centimeters from sternal angle to right atrial mean pressure in mm Hg, the following formula can be used: (JVP height in cm + 5 cm) × 0.75 = in mm Hg. In general, "a" waves are normally taller and "x" descent is the more prominent descent. **Box 3** lists common causes of elevated JVP. Abnormalities in waveforms are listed in **Figure 1**.

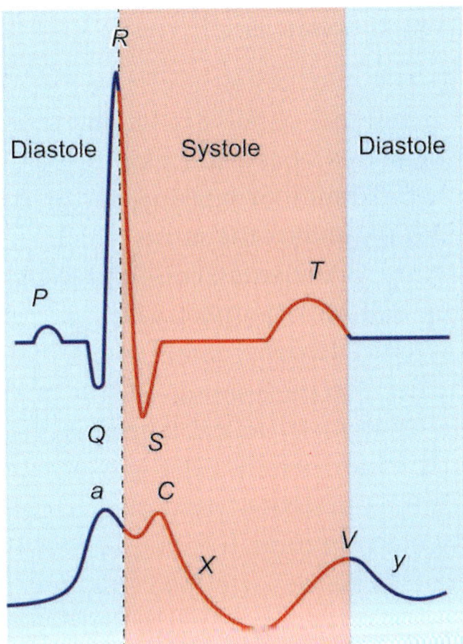

Fig. 1: Physiologic correlates of the jugular venous pressure waveforms. The ECG is shown above and the jugular venous pressure trace below.

Hepatojugular Reflux (Abdominojugular Test)

To assess incipient right HF, sustained pressure is applied by palm of hand over periumbilical area or right upper abdomen for 10–15 seconds when patient lies down with quiet breathing with an inclination of 45°. The normal response is a transient elevation of JVP to <3 cm that is not sustained. Incipient HF is suggested by elevation of JVP of >3 cm that is sustained elevation as long as pressure is applied. This is because the excessive venous blood that reaches thorax on abdominal compressions cannot be accommodated by the right ventricle without an increase in filling pressures.[13,14]

Kussmaul sign: This refers to an increase in JVP during inspiration. The list of conditions where this sign is positive include certain conditions:

- Constrictive pericarditis
- Pericardial effusion
- Severe congestive HF

TABLE 13: Differences between jugular venous pressure (JVP) and carotid pulsation.

Jugular venous pulsations	*Carotid pulsations*
• Better seen than felt	• Easily felt
• Has two waves with descents being more prominent	• Single prominent upstroke
• Has a definite upper level	• No definite upper level
• Changes with position and respiratory cycle	• No change
• Gentle compression of root of neck can obliterate pulsations	Gentle compression has no effect

BOX 3: Causes of elevated jugular venous pressure (JVP).

- Right heart failure due to any cause
- Abnormal right ventricular compliance as a result of hypertrophy: Here, the "a" waves are characteristically prominent.
- Pericardial diseases
- Tricuspid stenosis and regurgitation
- *Noncardiac causes*: Fluid overload; increased abdominal pressure
- Nonpulsatile engorgement of neck veins result from obstruction to the superior vena cava and in some instances after the Glen (cavopulmonary) shunt

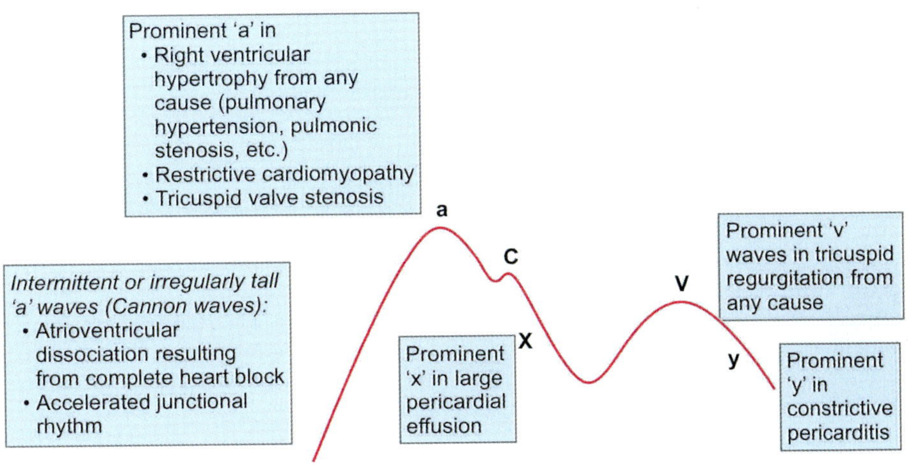

Fig. 2: The various causes of abnormal waveforms in jugular venous pressure.

- Restrictive cardiomyopathy
- Massive pulmonary embolism.

Examination of Precordium

Precordium is the chest wall which overlies the heart. Inspection, palpation, and, in some situations, percussion form the preliminary evaluation prior to auscultation.

Inspection

This includes the following items:

- *Chest wall symmetry*: Precordial prominence will distort precordial symmetry. Additionally, underdeveloped or persistent collapsed lung on one side can result in chest wall asymmetry as well.
- *Chest wall deformity*: A significant proportion of patients with CHD can have associated skeletal anomalies, many of which are in the thorax. They include pectus excavatum, pectus carinatum, kyphosis, and scoliosis. Harrison's sulcus results from persistent tachypnea in infancy.
- Scars of previous cardiac surgeries may be important (**Fig. 3**). *Left anterior thoracotomy indications.*
- *Pulsations*: These include apical impulse, epigastric pulsation, suprasternal, and IC pulsations including 2nd and 3rd interspace pulsations.

Palpation

A number of important clues to the underlying heart disease can be ascertained from palpation alone.[15]

Apical Impulse

Palpable apical impulse in a normal child is produced by an anterior movement of left ventricle during early systole. Apex beat is clinically the lowermost and outermost definite cardiac impulse felt over precordium and generally reflects LV activity. One usually examines for the apex beat with the patient in supine position or in upright position. If apex beat is not palpable, it is palpated in the left lateral position. It is important not to overlook the possibility dextrocardia.

Normal Apex Beat

Until the age of 2 years, the normal location of the apex beat is in the 4th left IC space in midclavicular line and beyond 4 years it is in the 5th left intercostal space 1 cm media to the midclavicular line. Between the ages of 2 and 4 years, apex beat can be either in the 4th or 5th space. It typically occupies only one IC space with a diameter of <2.5 cm. The normal character is a gentle nonsustained tap that lasts for less than half of systole. Normally, no sound or thrill is palpable at apex.

Abnormal Apex

Displacement: A displaced apex generally indicates cardiomegaly, usually of LV type. Lateral displacement can also occur in scoliosis, straight back syndrome, or any intrathoracic pathology such as pleural effusion, pneumothorax, congenital lobar emphysema, and without true cardiomegaly.

Forcefulness: The apical impulse is forcible and usually lifts examiner's finger tips above the plane of ribs. A forceful apex can be hyperkinetic or heaving. In the *hyperdynamic apex,* the duration remains the same—<50% systole. This is seen in LV volume overloading conditions such as a mitral or aortic regurgitation, large post-tricuspid shunt (VSD or patent arterial duct), hyperdynamic states such as anemia, thyrotoxicosis, beriberi, or systemic arteriovenous fistula.

A *heaving (sustained)* apical impulse lifts the fingers markedly and duration of outward impulse is >50% systole—it is sustained. The duration of sustained apical impulse is a function of LV ejection time. It is due to pressure overload. The causes of pressure overload include LV outflow tract obstructions such as aortic stenosis and systemic

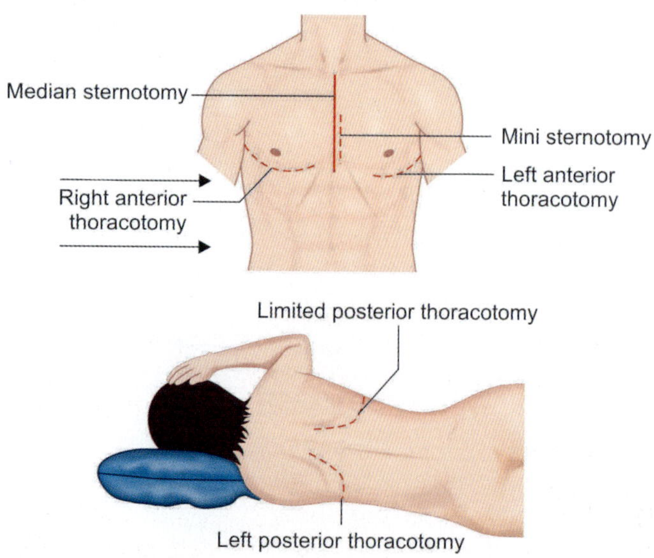

- *Right anterior thoracotomy (inframammary)*: ASD closure in older patients
- *Left anterior thoracotomy*: Closed mitral valvotomy
- *Right posterior thoracotomy*: Right BT shunt; ASD closure via limited posterior thoracotomy approach
- *Left posterior thoracotomy*: Left BT shunt, PDA ligation, coarctation repair and rarely, PA banding
- *Median sternotomy*:
  - Most corrective open heart operations
  - Central shunt
  - Infundibular resection
  - PA banding
  - Glenn shunt and intracardiac repairs

Fig. 3: Scars of previous cardiothoracic surgery.

hypertension. It is often associated with an audible or palpable fourth heart sound (also referred to as a double apical impulse).

In LV enlargement resulting from dysfunction such as in DCM, the apex occupies more than one IC space and may appear to thrust forcefully because of enlargement. It is characteristically ill-sustained and often associated with an audible or palpable third heart sound.

A "tapping apex" refers to a palpable first heart sound (S1) and is always associated with a loud S1 as in MS.

Right Ventricular Activity

Right ventricular activity can be assessed by parasternal heave and epigastric impulse.[16,17] The former is useful in older patients and the latter in infants. Parasternal heave or lift can be graded empirically based on amplitude of the lift.

Grade I: Very mild lift. Pressure applied by hand easily abolishes it. It can be seen tangentially looking at it.

Grade II: Obvious, well palpable lift.

Grade III: A very prominent lift. Pressure applied by hand cannot abolish it.

The lift is sustained as in severe pulmonic stenosis or PAH and less well-sustained as in volume loaded right ventricle such as ASD or tricuspid or pulmonary regurgitation. Left parasternal lift or heave can also be due to severe MR when the systolic rise in LA results in an impulse which can be transmitted to anterior chest wall. It is more diffuse and late systolic in timing.

Impulses in Other Locations

Suprasternal: This results from aortic enlargement or forceful aortic expansion as in aortic aneurysm, coarctation, and AR.

2nd left space: Systolic pulsation in the left 2nd interspace close to the sternum can result from PAH. This characteristically ends with a palpable P2. Additionally, leftward and anterior location of the ascending aorta (L-malposition) results in systolic pulsations in the same location.

Intercostal spaces in the precordium: This results from a variety of hyperkinetic cardiac states.

Palpable Murmurs or Thrills

They can be felt in anywhere, at the apex, left sternal border either lower, mid or upper, right upper sternal border and infraclavicular. It is essential to accurately time the thrill (systolic, diastolic, or continuous). Any murmur that acquires sufficient intensity can potentially result in a thrill. However, certain murmurs that are of a high frequency may be very loud with an associated thrill. A good example is the high frequency murmur of MR.

Percussion

This has very little value, if any, in infants and small children. They may help identify situs and right heart border in pericardial effusion or right atrial enlargement. The diagnostic utility has not been validated.

Cardiac Auscultation

Of Sound, Cardiac Sound and Cardiac Auscultation

The human ear is capable of detecting sound with frequency ranging from 20 to 20,000 Hz. Optimal hearing acuity for human ear is for sound with frequency ranging from 2,000 to 3,000 Hz. But most cardiac sounds are below that frequency, i.e., between 30 and 800 Hz. Low frequency heart sounds (S3/S4) are <150 Hz, high frequency sounds are >300 Hz (MR and AR) and medium frequency sounds have a range between 150 and 300 Hz. Background noise in an ordinary hospital setting will be around 60–75 decibels whereas an optimal setting should have 35 dB as ambient noise level. With aging, people tend to have high frequency deafness—fortunately most cardiac sounds and murmurs are of low and medium frequency, i.e., <1,000 Hz.[18-21]

The stethoscope should have a bell and a diaphragm. The bell is best suited for hearing low-pitched sounds and murmurs (30–150 Hz) and diaphragm is for hearing high-pitched sounds and murmurs (>300 Hz). The bell should be applied with a light touch lest, low-pitched sounds may be missed. It should have a large diameter (~2.5 cm). Diaphragm should shut out low frequency sounds when tightly applied. Tube should be 25–30 cm long and it is ideal to have a double tubing.

Listening for Cardiac Sounds

- Identification of systole and diastole using carotid pulse and apex beat
- "Inching" technique by which stethoscope is slowly moved or inched from one site where systole and diastole are easily identified to other areas of chest wall.
- Progress from apex beat (mitral area) to left lower sternal border to left upper sternal border and then to right upper sternal border. Unlike in adults many cardiac murmurs due to CHD such as VSD, TOF, etc., are found maximally over nontraditional areas. The other auscultatory area in infants and children are—both infraclavicular areas, axilla, back, and carotids
- "Selective" listening is very crucial for accurate and meaningful cardiac auscultation. Try to focus on one event at a time, e.g., concentrate on S_1 first and then S_2 and systole alone, diastole alone, etc.

The inching technique and technique of selective listening has been popularized by Levine and Harvey.

Sound is the organized movement of molecules caused by vibrating body in some medium. In CVS, the medium is

TABLE 14: Components of cardiac auscultation.

Sound type	*Specifics*
Basic heart sounds	S_1, S_2, S_3, and S_4
Additional sounds	Clicks, knock, rub, and prosthetic sounds
Murmurs	Systolic, diastolic, and continuous

blood and the body is cardiovascular structures. The sounds produced can be short or long. Short sounds are called plainly sounds and long ones are called murmurs (**Table 14**).

First Heart Sound (S_1)

It is a medium-high-pitched sound that results from mitral valve closure (M_1) and TV closure (T_1).[22] Normally, M_1 is the dominant component and S_1 is best appreciated at apex (mitral area). M_1-T_1 time difference is <20 ms and the human ear cannot separate them out, and hence S_1 is heard normally as a single sound. S_1 is maximally heard at apex and S_2 at pulmonary area. If S_1 heard at apex is louder or equal to intensity of S_2 at left second interspace, it is loud. It is often subjective in evaluation. S_1 is affected by integrity and mobility, velocity of closure, and distance covered on closing of the mitral valve, ventricular contractility, heart rate, PR interval, and transmitting medium that includes pericardial space and chest wall. S_1 is louder in tachycardia, is louder with short PR interval (<130 ms) and soft in long PR interval (>200 ms). A soft S_1 is found in AR, chronic MR, ventricular dysfunction, left bundle branch block, and calcific MS. Extracardiac factors such as obesity, emphysema, and pericardial effusion can also reduce S_1 intensity.

A loud S_1 is found in tachycardia, MS, MVP, short PR interval, and ASD (due to T_1). *Split S_1 is classically found in* Ebstein anomaly and right bundle branch block.

Second Heart Sound (S_2)

Normally, S_2 is best heard at left upper sternal border and is split in inspiration and single in expiration and the first component, A_2 is louder than the second component, P_2. P_2 is normally not audible at the apex. In inspiration A_2-P_2 distance is >20–30 ms and is appreciated as two components while in expiration the A_2-P_2 distance is <20 ms and is appreciated as a single sound. S_2 is a relatively high-pitched sound, best appreciated by diaphragm. The physiological inspiratory widening of S_2 split is due to:

- Increased pulmonary artery hang out interval (*see* **Fig. 3**)
- Increased RV ejection time
- Decreased Q—A_2, i.e., early A_2. The most significant factor is increased PA hangout interval and least significant is increased RV ejection time.

A split is perceived as wide if it is >60 ms during inspiration and >40 ms during inspiration. It is important to understand the concept of "hang-out interval" (*see* **Fig. 3**). The hang-out interval time results because the actual reversal of flow

Flowchart 1: Causes of single second heart sound.

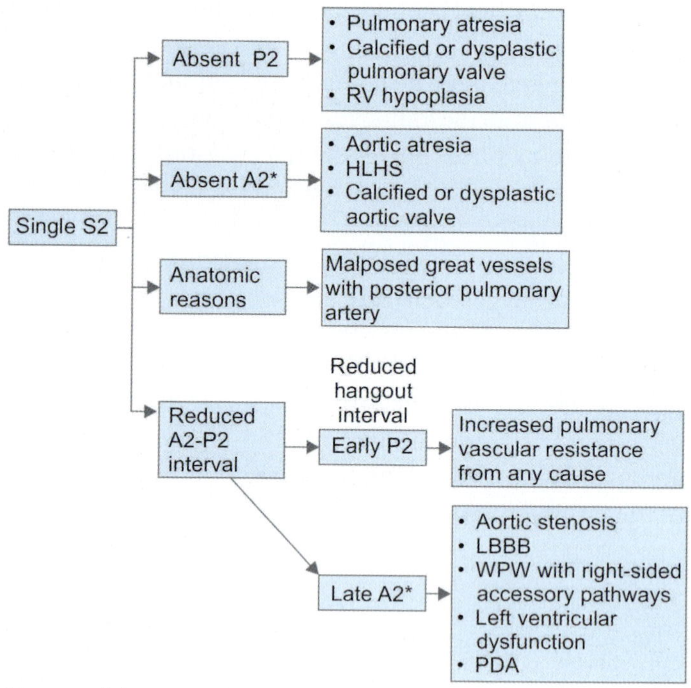

*Extreme delay in A2 can result in reversed or paradoxical splitting (LBBB: left bundle branch block; PDA: patent ductus arteriosus; HLHS: hypoplastic left heart syndrome)

in the great vessels that result in closure of the semilunar valves occurs a little after the crossover of the pressures in ventricle and in the great vessel. The hang-out interval is largely determined by the vascular resistance. Because of the systemic vascular resistance is much higher than the pulmonary vascular resistance the hang out interval is substantially shorter for the systemic side. A substantially lower pulmonary vascular resistance allows blood to continue to flow peripherally even after the crossover of the RV and pulmonary arterial tracings. This is because of inertia. Eventually, the flow direction briefly reverses to allow closure of the pulmonary valve.[23,24]

It is often possible to identify the individual components of the second heart sound in newborns about 48 hours after birth. A normally split second heart sound is often reassuring in newborns because it rules out most serious congenital heart defects (**Flowchart 1**).

Describing the second sound correctly: It is essential to try and answer the following questions:

- Does the sound split or is S_2 Single? This is a fundamental skill that is worth acquiring. After some practice, it is often possible to accurately identify the splitting of S_2.
  - If it splits, is it normally split, widely split (wider in inspiration) or paradoxically split (wider in expiration)?
  - If wide, is it fixed or variable?
- Which component is louder, A_2 or P_2?

  Correct description of S_2 involves use of one of the following standard terms:

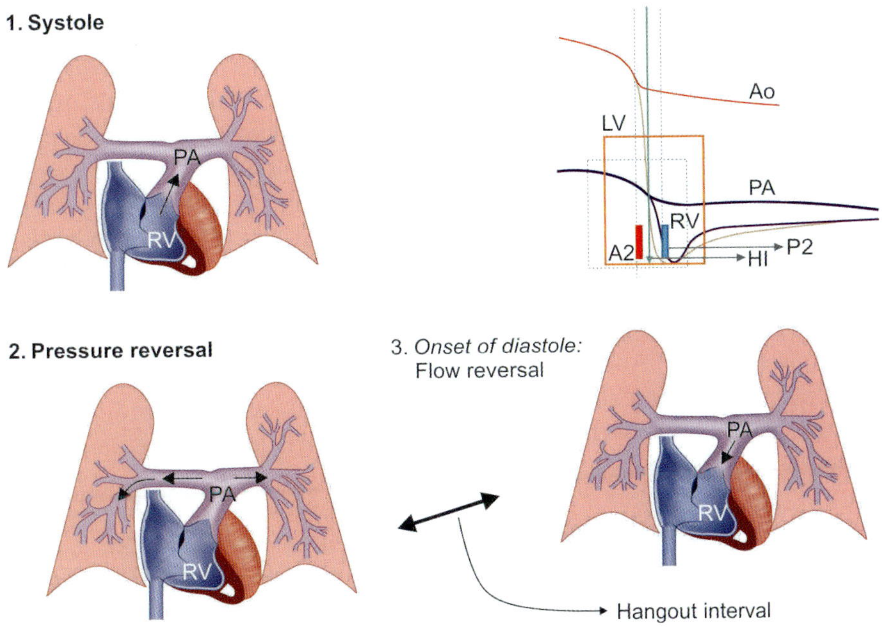

Fig. 4: The physiological basis of delayed closure of the pulmonary component of S2 (P2). In systole, blood is ejected into the pulmonary artery after pulmonary valve opens. In the second insert (pressure reversal), the inertia carries blood forward into the pulmonary arteries even after the pressure in the right ventricle falls below the pulmonary artery because the pulmonary vasculature normally offers little resistance. In insert 3 (flow reversal), the flow direction reverses and the pulmonary valve closes. The interval between pressure reversal and flow reversal with closure of the semilunar valve is the hangout interval. These intervals are illustrated in the insert with pressure traces.
(A2: aortic component of S2; Ao: aorta; LV: left ventricle; PA: pulmonary artery; RV: right ventricle)

Flowchart 2: Causes of widely split second heart sound.

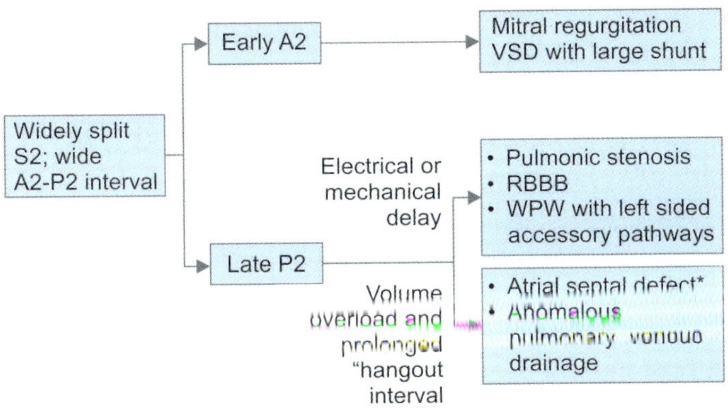

*Atrial septal defect results in wide-fixed splitting because normal respiratory influence on right-sided filling is largely eliminated.
(RBBB: right bundle branch block, WPW: Wolf-Parkinson White syndrome; VSD: ventricular septal defect)

- *Normally split*: Split in inspiration and single in expiration
- *Wide fixed*: Split both in inspiration and expiration with no discernable difference in timing
- *Wide variable*: Split in both inspiration and expiration. Split distinctly wider in inspiration
- *Single*: only one component made out
- *Reversed or paradoxically*: Split in expiration and single in inspiration.

Terms such as "narrow split" or "closely split" S_2 should be used with caution. **Figure 4 and Flowchart 2** summarize the causes of abnormal splitting of S_2.

Third Heart Sound (S_3)

It is a low-pitched sound occurring during the rapid filling phase of diastole. It is also called a filling sound, ventricular diastolic gallop, or protodiastolic gallop. It is best heard at the apex for the LV S_3 and less commonly in the left parasternal region for the RVS_3. The A_2-S_3 interval is between 120 and 200 ms, and hence it is not a very early diastolic sound. It is often normally heard in infancy, childhood, and adolescence. However, a normal or physiological S_3 can be distinguished from a pathological S_3 of LV dysfunction by the intensity of S_1 which is soft in the presence of LV dysfunction. In addition to LV dysfunction from any cause, S_3 is found in volume overload of the ventricle as in chronic MR or AR, post-tricuspid shunts such as VSD, patent ductus, anemia, and thyrotoxicosis. A right ventricular third heart sound (RVS_3) is associated with severe tricuspid regurgitation and RV dysfunction from any cause. The RVS_3 is localized in the left parasternal region and may be better heard during inspiration.

In constrictive pericarditis, S_3 occurs earlier and acquires a relatively high-pitched character due to marked elevation of filling pressures associated with increased velocity of rapid filling phase. These features are distinctive enough to merit a specific term, *the pericardial knock.*

Fourth Heart Sound

Unlike S_3, the presence of S_4 is almost always abnormal.[25] It is seen in situations where the atrium forcefully contracts to enable filling of a relatively noncompliant ventricle as a result of fibrosis or marked hypertrophy. It is low-pitched and heard just prior to the first heart sound. It is sometimes better felt than heard as an additional thrust just prior to the palpation of the apical impulse. The most common associations with S_4 include LV hypertrophy from systemic hypertension or outflow tract obstruction or hypertrophic cardiomyopathy.

Clicks

Clicks are sharper, higher pitched sounds heard in systole. Clicks can be ejection click and nonejection clicks. Ejection clicks that originate from semilunar valves as a result of aortic or pulmonary valve stenosis or great vessels are known as valvular clicks.

Valvar ejection clicks are due to sudden doming and snapping of semilunar valve during ejection and vascular clicks are due to distension of dilated great vessels.

The aortic valve ejection click is a consistent finding in bicuspid aortic valve. It can be present even when the valve is not stenotic. Its intensity is constant in expiration and inspiration, i.e., a constant ejection click. It can also be seen in persistent truncus arteriosus perhaps because the truncal valve is often abnormal. The aortic click is often best heard at apex but can be heard at other locations in the precordium including the right second interspace (aortic area).

Pulmonary valve ejection click is phasic of "inconstant" in nature, i.e., increases on expiration and decreases in intensity in inspiration unlike other right-sided cardiac auscultatory events that increase in inspiration. The interval between S_1 and the ejection click distance progressively decreases as PS progresses and in severe cases, the presence of valvar pulmonic stenosis is suggested by a perceived variation in intensity of first heart sound that becomes louder and sharper with expiration. Unlike the aortic ejection click, the pulmonary click is usually localized to the left second interspace.

Clicks that result from a dilated pulmonary artery in PH are constant and occur after a slightly longer interval after S_1.

Nonejection clicks are usually mid- or late systolic in timing and classically found in mitral or tricuspid valve prolapse.

Opening Snap

Rheumatic mitral valve stenosis is associated with an opening snap (OS). Its presence suggests that the valve is pliable. It is most unusual for congenital MS to be associated with OS. The OS is the result of sudden downward movement of the anterior mitral valve leaflet. It may be widely conducted if severe MS is present. It represents mobility of the valve and is due to sudden arrest of doming mitral valve. The interval between the second heart sound and OS (A_2-OS interval) interval is 40–160 ms, and it is the earliest diastolic sound. As MS becomes severe A_2-OS interval shortens.

Prosthetic Valve Sounds

Usually from mechanical valves, occurs in children who had replacement of the aortic or mitral valves with a metallic prosthetic valve. Sounds can be opening and closing, and is more prominent with ball and cage valves than disk valves. Sharpness of the valve clicks indicates that the valves are functioning well and are likely to be unobstructed.

Pericardial Rub

It is a high-pitched, leathery, scratchy murmur best heard over left lower sternal border. It can have three components (presystolic, systolic, and late diastolic) that produce a characteristic cadence that is quite unlike any heart murmur. The presence of a rub indicates friction between the two layers of the pericardium that usually results from inflammation (pericarditis). A sound quite similar to a pericardial rub can also result from the presence of air and fluid in the pericardial space early after cardiac surgery.

Cardiac Murmurs

A murmur is a prolonged series of auditory vibrations which often contain mixed elements of sound. The murmur is intimately related to turbulence. The turbulence is a function of the medium, vibrating structures, etc. A number called *Reynolds number* encompasses the factors which determine turbulence and therefore, murmur.[26,27]

$$\text{Reynolds number (Re)} = \frac{\text{(Density of fluid) (Velocity) (Tube diameter)}}{\text{Viscosity of fluid (blood)}}$$

When Re exceeds 2000, a murmur is heard. An increased velocity, lower viscosity of blood, increased stroke volume, and narrowing of blood passage will cause a higher Re, and hence murmur.

Murmur is the most frequent reason for referral of a child or infant with suspected heart disease—whether congenital or acquired. Yet many CHD, both benign and malignant, can present with no murmur whatsoever. In some CHDs, a cardiac murmur is either essential useful for the diagnosis, example being ASD and coarctation of aorta. But a murmur still continues to be the major marker for heart disease and also has significant localizing value—in localizing the clinical diagnosis. In infants with cardiac murmur, one-fourth presented before 2 weeks and one-third presented only after 3 months. Detection of a heart murmur should prompt one to initiate a complete evaluation of an infant or child.

Murmurs can be:

- Systolic (between S_1 and S_2)
- Diastolic (between S_2 and S_1)
- Continuous.

Aubrey Leatham in 1958 had classified systolic murmurs into ejection systolic murmurs and pansystolic murmurs and diastolic murmurs into early, mid, and late diastolic murmurs. Ejection murmurs are generated by turbulent flow across abnormal semilunar valves, increased flow through

BOX 4: Murmur likely organic when.

- There is a diastolic murmur
- There is a continuous murmur
- Murmur is of Gr 3/6 or more
- Murmur is either pansystolic or early systolic
- When S_2 is abnormal
- When associated findings suggest the presence of heart disease

normal semilunar valves, and abnormal flow through great vessels. Pansystolic murmurs are due to a holosystolic flow of blood from a high pressure chamber to a low pressure chamber. Murmurs can be classified as organic or innocent. The features of organic murmurs are listed in **Box 4**.

Timing of Murmurs

Systolic Murmurs

I. *Early systolic murmur*: It starts with S_1 (S_1 coincident) and extends variably into systole and stops short of S_2. It is usually decrescendo. Causes are:
   (a) Acute MR
   (b) Tricuspid regurgitation (TR) with a normal RV pressure
   (c) Very small, restrictive VSD, especially muscular
   (d) Very large, unrestrictive VSD with significant PAH.

Note: The quality of murmur in (c) differs from (d) in that the former is high pitched.

In acute MR, LA pressure equalizes with LV pressure much before the end of systole. Hence, the murmur is early systolic and decrescendo. In acute TR also, similar phenomenon leads to an early systolic murmur. In small VSD, the defect closes by the middle of systole and generates an early high-pitched systolic murmur. In large VSD, RV systolic pressure is high and quickly equalizes with LV pressure, and hence the early systolic timing and low pitch.[28]

II. *Mid systolic murmur*: The murmur starts a little after S_1 and usually ends before S_2. Majority of such mid-systolic murmurs are ejection systolic murmurs, i.e., it is due to phasic flow through LV and RV outflow tract and the onset of murmur coincides with the beginning of ejection. The intensity increases in early systole and decelerates in latter half. So, the murmur is often crescendo-decrescendo. Examples are many.
   i. Aortic or pulmonic stenosis
   ii. Aortic root dilatation or main pulmonary artery dilation as in PH. Here, the murmur is characteristically very short in duration
   iii. ASD
   iv. Innocent murmurs—Still's murmur

III. *Late-systolic murmur:* The murmur begins well after S_1, begins in mid or late systole and travels variably into systole. It is classically found in mitral or tricuspid valve prolapse and often follows the nonejection click.

IV. *Pansystolic murmur (Holosystolic)*: It begins with S_1 (S_1 coincident) and occupies all of the systole up to S_2 (or S_2 on its side of origin) and is constant is shape and amplitude usually. Examples are:
   - VSD
   - MR
   - TR.

Diastolic Murmurs

Early diastolic murmur: It begins with S_2, travels variably into diastole, and is decrescendo in nature. Examples are AR and hypertensive pulmonary regurgitation (Graham-Steell murmur of PAH).

Mid-diastolic murmurs: It starts in mid diastole and occupies variable phase of diastole. They are usually low-pitched murmurs. It occurs in:

- Mitral and tricuspid valve stenosis and left atrial myxoma. MS is characterized by a presystolic accentuation.[29]
- Exaggerated diastolic flow across a normal mitral or tricuspid valve; these murmurs are not associated with a presystolic accentuation and are localized to the apex (mitral flow murmurs) or left lower parasternal area (tricuspid flow murmurs).
   i. Post-tricuspid shunts (VSD and PDA) result in exaggerated flow across the mitral valve
   ii. Pre-tricuspid shunts result in exaggerated flow across the TV
   iii. Severe valve regurgitation (mitral or tricuspid).
- Austin Flint murmur of AR that result from vibrations generated by the AR jet striking the mitral valve together with some flow restriction because of premature closure.
- Nonhypertensive pulmonary regurgitation such as in absent pulmonary valve or after a tetralogy repair.

Late diastolic murmur: It is also called presystolic murmur which ends with S. It commonly occurs only in sinus rhythm and is associated with mitral or tricuspid valve stenosis. When the stenosis is mild, the murmur is largely limited to late diastole.

Pan-diastolic murmur: This is typically associated with hypertensive pulmonary regurgitation. The jet of regurgitation from anteriorly located structures and can be very loud. Both duration and intensity do not indicate the severity of pulmonary regurgitation.

Continuous Murmur

Continuous murmur is a murmur which begins in systole, continues without interruption into diastole—into all or part of diastole. It usually peaks around S_2. Continuous murmurs are generally generated when blood flows from one (high pressure) vascular bed to another (low pressure) vascular bed without interruption. To and fro murmurs result from two distinct physiological events (e.g., VSD and AR). While it may be difficult to identify the gap between the two events, it is often possible to identify an abrupt change in the character of the murmur at S_2.

Table 15 lists the causes of continuous murmurs and their distinguishing characteristics.

Grading of Murmurs

Grading of murmurs was originally described by Levine and Freeman in 1933 for systolic murmur. Now it is applied for systolic and diastolic murmurs.

Intensity: Murmurs are graded as follows:

- *Grade 1*: Heard only with intense concentration after a period of "tuning in"
- *Grade 2*: Faint but heard immediately
- *Grade 3*: Easily heard, of intermediate intensity
- *Grade 4*: Easily heard and loud (may be associated with a thrill)
- *Grade 5*: Very loud, thrill present, and audible with the edge of the stethoscope on the chest
- *Grade 6*: Audible with the stethoscope off the chest.

The difference between Grades 2 and 3 or Grades 5 and 6 may be somewhat subjective.

Quality and Character of Murmurs

Quality or character of the murmur is many times diagnostic. With increasing experience one identifies the lesion associated with a murmur, e.g., early systolic, harsh murmur of a small VSD and high-pitched pan systolic murmur of rheumatic mitral valvulitis and musical murmur of MVP.

Conduction can be often useful in diagnosis:

- MR—conducts to axilla, back and occasionally to base
- PS—conducts along supraclavicular area to acromion, base of neck
- AS—conducts to carotids
- VSD—conducts along sternal border, widely heard in infants.

Maneuvers (Hemodynamic Auscultation)

While using maneuvers to improve the diagnostic yield of clinical evaluation, it is important to understand the physiology. In general right-sided auscultatory events (with the exception of the pulmonary valve click) increase in intensity on inspiration and, to a lesser extent, left-sided events increase on expiration.[30]

A reduction in the LV cavity size can result from reduced venous return as a result of standing. This exaggerates the murmur of hypertrophic obstructive cardiomyopathy and MVP. An increase in LV cavity size as a result of increased afterload from squatting, isometric handgrip, and Valsalva strain reduces the intensity of these murmurs.

TABLE 15: Continuous murmurs.

Condition	*Location*	*Character*
Patent ductus arteriosus (PDA)	Left first interspace, sometimes second interspace	Harsh with eddy sounds (machinery) that results from the PDA jet colliding with forward flows from the pulmonary valve. A palpable thrill usually indicates a large shunt. Large PDAs often have a relatively soft diastolic component. Very small PDAs may also result in a systolic murmur. Diastolic component may not be heard in newborns
PDA in presence of pulmonary atresia	Left first interspace, sometimes second interspace	Relatively soft, no eddy sounds. Murmur intensity reduces as the PDA closes. Newborns with duct-dependent pulmonary atresia and significant cyanosis often do not have audible murmurs
Aortopulmonary shunts or Blalock–Taussig (BT) shunt	On the side of the BT shunt in the infraclavicular region and over the back	Relatively softer unless the shunt is large. Eddy sounds are characteristically absent. In the early postoperative period, the murmur of the right BT shunt is well heard on the endotracheal tube
Aortopulmonary collaterals	Anywhere but most typically over the back since they mostly originate from the descending thoracic aorta	Very much like that of aortopulmonary shunts
Ruptured sinus of Valsalva aneurysm to right ventricular outflow	Left second interspace	Harsh, often associated with a thrill
Rupture of sinus of valsalva to right atrium	Left lower sternal border	Harsh, often associated with a thrill
Coronary arterial fistula	Anywhere over precordium depending on the drainage site. Common sites of drainage include the right atrium (murmur best heard in the right sternal border) and right ventricle	"Superficial" character. Usually harsh
Pulmonary arteriovenous malformation	Anywhere in the chest, often away from precordium	Soft with predominantly low frequencies. Associated cyanosis
Coarctation	Best over back in the interscapular region	Relatively soft, diastolic component tends to be very short and soft. Often the murmur is heard only during systole
Venous hum	Right or left first intercostal space or at the sites of insertion of the sternomastoid	Soft, louder on sitting up and eliminated by pressure on the internal jugular vein. Exaggerated by anemia. Often heard in young children between 3 and 6 years

Describing a Murmur

- Timing—systole, diastole, continuous, to and fro
- Timing within the cycle—early, mid, late, throughout (pan)
- *Grading*: I–VI for systolic and I–IV for diastolic
- Length of murmur—short, long
- Pitch—low, medium, high, mixed
- Character—quality of (soft/harsh)
- Area of maximum intensity
- Conduction (selective propagation)
- Response to maneuvers.

REFERENCES

1. Shakespeare W. The Tempest. London: Cassel and Company Ltd; 1887.
2. McMullen SM, Patrick W. Cyanosis. Am J Med. 2013;126(3):210-2.
3. Wood P. Attacks of deeper cyanosis and loss of consciousness in Fallot's tetralogy. BHJ. 1958;20(2):282-6.
4. Ducharme-Crevier L, Wainwright MS. Childhood stroke and congenital heart disease. Pediatr Neurol Briefs. 2015;29(3):18.
5. NYHA. Nomenclature and Criteria for Diagnosis, 6th edition. Boston: Little Brown; 1964.
6. Hurst JW. The value of using the entire NYHA classification of heart and vascular disease. Clin Cardiol. 2006;29(9):415-7.
7. Ross RD. The Ross classification for heart failure in children after 25 years: a review and age stratified revision. Ped Cardiol. 2012; 33(8):1295-300.
8. Myers KA, Farquhar DF. Does this patient have clubbing? JAMA. 2001;286(3):341-7.
9. Gersh BJ. Examination of the arterial pulse. InOtto CM, Yeon SB (Eds). UpToDate; 2010.
10. Seth R, Magner P, Matzinger F, van Walraven C. How far is the sternal angle from the mid right atrium? J Gen Intern Med. 2002;17(11):852-6.
11. Meyer TE. Examination of jugular venous pulse. In: Drazner MH, Yeon SB (Eds). Massachusetts: UpToDate Inc.; 2020.
12. Sinisalo J, Rapola J, Rossinen J, Kupari M. Simplifying the estimation of jugular venous pressure. Am J Cardiol. 2007;100(12):1779-81.
13. Ewy GA. The abdominojugular test: technique and hemodynamic correlates. Ann Intern Med. 1988;109(6):456-60.
14. Ahmad ZS. Clinical sign: the hepatojugular reflux in Kerala J Cardiol. 2017;1(1).
15. Gersh BJ, Otto CM, Yeon SB. Examination of the Precordial Pulsation. Massachusetts: UpToDate Inc.; 2020.
16. Armstrong TG, Gotsman MS. The left parasternal lift in tricuspid incompetence. Am Heart J. 1974;88(2):183-90.
17. Gillan PMS, Deliyannis AA, Mounsey JPD. The left parasternal impulse. Br Heart J. 1964; 26(6):726-36.
18. Montinari MR, Minelli S. The first 200 years of cardiac auscultation and future perspectives. J Multidiscip Healthc. 2019;12:183-9.
19. Tavel ME. Cardiac auscultation: a glorious past and it does have a future! Circulation. 2006; 113(9):1255-9.
20. Leon DF, Shaver JA (Eds). Physiologic Principles of Heart Sounds and Murmurs. New York: American Heart Association; 1975.
21. Chizner MA. Cardiac auscultation: rediscovering the lost art. Curr Probl Cardiol. 2008; 33(7):326-408.
22. Leatham A. Splitting of the first and second heart Sounds. Brit Heart J. 1968;30:739.
23. O'toole JD, Reddy PS, Curtiss EI, Shaver JA. The mechanism of splitting of the second heart sound in ASD. Circulation. 1977;56(6):1047-53.
24. Sutton G, Harris A, Leatham A. Second heart sound in pulmonary hypertension. BHJ. 1968;30(6):743-56.
25. Tavel ME. The fourth heart sound: a premature requiem? Circulation. 1974;49:4.
26. Geggel RA, Fulton DR, Armsby C. Approach to the infant or child with a cardiac murmur. Massachusetts: UpToDate (Wolters Kluwer); 2020.
27. Pelech AN. Evaluation of the pediatric patient with a cardiac murmur. Pediatr Clin North Am. 1999;46(2):167-88.
28. Freeman AR, Levine SA. The clinical significance of the systolic murmur. A Study of 1000 consecutive non-cardiac cases. Ann Intern Med. 1933;6:1371.
29. Wood P. An appreciation of mitral stenosis. I. Clinical features. BMJ. 1954;1(4870):1051-63.
30. Gersch BJ, Otto CM, Yeon SB. Physiological and pharmacological maneuvers in the differential diagnosis of heart murmurs and sounds. Massachusetts: UpToDate (Wolters Kluwer); 2019.

SUGGESTED READING

Here is a list of excellent resources for the student interested in delving further into the art and science of clinical cardiology.

1. Abrams J. Essentials of Cardiac Physical Diagnosis. Philadelphia: Lea and Febiger; 1987.
2. Cassidy SC, Allen HD, Phillips JR. History and physical examination. In: Allen HD, Driscoll DJ, Shaddy RE, Feltes TF (Eds). Moss and Adams' Heart Disease in Infants, Children and Adolescents, 9th edition. Philadelphia: Wolters Kluwer Lippincott Williams & Wilkins; 2016.
3. Constant J. Bedside Cardiology, 5th edition. Philadelphia: Lippincott Williams and Wilkins; 1999.
4. Constant J. Essentials of Bedside Cardiology, 2nd edition. New Jersey: Humana Press; 2003.
5. Duff DF, Mac Namara DG. History and physical examination of the cardiovascular system. In: Garson A, Bricker JT, Fisher DJ, Neish SR (Eds). The Science and Practice of Pediatric Cardiology, 2nd edition. Philadelphia: Lippincott Williams and Wilkins; 1998.
6. Fang JC, O'Gara PT. History and physical examination: an evidence-based approach. In: Zipes DP, Libby P, Borrow RO, Mann DL, Tomasell G. Braunwald's Heart Disease (e-book), 11th edition. Amsterdam: Elsevier; 2018. pp. 83-101.
7. Felner JM. Chapter: an overview of the cardiovascular system. In: Walker HK, Hall WD, Hurst JW (Eds). Clinical Methods, 3rd edition. Boston: Butterworths; 1990.
8. Grubb N, Spratt J, Bradbury A. The cardiovascular system. In: Douglas G, Nicol F, Robertson C (Eds). Mcleods' Clinical Examination, 13th edition. London: Churchill Livingstone Elsevier; 2013.
9. Kaplan NM. Kaplan's Clinical Hypertension, 9th edition. Philadelphia: Lippincott Williams and Wilkins; 2005.
10. Kleigman RM, St Geme, Blum NJ, Shah SS, Tasker RC, Wilson KM. Nelson's Textbook of Pediatrics, 21st edition. Amsterdam: Elsevier; 2019.
11. Levine GN. Cardiology Secrets, 5th edition. Amsterdam: Elsevier; 2018.
12. Perloff JK, Marelli AJ. Perloff's Clinical Recognition of Congenital Heart Disease, 6th edition. Amsterdam: Elsevier; 2012.
13. Rudolph A. Congenital Diseases of the Heart: Clinical-Physiological Considerations, 3rd edition. Hoboken: Wiley Blackwell; 2009.
14. Soma Raju B. Clinical Methods in Cardiology. Cambridge: Universities Press; 2002.
15. Tandon R. Bedside Approach in the Diagnosis of Congenital Heart Disease. London: Churchill Livingstone; 1998.
16. Timmis AD, Archbold A. Cardiovascular system. In: Glynn M, Drake WM (Eds). Hutchison's Clinical Methods, 23rd edition. Philadelphia: Saunders; 2012.
17. Walker HK, Hall WD, Hurst JW (Eds). Clinical Methods, 3rd edition. Boston: Butterworths; 1990.
18. White PD. A short history of cardiology. Book Review. Herrick JB. JAMA. 1942;202-3.
19. Zipes DP, Libby P, Bonow RO, Mann DL, Tomaselli GF. (Eds). Braunwald's Heart Disease, 11th edition. Amsterdam: Elsevier; 2019.
20. Zulfikar Ahamed M. Cardiovascular examination. In: Gupta P, Menon PSN, Ramji S, Lodha R (Eds). PG Textbook of Pediatrics, 2nd edition. Jaypee Brothers Medical Publishers; 2015.

6

CHAPTER

Screening for Congenital Heart Disease

Navaneetha Sasikumar

INTRODUCTION

Congenital heart disease (CHD) is one of the most common birth defects in the population. The prevalence of CHD is estimated to be 8 per 1,000 live births. CHDs account for 6–10% of infant mortality and 30–50% of infant mortality from congenital malformations.[1] Up to 10% of these are diagnosed at autopsy in settings where they are regularly performed.[2] Critical congenital heart diseases (CCHD) are structural malformations of the heart that are present at birth and require surgery or intervention in the first year of life, to survive.[3] They account for approximately 25% of CHD, and are the primary culprits for infant mortality as well as morbidity from heart disease.[4-6] Advances in surgical and interventional management of CHD in the past decades have ensured that today; most CHDs can be corrected or meaningfully palliated when detected in a timely fashion. Hence, timely detection of CCHD is imperative in decreasing infant mortality rate.

Do all babies with CCHD require intervention or surgery in neonatal period? The answer is no. Some of them can electively undergo surgery or intervention later in infancy. Tetralogy of Fallot is a good example. There is still significant room for subjectivity in judgment calls about the timing of surgery in these settings.

So what percentage of CCHDs would need surgery or intervention in the neonatal period, and thus would benefit greatly from screening? Estimates from the United States show that the birth prevalence of cyanotic CHDs and left-sided obstructive lesions are 1.75 and 1.15 per 1,000 live births, respectively. Among these 1.1 and 0.55 per 1,000 live births respectively are estimated to benefit from early detection and treatment.[7]

A significant number of newborns with CCHD will not show any obvious clinical signs, as they depend on flow through the ductus arteriosus for survival. Duct-dependent systemic circulation includes all hypoplastic left heart syndrome, interrupted aortic arch, critical coarctation of aorta, and aortic stenosis. Duct-dependent pulmonary circulations include all cases of pulmonary atresia with or without ventricular septal defect (VSD), some cases of tetralogy of Fallot, or similar physiology. Newborns are often not suspected to have CCHD until transitional events occur in their circulation. In these newborns, closure of the ductus arteriosus after discharge leads to a catastrophic situation. Hospital-based screening for CCHD, before discharge, is targeted at avoiding these unexpected deaths.

BOX 1: Rationale for screening newborns for congenital heart disease (CHD).

- Critical congenital heart disease is a significant contributor to infant mortality in most global settings
- Most babies with CHD show no signs or symptoms of heart disease in the newborn period
- *Physical examination is insensitive*: Of babies with congenital cardiac malformation, less than half have a murmur in the newborn period
- The most dangerous diagnoses (duct-dependent systemic circulation) usually only become symptomatic once they are already established on a rapidly deteriorating course which can lead to death in a matter of hours
- Prenatal diagnosis enables a newborn with critical CHD to be in the best possible condition prior to surgery

Further, multiple studies have confirmed that when prenatally diagnosed (which is a major opportunity for screening), CCHD surgery has lower surgical morbidity and mortality.[8-12] Presurgical cardiovascular collapse and attendant end-organ injury are risk factors for adverse immediate surgical outcomes. Also, a more stable perioperative status will help decrease perioperative neurological injury, which in turn would result in better long-term neurodevelopmental outcomes. **Box 1** summarizes the rationale for screening of newborns with CHD.

SCREENING: PRINCIPLES AND APPLICATION IN PEDIATRIC CARDIOLOGY

The 10 points of the public health classic "Wilson and Jungner Criteria" for screening are quite valid in CHD screening (**Box 2**).[13] Considering these in the background of critical CHD makes it clear that the disease (CCHD) qualifies to be screened. Obviously more challenging are the choice of the screening test and system principles. Performance characteristics of screening tests, interpretation of screening test results, and postscreening test options need careful consideration and planning. When a screening test is applied to a disease with a relatively low prevalence rate such as CCHD, it should be all the more accurate. As to the screening program, capacity of infrastructure not only to screen, but also to treat newborns that have been detected to have CCHD, coordination and integration into the pre-existent broader healthcare system, acceptability to participants, health professionals and society, ethics, benefits, and harms are all equally important aspects.[13] As primary caretakers of children and advocates of child health, pediatricians have a major role in understanding, implementing, and advocating for each of the above-mentioned aspects.

For these reasons, screening for CHD needs to be introduced to a region as a part of a comprehensive population-based plan to tackle CHD and not as an isolated exercise. It is necessary to be mindful of the care continuum for CHD (**Fig. 1**) and recognize that screening needs to be complemented by all the other elements in the care continuum.

OPPORTUNITIES FOR SCREENING FOR PEDIATRIC HEART DISEASE

Prenatal ultrasonography of the fetus, postnatal physical examination of the newborn, and pulse oximetry are currently being utilized for screening for CHD.

Prenatal Ultrasonography of the Fetus

Congenital heart disease can be identified by ultrasonographic examination of the fetal heart after 14–16 weeks of gestation. Screening for CHD is a part of the antenatal anomaly scan. With a four-chamber view alone, the sensitivity for CHD detection is approximately 30%. Conotruncal defects are particularly missed if only four-chamber view is evaluated. When outflow tract evaluation is added, sensitivity increases to 69–83%. Up to 90% major CHDs can be detected in the anomaly scan if the three vessels (3V) and 3V with trachea (3VT) views are added to cardiac screening.[14] When the screening suggests an abnormality, a comprehensive fetal echocardiographic study is indicated. Other fetal indications include arrhythmia, increased nuchal translucency, extracardiac structural malformations, genetic/chromosomal abnormalities, pericardial or pleural effusions or skin edema, nonimmune hydrops fetalis, monochorionic twins, and noncardiac abnormalities that can lead to heart failure. Fetal echocardiography is also recommended for maternal and familial indications such as family history of CHD or genetic syndromes, maternal metabolic diseases, exposure to teratogens or viruses, connective tissue disorder, and assisted reproduction. Sensitivity and specificity of fetal echocardiography is known to vary depending on the expertise of operator as well as the quality of equipment.

Prenatal detection appears to be ideal for early detection as this will allow in utero transport of babies with CCHD. These babies can then be delivered at a facility capable of promptly managing CCHD. If detected before 20 weeks of gestation (or before the legal temporal limit of medical termination of pregnancy), family will have the option of termination of pregnancy in disease conditions where outcomes are known to be poor. Even with high-end equipment and expert hands, many disease situations are technically challenging when it comes to confirming detailed anatomy and providing the best possible management plan in early pregnancy. Sociocultural aspects such as stigma associated with CHD and potential financial considerations significantly complicate this situation. The decision to terminate should always be taken in careful consultation with a pediatric cardiologist. The parents should completely understand the implications of the fetal diagnosis and prognosis and no effort should be spared to ensure this. Another important consideration is the psychological trauma to the family that comes with a fetal diagnosis of a CHD. It is imperative that comprehensive and thoughtful counseling accompanies fetal echocardiography.

The reported prenatal detection rates of CHD in low-risk populations does not exceed 35–40%.[15] The introduction of a mandatory nationwide screening program in the

BOX 2: Wilson and Jungner's principles of screening

1. The condition sought should be an important health problem
2. The natural history of the condition, including development from latent to declared disease, should be adequately understood
3. There should be a recognizable latent or early symptomatic stage
4. There should be a suitable test or examination
5. The test should be acceptable to the population
6. There should be an agreed policy on whom to treat as patients
7. There should be an accepted treatment for patients with recognized disease
8. Facilities for diagnosis and treatment should be available
9. The cost of case-finding (including diagnosis and treatment of patients diagnosed) should be economically balanced in relation to possible expenditure on medical care as a whole
10. Case-finding should be a continuing process and not a "once and for all" project

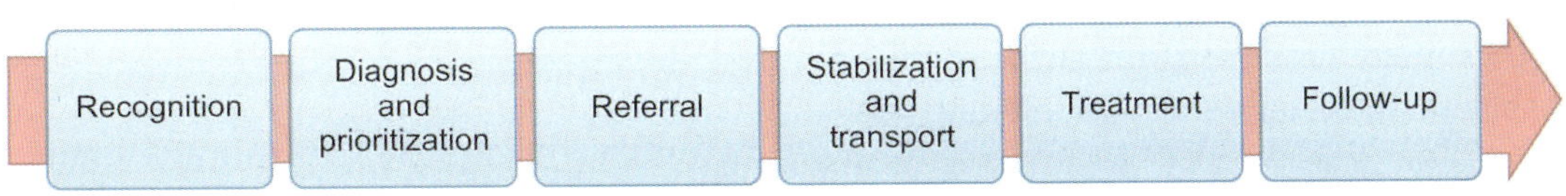

Fig. 1: The care continuum for congenital heart disease; screening is an integral part of the first step, i.e., recognition. It is essential to have all the elements of the continuum to be in place without which screening is likely to be ineffective.

Netherlands resulted in an improved detection rate of 59.7%.[16] This underscores the fact that detection rates are substantially improved where there is a preexistent centralized, well-organized national healthcare system with uniform practices; policy changes, rigorous training, and attention to quality.

Pitfalls of fetal echocardiography include unfavorable fetal position or maternal habitus, late onset or progressive cardiac lesions such as valve stenosis, coarctation of aorta, endomyocardial fibroelastosis, hypertrophic cardiomyopathy, rhabdomyoma, and difficult to diagnose lesions such as pulmonary venous or coronary abnormalities. Screening only "high risk" pregnancies is unlikely to increase yield as the prevalence in this population is only marginally high compared to "low-risk" pregnancies[17] because the vast majority of babies with CHDs are born to "low-risk mothers." The best foot forward is enhancing cardiac screening during anomaly scan and offering fetal echocardiography to those with abnormal scans. The cost effectiveness of this strategy as a nationwide screening program will remain a major challenge at least for low- and middle-income countries.

Postnatal Physical Examination of the Newborn

Only a relatively small proportion of newborns with CHD present with readily identifiable pointers, e.g., multiple congenital anomalies, family history of CHD, or cytogenetic abnormalities. Physical examination of a newborn is particularly known to have limitations in identifying CCHD. Some of these include, lack of specificity of murmurs (half of newborns with murmur do not have CHD) and absence of any cardiac findings including murmur in nearly half of all infants with CCHD. Of particular importance is the fact that neonatal emergencies such as transposition of great arteries and pulmonary atresia often do not present with a murmur. On the other hand, flow murmurs of the transitional circulation, transient tricuspid regurgitation, peripheral pulmonary stenosis of the newborn, and small ventricular septal defects are common and these conditions are of little clinical significance in the newborn. Difficulty in differentiating innocent from pathological murmur and suboptimal visual assessment of cyanosis adds to the limitations. In addition, physical examination skills are perhaps declining with each generation of trainees.

Electrocardiogram, Chest X-ray, and Echocardiography

Identification of CCHD is aided by electrocardiogram, and chest radiograph in many cases, but they lack sufficient sensitivity and specificity to be used as screening tools. Echocardiography also has serious limitations when considered as a primary screening tool for CCHD. The cost in itself is a significant deterrent. Additionally, availability of trained personnel to screen all neonates, with a reasonable degree of accuracy to detect CCHD, will also remain a humungous challenge. High rate of false positives (normal features of transitional circulation like a patent foramen ovale and a patent ductus arteriosus) and detection of nonsignificant defects (small muscular ventricular septal defects which are statistically more common) are also major concerns when echocardiography is considered as a screening tool.

Pulse Oximetry Screening of the Newborn

Pulse oximetry rightly has the status of a vital sign in contemporary clinical practice. Hypoxemia is a common feature of many CCHDs. The differential absorption spectra of oxygenated hemoglobin (Hb) (infrared band—850–1,000 nm) and deoxygenated Hb (red band—600–750 nm) forms the basis for pulse oximetry. The ratio of light absorbance in these two wavelengths correlates with oxygen saturation in the capillaries. Pulse oximetry can be particularly useful in detecting hypoxemia that is not visible to human eye (85–95% SpO_2), more so when newborns are dark skinned. Data from studies prior to the pulse oximetry screening era show that up to 30–50% of newborns with CCHD in US went home undiagnosed and nearly 10% of babies with CCHD died before a timely diagnosis was made.[15] The numbers are expected to be worse in low-middle income countries. Universal pulse oximetry screening before hospital discharge targets timely detection of CCHD in these group of babies thereby bridging the diagnostic gap. It is a good practice to make sure that no newborn leaves the hospital without SpO_2 values documented on the discharge summary (**Flowchart 1**).

Efficacy of pulse oximetry screening: A meta-analysis that included 13 newborn pulse oximetry screening studies with 230,000 newborns showed moderate sensitivity (~76.5%) and high specificity for detection of CCHD with a very low false positive rate of 0.14% (14 false positive cases per 10,000 screened infants).[18] Universal pulse oximetry screening is expected to detect nearly 50–70% of asymptomatic

Flowchart 1: Approach to a patient who fails pulse oximetry screening. Prompt initial clinical assessment is followed by work up based on the assessment.

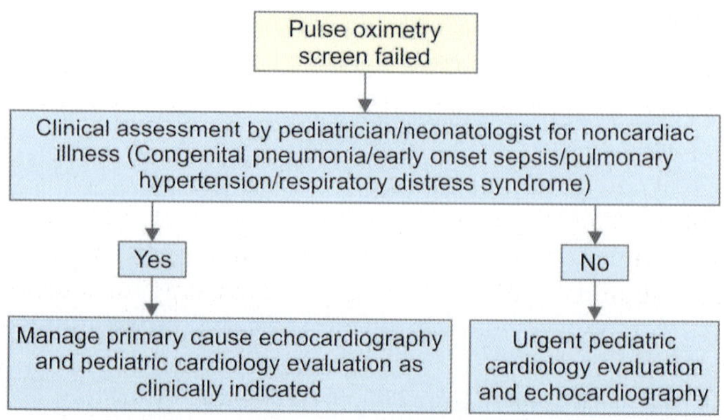

infants born with CCHD, after excluding babies with prenatal diagnosis. Accordingly, the United States and many European countries have implemented mandatory universal pulse oximetry screening for all newborns prior to their discharge from hospital. Within India, universal pulse oximeter screening is now recommended in Kerala as a part of the Hridyam initiative for diagnosis and treatment of CHD *(www.hridyam.net)*.

Typically, when a newborn is screened and found to be positive, the baby is evaluated by a pediatrician or a neonatologist first. Further work up is tailored to clinical assessment. Except in the presence of an obvious noncardiac diagnosis that can explain hypoxia, this typically includes an echocardiogram and/or pediatric cardiology consultation (*see* **Fig. 1**). Major variations in screening protocols exist which include pre and postductal saturations (right hand and either foot) versus single postductal measurement (foot only) and timing of screening (screening before 24 hours of age vs. after 24 hours of age). The sensitivity of pulse oximetry screening has not been found to be substantially affected by either.[18] However, the false positive rate was significantly high when screening was done before vs. after 24 hours of age (0.50 vs 0.05%).[18] Screening is done after 24 hours of age in the US and before 24 hours in the UK and Nordic countries.

Although "false positive" babies might not have an underlying CCHD, 30–80% of them have alternative life-threatening noncardiac disease such as congenital pneumonia, early-onset sepsis, or pulmonary hypertension. Early detection of these diseases is considered an advantage. Evaluation of the real false positives (with no cardiac or noncardiac illness that can explain hypoxia) would pose a major challenge, more so in resource constrained healthcare systems. In addition, the time from announcing screen positive (likely to have CCHD with attendant lifelong financial and social implications) to completion of evaluation can turn out to be psychologically distressing to the parents. The false negatives also would get amplified proportionate to the size of the population screened. Large proportion of patients missed by pulse oximetry screening have duct-dependent systemic circulation such as coarctation of aorta and aortic stenosis. This contrasts with physical examination where more than half the missed cases are cyanotic lesions, thereby justifying combining physical examination and pulse oximetry.

Universal pulse oximetry screening in low- and middle-income countries: Political commitment to the cause, capacity building of the healthcare system, and maintaining quality are equally important links when a nationwide pulse oximetry screening program is being introduced. The primary consideration would be to analyze the major contributors to infant mortality in each geopolitical region. When the infant mortality rate has substantially decreased (<15–20), congenital malformations can be perceived as important enough to justify systemic intervention.

The sensitivity of pulse oximetry screening is reportedly low in low resource settings.[19,20] When the above-mentioned statistics are applied to populations as large as India and China, the false positives and false negatives get amplified. The low sensitivity will translate to a large number of CCHDs still being missed. A small false positivity rate will end up in a large number of unnecessary echocardiograms being performed. This apart, the bottle neck would essentially be capacity of healthcare infrastructure to do screening with reasonable accuracy, and to provide for timely work up and treatment of screen positive cases. Screening will have to be conducted by trained personnel and continued training and quality assurance will have to be in place. At each point of screening, pediatricians and neonatologists should be designated for primary evaluation of screen positive cases. A pathway for cardiac assessment should be prespecified. Availability of trained personnel to perform and interpret neonatal echocardiograms with a reasonable degree of accuracy should be ensured (*see* **Fig. 1**). Once diagnosed with a CCHD, facilities for safe transport to a pediatric cardiac center capable of managing CCHD in the newborn should be available. Above all, pediatric cardiac care systems capable of managing CCHD in the newborn should be made available, accessible, and affordable to the large number of additional CCHD cases that would be picked up by screening. In India, for example, all currently running pediatric cardiac programs together can cater to only <10% of infants with CCHD. Implementing nationwide screening without strengthening this network would only bring the healthcare system to a challenging situation where meaningful treatment cannot be offered to the large number of babies with CCHD picked up by screening.[17] Each of the above steps mandates trained manpower and finances which would indeed pose a major challenge to the low-middle income countries. However, with progressive improvements in human development indices, it is only to be expected that the overall scenario in many low- and middle-income counties will change for the better. In the coming decades, more and more parts of the world will introduce mandatory pulse oximeter screening in neonates.

Peripheral Perfusion Index

A significant number of CCHDs missed by pulse oximetry screening are the left heart obstructive diseases, all of which when severe has the potential to compromise cardiac output and peripheral perfusion. The peripheral perfusion index (PPI) is measured by new generation pulse oximeters and the values can be obtained simultaneously with pulse oximetry. PPI is the ratio of pulsatile (AC) to nonpulsatile (DC) components of the infrared signal used in the pulse oximeter and corresponds to the relationship of the pulsatile to the nonpulsatile amounts of blood at the measuring site. The numerical value is displayed on the monitor and reflects real time changes in peripheral blood flow. A decrease in stroke volume can be picked up by measuring PPI. PPI is dependent on physiologic conditions and varies from patient to patient and also from site to site.[21] Limited work has been done in this area. Available data from a case control study suggests that a PPI <0.7 could be used as an additional screening tool along with pulse oximetry.[21]

Hyperoxia Test

Earlier, the hyperoxia test was recommended for neonates with resting desaturation (oxygen saturation <95%). Arterial blood gas at baseline and after administration of 100% oxygen for 5–10 minutes is measured. Classically, if the PaO_2 is >250 mm Hg in both upper and lower extremities with 100% oxygen, it mostly rules out critical cyanotic CHD. Hypoxia in this setting is attributed to lung disease. PaO_2 <100 mm Hg, in the absence of clear-cut lung disease, points to right-to-left shunting from a cyanotic CHD. PaO_2 100–250 mm Hg could be due to cyanotic CHD with intracardiac mixing and increased pulmonary blood flow. Limitations of the test have been long recognized as summarized below.

- Lung disease with large intrapulmonary shunt might not respond to oxygenation.
- Persistent pulmonary hypertension can mimic cyanotic CHD. The hyperoxia-hyperventilation test is advised in the situation. This requires mechanical ventilation at high respiratory rates for failed hyperoxia test. If the PaO_2 increases, at a critical PCO_2, often to <25 mm Hg, it suggests persistent pulmonary hypertension. Still, persistent pulmonary hypertension with nonlabile pulmonary vascular resistance cannot be ruled out.
- Some critical CHDs such as total anomalous pulmonary venous connection and hypoplastic left heart syndrome (which have a significant component of pulmonary venous hypertension and pulmonary edema) might respond to oxygenation.
- In patients with respiratory distress and acidosis, providing cardiorespiratory support and resuscitation is more important than the test itself.
- It is less reliable than an echocardiogram done by trained personnel.

When performing hyperoxia test, pulse oximetry cannot be used instead of PaO_2. This is because a pulse oximetry reading of 100% can reflect a PaO_2 ranging anywhere from 80 to 680 mm Hg. The test itself is cumbersome, and yet does not provide a definitive diagnosis. Hence, hyperoxia test is not recommended as a part of work up in any universal pulse oximetry screening program. However, in a ventilated baby, the above principles can be applied to interpreting arterial blood gases. A postductal PO_2 in excess of 250 mm Hg makes critical CHD unlikely.

Screening beyond the Neonatal Period

It needs to be underscored that there would still be a large number of babies who escape newborn screening. Large left-to-right shunts such as large ventricular septal defects will not screen positive in pulse oximetry. Moreover, the murmur as well as symptoms develop only over 4–6 weeks of life when the pulmonary vascular resistance falls and the shunt sets in. Immediate surgery or intervention is not warranted in these infants, unlike in duct-dependent lesions, but they do need correction by 4–6 months of age. Statistically, they pose large numbers to deal with, and are associated with substantial morbidity and mortality from congestive heart failure and intercurrent serious infections such as pneumonia and sepsis. Every contact of the healthcare system with infants should be utilized for continued surveillance for CCHD. To the advantage is the fact that infants with CCHD generally pronounce patterns of presentation. Large left-to-right shunts present with feeding difficulties and failure to thrive. Cyanotic CHDs present with desaturation and or spells. Immunization visits are an excellent opportunity to ask a few questions, repeat pulse oximetry, and physical examination, to detect CCHDs. Screening for CCHD in school age children is not expected to prevent significant mortality and morbidity as the majority of CCHD cases would have either died or become inoperable by this age. Questionnaires and physical examination can help detect less critical CHDs in these settings.

Role of Technology and Artificial Intelligence

Nonavailability of skilled personnel for training of health-care workers locally can be overcome by remote training and online modules (e Classes). Universal pulse oximetry screening algorithms, and the correct technique of obtaining values can be challenging for healthcare workers to understand, remember, and reproduce; for every single baby being screened. Similar is the case for screening during immunization visits. What to ask and what to look for in every single child can be challenging for healthcare workers to remember and reproduce offhand. Smartphone applications with screening pulse oximetry algorithms, visual guides as to the correct technique of obtaining values, and simple questionnaire and physical examination-based protocols can assist this process.[22] An important limitation in low resource settings is availability of echocardiography. Smartphone applications with artificial intelligence have been developed to empower pediatricians and neonatologists to do neonatal echocardiograms and reach a provisional diagnosis.[22] These will have to be evaluated in field studies before they can be incorporated into nationwide screening programs.

CONCLUSION

Universal screening for CHD deserves serious consideration in geopolitical regions where infant mortality rate has

TABLE 1: A simple recommendation for neonatal screening that combines physical examination and pulse oximeter.

See	• Cyanosis • Respiratory rate
Feel	• Pulse • Perfusion
Hear	• Second heart sound • Murmur
Do	• Pulse oximetry

substantially decreased, so that congenital malformations are considered to be important. Prenatal detection appears to be ideal for early detection of critical CHD. This ensures that babies with CCHD are safely transported in utero and delivered at a center capable of managing CCHD in the newborn. Physical examination of the newborn in itself cannot be relied upon as a screening method for CCHD. Universal pulse oximetry screening has been widely utilized for this purpose. Combining same with physical examination and newer methods such as peripheral perfusion index has the potential to identify a large number of newborns with CCHD in a timely fashion (**Table 1**). Screening is meaningful only when a system for further work up, safe transport, timely management, and follow-up of these babies is in place. Ongoing surveillance for CCHDs that are missed in the newborn period at every contact with the health system is important. Technology and artificial intelligence can help a long way in the path toward universal screening and follow-up. Any nationwide screening program for CCHD requires strong political commitment and financial support for its success.

REFERENCES

1. Rosano A, Botto LD, Botting B, Mastroiacovo P. Infant mortality and congenital anomalies from 1950 to 1994: an international perspective. J Epidemiol Community Health. 2000;54(9):660-6.
2. Kuehl KS, Loffredo CA, Ferencz C. Failure to diagnose congenital heart disease in infancy. Pediatrics. 1999;103(4 Pt 1):743-7.
3. Olney RS, Ailes EC, Sontag MK. Detection of critical congenital heart defects: review of contributions from prenatal and newborn screening. Semin Perinatol. 2015;39(3):230-7.
4. Hoffman JI, Kaplan S. The incidence of congenital heart disease. J Am Coll Cardiol. 2002; 39(12):1890-900.
5. Oster ME, Lee KA, Honein MA, Riehle-Colarusso T, Shin M, Correa A. Temporal trends in survival among infants with critical congenital heart defects. Pediatrics. 2013;131(5):e1502-8.
6. Reller MD, Strickland MJ, Riehle-Colarusso T, Mahle WT, Correa A. Prevalence of congenital heart defects in metropolitan Atlanta, 1998-2005. J Pediatr. 2008;153(6):807–813.
7. Liske MR, Greeley CS, Law DJ, Reich JD, Morrow WR, Baldwin HS, et al. Tennessee Task Force on Screening Newborn Infants for Critical Congenital Heart Disease. Report of the Tennessee task force on screening newborn infants for critical congenital heart disease. Pediatrics. 2006;118(4):e1250-6.
8. Bonnet D, Coltri A, Butera G, Fermont L, Le Bidois J, Kachaner J, et al. Detection of transposition of the great arteries in fetuses reduces neonatal morbidity and mortality. Circulation. 1999;99(7):916-8.
9. Tworetzky W, McElhinney DB, Reddy VM, Brook MM, Hanley FL, Silverman NH. Improved surgical outcome after fetal diagnosis of hypoplastic left heart syndrome. Circulation. 2001;103(9):1269-73.
10. Franklin O, Burch M, Manning N, Sleeman K, Gould S, Archer N. Prenatal diagnosis of coarctation of the aorta improves survival and reduces morbidity. Heart. 2002;87(1):67-9.
11. Gaynor JW, Stopp C, Wypij D, Andropoulos DB, Atallah J, Atz AM, et al. Neurodevelopmental outcomes after cardiac surgery in infancy. Pediatrics. 2015;135(5):816-25.
12. Goldberg CS, Lu M, Sleeper LA, Mahle WT, Gaynor JW, Williams IA, et al. Factors associated with neurodevelopment for children with single ventricle lesions. J Pediatr. 2014;165(3):490-6.e8.
13. Dobrow MJ, Hagens V, Chafe R, Sullivan T, Rabeneck L. Consolidated principles for screening based on a systematic review and consensus process. CMAJ. 2018;190(14):E422-9.
14. Yoo SJ, LeeYH, Kim ES, Ryu HM, Kim MY, Choi HK, et al. Three-vessel view of the fetal upper mediastinum: an easy means of detecting abnormalities of the ventricular outflow tracts and great arteries during obstetric screening. Ultrasound Obstet Gynecol. 1997;9(3):173-82.
15. Kumar P. Universal pulse oximetry screening for early detection of critical congenital heart disease. Clin Med Insights Pediatr. 2016;10:35-41.
16. Dudley DJ, Schneider D. Prenatal detection of congenital heart disease: the case for improved training. BJOG. 2016;123(3):408.
17. Kumar RK. Screening for congenital heart disease in India: rationale, practical challenges, and pragmatic strategies. Ann Pediatr Cardiol. 2016;9(2):111-4.
18. Thangaratinam S, Brown K, Zamora J, Khan KS, Ewer AK. Pulse oximetry screening for critical congenital heart defects in asymptomatic newborn babies: a systematic review and meta-analysis. Lancet. 2012;379(9835):2459-64.
19. Vaidyanathan B, Sathish G, Mohanan ST, Sundaram KR, Warrier KK, Kumar RK. Clinical screening for congenital heart disease at birth: a prospective study in a community hospital in Kerala. Indian Pediatr. 2011;48(1):25-30.
20. Saxena A, Mehta A, Ramakrishnan S, Sharma M, Salhan S, Kalaivani M, et al. Pulse oximetry as a screening tool for detecting major congenital heart defects in Indian newborns. Arch Dis Child Fetal Neonatal Ed. 2015;100(5):F416-21.
21. de-Wahl Granelli A, Östman-Smith I. Noninvasive peripheral perfusion index as a possible tool for screening for critical left heart obstruction. Acta Pædiatrica. 2007;96(10):1455-9.
22. Smiling Heart. [online] Available from: https://play.google.com/store/apps/details?id=com.smilingheart.smiling_heart. [Last accessed September, 2020].

7 CHAPTER

The Electrocardiogram, Ambulatory ECG and Exercise Testing

Mani Ram Krishna

THE ELECTROCARDIOGRAM

The electrocardiogram (ECG) is a simple and inexpensive tool for cardiac evaluation. Before the current era of noninvasive cardiac imaging, the ECG was (along with clinical examination and the chest X-ray) considered a key leg in the tripod of congenital heart disease (CHD) diagnosis. Its utility in the diagnosis of CHD is limited by a poor sensitivity and moderate specificity. However, the ECG remains a very important tool in the follow-up of children with corrected and palliated CHD as well as the evaluation of common clinical symptoms such as chest pain, breathlessness, palpitation, and syncope. As the utility of ECG in the pediatric age group is greatly limited compared to adults, pediatricians lack familiarity about the systematic interpretation of ECG. In this section, we will briefly discuss the vectorial approach in the ECG, the calculation of intervals, and axis as well as recognition of abnormalities.

The Vectorial Approach to ECG

In mathematics, a scalar is a quantity that provides only magnitude while a vector provides both magnitude and direction. The vectorial approach hence allows to understand the electrical activation of the heart from a three-dimensional perspective if the leads are placed appropriately. Information about the superior-inferior and left-right axis can be obtained from the limb leads (leads I, II, III, aVR, aVF, and aVL). Information about the anteroposterior and left-right axis can be obtained from the chest leads (V1-V6). The standard position of chest leads is depicted in **Figure 1**. Additional chest leads such as V3R, V7, and V8 can be used in selected cases to obtain specific information. The alignment of the limb leads is the hexaxial reference system and that of the chest leads is referred to as the horizontal reference system.

Hexaxial Reference System

The hexaxial reference systems compromise the limb leads (**Fig. 2**). These include the augmented unipolar limb leads aVR, aVF, and aVL and the bipolar leads I, II, and III. The leads I and aVF are perpendicular to each other and their positive poles represent 0° and 90°. This angle represents the direction of positive deflection. The negative deflection is at a 180° opposite direction. The negative deflection of lead I is hence at 180° and that of lead aVF at –90°. These two leads are

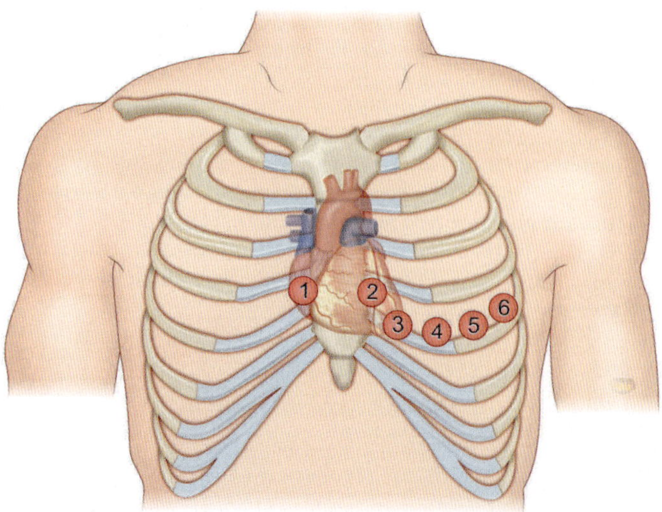

Fig. 1: Illustration depicting the placement of the chest leads V1 to V6.

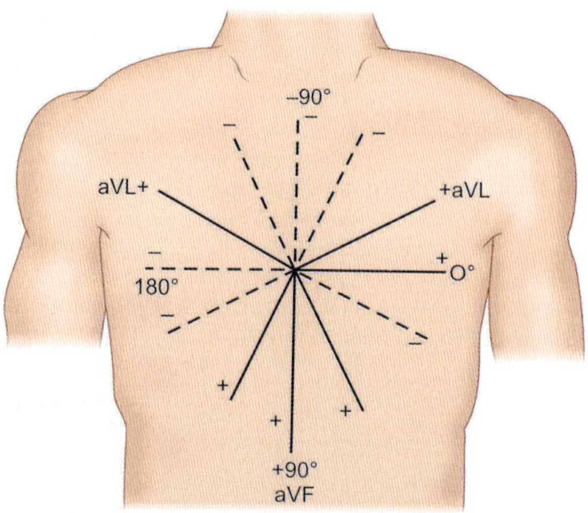

Fig. 2: Illustration depicting the frontal projection of the hexaxial reference system.

frequently used to calculate the hexaxial axis of the various ECG waves. The bipolar leads are arranged in a clockwise direction at an angle of 60° from the previous lead. As lead I represents 0°, lead II represents 60°, and lead III represents 120°, the unipolar leads are separated from each other by 120°. Hence, while aVF represents 90°, aVR represents –150° and aVL –30°. The R wave in each lead represents deflection toward the positive pole of that electrode while the S wave represents deflection toward the negative pole.

Horizontal Reference System

The horizontal reference system compromises the chest leads (**Fig. 3**). The lead V2 represents the anteroposterior axis and V6 the left-right axis. These leads are perpendicular to each other. The horizontal axis of the various ECG waves is not routinely calculated unlike the hexaxial waves.

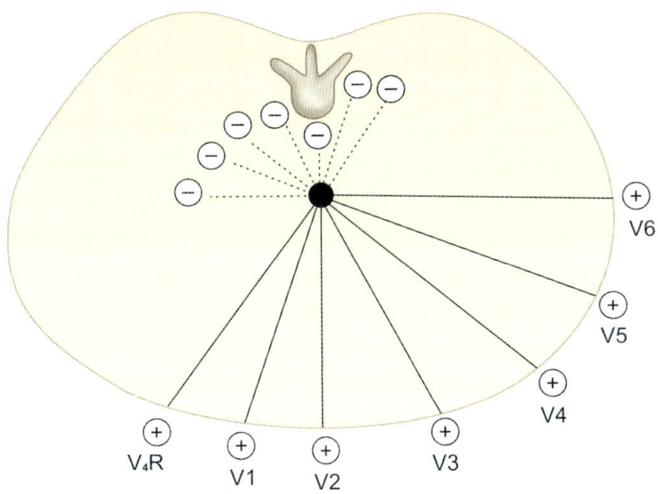

Fig. 3: Illustration depicting the vector loop of the horizontal reference system.

Systematic Interpretation of the Pediatric ECG

The ECG Strip

The ECG is usually recorded on a standardized graph strip, which consists of large as well as small squares. The large squares measure 5 millimeter (mm) on each side. The large squares are divided into 25 small squares with a side of 1 mm each. The x-axis of the graph represents time and the y-axis, amplitude.

ECG Standardization

Before attempting to interpret an ECG, it is important to ensure that this is standardized for amplitude and duration of signals. In a standard ECG, a 10-mm deflection in the y-axis (vertical) denotes a 1 mV amplitude while a 25-mm deflection in the x-axis (horizontal) takes 1 second for completion. A standardized ECG recording hence represents 10 seconds of cardiac electrical activity. A systematic interpretation of the ECG is possible only if the standardization is known. Standardization in an ECG can be verified by two methods (**Fig. 4**): The speed and amplitude of the deflections are printed at the bottom of the strip (a standardized ECG has 10 mm/mV amplitude and 25 mm/s speed of deflection). Alternatively in more basic ECG machines, a standard rectangular deflection is provided at the start or end of each lead. This rectangular deflection should cover two large squares in the vertical direction and one large square in the horizontal direction. On rare occasions, nonstandardized ECG at faster speeds or lower amplitudes are ordered by cardiologists when adequate information cannot be obtained from a standardized ECG.

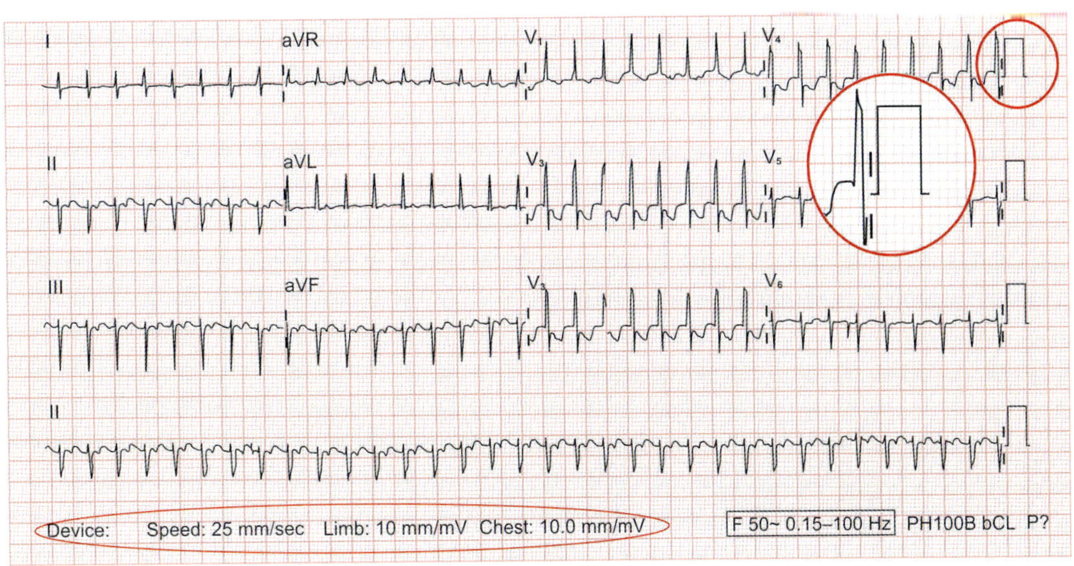

Fig. 4: A standardized 12-lead ECG. The red circle and the inset highlight the graphical depiction of standardization by a rectangle 10 mm tall and 5 mm wide. The red oval highlights the textual depiction of the standardization.

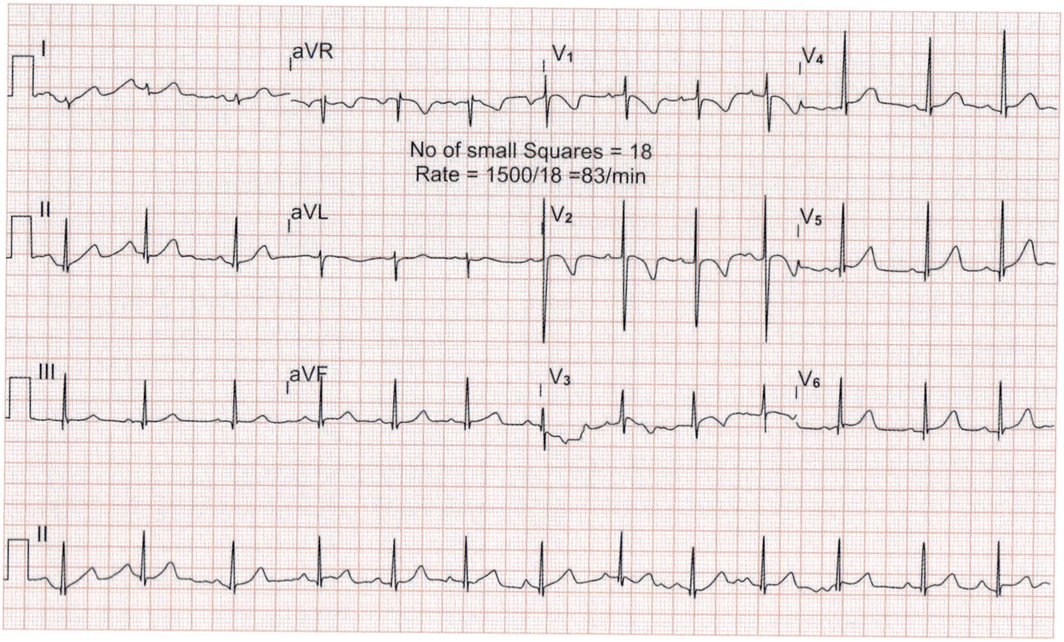

Fig. 5. This is a standardized 12-lead ECG. The R-R interval measures 18 small squares and the heart rate by the formula 1500/small squares is 83 beats per minute.

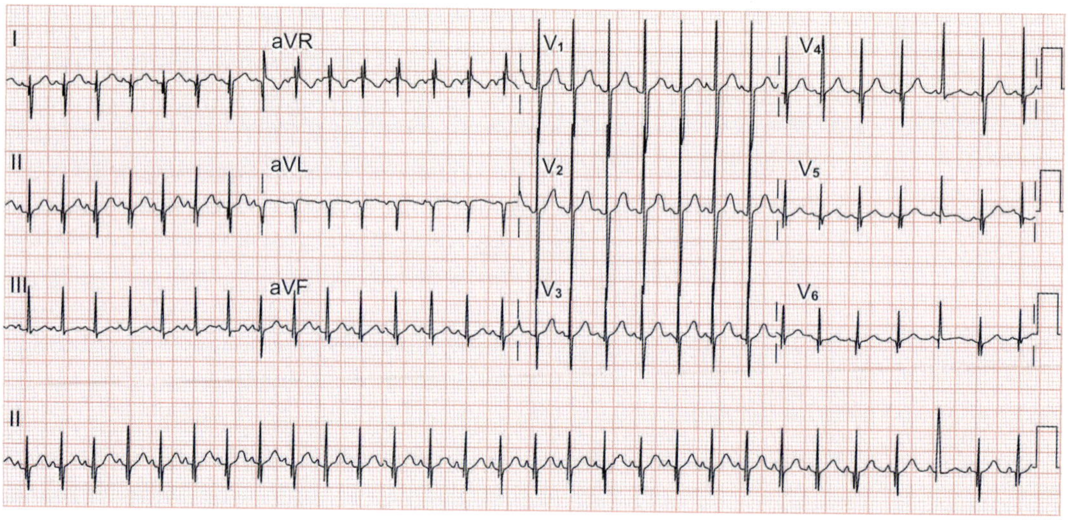

Fig. 6. A standardized 12-lead ECG of an infant. Every QRS complex is preceded by a P wave which is positive in lead I and avF. The infant is thus in sinus rhythm

The Heart Rate

Before calculating the heart rate, it should be ensured that the ECG is standardized to time. A rapid way to calculate the heart rate is to calculate the number of large squares between two consecutive R waves (R-R interval). The heart rate is then obtained by dividing the number of large squares from 300. This method is usually adequate to calculate the heart rate in adults. However, the normal heart rate in infants and toddlers is above 100 per minute and the rapid method is inadequate at such fast heart rates. A more appropriate method for calculating the heart rate is measuring the number of small squares between two consecutive R waves and utilizing the formula 1500/number of small squares. An example for heart rate calculation is provided in **Figure 5**.

The Rhythm

The electrical activity of the heart is initiated at the sinus node and after depolarization of the atria is conducted to the ventricles through the atrioventricular node. This is termed as sinus rhythm. An ECG is said to be in sinus rhythm (**Fig. 6**) when:

- Each QRS complex is preceded by a P wave.
- The P wave axis is normal (the P wave deflection is positive in both leads I and aVF).

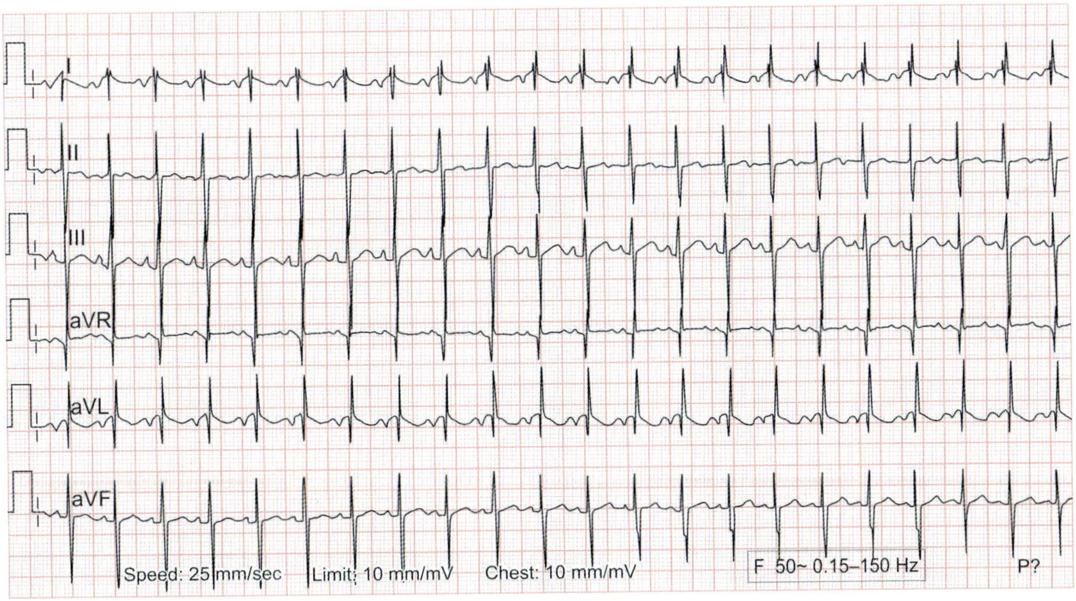

Fig. 7: A standardized 12-lead ECG of an infant with situs inversus totalis. Every QRS complex is preceded by a P wave. The P wave in situs inversus is negative in lead I and positive in aVR.

TABLE 1: Method of determining QRS axis using leads I and aVF and its clinical significance.

QRS Axis	*Net vector in lead I*	*Net vector in lead aVF*	*Comments*
Normal axis	Positive	Positive	Can be abnormal in neonates and young infants
Right axis deviation	Negative	Positive	Normal finding in early infancy but abnormal in older children
Left axis deviation	Positive	Negative	Always abnormal in the pediatric age group Common finding in Noonan's syndrome, cardiomyopathies and certain CHD–tricuspid atresia
Extreme axis/ Indeterminate axis	Negative	Negative	Children with AVSD

(AVSD: atrioventricular septal defect; CHD: congenital heart disease)

However, in a child with situs inversus totalis, the sinus node is located to the left of the body and the P wave is hence negative in lead I but positive in aVF and aVR (**Fig. 7**).

The QRS Axis

The simplest way to assess the QRS axis is the successive approximation method in which the axis is determined by looking at the deflections in two perpendicularly oriented leads—I and aVF. The determination of axis is represented in **Table 1**. It is important to remember that right axis deviation is normal in neonates and young infants. In fact, a normal axis in a neonate should raise the suspicion of an associated heart disease. Examples of normal and abnormal axis are provided in **Figures 8A to D**. The utility of axis in a pediatric ECG include the following:

- Left axis deviation is always abnormal in a young child. This can be present in children with Noonan syndrome as well as some form of inherited cardiomyopathies. It can also be seen in children with posterior muscular ventricular septal defect as well as tricuspid atresia.
- Extreme axis deviation is typical of atrioventricular septal defect (AVSD) and its presence in a child with trisomy 21 raises the suspicion of associated AVSD.

The ECG Intervals

The normal ECG intervals in children are generally much shorter than the accepted ranges in adults. Published references are available for each of the intervals in each age group.[1]

P-R interval: The P-R interval is measured from the start of the P wave to the start of the QRS complex. The P-R interval represents conduction of electrical activity from the sinus node to the ventricles and can be prolonged due to abnormalities in conduction at multiple levels. However, the P-R interval is contributed predominantly by delay in atrioventricular (A-V) conduction and hence prolongation in P-R interval is almost synonymous with A-V conduction delay. The normal P-R interval in adults is 120–200 milliseconds (ms). The P-R interval is measured by counting the number of small squares from the beginning of the P wave to the beginning of the QRS complex and multiplying by 40 ms (**Fig. 9**). In infants, the normal interval is generally 80–100 ms and reaches the adult values only in adolescence. Although there are no standard definitions a P-R interval of 160 ms in a young child should be considered prolonged.

A prolonged P-R interval is seen in lower degrees of A-V block, rheumatic carditis, dyselectrolytemia as well as in certain postoperative states. A short P-R interval is seen in Wolff–Parkinson–White (WPW) syndrome as well as in certain glycogen storage disorders such as Pompe disease and mutation in the *PRKAG2* gene.

QRS duration: The normal QRS duration in an adult is 80 ms (two small squares) and a QRS duration of greater than 90 ms is considered wide complex. However, the normal QRS duration is between 50 and 60 ms in neonates and infants and <70 ms in children.

QTc interval: The T wave represents ventricular repolarization. The QTc interval is the most commonly measured index of repolarization. The duration varies with the heart rate and hence to compare the interval at different heart rates, it has to be "corrected" for the heart rate. A number of formulas exist for heart rate correction. Of these, the Bazett's formula

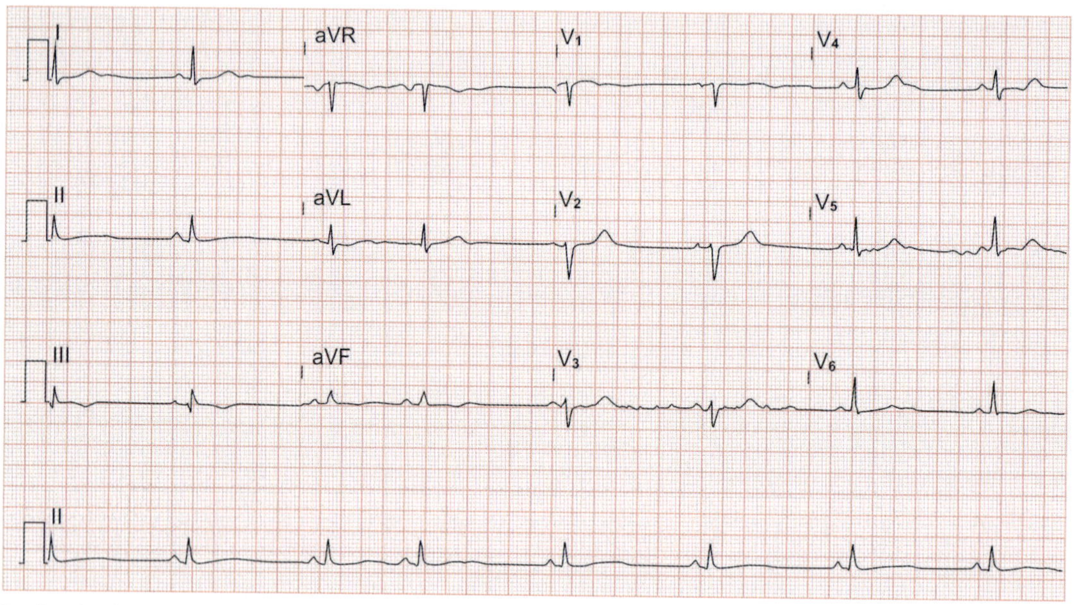

Fig. 8A: Standardized 12-lead ECG in sinus rhythm. The QRS complex is positive in I and aVF and hence the QRS axis is normal.

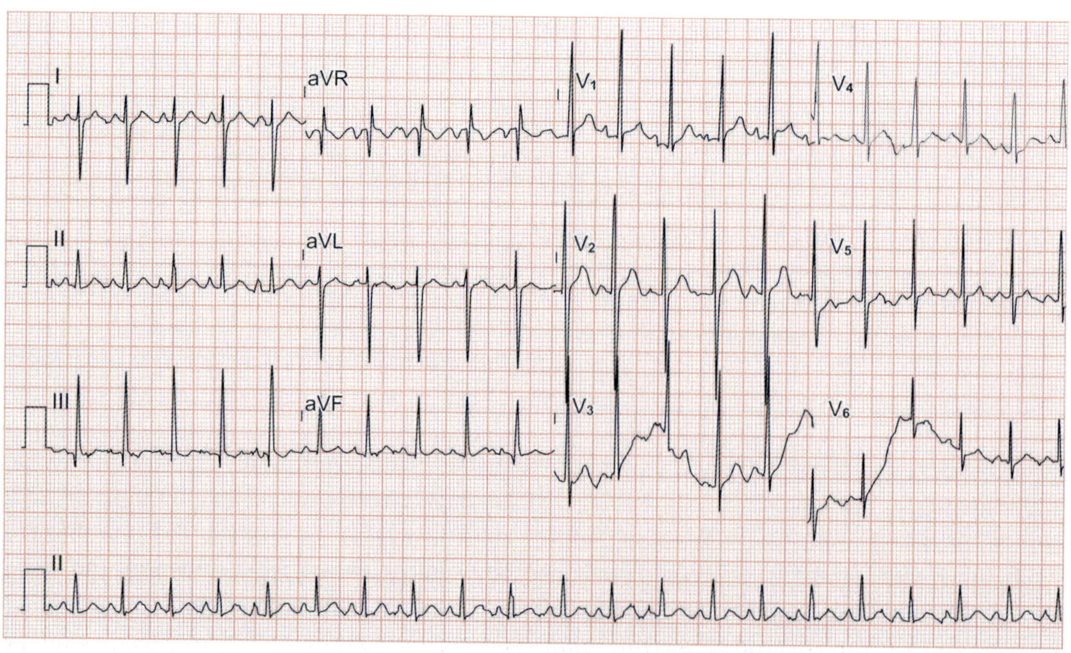

Fig. 8B: The QRS complex is negative in lead I and positive in aVF and hence there is right axis deviation.

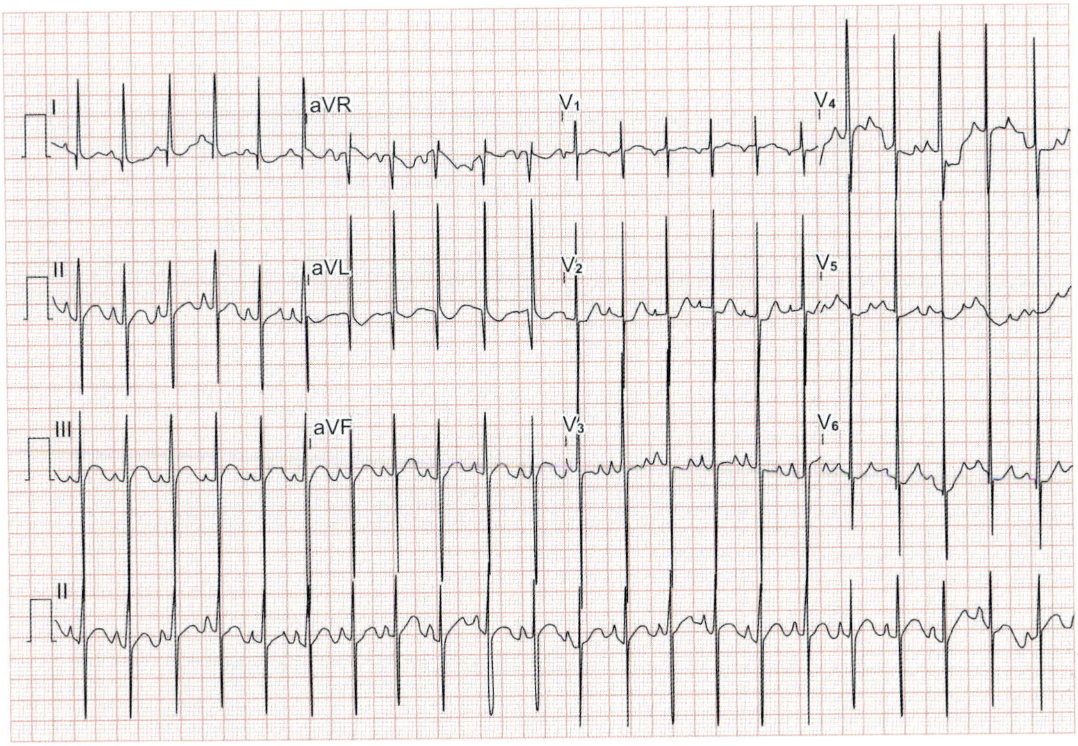

Fig. 8C: The QRS complex is positive in lead I and negative in aVF and hence there is left axis deviation.

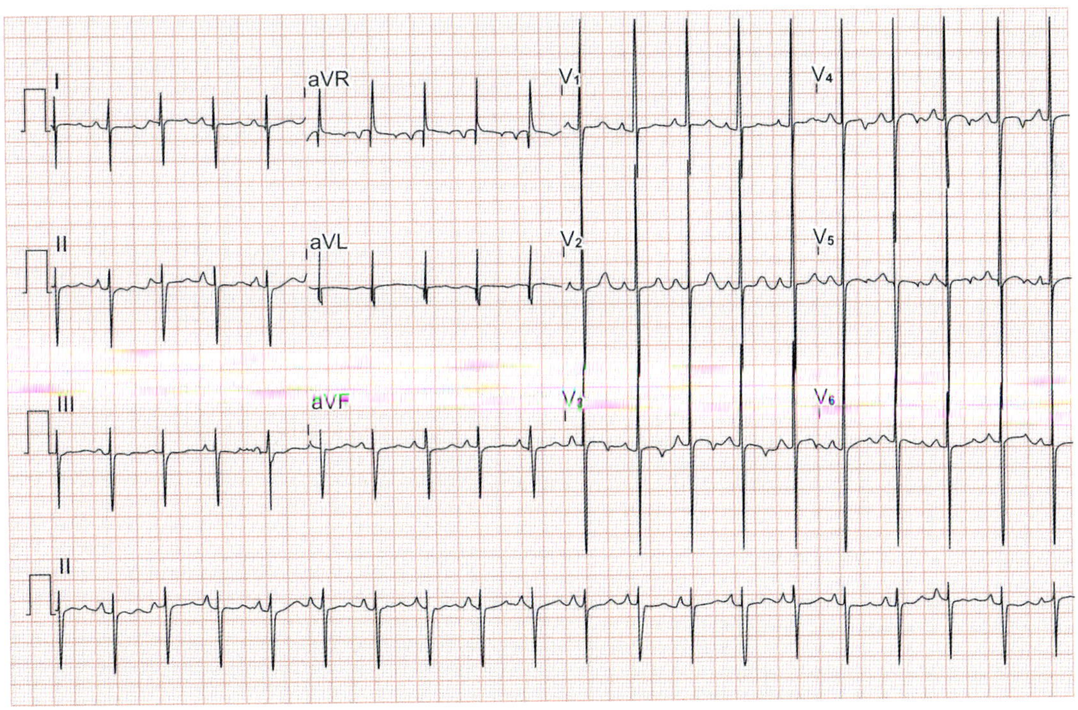

Fig. 8D: The QRS complex is negative in lead I and positive in aVF and hence there is extreme axis deviation.

is the most widely used and validated in children.[2] According to this formula,

QTC = QT interval (in ms)/square root of RR-interval (in seconds)

The normal QTc interval does not vary between males and females during childhood and a value greater than 460 ms is widely considered to be abnormal.

Chamber Enlargement

Right atrial enlargement: The right atrial enlargement is evident by tall P waves (**Fig. 10A**) usually best seen in lead II. The adult criteria of more than three small squares is widely used in children as well.

Left atrial enlargement: The left atrial enlargement is evidenced by broad P waves. The width of the P waves should be

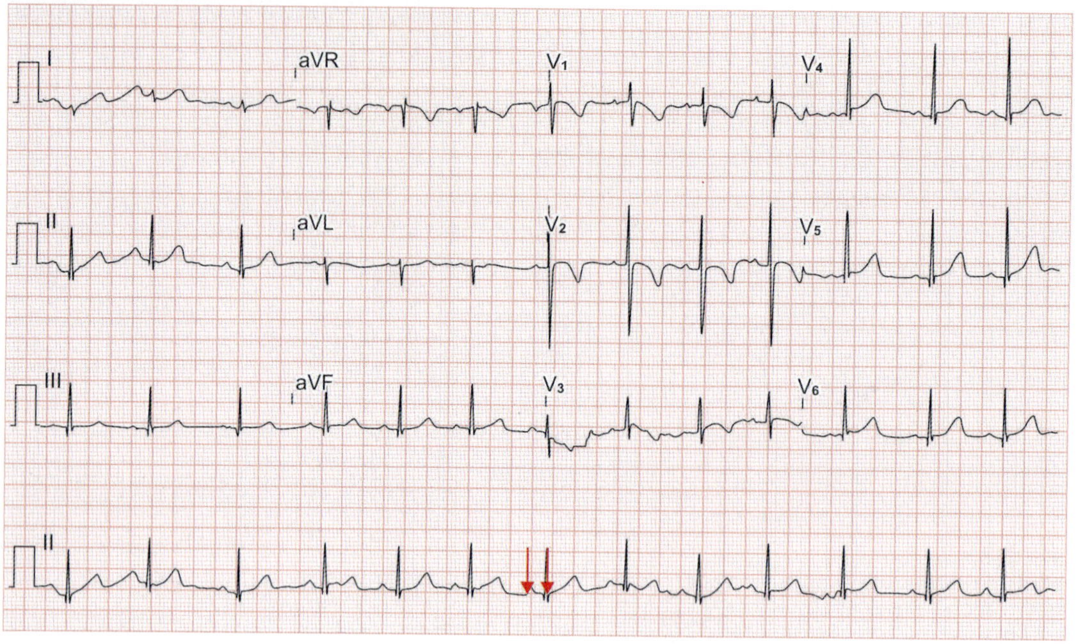

Fig. 9: A standardized 12-lead ECG in sinus rhythm. There are 3 small squares from the start of the P wave to the QRS complex. The P-R interval is hence 120 ms.

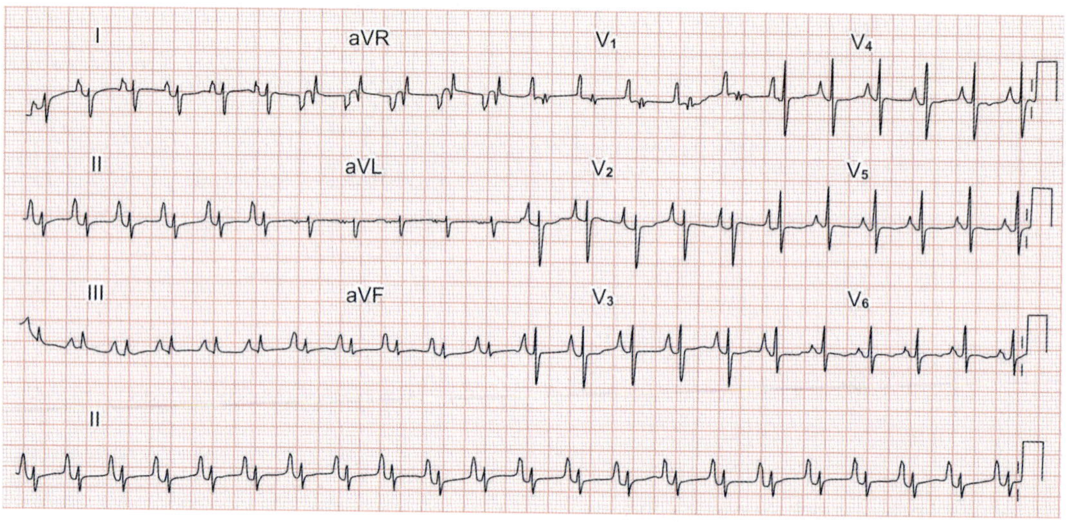

Fig. 10A: A standardized 12-lead in ECG in sinus rhythm. The P wave is tall and peaked suggesting significant right atrial enlargement.

more than 2 to 2½ small squares (80–100 ms). In lead V1, the P wave is frequently biphasic and a broad negative deflection is indicative of left atrial enlargement (**Fig. 10B**).

Right ventricular hypertrophy (RVH): RVH is a normal finding in the ECG of neonates and young infants. However, it rarely persists beyond 2–3 years of life and a finding of RVH beyond this age group should prompt further evaluation. The findings favoring RVH include the following:

- Right axis deviation
- Tall R wave in leads V1/V2 and a deep S wave in V6. An abnormal R/S ratio (greater than normal for age in lead V1 and <1 in V6)
- Monomorphic R wave in lead V1
- Upright T wave in lead V1 in children <7 years of age.

Left ventricular hypertrophy: Children have compliant chest walls and hence the amplitudes recorded in the chest leads are usually higher than that in adults. The use of traditional voltage criteria for detecting LVH in children has hence been challenged. The Sokolow–Lyon criteria is still widely used where the sum of the S-wave in lead V1 and R wave in V6 is above the normal for age. An additional criteria using a right-sided lead (lead V3 placed to the right of the sternum instead of the left) instead of V1 has been shown to be more specific for LVH in children.[3]

Ventricular Pre-excitation

The most common tachyarrhythmia in children is the atrioventricular re-entrant tachycardia where an abnormal accessory pathway exists between the atria and ventricles. This accessory pathway is capable of conducting from the ventricles to the atria (retrograde conduction) in all cases. In some, it is capable of conducting from the atria to the ventricles (antegrade conduction). This is usually evident on a baseline ECG as ventricular pre-excitation. Wolff, Parkinson, and White in 1930 first described the association of a short P-R interval and a broad QRS in children prone to develop recurrent palpitation[4] and the entity is hence commonly referred to as WPW syndrome.

In WPW syndrome, the ventricles are activated by both the A-V node as well as the accessory pathway (**Fig. 11A**). As there is no delay in conduction through the accessory pathway unlike the A-V node, the P-R interval is shorter than normal. Ventricular excitation through the accessory pathway is abnormal and is hence broad. When the activation fronts through the normal and pathways intersect, this results in a sharp deflection of the QRS complex referred to as the delta wave. As the ventricles are depolarized (activated) earlier than would normally occur, this phenomenon is referred to as pre-excitation.

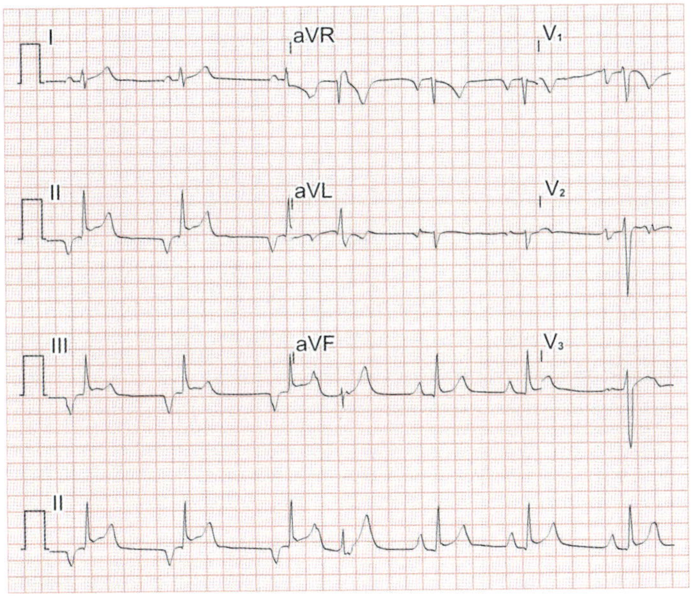

Fig. 10B: Standardized ECG of an adolescent with severe mitral stenosis. The biphasic P wave in V1 with a deep negative component suggests left atrial enlargement.

The criteria for ventricular pre-excitation in the ECG include the following (**Fig. 11B**):

- A short P-R interval (lower than the normal limit for age)
- Broad QRS complex (>70 ms in infants and 80 ms in older children)
- Slurring of the initial segment of the QRS complex (delta wave)
- Although not an absolute criteria, the T wave is frequently discordant to the QRS complex (a positive QRS complex deflection is accompanied by a negative T wave and vice-versa).

Systematic Interpretation of the ECG

A checklist for systematic interpretation of the pediatric ECG should be as follows:

- Is the tracing appropriately standardized?
- What is the heart rate?
- Is the rhythm a normal sinus rhythm?
- What is the P-R interval?
- What is the QRS axis? Is the morphology of the QRS complex normal?

A more advanced interpretation of the ECG should also include any abnormalities of repolarization evidenced by changes in the ST-T segment of the ECG. An appropriate interpretation of an ECG is provided in **Figure 12**.

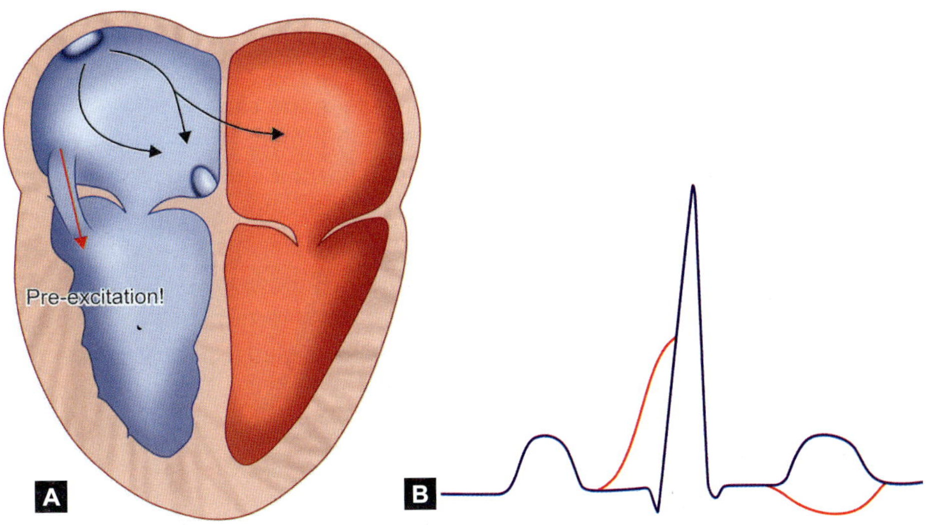

Figs. 11A and B: Pictorial depiction of the accessory pathway in WPW syndrome. The ventricle is depolarized through both the AV node as well as the accessory pathway; (B) The ECG changes in WPW syndrome (red) against the normal ECG (blue)—note the short P-R interval, broad QRS, sharp deflection in the primary component of the (delta wave) and the T wave changes.

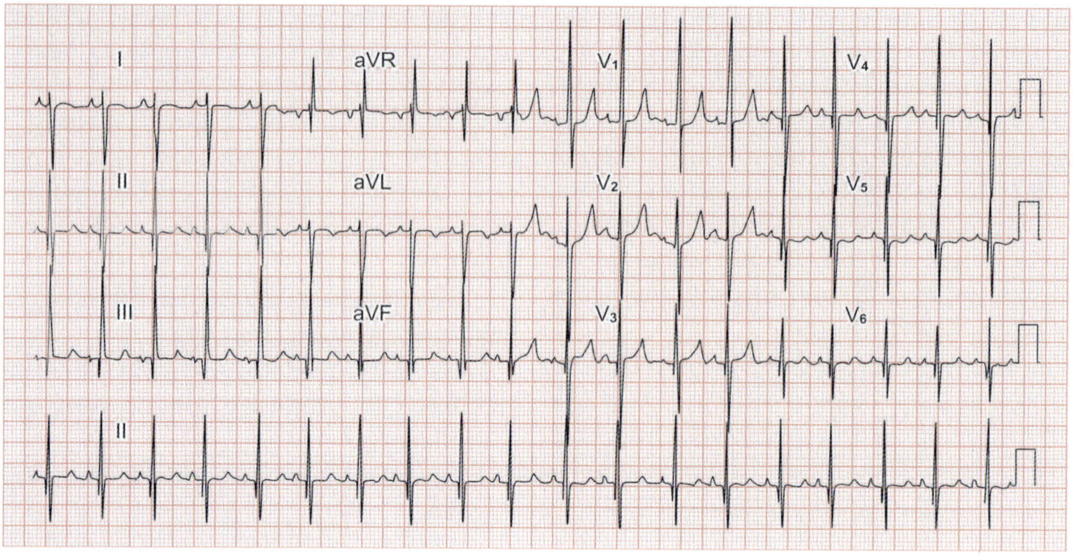

Fig. 12: This is a standardized 12-lead ECG from an infant in sinus rhythm with a PR interval of 120 ms. There is right axis deviation. There is no evidence of significant chamber hypertrophy and the QTc measures 450 ms.

Role of ECG in Congenital Heart Disease

The low sensitivity of the ECG has meant that it is no longer a first line investigation in the diagnosis of CHD. ECG however continues to remain a relevant and important investigation in this era of echocardiography and noninvasive imaging. Its primary role in the current era varies vastly from the time when Alexander Nadas termed it as an indispensable investigation for recognition of CHD. The major role of ECG in the management of CHD include the following:

- Recognition of CHD in a high-risk neonate or young infant (e.g., Trisomy 21) when access to echocardiogram is not available in a timely fashion
- Identification of a substrate for arrhythmia in CHD (e.g., ventricular pre-excitation in Ebstein anomaly and varying degrees of heart block)
- Decision-making on operability in an older child with a large left-to-right shunt [ventricular septal defect/patent ductus arteriosus (VSD/PDA)] and severe pulmonary arterial hypertension.
- Postoperative follow-up of children with repaired or palliated CHD.

AMBULATORY ELECTROCARDIOGRAM RECORDING

A standard 12-lead ECG records the cardiac rhythm for a period of 10 seconds. Arrhythmias in children can frequently be self-limiting. It is hence not uncommon for children to present to the pediatrician after the symptoms have subsided. Children who present with symptoms potentially related to an arrhythmia such as palpitation, syncope, or chest pain should be evaluated with an ECG. The detection of ventricular pre-excitation or a prolonged QTc interval will provide the diagnosis even after symptoms have subsided. However, in a majority of cases, the interval ECG is normal. It hence becomes imperative to obtain an ECG when symptoms are present. The American physicist Norman Holter pioneered the ambulatory ECG recording on a cathode ray tube in the late 1950s.[5] Subsequently commercial Holter monitors have been available for clinical use from the 1960s. A number of devices are currently available for prolonged ECG recording. In this section, we will discuss briefly the indications, type of devices available, and their relative advantages and disadvantages.

Methods Available for Ambulatory ECG Recording

The various modalities available for ambulatory ECG recording as well as their relative merits and disadvantages are summarized in **Table 2**.

Holter Monitor

The Holter is the most widely used method for ambulatory ECG recording. The current generation devices are lightweight and can be carried on a hip-pouch or strapped to the abdomen. They are inconspicuous. The wires are attached to the child's chest wall by the soft gel electrodes utilized for obtaining ECG (**Fig. 13**). The commonly available Holter are either three-channel (where three electrodes are used, and three leads will be visible in the report) or a five-channel EASI format [five electrodes are used in this format (**Fig. 14**) and if placed appropriately, this can be converted into a 12-lead ECG]. They are capable of recording ECG for a 24–48-hour period. The quality of the recording is excellent across all age groups. However, Holter does not provide real-time data. The child wears the device for the prescribed period and returns the device to the hospital where a cardiac physiologist or cardiologist analyzes the recordings. The family is usually provided with a diary in which the important

TABLE 2: Comparison of the various modalities of ambulatory electrocardiogram monitoring which are commonly used in the pediatric population.

Modality	*Duration*	*Advantages*	*Disadvantages*
Holter	24–48 hours	• Standardized method with wide experience and ready availability • Good quality of recordings • Ability to obtain 12 lead recordings	• Short duration negates its use when symptoms are infrequent • Small children get frightened by the wires attached to the body • Family have to stay near the hospital to return equipment for analysis
Patch recorders	3–30 days	• Wireless connectivity • Capability for real time monitoring • Disposable patches means that the family need not return to the hospital	• Not widely available in our country • Limited number of channels available • Quality of signals may be poor in neonates and infants
Implantable loop recorder	2–3 years	• Longest duration of recording and hence ideal for children with infrequent symptoms • Capability for real time monitoring	• Need for an interventional procedure for placement and removal • Limited number of channels
Wearable devices		• 24/7 usage • Hassle free use • In devices with superior hardware, good quality images can be obtained	• Expensive • Only single channel recording is possible • Not well standardized

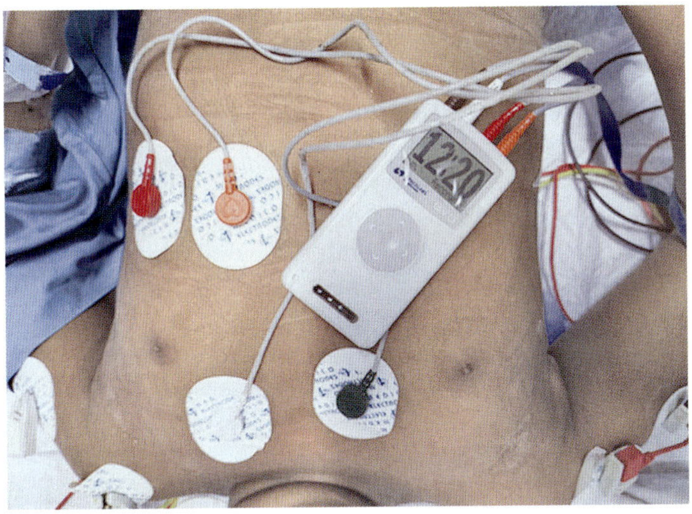

Fig. 13: Placement of a traditional Holter in a child using conventional gel electrodes

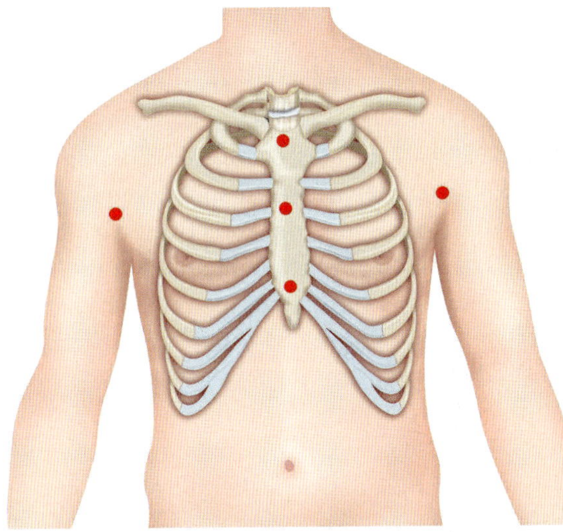

Fig. 14: Illustration depicting the placement of Holter leads in the EASI format. If appropriately placed this 5 channel Holter can be utilized to obtain a 12 lead ECG.

events such as physical activity, sleep as well as the presence of symptoms are recorded along with time. This will permit matching the rhythm to the patients' symptoms. The use of wires makes it cumbersome to apply in young children and the devices are not water resistant

Patch Recorders

The miniaturization of electronic circuits as well as improvements in rapid wireless technology such as Bluetooth have permitted the development of patches, which can be stuck on the left pectoral region and can continuously monitor cardiac electrical activity. These are available as two- and three-channel monitors. These can be used for periods ranging from 3 to 30 days. Current day advanced patch monitors are water resistant and permit bathing as well as water sports. There are two kinds of patch monitors. Devices, which provide real-time data, are more expensive and not widely available. The device constantly transmits data to an online database, which is monitored to detect abnormal rhythms. In our unit, we utilize a nonreal-time system available for 3 and 7 days. The patch is placed on the child's chest and activated by connecting it via Bluetooth to a mobile application which can be downloaded to Android or iOS-based smartphones (**Fig. 15**). At the end of the designated period, the recordings are transmitted to a secure cloud database where a cardiac physiologist analyzes the tracings and provides a report similar to a traditional Holter. In the authors' experience, these systems provide reliable recording beyond infancy.

Implantable Loop Recorders

The implantable loop recorder (ILR) is a small box about the size of a USB flash drive (**Fig. 16**) capable of recording two-channel ECG. The battery life of most available ILR

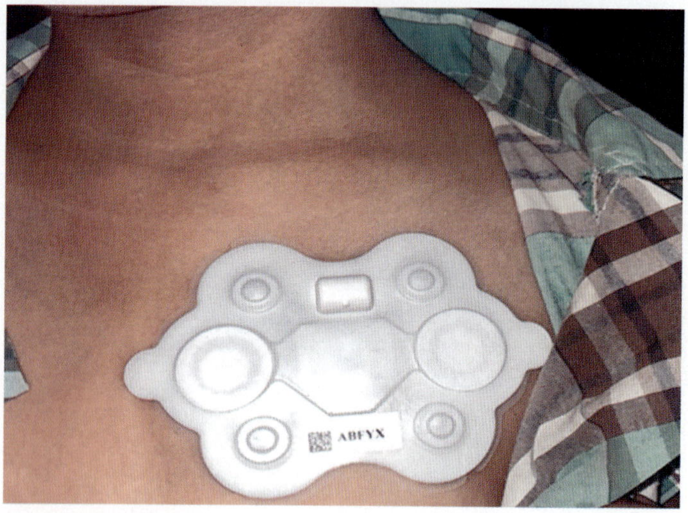

Fig. 15: A patch recorder placed in a 3-year-old boy.

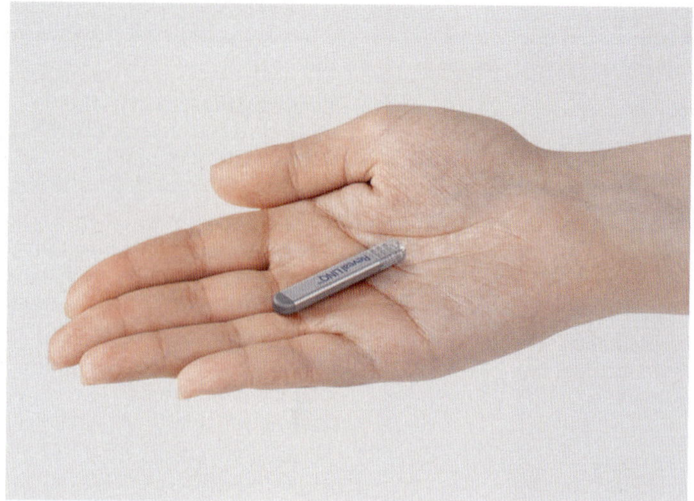

Fig. 16: An implantable loop recorder.

is 3 years. The ILR has to be placed surgically on the chest wall. A pocket is created in the left chest wall to place the device. The device is connected to an external transmitter or a mobile application by WiFi technology and continuously monitors the ECG. It can store ECG for a period of up to 7 minutes. Storage can be activated spontaneously whenever an abnormal rhythm is recorded or activated by the patient.

The most common indication for an ILR is the evaluation of recurrent syncope. In our unit, we utilize commercially available loop recorders which are available in varying sizes and battery lives.[6] ILR are an invasive option requiring a surgical procedure for implantation as well as removal and are hence not routinely used as a first-line investigation. They also carry a small risk of pocket site infection.

Wearable Technology

In recent years, there has been a rapid increase in the adoption of wearable technology capable of recording the heart rate and rhythm in addition to a number of other physiological parameters. These devices include smartwatches, heart rate monitoring belts, and electronic vests. Most of these "smart" devices utilize photoplethysmography to detect the heart rate.[7] This is considered inferior to electrograms in detection of the heart rhythm. However, a reasonably accurate diagnosis is possible in close to 80% of cases. A commercially available wearable device is shown in **Figure 17A**. An example of a single lead ECG recording from this wearable device, which resulted in diagnosis of arrhythmia in a child, is provided in **Figure 17B**.

Indications for Ambulatory ECG Recording

The common indications for ambulatory ECG recording in children are:

- Evaluation for a possible arrhythmia as the cause of chest pain, syncope, or palpitation in children
- Evaluation of the response to treatment in arrhythmia, e.g., adequacy of beta-blockade in children with long QT syndrome (LQTS)
- Evaluation of intermittent arrhythmias in high-risk groups (e.g., children with hypertrophic cardiomyopathy, postoperative children after high-risk surgeries such as the Senning's operation)
- Evaluation of children with A-V conduction disorders such as CHB. The average heart rate as well as intermittent long pauses can only be detected by a Holter
- As an alternative to an exercise stress test in children with exertion induced symptoms who cannot safely undergo an exercise test.

Clinical Utility of Ambulatory ECG Recording

The three most common symptoms for which a Holter or other forms of ambulatory ECG recordings are utilized are chest pain, palpitations, and syncope. The diagnostic yield of these modalities has been estimated to be between 5 and 20%. Whenever symptoms are infrequent, a modality with a longer duration of monitoring improves the yield dramatically. Hence, patch monitors are rapidly replacing the traditional Holter as the modality of choice for ambulatory ECG recording because of the ease of use, convenience as well as longer duration of monitoring. In a large study, looking at the utility of patch monitors in the pediatric age group, the diagnostic yield was 12%. More importantly, >50% of these positive findings were recorded after the third day, a period which is beyond the capability of the traditional Holter.[8]

CARDIOPULMONARY EXERCISE TESTING

Exercise Stress Testing

The response of the cardiopulmonary system to exercise is an important estimate of the health of these two organ systems. Clinical exercise stress testing (EST) has been available for a

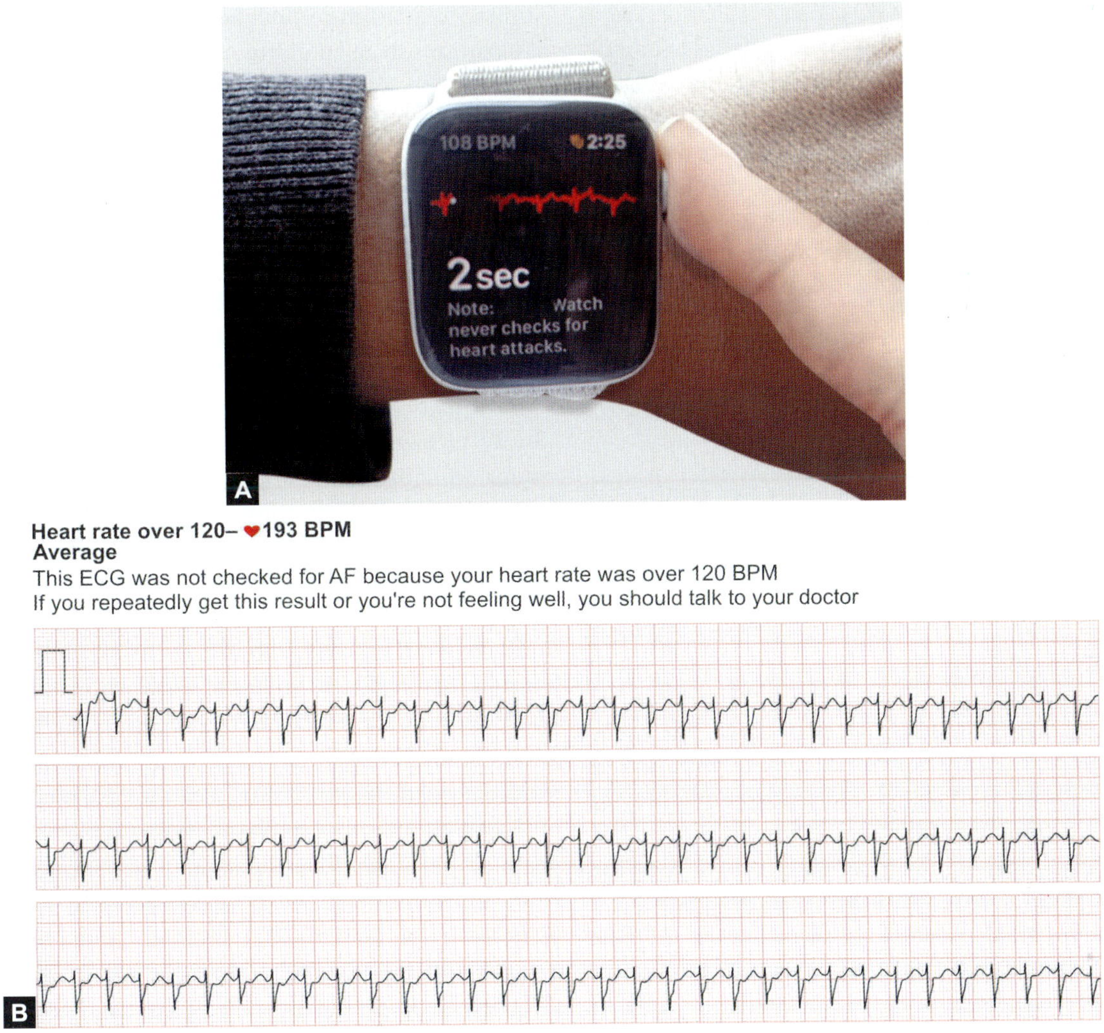

Figs. 17A and B: (A) A smart watch the most widely used device among the current generation wearable technology; (B) A sample single channel ECG obtained using a smart watch from a child with supraventricular tachycardia.

number of decades and is considered a routine investigation during a hospital visit for most adults with a suspected or proven heart disease. However, this modality is less commonly used for children. In this section, we discuss the exercise physiology in brief along with the test modalities available, indications in children as well as interpretation of test results.

Exercise Physiology

The cardiovascular and respiratory responses to exercise have been well characterized. The cardiovascular response to exercise is an augmentation of cardiac output. The maximal increase is 6–8 times the basal output. This is achieved through increase in both the heart rate as well as the stroke volume. Unlike adults, where the increased cardiac output is predominantly provided by an increase in stroke volume during the early phase of exercise, children have smaller maximal left ventricular volumes and hence the cardiac output is primarily increased by an increase in the heart rate.[9] The maximal heart rate achieved in children is usually around 200 per minute. There is an increase in the systolic as well as mean blood pressure (BP). However, there is very little change in the diastolic pressure. There is also redistribution of blood flow with increased perfusion of the heart, the skeletal muscles involved in the exercise, and the skin (as body temperature increases with exercise). The respiratory response to exercise comprises of an increase in the tidal volume at lower intensities and an increase in the respiratory rate as the intensity increases. Both of these result in an increase in oxygen compensation and minute ventilation. These compensatory mechanisms ensure increased oxygen delivery to the skeletal muscles to maintain aerobic metabolism. However, when the maximal capacity of the cardiorespiratory system is reached, further energy production is achieved by anaerobic metabolism. The point of switchover from aerobic to anaerobic metabolism is referred as the lactate threshold. The physiological parameters, which can be measured by a cardiopulmonary exercise test (CPET), include:

- *Maximal heart rate*: Inability to achieve a heart rate above 80% of the maximal heart rate suggests an impaired chronotropic response.

- *Peak oxygen consumption (VO_2 max)*: The maximum oxygen uptake achieved during exercise (this is usually averaged over a 30-second period of peak exercise).
- *Ventilatory anaerobic threshold (VAT/AT)*: This is the volume of oxygen consumption at which a switch happens to anaerobic metabolism from aerobic metabolism. A significant decrease in VO_2 max or VAT suggests impaired cardiorespiratory reserve or very poor exercise conditioning.
- *Peak partial pressure of end-tidal carbon dioxide ($PETCO_2$)*: This is the maximal value of $ETCO_2$ measured during exercise.

Types of Exercise Stress Testing

Exercise testing is commonly performed by two methods—the treadmill and the cycle ergometer (CE). The relative advantages and disadvantages of these methods are discussed in **Table 3**. The most common protocol used in treadmill testing is the Bruce protocol. The Bruce protocol involves stages of 3 minutes each. The treadmill test starts at 10% incline and a pace of 2.7 kilometer per hour (km/h). There is an increase of 2% incline with every stage. The speed of the treadmill also progressively increases to 4 km/h, 5.5 km/h, 6.8 km/h, and 8 km/h. The McMaster protocol is the most studied CE protocol in children and involves increase in workload every 2 minutes. The James protocol provides increase in workload every 3 minutes. All these protocols are based on a multistage incremental principle and aim to achieve maximum effort from the subject. A number of other protocols exist including progressive incremental (ramp) protocols on CE, submaximal efforts, constant work rate protocols, and sprint protocols. Each type has its proponents who claim physiological superiority. However, because of their widespread use, clinical experience, and similarity to adult protocols, the Bruce and James protocols are commonly used in Indian exercise laboratories.

Exercise Stress Laboratory

There are published guidelines available regarding the requirements of a pediatric exercise stress laboratory. It is important that adequate space is available to accommodate all the equipment necessary for safe conduction of the test. A minimum requirement is 250 square feet of area. It is also important to ensure adequate lighting, temperature control (20–24°C), and humidity (<60%).

The equipment required for the laboratory depends on the services available. A majority of exercise laboratories in India offer only cardiac stress testing where chronotropic response and arrhythmia/ischemia risk are assessed. Cardiopulmonary testing, which involves assessment of exercise tolerance by ventilatory parameters including VO_2 max, is available only in select tertiary care centers. In addition to the treadmill and cycle ergometer, equipment should be available to record the ECG, BP, and oxygen saturation by a pulse oximeter. The BP is frequently recorded by a manual mercury-based sphygmomanometer. However, in recent years, a number of laboratories have moved toward automated BP measurement systems. These systems are typically based on the oscillometer principles and accurately measure the mean blood pressure. However, they only calculate the systolic and diastolic pressure utilizing the oscillations which were detected. The oscillations may be affected by the constant motion of the hand while running on the treadmill and hence there is a possibility of error in recording the systolic and diastolic BP although the mean BP is usually accurate. Irrespective of the method utilized, BP cuffs of varying sizes should be available. It is important

TABLE 3: Comparison of the advantages and disadvantages of the two common modalities for exercise stress testing.

Exercise stress method	*Advantages*	*Disadvantages*
Treadmill	· More widely available · Greater clinical experience throughout the world · Can be safely performed from 3–4 years of age (with additional safety features like a harness rope) · Involves the largest group of muscles and hence results in higher heart rate as well as maximum oxygen consumption (VO_2 max)	· Difficulty in obtaining accurate blood pressure measurements and risk of ECG artifacts due to constant motion · Bruce protocol – the commonest protocol followed worldwide involves larger increments which may be difficult for children · The long time period of 3 minutes per stage in the common protocols carries a risk of boredom and premature termination in children
Bicycle ergometry	· More comfortable for children to perform · Relatively inexpensive equipment compared to a treadmill · Easier to obtain blood pressure measurements and ECG recordings · More comfortable to obtain stress echocardiographic studies as well as combined exercise MRI or PET imaging	· Involves lesser group of muscles and hence the peak VO_2 obtained is lesser than that on treadmill testing · The poorly developed knee extensors in children does not permit testing in children younger than 6 years of age

(ECG: electrocardiogram; MRI: magnetic resonance imaging; PET: positron emission tomography; VO_2: volume of oxygen consumed). This is usually indexed to time and body surface area.

to use an appropriate size cuff to accurately record BP. The ideal cuff should have a width of around 40% of the mid-arm circumference.[10] The ECG recording apparatus should also be fitted with appropriate filters to ensure that chest muscle twitching does not result in an artifact. When cardiopulmonary testing is offered, a metabolic cart becomes necessary. In the early years of cardiopulmonary testing, ventilatory parameters were obtained using a Douglas Bag and a Tissot spirometer. This method although very accurate is cumbersome and impractical in a large-scale clinical setting. The development of sensors to detect air flow as well as the capability to measure the partial pressure of various gases in an air sample rapidly has permitted the development of automated systems where the air volume and partial pressure of oxygen as well as carbon dioxide can be measured in real time from a mask, fed into a computer and the results made available to the technician within seconds. These automated systems are referred to as metabolic carts and have replaced the Douglas bag. Commercially available metabolic carts have been used in clinical practice for more than three decades and have been validated in pediatric settings. The systems have been automated to such an extent that very little understanding of the respiratory physiology is necessary for a technician to perform these tests.[11]

In addition to the equipment necessary for conducting the test, age appropriate equipment for resuscitation should be available in an emergency cart. This should include emergency drugs including adrenaline, ventilatory bags, and masks of various pediatric sizes. Endotracheal tubes of appropriate sizes should ideally be available. The laboratory should have access to oxygen as well as a system to provide suction. It is important that the cardiac physiologists performing the test are trained in pediatric basic life support.

Pediatric EST can be classified into high-risk and low-risk tests. The high-risk category include children with pulmonary arterial hypertension, inherited arrhythmias, symptomatic cardiomyopathy, arrhythmia or syncope provoked by exercise, Marfan syndrome, and significant airway obstruction.[12] The high-risk category should be tested only in the presence of a physician familiar with the patient's cardiac physiology and trained in pediatric advanced life support. The low-risk category can be safely tested without the direct supervision of a physician when appropriately trained technicians are available.

Indications for Exercise Stress Testing in Children

Exercise stress testing in children is used for assessment of symptoms such as chest pain and syncope which could potentially be provoked by exercise, assess the functional capacity of children with heart disease or to assess the efficacy of an intervention in children with CHD (for example, pulmonary valve replacement in children with repaired tetralogy of Fallot). It is not typically used for recognition of coronary ischemia, the most common indication for EST in the adult population. The common conditions in which an EST is used in the pediatric population have been published[13] and are summarized in **Table 4**.

TABLE 4: Conditions for which an exercise stress test is frequently performed in the pediatric age group.
Unrepaired congenital heart disease
Aortic stenosis – assessment for severity and need for intervention
Repaired/Palliated congenital heart disease
• **Transposition of great arteries** – to assess potential problems related to coronary transfer after the arterial switch operation • **Tetralogy of Fallot** – to assess functional capacity in children with pulmonary insufficiency before and after pulmonary valve replacement • **Anomalous left coronary artery from the pulmonary artery** – to assess sub-clinical coronary insufficiency • **Fontan physiology** – to assess functional capacity in children who have underwent single ventricle palliation
Other heart diseases
• **Kawasaki disease** – to assess for exercise induced coronary ischemia • **Hypertrophic cardiomyopathy** – to assess for arrhythmias as well as an abnormal blood pressure response to exercise which is an indication for intervention • **Inherited arrhythmias** – arrhythmias in long QT syndrome and catecholaminergic polymorphic ventricular tachycardia are frequently precipitated by exercise. Stress testing is useful both in the diagnosis as well as evaluation of response to treatment in these conditions • **Heart transplant recipients**
Non-cardiac conditions
• Exercise induced asthma • Assessment of athletes

Clinical experience has shown that EST can be safely performed in children with a very low risk of serious adverse events. The safety of testing can further be improved by recognizing high-risk individuals. There are no absolute contraindications to EST in children. It is important that each laboratory device has its own contraindications based on the available equipment, training level of the cardiac physiologists, and ability to provide emergency management in the exercise laboratory. Historically, the subgroups thought to be of very high risk include children with active cardiac inflammation (including rheumatic carditis), severe valvular stenosis, decompensated heart failure, unstable arrhythmias, and fixed pulmonary vascular disease.[14] The American Heart Association recommends that the EST should be terminated whenever the required diagnostic information is obtained, when there is failure of the monitoring equipment or when it is felt that further testing may compromise the safety of the child.[12] Signs that may raise concern about the safety of the patient include:

- Extreme fatigue, dizziness, or breathlessness
- Severe hypertension or hypotension
- A >10% drop in oxygen saturation

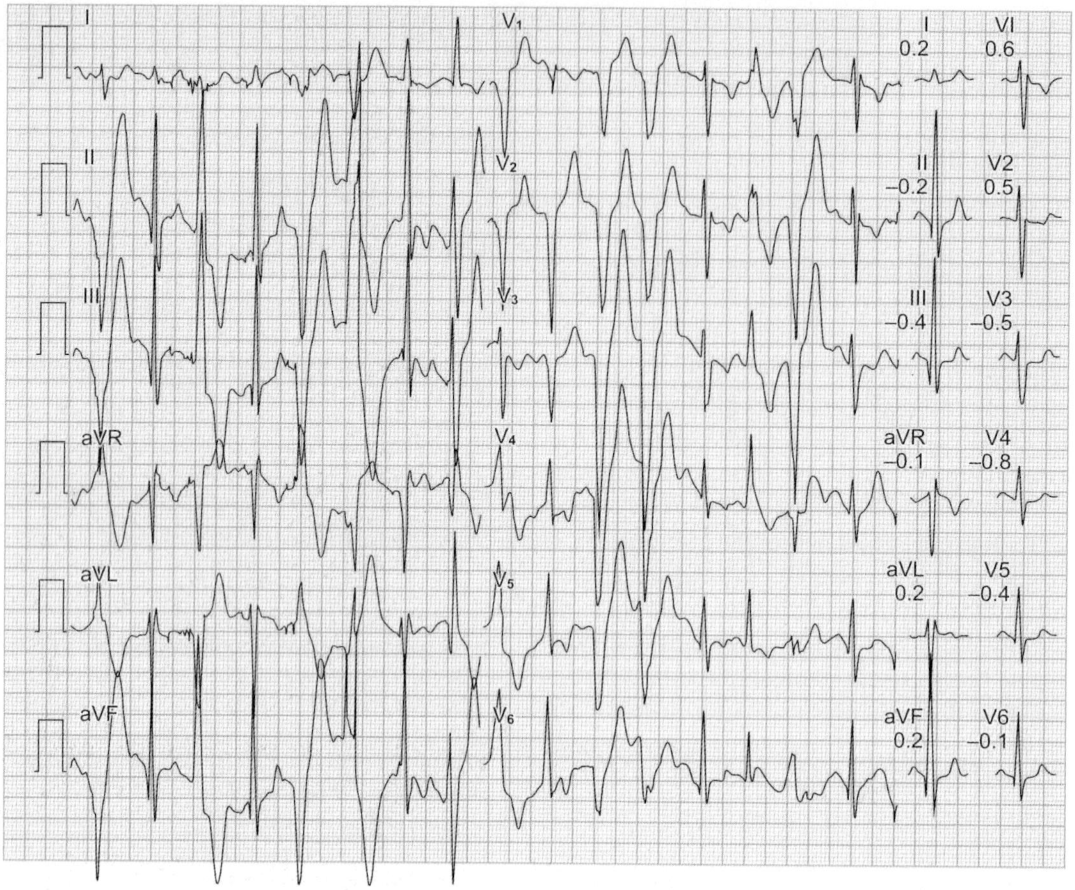

Fig. 18: Exercise stress test of a girl with recurrent exercise induced seizures demonstrating bidirectional ventricular ectopy characteristic of catecholaminergic polymorphic ventricular tachycardia.

- Symptomatic arrhythmias or increase in ventricular ectopy
- ST segment depression which satisfies the adult criteria for exercise-induced ischemia.

Case Examples

In this section, we endeavor to present a few case examples where the utility of an EST resulted in the accurate diagnosis of the cardiac condition in children.

Case 1

An 8-year-old girl was referred with recurrent episodes of exertion-induced syncope. The child did not have any other medical conditions and there was no family history of cardiac conditions. Her cardiac evaluation including echocardiogram and ECG were normal. As her symptoms were related to exertion, an exercise stress test was performed. During the early stages of exercise, there was occasional ventricular ectopy. As the stress progressed, there was bidirectional ventricular ectopy **(Fig. 18)** and this disappeared on recovery. The bidirectional ectopy was diagnostic of catecholaminergic polymorphic ventricular tachycardia (CPVT), an inherited arrhythmia characterized by exercise-induced ventricular arrhythmias, syncope, and sudden death.

Case 2

A 13-year-old athletic boy was referred by his pediatrician who noticed a low heart rate. His clinical examination was unremarkable except for bradycardia. His effort levels were normal. His baseline ECG showed a low heart rate with regular QRS complexes but no clear P wave. Sinus node dysfunction was suspected. However, on an exercise stress test, his heart rate increased normally with reappearance of P waves with an increase in the heart rate (**Figs. 19A and B**). Hence, it was apparent that the absence of P waves was due to physiological sinus slowing at rest.

Other Modalities of Cardiopulmonary Exercise Test

6-minute Walk Test

Children with decompensated heart disease will not tolerate running on the treadmill or bicycling. The 6-minute walk test (6MWT) was specifically designed for testing cardiopulmonary capacity in children and adults with severe restriction of physical activity. The standardized protocol for testing has been reported. The test should be performed indoors. A corridor of 100 feet should be identified and a 30-meter walking track with markings every 3 m should be charted.[15] Supplemental oxygen should be available in the test area.

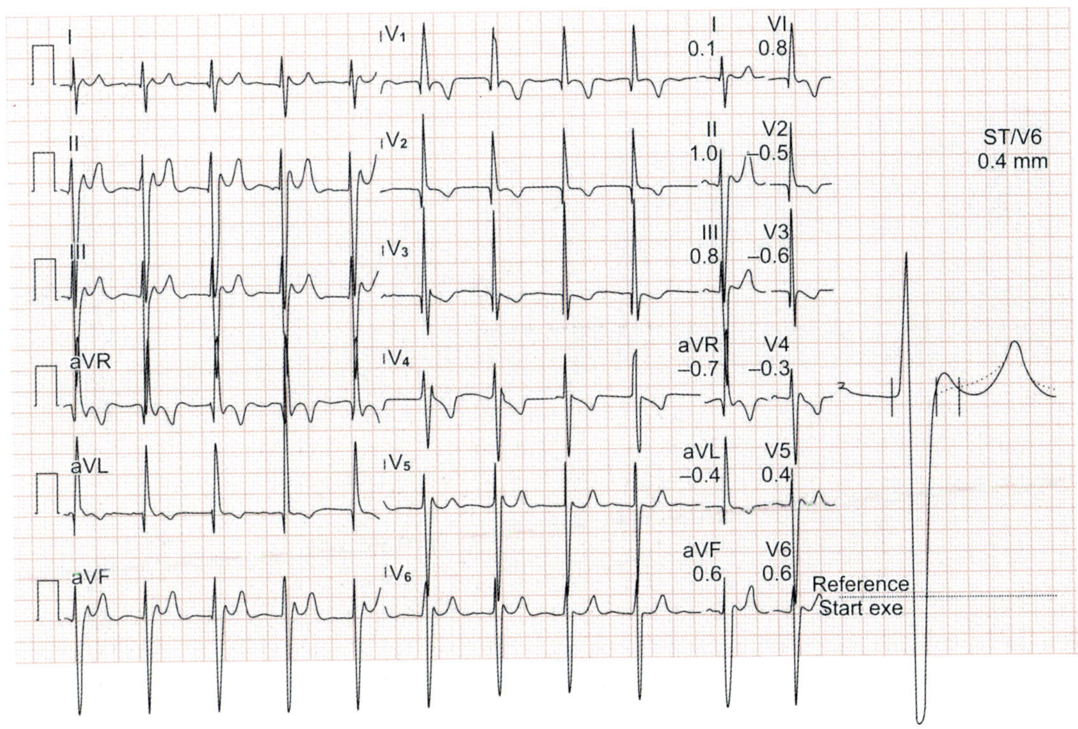

Fig. 19A: Electrocardiogram (ECG) of a 13-year-old boy pre-exercise demonstrating a junctional rhythm. No clear P waves are seen preceding the QRS complex.

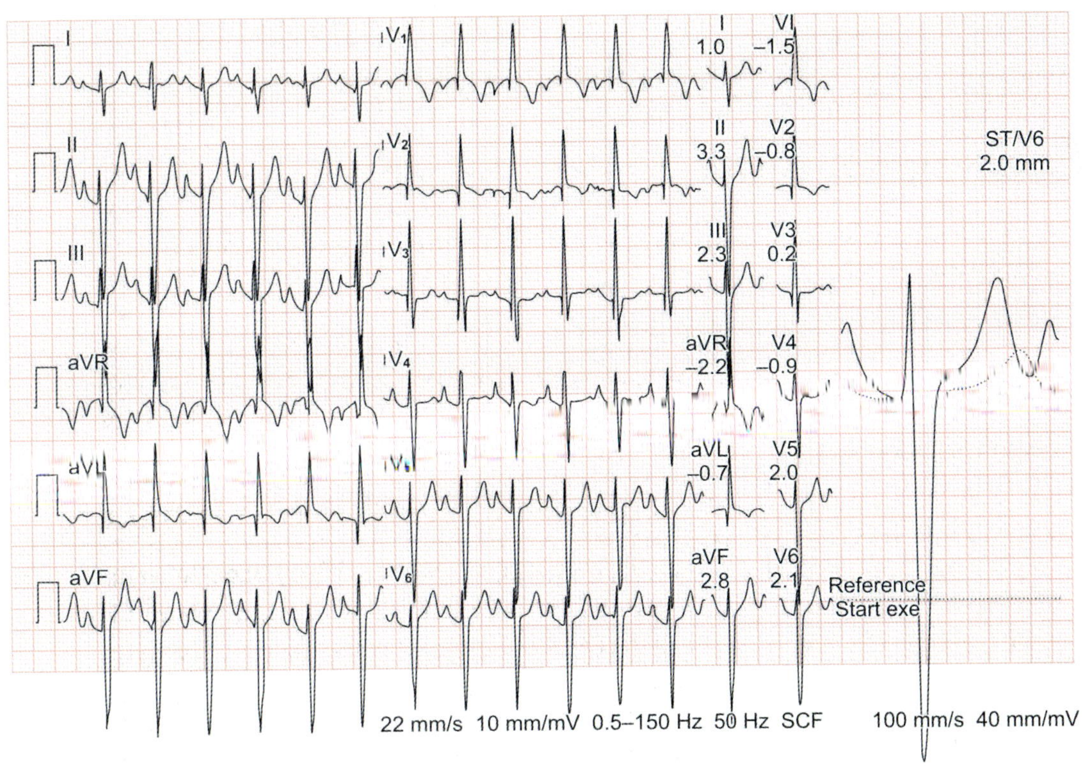

Fig. 19B: Electrocardiogram (ECG) of the same boy during stage II of treadmill exercise stress testing. There is an increase in heart rate with exercise and the rhythm now is a normal sinus rhythm.

The test is performed in environmental conditions similar to EST with a comfortable temperature and humidity. The baseline heart rate and oxygen saturation are recorded. The child is then asked to complete as many laps of the walking track as possible during a 6-minute period. When possible, the heart rate and oxygen saturation should be continuously recorded during the test period and a final recording should be made at the completion of the test.

6 Minutes walk test - (1 LAPSE-100 meters)

Patient name: MRD:

Date of birth: Sex:

Date: 13/09/2019 Doctor:

Ht: 163 cm Wt: 45 kg

	HR	SPO_2	Distance covered	Dyspnea Borg scale	Fatigue Borg scale
6 mt walk test	100/minute	99%			
3 mt walk test	122/minute	97%	480 meters	0.5 (very slight)	Nil
10 mt recovery	108/minute	100%			

Stopped before 6 minutes: No

Fig. 20: A model reporting format for the 6-minute walk test.

The child should be encouraged constantly during the test period. A chair should be made available which can be moved easily along with the child. This allows the child to rest when fatigued during the test. The number of laps covered during the test period is recorded and used to calculate the total distance walked. There are published normative data for children of various age groups and ethnicities. A very low distance covered (typically < 380 m in adolescents) has been shown to predict adverse outcomes in children and adults with severe pulmonary arterial hypertension. Subjective symptoms including fatigue and dyspnea are recorded by the use of the Borg scale. A model reporting format for the 6MWT is shown in **Figure 20**.

The 6MWT hence provides a standardized and reproducible method for the assessment of functional capacity in children with severe heart disease who cannot withstand the rigors of an EST. However, the major limitation of the test is that it is self-paced and hence it is possible that the child may not exert himself or herself to the maximum capacity despite adequate encouragement.

Field Exercise Testing

A major limitation of EST in children is that a majority of children are not accustomed to running on the treadmill or bicycling. The extensors of the knee, which are the most important muscle group in both these exercises, are underdeveloped in children.[16] There are also important safety concerns with performing EST in preschool children. Preschool children however are able to run and play in normal life and can frequently outperform even adults while running on the field. The motivation levels are probably higher on the field than in the claustrophobic settings of the exercise laboratory. An interest in testing the exercise capacity of children on the field has hence existed for a long time. The recent advancements in miniaturization of the metabolic cart have permitted measurement of ventilation parameters as well as the work capacity in the field. These tests have been validated in select groups of children and the results have been found to be comparable with established modalities of EST.[16] However, the equipment for the same is not widely available. The testing methodology is cumbersome requiring special training of personnel and longer time period for performing the test. It is hence not practical to perform these tests outside the research setting.

Pharmacological Stress Testing

It is often not practical to perform EST in certain groups of children. These include the very young as well as the very sick. In these groups of children, when it is necessary to understand the cardiac response to stress, pharmacological agents can be utilized. The cardiac response is analyzed by echocardiography or nuclear imaging. Testing may be performed by using either of two groups of agents—medications that increase myocardial oxygen demand (dobutamine or isoprenaline) or those which cause coronary vasodilation (adenosine).[12]

Dobutamine is usually started as a dose of 10 microgram per kilogram per minute (μg/kg/min) and increased to a maximum of 50 μg/kg/min every 3–5 minutes. Atropine can be administered to increase the heart rate. Esmolol should be available to reverse the effects of dobutamine emergently if there is ischemia. Adenosine is administered at a dose of 140 μg/kg/min for 6 minutes with continuous echocardiographic assessment. Myocardial perfusion imaging can also be performed through nuclear studies based on the single photon emission computed tomography (SPECT) or photon emission tomography (PET) scans.

REFERENCES

1. Davignon A, Rautaharju P, Boisselle E, Soumis F, Mégélas M, Choquette A. Normal ECG standards for infants and children. Pediatr Cardiol. 1980;1(2):123-31.
2. Phan DQ, Silka MJ, Lan YT, Chang RK. Comparison of formulas for calculation of the corrected QT interval in infants and young children. J Pediatr. 2015;166(4):960-4.e1-2.

3. Rijnbeek PR, van Herpen G, Kapusta L, Ten Harkel AD, Witsenburg M, Kors JA. Electrocardiographic criteria for left ventricular hypertrophy in children. Pediatr Cardiol. 2008; 29(5):923-8.
4. Richardson JM. Ventricular preexcitation.Practical considerations. Arch Intern Med. 1983;143(4):760-4.
5. Del Mar B. The history of clinical Holter monitoring. Ann Noninvasive Electrocardiol. 2005;10(2):226-30.
6. Sakhi R, Theuns D, Szili-Torok T, Yap SC. Insertable cardiac monitors: current indications and devices. Expert Rev Med Devices. 2019; 16(1):45-55.
7. Sajeev JK, Koshy AN, Teh AW. Wearable devices for cardiac arrhythmia detection: a new contender? Intern Med J. 2019;49(5):570-3.
8. Bolourchi M, Batra AS. Diagnostic yield of patch ambulatory electrocardiogram monitoring in children (from a national registry). Am J Cardiol. 2015;115(5):630-4.
9. Takken T, Bongers BC, van Brussel M, Haapala EA, Hulzebos EHJ. Cardiopulmonary exercise testing in pediatrics. Ann Am Thorac Soc. 2017;14(Supplement_1):S123-S8.
10. Falkner B, Daniels SR. Summary of the Fourth Report on the diagnosis, evaluation, and treatment of high blood pressure in children and adolescents. Hypertension. 2004;44(4):387-8.
11. Macfarlane DJ. Automated metabolic gas analysis systems: a review. Sports Med. 2001; 31(12):841-61.
12. Paridon SM, Alpert BS, Boas SR, Cabrera ME, Caldarera LL, Daniels SR, et al. Clinical stress testing in the pediatric age group: a statement from the American Heart Association Council on Cardiovascular Disease in the Young, Committee on Atherosclerosis, Hypertension, and Obesity in Youth. Circulation. 2006;113(15): 1905-20.
13. Stephens P Jr, Paridon SM. Exercise testing in pediatrics. Pediatr Clin North Am. 2004; 51(6):1569-87, viii.
14. Washington RL, Bricker JT, Alpert BS, Daniels SR, Deckelbaum RJ, Fisher EA, et al. Guidelines for exercise testing in the pediatric age group. From the Committee on Atherosclerosis and Hypertension in Children, Council on Cardiovascular Disease in the Young, the American Heart Association. Circulation. 1994; 90(4):2166-79.
15. Laboratories ATSCoPSfCPF. ATS statement: guidelines for the six-minute walk test. Am J RespirCrit Care Med. 2002;166(1):111-7.
16. Schoffl I, Ehrlich B, Stanger S, Rottermann K, Dittrich S, Schoffl V. Exercise field testing in children: a new approach for age-appropriate evaluation of cardiopulmonary function. Pediatr Cardiol. 2020.

8
CHAPTER

The Chest X-ray

Munesh Tomar

INTRODUCTION

Cardiac anomalies impart significant changes on the chest X-ray in a number of situations and useful inferences on anatomy and physiology can be made. These inferences can meaningfully impact clinical decisions in a variety of circumstances. The chest X-ray (frontal and lateral views) provides considerable information about severity of cardiac disease if read systematically with clinical information in mind. Before the development of echocardiography and other imaging modalities, the chest X-ray served an important role in diagnosis and periodic evaluation of a patient with heart disease. With advancement in diagnostic techniques, the role of chest X-ray in diagnosis has, undoubtedly, declined. However, there is still independent value to this simple, accessible, and inexpensive investigation in pediatric cardiovascular disease. The chest X-ray provides an independent perspective on enlargement of the heart and its chambers, pulmonary vascularity, pulmonary venous hypertension, condition of the lung parenchyma, and also provides information on mediastinum, spine, and the rib cage. It is important to make correct use of the X-ray in today's times where more accurate imaging tools are available. The purpose is not to arrive at a precise diagnosis of the underlying heart disease but to ensure that those features that are of independent value in a chest X-ray are correctly identified. It is also important to acknowledge that there are very few systematic studies formally evaluating the sensitivity and specificity of the chest X-ray for the evaluation of pulmonary blood flow, pulmonary venous hypertension and asymmetric lung vascularity.

The chest X-ray has considerable value in the primary care setting or at the level of the district hospital where a child with heart disease first presents. The chest X-ray can be complementary to clinical evaluation in order to suspect or rule out heart disease.

Here in this chapter, the chest X-ray will be described under following headings:

- Technical quality
- Situs and cardiac position
- Physiologic interpretations:
  - Cardiac silhouette (cardiac size and ventricular configuration)
  - Pulmonary vasculature:
    - Pulmonary trunk
    - Pulmonary blood flow
    - Pulmonary venous hypertension
  - Mediastinum
  - Chest X-ray in different cardiac lesions
- Lung parenchyma and bony thorax
- Chest X-ray postcardiac intervention.

TECHNICAL QUALITY

Before reading a chest X-ray film, it is important to ascertain the quality of X-ray and this should be mentioned in the report. A checklist for the technical elements is presented further.

Position

A properly centered X-ray allows correct interpretation of heart size, cardiac position, chamber enlargement, and lung volumes. In a well centered X-ray, the medial ends of the clavicle are equidistant from the midline (**Fig. 1**). Rotation of the torso in relation to the direction of the X-ray beam results in unequal distances from the midline. A rotated X-ray often results in erroneous interpretation of cardiac position, cardiac silhouette, chamber sizes, and lung volumes (**Fig. 2**).

Exposure

A chest X-ray may be adequately exposed, overexposed, or underexposed and this seriously impacts the interpretation of lung vasculature and pulmonary venous hypertension.

The exposure is considered adequate if it shows the intervertebral disks spaces up to tracheal bifurcation (usually the first four disk spaces) and not below it (**Fig. 1**).

If vertebral bodies are visible clearly through the cardiac shadow, the X-ray is overpenetrated or overexposed. The lung parenchyma will appear darker and soft tissue shadows such as lung infiltrates, and pulmonary blood flow will be underestimated in an overpenetrated film (**Fig. 2**).

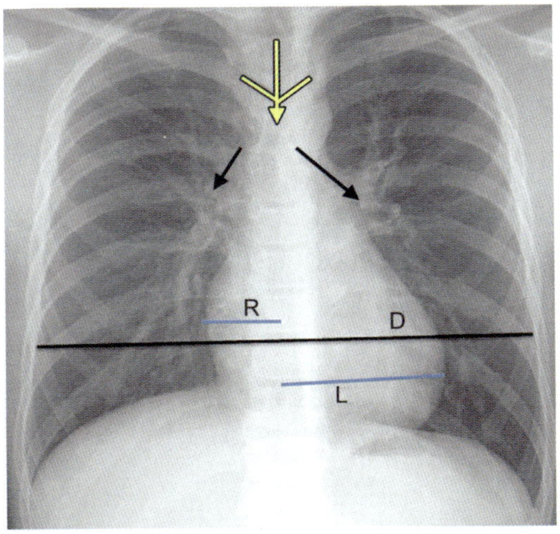

Fig. 1: Chest X-ray frontal view of a 16-year-old male patient fulfilling all criteria of "good quality X-ray." The film is at end of inspiration with adequate penetration, proper centering (marked by central line and equidistant between central line and medial end of both clavicles). Black arrows mark the difference in the length of right and left bronchi (right bronchus is shorter and more in line with trachea than left). There is situs solitus, levocardia, no cardiomegaly with normal pulmonary vasculature, and lung parenchyma. Cardiothoracic ratio also being measured for demonstration (CT ratio = R + L/D).

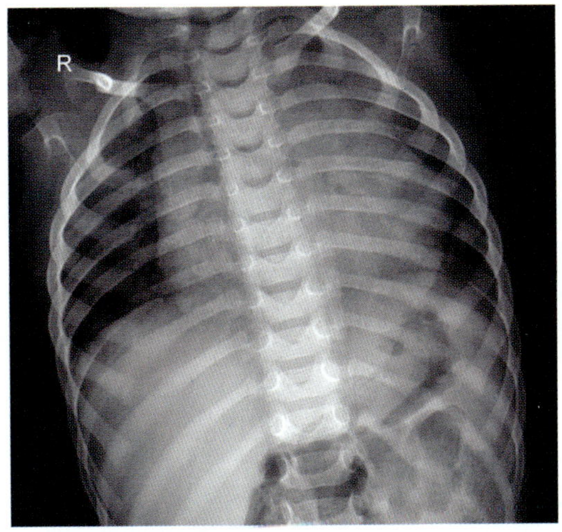

Fig. 2: Poor quality film in an infant with large ventricular septal defect. The film is rotated with over penetration. There is cardiomegaly but it is difficult to comment on pulmonary blood flow due to poor quality of X-ray.

On the other hand, in an underpenetrated or under-exposed film, the vertebral bodies are not visible at all and one cannot differentiate between vertebral bodies and intervertebral disks. The lung parenchyma will appear whiter and with possible overestimation of the pulmonary vascular markings.

In neonates, even with adequate exposure, fluid in the lungs may mimic pulmonary vascular congestion. Premature infants have fewer peripheral pulmonary arteries per gram of lung tissue than a term neonate leading to darker lung fields.[1]

Phase of Respiration

Ideally, the film should be taken at the end of inspiration but this may be unrealistic in small children.

If film is taken at the end of inspiration, the right hemidiaphragm crosses 6th rib in midclavicular line, 8th rib in midaxillary line, and 10th rib posteriorly. The right diaphragm is slightly higher than left (1–2 cm) in situs solitus (*see* **Fig. 1**).

If right hemidiaphragm is higher than 8th rib posteriorly, the film is likely to have been taken in expiration. In that case, cardiac shadow appears larger (impression of cardiomegaly) and lung parenchyma appears hazy giving impression of increased pulmonary vascularity.

DEFINING SITUS AND CARDIAC POSITION

While analyzing the chest X-ray with congenital heart defects, it is of utmost importance to start with situs and cardiac position (**Figs. 1 and 3A to C**).

Situs

The situs can be defined by the following criteria:

- *Abdominal*: In situs solitus, the stomach gas bubble is on the left side and the liver shadow on the right side with the right dome of the diaphragm at a higher position than the left dome (**Figs. 1 and 3A**), while in situs inversus, the stomach gas bubble is seen on the right side and the liver shadow with the higher hemidiaphragm is seen on the left side (**Fig. 3B**). In some cases, the liver is in the mid line (**Fig. 3C**), suggestive of situs ambiguous with either right or left isomerism (asplenia or polysplenia syndrome) and the possibility of a relatively complex congenital heart disease (CHD).
- *Bronchial*: Division of bronchus can sometimes be seen on routine chest X-ray and this can give a clue to the situs (*see* **Fig. 1**). The left main bronchus is longer and has a more acute angle with trachea as compared to the right main bronchus. If the right and left bronchi are lateralized normally, it indicates normal situs and if vice versa, i.e., inversely lateralized, it will indicate situs inversus (**Fig. 3B**).

If both the bronchi are of similar morphology (bilateral right-sided or left-sided), it suggests situs ambiguous with right or left isomerism. Bronchial arrangements are often better seen with overexposed films. However, overexposed films are seldom obtained for this specific purpose.

Cardiac Position

Normally, there is situs solitus and heart is in left hemithorax (levocardia), but it can be in midline (mesocardia) or in right hemithorax (dextrocardia). It is important to note the relation between situs and cardiac position as discrepancy between situs and cardiac position points toward complexity of cardiac malformation. Also, it is important to note associated

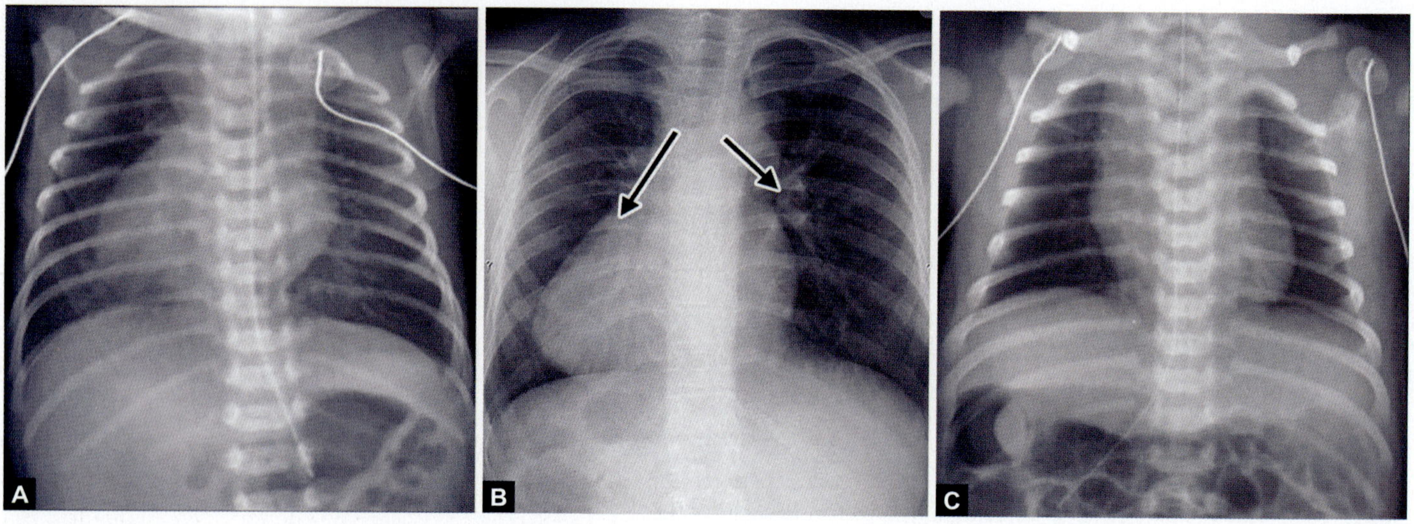

Figs. 3A to C: Chest X-rays showing situs and cardiac position. (A) Situs solitus with dextrocardia. Think of associated complex cardiac defect. Note the presence of stomach bubble on the left side and liver shadow on the right side; (B) Situs inversus with dextrocardia. Also called as situs inversus totalis. Note the presence of stomach bubble on the right side and liver shadow on the left side. The pattern of bronchial bifurcation is also suggestive of situs inversus; (C) Centrally placed liver (feature of isomerism left/right) with mesocardia. High chances of complex congenital cardiac defects.

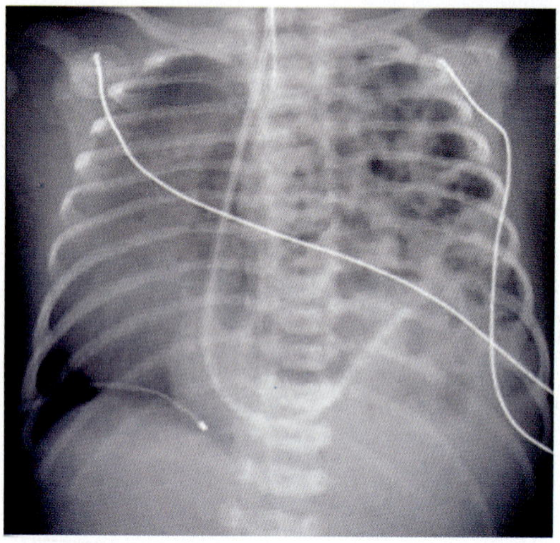

Fig. 4: Chest X-ray in a neonate with cyanosis and severe respiratory distress. X-ray shows left-sided diaphragmatic hernia and dextroposed heart. Diaphragmatic hernia is the cause of cyanosis and severe pulmonary arterial hypertension. Nasogastric tube is seen in left hemithorax.

lung pathology or malformation (e.g., diaphragmatic hernia, mass, tension pneumothorax, and lung hypoplasia) which can be the cause of cardiac malposition (**Fig. 4**).

PHYSIOLOGIC INTERPRETATIONS

The chest X-ray provides independent information on the physiology of the heart condition and this is perhaps of greater value than the anatomic information in many circumstances. Serial X-rays offer valuable insights about the progression of the lesions or their regression in response to therapy.

Cardiac Silhouette

Description of the cardiac silhouette includes cardiac position as described earlier, cardiac size (cardiomegaly or not), and its configuration. It is necessary to be familiar with normal structures forming the cardiac borders in order to correctly interpret enlargement of individual chambers or vessels. Familiarity with specific anatomical variations of some of the structures in CHD is also needed to identify them.

The normal cardiac borders are formed by the following structures:

- The right border, from above downward, is formed by superior vena cava (SVC), ascending aorta, and right atrium (RA).
- Likewise, the left border is formed by aortic knuckle, the main pulmonary artery (MPA), left atrial appendage (LAA), and left ventricle (LV). The medial two-thirds of the inferior border is formed by the right ventricle (RV) and lateral one-third is formed by the LV.
- In the lateral view, anterior border is formed by RV.

Heart Size

For the assessment of heart size, cardiothoracic ratio (CTR) is calculated. The cardiac dimension is measured from the middle of the spine to the maximum convexity on right and left side (R and L). The thoracic dimension is the widest internal thoracic dimension (D). A CTR (CTR = L + R/D) of >60% in neonates, 55% in infants, and 50% in children is taken as cardiac enlargement. A higher CT ratio in neonate and infants is due to more horizontally placed heart. While calculating this ratio, it is necessary that the chest X-ray is well-centered and a good inspiratory film has been taken. Expiratory film causes falsely increased CT ratio. Also, in neonates and infants, one should remember not to include thymic shadow in the heart borders (**Figs. 1 and 5**).

Cardiac Configuration

The value of cardiac configuration in arriving at a precise anatomic diagnosis is quite limited. While certain cardiac

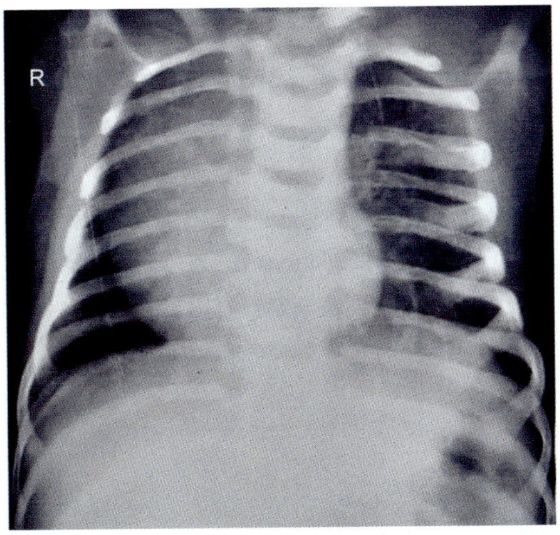

Fig. 5: A 1-month-old neonate referred for cardiac evaluation with the impression of dextrocardia in chest X-ray. Enlarged thymus (right lobe) is giving false impression of dextrocardia and cardiac enlargement. It is important to note that the rotated film is further contributing to "dextrocardia."

configurations can point accurately to the specific cardiac conditions, deviations are very common indeed. With the advent of echocardiography, the chest X-ray is no longer relied upon to arrive at a specific anatomic diagnosis of the underlying heart defect. However, there is value to carefully looking at the cardiac configurations not merely to look at specific patterns but, more importantly, to identify enlargements of individual chambers. At all times, it is important to keep in mind the very limited sensitivity and specificity of chest X-ray in diagnosing chamber enlargement.

- *Left ventricular enlargement*: When the apex of the heart is down and out with a rounded configuration, it suggests left ventricular enlargement. It is important to recognize that considerable LV enlargement is often needed to cast a shadow in the posteroanterior (PA) view and to create a LV configuration.
- *Right ventricular enlargement*: If the apex is lifted up and rounded (clockwise rotation of heart), it suggests RV enlargement. In the lateral view, obliteration of retrosternal space (**Figs. 6A to C**) is also a feature of RV enlargement. However, lateral views are seldom performed for this purpose.
- *Enlargement of the RA* (**Fig. 6A**):
  - Enlargement of right heart border (become more convex and elongated) which is formed by the RA.
  - When RA is enlarged the contour of the right heart border usually occupies more than 2½ intercostal spaces.
  - Dilatation of SVC
  - Distance from midline to maximum convexity of right heart border >5 cm in adult and >4 cm in children.
- *Enlargement of left atrium* (**Fig. 7**):
  - Double density on the right side. The left atrial shadow is more inferior/horizontal, and the curvature is increased with increased density
  - Widening of the angle of carina which is due to the elevation of the left bronchus. Normally, it is <70° and it increases with left atrial enlargement. If the carinal angle is 90° or more, it is more specific for left atrial enlargement.
  - Right border of left atrium projects outside the right heart border; this happens only if the left atrium is severely enlarged.
  - Atelectasis in left lung may result as a consequence of compression of the left main bronchus; again, this is seen in extreme left atrial enlargement.

Pulmonary Vasculature

Accurate assessment of the pulmonary vasculature is critical to correctly classify physiologic categories of CHD. While describing the pulmonary vasculature, one need to start from central pulmonary arteries and veins and then analyze these structures up to the periphery.

Causes of dilatation or prominence of central pulmonary arteries:

- Increased pulmonary blood flow
- Pulmonary arterial hypertension (PAH)
- Idiopathic and poststenotic dilation of the pulmonary arteries
- Pulmonary regurgitation
- Absent pulmonary valve syndrome.

Above listed causes point to the fact that dilatation of pulmonary artery (PA) could be a benign entity or could be manifestation of severe cardiac disease. Therefore, the size of the pulmonary trunk has absolutely nothing to do with the type of vascularity.[2]

Pulmonary Plethora (Increased Pulmonary Blood Flow)

Vascular shadows which we see on chest X-ray are contributed by both pulmonary arteries and veins and increased vascularity is contributed by both. For the pulmonary vasculature to appear abnormal on the plain X-ray film, the amount of blood contributed by the shunt must be at least 40% of the total pulmonary blood flow.[2] Following features point to increased pulmonary vascularity on chest X-ray.[3,4]

- Vascular shadows that can be traced to lateral one-third of lung field
- Increased end-on vessels (>3 in one lung field, >5 in both lung fields)
- End-on vessel diameter more than that of the accompanying end on bronchus.

Oligemia (Decreased Pulmonary Blood Flow)

Following features point to decreased pulmonary blood flow:

- With decreased pulmonary blood flow, vascular shadows will be reduced and lung fields appear darker.
- Central pulmonary arteries are of small size.
- Vascularity can be traced up to middle one-third of the lung fields only.

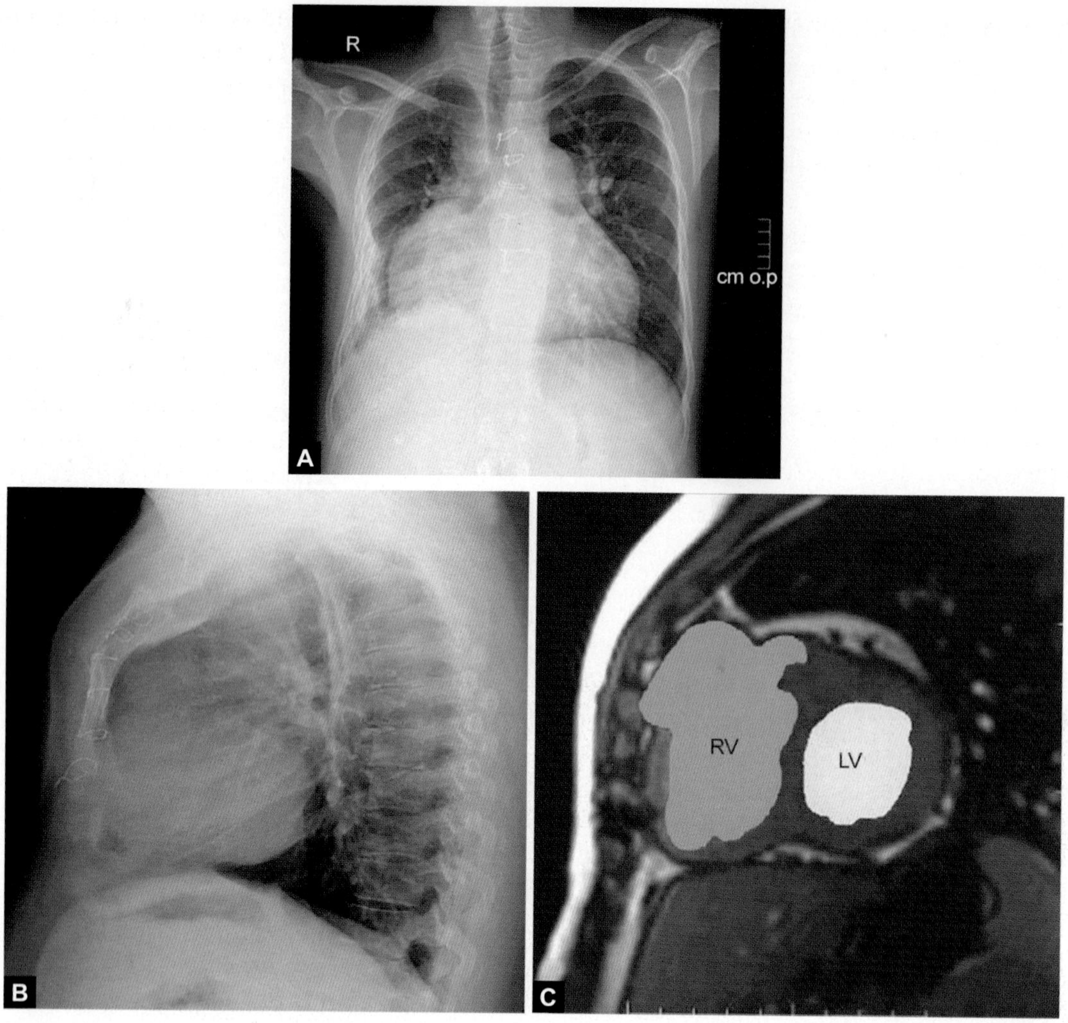

Figs. 6A to C: Chest X-ray in a 34-year-old adult patient who underwent total correction for tetralogy of Fallot in early childhood. He was not on regular cardiology follow-up and now presented with atrial flutter and congestive cardiac failure. The presentation is due to severe pulmonary regurgitation leading to right heart failure. (A) Frontal view showing gross cardiomegaly, dilated right atrium. Main pulmonary artery segment is dilated; (B) Lateral view showing RV enlargement occupying retrosternal space; (C) Cardiac MRI (magnetic resonance imaging) image in lateral view marking enlargement of right ventricle (RV). Left ventricle (LV) is seen in short axis posterior to RV.

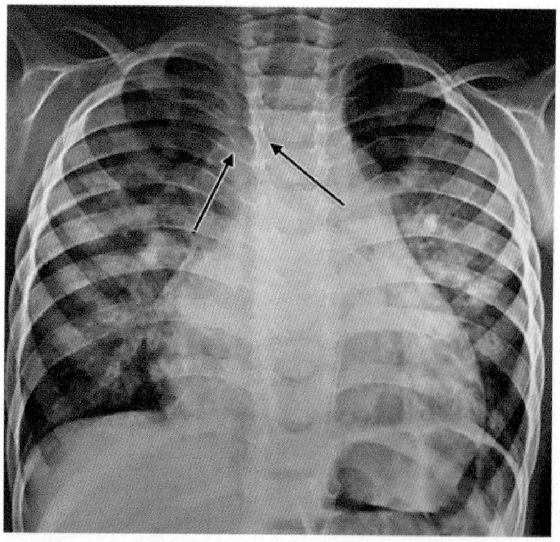

Fig. 7: A 2-year-old child with a large patent ductus arteriosus (PDA) presented with congestive cardiac failure.. Chest X-ray shows cardiomegaly with left ventricular configuration (apex down and out), dilated left atrium, left ventricle, and pulmonary arteries with increased pulmonary vascular markings. LA dilatation is evident by wide angle of carina (marked by arrows) and double density in the right atrium.

Pulmonary Arterial Hypertension

- The MPA dilates with the increase in the PA pressures and this can be seen on a chest X-ray, if the great vessels are normally related.
- In addition, the proximal right and left pulmonary arteries are also enlarged. In an adult, the absolute caliber of the right lower PA has been measured on chest X-ray and the upper limit of normal has been to be 17 mm. If the right lower PA is <14 mm, significant increase in pulmonary blood flow or pulmonary pressure is unlikely.
- *"Peripheral pruning"*: In case of Eisenmenger syndrome, dilated central pulmonary arteries with abrupt reduction in diameter. Pruning is defined as >50% loss of vessel diameter at branching points.[3]
- Calcification in proximal pulmonary arteries. Presence of calcium suggests severe and long-standing hypertension.

Pulmonary Venous Hypertension

While pulmonary vasculature is uniformly distributed throughout the lung, intrapulmonary vessels coursing in the lower lobe are relatively large perhaps because of upright posture and increased amount of lung tissue forming lower lobe. As a result, the lower lobe receives most of the blood leading to larger size of lower lobe branches of PA and vein.

Once pulmonary venous hypertension (regardless of cause) develops, changes appear in chest X-ray depending upon degree and duration of pulmonary venous hypertension. Elliot[2] has described four progressive stages of pulmonary venous hypertension.

1. *Stage I*: *Redistribution of blood flow*: One of the early signs of pulmonary venous hypertension may be decrease in size of lower lobe pulmonary arteries and veins which is termed as "equalization" of pulmonary vessels. Pulmonary venous pressure is mildly elevated above the normal upper limit of 12 mm Hg.
2. *Stage II*: Overt signs of interstitial edema that begins in the interstices of the lung, adjacent to the arterioles, arteries, bronchi, and in the interlobular septa (Kerley B lines). The pulmonary venous pressure is usually between 18 and 25 mm Hg.
3. *Stage III*: Edema in the alveolar spaces (pulmonary venous pressure >25 mm Hg) (**Fig. 8**), with evidence of pulmonary parenchymal densities.
4. *Stage IV*: Severe and chronic changes: These include changes such as deposits of hemosiderin and ossification (pneumonitis). It produces a stippled effect on X-ray film.

This is largely valid for relatively older patients and not applicable to neonates and infants and in settings such as early postoperative period after heart surgery. In these settings, features of pulmonary edema may set in early. Additionally, in children where the pulmonary venous hypertension sets in very slowly as in rheumatic mitral valve stenosis, the compensatory vasoconstriction and drainage of interstitial fluid via lymphatic pathways may not allow engorgement of pulmonary veins or development of parenchymal shadows. Instead these patients have features of PA hypertension that dominates the chest X-ray appearance.

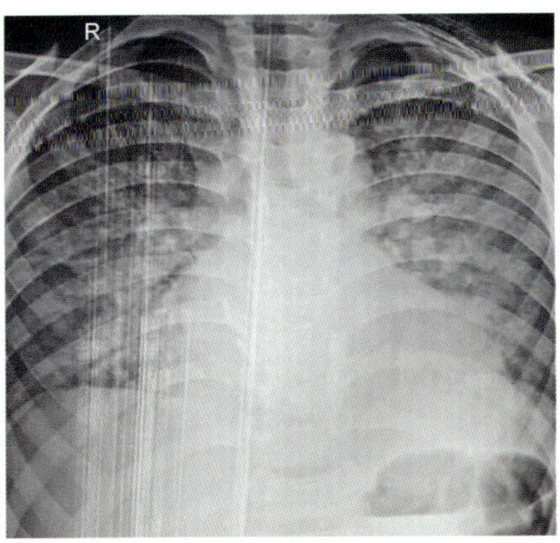

Fig. 8: Chest X-ray frontal view of an 8-year-old child with features of congestive cardiac failure showing cardiomegaly (CT ratio 65%), increased pulmonary vascular markings and features of pulmonary venous hypertension. The cause of congestive heart failure (CHF) in this child was severe systemic arterial hypertension leading to severe LV dysfunction and pulmonary venous hypertension.

MEDIASTINUM

Vascular structures (aortic arch, SVC, and pulmonary trunk) contribute to the mediastinum and should be looked at carefully. Additionally, the thymus is important because it could obscure everything else. The absence of a thymic X-ray shadow is characteristic of patients with severe cyanosis, such as in transposition. Here, thymic tissue is present but not visible. In some patients with 22 q11 deletion it is absent altogether, although the chest X-ray cannot make a distinction between the two.

- *Aortic arch sidedness*: Normally, aortic arch is left-sided but in a small percentage of individuals, arch can be right-sided with mirror image branching. It is the norm for patients with situs inversus, particularly if they do not have heart disease. In isolation, right-sided aortic arch does not carry any significance. Association of right aortic arch is higher with CHDs such as tetralogy of Fallot (TOF) and truncus arteriosus. Aortic arch sidedness is important at the time of surgery related to aortic arch such as coarctation of aorta repair, Blalock–Taussig (BT) shunt, patent ductus arteriosus (PDA) ligation, and also while repairing tracheoesophageal fistula. Arch sidedness is most reliably identified by the side of indentation of the arch on the trachea (**Fig. 9**).
    - *Double aortic arch*: Here, both limbs of double aortic arch pass on either side of trachea and esophagus and join as a single descending aorta forming a complete

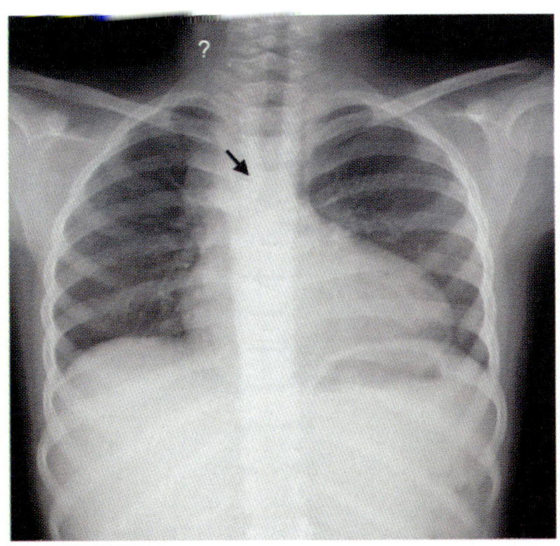

Fig. 9: Chest X-ray frontal view in a 3-year-old child with cyanosis showing situs solitus, levocardia, right ventricle (RV) type apex (upturned apex "boot-shaped heart"), pulmonary bay, and decreased pulmonary blood flow. Note indentation of trachea (arrow) by right aortic arch.

vascular ring.[5] In the frontal view, right arch is higher and larger than left and right arch causes tracheal indentation in most instances as it is the dominant arch in the vast majority. The lateral view shows narrowing and anterior displacement of trachea.

- *Systemic venous dilatation*: Systemic veins should be looked at while reading a chest X-ray as dilated vena cava or azygos vein point towards either a high right atrial pressure or anomalous vein joining SVC or azygos vein [total anomalous pulmonary venous connection (TAPVC), interrupted inferior vena cava with azygos continuation].
- The MPA (pulmonary trunk) consistently casts a shadow in the upper left heart border whenever the great arteries are normally related to each other (PA anterior and to the left of aorta). A narrow mediastinum suggests one of the following:
    - Malposed great vessels where aorta is in front of the PA (transposition of great arteries)
    - Single outlet (pulmonary atresia and persistent truncus arteriosus).

CHEST X-RAY IN SPECIFIC CARDIAC LESIONS

Left-to-Right Shunts

The chest X-ray can be useful in identifying the site of shunt and quantifying it. The chest X-ray helps in making the critical distinction between pulmonary hypertension that is the result of increased pulmonary blood flow (hyperkinetic PAH) from elevated pulmonary vascular resistance (pulmonary vascular obstructive disease). The left-to-right shunts can be at a pretricuspid (i.e., atrial septal defect, anomalous pulmonary venous drainage) or post-tricuspid [ventricular septal defect (VSD), aortopulmonary window, and patent ductus arteriosus] level, or at both levels (atrioventricular septal defect). Chest X-ray findings will depend upon the quantity of shunt and will vary from normal sized heart with small shunt to gross cardiomegaly with large shunt.[6] All the lesions causing moderate-to-large left-to-right shunt will result in X-ray evidence of increased pulmonary blood flow; the heart size correlates with the degree of shunt. The larger the shunt quantum, the larger will be the heart size as long as there is no other reason for increase in heart size like anemia or leakage of the atrioventricular valve. Pretricuspid shunts result in enlargement of the RA and the RV; post-tricuspid shunts result in left atrial and left ventricular enlargement.[6] The atrial level shunts are mostly due to atrial septal defect (**Fig. 10**) or occasionally due to partial anomalous pulmonary venous drainage or both (sinus venosus type of ASD).

With increasing pulmonary arterial pressure, RA and RV continue to dilate often with the development of progressive tricuspid regurgitation. All these factors contribute to persistence or increase in cardiomegaly in atrial septal defect with PAH unlike in post-tricuspid shunts that show a reduction in heart size as pulmonary vascular resistance increases (**Figs. 11 and 13B**).

The Scimitar (the word "Scimitar" refers to a Turkish sword) syndrome is a group of anomalies, most important anomaly being right pulmonary vein(s) anomalously joining inferior vena cava. The descending venous channel creates a "scimitar sword-shaped" shadow parallel to RA on the frontal chest X-ray (**Fig. 12**). This is usually associated with varying degree of right lung and right PA hypoplasia, shift of the cardiac shadow to the right side due to right lung hypoplasia. Children usually present with recurrent chest infections as a result of sequestration of a part of the right lower lobe or with features of PAH.

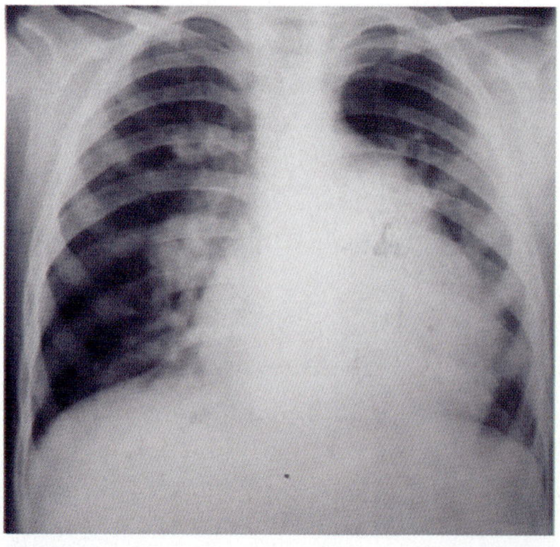

Fig. 10: Chest X-ray frontal view in a child with large atrial septal defect. The X-ray of chest shows moderate cardiomegaly with dilatation of the right atrium and enlargement of main pulmonary artery. Also, notice prominent hilar pulmonary arteries with evidence of increased pulmonary blood flow indicative of large shunt at atrial level.

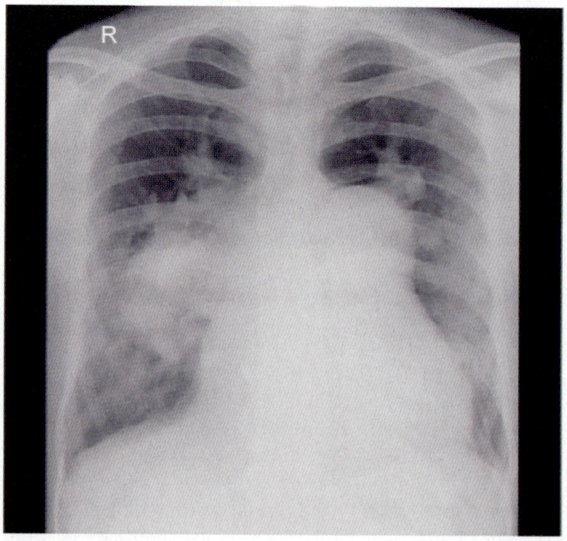

Fig. 11: Chest X-ray frontal view of a 36-year-old patient with large atrial septal defect and pulmonary arterial hypertension. Note the persistence of cardiomegaly and aneurysmal dilatation of pulmonary arteries.

Shunts at ventricular and aortopulmonary level will result in enlargement of left atrium, LV, and pulmonary arteries along with features of increased pulmonary blood flow (**Figs. 7 and 13A**).

Chest X-ray in a child with a large VSD[7] may show normalization of cardiac dimension on follow-up and this could be due to:

- Development of pulmonary vascular obstructive disease (Eisenmenger syndrome) with severe elevation of pulmonary vascular resistance. Chest X-ray shows normalization of heart size but central pulmonary arteries remain dilated with the presence of peripheral pruning (**Fig. 13B**).
- Some children develop progressive infundibular pulmonary stenosis (TOF physiology).
- Spontaneous reduction in size of the VSD.

It is easy to distinguish between these three situations by clinical examination.

A restrictive VSD with no cardiomegaly on chest X-ray may show cardiomegaly on follow-up[7] and this could be due to the following:

- Development of significant aortic regurgitation due to aortic valve prolapse or bacterial endocarditis
- *Rupture of sinus of Valsalva*: This is a relatively rare event and is seen in selected patients with a subpulmonic VSD with progressive prolapse of the aortic valve that eventually develops into an aneurysm and ruptures. These patients are usually older and chest X-ray is suggestive of large left-to-right shunt with left atrium and left ventricular enlargement together with dilatation of the aorta.

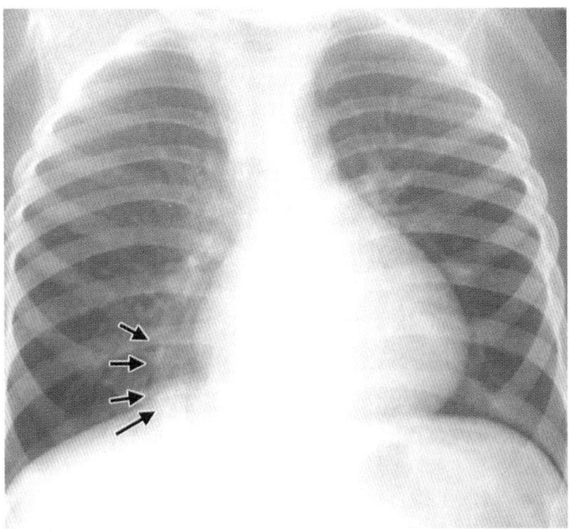

Fig. 12: Chest X-ray frontal view in an infant with features of atrial septal defect with pulmonary arterial hypertension. X-ray shows sword-shaped shadow parallel to right atrium "Scimitar syndrome" (marked by arrows). Shadow is produced by right lower pulmonary vein descending to join inferior vena cava.

Atrioventricular Septal Defect

These patients have shunts at atrial and ventricular levels. The X-ray appearance varies depending on the relative sizes of the shunts. Typically, there is cardiomegaly and increased pulmonary blood flow and individual chamber enlargement is not clearly evident.

Patent Ductus Arteriosus

Shunt at ductal level also leads to dilatation of aorta in addition to changes described with VSD (*see* **Fig. 7**). Rarely, there is aneurysmal dilatation of ductal ampulla with a well-defined homogeneous opacity in the left mediastinum.

Aortopulmonary Window

Chest X-ray with large aortopulmonary window similar to that of a large VSD.

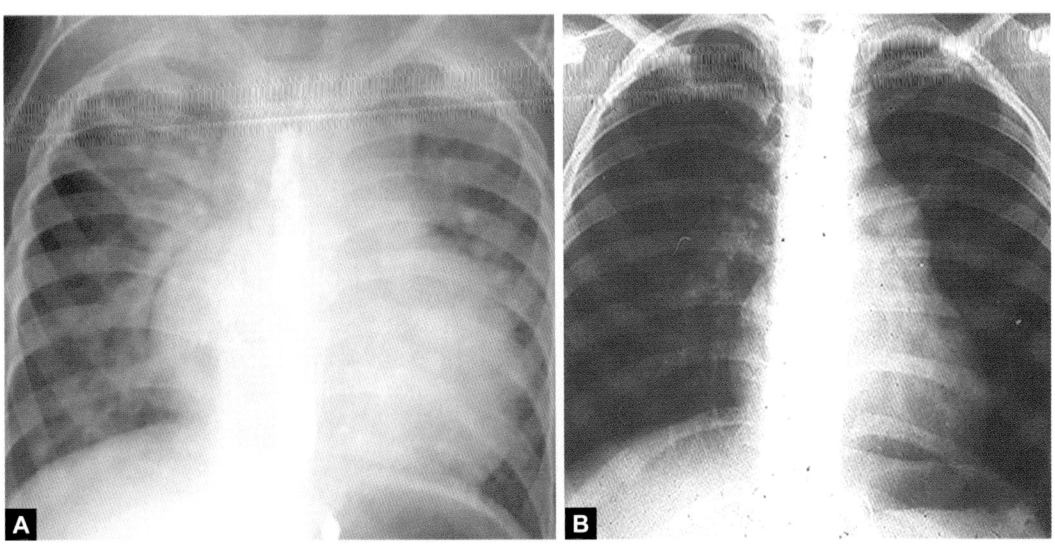

Figs. 13A and B: X-ray of chest from a patient with large ventricular septal defect. (A) X-ray was taken when child was 8 months old and was having features of large left-to-right shunt. X-ray of chest shows cardiomegaly (LV type apex) with enlargement of main pulmonary arterial (MPA) segment. Pulmonary vasculature is markedly increased. All findings indicative of large post-tricuspid shunt; (B) This unfortunate child could not be operated and came for follow-up at 12 years of age. Chest X-ray here shows absence of cardiomegaly, prominent main pulmonary artery with peripheral pruning suggestive of development of pulmonary vascular obstructive disease.

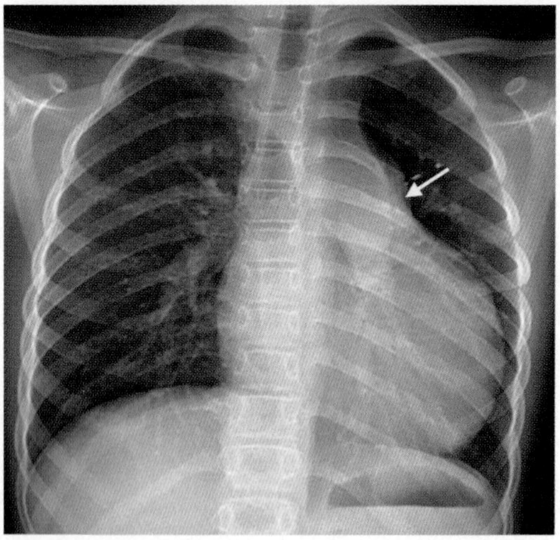

Fig. 14: Chest X-ray frontal view of an 8-year-old child with valvular pulmonary stenosis (PS). Notice normal heart size with dilated main pulmonary artery (MPA) (arrow) and left pulmonary artery (LPA) with normal pulmonary vascular markings.

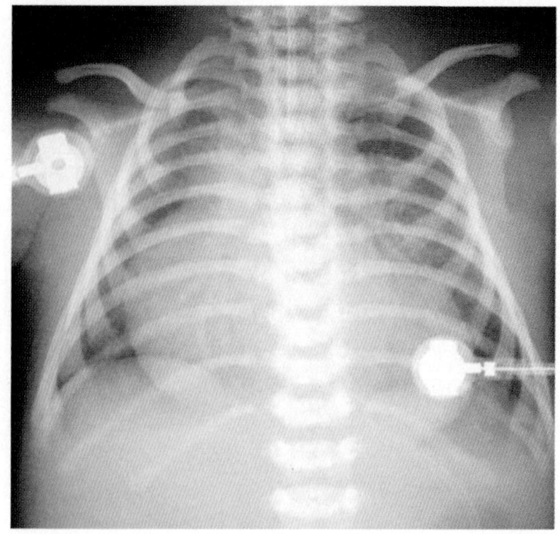

Fig. 15: Chest X-ray frontal view in a 4-day-old with cyanosis and respiratory distress showing gross cardiomegaly with right atrial enlargement. Baby was having critical pulmonary stenosis, severe tricuspid regurgitation with RA, and RV dilatation.

Obstructive Lesions

The chest X-ray has a limited diagnostic value in obstructive lesions. Critical narrowing of the aortic or pulmonary valve in the neonate may be associated with cardiomegaly.

Pulmonary Stenosis

- *Valvar pulmonary stenosis*: Dilated MPA and left pulmonary artery (LPA) are hallmarks for the diagnosis of pure valvular pulmonary stenosis (**Fig. 14**). If the pulmonary valve is dysplastic as in Noonan syndrome, the poststenotic dilation is noticeably absent. The heart size is usually normal. In case of critical pulmonary stenosis, associated right ventricular dysfunction and significant tricuspid regurgitation results in cardiac enlargement with a prominent RA and SVC with reduced lung vasculature (**Fig. 15**).
- In case of infundibular (subvalvar) and supravalvar pulmonary stenosis, the MPA is not dilated.
- Peripheral PA stenosis can result in dilatation of main and proximal pulmonary arteries which may sometimes become evident on the chest X-ray.

Valvular Aortic Stenosis

Dilated ascending aorta is the hallmark of valvular aortic stenosis, particularly in older children[8] (**Fig. 16**). The degree of dilatation is not related to severity of stenosis. There is often no cardiac enlargement. With critical aortic stenosis, left ventricular dysfunction results in left ventricular enlargement and pulmonary venous hypertension.

Coarctation of Aorta

Neonatal coarctation often presents early as a duct-dependent systemic circulation with right ventricular dominance. The chest X-ray often does not offer specific diagnostic clues here.

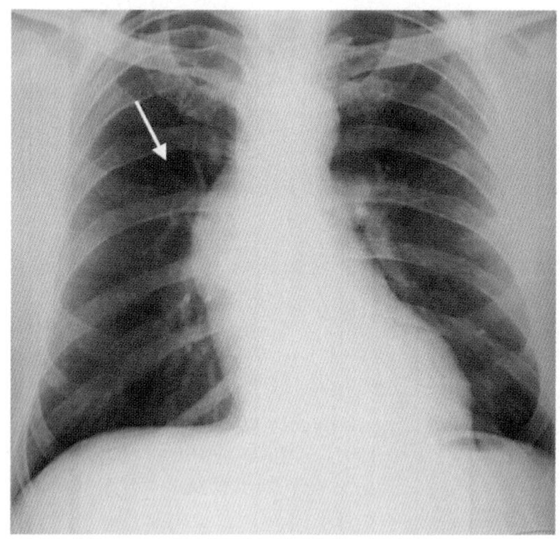

Fig. 16: Characteristic X-ray findings in a patient with bicuspid aortic valve, valvular aortic stenosis with preserved left ventricular function. Note the presence of dilated ascending aorta (arrow) suggestive of the diagnosis of bicuspid aortic valve.

Selected patients present with left ventricular dysfunction and chest X-ray shows cardiomegaly with pulmonary venous congestion. In older children with coarctation, chest X-ray shows a dilated ascending aorta. These children often also have an associated bicuspid aortic valve. In classical coarctation of aorta without arch hypoplasia, a notch at the site of coarctation may be seen on chest X-ray between the dilated proximal and distal segments—"3 sign" (**Fig. 17**). Before the era of echocardiography, this sign, along with "E/reversed 3 sign" on barium swallow, was used in the diagnosis of coarctation. E/reversed 3 sign is produced by indentation of dilated proximal aorta and the distal aorta and the distal aorta adjacent to the coarctation on barium filled esophagus. In older children, rib notching may be seen as a wavy indention at the lower border of 3–8th ribs on either or both sides due to augmented collateral flow

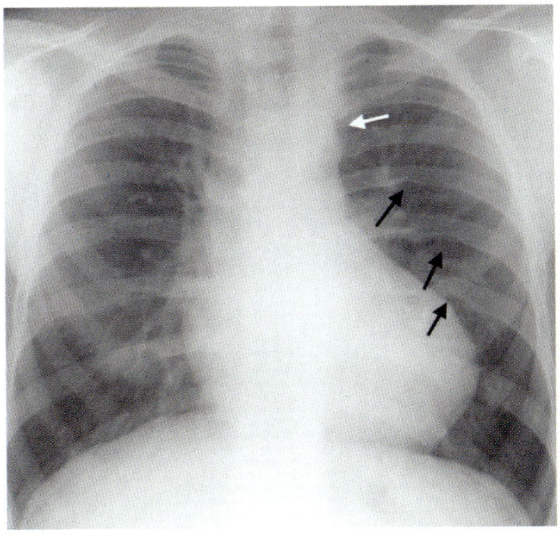

Fig. 17: Characteristic radiographic findings in a patient with coarctation of aorta. X-ray chest frontal view showing characteristic "3 sign" (white arrow at the site of coarctation) with rib notching (black arrows) in presence of long-standing coarctation of aorta.

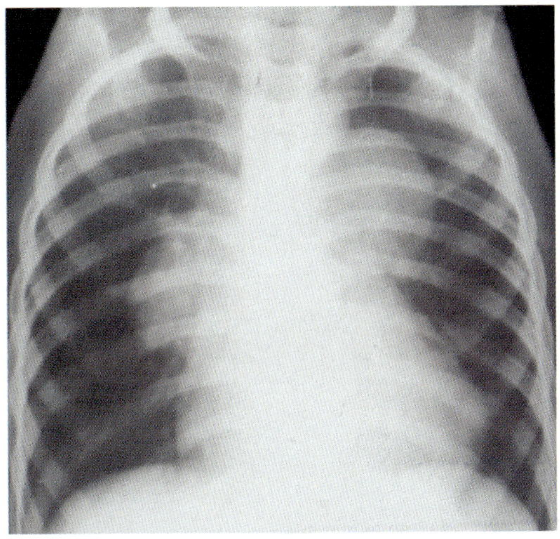

Fig. 18: Chest X-ray frontal view of a child with tetralogy of Fallot with absent pulmonary valve. Notice the markedly enlarged hilar pulmonary arteries. Rest of features are same as in tetralogy of Fallot (RV type venticular apex, decreased pulmonary blood flow).

through the dilated and tortuous intercostal arteries (**Fig. 17**).[9] If the left subclavian artery arises below the coarctation, the rib notching is seen only on the right side. In case there is aberrant right subclavian artery below the coarctation, the rib notching is seen on the left side.

Other causes of rib notching include a classical BT shunt, major aortopulmonary artery collaterals in cyanotic heart diseases, and neurofibromatosis.

Cyanotic Heart Disease

Cyanotic CHD is traditionally classified into two categories based on the pulmonary blood flow:

- Cyanotic CHD with reduced pulmonary blood flow
- Cyanosis with increased pulmonary blood flow.

Chest X-ray is helpful in categorizing the patient in different disease groups.

Cyanotic Congenital Heart Disease with Decreased Pulmonary Blood Flow

TOF: The cardiac size is usually normal with right ventricular configuration (lifted, upturned, and rounded apex). The ascending aorta and the aortic arch are usually enlarged and a concavity may be seen in the region of the MPA—referred to as "pulmonary bay" (*see* **Fig. 9**). When there is predominant valvar pulmonary stenosis, the MPA may be dilated. The hilar vessels and their branches are often small with dark lung fields. In 20% of these patients, aortic arch is right-sided that is identified by the indentation on the right border of tracheal shadow (*see* **Fig. 9**).[10] In TOF with pulmonary atresia, the chest X-ray is often indistinguishable from TOF with pulmonic stenosis. Similar finding can also be seen in patients with double outlet RV with VSD and pulmonary stenosis.

In D-transposition with VSD and pulmonary stenosis, the malposed great vessels may result in a relatively narrow pedicle.

In tetralogy and similar condition, the heart size is normal. Heart size may enlarge if there is associated anemia, valvular regurgitations that may result from endocarditis, ventricular dysfunction, with severe hypoxia.

Major aortopulmonary collaterals in TOF physiology are relatively common in older patients with TOF physiology; they help to supplement the reduced pulmonary blood flow. Chest X-ray may provide some clue to the presence of significant collaterals:

- Small end-on vessels and shadows in the lung fields that do not conform to the normal branching pattern (arborization) of the pulmonary arteries may suggest the presence of these collaterals.
- Rarely these collaterals can also produce rib notching which is common at the site of a previous thoracotomy such as in a BT shunt.
- In patients with very large collaterals, cardiac enlargement may result from the volume overload.

Tetralogy of Fallot with absent pulmonary valve syndrome: This variant of TOF is characterized by aneurysmal dilation of the proximal branch pulmonary arteries that is visible on the chest X-ray. Cardiomegaly is sometimes seen if the overall pulmonary blood flow is increased (**Fig. 18**). Aneurysmal pulmonary arteries lead to compression of bronchi leading to severe respiratory symptoms and early presentation in neonates. The chest X-ray in these patients shows air trapping as well as atelectasis.

The other rare association of TOF is absent left or right PA. This may produce hypoplasia and/or markedly decreased vasculature on the side with absent PA. Rarely one of the pulmonary arteries may arise directly from the aorta, in which case there will be plethoric lung field on the side with ectopic aortic origin of PA.

Here is a list of causes of differential pulmonary blood flow on chest X-ray (**Fig. 19**).

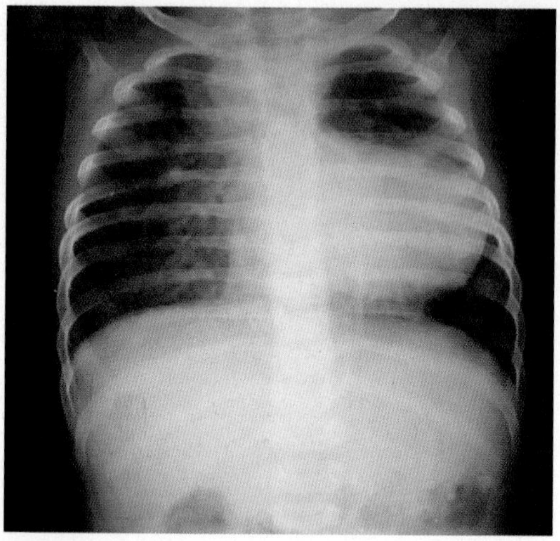

Fig. 19: Chest X-ray frontal view of a child with tetralogy of Fallot showing "boot-shaped" heart and decreased pulmonary blood flow. Main pulmonary artery (MPA) segment is concave (pulmonary bay) due to hypoplastic main pulmonary artery. Also, note differential flow in both lungs due to severe stenosis of left pulmonary artery.

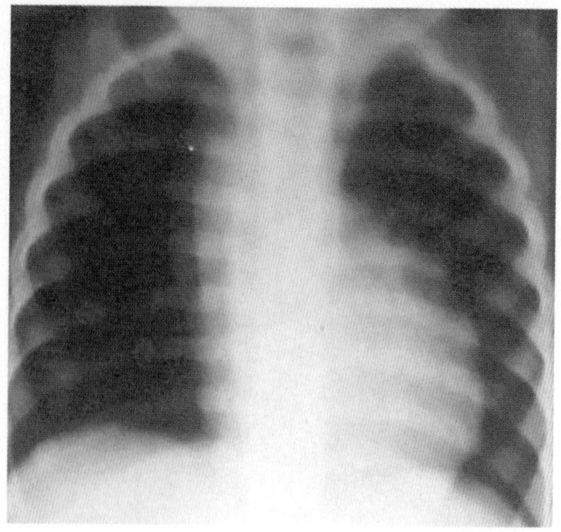

Fig. 20: Chest X-ray frontal view in a 2-year-old child with tricuspid atresia. Showing classical "box-shaped" heart and decreased pulmonary blood flow. Superior vena cava is dilated due to high right atrial pressure.

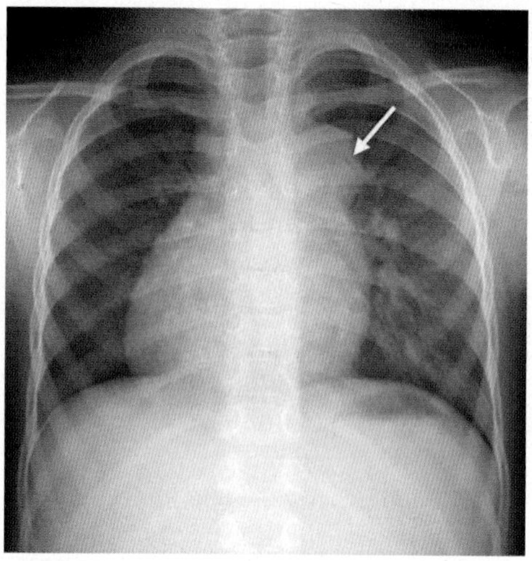

Fig. 21: Chest X-ray frontal view in a child with complex congenital cardiac defect. There is situs solitus, dextrocardia, and L-malposed aorta (marked by arrow). Pulmonary blood flow is reduced.

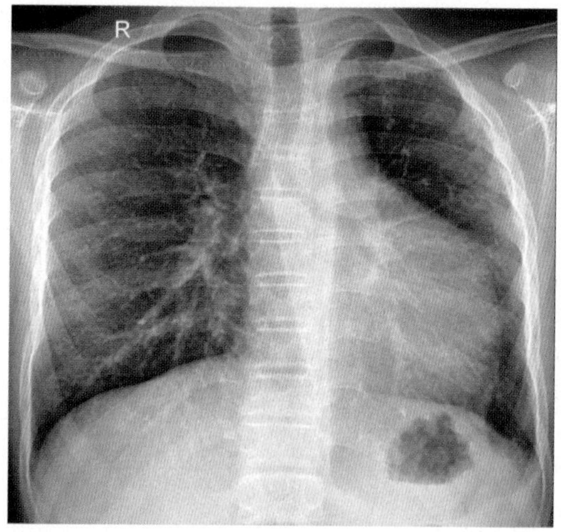

Fig. 22: Chest X-ray frontal view showing straightening of right heart border with prominent shadow at left heart border below MPA area—suggestive of diagnosis of juxtaposed right atrial appendage. Also, notice normal heart size with decreased pulmonary blood flow. This finding should suggest presence of single ventricle physiology with pulmonary stenosis.

- Absence, stenosis, or significant hypoplasia of one PA
- Origin of one branch PA from ascending aorta
- BT shunt or PDA dominantly flowing to one branch PA often with stenosis of the PA to the opposite side
- Major aortopulmonary collaterals to one lung.

Tricuspid atresia with pulmonary stenosis: The heart size is usually normal with left ventricular configuration, straight right heart border (dilated SVC), prominent aorta, and absence of MPA shadow. The lung fields show decreased vascularity (**Fig. 20**). The cardiac shadow in tricuspid atresia has been described as "box-shaped". If interatrial communication is restrictive, the RA and SVC dilate significantly and this becomes apparent on the chest X-ray.

Corrected transposition with VSD and pulmonary stenosis: In corrected transposition, aorta is left and anterior (L-posed) which produces a characteristic X-ray appearance a smooth shoulder on the left heart border due to enlarged left-sided aorta. The heart size is normal and often toward the midline (mesocardia) with decreased pulmonary blood flow (**Fig. 21**). The characteristic shadow of the aorta is seen with all situations with the L-posed aorta.

Univentricular physiology with pulmonary stenosis: There is no specific X-ray pattern that points to the diagnosis of a univentricular heart; the heart size is usually normal with decreased pulmonary blood flow. Associated juxtaposed right atrial appendage may result in lack of right atrial shadow and prominent shadow just below the area of MPA (**Fig. 22**).

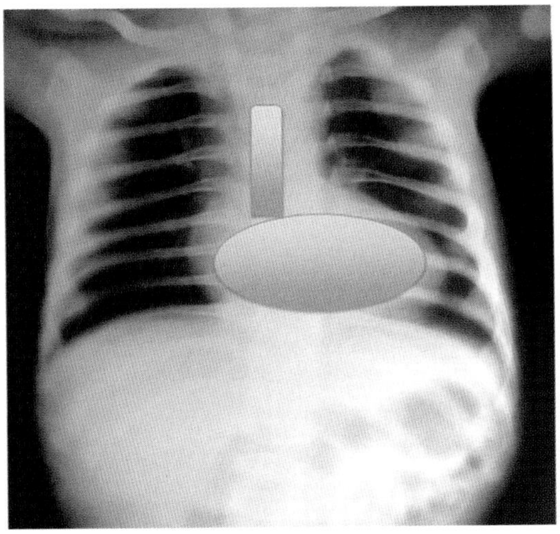

Fig. 23: Chest X-ray frontal view of a 1-month-old infant with complete transposition of great vessels. Note the narrow mediastinum due to malposed great vessels giving "egg on side" appearance.

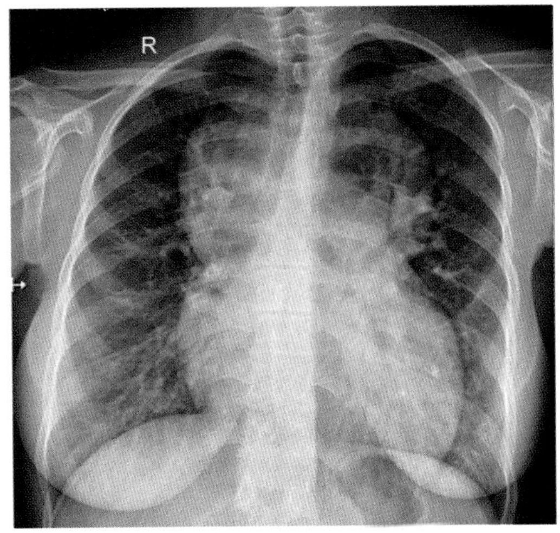

Fig. 24: A 34-year-old patient with supracradic total anomalous pulmonary venous connection (TAPVC). Characteristic "Snowman appearance" or "Figure of 8". Note the prominent upper circle due to aneurysmal dilatation of venous channel and superior vena cava.

Cyanosis with Increased Pulmonary Blood Flow

Transposition of great vessels: Presentation is in neonatal period or early infancy with severe cyanosis. Chest X-ray may show cardiac enlargement, increased pulmonary blood flow, and narrow pedicle giving the typical appearance of "egg on side" **(Fig. 23)**.

TAPVC: The chest X-ray shows cardiomegaly with enlarged right heart chambers and increased pulmonary blood flow. There are some typical X-ray features in TAPVC.

- *Figure of "8" or snow man's appearance*: Seen in older patients with total anomalous pulmonary venous drainage via the left vertical vein to innominate vein (**Fig. 24**). The lower circle is formed by cardiac shadow while upper circle will be formed by dilated left vertical vein on left side, dilated SVC on right and dilated innominate vein superiorly. This pattern is seldom seen in infants.
- *Vertical vein on right (TAPVC to SVC)*: Chest X-ray shows cardiomegaly with increased pulmonary blood flow (as in previous case) along with dilatation of SVC (**Fig. 25**).
- In case of cardiac type TAPVC (to coronary sinus or to RA), chest X-ray will show evidences of large atrial shunt with right atrial enlargement.
- *Obstructed TAPVC*: Presentation is in neonatal period with severe cyanosis and respiratory distress. The chest X-ray is very useful and often enables the diagnosis. The lung fields are diffusely hazy with a ground glass appearance like in hyaline membrane disease. However, the clinical circumstances are quite unlike hyaline membrane disease (**Fig. 26**).

In a neonate with unexplained cyanosis, the characteristic appearance should merit a careful search for obstructed TAPVC. Often this is infracardiac to the portal vein. A high index of suspicion warrants a thorough and meticulous echocardiography to specifically look for TAPVC.

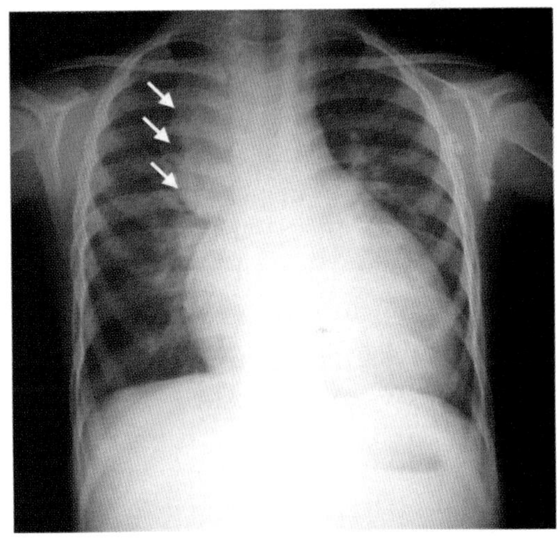

Fig. 25: Another patient with supracardiac total anomalous pulmonary venous connection (TAPVC) to right superior vena cava (SVC). Note the prominent right SVC shadow (arrows) along with cardiomegaly, right atrial (RA) enlargement, and increased pulmonary vasculature.

Persistent truncus arteriosus: The chest X-ray will show cardiomegaly of left ventricular configuration, increased heart size, prominent aorta (truncus), and absence of MPA shadow and increased pulmonary vasculature.

Some cases may show higher shadow of the hilar pulmonary arteries causing the waterfall appearance. In 30–40% cases, a right aortic arch may be seen.[11]

Miscellaneous

Severe Ebstein anomaly of tricuspid valve: The classical features being cardiomegaly with right ventricular configuration and right atrial enlargement. The MPA segment will not be prominent, giving an appearance of pencil sharp outline with decreased pulmonary blood flow (**Fig. 27**).[12] Differential diagnosis to Ebstein anomaly would be large pericardial effusion and dilated cardiomyopathy. In both

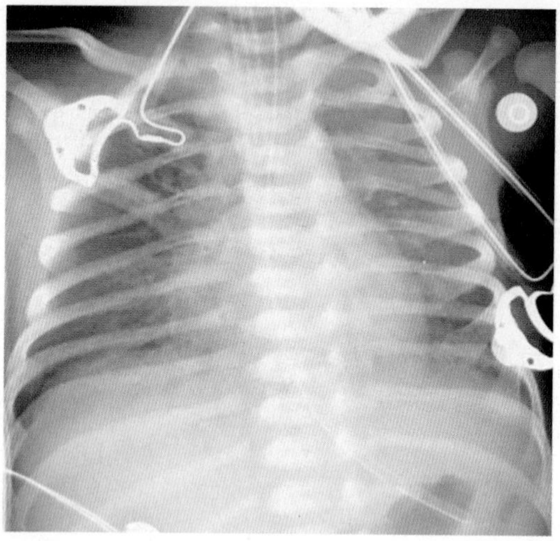

Fig. 26: Chest X-ray frontal view in a 3-day-old neonate with cyanosis, severe respiratory distress. X-ray shows ground glass apperance (pulmonary venous hypertension) of both lungs in obstrructed TAPVC.

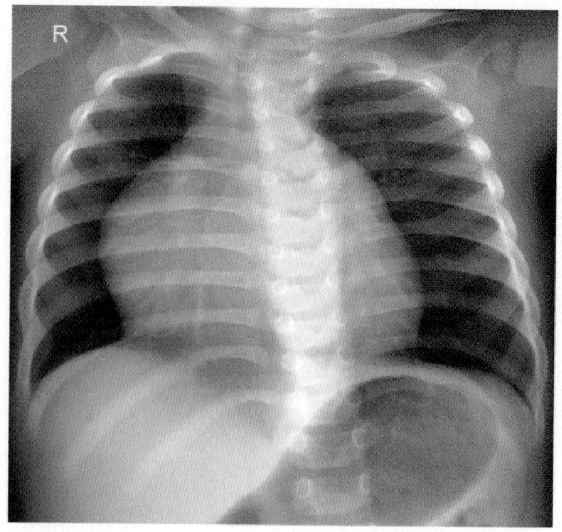

Fig. 27: Typical X-ray chest findings in patient an infant with severe Ebstein anomaly of tricuspid valve showing severe cardiomegaly, absent main pulmonary artery shadow, gross RA enlargement, and diminished pulmonary vascular markings.Infant presented with severe cyanosis (SpO_2 60%).

conditions, pulmonary conus shadow will remain normal. Those with cardiomyopathy will show features of pulmonary venous hypertension.

Pulmonary arteriovenous (AV) malformations and fistulae: Pulmonary AV fistula creates right-to-left shunt from PA to pulmonary veins and is one of the causes of central cyanosis. Fistula(s) can be diffuse or localized involving one or more than one PA branches (also known as a pulmonary AV malformation). It can be unilateral or bilateral. On chest X-ray, cardiac size and configuration are usually normal. Pulmonary AV malformations are suspected when one or more round or lobular opacities are apparent. These are usually peripheral, homogeneous, noncalcified, and well circumscribed. The dilated afferent and efferent vessels may resemble cord-like stalks connecting to the hilum and left atrium (**Fig. 28**).[13,14] In case of diffuse lesions, the chest X-ray may be unremarkable.

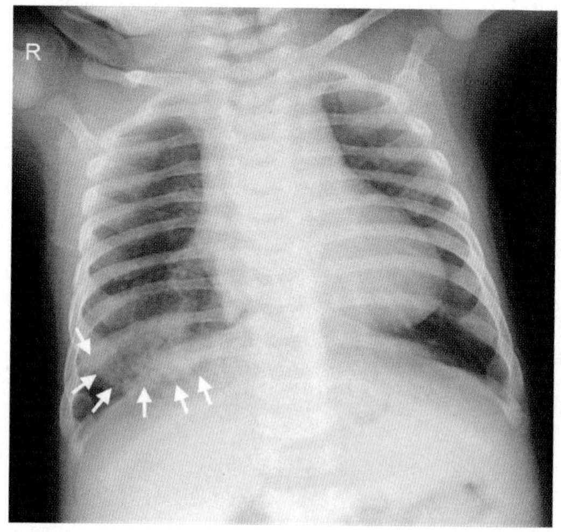

Fig. 28: A 5-month-old baby with severe cyanosis (SpO_2 55%). Chest X-ray shows normal sized heart, homogenous shadow in right lower zone (marked by arrows) with pulmonary arteriovenous fistula (multiple fistula from lower branch of right lower pulmonary artery).

LUNG PARENCHYMA AND THORAX (BONY AND SOFT TISSUE STRUCTURES)

One should always look at the lung parenchyma (collapse/consolidation/pneumothorax/pleural effusion/lung mass, etc.) and bony structures (ribs/spine/sternum) in detail. A checklist for assessment of extracardiac structures while looking at a chest X-ray is presented further:

- *Ribs*:
  - *Numbers*: 11 ribs/floating ribs in Down syndrome
  - *Rib fracture*: Accidental trauma and post-thoracotomy
  - Rib crowding as a result of lung hypoplasia or spinal deformity
  - *Rib notching*: *Causes*:
    - Coarctation of aorta, BT shunt, collaterals, and neurofibromatosis
- *Sternum*:
  - *Sternal hypoplasia*: Syndromic association
  - Pectus excavatum - Marfan syndrome and mitral valve prolapse (lateral view)
- *Spine*: It is very important to look for spine and comment. Bony deformity may cause difficulty in anaesthesia during cardiac surgical intervention. Extreme degree of spine deformities will limit lung capacity and may require specific intervention.
  - *Scoliosis (frontal view)*: The incidence is as high as 66% in grown-up cyanotic heart disease and 20% in acyanotic CHDs. Also, seen with Marfan syndrome and other musculoskeletal disorders.[3]
  - *Kyphosis and straight back syndrome (lateral view)*: A thoracic deformity characterized by normal loss of kyphosis of upper thoracic spine. This leads to reduced anteroposterior diameter of chest causing

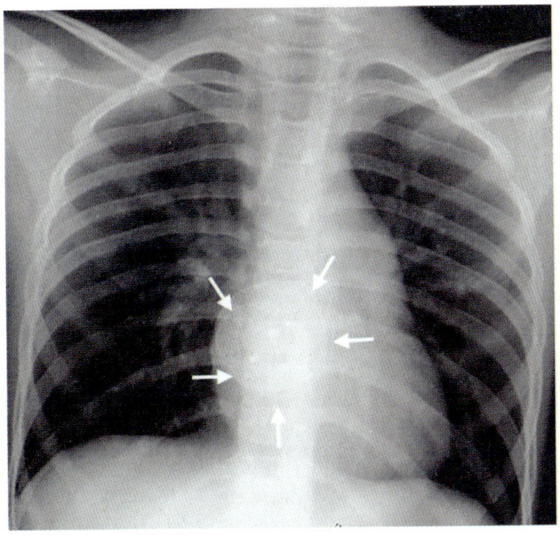

Fig. 29: Chest X-ray frontal view in a child postdevice closure of atrial septal defect. Device marked by arrows.

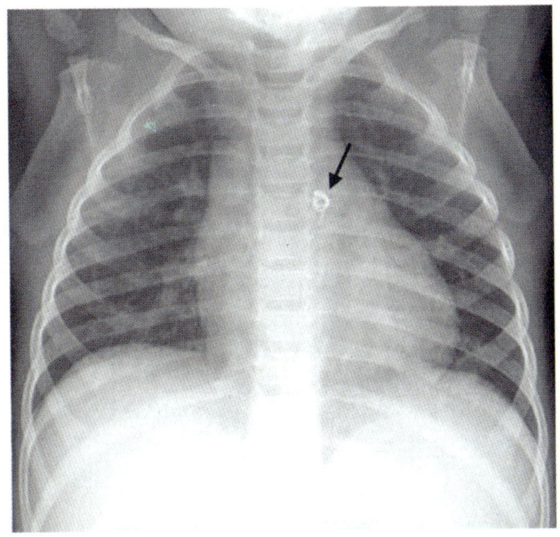

Fig. 30: Chest X-ray frontal view in child postcoil closure of PDA. PDA coil is marked by arrow.

compression of heart and great vessels. Cardiac shadow appears larger giving impression of cardiomegaly. Straight back syndrome has an association with mitral valve prolapse.

- *Previous surgery*: A sternotomy is often identified by metallic sternal wires.
- *Hypoplastic lung*:
    - Scimitar syndrome
    - Congenital bronchial agenesis
    - Chronic hypoperfusion.

CHEST X-RAY POSTCARDIAC SURGERY OR INTERVENTION

Chest X-ray is of vital importance in postsurgical period for the evaluation of the lungs and pleura as lung collapse, consolidation, atelectasis, pneumothorax, and pleural effusion are all common in this setting. The X-ray enables identification of endotracheal tube position, intracardiac lines, pacemaker wires, position of occlusive devices, and stents (**Figs. 29 and 30**).

Following removal of chest tubes and pacing wires, it is mandatory to get an X-ray done as there in chance of accumulation of air or blood in the pleural or pericardial spaces (**Fig. 31**).

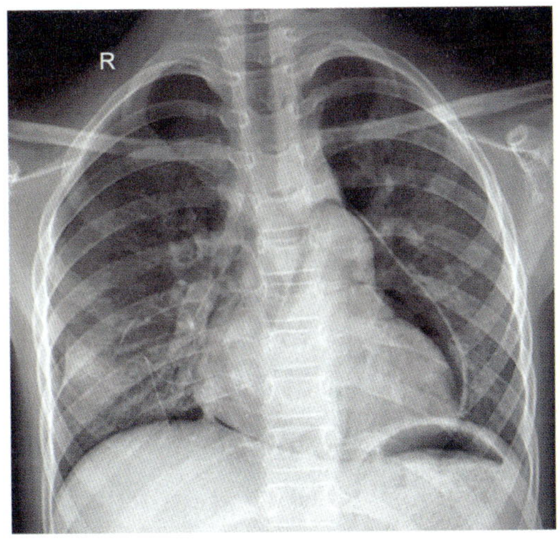

Fig. 31: Chest X-ray frontal view in child postsurgical closure of atrial septal defect. Postopen heart surgery pacing wires were put. Pacing wires were removed on 5th postoperative day. Chest X-ray shows pneumopericardium after removal of pacing wire.

CONCLUSION

- Radiological examination comes handy, particularly when other investigations like echocardiography are not available. However, radiology must not be considered for diagnosis in isolation.
- Cardiac anomalies impart significant changes on the chest X-ray in a number of structural and functional abnormalities.
- The chest X-ray provides an independent perspective on enlargement of the heart and its chambers, pulmonary vascularity, pulmonary venous hypertension, lung parenchyma, mediastinum and bony cage.
- X- ray chest when assessed after a careful clinical evaluation provides important clues required for management in a secondary care set-up.
- The purpose is not to arrive at a precise diagnosis of the underlying heart disease but to ensure that those features that are of independent value in a chest X-ray are correctly identified.

REFERENCES

1. Amplatz K, Molles JH, Castenda-Zuniga WR. Radiology of congenital heart disease, Volume 1. New York: Thieme Medical Publishers; 1986.
2. Hulett RL, Ovitt TW. The chest roentgenogram In: Allen HD, Gutgesell HP, Ckark EB, Driscoll DJ, (Eds). Moss and Adams' Heart Disease in Infant, Children, and Adolescent, 6th edition: Lippincott Williams & Wilkins, 2001:162-70.

3. Elliot LP. Pulmonary vascularity on the plain chest radiograph. Cardiology Clinics. 1983;1(4): 545-64.
4. Hegde M, Vijayalakshmi IB. Role of radiography in congenital heart diseases In: Vijayalakshmi IB, Rao S, Chugh R, (Eds). A Comprehensive Approach to Congenital Heart Diseases, 1st edition. New Delhi: Jaypee Brothers Medical Publishers (P) Ltd; 2013. pp. 190-202.
5. Coussement AM, Gooding CA. Objective radiographic assessment of pulmonary vascularity in children. Radiology. 1973;109(3): 649-54.
6. Kaplan S. Clinical and hemodyanamic basis of the roentgenographic findings in left to right shunting. Semin Roentgenol. 1966;1(1):34-46.
7. Freedom RM, Yoo S, Coles GJ, Konstantinov I. Ventricular septal defect In: Freedom RM, Yoo S, Mikailian H, Williams WG, (Eds). The Natural History and Modified History of Congenital Heart Disease, 1st edition. Hoboken: Blackwell Publishing; 2004. pp. 16-30.
8. Batson GA, Urquhart W, Sideris DA. Radiological features in aortic stenosis. Clin Radiol. 1972;23(2):140-4.
9. Tonkin IL. Coarcation of the aorta. In: Theros EG, Colley RN, Capp MP, et al. (Eds). Plain Film Diagnosis of Cardiovascular Disease Syllabus. Chicago: American College of Radiology; 1979. pp. 260-71.
10. Wilson WJ, Amplatz K. Unequal vascularity in tetralogy of Fallot. Am J Roentgenol Radium Ther Nucl Med. 1967;100(2):318-21.
11. Hoeffel JC, Mounton JN, Worms AM, Pernot C. Radiological patterns of truncus arteriosus in plain roentgenography. ROFO. 1981;135(6):686-91.
12. Amplatz K, Lester RG, Schiebler GL, Adams P, Jr Anderson RC. The roengenographic features of Ebstein anomaly of the tricuspid valve. Am J Roentgenol Radium Ther Nucl Med. 1959;81:788-94.
13. Quero Jimenez M, Acerete Guillen F. Arteriovenous fistulas. In: Adams FH, Emmanouilides GC, Riemenshneider TA, (Eds). Moss' Heart Disease in Infant, Children, and Adolescent, 4th edition. Baltimore: Williams & Wilkins; 1989. pp. 617-26.
14. Chilvers ER. Clinical and physiologic aspects of pulmonary arteriovenous malformations. Br J Hosp Med. 1988;39(3): 188-92.

CHAPTER 9

Echocardiography: What Pediatricians Should Know?

Praveen Kumar K, Sunita Maheshwari, Sejal Shah

INTRODUCTION

India has an enormous burden of pediatric cardiac disease—both congenital and acquired. Limited human resources as well as financial constraints pose considerable challenge to the field. As pediatricians, clinical history, examination, and investigations such as chest X-ray, and electrocardiogram (ECG) form the basis for suspecting heart disease and narrowing down the differentials, *echocardiography* is currently the primary diagnostic modality for congenital heart disease. It is also the invaluable first step for planning surgery/intervention as well as to assess adequacy of treatment. Pediatricians with echocardiographic skills can help balance the lack of human resources, at least from a diagnostic perspective. Additional knowledge of echocardiogram would also turn out to be valuable for day-to-day bedside management of children with heart disease, more so when pediatric cardiac support is not available. This chapter will discuss "Echocardiography" from "A to Z" to enable the pediatricians to help diagnosing heart disease better.

INTRODUCTION TO ECHOCARDIOGRAPHY

Echocardiogram Machine: Principle, How to Use, and Probe Selection

Echocardiography or cardiac ultrasound uses high-frequency sound waves to produce a real-time image of the heart. It provides detailed anatomic and physiologic information about the heart. Following are few terminologies commonly used while handling the echocardiography machine (**Figs. 1A and B**).

- *Frequency*: Sound waves are mechanical vibrations that are described in terms of frequency. The number of vibrations per unit time is called frequency, which is expressed in Hertz, 1 Hz = 1 vibration per second. The ability of ultrasound waves to penetrate human tissue is inversely proportionate to the frequency of transmitted waves. In pediatric and neonatal settings, the imaging frequency ranges between 4 and 12 MHz. The higher the frequency, the better is the resolution but lesser is the penetration. Hence, higher frequency probe is used for neonates and lower frequency for adults. For Doppler

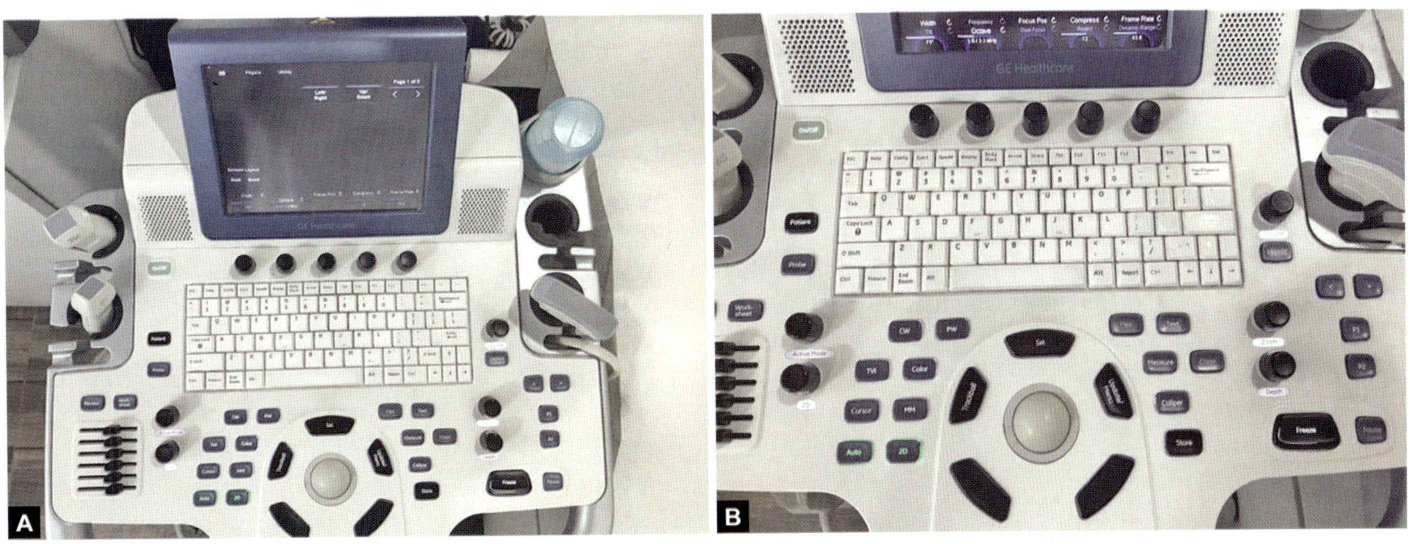

Figs. 1A and B: Echocardiogram machine panel showing important knobs namely width, compression, frame rate, and focus position.

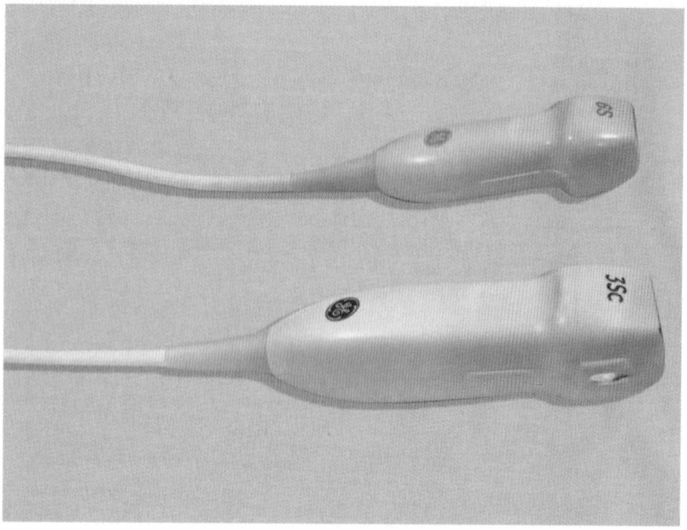

Fig. 2: Common probes used in pediatric echocardiography. 6S probe is of higher frequency, hence has poor penetration and better resolution. 3Sc probe is of low frequency, hence has better penetration.

and color flow mapping, lower frequency provides better information (**Fig. 2**).

- *Grayscale*: It reflects the different amplitudes detected by the ultrasound imaging system. High-amplitude signals are usually bright, low-amplitude signals are dark gray and when there is no signal, it will be black. In the machine, there will be different grayscale and color B mode settings preloaded which can be used for better image quality depending on the patient.
  Dynamic range is used to increase or decrease the gray shades displayed on B mode.
- *Depth and sector*: Depth allows to adjust the size of the image on the screen and sector indicates the scan area width. Depth and sector both influence the frame rate. The higher the frame rate, the greater the resolution and the lesser the penetration.
- *Gain and time gain composition (TGC)*: Gain regulates the overall brightness of the image. TGC helps to increase or decrease the brightness at different depth level.
- *Zoom*: There are two types of zoom: Preprocessing and postprocessing. Preprocessing zoom can be used to image region of interest (ROI) in a live image without affecting the number of pixels displayed, with a better image resolution and can increase the frame rate. In postprocessing zoom, the image is frozen and the ROI can be selected and zoomed which results in simple magnification of the anatomic structure and the image resolution may be tampered.
- *Focus*: Focus improves image quality in the focal area.
- *Frame rate*: The higher the frame rates, the better the temporal resolution. Frame rate can be increased by decreasing the depth, narrowing the sector width, or using live zoom.
- *Doppler*: In ultrasound, Doppler is used to detect moving structures or blood cells and measure their direction and speed. Doppler effect is used to measure the change in frequency of echoes reflected from the moving structure. In cardiac ultrasound, three types of Doppler are used: color Doppler, spectral Doppler, and tissue Doppler. In color Doppler, the array of color is combined with the standard B mode picture of a blood vessel or a cardiac chamber to show the speed and direction of blood flow. Flow that is moving away from the transducer is blue and the flow that is moving toward the transducer is red. Spectral Doppler (pulsed wave—PW and continuous wave—CW) displays graphically the blood flow measurements through flow velocities and time. PW Doppler is used to obtain velocity information for low-velocity flows at a specific location in the heart or blood vessel. With CW Doppler, we can interrogate higher velocities. However, we cannot determine the location of maximal velocity along the line of ultrasound beam. When we are using the PW or CW Doppler, we can further adjust the Doppler gain, velocity, sample volume, speed, and the wall filter in order to receive the correct information. Tissue Doppler is used to measure the velocity of myocardial motion.

Image Optimization

The quality of an image does depend on the skill of the operator, the settings in the echocardiogram machine, and the body habitus of the patient. Turning the patient to left lateral position for chest views or flexing the knees for relaxing the abdominal muscles and working the parameters described above like selection of an ideal probe or adjusting the focus would help in improving the image quality.

Preparation of Patient

Pediatric echocardiography is a challenging proposition. First, there can be innumerable permutations and combinations of abnormalities in all the anatomical segments of the heart. A complete study is needed so as none of the abnormalities are missed. Second, the patient should be still during the study. Sedation as per hospital protocol will be needed for those who are unable to co-operate. Toys, games, and videos could be used for older kids. Parents should be allowed to accompany the child during the entire course of examination.

Patient should be placed in resting position with comfortable environment. The gel should be warmed to the patient body temperature before the starting of examination. During intensive care unit (ICU) echocardiograms, vitals should be monitored continuously, and focused echocardiography rather than a comprehensive study should be considered.

BASIC VIEWS AND SEQUENTIAL SEGMENTAL APPROACH: THE STRUCTURAL ASSESSMENT

Building Blocks: Recognition of Structures

This section will explain how to recognize different cardiac structures while performing an echocardiogram. A cardiac chamber is not diagnosed based on its position but based on its anatomical features, e.g., right ventricle (RV) is not so as it is on the right side but is decided based on the unique right ventricular morphological features. Based on this understanding, step by step, the connections inside the heart are understood and the final diagnosis is made. It starts with the visceral situs and ends with the great arteries.

- *Abdominal visceral situs*: Solitus is a normal arrangement where the spleen and stomach are on the left side and liver is on the right side (**Figs. 3A and B**). Inversus is exactly the mirror image of solitus where the stomach and spleen are on the right side and liver on the left side. Ambiguous situs is where situs cannot be defined, e.g., liver is in the midline.
- *Cardiac position*: Levocardia is where the heart is positioned predominantly in the left hemithorax and the apex can be seen pointing to the left side (**Fig. 4**). Dextrocardia is where the heart is positioned predominantly in the right hemithorax with apex pointing to the right side.

  Mesocardia is a midline heart with equal proportion of cardiac masses on each side of the sternum and the apex pointing either anteriorly or inferiorly.
- *Atrial situs*: Solitus is when the morphological right atrium (MRA) is on the right side of morphological left atrium (MLA) (**Figs. 5 and 6**). Inversus is when the MRA is on the left side of MLA. Ambiguous is when we cannot determine which is the morphological right or left atrium.

Morphological right atrium has a broad-based, triangular-shaped anterior appendage. Septum secundum has the limbus of fossa ovalis on the right atrial wall. Right atrium (RA) receives inferior vena cava (IVC), superior vena cava (SVC), and coronary sinus (CS) into it and has Eustachian valve and crista terminalis.

Morphological left atrium receives all four pulmonary veins. It has a long narrow (finger-like) posterior appendage and the primum septum with foramen ovale valve flap on its side.

- *Ventricular loop*: D-loop is in normal hearts where morphological right ventricle (MRV) is on the right side and morphological left ventricle (MLV) is on the left side. L-loop is when MRV is on the left side and MLV is on the right side.

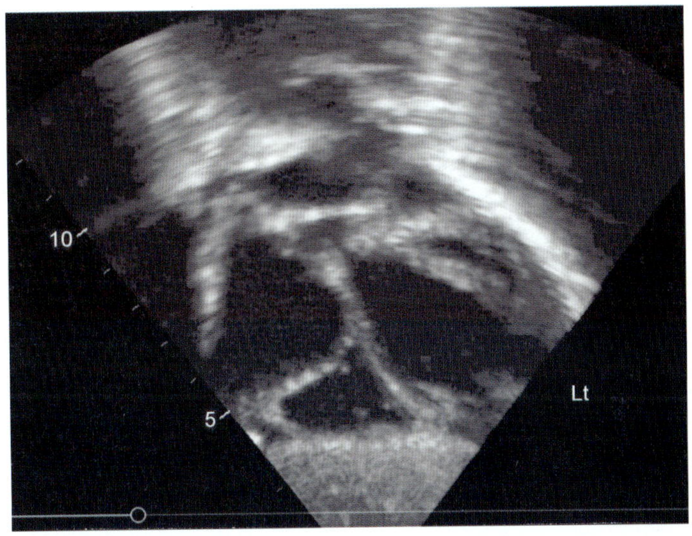

Fig. 4: Subcostal coronal view showing the cardiac apex pointing toward the left side of the patient suggesting the cardiac position to be levocardia.
(Lt: left)

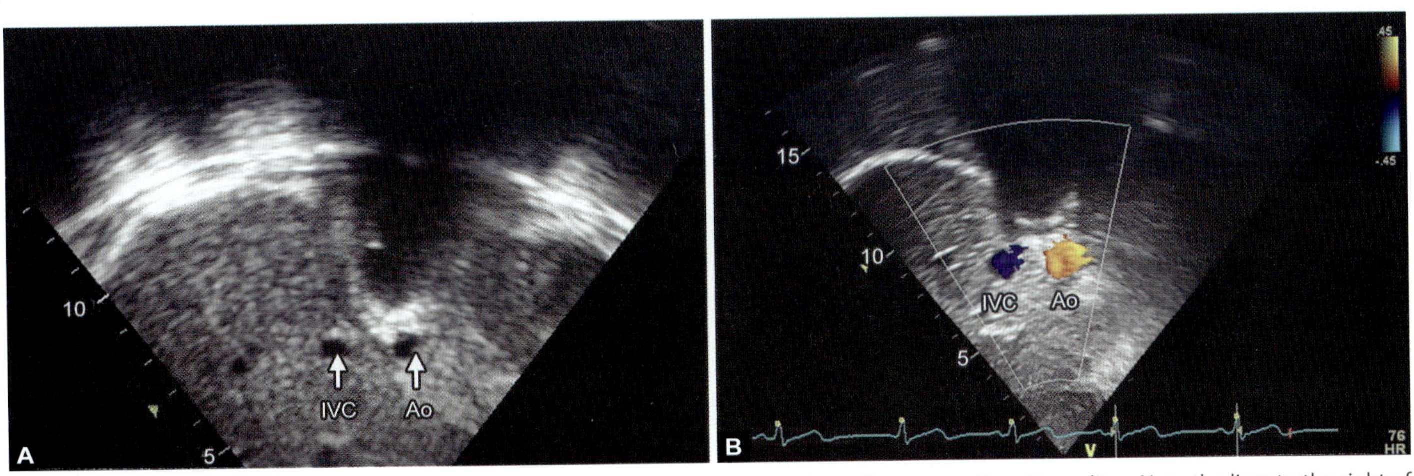

Figs. 3A and B: Subcostal view with aorta to the left of midline and IVC to the right midline suggesting situs solitus. Note the liver to the right of midline. Figure B shows the color Doppler in IVC and aorta. IVC is showing blue color as the flow is away from the probe, aorta is showing red color as the flow is toward the probe.
(Ao: aorta; IVC: inferior vena cava)

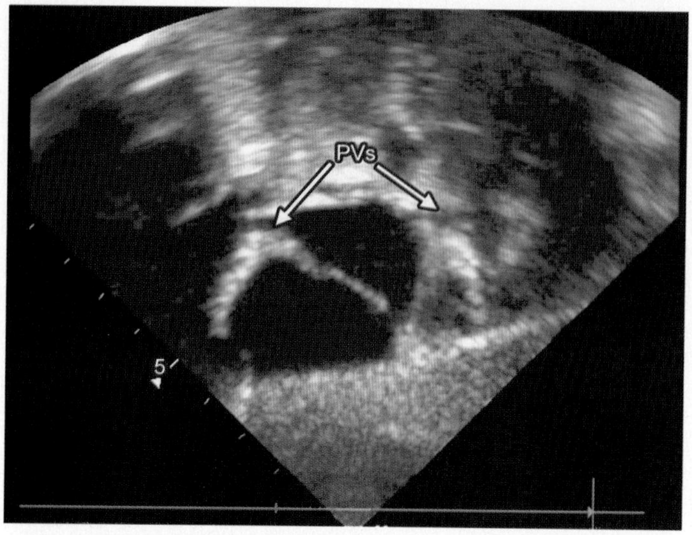

Fig. 5: Subcostal coronal view with pulmonary veins on two-dimensional (2D) into left sided atrium suggesting the possibility of atrial situs solitus.
(PVs: pulmonary veins)

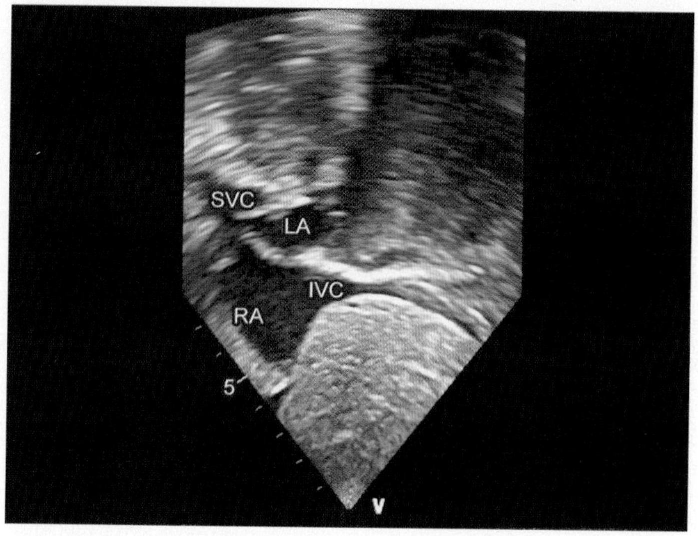

Fig. 6: Subcostal sagittal view showing atrial situs solitus with SVC and IVC draining into the right atrium.
(IVC: inferior vena cava; LA: left atrium; RA: right atrium SVC: superior vena cava)

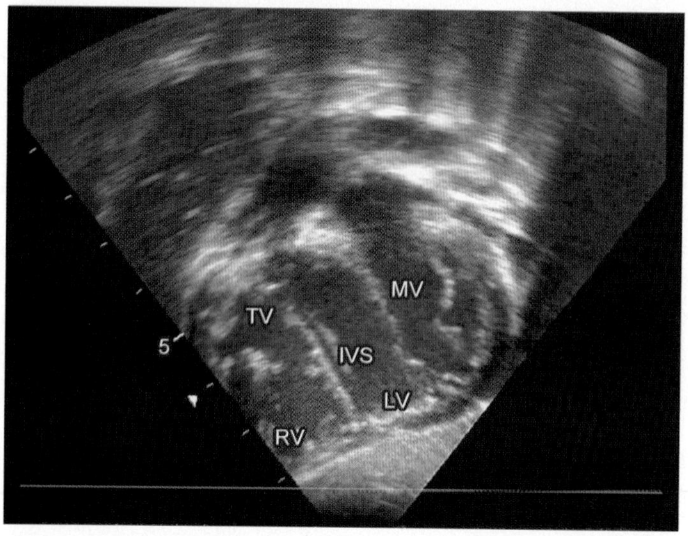

Fig. 7: Subcostal coronal view showing the mitral valve away from the septum, tricuspid valve closer to the septum, the morphological right ventricle on the right of morphological left ventricle suggestive of d-looped ventricles.
(IVS: interventricular septum; LV: left ventricle, MV: mitral valve, RV: right ventricle, TV: tricuspid valve).

Morphological right ventricle is triangular externally. Internally, RV is characterized by distinct septal surface including septal and moderator band and an infundibulum. The atrioventricular valves always go with the ventricles. The tricuspid valve (TV) leaflets have septal attachments (septophilic) and TV has a triangular orifice.

Morphological left ventricle is cone-shaped externally. Left ventricle (LV) has smooth and fine apical trabeculations and has aortomitral continuity. The mitral valve leaflets have attachment to LV free wall (septophobic), have two distinct papillary muscle, and the mitral valve orifice is elliptical (**Fig. 7**). The TV leaflets are attached more apically than the mitral valve leaflets to the interventricular septum (IVS).

- *Atrioventricular connections*: Concordance is normal connection wherein the MRA is connected to the MRV and MLA is connected to MLV. Discordance is when MRA is connected to MLV and MLA is connected to MRV. Other abnormalities include atresia of one of the atrioventricular valves, double-inlet LV, straddling of atrioventricular valve, etc.
- *Ventriculoarterial connections*: Concordance is where the aorta is connected to the MLV and pulmonary artery (PA) is connected to the MRV. Discordance is where aorta is connected to the MRV and PA is connected to the MLV. Examples of ventriculoarterial connection abnormalities include transposition of great arteries (TGA), double-outlet RV, etc.
- *Great artery relationship*: Normally, related great arteries are when aorta is right and posterior and pulmonary artery is left and anterior (**Fig. 8**). D-malposed great arteries are when aorta is right and anterior and PA left and posterior. L-malposed great arteries when aorta is left and anterior and PA right and posterior.

Views

Pediatric echocardiogram is done from the subcostal, apical, parasternal, and suprasternal views. It is advisable to start from the subcostal view. This view is expected to give most of the information in children. Most of the views have two planes and a complete sweep of the transducer needs to be done in each plane, on two-dimensional (2D), and on color.

Subcostal View

- The transducer is placed in the subxiphoid region.
  - Coronal plane (longitudinal view) (**Fig. 9A**):
    - The pointer is toward 3 o'clock position

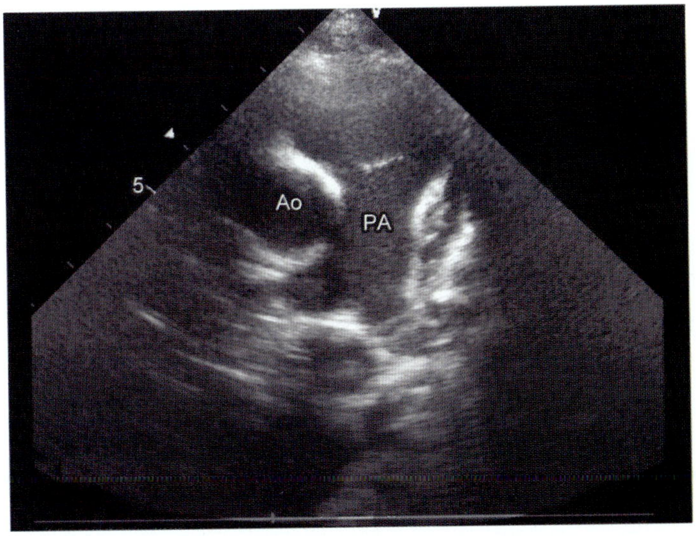

Fig. 8: Pulmonary artery (PA) is left and anterior to aorta (Ao) in a normal heart which is shown in the parasternal short axis view.

- Sweep the transducer from posterior to anterior and then again anterior to posterior
- Orientation of structures is:
  - *Top*: Superior and Bottom: Inferior
  - *Left side of the screen*: Left-sided structures: Right side of the screen: right-sided structures

Structures visualized in coronal plane (see **Fig. 7***)*: Visceral situs, cardiac position and base apex axis of the heart, IVC and hepatic veins and right SVC entry to RA, interatrial septum, selected pulmonary veins entering the left atrium (LA), mitral valve papillary muscles and its attachment to left ventricular free wall, TV and its attachment to the septum, LV and its outflow tract, and RV and its outflow tract.

- Sagittal plane (short axis view):
  - The probe is rotated clockwise from the coronal plane and the pointer is toward 6 o'clock position (**Fig. 9B**).
  - Sweep the transducer from the left side to the right side and then from the right side to the left side.
  - Orientation of the structures is:
    - *Top*: Superior and Bottom: Inferior
    - *Left side of the screen is*: Posterior structures, right side of the screen: anterior structures

Structures visualized (see **Fig. 6***)*: IVC-RA junction, IVC and SVC entering to RA, interatrial septum, selective pulmonary veins draining to LA, right atrial appendage, Eustachian valve, mitral valve, TV, papillary muscles, interventricular septum, right ventricular outflow tract (RVOT), left ventricular outflow tract (LVOT), and descending abdominal aorta.

Apical View

- The transducer is in 4th to 5th intercostal space midclavicular line or at the point of maximal impulse (**Fig. 10**). Sweep from anterior to posterior and posterior to anterior.

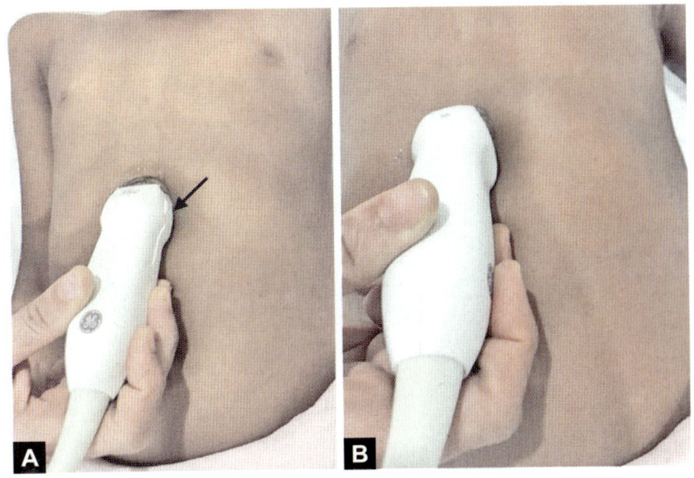

Figs. 9A and B: Probe position and the cursor position for subcostal coronal (A) and sagittal (B) views. Note that the cursor or the pointer (shown by an arrow) is facing the left side in the coronal view and toward the umbilicus in the sagittal view.

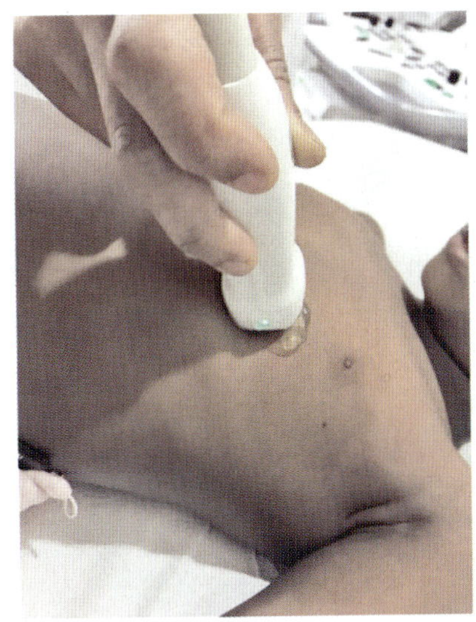

Fig. 10: For the apical view, the probe is positioned at the apex with the pointer toward the left side of the patient.

- Orientation:
  - *Top*: Superior and Bottom: Base/inferior
  - *Left side of the screen*: left-sided structures, right side of the screen: right-sided structures

*Visualized structures (***Fig. 11***)*: RA, TV and its septal attachment, interventricular septum, interatrial septum, RV, moderator band, RVOT (infundibulum), pulmonary valve and main PA, LA, mitral valve and its leaflets attachment to left ventricular free wall, papillary muscles, LVOT, aortic valve and its proximal root, CS, and descending aorta behind the LA.

Parasternal View

- *Long axis*: The transducer is placed on the upper to mid-left sternal border with the transducer notch toward the right shoulder (10–11 o'clock) (**Fig. 12A**).

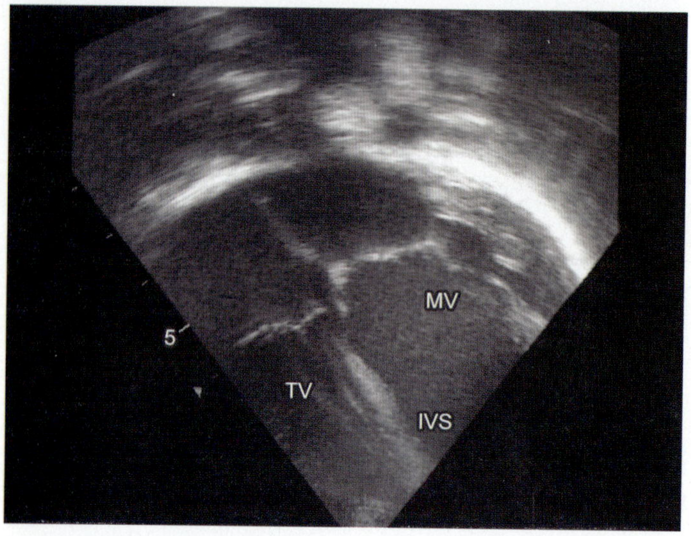

Fig. 11: Apical four-chamber view showing the atrioventricular valves with its differential insertion pattern.
(IVS: interventricular septum; MV: mitral valve; TV: tricuspid valve)

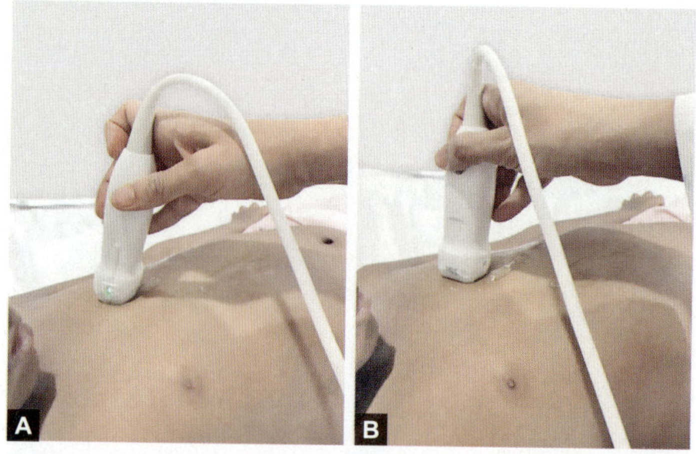

Figs. 12A and B: Probe position in the parasternal views. (A) The position of the cursor toward the right shoulder for the long axis view; (B) The position of the cursor toward the left shoulder for the short axis view.

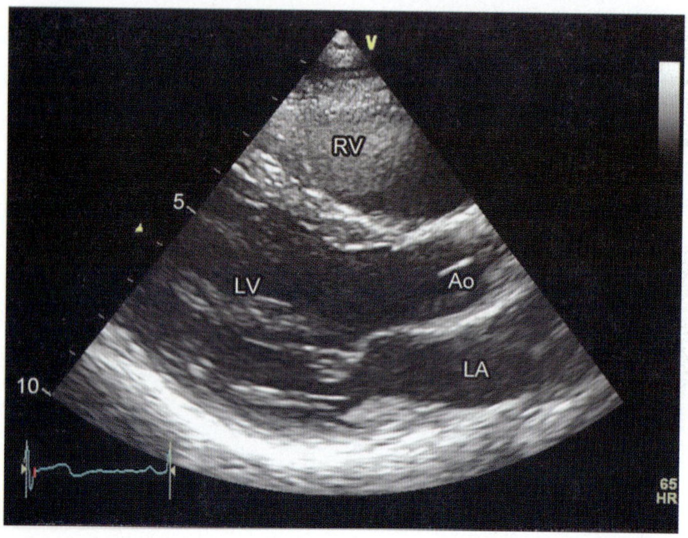

Fig. 13: Parasternal long axis view showing the aortomitral continuity. The left atrium, the left ventricle, and the aorta can be seen together in one image. The interventricular septum can be seen between the left and the right ventricles.
(Ao: aorta; LA: left atrium; LV: left ventricle; RV: right ventricle)

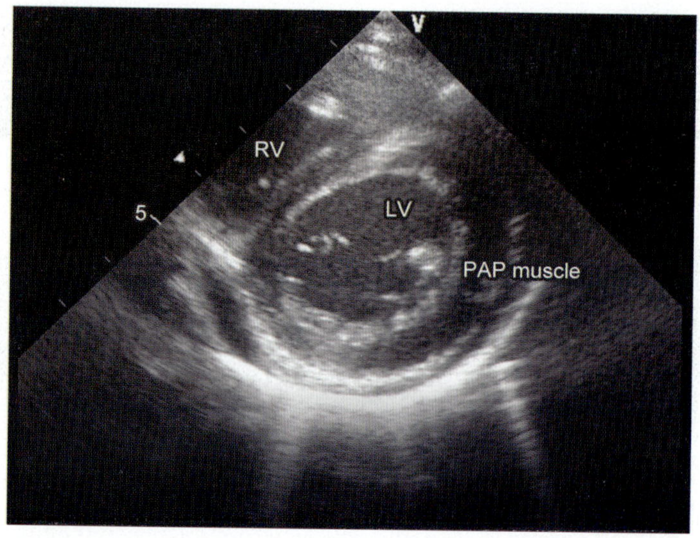

Fig. 14: Parasternal short axis view showing the left and the right ventricles. The left ventricle has characteristically two papillary muscles.
(LV: left ventricle; Pap muscle: papillary muscle; RV: right ventricle).

- Sweep is from posterior to anterior and anterior to posterior (and from right to left and left to right).
- Orientation:
  - *Top*: Anterior and Bottom: Posterior
  - Right side is more inferior and apical, left side is more posterior and basal (right-sided structures are more toward the left side, left-sided structures are more toward the right side).

*Structures visualized (**Fig. 13**)*: LA, mitral valve, LV, LVOT, aortic valve, aortic sinus, sinotubular junction, ascending aorta, interventricular septum, RV and its free wall, descending aorta, CS, TV and RA, pulmonary valve, main PA, and IVC.

- *Short axis view*: The transducer is rotated clockwise from parasternal long axis view (almost by 90°) with the pointer toward the left shoulder (**Fig. 12B**).
  - Sweeping from base of the heart to apex of the heart and apex to base
  - Orientation:
    - *Top*: Anterior and Bottom: Posterior
    - Right side of the screen is right-sided structures, left side of the screen is left-sided structures.

*Structures seen (**Fig. 14**)*: While sweeping toward the apex of the heart: Mitral valve, ventricular septum, LV, RV, papillary muscles, and regional and global function.

While sweeping toward the base of the heart (aortic short axis view): LA, IVC, RA, interatrial septum, pulmonary veins, TV, RVOT, ventricular septum, aortic valve leaflets, pulmonary valve leaflets, coronary arteries, main PA and branch pulmonary arteries, and descending aorta.

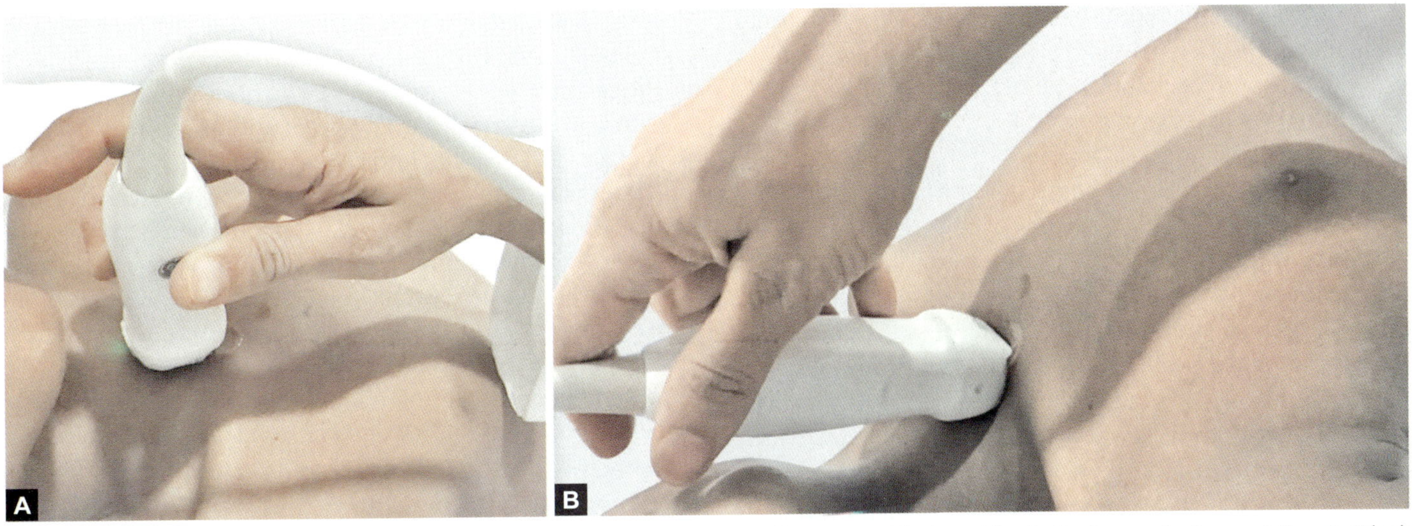

Figs. 15A and B: Probe position in the suprasternal notch. The cursor is placed facing 12 o'clock position in the long axis view and then 3 o'clock position in the short axis view.

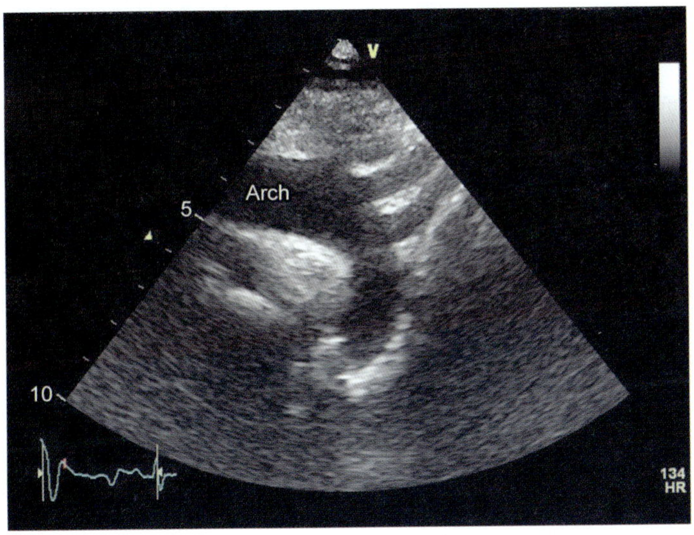

Fig. 16: Suprasternal long axis view showing arch and its vessels. Note the right pulmonary artery seen under the arch.

Suprasternal View

- *Long axis view*: Transducer is kept in the suprasternal notch with cursor at 12 o'clock position (**Fig. 15A**).
  - Sweep is from left to right and right to left
  - Orientation:
    - *Top*: Superior and Bottom: Inferior
    - Right-sided structures on right of the patient, left-sided structures on the left of the patient

Structures visualized (***Fig. 16***): Aortic arch and its sidedness, isthmus, descending aorta, right and left pulmonary arteries, right innominate, left common carotid and left subclavian arteries, and right SVC.

Short Axis View (Crab View)

- Short axis view is obtained by rotating the transducer by 90° so that the cursor is at 3 o'clock position (**Fig. 15B**).
- Sweep is from neutral to posterior and posterior to neutral.
- Orientation:
  - *Top*: Anterior and Bottom: Posterior
  - Left-sided structures on patient's left, right-sided structures on patient's right.

Structures visualized: SVC, LA, pulmonary veins, aorta, and main and branch pulmonary arteries.

FUNCTIONAL ECHOCARDIOGRAPHY: ASSESSMENT OF SYSTOLIC AND DIASTOLIC FUNCTION

Use of point-of-care echocardiography has been gaining interest among the neonatologists, intensivists, and pediatricians. The structural and the hemodynamic information gathered from echocardiography helps in taking crucial decisions like the amount of fluid to be given, the type of inotrope to be used, to start a pulmonary vasodilator, and need for higher pediatric cardiac care. Echocardiogram also has the advantage of providing longitudinal functional assessment, which helps in monitoring the progress of the baby. This investigation modality should be used in addition to the basic tools available like taking a detailed history, performing a complete clinical examination, and should not be a replacement for the clinical parameters. In order to ensure optimum utilization of this diagnostic tool, it is important to be clear with the basic views, the interpretation of structures seen, and what is abnormal.

With better ultrasound technology, we have much superior portable machines available. In order to ensure that this technology is used in a judicious way, it is important to have in-depth training about the use and limitations of bedside echocardiogram, the basic hemodynamic and most important to use it with a "problem-oriented approach."

A few requirements for bedside functional echocardiogram include:

- An ultrasound machine with 2D, PW, and CW Doppler and color flow mapping
- Cardiac preset in the machine
- ECG gating to decide the phase of cardiac cycle—systole or diastole
- Storage system to evaluate the images in the future.

The major goals of functional echocardiogram include an understanding of the cardiac anatomy, check the direction of blood flow across the physiological shunts, estimate pressure gradients across the valves/vessels/shunts, estimate the filling pressure and PA pressure, to rule out vegetation/thrombus and pericardial effusion, and quantify systolic-diastolic function. This information is gathered by 2D, M-mode, and Doppler techniques. This chapter will provide an overview of the basics for ventricular function assessment, which can be applied bedside in clinical practice.

Assessment of Left Ventricular Systolic Function

The common parameters used to assess left ventricular function are fractional shortening (FS) and ejection fraction (EF). FS is obtained from M-mode of the LV in parasternal long/short axis views (**Fig. 17**). EF can be obtained from M-mode of the LV in parasternal long/short axis or by biplane measurement of left ventricular volumes by Modified Simpson's method in apical four chamber and modified two chamber views. In this method, the endocardial border of LV is manually traced at end-diastole and end-systole. Any change in the geometry of the LV will affect the FS and EF. FS and EF are also affected by preload and afterload conditions.

Although the biplane Simpson's method is more accurate, M-mode is routinely used to calculate EF in most pediatric echo laboratories. Left ventricular EF is classically calculated based on the left ventricular dimensions, which are measured on M-mode of LV in parasternal long axis or short axis views. The cursor of the M-mode is placed perpendicular to the interventricular septum and the posterior wall at the level of the posterior mitral valve leaflet (**Fig. 17**). Ideally, the end-diastolic measurement of LV needs to be done at the "R" wave on ECG and end-systolic measurement at the end of "T" wave on ECG. However, for quicker results, the maximum and minimum ventricular diameters can be taken. For accurate measurements, the leading edge – to leading edge technique should be used. For individual cardiac dimensions, the values need to be indexed to the body surface area as the size changes with age in children and these values need to be expressed as Z scores. On 2D echocardiogram, eyeballing can give an approximate idea of left ventricular function before M-mode is taken.

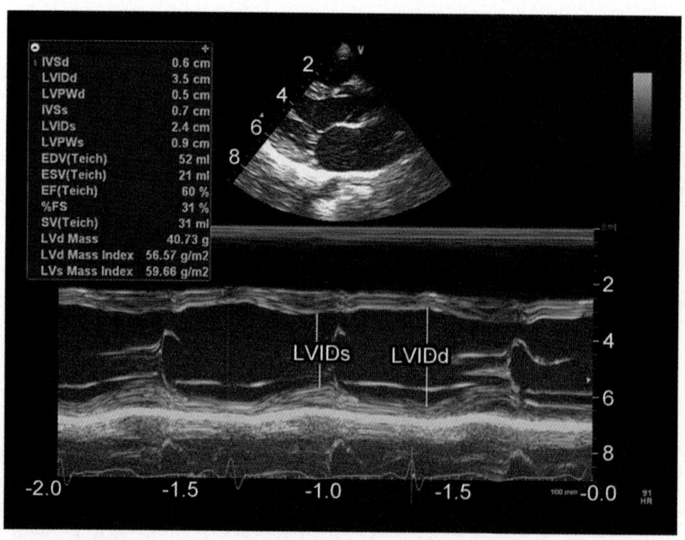

Fig. 17: Parasternal long axis showing M-mode of the left ventricle with assessment of left ventricular function. Note the left ventricular ejection fraction, fractional shortening, and the mass calculated.

$$FS\ (\%) = \frac{LVEDD - LVESD}{LVEDD} \times 100$$

where

LVEDD = left ventricular end-diastolic dimension

LVESV = left ventricular end-systolic dimension

Normal FS in children is 28–40%.[1]

$$EF\ (\%) = \frac{LVEDV - LVESV}{LVEDV} \times 100$$

Where

LVEDV = left ventricular end-diastolic volume

LVESV = left ventricular end-systolic volume

Normal EF in children is 55–65%. EF of 45–55% is mild dysfunction, 31–44% is moderate dysfunction, and ≤30% is severe dysfunction.

Assessment of Left Ventricular Diastolic Function

Diastolic dysfunction is commonly found along with other diseases but can rarely be the primary pathology as in restrictive cardiomyopathy. There is no single marker of diastolic dysfunction like the EF for systolic dysfunction. In the appropriate clinical setting, it requires assessment of several parameters from PW and tissue Doppler of mitral valve, left atrial volume, PW Doppler of pulmonary vein flow and assessment of pulmonary hypertension to reach a conclusion. Assessment of diastolic function is an exhaustive topic and details are beyond the scope of this chapter. Pulsed wave Doppler is used to record the velocity across the mitral valve where the cursor is positioned slightly proximal to the valve. The mitral valve has flow in diastole, with E wave in early diastole representing the early passive ventricular filling, followed by A wave representing late ventricular filling due to atrial contraction (**Fig. 18**). The mitral peak velocity is slightly higher than tricuspid peak velocity. Normally, E wave velocity is higher than the A wave velocity (**Fig. 18**).

In diastolic dysfunction, the mitral E/A ratio, the velocity of E and A waves and the deceleration time of the E wave can be altered.

In tissue Doppler imaging (TDI), the myocardial velocities are measured with a PW Doppler placed on the medial and lateral mitral annulus. It is relatively independent of preload conditions. Normally, there is a peak-systolic (S') wave, early-diastolic (E') wave, and end-diastolic (A') which is the atrial contraction (**Figs. 19A and B**). The S' wave velocity indicates systolic function, the E' and A' waves indicated diastolic function. Z scores are available for normal pulse wave Doppler and TDI for pediatric population.

The normal flow in the pulmonary veins is continuous with three waves—the S wave in systole, the D wave in diastole, and the A wave in late diastole when there is flow due to atrial contraction. The peak diastolic velocity is usually higher than the peak systolic velocity. These velocities do not change with respiration. In diastolic dysfunction, the ratio of S/D waves, A wave velocity/duration may be altered.

Diastolic dysfunction of the LV can be graded on echocardiogram as given in **Table 1**.[2]

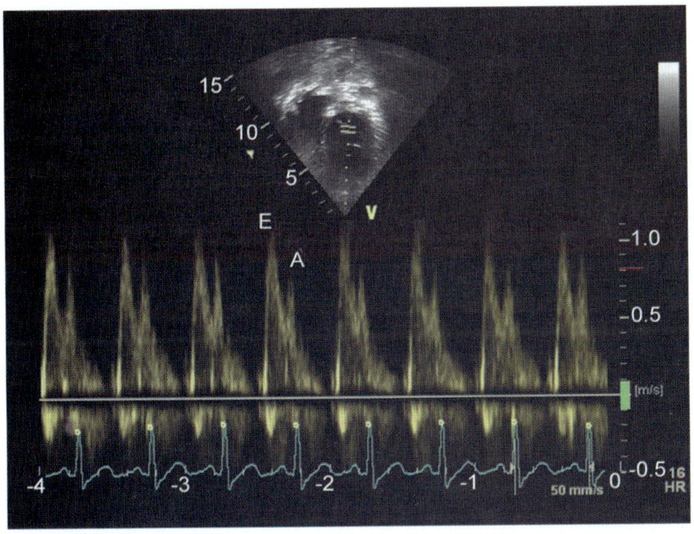

Fig. 18: Mitral inflow Doppler showing E and A waves, E wave velocity being higher than A wave.

Assessment of Right Ventricular Systolic Function

Evaluation of right ventricular function is difficult and less reliable compared to the LV as it has a different geometrical shape and its position in the chest. This makes the volume assessment on 2D technique not an ideal way to calculate the function. The muscle fibers of the RV are also oriented in a longitudinal way and hence, the systolic function needs to be determined by longitudinal shortening. Generally, eyeballing of right ventricular function is practiced as a bedside technique.

Right ventricular function can be assessed by getting the right ventricular end-diastolic and end-systolic area in the apical four-chamber view by manually tracing the endocardial border in diastolic and systole.

$$\text{FAC (\%)} = \frac{\text{RVEDA} - \text{RVESA}}{\text{RVEDA}} \times 100$$

Where

FAC = fractional area change

RVEDA = right ventricle end-diastolic area

RVESA = right ventricle end-systolic area

Normal FAC is from 43 ± 18% and <35% is systolic dysfunction.[3]

Another measure for right ventricular function, which is a marker for longitudinal function, is tricuspid annular plane systolic excursion (TAPSE), which is measured in apical four-chamber view by placing the M-mode cursor through the lateral TV annulus (**Fig. 20**). The excursion of the tricuspid annulus during the cardiac cycle is measured. A value of <16 mm in adults and <10 mm in children is systolic dysfunction.[4]

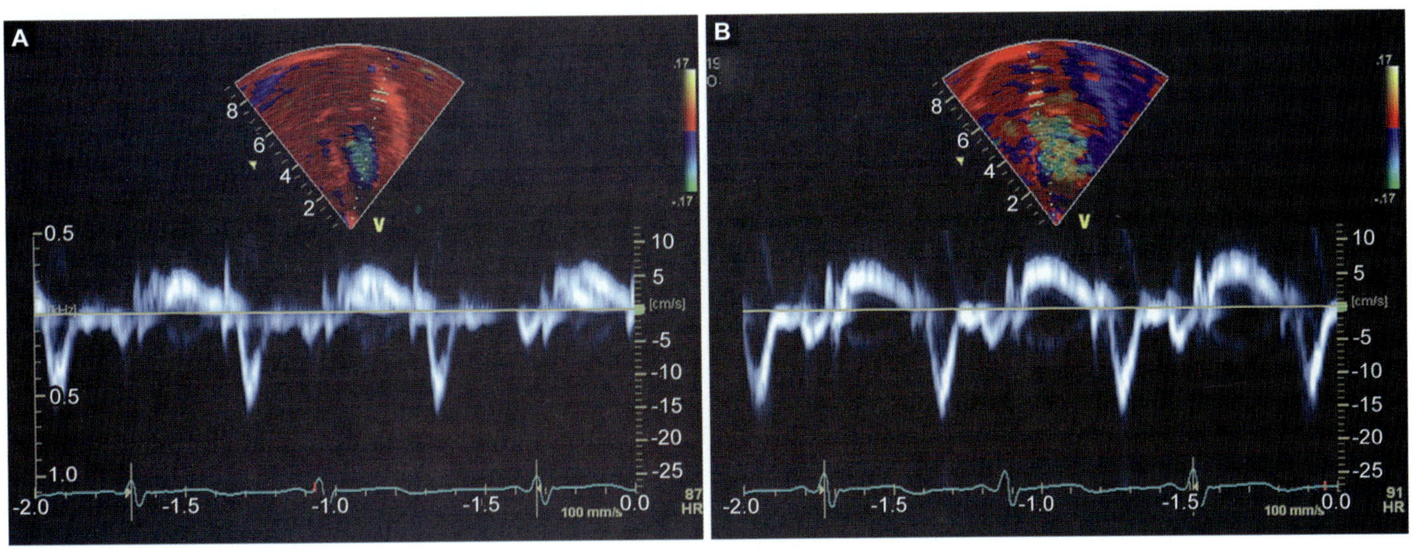

Figs. 19A and B: Tissue Doppler tracing of mitral valve (lateral and septal) showing E', A', and S' waves.

TABLE 1: LV relaxation, filling pressures and 2D and Doppler findings according to LV diastolic function based on ASE guidelines.[2]

	Normal	*Grade I*	*Grade II*	*Grade III*
LV relaxation	Normal	Impaired	Impaired	Impaired
LAP	Normal	Low or normal	Elevated	Elevated
Mitral E/A ratio	≥0.8	≤0.8	>0.8 to <2	> 2
Average E/e' ratio	<10	<10	10–14	> 14
Peak TR velocity (m/sec)	<2.8	<2.8	>2.8	>2.8
LA volume index	Normal	Normal or increased	Increased	Increased

(LA: left atrium; LAP: left atrial pressure; LV: left ventricle; TR: tricuspid regurgitation)

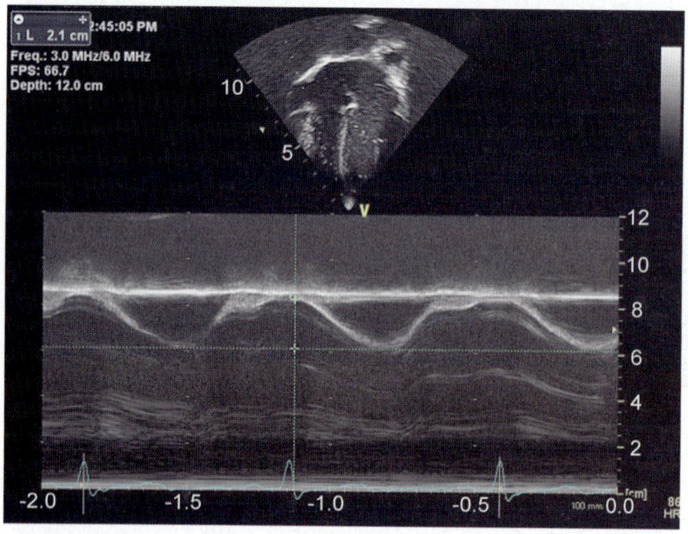

Fig. 20: Tricuspid annular plane systolic excursion (TAPSE) measured by using M-mode cursor on the tricuspid valve showing right ventricular function.

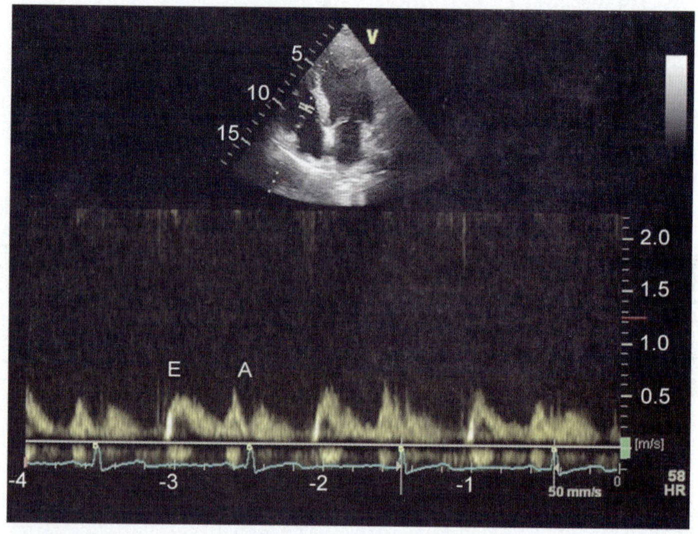

Fig. 21: Tricuspid valve inflow Doppler using pulsed wave (PW) showing E and A waves, like mitral valve in flow Dopplers.

Assessment of Right Ventricular Diastolic Function

This is done in a similar way as LV by PW Doppler of the TV and tissue Doppler at the lateral tricuspid annulus (**Figs. 21 and 22**). Grading of RV diastolic dysfunction should be done as follows: tricuspid E/A ratio <0.8 suggests impaired relaxation, a tricuspid E/A ratio of 0.8–2.1 with an E/E' ratio >6 or diastolic flow predominance in the hepatic veins suggests pseudonormal filling, and a tricuspid E/A ratio >2.1 with a deceleration time <120 ms suggests restrictive filling (as does late-diastolic antegrade flow in the PA).[4,5]

Inferior vena cava is also used for estimation of preload and fluid responsiveness (**Fig. 23**). As the diameter of IVC is variable with weight and height, it is a poor indicator for fluid responsiveness. Hence, its diameter change with respiration is a reliable marker for volume responsiveness when the child is mechanically ventilated. The greater the respiratory changes in IVC, the higher is the increase in cardiac output with fluid replacement.

Assessment of Pulmonary Artery Pressures

This is done by Doppler data, which is displayed as velocity. Based on the modified Bernoulli's equations, the velocity

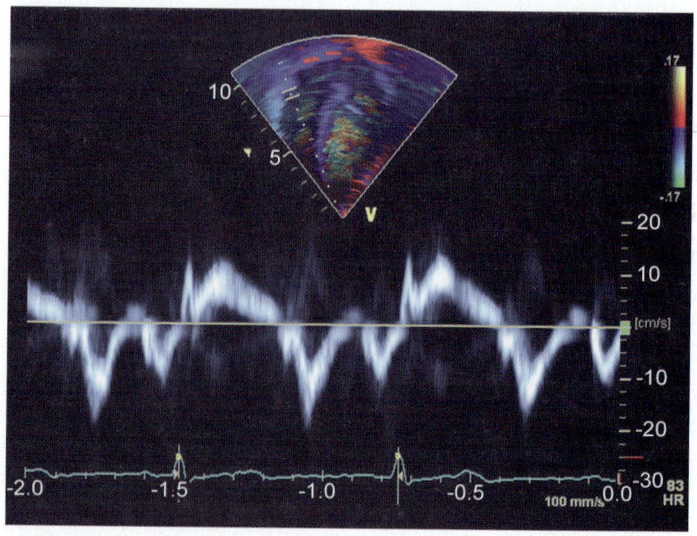

Fig. 22: Tissue Doppler at lateral tricuspid annulus showing E', A', and S' waves.

can be converted into pressure data (which the machine does automatically).

Pressure gradient = $4\,(V_{max})^2$

This principle is used for estimating the PA pressure. The tricuspid regurgitation (TR) gradient is the pressure

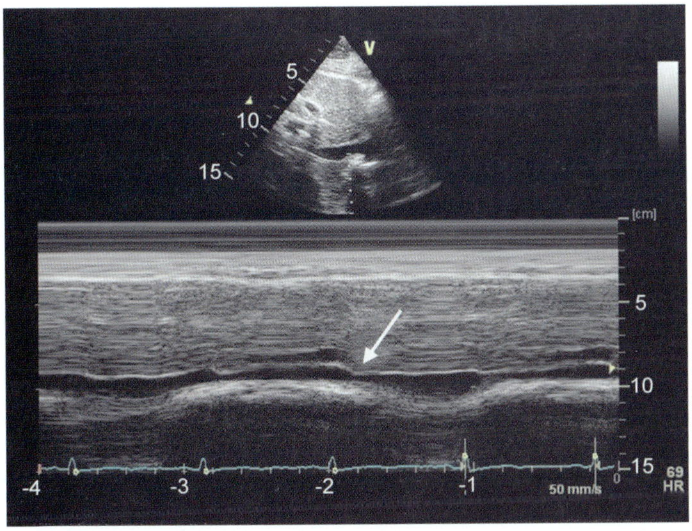

Fig. 23: Inferior vena cava (IVC) M-mode showing normal respiratory variations in subcostal view.

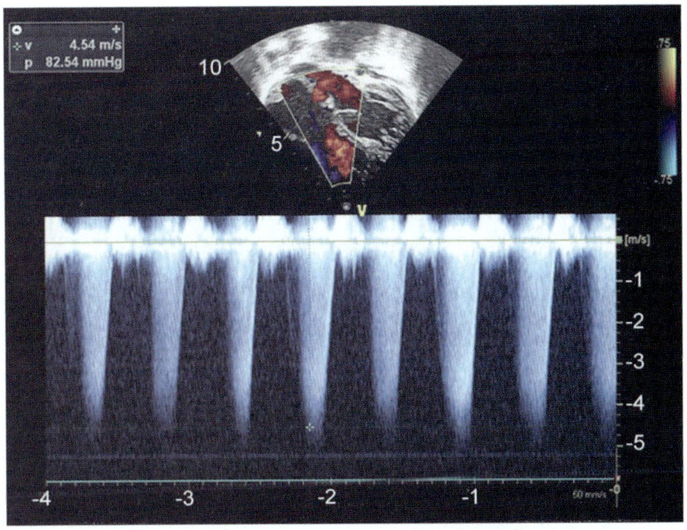

Fig. 24: Doppler (CW) tracing of tricuspid regurgitation jet showing severe pulmonary hypertension (pulmonary artery pressures are equal to right ventricular pressures in absence of right ventricular outflow obstruction).

difference between RV and RA in systole. Hence, pressure in RV = TR gradient + pressure in RA. In absence of pulmonary stenosis (PS), RV pressures reflect the PA systolic pressures (**Fig. 24**).

The same principle is used to calculate PA pressure in the presence of a shunt, which is shunting in systole, e.g., ventricular septal defect (VSD), or a patent ductus arteriosus (PDA). The gradient across the VSD is going to be the systolic pressure difference between the left and right ventricles, i.e., between the aorta and PA. Hence, the pulmonary artery pressure = aortic pressure (BP) – the gradient across the VSD (**Fig. 25**).

ECHOCARDIOGRAPHY IN CONGENITAL HEART DISEASE

Congenital Heart Disease: Intensive Care Unit Setting

Echocardiogram plays a critical role in the ICU setting in two aspects: (1) Diagnosis and (2) postoperative assessment.

Newborn Diagnosis

An echocardiogram is very useful when a sick newborn is admitted to the ICU with heart failure, shock, or cyanosis. In a newborn, such a presentation is highly suggestive of a duct-dependent pulmonary/systemic or mixing lesion. It is acceptable to start prostaglandin infusion based on clinical suspicion only, without echocardiographic confirmation of diagnosis in such a situation. However, an echocardiographic diagnosis makes choice of additional supportive measures less cumbersome and aids in quicker transport to a pediatric cardiac center capable of managing critical congenital heart disease (CCHD) in the newborn.

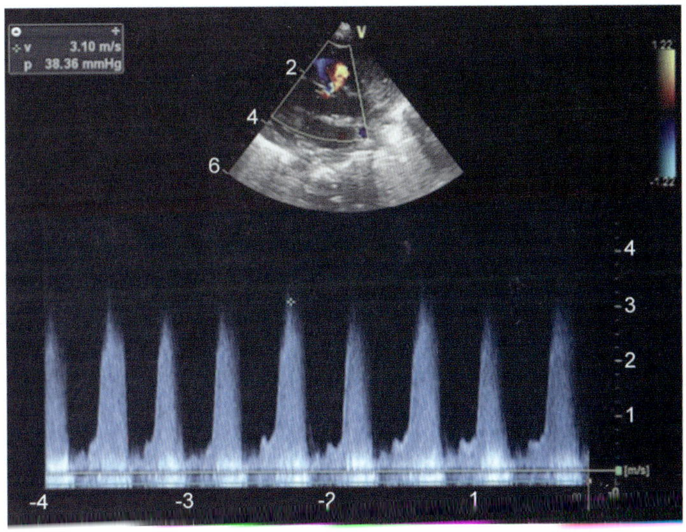

Fig. 25: Doppler tracing across the ventricular septal defect shunting from left-to-right ventricle showing a gradient of 38 mm Hg. Hence, the right ventricular pressures and the pulmonary artery pressures would be systolic pressure minus 38 mm Hg.

Shock/heart failure: The differential diagnosis includes myocardial disease or left heart obstruction, e.g., critical aortic stenosis (AS), hypoplastic left heart syndrome (HLHS) (**Fig. 26**), or coarctation. An echocardiogram can rapidly distinguish these entities. In myocarditis, there would be evidence of reduced left and right ventricular function without detectable structural abnormality. Critical AS presents with a thick abnormal aortic valve with minimal opening resulting in a dilated, dysfunctional LV. In HLHS on the other hand, the LV would be small. The diagnosis of neonatal coarctation is tricky even in expert hands. Neonatal coarctation should be suspected when the presentation is shock or heart failure. A dysfunctional LV without any intracardiac structural

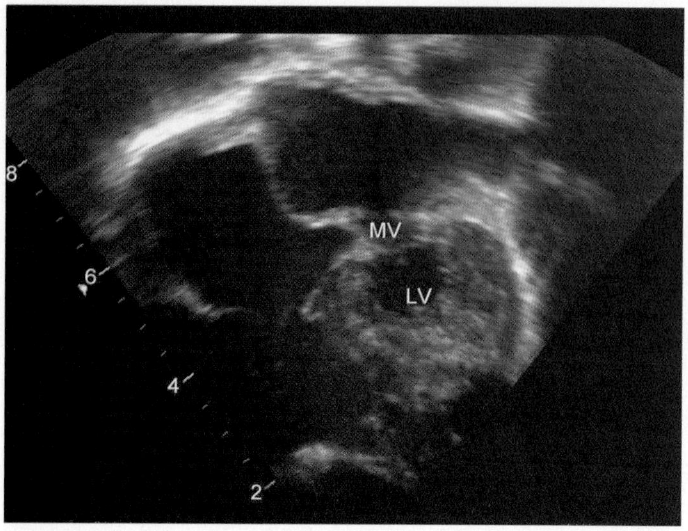

Fig. 26: Apical four-chamber view showing hypertrophied hypoplastic left ventricle with small mitral valve annulus and leaflets of the mitral valve not opening. Note that the interatrial septum is bulging to the right side indicating high left atrial pressures.
(LV: left ventricle; MV: mitral valve)

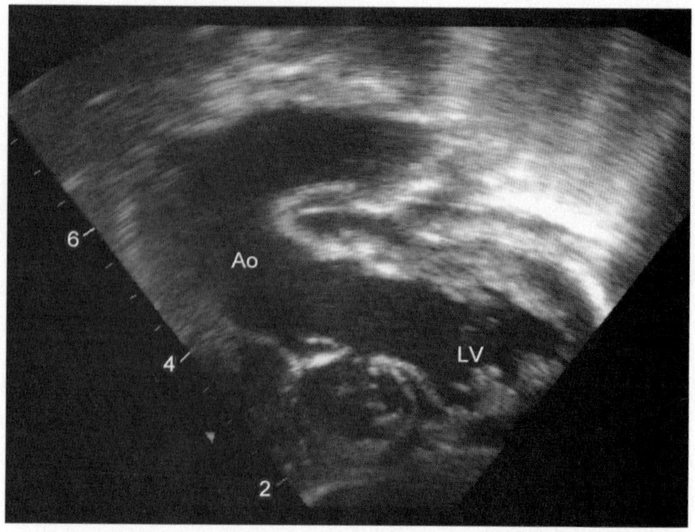

Fig. 27: Subcostal coronal view showing aorta overriding the interventricular septum with a large subaortic ventricular septal defect, small pulmonary artery underneath aorta is seen.
(Ao: aorta; LV: left ventricle)

abnormality should direct toward thorough assessment for coarctation. Left ventricular hypertrophy adds to the suspicion. The RV can also be affected when the ductus is open, and the former ejects blood through the latter to the lower part of the body. The suprasternal long axis views are diagnostic, where the narrowed isthmus as well as the frequently associated arch hypoplasia can be identified.

Cyanosis: The cardiac differential diagnosis of a newborn with cyanosis commonly includes right heart lesions with reduced pulmonary blood flow (**Fig. 27**). An echocardiogram can differentiate between critical PS [thickened abnormal pulmonary valve with reduced opening and a poorly functional RV with an atrial septal defect (ASD) shunting right to left] or lesions with pulmonary atresia where there is no flow across the pulmonary valve to the PA. Other causes of newborn cyanosis such as transposition of the great arteries (d-TGA) or Ebstein anomaly (**Fig. 28**) (the septal leaflet of the TV is apically displaced and there are varying degrees of TR and ASD) can also easily be differentiated on an echocardiogram. In d-TGA, an echocardiogram can help determine if the ASD is restrictive and whether the patient needs a balloon atrial septostomy or not. If the baby is blue and in right heart failure but no structural lesion is detected, a Doppler of the tricuspid regurgitant jet may enable persistent pulmonary hypertension to be diagnosed and work up and therapy accordingly planned.

Heart failure and cyanosis: Lesions such as truncus arteriosus and total anomalous pulmonary venous connection (TAPVC) which cause both cyanosis and can present with heart failure symptoms can easily be differentiated on an echocardiogram in the ICU setting in the neonatal period.

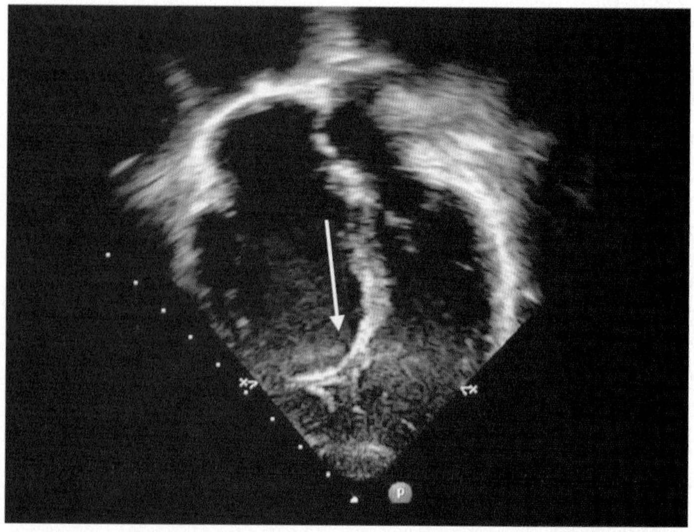

Fig. 28: Tricuspid valve—anterior leaflet is tethered and displaced in apical four-chamber view (arrow shows the displacement of anterior tricuspid leaflet).

Thus, an echocardiogram in a sick newborn in the ICU can very quickly identify the cause of the symptoms—from complex left or right heart disease to a structurally normal heart with reduced ventricular function. Accordingly, the line of management can be decided upon.

Postoperative

In the postoperative cardiac patient, bedside echocardiography is the mainstay of assessing the adequacy of repair, documenting the presence or absence of residual lesions, and as well as the first step to investigate cause of an unsatisfactory postoperative course. As in any ICU, the postoperative echocardiogram provides functional assessment as well.

Echocardiography for Congenital Heart Disease: Outpatient Department Setting

A thorough history and physical examination remains the building blocks of evaluation of any pediatric patient for congenital heart disease. Not only do they help in anticipating what to expect on the echocardiogram, but they also help in deciding the need and timing of surgical or interventional management. An echocardiographic study is best considered an extension of the clinical evaluation.

Left-to-Right Shunts

In left-to-right shunt lesions, an echocardiogram helps determine the size, and type of the defect along with the presence or absence of pulmonary hypertension. In pretricuspid shunts (all types of ASDs and partial anomalous pulmonary venous connections), the RA and RV are dilated. Pulmonary hypertension generally does not develop in early childhood. Post-tricuspid shunts [VSD, PDA, aortopulmonary (AP) window] are characterized by dilation of the left atrium and ventricle, when the shunt is significant (**Fig. 29**). In large defects, there is no restriction to flow at the defect and hence the pulmonary pressures are systemic. Moderate defects have some restriction, but the pulmonary pressures may not be normal. Small left-to-right shunts are not accompanied by chamber dilation or pulmonary hypertension. Atrioventricular septal defects comprise another group of left-to-right shunts, with different subtypes such as partial, complete, intermediate, and transitional. Within each subtype itself is an array of anatomic variations, each of which impacts surgical approach and timing. Complete atrioventricular septal defect is one of the easiest diagnosis on echocardiogram, as the four-chamber view makes the absence of the crux of the heart very evident. All subtypes of atrioventricular septal defects can be associated with atrioventricular valve regurgitation. This can primarily be from a "cleft" of the left atrioventricular valve component, which is a developmental abnormality, or from a variety of other pathoanatomies. Often times, this can explain the heart failure presentation in infancy encountered in partial atrioventricular septal defects. Quantifying the regurgitation as well as delineating its underlying pathology is an important step in surgical planning for atrioventricular septal defect correction.

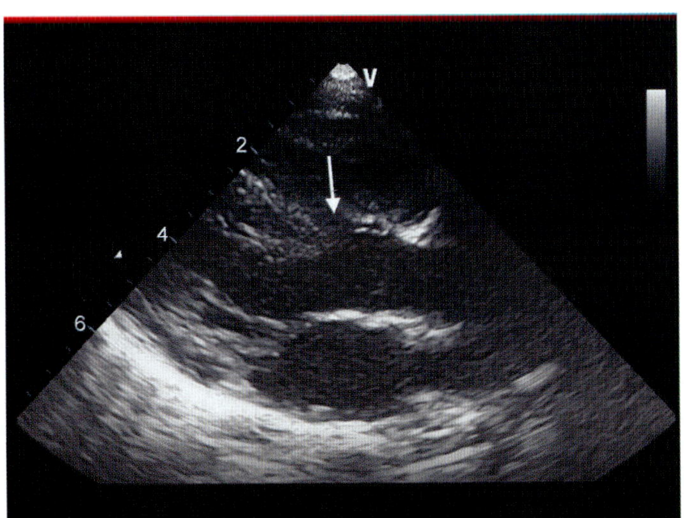

Fig. 29: Parasternal long axis view showing a ventricular septal defect below the aortic valve (shown by arrow).

Valvular Heart Disease

These patients generally remain asymptomatic for a long period and are generally picked up by virtue of their loud murmurs. By the time they develop symptoms, the disease would have invariably progressed to the severest of stages. Echocardiography helps in quantification of the severity of the lesions and in interrogating the hemodynamic consequences. Severity of stenotic lesions is assessed by continuous wave Doppler echocardiography. Regurgitant lesions on the other hand are assessed primarily by color Doppler imaging. Several supportive findings also need to be looked at before deciding the severity. Severe stenotic lesions are accompanied by hypertrophy of the corresponding ventricle, left ventricular hypertrophy in AS and coarctation of aorta, right ventricular hypertrophy in PS. Regurgitant lesions of the left-sided valves when significant are invariably associated with dilation of the LV. Similarly, the right-sided regurgitant lesions are accompanied by dilation of the RV.

Bicuspid aortic valve is a common abnormality in the population, this is often the underlying pathology for AS. Presence of AS warrants evaluation of other left-sided abnormalities such as congenital mitral stenosis and coarctation of the aorta as part of Shone's complex. Coarctation of aorta tends to be particularly missed if not specifically looked for. The suprasternal views should be used for this. Aortic regurgitation from bicuspid aortic valve generally presents later in life but can present in childhood too. Assessment of severity as well as its mechanism is important for management decisions. Width of the jet relative to the left ventricular outflow tract, width of the "vena contracta", reversal of flow in descending aorta are some of the important Doppler criteria for assessment of severity. PS is another common abnormality. The level of right ventricular outflow tract obstruction (infundibular/valvar/supravalvar), severity of obstruction, and presence or absence of associated abnormalities (commonly a VSD) determines the approach to management, all of which are assessed by echocardiography. Isolated congenital pulmonary regurgitation is extremely rare.

Cyanotic Congenital Heart Disease

In a cyanotic baby, echocardiograms help in pin-pointing the diagnosis, as well as in planning management as per the anatomy. Anomalies under the category of "Tetralogy of Fallot (TOF) Physiology" are all characterized by a large nonrestrictive VSD and PS. Echocardiography confirms the specific diagnosis (TOF/double-outlet RV, L-TGA with VSD and PS, D-TGA with VSD and PS, single ventricle with PS). In the large majority of cases, a thorough echocardiographic study is all that is needed to decode the anatomic details and plan the timing and approach to surgery. The group of cyanotic congenital heart diseases with no restriction to pulmonary blood flow includes TGA with VSD and no PS, double-outlet RV with no PS, truncus arteriosus, TAPVC, and single ventricle with no PS.

ECHOCARDIOGRAPHY IN ACQUIRED HEART DISEASE: RHEUMATIC HEART DISEASE, KAWASAKI DISEASE, AND INFECTIVE ENDOCARDITIS

Rheumatic Heart Disease

In rheumatic heart disease (RHD), primarily the valves are impacted, either presenting with regurgitation in the early phases or a combination of thickening, impaired mobility, regurgitation, and narrowing in the chronic stages. Some classic features can be noted on echocardiogram, e.g., hockey stick appearance of the mitral valve (**Fig. 30**). Echocardiogram can help diagnose RHD and determine the severity of the valve lesions (mild, moderate, or severe) along with helping determine timing of intervention.

Kawasaki Disease

In Kawasaki disease, without intravenous immunoglobulin (IVIG) 50% of the patients develop coronary artery aneurysms (**Fig. 31**); if IVIG is given within the first 10 days, the incidence drops to <5%. Echocardiography is the primary imaging modality for detection of coronary artery abnormalities in Kawasaki disease. It has a high sensitivity and specificity for the detection of abnormalities of the proximal coronary artery segments. It is important to know that initiation of treatment should not be delayed for echocardiographic assessment. The initial study establishes a baseline for longitudinal follow-up monitoring of coronary artery sizes. The initial echocardiogram in the first week of illness is typically normal and does not rule out the diagnosis. Echocardiography is particularly helpful in late presentation (>10 days), wherein coronary artery abnormalities would qualify the patient for IVIG therapy along with evidence of ongoing systemic inflammation in the form of elevated erythrocyte sedimentation rate (ESR) or C-reactive protein (CRP). It is also quite helpful in confirming diagnosis and planning treatment when the presentation is atypical. Echocardiographic detection of coronary artery abnormalities in Kawasaki disease is based on Japanese criteria/Z scores. Z scores take into account the body size of the patient and are more sensitive than Japanese Criteria, hence recommended. If the baseline echocardiography is normal, it is recommended to repeat within 1–2 weeks and 4–6 weeks after treatment. If an abnormality (Z score >2.5) is detected during the acute illness, more frequent echocardiography (at least twice per week) is recommended until luminal dimensions have stopped progressing to determine the risk for and presence of thrombosis. Expanding large or giant aneurysms need frequent, twice per week examinations while dimensions are expanding rapidly and at least once weekly in the first 45 days of illness, and then monthly until the 3rd month after illness onset. This is because the failure to escalate thromboprophylaxis in time with the rapid expansion of aneurysms is a primary cause of morbidity and mortality.[6]

Infective Endocarditis

The varied presentation and changing epidemiological profile of infective endocarditis (IE) continues to pose

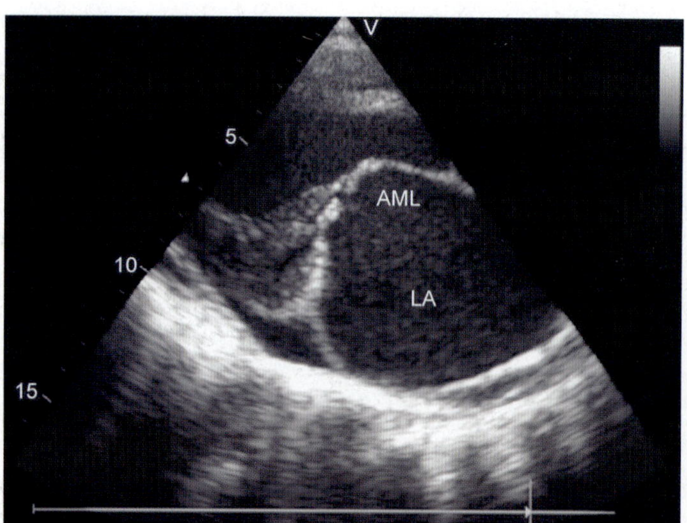

Fig. 30: Parasternal long axis view showing the hockey stick anterior mitral valve leaflet in rheumatic heart disease.
(AML: anterior mitral valve leaflet; LA: left atrium)

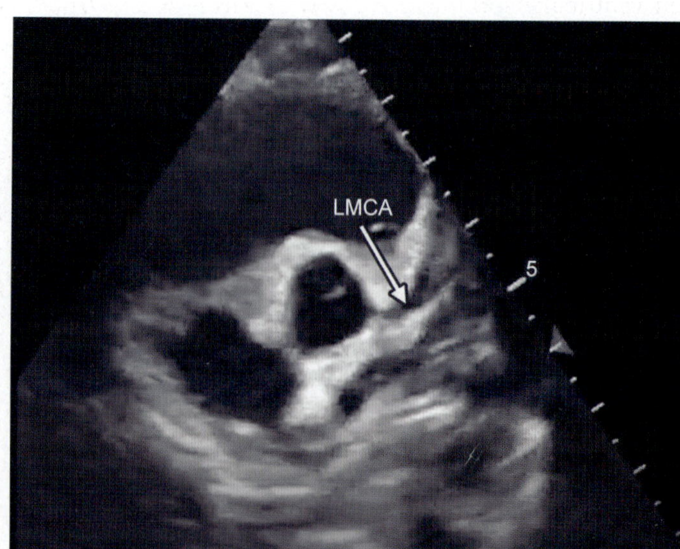

Fig. 31: Left main coronary artery (LMCA) dilatation is seen in parasternal short axis view.

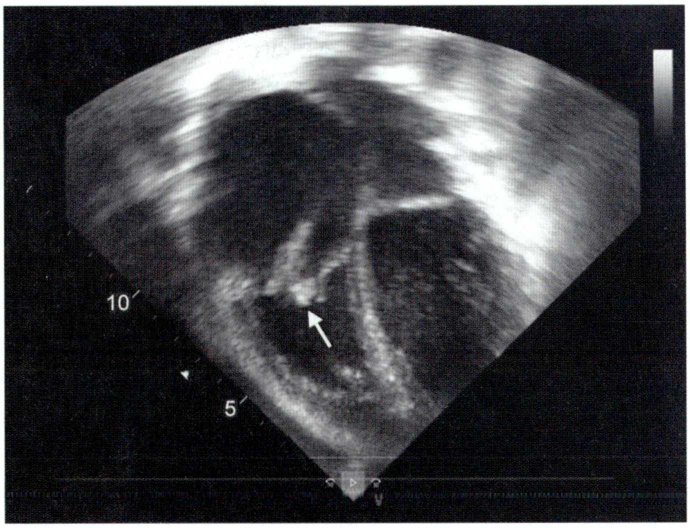

Fig. 32: Tricuspid valve endocarditis as shown in apical four-chamber view with vegetation (arrow) attached to the inferior surface of the anterior tricuspid leaflet.

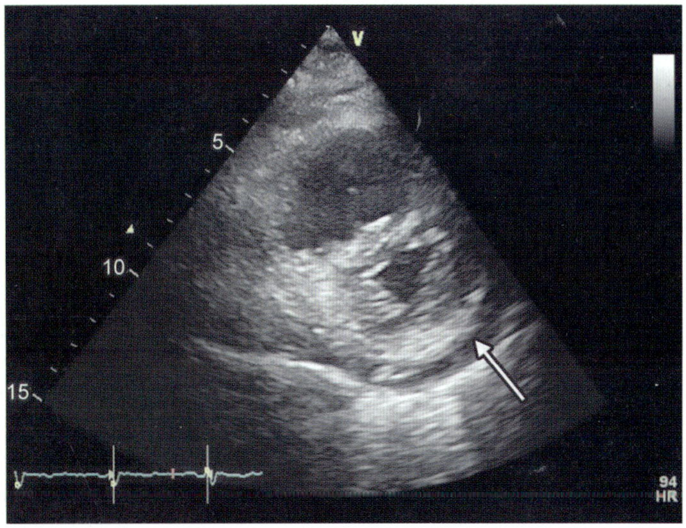

Fig. 33: Parasternal short axis view showing mild pericardial effusion (clear fluid).

challenges in diagnosis (**Fig. 32**). The currently recommended modified Duke criteria for diagnosis of IE combines echocardiographic findings with clinical and microbiological data. Echocardiogram positive for IE is a major criterion for diagnosis. This is defined as an oscillating intracardiac mass on valve or supporting structures, in the path of regurgitant jets, or on implanted material in the absence of an alternative anatomic explanation (implying a vegetation); abscess; or new partial dehiscence of prosthetic valve or new valvular regurgitation.[7] While valve regurgitation can be easily noted, vegetations are harder to pick up. Only 25% of vegetations <5 mm can be picked up on transthoracic echocardiogram (TTE). Transesophageal echocardiography (TEE) is more sensitive in this regard. TTE sensitivity ranges between 40 and 60% and that of TEE between 90 and 100%.[8] TEE is superior to TTE in diagnosing paravalvular leakage or dehiscence, left ventricular outflow tract complications, including root abscesses; involvement of the sinuses of Valsalva, prosthetic valve endocarditis, and for infants and children in whom TTE views may be limited (those who have had chest wall disruptions from previous surgery or from trauma, who have had placement of intracardiac prosthetic material, or who have congenital or acquired anomalies of the thoracic cage, patients with chronic lung disease of various pathogeneses). Children >10 years of age and weighing >60 kg, the TEE, as in adults, has been shown to be a more sensitive tool.[9]

ECHOCARDIOGRAPHY IN PERICARDIAL DISEASES, MYOCARDIAL DISEASES, AND ARRHYTHMIAS

Pericardial Diseases

Normally, pericardium is an inelastic fibrous sac that constricts the heart in position, limits the distension of cardiac chambers, and protects it from infections. The space between the inner layers of pericardium—the visceral and parietal pericardium, has a small amount of fluid.

Pericardial effusion is characterized by increase in the amount of fluid within the pericardial space (**Fig. 33**). The increase in the pericardial fluid increases the pressure in the pericardial space. The effect of fluid on the clinical presentation will depend on the cause of pericardial effusion, the amount of fluid, and the rapidity with which the fluid collects.

Echocardiography is a safe, bedside, quick, and reliable technique for diagnosing pericardial effusion. Following is the checklist to be focused on in a child with pericardial effusion. 2D, M-mode, and Doppler techniques are used in the subcostal, apical, and parasternal views.

- *The amount of pericardial effusion*: This is measured at end-diastole, in multiple views. This is important for serial monitoring of effusion. Large effusions can cause tamponade. However, volume alone may not necessarily correlate with symptoms. The rate of increase in the accumulation is equally important as rapid collection of even small amounts of effusion can lead to faster cardiac tamponade.
- *Appearance of the fluid*: Whether the fluid is clear or with strands, might give an idea about the etiology of pericardial effusion. Transudate will give an echo-free signal whereas an exudate (e.g., tuberculous pericardial effusion or pyogenic pericardial effusion) likely would have fibrinous strands.
- *Location of fluid*: The fluid might be localized to a part of the pericardial cavity or generalized seen throughout the pericardial cavity. Pyogenic exudates tend to loculate the effusion.
- *Presence of any hemodynamic compromise*: See cardiac tamponade.

Cardiac tamponade is caused by accumulation of fluid in the pericardial space causing compression on the cardiac chambers and restriction of filling. This increase in pericardial pressure nullifies the normal respiratory variation in intracardiac pressures. Even though cardiac tamponade is a clinical diagnosis, the following signs need to be assessed on echocardiography.

- *Collapse of RA and RV*: The collapse happens during the relaxation phase when the intracardiac pressures are lower than the intrapericardial pressures. Right atrial collapse is seen during systole. The duration of atrial collapse (longer than 1/3rd of cardiac cycle) is a sensitive and specific sign of cardiac tamponade.[10] Collapse of both the atria also increases the sensitivity and specificity of tamponade. Right ventricular collapse is seen during diastole, initially during expiration and then throughout the respiratory cycle. Duration of right ventricular collapse is an indicator for severity. In the sequence of progression, right ventricular collapse is seen after the right atrial collapse.
- *Exaggerated ventricular interdependence*: In diastole, during inspiration, the normal increase in the size of RV and decrease in the size of LV are exaggerated.

Septal bounce, a paradoxical bouncing motion of the interventricular septum initially directed toward and then away from the LV during early diastole owning to exaggerated interventricular dependence, can be seen in cardiac tamponade, although this is more classically described in constrictive pericarditis.

In constrictive pericarditis, an abnormal atrial systolic notch in the interventricular septum on M-mode is an additional useful sign (in addition to the early diastolic notch) to differentiate constrictive pericarditis from restrictive cardiomyopathy. The mechanism is thought to be related to transient late-diastolic pressure gradients between both ventricles resulting from asynchrony of left and right atrial contractions.[11]

- *IVC*: IVC is dilated with reduced physiological collapsibility during inspiration.
- *Doppler study*: There is an exaggerated increase in velocities of tricuspid (at least 40%) and pulmonary valves and decrease in velocities of mitral and aortic (at least 25%) valves during inspiration.[12] Doppler of hepatic veins will show an increased flow with inspiration and decrease/reversal of diastolic flow in expiration.

Myocardial Diseases

Cardiomyopathy can be of different subtypes—dilated cardiomyopathy, restrictive cardiomyopathy, hypertrophic cardiomyopathy, and less common forms such as arrhythmogenic right ventricular dysplasia and noncompaction cardiomyopathy. Echocardiogram is the first-line imaging modality for the diagnosis of cardiomyopathy. Serial echocardiography in heart failure patients provide invaluable hemodynamic information for titration after the failure medications.

Dilated Cardiomyopathy

Dilated cardiomyopathy is characterized by contractile dysfunction of the ventricle in absence of a structural abnormality of the heart. Hence, on echocardiogram, it is important to rule out other etiologies for ventricular dysfunction like hidden coarctation or anomalous origin of left coronary artery from PA, before dilated cardiomyopathy diagnosis is established. Following parameters are documented in this situation.

- *2D features*: There is marked left atrial and left ventricular enlargement (**Fig. 34**) and poor contractility easily recognized on 2D echocardiogram. The hypokinesia is global. Spontaneous echocardiographic contrast/smoke is frequently seen due to stasis of blood in the left atrium and ventricle.[13] There is also increased risk for thrombus formation in the left ventricular apex and left atrial appendage both of which are difficult to diagnose.
- *M-mode technique*: Reduced EF and FS are calculated as mentioned in the section "Functional Echocardiography" with the measurements of LV dimensions, volumes, and thickness of the walls.
- *Doppler features*: Mitral regurgitation is usually secondary to the disease of LV and dilatation of LV. It can sometimes be challenging to decide the primary versus secondary role of mitral regurgitation, and it is best done by experts. TR jet can give an idea regarding PA pressures. Peak velocity of >2.5 m/sec may indicate higher mortality and morbidity. CW Doppler of the mitral regurgitation jet shows peak velocity of the jet in midsystole compared to early systole in a normal heart, indicating slow rate of

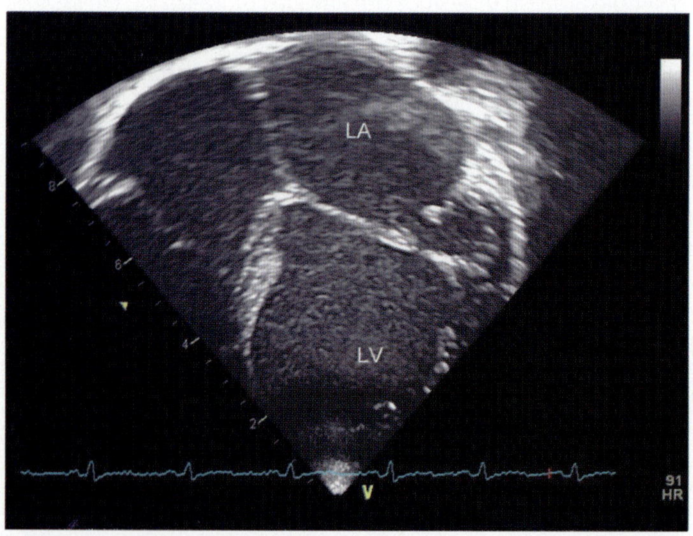

Fig. 34: Apical four-chamber view with dilated left atrium and ventricle. (LA: left atrium; LV: left ventricle)

rise in left ventricular pressure (mean ventricular dP/dT). Using a PW Doppler on the ascending aorta, peak aortic flow velocity, velocity time integral, acceleration time, and deceleration time are calculated, all of which are reduced in patients with cardiomyopathy. Diastolic dysfunction might be also seen in patients with dilated cardiomyopathy, which can be masked by presence of mitral regurgitation.

Restrictive Cardiomyopathy

Restrictive cardiomyopathy is characterized by impaired diastolic function with restrictive pattern of filling on assessment of diastolic function as mentioned earlier. Usually, the systolic function of the ventricles is preserved. As the myocardium is stiff, a small increase in the volume leads to significant increase in the pressure in the ventricles and abrupt cessation of filling in the first third of diastole.[14] Following points are important for diagnosing restrictive cardiomyopathy (**Figs. 35A to D**).

- *2D echocardiogram and M-mode features*: There is characteristically biatrial enlargement (owl-eye appearance) due to chronic rise in filling pressures. Myocardium may appear hyper-refractile, not always. There is normal biventricular volume, normal or low systolic function, and normal or increased ventricular wall thickness. The atrioventricular valves are frequently thickened.
- *Doppler technique*: Assessment of LV diastolic function shows characteristic restrictive pattern as described previously. AV valve regurgitation and pulmonary hypertension are frequently seen in restrictive cardiomyopathy as well.

Hypertrophic Cardiomyopathy

Hypertrophic cardiomyopathy is usually asymmetric. Diastolic dysfunction is related to impaired relaxation and poor chamber compliance. Systolic dysfunction sets in late in the course of disease and indicates poor prognosis.

- *2D echocardiogram features*: The hypertrophy is usually of the LV (commonly of the interventricular septum) but can also involve the RV and is obvious on 2D echocardiogram (**Fig. 36**). Additionally, 2D echocardiogram provides an understanding of mitral valve abnormalities, mechanism of mitral regurgitation, and left ventricular obstruction.
- *M-mode technique*: It shows hypertrophy of the ventricles, more of the ventricular septum. The ratio of the septum thickness to the posterior wall thickness in diastole would exceed 1.3. Usually, they have normal left ventricular end-diastolic volume, smaller left ventricular end-systolic volume, and higher EF.[15] Systolic anterior motion of the anterior mitral leaflet can be demonstrated.
- *Doppler technique*: The degree and magnitude of mitral regurgitation can give an idea about the mitral valve

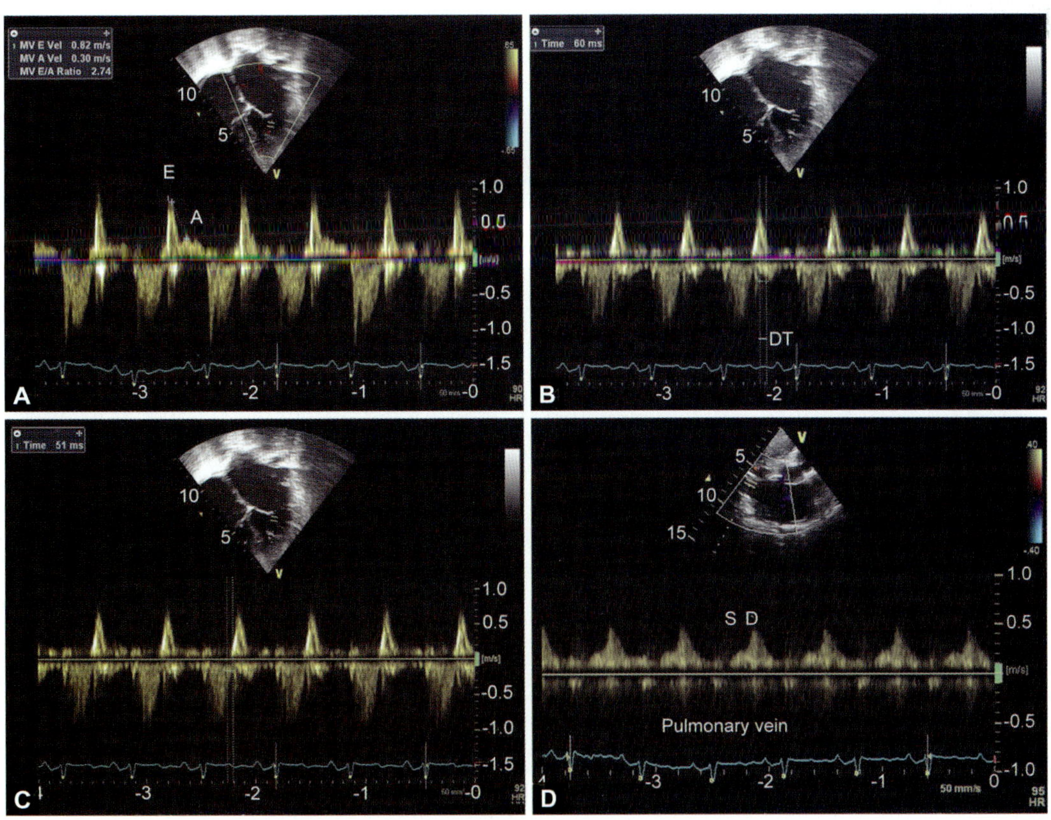

Figs. 35A to D: Four-chamber view with MV Doppler showing E/A velocity >2, deceleration time <150 ms, isovolumic relaxation time <60 ms, and pulmonary vein Doppler showing reduced S velocity and most of the flow occurring in diastole.

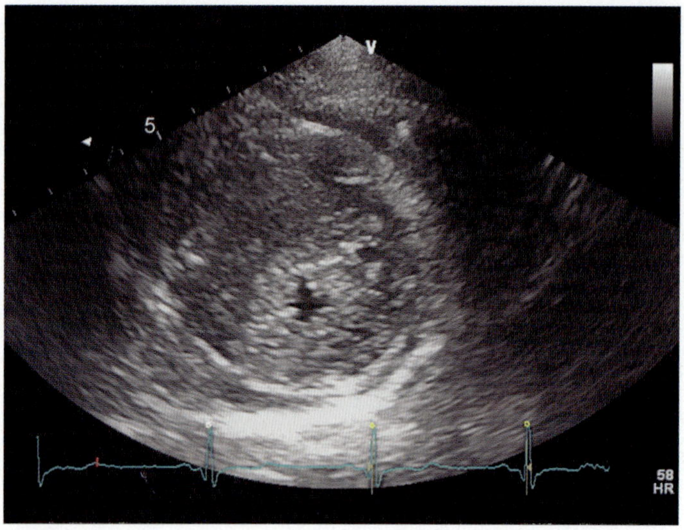

Fig. 36: Parasternal short axis view with hypertrophied left ventricle and small left ventricular cavity.

abnormality and the left ventricular pressures. The left ventricular outflow tract obstruction can be documented by CW Doppler and the tracing is typically "dagger"-shaped. LV diastolic function is abnormal and can be assessed as described previously.

Left Ventricular Noncompaction

Left ventricular noncompaction is characterized by prominent trabeculations in the left ventricular myocardium with prominent intertrabecular recesses as the normal process of condensing of the myocardium is arrested. It can occur in isolation or along with a congenital heart condition. This situation can lead to formation of thrombus in the intertrabecular recesses and can cause reduced systolic function.

ROLE OF ECHOCARDIOGRAPHY IN CARDIAC ARRHYTHMIAS

Echocardiogram is an important diagnostic and prognostic tool. Echocardiogram can sometimes help in differentiating the type of rhythm abnormality, e.g., ventricular ectopic and atrial ectopic. Echocardiography has a role in revealing a potential etiology for cardiac arrhythmia like a structural heart disease and to rule out any secondary effects of arrhythmia like a clot in the atria or reduced ventricular function. Following are the points to be pondered whenever there is a tachyarrhythmia, bradyarrhythmia, or irregular rhythm.

- *Rule out a structural heart disease*: Ebstein anomaly of TV, cardiac tumors such as rhabdomyomas, and myocarditis can have associated supraventricular tachycardia. Corrected TGA, atrioventricular septal defect, and left-sided isomerism syndrome are known to have associated bradycardia. Rheumatic heart disease with chronic valvular heart disease can also precipitate an abnormal rhythm. Presence of a structural heart disease would change the further management and long-term prognosis of the child. Arrhythmias can happen in postoperative situations also.
- *Ventricular function—size and volume assessment*: Ventricular dysfunction can be a result of persistent tachyarrhythmia (tachycardiomyopathy) or chronic bradyarrhythmia due to dilatation of cardiac chambers. Rarely, myocarditis can be a primary pathology causing both ventricular dysfunction and arrhythmias. Pre-existing cardiomyopathy can present with an arrhythmia as well.

THE ECHOCARDIOGRAM REPORT AND ITS INTERPRETATION

So far, we have understood that bedside echocardiography in children includes 2D technique, M-mode, color Doppler, PW Doppler, CW Doppler, and TDI. Echocardiogram provides us with anatomical and functional information of the heart. The study should be done in sequential segmental manner starting from the visceral situs, to the atrial situs—ventricular looping—great arterial relationship building up an understanding of atrioventricular and ventriculoarterial relationship. These sequences are done on 2D and color with complete sweeps. While doing this, it is important not to forget the pericardium, the myocardium, and to check if there is any evidence of arrhythmia. M-mode of the left heart is included as a routine in all echocardiograms. Additional measurement of cardiac structures is done whenever needed. Doppler study is included in situations like presence of TR or PDA for pressure data. Functional assessment including TDI is done whenever situation demands.

It is important to gather all the information while doing the study. Height, weight, body surface area, and systemic blood pressure measurement of the child preferably should be mentioned. At the same time, there is an art to represent all that information into the report in a clear way. At the end, the report needs to be correlated with the clinical findings. An echocardiogram can be reported in the following sequence:

- Situs and position of the heart—levocardia/mesocardia/dextrocardia
- Visceral situs—solitus/inversus/ambiguous
- Atrial situs—solitus/inversus/ambiguous (including systemic and pulmonary venous drainage)
- Atria—normal/dilatation
- Interatrial septum—intact/ASD—position and size
- Atrioventricular valves—annuli size, offset seen/common atrioventricular valve, patent tricuspid and mitral valves/stenotic or atretic or regurgitant
- Ventricular looping—D-looped/L-looped
- Ventricles—normal/dilatation or hypoplastic or dysfunctional or hypertrophied

- Atrioventricular concordance—concordant/discordant
- Interventricular septum—intact/VSD—position, size, and gradient
- Great artery relationship—normally related: S—solitus/D-malposed/L-malposed/I malposed
- Ventricular arterial relationship—concordant/discordant/double-outlet RV
- Semilunar valves—annuli size, normal/stenotic or regurgitant
- Great arteries—normal/dilated or small size
- Branch pulmonary arteries—confluent/nonconfluent or absence of one PA, size
- PDA—absent/present—size and gradient
- Arch-sidedness—left/right, normal/narrowed—size and gradient
- Doppler study—(including tissue Doppler if done)
    - *Mitral valve*: E velocity, A velocity, DT, isovolumic relaxation time (IVRT), mean gradient
    - *Tricuspid valve*: E velocity, A velocity, TR gradient
    - *Aortic valve*: Peak velocity, acceleration time, pressure half time for aortic regurgitation
    - Pulmonary valve
- Pericardium—normal/effusion or thickened
- Miscellaneous—including any rhythm disturbances, clots, and vegetations.

Final Impression of Echocardiogram Report

If possible, the indication of the study needs to be mentioned with the echocardiogram report. The measurements of cardiac struc-tures such as the valve sizes, chamber dimensions can be taken on 2D and M-mode, and need to be normalized for body surface area (Z score values). The outflow measurements are taken during ventricular systole and inflow measurements in ventricular diastole. Any technical limitations, e.g., chest deformity that might compromise on the diagnostic accuracy, need to be mentioned in the report. The location where the study was performed, e.g., bedside or in the outpatient department, also needs to be mentioned.

Now, let us take some examples of echocardiogram reports to understand how to interpret the findings and use them in clinical management.

Echo report 1: This is a bedside echocardiogram done for a preterm baby delivered at 30 weeks of gestation, on day 21 of life. As there is left heart dilatation, pan diastolic flow reversal in abdominal aorta and increased flow across the mitral valve, we can say that the pulmonary vascular resistance has reduced and there is some evidence of increased pulmonary blood flow. This PDA will need monitoring closely.

Echo report 2: This is an echocardiogram done for a 2-month-old child referred for an incidental detection of a systolic murmur. The VSD is considered moderate sized as there is left heart dilatation. The VSD is restrictive and has a gradient of 80 mm Hg, hence the right ventricular pressures (and the PA pressures) are normal. As the child has no cardiac failure and has normal PA pressures, it does not need any intervention at this stage. Additionally, perimembranous VSD can reduce in size spontaneously over time.

Patient Name: **Medical Record Number:** ☐
Age: **Gender:**
Date of Exam:

Echo Report

Situs	:	Solitus
Cardiac Position	:	Levocardia
Systemic Venous Drainage	:	Normal
Pulmonary Venous Drainage	:	Normal
Right Atrium	:	Dilated
Left Atrium	:	Dilated
IAS	:	PFO, L-R shunt with peak gradient of 15 mm Hg
Tricuspid Valve	:	Normal
Mitral Valve	:	Inflow increase
Av-Connection	:	Concordance
Ventricular Loop	:	d-loop
Right Ventricle	:	Dilated
Left Ventricle	:	Dilated
IVS	:	Intact and moving with LV
VA-Connection	:	Concordance
Great Artery Relationship	:	Normally related
Aortic Valve	:	Normal
Pulmonary Valve	:	Normal
Aorta	:	Pan diastolic flow reversal in abdominal aorta
Pulmonary Artery	:	Normal
PDA/Collaterals	:	3.8 mm PDA L-R shunt continuous flow with PSG/EDG – 40/15 mmHg
Aortic ARCH	:	Left no coarctation
Coronary Arteries	:	Normal
Pericardium	:	Normal
Miscellaneous	:	Nil

Impression

Moderate PDA, L.R Shunt
Moderate PAH

Echo report 1

Echo report 3: This is an echocardiogram done for a 5-year-old child with an ejection systolic click and ejection systolic murmur (ESM) 2/6 heard at the left upper sternal border and apex. It shows a bicuspid aortic valve which is reasonably functioning well which goes with the clinical findings. The parents need to be reassured and counseling needs to be done for the need for follow-up.

The interpretation of the echocardiogram report needs to be done in the clinical context, e.g., the age of the baby, maturity, symptoms, etc. For example, presence of patent foramen ovale/fossa ovalis ASD and PDA might be acceptable in the neonatal period. Diagnosis of bicuspid aortic valve with no AS or regurgitation needs counseling of parents and reassurance. Presence of mitral valve prolapse might be pointing toward the child having Marfan syndrome, etc.

FETAL ECHOCARDIOGRAPHY

Introduction

A significant number of newborns with CCHD will not show any obvious clinical signs, as they depend on flow through

Patient Name: **Medical Record Number:** ☐
Age: **Gender:**
Date of Exam:

Echo Report

Situs	:	Solitus
Cardiac Position	:	Levocardia
Systemic Venous Drainage	:	Normal
Pulmonary Venous Drainage	:	Normal
Right Atrium	:	Normal
Left Atrium	:	Minimal dilatation
IAS	:	Intact
Tricuspid Valve	:	Tricuspid regurgitation—mild
Mitral Valve	:	Normal
AV-Connection	:	Concordance
Ventricular Loop	:	d-loop
Right Ventricle	:	Normal
Left Ventricle	:	Minimal dilatation
IVS	:	3.8 mm perimembranous VD partially closed by septal aneurysm with fenestration shunting L-R with peak gradient of 80 mm Hg
VA-Connection	:	Concordance
Great Artery Relationship	:	Normally related
Aortic Valve	:	Normal
Pulmonary Valve	:	Normal
Aorta	:	Normal
Pulmonary Artery	:	Normal
PDA/Collaterals	:	Absent
Aortic Arch	:	Left
Coronary Arteries	:	Normal
Pericardium	:	Normal
Miscellaneous	:	Nil

Impression

Moderate Fenestrated PM VSD L-R
No PAH

Echo report 2

Patient Name: **Medical Record Number:** ☐
Age: **Gender:**
Date of Exam:

US Echo Report

Situs	:	Solitus
Cardiac Position	:	Levocardia
Systemic Venous Drainage	:	Normal
Pulmonary Venous Drainage	:	Normal
Right Atrium	:	Normal
Left Atrium	:	Normal
IAS	:	Intact
Tricuspid Valve	:	Tricuspid regurgitation—trivial; gradient—20 mm Hg
Mitral Valve	:	Normal
AV-Connection	:	Concordance
Ventricular Loop	:	d-loop
Right Ventricle	:	Normal
Left Ventricle	:	Normal
IVS	:	Sigmoid-shaped IVS, IVS 7 mm in upper part
VA-Connection	:	Concordance
Great Artery Relationship	:	Normally related
Aortic Valve	:	Normal
Pulmonary Valve	:	Normal
Aorta	:	Functionally bicuspid, fused raphe between RCC and NCC, Ann. 12 mm, ascending aorta 17 mm, PPG/MPG–35/21 mm Hg
Pulmonary Artery	:	Normal
PDA/Collaterals	:	Absent
Aortic Arch	:	Left
Coronary Arteries	:	Normal
Pericardium	:	Normal
M-mode	:	LVIDd–27 mm, LVIDs–15 mm, IVSd–6 mm, PW–5 mm, EF–70%, Ao–14 mm, LA–17 mm

Impression

Bicuspid Aortic Valve
NO/Mild AS, NO AR
Sigmoid Shaped IVS
NO Concentric LVH
Good BVF

Echo report 3

the ductus arteriosus for survival. In these newborns, closure of the ductus arteriosus after discharge leads to a catastrophic situation. Prenatal ultrasound is on way of identifying cyanotic congenital heart diseases well before this occurs. Prenatal diagnosis of congenital heart disease gives us an opportunity for parenteral counseling, planning delivery at a center capable of managing CCHD, and provides a window to offer fetal treatment. Furthermore, babies with prenatally diagnosed CCHD have been found to have more favorable outcomes after neonatal cardiac surgery compared to those with a postnatal diagnosis. As a pediatrician, it would be imperative to understand when a fetal echocardiogram is considered in pregnancy, how to interpret a fetal echocardiogram report, understand its limitations, and how to plan the postnatal management of the baby.

Indications of Fetal Echocardiogram

The list of indications of fetal echocardiogram has been summarized in **Box 1**.[16] A full fetal study is done when an abnormality is picked up during cardiac screening done as a part of routine anomaly scan or for any of the indications as mentioned.[16] Timing of fetal echocardiogram is conventionally at 18–22 weeks of gestation, a time when most of the obstetric scans are performed. It may be difficult to obtain satisfactory images later in gestation due to increase in the amniotic fluid and shadowing from the thoracic cage. This single midtrimester scan has a possibility of missing lesions, which could evolve later in pregnancy, e.g., cardiac chamber hypoplasia, arrhythmias, and cardiomyopathy. An early fetal echocardiogram by 14–16 weeks is recommended in extremely high-risk cases like previous child with complex congenital heart disease, increased nuchal translucency (NT) or a fetus at risk for chromosomal abnormalities. In such situations, a repeat fetal echocardiogram is recommended at 18–22 weeks of gestation. There are situations where fetal echocardiogram is repeated, e.g., to monitor the progression of atrioventricular valve regurgitation or semilunar valve steno-sis or aortic arch hypoplasia, arrhythmias, and heart failure. The timing and frequency of repeat echocardiograms is individualized based on the lesion diagnosed and the course expected.

Views

Steps for Fetal Cardiac Screening

- Identification of fetus lie is the initial step to decide the fetal head and spine.

BOX 1: Common indications for fetal echocardiogram.

Indications with higher risk profile (estimated >2% absolute risk)

- Maternal diabetes mellitus pregestational/diagnosed in the first trimester
- Maternal phenylketonuria (uncontrolled)
- Maternal autoantibodies (SSA/SSB$^+$)
- Maternal medications:
  - ACE inhibitors
  - Retinoic acid
  - NSAIDs in third trimester
- Maternal rubella infection in the first trimester
- Maternal infection with suspected fetal myocarditis
- Assisted reproduction technology
- CHD in first-degree relative of fetus (maternal, paternal, or sibling with CHD)
- First- or second-degree relative with disorder with Mendelian inheritance with CHD association
- Fetal cardiac abnormality suspected on obstetrical ultrasound
- Fetal extracardiac abnormality suspected on obstetrical ultrasound
- Fetal karyotype abnormality
- Fetal tachycardia or bradycardia, or frequent or persistent irregular heart rhythm
- Fetal increased NT >95% (≥3 mm)
- Monochorionic twinning
- Fetal hydrops or effusions

Indications with lower risk profile (estimated >1% but <2% absolute risk)

- Maternal medications:
  - Anticonvulsants
  - Lithium
  - Vitamin A
  - SSRIs (only paroxetine)
  - NSAIDs in first/second trimester
- CHD in second-degree relative of fetus
- Fetal abnormality of the umbilical cord or placenta
- Fetal intra-abdominal venous anomaly

(ACE: angiotensin converting enzyme; CHD: congenital heart disease; NSAID: nonsteroidal anti-inflammatory drug; NT: nuchal translucency; SSRI: selective serotonin reuptake inhibitor)

- *Visceral (and cardiac) situs and right left orientation*: In the sagittal view, the baby's head is positioned to the right side of the screen. Then, the transducer is rotated 90° clockwise. Once we get the transverse view, the spine and the sternum of the fetus are located and then the right and left sides of the fetus are decided (**Figs. 37A and B**).
- *Cardiac axis*: In the transverse view of the chest, at the level of four-chamber view, an imaginary line is drawn from the spine to the sternum. Cardiac axis is the angle, which the interventricular septum makes with this line (**Fig. 38**). Normal cardiac axis is 45 ± 20°.
- *Cardiac size*: In the same view, the cardiac size is assessed by the ratio of the cardiac circumference to the chest circumference (**Fig. 38**). Normal cardiac size is 0.38–0.45.
- *Cardiac position*: Normally, the heart is situated in the left side of the chest (**Fig. 38**).

- Structural evaluation of heart:
  - *Four-chamber view*: The transverse section just above the diaphragm will give the four-chamber view (**Fig. 39**). This view gives us information about the atria (size of atria and pulmonary venous drainage), the foramen ovale (size and direction of the flap), the crux of the heart (offset of atrioventricular valves, tricuspid and mitral valves), the ventricles (size and morphology), interventricular septum, and pericardium.
  - *Left ventricular outflow tract view*: Further sweep from four chamber opens the left ventricular outflow tract (**Fig. 40**). This shows the continuity between the ventricular septum and the anterior wall of aorta. Outlet part of interventricular septum can be seen in this view in addition of abnormalities of the left ventricular outflow tract.
  - *Right ventricular outflow tract view*: Further sweep from the left ventricular outflow view will open the

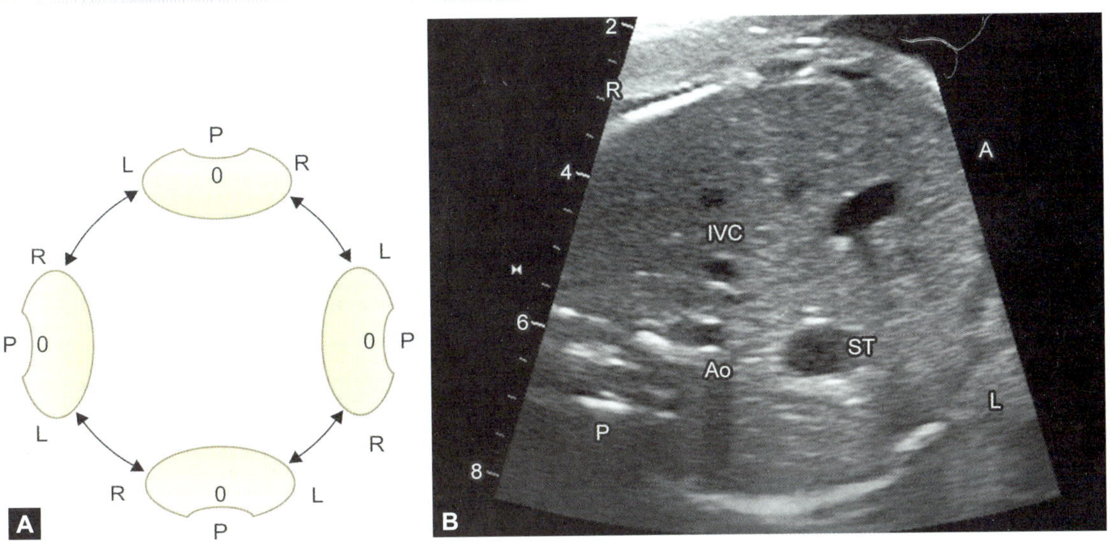

Figs. 37A and B: (A) Diagram used to decide left and right in a fetus (L: left, P: posterior; R: right); (B) Showing stomach bubble (ST) and aorta (Ao) to the left and inferior vena cava (IVC) to the right side.

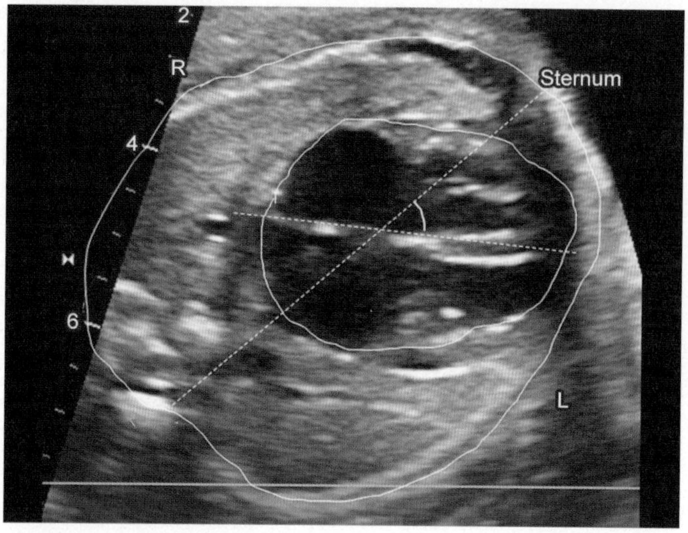

Fig. 38: Cardiac position is shown in the left chest with base apex axis toward the left side of the fetus. Cardiac axis is calculated by two imaginary lines and cardiac size by comparing the circumference of the heart to the chest.

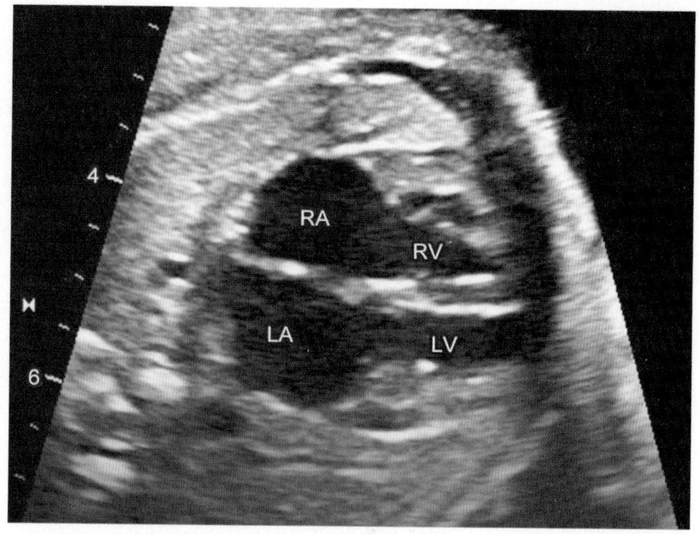

Fig. 39: Transverse section of the heart just above the diaphragm shows the four-chamber view of the fetal heart.
(LA: left atrium; LV: left ventricle; RA: right atrium; RV: right ventricle).

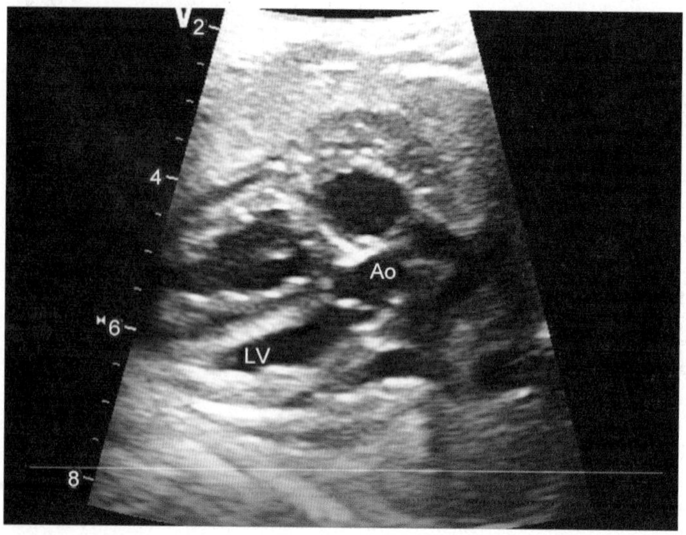

Fig. 40: Anterior sweep from the four-chamber view opens up the left ventricular outflow tract.
(Ao: aorta; LV: left ventricle)

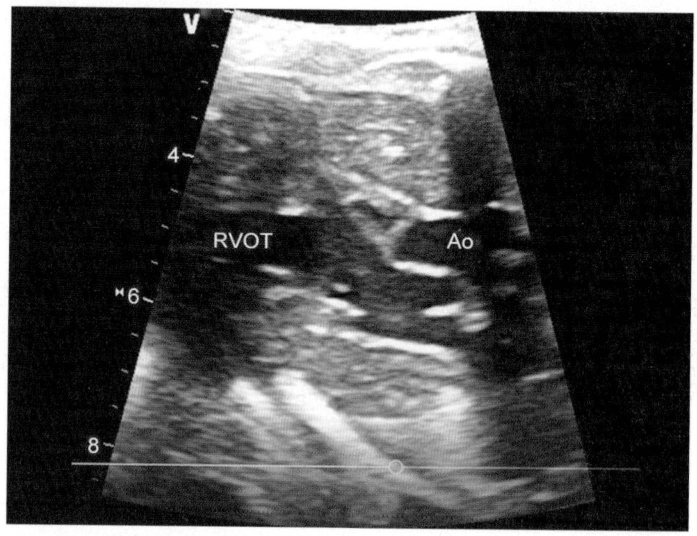

Fig. 41: Further anterior sweep from the left ventricular outflow tract shows the right ventricular outflow tract with the branch pulmonary arteries.
(Ao: aorta; RVOT: right ventricular outflow tract)

right ventricular outflow tract view (**Fig. 41**). This view would show the main PA from RV, crossing the aorta and bifurcating into branch pulmonary arteries.
- *Three-vessel view*: Further cephalad sweep in the transverse plane will show the three-vessel view (**Fig. 42**). The three vessels from left to right are PA, aorta, and SVC with gradual decrease in their sizes.
- *Sagittal plane*: This is useful for evaluating the systemic veins, the ductal and the aortic arches (**Fig. 43**).

- *Assessment of heart rate and rhythm*: This can be performed by Doppler or M-mode technique using simultaneous atrial and ventricular activities.
- *Cardiac biometry*: 2D or M-mode techniques can be used for measurements of cardiac structures. These measurements can be compared with the Z scores for the respected gestational age. Sometimes, the comparison of diameters of right and left heart structures might be useful.

Limitations and Strengths

Fetal echocardiogram can diagnose complex cardiac conditions with reasonable accuracy. Major cardiac defects such as TGA, pulmonary atresia, truncus arteriosus, common atrioventricular septal defect, Ebstein anomaly of TV are malformations that do not evolve in pregnancy and can be picked up in fetal echocardiogram.

Like any other investigation modality, fetal echocardiogram has limitations, which we need to keep in mind

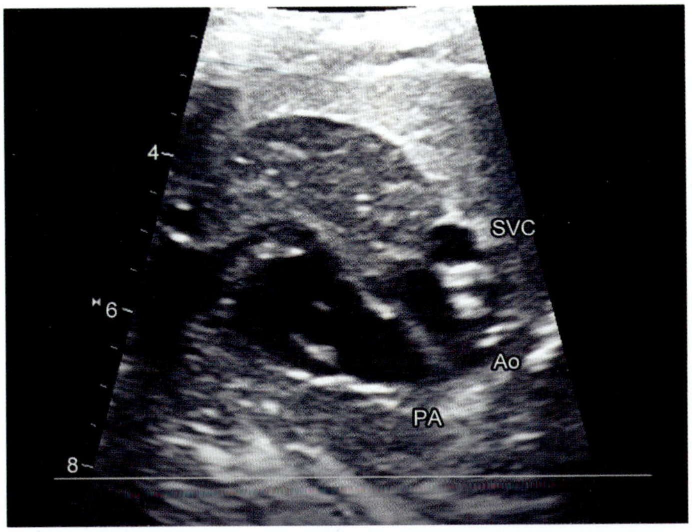

Fig. 42: The three-vessel view showing superior vena cava, aorta, and pulmonary artery from left-anterior aspect to right-posterior aspect.
(Ao: aorta; PA: pulmonary artery; SVC: superior vena cava)

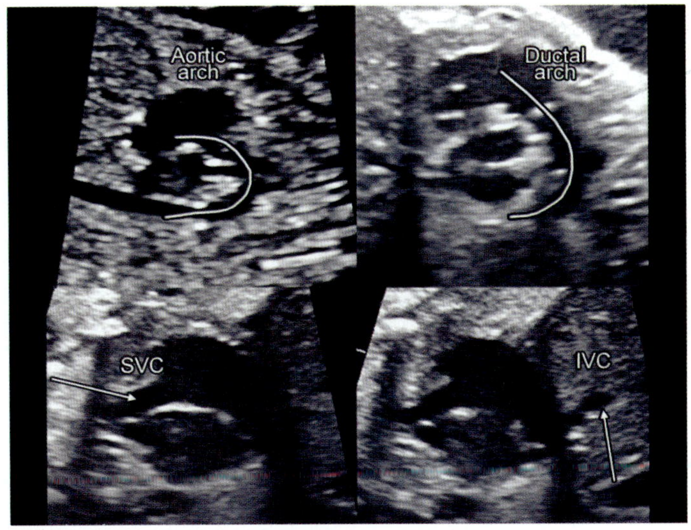

Fig. 43: The sagittal view showing the arches (ductal and aortic) and the vena cavas.
(IVC: inferior vena cava; SVC: superior vena cava).

while interpreting the report. These limitations are either due to technical factors or related to the interpretation.

- *Technical factors*: Technical limitations, which could prevent us getting the correct information, could be related to the mother or the fetus or the machine.

Poor maternal habitus/maternal obesity can cause poor penetration of ultrasound beam giving suboptimal images. Fetal position is another crucial aspect as multiple views are needed (apical, lateral, transverse views) to have a complete cardiac understanding. Hence, if the fetus position is not ideal and the movements are less, than the study may not be complete. Less amniotic fluid can cause reduced acoustic windows and less fetal movements and more amniotic fluid can cause increased fetal movements. Fetal echocardiogram done early in gestation can be technically difficult. Late third-trimester scan also can be difficult due to shadowing of the thoracic cage and reduced fetal movements. Finally, if the technical settings are not optimized, then an ideal quality of image may not be obtained.

- *Incorrect diagnosis*: Underdiagnosis or overdiagnosis—false drop out in the interventricular septum, especially the membranous septum, is not uncommon and is dependent on the transducer placement. Paradoxically, VSD, especially small-sized, is the most common missed lesion as the right and left ventricles are at same pressures. As the pulmonary venous drainage is too little, partial pulmonary venous drainage is difficult to diagnose in fetal life. Lesions such as bicuspid aortic valve and abnormal coronaries are also unlikely to be picked up in fetal life. Transient bradycardia which can happen due to pressure on the maternal abdomen might be misinterpreted as arrhythmia.
- *Evolving lesions or lesions of late pregnancy*: There are lesions, which become apparent later in pregnancy such as discrepancy in the chamber size, discrepancy in the great artery size, stenosis in semilunar valve, cardiac tumors, hypertrophic cardiomyopathy, and premature ductal and foramen ovale closure.
- *Lesions evident only after birth*: Fetal echocardiogram cannot let us know if the ductus arteriosus or foramen ovale will close postbirth or not. Hence, ASD and PDA cannot be diagnosed in fetal life.

Hence, the importance of counseling of the family as to what to expect out of fetal echocardiogram cannot be undermined (**Table 2**).

Correlation of Fetal Echocardiogram with Postnatal Management

Fetal diagnosis of congenital heart disease may alter the way the pregnancy is managed. These changes might be in the antenatal period, at delivery, or in the postnatal period. These changes are made with an intention of making the outcome of the baby more favorable. Most importantly, the safest mode of transport is in utero, hence a diagnosis of critical CHD mandates that the baby be delivered in a center where postnatal management of the baby is possible. It is to be emphasized that a diagnosis of complex congenital heart disease does not justify termination of pregnancy as such. The decision for termination should only be taken after a complete diagnosis and discussion with a pediatric cardiologist as to the postnatal outcome of such a condition. Only when reasonable correction is not available, termination is justified, e.g., a fetal diagnosis of TOF, TGA, TAPVC, etc., does not justify termination. On the other hand, in conditions such as heterotaxy, single ventricle, etc., where long-term outcomes are not satisfactory, it is justifiable. Also, the psychological trauma that comes with the fetal diagnosis of CHD should be given due importance. The family should be counseled with all available information and support offered.

TABLE 2: Impact of fetal cardiac diagnosis on management.

Antenatal	Natal	Postnatal
Counseling	Changing place of delivery	PGE1 and transport to be ready if in utero transport was not feasible
Termination	Changing time of delivery (early delivery only when baby is expected to do worse in utero)	
Work up for other anomalies, Genetic tests	Changing mode of delivery (CS only needed when fetus is compromised as in complete heart block)	
Transplacental therapy as in fetal arrhythmias		
Fetal intervention—critical AS/PS, restricted foramen ovale		

(AS: aortic stenosis; CS: coronary sinus; PGE1: prostaglandin E1; PS: pulmonary stenosis)

TELE-ECHOCARDIOGRAPHY

Echocardiograms need experts interpreting them to arrive at an accurate diagnosis. While technicians and physicians can be trained[17] to acquire echocardiographic images, many times a skilled pediatric cardiologist is needed to give an interpretation and plan management. In places where there are no specialists available, tele-echocardiography is a solution that can enable diagnosis at a distance.

Most recent echocardiogram machines are DICOM compliant, so transmission of these images is possible using a Cardiovascular Picture Archiving and Communication Systems (PACS). One issue in the transmission of echocardiogram images is its size as many are large cine files. This requires robust compression techniques without loss of image quality. Newer technologies address this issue and today, even cloud-based tele-echocardiography is available for use in India.

Imagine a pediatric cardiologist in a traffic jam in a major city of India utilizing his or her time to review an echocardiogram of a baby in a remote town, giving a diagnosis and directing therapy. With tele-echocardiography and teleconsultations, this is now possible.

REFERENCES

1. Gutgesell HP, Paquet M, Duff DF, McNamara DG. Evaluation of left ventricular size and function by echocardiography. Results in normal children. Circulation. 1977;56(3):457-62.
2. Nagueh SF, Smiseth OA, Appleton CP, Byrd BF, Dokainish H, Edvardsen T, et al. Recommendations for the evaluation of left ventricular diastolic function by echocardiography: an update from the American Society of Echocardiography and the European Association of Cardiovascular Imaging. J Am Soc Echocardiogr. 2016;29(4):277-314.
3. Kjaerjaard J, Kjaer A, Flachskampf PA, Foster E, Pelikka PA. Evaluation of right ventricular volume and function by 2D and 3D echocardiography compared to MRI. Eur J Echocardiogr. 2006;7(6):340-8.
4. Rudski LG, Lai WW, Afilalo J, Hua L, Handschumacher MD, Chandrasekaran K, et al. Guidelines for the echocardiographic assessment of the right heart in adults: a report from the American Society of Echocardiography endorsed by the European Association of Echocardiography, a registered branch of the European Society of Cardiology, and the Canadian Society of Echocardiography. J Am Soc Echocardiogr. 2010;23(7):685-713.
5. DiLorenzo MP, Bhatt SM, Mercer-Rosa L. How best to assess right ventricular function by echocardiography? Cardiol Young. 2015; 25(8):1473-81.
6. McCrindle BW, Rowley AH, Newburger JW, Burns JC, Bolger AF, Gewitz M, et al. Diagnosis, treatment, and long-term management of Kawasaki disease: a scientific statement for health professionals from the American Heart Association. Circulation. 2017;135(17):e927-99.
7. Baddour LM, Wilson WR, Bayer AS, Fowler Jr VG, Tleyjeh IM, Rybak MJ, et al. Infective endocarditis in adults: Diagnosis, antimicrobial therapy, and management of complications: a scientific statement for healthcare professionals from the American Heart Association. Circulation. 2015;132(15):1435-86.
8. Evangelista A, Gonzalez-Alujas MT. Echocardiography in infective endocarditis. Heart. 2004;90(6):614-7.
9. Baltimore RS, Gewitz M, Baddour LM, Beerman LB, Jackson MA, Lockhart PB, et al. Infective Endocarditis in Childhood: 2015 Update: A Scientific Statement from the American Heart Association. Circulation. 2015;132(15):1487-515.
10. Gilliam LD, Guyer DE, Gibson TC, King ME, Marshall JE, Weyman AE. Hydrodynamic compression of the right atrium: a new echocardiographic sign of cardiac tamponade. Circulation. 1983;68(2):294-301.
11. Tei C, Child JS, Tanaka H, Shah PM. Atrial systolic notch on the interventricular septal echogram: an echocardiographic sign of constrictive pericarditis. J Am Coll Cardiol. 1983;1(3):907-12.
12. Merce J, Sagrista-Sauleda J, Permanyer-Miralda G, Evangelista A, Soler-Soler J. Correlation between clinical and Doppler echocardiographic findings in patients with moderate to large pericardial effusion: implications for the diagnosis of cardiac tamponade. Am Heart J. 1999;138(4 Pt 1):759-64.
13. Black IW, Hopkins AP, Lee LC, Walsh WF. Left atrial spontaneous contrast: a clinical and echocardiographic analysis. J Am Coll Cardiol. 1991;18(2):398-404.
14. Appleton CP, Hatle LK, Popp RL. Demonstration of restrictive ventricular physiology by Doppler echocardiography. J Am Coll Cardiol. 1988; 11(4):757-68.
15. Gotsman MS, Lewis BS. Left ventricular volumes and compliance in hypertrophic cardiomyopathy. Chest. 1974;66(5):498-505.
16. Donofrio MT, Moon-Grady AJ, Hornberger LK, Copel, JA, Sklansky MS, Abuhamad A, et al. Diagnosis and treatment of fetal cardiac disease - a scientific statement from American Heart Association. Circulation. 2014;129(21):2183-242.
17. Singh S, Bansal M, Maheshwari P, Adams D, Sengupta SP, Price R, et al. American Society of Echocardiography: Remote echocardiography with web-based assessments for referrals at a distance (ASE-REWARD) study. Am Soc Echocardiogram. 2013;26(3):221-33.

10 CHAPTER

Advanced Cardiac Imaging: Computed Tomography and Magnetic Resonance Imaging

Mahesh Kappanayil

INTRODUCTION

Congenital heart disease (CHD) spans a wide spectrum of lesions that range from simple lesions to complex malpositions with variable combinations of intracardiac or extracardiac defects, and visceral abnormalities. Cardiovascular assessment hinges on accurate identification, characterization, and 3D spatial understanding of all these abnormalities.

Echocardiography is the mainstay of cardiovascular imaging in the assessment of CHD, it is dynamic, noninvasive, inexpensive, available at point-of-care, and capable of providing excellent anatomical as well as functional information. It is a "safe" modality—with no exposure to ionizing radiation or need for deep/prolonged anesthesia. Interpretation and reporting are quick (almost real-time), and the findings are highly reproducible. Echocardiography can provide efficient and accurate imaging, sufficient for clinical decision-making in most simple cardiac lesions and even some of more complex ones.

It does however have important limitations, which include the following:

- *Dependence on the acoustic window for imaging*: While usually excellent in most neonates and young children, acoustic windows typically become progressively worse in older, bigger patients. Postcardiac surgery patients also tend to have worse acoustic windows.
- *Limited field of visualization*: Structures of interest need to be in the narrow field of the ultrasound beam. Frequency, penetration, and other parameters of the ultrasound determine image quality.
- *Dependence on operator skill*: Acquisition of information depends upon the operator's ability to obtain specific views and sweeps from specific locations, and his/her ability to understand and integrate the anatomical and physiological cues.
- *Predominantly two-dimensional imaging*: Much of the routine transthoracic as well as transesophageal echo imaging is two-dimensional (2D), with visualization of slices of imaging data. The operator is required to mentally reconstruct the three-dimensional (3D) spatial relationships between structures. Even though contemporary 3D ultrasound technologies have led to be better spatial visualization, echocardiogram is still not the ideal tool for 3D visualization over large regions of interest.

Cardiac catheterization is the other traditional modality used for anatomical and physiological assessment of CHD. It provides excellent fluoroscopic and angiographic imaging along with vital hemodynamic data (pressures, flows, and vascular resistances). The trade-off is in being an invasive procedure with exposure to ionizing radiation. The anatomic information obtained is again 2D.

COMPUTED TOMOGRAPHY AND MAGNETIC RESONANCE IMAGING

Computed tomography (CT) and magnetic resonance imaging (MRI) are well-established noninvasive radiological imaging techniques used for wide range of imaging needs. Optimization of these techniques for cardiovascular assessment has spawned the specialized area of *cardiac radiology*, which lies at the convergence of cardiology and radiology. Both CT and MRI have their own distinct advantages and disadvantages in cardiovascular imaging, particularly with reference to CHD.

Computed Tomography

Allan M Cormack and Godfrey N Hounsfield were jointly awarded the Nobel Prize in Physiology or Medicine in 1979 for their work in developing computer-assisted tomography (CAT). This technique uses multiple X-rays taken from different angles to produce cross-sectional images. Digital reformatting and geometry-processing of these multiple contiguous or helical scans generates volumetric images that are amenable to multiplanar reconstructions and 3D viewing. CT has high-contrast resolution, capable of differentiating between tissues with 1% difference in physical density.

Heart being a constantly moving object, offers considerable challenges to all imaging modalities. Early CT scanners had a single detector translating around the patient as the patient-table moved in cephalocaudal direction (z-axis). Subsequently, as technology developed, more and more detector channels were added [multidetector computed tomography (MDCT)], gantry rotations and patient-table movements became faster, and electrocardiographic gating techniques were developed.[1] All of these developments led to exponential improvement in the quality of CT imaging of cardiovascular anatomy. Current MDCT scanners can have up to 640 detector channels, making for extremely fast acquisitions and high resolution imaging with reduced radiation doses. ECG gating enables acquisition and construction of imaging data at precise points during the R-R interval (enhancing temporal resolution), and can be either prospective or retrospective. Prospective ECG gating enables acquisition at predetermined segments of the R-R interval (usually 70–80% of the R-R interval), every other heartbeat, one slice at a time, and subsequent stacking-up of the image slices. Retrospective ECG gating involves acquisition through several cardiac cycles and subsequent division and viewing in blocks of time. Retrospective gated scans use more radiation, but can potentially give functional information and cine renderings in addition to the static imaging. Dual-source MDCT scanners can further reduce scan times and radiation dose by acquiring scans twice as fast as single-source scanners. CT assessment of most CHD requires the administration of iodine-based radiocontrast (contrast-enhanced CT), optimize the field of view, and timing the acquisition appropriately, in order to optimally image the cardiovascular structures of interest.

Advantages of Computed Tomography Imaging for Congenital Heart Disease Assessment

The most striking advantages of CT imaging are summarized as follows:

- Rapid acquisition
- Excellent spatial and temporal resolution
- Wide field of view
- Excellent visualization of extracardiac vascular structures such as distal pulmonary arteries, pulmonary arborization, pulmonary veins, aortic malformations, and aortopulmonary collaterals
- Excellent visualization of airways and other viscera in relation to cardiovascular structures
- Volumetric imaging data that can be viewed in infinite planes using multiplanar reconstruction techniques
- Amenable to 3D printing.

Indications for Cardiac Computed Tomography in Assessment of Neonates, Infants, and Children with Congenital Heart Disease

Some important examples of cardiac CT applications are shown in **Figures 1A to D**.

- Complex intracardiac anatomical defects, e.g., criss-cross heart with associated defects, complex double outlet right ventricle (DORV), and anatomically corrected malposition of great arteries
- Assessment of pulmonary venous anomalies, particularly, in complex or mixed forms of total anomalous pulmonary venous connections (TAPVC)
- Assessment of pulmonary artery anatomy and aorto-pulmonary collaterals in cases with pulmonary atresia with hypoplastic or nonconfluent central pulmonary arteries
- Aortic and aortic arch anomalies such as interrupted aortic arch, double aortic arch, aortic aneurysm, and aortic tortuosity
- Coronary anomalies, e.g., coronary arteriovenous fistula, aneurysm, and anomalous origin
- Vascular ring and vascular sling anomalies with airway compression
- CHD with other associated complex visceral anomalies, e.g., heterotaxy syndrome
- Postoperative residual or secondary lesions, e.g., branch pulmonary artery or vein stenosis and postvascular stenting
- Assessment of pericardial pathology, e.g., pericardial thickening/constriction
- Conditions where MRI is not useful or is contraindicated, e.g., presence of metallic implants/coils, older generation pacemakers, and defibrillators.

Disadvantages of Computed Tomography in Patients with Congenital Heart Disease

It is important to be aware of the disadvantages and limitations of CT imaging

- Exposure to ionizing radiation—not suitable for frequent or serial evaluations
- Static anatomical imaging with little or no dynamic or functional information
- ECG-gating is challenging in neonates and young infants/children due to fast heart rates
- Expensive and the quality of imaging depends upon the scanner hardware and software
- Interpretation and reporting needs understanding of tomographic anatomy in addition to knowledge of tenets of CHD anatomy/physiology.

Magnetic Resonance Imaging

Magnetic resonance imaging or MRI is based on the phenomenon of "nuclear magnetic resonance" or NMR, a phenomenon first described by Isidor Rabi in 1938. Rabi was awarded the Nobel Prize in Physics in 1944 for his discovery. Edwards Purcell and Felix Bloch expanded this technique to develop NMR "spectroscopy" for which they shared the Nobel Prize in Physics in 1952. The fundamental principle underlying these phenomena is the behavior of

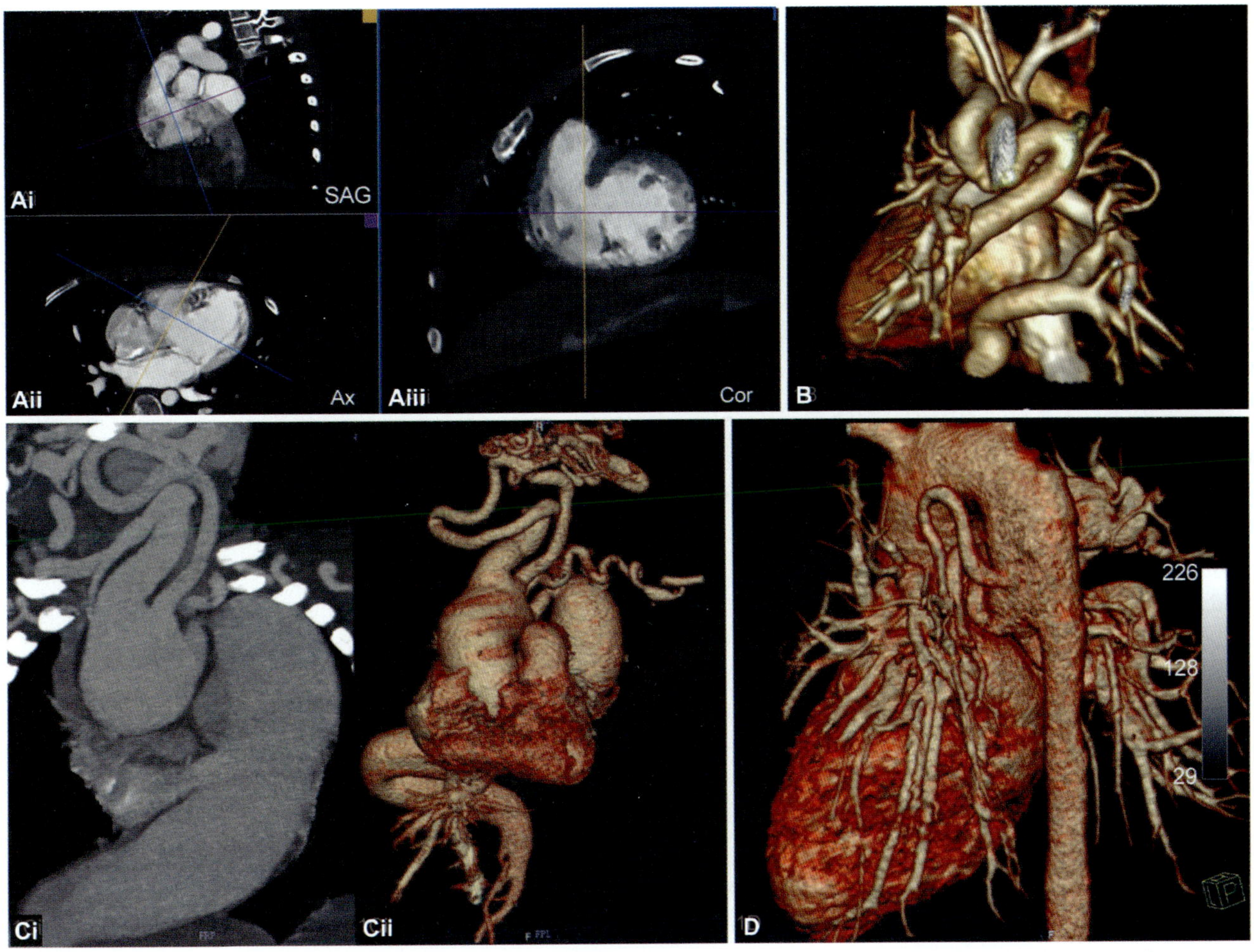

Figs. 1A to D: Panel showing some of the applications of computed tomography (CT) in cardiovascular imaging. (A) Multiplanar imaging using CT—the same image of a ventricular septal defect simultaneously in three orthogonal planes: (Ai) sagittal (SAG), (Aii) axial (Ax), and (Aiii) coronal (Cor) projections; (B) A 3D rendition of CT showing a complex mixed variety of total anomalous pulmonary venous connection; (Ci) Coronal slice of CT in an infant with severe aortic dilatation and tortuosity in a patient with FBLN4 mutation-related arteriopathy (Kappanayil M, et al. Orphanet J Rare Dis. 2012;7:61), (Cii) the 3D rendering of the same CT data; (D) 3D rendered image of aortopulmonary collaterals in a patient with pulmonary atresia.

certain magnetic nuclei when placed in a magnetic field and subjected to radiofrequency (RF) energy. The nuclei tend to absorb this RF energy when it is of a frequency specific to the identity of the nuclei, and when this absorption happens, the nuclei are said to be in "resonance". Different atomic nuclei within the same molecules may resonate at different frequencies of RF energy, depending upon the differences in their structure and chemical properties.

Magnetic resonance imaging uses these principles for structural and functional imaging of various tissues and organs noninvasively and without the use of any ionizing radiation. The hydrogen atoms (protons) ubiquitous in all body organs and tissues as part of water and fat act as magnets. When the patient is laid within the powerful magnetic field of an MRI machine, the protons align themselves along the field. Then, these protons are stimulated and spun out of their equilibrium by applying RF energy. When the RF field is subsequently turned off, the protons realign themselves to their state of equilibrium, emitting RF energy as they do so, which in turn is picked up by sensors or "coils" and finally transformed into images. The time taken for the protons to thus realign as well as the amount of energy released during the process depends upon the tissue characteristics. By varying the parameters of the excitation pulses, different contrasts may be generated among tissues.

Cardiac magnetic resonance imaging (CMRI) uses these same principles for imaging the cardiovascular system.

It is important to understand that CMRI is not a single homogeneous modality, rather it comprises of *multiple* NMR-based techniques or "pulse sequences", which provide different forms of morphological and physiological information. Pulse sequences are different software programs that encode magnitude and timing of RF pulses emitted by the MR scanner, switching of the magnetic field gradient, and data acquisition, each one tailored for a specific purpose. Each CMR study, typically, is comprised of a set of different sequences that are chosen to answer the specific study questions of the particular case. Some of the commonly used CMRI sequences and their specific uses are as listed here.

- *For morphological imaging*: Black blood (static images), bright blood, or gradient recalled sequences (GRE) (static or cine), gadolinium contrast-enhanced magnetic resonance angiography (MRA)
- *For ventricular function assessment*: Cine steady state free precession (SSFP)
- *For blood flow quantification*: Phase contrast magnetic resonance imaging (PC-MRI)
- *For myocardial imaging*: Myocardial perfusion imaging, myocardial delayed enhancement (MDE), and myocardial tissue tagging, T2*.

Specific Applications of Cardiac Magnetic Resonance Imaging in Congenital Heart Disease

The versatility of MRI allows comprehensive investigation in a wide variety of CHDs (**Figs. 2A to C**).

Comprehensive assessment of complex CHD: For detailed assessment of anatomical details, ventricular functions, adequacy for biventricular repair, and blood flow dynamics.[2]

Postoperative follow-up after tetralogy of Fallot repair: For decision-making regarding requirement for pulmonary valve replacement or other interventions.

Long-term follow-up after other CHD surgeries such as arterial switch operation and Fontan operation.

Diagnosis and serial follow-up of extracardiac vascular abnormalities in Marfan syndrome, Loeys–Dietz Syndrome, and other inherited connective tissue disorders.

Imaging and tissue characterization of cardiac tumors.

Advantages of Cardiac Magnetic Resonance Imaging

The following advantages of cardiac MRI are widely accepted:

- Noninvasive
- No exposure to ionizing radiation or iodine-based contrast
- True 3D volumetric imaging—amenable to customized acquisitions and multiplanar viewing
- Flexible modality with multiple modules or sequences that can be customized according to requirement
- Excellent dynamic and cine imaging with good tissue/blood-pool contrast
- Excellent and robust hemodynamic and functional information—blood flows, ventricular functions. Scope for internal validation of hemodynamic data

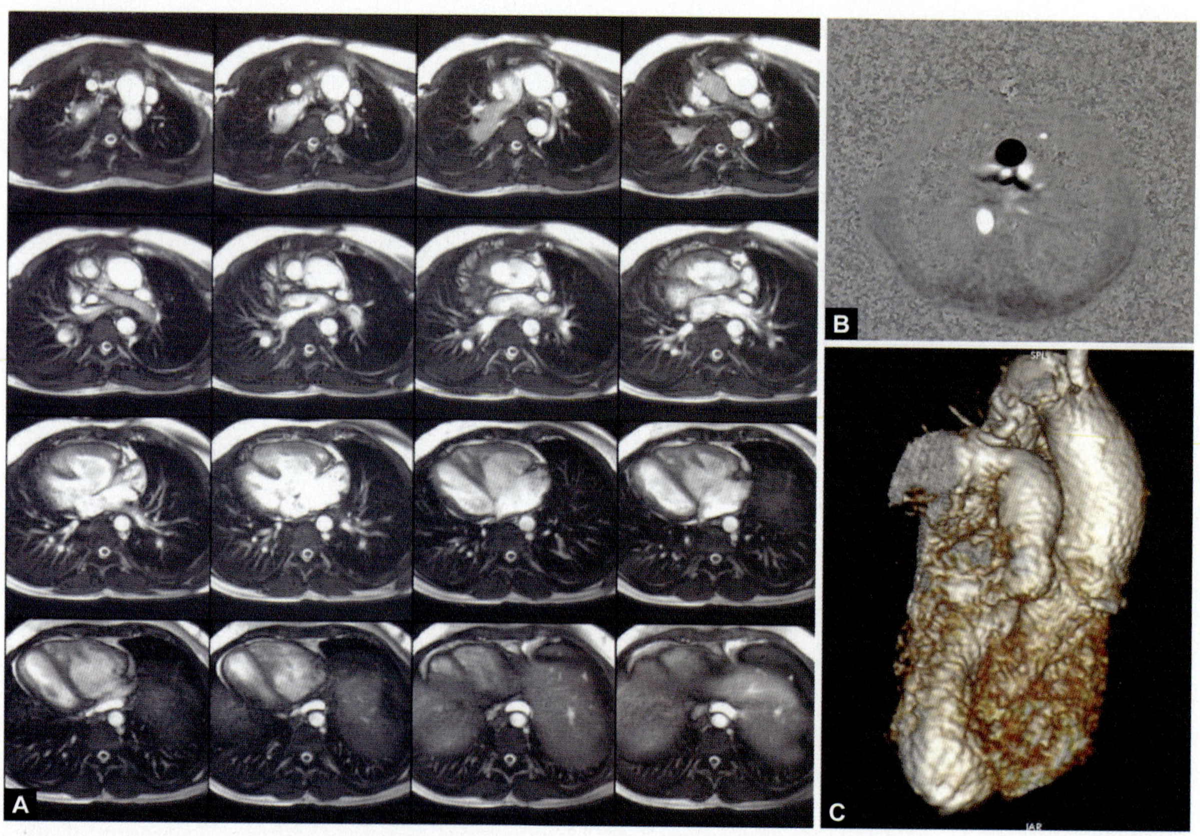

Figs. 2A to C: Panel showing some of the imaging sequences commonly used in cardiac magnetic resonance imaging (MRI) studies. (A) A frozen frame from the axial "stack" of cine bright blood cardiovascular images ("Steady State Free Precession" or SSFP sequence) in a patient with dextrocardia with complex DORV. This sequence provides excellent dynamic anatomical information, and can also be used for accurate estimation of cardiac chamber volumes and functions; (B) A "phase contrast" or PC sequence imaging of a cross-section of aorta, which yields accurate flow information. PC is accepted as the "gold standard" in vascular flow assessments; important applications include calculation of pulmonary regurgitation (PR) fraction in post-tetralogy repair assessment for pulmonary valve replacement, and Qp:Qs estimations in complex CHD; (C) A 3D volume rendition of the cardiac anatomy in a case of dextrocardia, DORV, derived from gadolinium-enhanced "magnetic resonance angiography" or MRA.

by comparison of information acquired via different sequences
- Gold standard for assessment of right ventricular dimensions/functions and blood flow assessment (e.g., pulmonary regurgitation fractions and differential pulmonary blood flows after tetralogy repair)
- Assessment and quantification of myocardial scarring
- Noncontrast 3D angiographic sequences
- Amenable to postprocessing for wide range of anatomical and functional information
- Potential for radiation-free MRI-based cardiac interventions
- Ideally suited for serial evaluations in the long-term follow-up of postoperative CHD
- Amenable to 3D printing, computational fluid dynamic, and simulation studies.

Disadvantages of CMR

- Expensive (costs comparable to cardiac CT)
- Limited availability of facilities with the hardware, software, and expertise
- Time-consuming and requires patient cooperation with breath-holds
- Children younger than 7 years, uncooperative patients, and those with claustrophobia may require general anesthesia
- Spatial resolution less than CT
- Not ideal for evaluation of distal coronaries or calcific lesions
- Metal artefacts with objects such as MRI-incompatible vascular embolization coils
- Contraindicated in patients with MRI-incompatible devices (implantable pacemakers and defibrillators) or implants
- Potential risk of gadolinium-induced nephrogenic systemic fibrosis in patients with end-stage renal failure.

3D plus technologies: Volumetric data obtained through CT or MRI can be converted into physical replicas using the technology of 3D printing. 3D printing involves creation of a physical 3D object from a computer-aided design (CAD) model by successive addition of material layer-by-layer, under precise computer control. This cutting-edge technology is beginning to dramatically alter the way we interact with medical imaging data.

Conventionally, the CT and MRI 3D data is viewed on the 2D screen of workstations. This volumetric DICOM (digital communication in medicine) data can be imported into specialized software, and converted into digital 3D models and exported out in special formats (.stl, .obj, etc.) that can be read by machines called "3D Printers". 3D printers can then convert these digital 3D models into a physical prototypes through a precise computer-controlled process by adding layer-after-layer of material.

The 3D printed cardiovascular models, derived from patients' own imaging data, are precise replicas of the actual anatomy, and can greatly enhance the understanding of complex pathology (**Fig. 3**). This in-turn can significantly

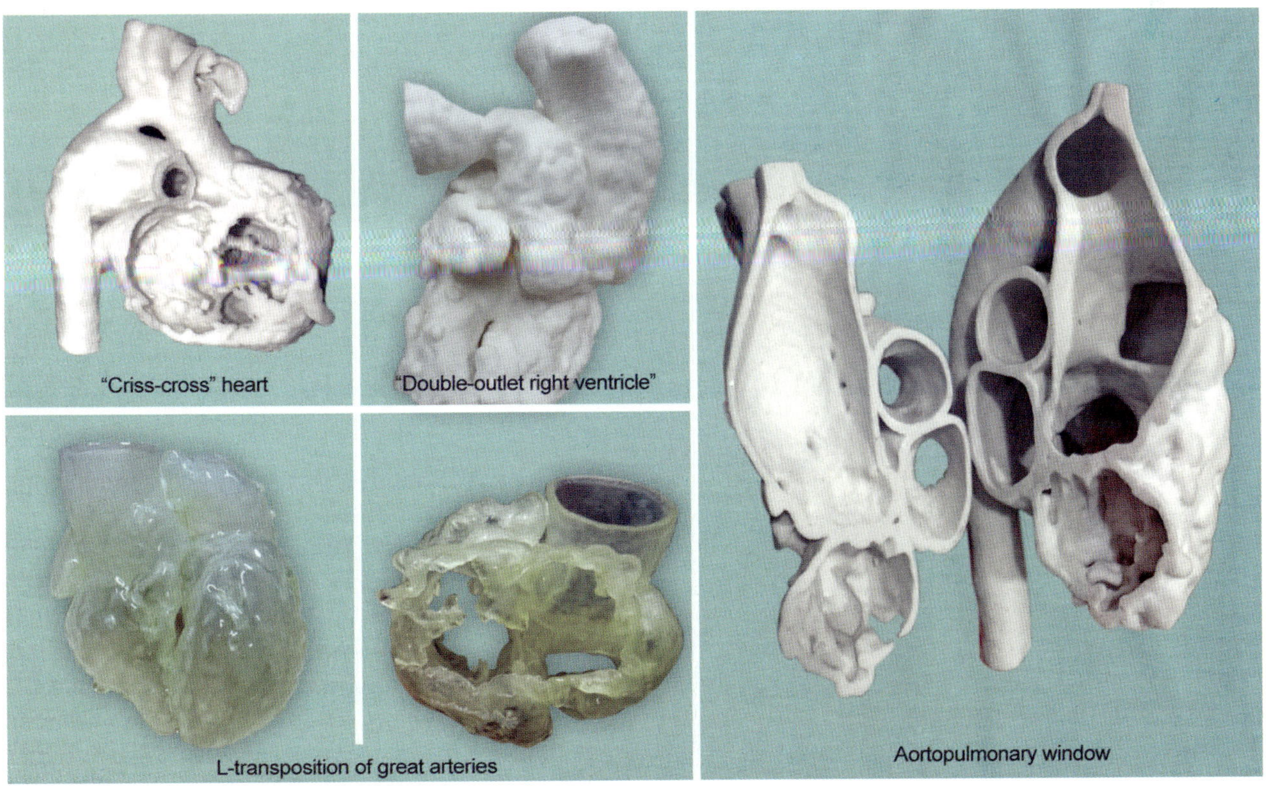

Fig. 3: Panel showing 3D-printed heart models derived from either computed tomography (CT) or magnetic resonance (MR)-based 3D angiographic techniques. These 3D prints allow the observer to physically handle and manipulate precise replicas of the intracardiac as well as extracardiac defects, allowing deep and realistic understanding.

aid planning and safe execution of complex heart surgeries for CHD. 3D-printed replicas can also serve as invaluable tools for communication, education, simulation, and research.[3-5] Virtual reality (VR) and augmented reality (AR) tools are exciting new developments in the visualization of cardiovascular imaging data that will allow physicians to immersively interact with the images in new and unique ways.

Together, these 3D+ technologies are poised to transform the visualization of cardiovascular imaging.

CONCLUSION

Cardiovascular imaging is challenging and complex. Echocardiography will continue to be the primary imaging tool for imaging CHD. CT and MRI are powerful and versatile tools that must be used judiciously. Majority of patients with complex lesions and those requiring long-term follow-up with in-depth imaging will require multimodality imaging. Choice of imaging modalities in isolation or in conjunction with others must be tailored to answer the specific study questions of the case. 3D printing, AR, VR, artificial intelligence (AI), and other evolving technologies will revolutionize the way clinicians of the future view medical imaging.

REFERENCES

1. Bardo DM, Brown P. Cardiac multidetector computed tomography: basic physics of image acquisition and clinical applications. Curr Cardiol Rev. 2008;4(3):231-43.
2. Kappanayil M, Kannan R, Kumar RK. Understanding the physiology of complex congenital heart disease using cardiac magnetic resonance imaging. Ann Pediatr Cardiol. 2011;4(2): 177-82
3. Opfer E, Shah S. Advances in pediatric cardiovascular imaging. Mo Med. 2018;115(4):354-60.
4. Yoo SJ, Thabit O, Kim EK, Ide H, Yim D, Dragulescu A, et al. 3D printing in medicine of congenital heart diseases. 3D Print Med. 2016;2:3.
5. Kappanayil M, Koneti NR, Kannan RR, Kottayil BP, Kumar K. Three-dimensional-printed cardiac prototypes aid surgical decision-making and preoperative planning in selected cases of complex congenital heart diseases: early experience and proof of concept in a resource-limited environment. Ann Pediatr Cardiol. 2017;10(2):117-25.

11

CHAPTER

Diagnostic Cardiac Catheterization and Angiography

Arun Gopalakrishnan

INTRODUCTION

With improvements in echocardiography and imaging modalities, the need for diagnostic cardiac catheterization for structural heart diseases in children has considerably dwindled over the past decade. While the diagnosis of several congenital heart diseases depended largely on carefully conducted cardiac catheterizations even into the early 90s, echocardiographic imaging can accurately delineate most structural heart diseases in even in fetal and neonatal life. The application of the principles of Doppler imaging facilitates considerable understanding of hemodynamics without invasive catheterization. Ventricular septal defect (VSD), tetralogy of Fallot (TOF), transposition of the great arteries, total anomalous pulmonary venous connections (TAPVCs), Ebstein anomaly, hypoplastic left heart syndrome, and endocardial cushion defects are some of the conditions where diagnostic catheterization used to be done in the past but is nearly obsolete in the current era. Even in complex heart diseases, cardiac magnetic resonance imaging (MRI) and computed tomography (CT) can give diagnostic clarity similar to a virtual dissection in the current era.[1] However, cardiac catheterization does play a role in several specific instances where accurate hemodynamic assessment guides therapeutic decision-making.

INDICATIONS FOR CARDIAC CATHETERIZATION IN CHILDREN

The indications for diagnostic cardiac catheterization as recommended by the American Heart Association in 2011 are as follows:[2]

Class I (Strong Recommendation)

- It is recommended that hemodynamic and anatomic data be obtained (via angiography when necessary) at the time of a planned interventional cardiac catheterization. It would be reckless to perform a catheter intervention without obtaining the necessary anatomic and physiologic information.
- It is recommended that cardiac catheterization be used to assess pulmonary resistance and reversibility of pulmonary hypertension in patients with congenital heart disease (CHD) or primary pulmonary hypertension when accurate assessment of pulmonary resistance is needed to make surgical and medical decisions. Cardiac catheterization is the only means to obtain an accurate recording of mean pressures in any location. This enables calculations of resistances in pulmonary and systemic circuits. Additionally, the acute responses to vasodilators can be tested with the catheters in place. This is very useful in planning long-term therapy in idiopathic pulmonary hypertension (*see* Chapter 18).
- Cardiac catheterization is indicated in patients with complex pulmonary atresia for the detailed characterization of lung segmental pulmonary vascular supply, especially when noninvasive imaging methods incompletely define pulmonary artery anatomy. Here, there may also be the opportunity to occlude collaterals that are supplying territories that overlap with native pulmonary arterial supply,
- Cardiac catheterization is indicated in delineation of coronary circulation in pulmonary atresia with intact septum. Here the specifics of coronary artery anatomy may not be obtained by other means (*see* Chapter 32).
- Cardiac catheterization is indicated in patients being assessed for cardiac transplantation unless the patient's risk for catheterization outweighs the potential benefit.
- Cardiac catheterization is recommended for surveillance of graft vasculopathy (involving the coronary arteries) after cardiac transplantation.

Class IIa (Moderately Strong Recommendation)

- It is reasonable to perform a cardiac catheterization to determine pulmonary pressure/resistance and transpulmonary gradient in palliated single ventricle patients before a staged Fontan procedure. Again the information on mean arterial pressures is not obtained by other means (*see* Chapter 39).

- Cardiac catheterization is reasonable in any CHD patient in whom complete diagnosis cannot be obtained by noninvasive testing or in whom such testing yields incomplete information.
- Cardiac catheterization is reasonable for the assessment of cardiomyopathy or myocarditis whenever endomyocardial biopsy is contemplated (*see* Chapter 43).
- Cardiac catheterization is reasonable for the assessment of coronary circulation in some cases of Kawasaki disease in which coronary involvement is suspected or requires further delineation or in the assessment of suspected congenital coronary artery anomalies (*see* Chapter 44).
- Cardiac catheterization is reasonable to perform for the assessment of anatomy and hemodynamics in postoperative cardiac patients when the early postoperative course is unexpectedly complicated and noninvasive imaging techniques [e.g., magnetic resonance angiography (MRA), CT angiography] fail to yield a clear explanation.

PRECATHETERIZATION ASSESSMENT

A detailed clinical evaluation and patient selection is the prerequisite for a good catheterization study. After meticulous history and clinical examination, all relevant noninvasive investigations should be studied, including oxygen saturation, electrocardiograms (ECGs), radiological investigations, data from surgical records and prior catheterization, and thorough echocardiographic evaluation. This will help in arriving at a comprehensive precatheterization diagnosis. The indications of catheterization and goals of the study need to be listed down and the entire team should be aware of the same before the patient is taken for the procedure.

The patient must be in the best possible physical condition when taken up for cardiac catheterization. All comorbid conditions such as anemia, acidosis, dyselectrolytemia, and arrhythmia need to be controlled for optimal assessment of hemodynamics.

Assessment of systemic veins and arteries is important to plan vascular access. The patient must be optimally hydrated as hemodynamics gets significantly altered in dehydrated states. Most pediatric catheterizations are performed under general anesthesia or with sedative agents. Anesthetic support must be available in all cases. The catheterization laboratory should have size-appropriate resuscitative equipment including defibrillator and temporary pacemaker.

MONITORING DURING CATHETERIZATION

Continuous ECG monitoring, peripheral oxygen saturation, and blood pressure recordings are required during catheterization. Temperature should be monitored particularly in infants and neonates, besides the use of external warming devices. Patients on ventilator should have end-tidal CO_2 monitoring and periodic blood gas monitoring. A defibrillator should be ready throughout the procedure.

VASCULAR ACCESS

The percutaneous femoral approach is standard for diagnostic cardiac catheterization for congenital heart disease. While vascular cut-down procedures were common in the past, the application of the Seldinger technique has made percutaneous vascular access possible in nearly all instances. This involves antegrade vascular puncture with a needle to introduce a wire into the target vessel. Ultrasound-guided approach now facilitates safe and quick access even in preterm neonates. The common femoral artery is best palpated against the femoral head at the mid-point between the anterior superior iliac spine and the pubic symphysis just below the inguinal ligament. The femoral vein lies immediately medial to the femoral artery.

The umbilical vein presents a readily available vascular access for bedside balloon atrial septostomy in the early neonate. However, it is rarely used for diagnostic cardiac catheterization.

Anterior cubital vein, axillary vein, internal jugular vein, and the subclavian veins are alternate venous approaches to diagnostic cardiac catheterization if the femoral approach is unavailable. Axillary and carotid artery approaches are occasionally used for interventions. Direct hepatic vein entry with a Chiba needle under ultrasound guidance is an option when the femoral veins are impassable.[3]

Systemic anticoagulation with unfractionated heparin is not routinely recommended for purely venous catheterization for brief procedures. For prolonged procedures and those involving arterial access, heparin at 50–100 IU/kg is recommended with periodic monitoring of activated clotting time (target 200–250 seconds).[4]

TECHNIQUE OF DIAGNOSTIC CARDIAC CATHETERIZATION

After obtaining vascular access and confirming patient stability by reviewing the vitals, cardiac catheterization is done using diagnostic catheters to obtain hemodynamic information in the form of pressure data and oximetry. All the catheters must be flushed with heparinized saline and the transducers zeroed before proceeding with data collection. During right heart catheterization, oxygen saturation and pressures are taken from the superior vena cava (SVC), inferior vena cava (IVC), right atrium, right ventricle, main pulmonary artery and the left and right pulmonary arteries, and pulmonary capillary wedge position. Left atrial and pulmonary venous saturation and pressures may be obtained in the presence of a patent foramen ovale or atrial septal defect. Left heart catheterization is most often done by retrograde approach from the femoral artery. Pressure and oximetry information is gathered from the descending aorta, ascending aorta, and the left ventricle.

PRESSURE MEASUREMENTS

Pressure recording from cardiac chambers involves identification of pressure wave changes using a fluid-filled system involving the diagnostic catheter, manifold, and tubings. At the other end, this is connected to a thin silicon diaphragm which serves as a pressure transducer converting the information into hemodynamic pressure recordings by oscillometry. The transducer should be positioned at the mid-chest level for zero reference. A higher position of the transducer would lead to falsely low pressure recordings and vice versa. Stability of the loading conditions and cardiac contractility as well as precise positioning of the catheter tip are crucial to obtain accurate pressure recordings on catheterization. The normal values of pressures in various cardiac chambers are given in **Table 1**. Side-hole catheters and balloon-tipped catheters give better stability to pressure recordings.

Types of Pressure Recordings

The atrial pressure recording is characterized by multiple positive waves for every cardiac cycle. Typically, it has three positive waves—"a," "c," and "v," and two troughs—"x" descent and "y" descent (**Fig. 1**). The "a" wave corresponds to atrial contraction and occurs in late diastole. It is followed by the "x" descent during atrial relaxation. Transient bulging of the atrioventricular valve apparatus into the atrium at the beginning of ventricular systole causes the "c" wave. During continued ventricular systole, the descent of the atrioventricular valve apparatus results in x' descent. Since the "c" wave is mostly inconspicuous, the x and x' descents are often fused. Venous return to the atrium during ventricular systole against a closed atrioventricular valve explains the "v" wave. Rapid inflow of blood into the ventricles during early diastole causes the "y" descent.

The ventricular pressure waveform consists of a systolic and diastolic phase. In early diastole (isovolumetric relaxation), the ventricular pressure tracing shows a transient steep decline to zero or even negative value—the dip diastolic phase (*see* **Figs. 4 and 5**). The diastasis phase of ventricular diastole is characterized by a gradual and steady rise in pressure. The ventricular end-diastolic pressure corresponds to the peak or nadir of the QRS complex. The steep rise in ventricular pressure occurs in isovolumetric contraction before ejection sets in with opening of the semilunar valves. The normal left ventricular pressure tracing has a "bullet-like" contour (**Fig. 2**), while the right ventricular waveforms tend to be more triangular (**Fig. 3**).

The arterial pressure tracing is the result of the forward and reflected waves upon ejection of blood (**Figs. 4 and 5**). The dicrotic notch in the descending limb of the arterial tracing corresponds to the closure of the corresponding semilunar valve and end of ejection. The dicrotic notch is relatively delayed in the arterial trace from a more distal artery as opposed to the ascending aorta (**Fig. 5**). The reflected waves are responsible for systolic pressure amplification in peripheral arteries as opposed to centrally located vessels. This must be kept in mind before estimating gradients across the aortic valve or at the site of coarctation.

The pulmonary capillary wedge pressure (PCWP) involves recording of pressure in the distal most pulmonary artery with an end-hole catheter facing the pulmonary capillary bed after eliminating additional flow. This is mostly done by end-hole balloon-tipped catheter (e.g., Swan-Ganz). This pressure recording reflects pulmonary venous pressure and therein left atrial pressure in the absence of intervening pathology (**Figs. 6A and B**). Thus, PCWP recording has an atrial contour. PCWP serves as an indirect means of recording left atrial pressures by right heart catheterization in the presence of intact atrial septum.

OXIMETRY

The aims of diagnostic cardiac catheterization include estimation of cardiac output, pulmonary and systemic blood flows (in shunt lesions), and resistance. It is very difficult to directly estimate the blood flow directly from the heart or blood vessels. This is most often done using the Fick principle, which states that that uptake or release of a substance by any organ is the product of the arteriovenous concentration difference of the substance and the blood flow to that organ. While Douglas bag method and polarographic methods can directly measure oxygen consumption (VO_2), they are not readily available. Hence, most often assumed values of VO_2 are used based on the formulas of Lafarge and Meittinen.[6]

Male patients: VO_2 (mL/min/m^2) =
138.1 – [11.49 × ln (age)] + (0.378 × *heart rate*)

TABLE 1: Normal pressures of the various cardiac chambers in children (mm Hg).[5]

Chamber	*Systolic (v wave for atria)*	*Diastolic (a wave for atria)*	*Mean*
Right atrium			3 ± 1
Right ventricle	25 ± 5	4 ± 2	
Pulmonary artery	22 ± 4	10 ± 3	13 ± 3
Left atrium (pulmonary capillary wedge)			8 ± 2
Left ventricle	110 ± 12	9 ± 2	

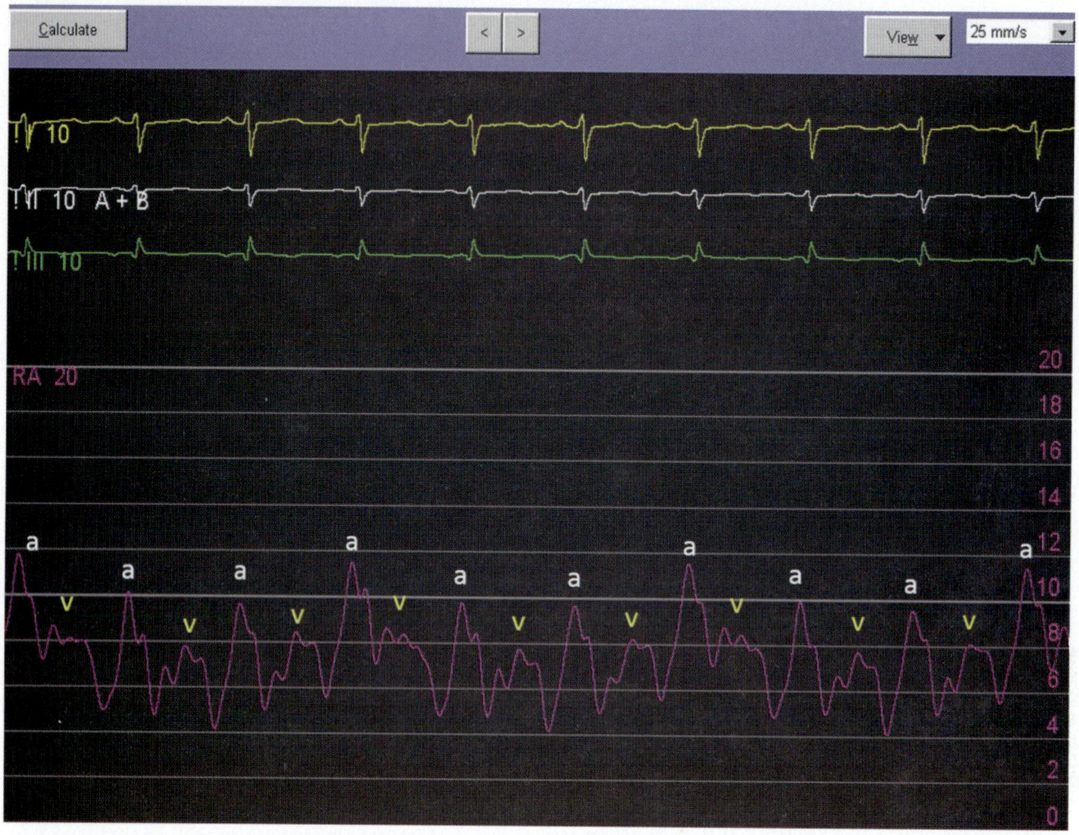

Fig. 1: Right atrial pressure trace of a 4-year-old with severe pulmonary stenosis upon catheterization for balloon pulmonary valvotomy. Prominent "a" wave is notable.

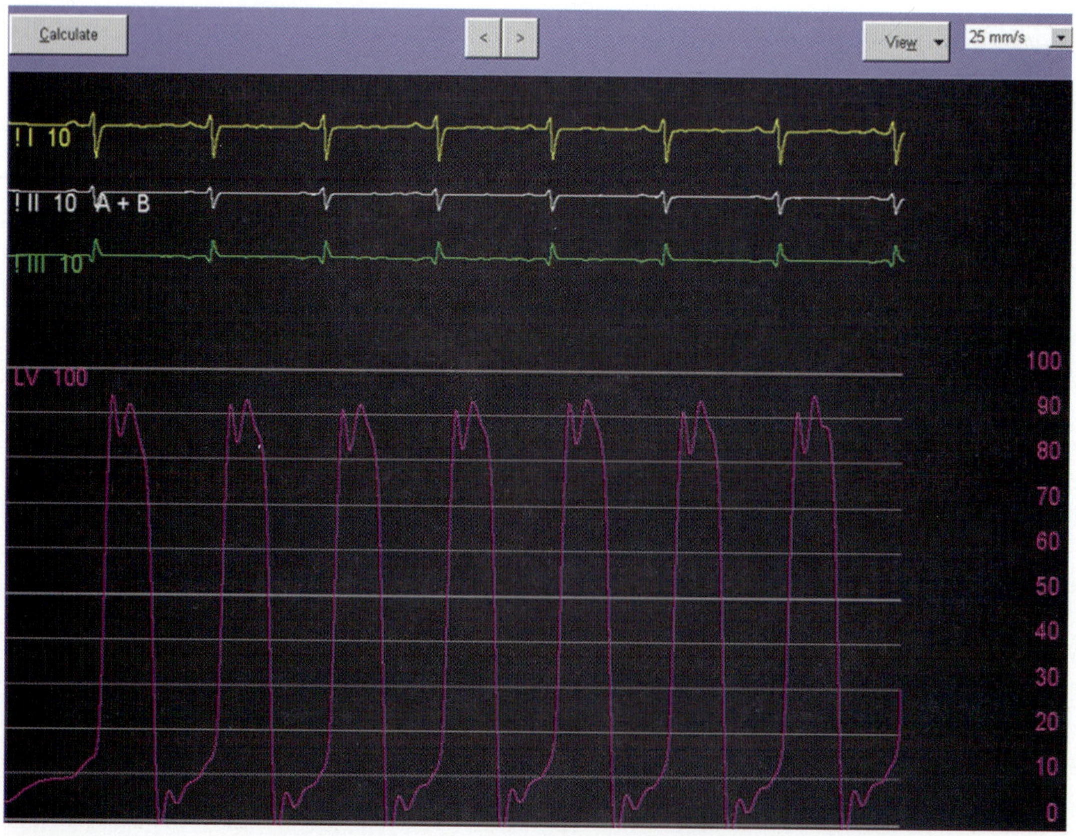

Fig. 2: Normal left ventricular pressure tracing of a 7-year-old child prior to Fontan completion.

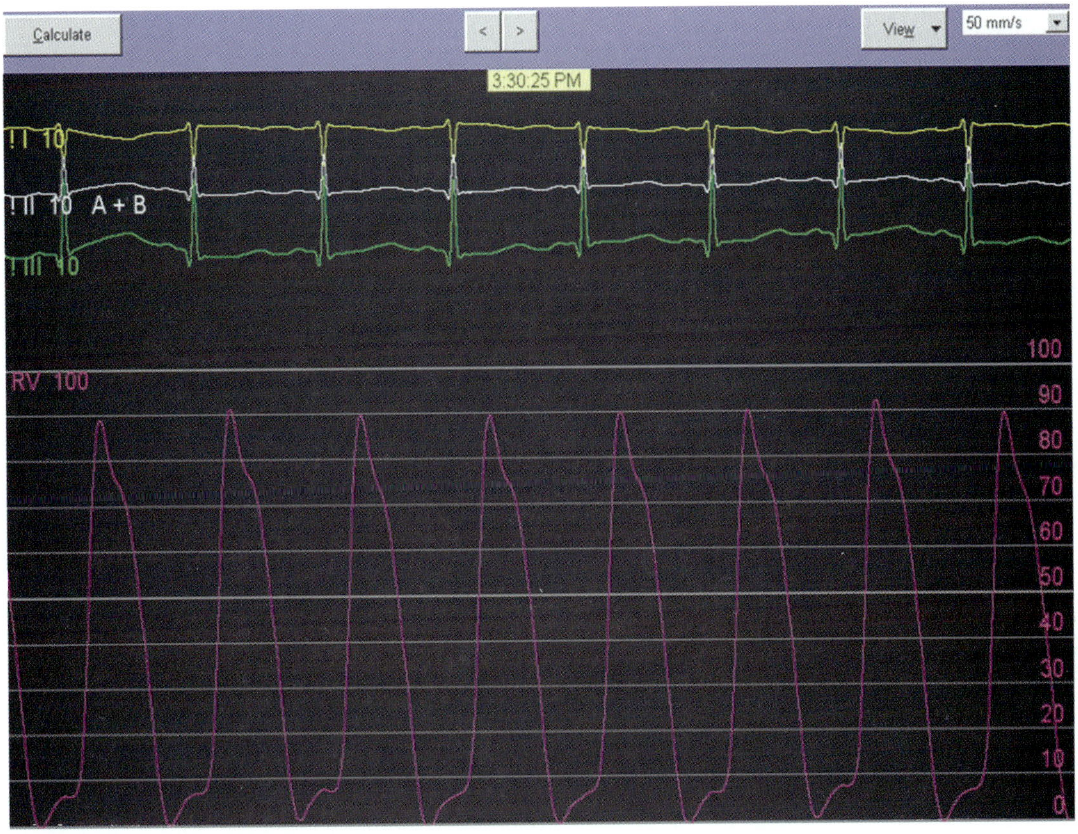

Fig. 3: Right ventricular pressure trace of a 10-year-old boy with atrial septal defect and severe pulmonary hypertension showing a right ventricular systolic pressure of 90 mm Hg.

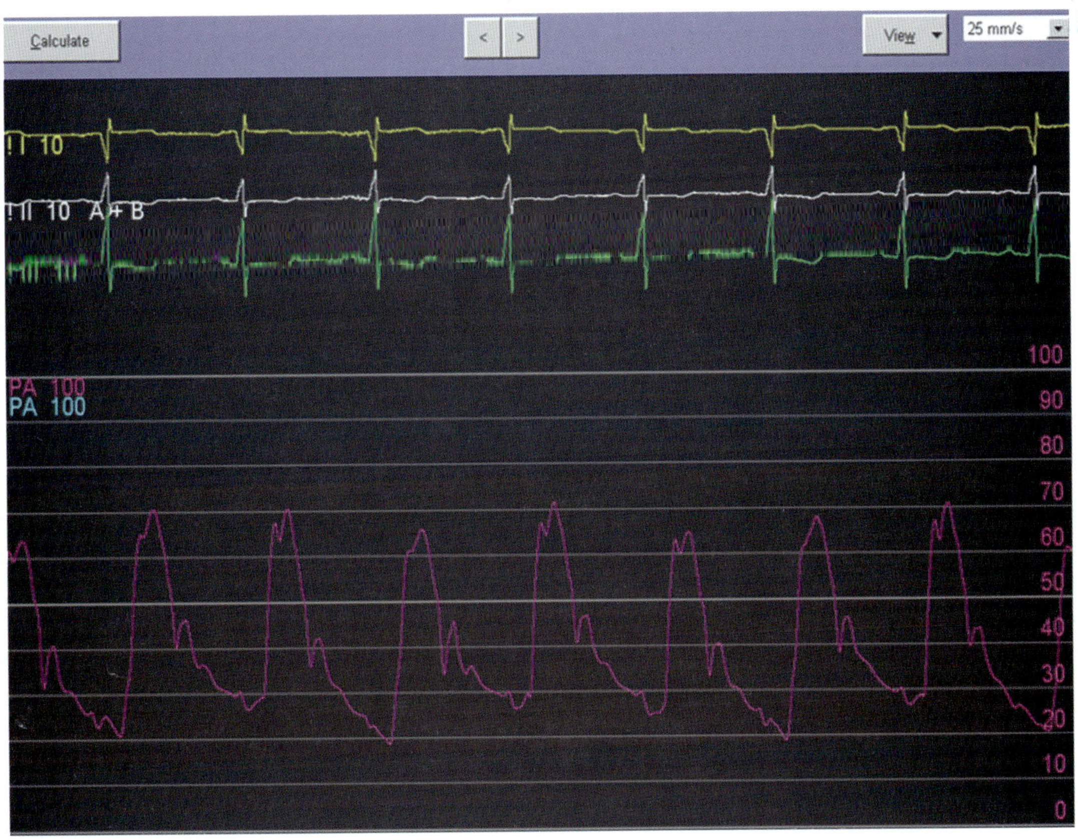

Fig. 4: Pulmonary artery pressure trace of a 10-year-old boy with atrial septal defect and severe pulmonary hypertension.

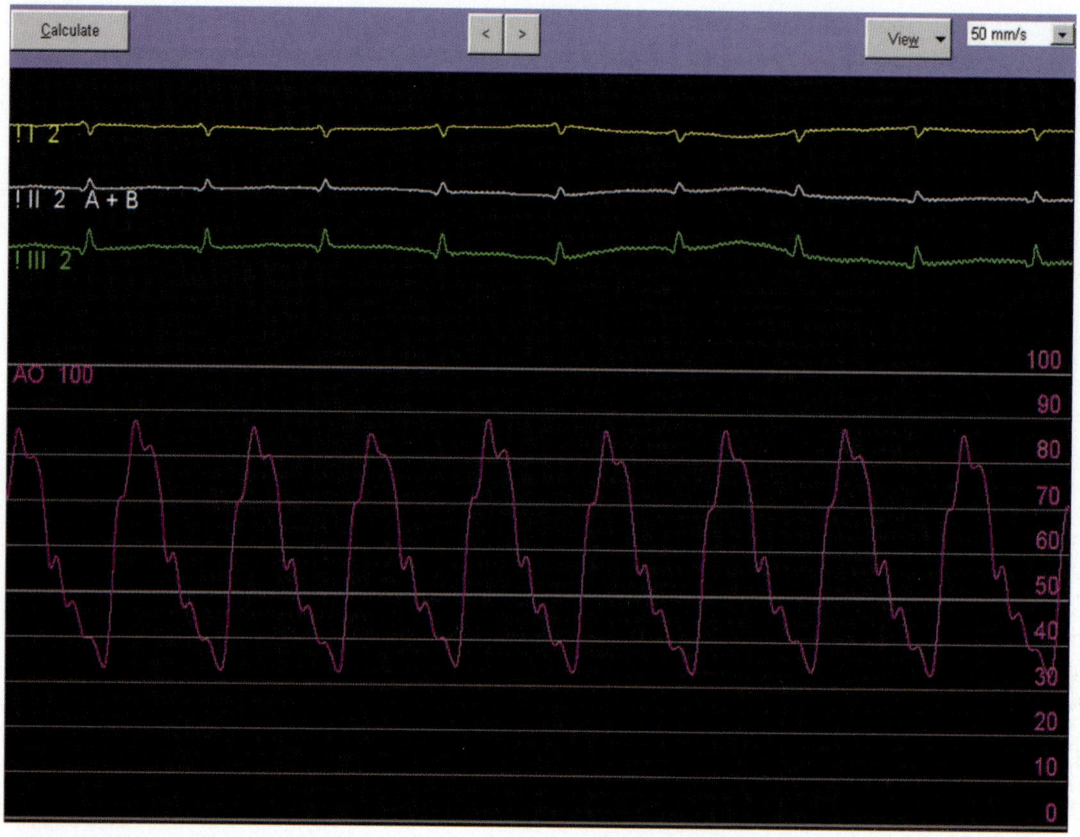

Fig. 5: Ascending aortic pressure recording of a 3-year-old child with a moderate patent ductus arteriosus.

Female patients: VO_2 (mL/min/m^2) =
138.1 – [17.04 × ln (age)] + (0.378 × *heart rate*)

However, these formulae tend to be less accurate in children below 3 years of life.[7] An alternate weight-based calculation of VO_2 is: (2–5 kg: 10–14 mL/min/m^2, 5–8 kg: 7–10 mL/min/m^2).[8] A commonly use rule of thumb is 125 mL/m^2 as the estimated VO_2 for children.

Oximetry runs must be carefully done to obtain valid hemodynamic information. To obtain a reliable oximetry run, blood samples should be taken from multiple sites with minimal intervening time. Erroneous recordings on modern oximeters are approximately ±2.5–3%.[9] Flow sampling related errors are accentuated with unstable catheter position and frequent ventricular ectopics. If the difference in oxygen saturation between the SVC and pulmonary artery is >7%, a left-to-right shunt must be suspected.[10,11] Ideally multiple samples should be taken to obtain a mean for the chamber. A step up of ≥7%, ≥5%, and ≥5% are considered significant for atrial, ventricular, and great artery level shunts, respectively.[11] The oxygen saturation in the IVC is higher than in the SVC because oxygen extraction of the internal organs and lower extremity muscles is lower in a fasting and resting state than that of the brain. So, the mixed venous saturation must be ascertained by accounting for the SVC, IVC, and the coronary sinus. The Flamm formula is the most frequently used formula used to determine the mixed venous saturation:

$$\text{Mixed venous } O_2 \text{ content} = \frac{3\,(\text{SVC } O_2 \text{ content}) + 1\,(\text{IVC } O_2 \text{ content})}{4}$$

Oxygen-carrying capacity of blood includes hemoglobin bound oxygen and dissolved oxygen. Oxygen saturation is the percentage of hemoglobin that is bound to oxygen. An absolute increase in oxygen saturation by >5% from the preceding chamber defines a significant step up. Shunt occurring at a given level is best assessed by sampling from the subsequent chamber along the direction of flow, rather than at the same level to allow for uniform mixing. In an ASD, left-to-right shunt is best estimated by sampling for step up in the right ventricle rather than in the right atrium. Erroneously high or low values may be obtained in samples taken at the same level.

SHUNT QUANTIFICATION

After the closure of the physiological shunts shortly after birth, human circulation is established in a series manner. This implies that, unlike in fetal life, the right and the left heart handle, the same volume of blood in the absence of a persistent or pathological "shunt". Shunt quantification involves estimation of the total pulmonary blood flow (Qp) and total systemic blood flow (Qs). Blood flow is calculated as the ratio of oxygen consumption to the arteriovenous oxygen difference across the concerned vascular bed.

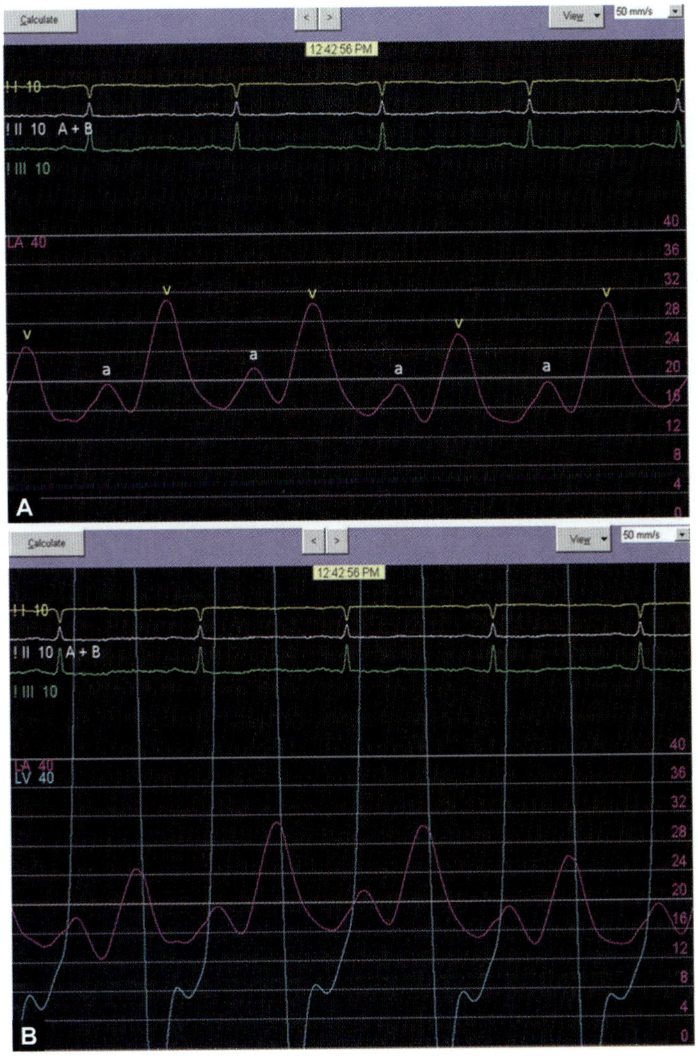

Figs. 6A and B: Hemodynamic traces of an 11-year-old boy with severe mitral stenosis prior to balloon mitral valvotomy. (A) Markedly elevated left atrial pressures; (B) The diastolic pressure gradient between the left atrial trace (purple) and left ventricular recording (light blue).

Total pulmonary blood flow (Qp) is the amount of blood that reaches the pulmonary vascular bed. Total systemic blood flow (Qs) is the amount of blood ejected from the heart into the systemic circulation. Effective pulmonary blood flow (Qep) is the amount of systemic venous return that reaches the pulmonary vascular bed. Normally, in the absence of intracardiac shunts, the blood volume entering the systemic circulation per unit time is the same as the blood volume entering the pulmonary circulation in the same time period. Mathematically, Qp = Qs. Since the deoxygenated blood entering the right heart is normally the volume that reaches the pulmonary circulation, Qp is equal to Qep. A left-to-right shunt implies that Qp > Qep, and the difference between the two is the quantum of the shunt. Estimation of the shunt fraction (Qp/Qs) is important in therapeutic decision-making.

The amount of oxygenated pulmonary venous return that reaches the systemic circulation is the effective systemic blood flow (Qes). Again, normally Qs = Qes. A right-to-left shunt is indicated by Qs > Qes. In a steady state, it is imperative that the volume of blood that flows to the lungs per unit time is equal to the volume of blood that flows out of the lungs and into the systemic circulation per unit time. In other words, Qep is always equal to Qes, failing which one circulation will end up emptying itself over time.

Some of the commonly used formulas used to analyze data from cardiac catheterization are summarized as follows:

- Oxygen content = [Hemoglobin (g/dL) × 1.36 (mL of O_2/g of Hb) × 10 × SaO_2 (saturation %] + [0.003 × pO_2 (partial pressure of oxygen in mm Hg)]
- Cardiac output (L/min) =
$$\frac{\text{Oxygen consumption } (VO_2)(\text{mL/min})}{\text{Arteriovenous oxygen difference (mL/L)}}$$
- Arteriovenous oxygen difference = (arterial O_2 content) – (mixed venous O_2 content)
- Qp (L/min) =
$$\frac{\text{Oxygen consumption } (VO_2)\ (\text{mL/min})}{\text{PV } O_2 \text{ content (mL/L)} - \text{PA } O_2 \text{ content (mL/L)}}$$
- Qs (L/min) =
$$\frac{\text{Oxygen consumption } (VO_2)\ (\text{mL/min})}{\text{Aortic } O_2 \text{ content (mL/L)} - \text{mixed venous } O_2 \text{ content (mL/L)}}$$
- Qep (L/min) =
$$\frac{\text{Oxygen consumption } (VO_2)\ (\text{mL/min})}{\text{PV } O_2 \text{ content (mL/L)} - \text{mixed venous } O_2 \text{ content (mL/L)}}$$
- Qp/Qs =
$$\frac{\text{Aortic } O_2 \text{ content (mL/L)} - \text{mixed venous } O_2 \text{ content (mL/L)}}{\text{PV } O_2 \text{ content (mL/L)} - \text{PA } O_2 \text{ content (mL/L)}}$$
- If dissolved oxygen is insignificant, Qp/Qs
$$= \frac{\text{Aortic } SaO_2 - \text{mixed venous } SaO_2}{\text{PV } SaO_2 - \text{PA } SaO_2}$$
- Left-to-right shunt = Qp – Qep
- Right-to-left shunt = Qs – Qep

VASCULAR RESISTANCE

Hydraulic resistance (vascular resistance) is defined as the ratio of pressure drop to flow across the vascular circuit, analogous to the Ohm's law. According to Poiseuille's law, flow is directly proportional to the pressure difference across the tube and the fourth power of its radius, and inversely proportional to its length and viscosity of the fluid medium. While these refer to steady state fluid mechanics, blood flow is pulsatile and the vascular bed is elastic. Though vascular resistance is dynamic and affected by several factors that are not routinely assessed, calculation of pulmonary and systemic vascular resistance from catheterization has significant importance in clinical decision-making.

Total pulmonary resistance (TPR) is the resistance to flow of blood from the pulmonary artery to the left ventricle in diastole, neglecting left ventricular diastolic pressure. TPR is a less useful tool to assess the pulmonary vasculature. Pulmonary vascular resistance (PVR) assesses pressure drop across the major pulmonary vessels, the precapillary arterioles, and the pulmonary capillary bed. PVR is a more useful tool to assess the precapillary component of pulmonary hypertension. Pulmonary vascular resistance index (PVRI) is to be used when the body surface area is less than one.

- Pulmonary vascular resistance (Wood units) = $\dfrac{\text{Mean PA pressure} - \text{LA pressure}}{\text{Qp}}$
- Systemic vascular resistance (Wood units) = $\dfrac{\text{Mean aortic pressure} - \text{RA pressure}}{\text{Qs}}$
- Total pulmonary resistance (Wood units) = $\dfrac{\text{Mean PA pressure}}{\text{Qp}}$
-
- PVRI (Wm^2) = PVR × body surface area (m^2)
- Systemic vascular resistance index (SVRI) (Wm^2) = SVR × body surface area (m^2)

Normal Values

PVR: 20 – 130 dynes.sec.cm^{-5}
SVR: 700 – 1600 dynes.sec.cm^{-5}
1 Wood unit (WU) = 80 dynes.sec.cm^{-5}

As mentioned earlier, since the pulmonary circulation is dynamic, measured PVR can vary depending on various mechanical and biochemical influences. Hypoxia, hypercapnia, acidosis, increased sympathetic tone, pulmonary emboli, and extrinsic factors such as pleural effusion, lung consolidation, and positive airway pressure can elevate PVR. PVR can be lowered by oxygen, adenosine, inhaled nitric oxide, prostacyclin infusion, high dose of calcium channel blockers, and alpha blockers.

In patients with pre- and post-tricuspid shunts, a decrease in PVRI below 4 Wood units WU.m^2 and/or in the ratio of pulmonary: systemic vascular resistance [PVRI:SVRI (SVR index)] below 0.3 indicates that shunt closure may be undertaken safely with a good long-term prognosis.[12] Test balloon occlusion of a hypertensive PDA may be useful in those with PVR between 4 and 8 WU.m^2.[13] Selected cases of VSD with pulmonary hypertension and a PVR of 6 - 8 WU.m^2 also do well with surgical closure.[14] However, immediate postoperative deaths are also common in 21% of this cohort, which limits generalization.[14] Patients with VSD and pulmonary arterial hypertension (PAH) with a shunt fraction >1.5 and PVR <2/3 of systemic values may benefit with closure along with targeted PAH therapy.[15] Though development of pulmonary hypertension is later in ASD as opposed to large post-tricuspid shunts, it is more often associated with pulmonary vascular disease. PAH may not regress and may even progress after ASD closure.[16] Acute vasoreactivity testing is recommended for shunt lesions with PVRI >6 WU.m^2 and PVR/SVR >0.3.[17] A positive vasoreactive response with short-term exposure to inhaled nitric oxide in children with higher baseline PVR (decrease of 20% in PVR, a decrease of 20% in PVR:SVR ratio, a final PVR index <6 WU.m^2 and a final PVR:SVR ratio of <0.33) may predict beneficial outcomes after surgery.[18,19] A resistance ratio of 0.3–0.50 indicates moderate pulmonary vascular disease, and values higher than 0.75 indicates severe pulmonary vascular disease.

SOURCES OF ERROR

The calculation of cardiac output on the basis of Fick principle is based on the assumption of steady state hemodynamics. This is often adulterated when catheterization is done under sedation rather than general anesthe-sia, with prolonged procedures, dehydration, frequent sampling, and arrhythmias.

Conventional oximeters use the principle of spectrophotometry to provide oxygen saturation. This is fairly accurate in the range of oxygen saturations between 45 and 98%, but falter in extremes, especially in very low cardiac output states. Presence of carboxyhemoglobin and other abnormal hemoglobin can also yield erroneous results.

Presence of bubbles in the syringe while sampling can alter oximetry results. Sampling adjacent to the site of shunt can fallaciously overestimate shunt fraction. This is particularly common with pulmonary artery sampling adjacent to the entry of a PDA, and in right atrial sampling for estimating shunt in ASD.

The average error in determining oxygen consumption has been estimated to be 6%.[20] The error for arteriovenous oxygen difference has been estimated at 5%. The Fick principle is most accurate in low cardiac output states with a wide arteriovenous oxygen difference. A total error of up to 10% is estimated with the use of Fick principle in the calculated cardiac output.[11]

ANGIOGRAPHY

Angiography is the technique of using contrast medium-enhanced fluoroscopy to delineate anatomical details of cardiovascular structures. Ventriculography is one of the means of delineating cardiac anatomy. In the era of advanced noninvasive imaging, ventricular angiograms are used only for specific indications rather than as a primary diagnostic tool.

Current systems for generating X-rays consist of a rotating rhenium–tungsten anode target and a cathode made from a tungsten filament housed in a focusing apparatus.

The X-ray generator of the C-arm in the catheterization laboratory would emit X-rays to the patient along the line of interrogation, while the image intensifier close to the patient converts them to conveniently bright visible light output. In fact, only ~1% of the original X-ray beam reaches the image intensifier through the patient. Denser structures such as bones absorb more radiation than soft tissue. Modern catheterization laboratories have several measures to reduce fluoroscopic radiation exposure to the patient and to maximize the information obtained from a given dose of radiation.

Iodinated contrast agents most often used for angiography include iohexol (a low osmolar agent) and iodixanol (an iso-osmolar agent). The maximum permissible contrast dose for a safe catheterization study is 5 mL/kg body weight. Biplane catheterization laboratories can help reduce contrast doses by permitting multiple angiographic projections during the same contrast injection. Automatic injection systems are used most often for ventriculograms and large vessel angiograms, while manual injections are used in smaller vessels. Cine angiography is mostly done at 30–60 frames/second in children and involves 10 times higher dose exposure than conventional fluoroscopy.

RADIATION SAFETY

The principle of ALARA (as low as reasonably achievable) governs all procedures done in the catheterization laboratory to limit the deterministic and stochastic effects of radiation.[21] Modern catheterization laboratories present several measures to reduce radiation exposure to the patient and to healthcare personnel. The use of safety equipment, radiation training procedural check lists, time out, procedural data recording, and quality control measures such as mock drills are some of the measures that are universally accepted to limit radiation exposure.[22-24] The typical radiation dose for a cardiac catheterization ranges from 3 to 10 milliSieverts (mSv).[25] The radiation exposure in absolute terms and adjusted for weight has been noted to be higher in older children during catheterization.[23]

Cataract, hair loss, and dermatitis are dose-dependent or *deterministic* effects of radiation. While skin erythema and peeling can occur within hours of radiation exposure, skin necrosis can occur over days or weeks. Neoplasms and genetic defects are stochastic effects of radiation exposure and do not have a threshold dose for their development. An approximation of the total X-ray energy delivered to the patient therefore serves as a measure of the risk for stochastic effects. This is expressed as the *dose-area product*, which is the absorbed dose to air (air kerma) multiplied by the cross-sectional area of the X-ray beam at the point of measurement.[21]

LESION SPECIFIC DIAGNOSTIC CATHETERIZATION AND ANGIOGRAPHY

Atrial Septal Defect

Cardiac catheterization is required only in cases of moderate–severe pulmonary hypertension for shunt quantification and estimation of PVR to decide on operability. Diagnostic angiography is obsolete in the modern era. Secundum ASD is profiled in left anterior oblique (LAO) 30° with 30° cranial tilt in the follow-through phase of injection from the pulmonary artery.

Ventricular Septal Defect

Ventricular angiography is often done prior to device closure as an adjunct to noninvasive imaging. Perimembranous and muscular defects are best profiled in the steep LAO projection (60–70°) with cranial angulation (20°) on left ventricular angiography.[11] Subarterial (subpulmonic or supracristal) VSD and high anterior muscular VSD are best delineated in 30° right anterior oblique view.[26]

Patent Ductus Arteriosus and Aortopulmonary Window

Aortic angiograms are occasionally done to confirm the size and anatomy of the patent ductus arteriosus and distal aortopulmonary window for device closure. PDA is best profiled in the 90° lateral and 30° right anterior oblique projections. Straight posteroanterior projection is best suited to delineate aortopulmonary window. Test occlusion of PDA and hemodynamic assessment may be required in pulmonary hypertension.

Atrioventricular Septal Defects

Routine cardiac catheterization is not indicated, except to assess for operability in severe pulmonary hypertension. While angiography is no longer the modality for diagnosis, inflow VSDs are best delineated in a "hepatoclavicular view" (45° LAO 45° cranial).

Coarctation of Aorta

Aortic angiograms in the LAO, right anterior oblique, and lateral projections are used during balloon/stent angioplasty for native coarctation of aorta in older children and in recoarctation.

Tetralogy of Fallot

Routine cardiac catheterization and angiography is obsolete in unrepaired TOF. Occasionally aortic angiograms are useful to demonstrate unusual coronary artery course, aortopulmonary collaterals, and unilateral agenesis of the pulmonary artery. In postoperative TOF, cardiac catheterization may be needed to close residual VSD and to optimize management of left or right ventricular dysfunction with hemodynamic inputs. A right ventricular angiogram in 30° right anterior oblique projection best delineates the right ventricular outflow tract obstruction in TOF.

Tetralogy of Fallot with Pulmonary Atresia

In TOF with pulmonary atresia, pulmonary blood flow is commonly provided by major aorto-pulmonary collaterals arteries (MAPCAs), especially when pulmonary arteries are nonconfluent. Cardiac CT is the most commonly used modality to delineate the anatomy of collaterals and native pulmonary artery anatomy. Diagnostic cardiac catheterization is recommended in MAPCA-dependent pulmonary circulation with confluent or nonconfluent pulmonary arteries.[27] Catheterization helps to identify the pulmonary artery pressures and pressures in the various lung segments.[28] Lung segments with single and dual blood supply (MAPCA and native pulmonary artery) can be delineated. Those presenting with large MAPCA or presenting late need catheterization to rule out pulmonary vascular disease.

Transposition of the Great Arteries

Diagnostic cardiac catheterization is useful to measure left and right ventricular pressures to assess for regression of the left ventricle in late presenters, to assess for suitability for arterial switch operation.[29] Aortic root angiogram in the posteroanterior projection with 45° caudal tilt is often used for delineating coronary artery origins in transposition of the great arteries (TGA).

Double Outlet Right Ventricle

Cardiac catheterization and ventricular angiography are needed only in select cases of double outlet right ventricle (DORV), as an adjunct to noninvasive imaging to plan surgical repair. Relative sizes of the ventricles, routability, level(s) of obstruction, and coronary anatomy can very well be appreciated by echocardiography and MRI in the current era. Catheterization is needed to assess for operability in late presenters with DORV with large VSD and moderate or severe pulmonary hypertension as the systemic saturation may not accurately reflect the pulmonary blood flow.[30]

Congenitally Corrected Transposition of the Great Arteries

Routine cardiac catheterization is not indicated in congenitally corrected transposition of the great arteries (ccTGA). It may be useful in selected cases to delineate coronary artery anatomy prior to double switch repair, and to assess for operability when associated with large hypertensive left-to-right shunts. Due to altered septal alignment, the straight posteroanterior projection is most useful to delineate VSD by ventricular angiogram in ccTGA.

Univentricular Hearts

Measurement of pulmonary artery pressures and vascular resistance, ventricular end-diastolic pressure, identification of additional sources of pulmonary blood flow, and delineation of pulmonary artery anatomy are important to plan a second/third surgery in staged univentricular palliation. The straight posteroanterior projection is most commonly employed to demonstrate bidirectional Glenn function and pulmonary artery anatomy prior to Fontan completion. A 30° caudal tilt with shallow LAO angulation can demonstrate the Glenn anastomotic site for obstruction.[26] A Fontan pathway is best delineated by injection from the IVC in the anteroposterior (AP) and lateral views. Functioning of fenestration and venovenous collaterals can be delineated in these views.

Pulmonary Arteriovenous Fistula

This is an occasional differential diagnosis of cyanosis in the absence of structural heart disease. Pulmonary angiography is highly sensitive in identification of these fistulas. In this condition, contrast injected into the pulmonary arteries immediately opacifies the pulmonary veins bypassing the capillary phase. Pulmonary venous desaturation is confirmative of the diagnosis.

Persistent Truncus Arteriosus

Cardiac catheterization is indicated in older patients beyond infancy with suspected pulmonary vascular disease, for the assessment of operability.

Total Anomalous Pulmonary Venous Connection

Diagnostic cardiac catheterization is very rarely required in patients with a primary diagnosis of TAPVC. It is occasionally required in late presenters with pulmonary hypertension to assess for operability.

SPECIAL CIRCUMSTANCES

Down Syndrome

The older child with Down syndrome frequently has several comorbidities such as thyroid dysfunction, gastroesophageal reflux, and dementia. They have airway issues and can pose specific challenges to catheterization, including higher risk of aspiration. They have earlier onset of pulmonary vascular disease and often have coexistent ventilatory abnormalities.[31] Mechanical ventilation is preferable in these children.

Coronary Artery Disease

Children with severe coronary artery lesions in Kawasaki disease, anomalous coronary artery origin or course (intramural), or in postoperative left ventricular dysfunction after arterial switch operation may require diagnostic coronary angiograms. Femoral artery is the most common approach used in small children. Judkins 4F and 5F catheters are most commonly used for this purpose.

Pulmonary Venous Wedge Angiography

This technique was used to delineate pulmonary artery anatomy by right heart catheterization in patients with pulmonary atresia. Contrast injection is done in pulmonary vein with a saline follow through while preventing run-off into the atrium. This causes retrograde opacification of the pulmonary capillary bed and pulmonary arteries. In the era of advanced noninvasive imaging, this technique is nearly obsolete.

Cardiac Transplantation

Cardiac catheterization is a mandatory investigation in the work up for cardiac transplantation in children to estimate PVR.[32] PVRI of >6 WU.m^2 is associated with poor survival with transplantation.

COMPLICATIONS OF CARDIAC CATHETERIZATION

Though the incidence of complications after cardiac catheterization has decreased over the years with improved techniques and miniaturization of equipment, they are still considerable as compared to adult procedures. A large study reported a complication rate of 7.3% in pediatric cardiac catheterizations, one-third of them being vascular complications.[33] 20% of the vascular complications were major complications. An Indian series reported minor complication rate of 17% but there were no major complications.[34] Young age and low body weight are associated with catheterization-related arterial thrombosis.[35] Some of the other major complications associated with cardiac catheterization include cerebral or systemic embolus, cardiac perforation potentially leading to tamponade, heart block, arrhythmia, hypercyanotic spells, pulmonary hypertensive crisis, and sepsis.

CONCLUSION

The indications for diagnostic cardiac catheterization in children are specific and highly refined in the current era. When appropriately used, it yields valuable hemodynamic information and is an invaluable tool in decision-making and patient management. With appropriate safety precautions and minimization of radiation to the patient and the operator, cardiac catheterization will continue to aid the congenital cardiac team for a long time.

REFERENCES

1. Gupta SK, Spicer DE, Anderson RH. A new low-cost method of virtual cardiac dissection of computed tomographic datasets. Ann Pediatr Cardiol. 2019;12(2):110-6.
2. Feltes TF, Emile B, Beekman RH, Cheatham JP, Feinstein JA, Gomes AS, et al. Indications for cardiac catheterization and intervention in pediatric cardiac disease. Circulation. 2011; 123(22):2607-52.
3. Ebeid MR. Transhepatic approach for rehabilitation of stenosed pulmonary arteries. Ann Pediatr Cardiol. 2010;3(1):25-30.
4. Saxena A, Gupta R, Kumar RK, Kothari SS, Wasir HS. Predictors of arterial thrombosis after diagnostic cardiac catheterization in infants and children randomized to two heparin dosages. Cathet Cardiovasc Diagn. 1997;41(4):400-3.
5. Allen HD, Shaddy RE. Moss & Adams' Heart Disease in Infants, Children, and Adolescents, Including the Fetus and Young Adult, 9th edition. Philadelphia: Lippincott Williams & Wilkins; 2016. p. 1900.
6. LaFarge CG, Miettinen OS. The estimation of oxygen consumption. Cardiovasc Res. 1970; 4(1):23-30.
7. Rutledge J, Bush A, Shekerdemian L, Schulze-Neick I, Penny D, Cai S, et al. Validity of the LaFarge equation for estimation of oxygen consumption in ventilated children with congenital heart disease younger than 3 years— a revisit. Am Heart J. 2010;160(1):109-14.
8. Hollinger I, Mittnacht A. Cardiac catheterization laboratory: catheterization, interventional cardiology, and ablation techniques for children. Int Anesthesiol Clin. 2009;47(3):63-99.
9. Shepherd AP, McMahan CA. Role of oximeter error in the diagnosis of shunts. Cathet Cardiovas Diagn. 1996;37(4):435-46.
10. Freed MD, Miettinen OS, Nadas AS. Oximetric detection of intracardiac left-to-right shunts. Br Heart J. 1979;42(6):690-4.
11. Moscucci M. Grossman & Baim's Cardiac Catheterization, Angiography, and Intervention, 8th edition. Philadelphia: Wolters Kluwer; 2013. p. 1168.
12. del Cerro MJ, Moledina S, Haworth SG, Ivy D, Al Dabbagh M, Banjar H, et al. Cardiac catheterization in children with pulmonary hypertensive vascular disease: consensus statement from the Pulmonary Vascular Research Institute, Pediatric and Congenital Heart Disease Task Forces. Pulm Circ. 2016; 6(1): 118-25.
13. Viswanathan S, Kumar RK. Assessment of operability of congenital cardiac shunts with increased pulmonary vascular resistance. Catheter Cardiovasc Interv. 2008;71(5):665-70.
14. Kannan BRJ, Sivasankaran S, Tharakan JA, Titus T, Ajith Kumar VK, Francis B, et al. Long-term outcome of patients operated for large ventricular septal defects with increased pulmonary vascular resistance. Indian Heart J. 2003;55(2):161-6.
15. Baumgartner H, Bonhoeffer P, De Groot NMS, de Haan F, Deanfield JE, Galie N, et al. ESC Guidelines for the management of grown-up congenital heart disease (new version 2010). Eur Heart J. 2010;31(23):2915-57.
16. Gabriels C, De Meester P, Pasquet A, De Backer J, Paelinck BP, Morissens M, et al. A different view on predictors of pulmonary hypertension in secundum atrial septal defect. Int J Cardiol. 2014;176(3):833-40.
17. Abman SH, Georg H, Archer SL, Ivy DD, Adatia I, Chung WK, et al. Pediatric pulmonary hypertension. Circulation. 2015;132(21): 2037-99.
18. Berner M, Beghetti M, Spahr-Schopfer I, Oberhansli I, Friedli B. Inhaled nitric oxide to test the vasodilator capacity of the pulmonary vascular bed in children with long-standing pulmonary hypertension and congenital heart disease. Am J Cardiol. 1996;77(7):532-5.
19. Jain S, Dalvi B. Atrial septal defect with pulmonary hypertension: when/how can we consider closure? J Thorac Dis. 2018;10(Suppl 24):S2890-8.
20. Barratt-Boyes BG, Wood EH. The oxygen saturation of blood in the venae cavae, right-heart chambers, and pulmonary vessels of healthy subjects. J Lab Clin Med. 1957;50(1): 93-106.

21. Naidu SS, Aronow HD, Box LC, Duffy PL, Kolansky DM, Kupfer JM, et al. SCAI expert consensus statement: 2016 best practices in the cardiac catheterization laboratory: (Endorsed by the cardiological society of india, and sociedad Latino Americana de Cardiologia intervencionista; Affirmation of value by the Canadian Association of interventional cardiology-Association canadienne de cardiologie d'intervention). Catheter Cardiovasc Interv. 2016;88(3):407-23.
22. Ali F, Qasim Mehdi M, Akhtar S, Aslam N, Abbas R, Shah I, et al. Impact of congenital cardiac catheterization project on outcomes-quality improvement (C3PO-QI) in LMICs. Heart Asia. 2019;11(1):e011105.
23. Borik S, Devadas S, Mroczek D, Lee KJ, Chaturvedi R, Benson LN. Achievable radiation reduction during pediatric cardiac catheterization: How low can we go? Catheter Cardiovasc Interv. 2015;86(5):841-8.
24. Shah P, Khanna R, Kapoor A, Goel PK. Efficacy of RADPAD protection drape in reducing radiation exposure in the catheterization laboratory—First Indian study. Indian Heart Journal. 2018;70:S265-8.
25. Vijayalakshmi K, Kelly D, Chapple C, Williams D, Wright R, Stewart MJ, et al. Cardiac catheterisation: radiation doses and lifetime risk of malignancy. Heart. 2007;93(3):370-1.
26. Sievert H, Qureshi SA, Wilson N, Hijazi ZM, Qureshi SA, Wilson N, et al. Interventions in Structural, Valvular and Congenital Heart Disease. London: CRC Press; 2015.
27. Saxena A, Relan J, Agarwal R, Awasthy N, Azad S, Chakrabarty M, et al. Indian guidelines for indications and timing of intervention for common congenital heart diseases: Revised and updated consensus statement of the Working group on management of congenital heart diseases. Ann Pediatr Cardiol. 2019;12(3): 254-86.
28. Dimopoulos K, Diller GP, Opotowsky AR, D'Alto M, Gu H, Giannakoulas G, et al. Definition and management of segmental pulmonary hypertension. J Am Heart Assoc. 2018;7(14):e008587.
29. Gopalakrishnan A, Sasidharan B, Krishnamoorthy KM, Sivasubramonian S, Dharan BS, Mathew T, et al. Left ventricular regression after balloon atrial septostomy in d-transposition of the great arteries. Eur J Cardiothorac Surg. 2016;50(6):1096-101.
30. Tharakan JA. Admixture lesions in congenital cyanotic heart disease. Ann Pediatr Cardiol. 2011;4(1):53.
31. Sharma M, Khera S, Sondhi V, Devgan A. A study to determine the prevalence of pulmonary arterial hypertension in children with Down syndrome and congenital heart disease. Med J Armed Forces India. 2013;69(3):241-5.
32. Mehra MR, Canter CE, Hannan MM, Semigran MJ, Uber PA, Baran DA, et al. The 2016 International Society for Heart Lung Transplantation listing criteria for heart transplantation: a 10-year update. J Heart Lung Transplant. 2016;35(1):1-23.
33. Mehta R, Lee K-J, Chaturvedi R, Benson L. Complications of pediatric cardiac catheterization: a review in the current era. Catheter Cardiovasc Interv. 2008;72(2):278-85.
34. Kumar P, Joshi VS, Madhu PV. Diagnostic pediatric cardiac catheterization: experience of a tertiary care pediatric cardiac centre. Med J Armed Forces India. 2014;70(1):10-6.
35. Brotschi B, Hug MI, Kretschmar O, Rizzi M, Albisetti M. Incidence and predictors of cardiac catheterisation-related arterial thrombosis in children. Heart. 2015;101(12):948-53.

12 CHAPTER

Essential Cardiovascular Pharmacology: Common Drugs in Pediatric Cardiac Practice

Balaganesh Karmegaraj, Alice Neetha, R Krishna Kumar

INTRODUCTION

Cardiovascular drugs are used in children for several specific circumstances. The fundamental concerns relating to cardiovascular medications in children are related to the fact that there is very little systematic evidence available on their safety and efficacy. Much of what is used in children is extrapolated from adult use. This practice is fundamentally flawed due to a number of reasons that include the fact that children have a completely different disease profile, response to medications and pharmacokinetics. However, it must also be acknowledged that gathering high-quality evidence on cardiovascular medications through randomized controlled trials is a rather difficult task. Drug trials are, in general, far more difficult to conduct in children as there is considerable diversity due to a wide age-range from neonates to adolescents and an even wider range of etiology for conditions such as heart failure and pulmonary hypertension.[1] Also, the number of affected patients that can be enrolled into trials tends to be much smaller than adults leading to inconclusive data. As a result, much of what is administered in children with heart disease tends to be empirical with limited support from case series and uncontrolled studies. This chapter will discuss the pharmacology of common medications used in pediatric cardiac practice. The readers should refer to a more detailed reference for a comprehensive treatise.[2] The individual chapters will deal with treatment plans for specific conditions in considerable detail.

β-BLOCKING AGENTS

The spectrum of actions include reduction of myocardial contractility, blood pressure, slowing of atrioventricular (AV) conduction, and suppression of automaticity that results in slowing of the heart rate (**Table 1**). As a result, beta-blockers are used in a wide variety of cardiovascular ailments in children (**Table 2**). The electrophysiological effects of beta-blockers find application in treatment of supraventricular tachyarrhythmias, selected ventricular tachycardias, and long QT syndrome. Slowing of resting and postexercise heart rates is desirable in situations such as mitral stenosis where the duration of diastole needs to be prolonged. The reduction in myocardial contractility is desirable in conditions such as hypertrophic cardiomyopathy, aortopathy from Marfan syndrome and related conditions, tetralogy of Fallot, and myocardial ischemia where a reduction in oxygen consumption is of particular value. Its use in heart failure is counterintuitive and stems for the vast adult experience.[3-5] Because of its widespread usage, it is necessary to be familiar with the basic pharmacology of the commonly used beta-blockers (**Table 3**).

Classification

The classification is based on the effect on the beta-receptor subtypes and whether or not there is an additional

TABLE 1: Actions of beta-blockers.

Cardiac effects of β-blockers	• Negative chronotropic/dromotropic/inotropic • Antiarrhythmic • Anti-ischemic
β-blockade on ischemic heart	• Decrease heart rate • Decrease afterload • Decrease O_2 wastage • Antiarrhythmic • Reduce contractility • Increase diastolic perfusion
Three major mechanisms for β-blocker side effects	• Smooth muscle spasm (especially β2-blocker bronchospasm) • Exaggeration of the cardiac therapeutic actions (bradycardia, heart block, and excess negative inotropic effect) • Central nervous system penetration (insomnia and depression)

TABLE 2: Indications for beta-blockers and mechanisms of action.

Indications	*Commonly used beta-blocker*	*Mechanism of action*
Cyanotic spells	Propranolol, metoprolol, and esmolol	Slowing of heart rate and improved diastolic ventricular filling with increased preload; reduction of infundibular spasm; increased SVR by antagonizing the vasodilating effects of beta-adrenergic stimulation
Tachyarrhythmias	• *Atrial flutter*: Propranolol/sotalol ectopic atrial tachycardia: Metoprolol, sotalol • *AV re-entrant tachycardia*: Propranolol and metoprolol • *PVC control*: Propranolol and metoprolol	Alters the electrophysiologic milieu by reducing conduction in one of the limbs of the ectopic atrial re-entrant circuit; reduced automaticity helps ectopic atrial tachycardia
Congenital long QT syndrome	Propranolol	Sympathetic blockade
HCM	Propranolol and metoprolol	Reduced contractility; reduction in gradients, improved diastolic function
Congestive heart failure	Carvedilol, metoprolol bisoprolol	Improved ventricular remodeling, increased beta-receptor density
Hypertension	Atenolol, bisoprolol, labetalol, metoprolol, and propranolol	Reduced contractility
Connective tissue disorders (Marfan syndrome)	Atenolol	Reduced contractility with reduced dP/dT
Infantile, cardiac, and other hemangiomas[10-12]	Propranolol	• *Early effects*: Vasoconstriction due to decreased release of nitric oxide • *Intermediate effects*: Blocking proangiogenic signals (vascular endothelial growth factor, basic fibroblast growth factor, matrix metalloproteinase, and result in growth arrest) • *Long-term effects*: Induction of apoptosis in proliferating endothelial cells, which results in tumor regression
Congenital or acquired mitral stenosis	Propranolol and metoprolol	Improved diastolic filling

(AV: atrioventricular; HCM: hypertrophic cardiomyopathy; PVC: premature ventricular complex; SVR: systemic vascular resistance)

TABLE 3: Doses of commonly prescribed beta-blockers.

Drug	*Dose*
Propranolol	• *Oral*: TOF prophylaxis to prevent cyanotic spell (2–3 mg/kg/day) • *Others*: 0.2–0.5 mg/kg 6–8 hours (adult 10–25 mg) • *Hemangioma*: 5 weeks to 5 months: 0.6 mg/kg week 1; 1.1 mg/kg week 2; then 1.7 mg/kg 12 hours oral with feed • *IV*: 0.1 mg/kg over 10 minutes them 0.1–0.3 mg/kg 3 hours (adult 5–15 mg)
Sotalol	• *Oral*: 1–4 mg/kg 8–12 hours (adult 50–160 mg) • *IV*: 0.5–2 mg/kg over 10 minutes 6 hours
Metoprolol	• *Oral*: 1–2 mg/kg 6–12 hours (adult 50–100 mg) • *IV*: 0.1 mg/kg over 5 minutes (adult 5 mg), repeat every 5 minutes to maximum three doses, then 1–5 mg/kg/min
Atenolol	• *Oral*: 0.5–1 mg/kg 12–24 hours (maximum 25–50 mg) • *IV*: 0.05 mg/kg (maximum 2.5 mg) every 5 minutes if required (maximum four doses), then 0.1–0.2 mg/kg (maximum 5–10 mg) over 10 minutes 12–24 hours
Bisoprolol	0.2–0.4 mg/kg daily oral (adult 10–20 mg)
Carvedilol	0.1 mg/kg 12 hours oral (adult 3.125 mg); if tolerating increase by 0.1 mg/kg every 1–2 weeks to maximum 0.5–0.8 mg/kg 12 hours (adult 25 mg)
Labetalol	• *IV intermittent bolus*: 0.2–0.5 mg/kg/dose over 2–3 minutes every 4–6 hours with a range of 0.2–1 mg/kg/dose has been suggested; maximum dose 20 mg/dose. • Treatment of pediatric hypertensive emergencies: • *Continuous IV infusion*: 0.4–1 mg/kg/hour with a maximum of 3 mg/kg/hour • *Alternate dosing*: Bolus 0.2–1 mg/kg followed by a continuous infusion of 0.25–1.5 mg/kg/hour. Oral: Initial: 1–2 mg/kg/day in two divided doses. Maximum dose 10–20 mg/kg/day

(IV: intravenous; TOF: tetralogy of Fallot)

vasodilatory effect from actions on alpha receptors. Based on these considerations, beta-blockers are classified as follows:

- *First generation*: Nonselective (β1 and β2)
- *Second generation*: Selective (β1)
- *Third generation*: Vasodilatory (β1, β2, and alpha-blocker).

First Generation

Non-selective β-blockers: Causes bradycardia, negative inotropy, and lower blood pressure with a risk of bronchospasm from its action on the bronchial smooth muscle β2 receptor. They include the following:

- Propranolol
- Sotalol.

Second Generation

β1-cardioselective blockers: These have a varying degree of selectivity to the β1 receptor. For this reason, this class of drugs causes less bronchospasm. They include the following:
- Metoprolol
- Atenolol
- Bisoprolol

  Bisoprolol is among the most selective.

Third Generation

Vasodilatory (β1, β2, and alpha-blocker): These include vasodilatory β-blockers that are specifically used for heart failure management and in conditions such as pheochromocytoma. They include the following:
- Carvedilol
- Labetalol

The actions, indications and drug dosage of beta-blockers are summarized in **Tables 1, 2 and 3** respectively.

Details on the commonly used beta-blockers are discussed here.

Propranolol

Mechanism of Action

It is a noncardioselective β-blocking agent (β1 cardiac and β2 receptors and a class II antiarrhythmic agent). It decreases heart rate, slows AV conduction, and decreases myocardial contractility, blood pressure, and myocardial oxygen demand.

Indications

Cyanotic spells, infantile cardiac and other hemangiomas, long QT syndrome, and tachyarrhythmias.

Pharmacokinetics

- *Onset of action*: 1–2 hours after oral administration and 2 minutes after intravenous (IV) administration
- *Duration of action*: 6 hours after oral dosing and 3–6 hours after IV dosing. It gets absorbed through gastrointestinal (GI) tract. It has extensive first-pass metabolism with a bioavailability of 30–40%. It is metabolized in the liver and eliminated in urine.
- *Half-life*: 4–6 hours.

Important Adverse Effects

Hypotension, impaired myocardial contractility, congestive heart failure (CHF), bradycardia, AV block, hypoglycemia, and bronchospasm.

Specific Precautions

It should be used with care in patients with reactive airway disease and neonates because of risk of hypoglycemia. Sudden discontinuation may result in withdrawal symptoms.

Monitoring

It is useful to monitor heart rate and this can help titrate the dose.

Key Interactions

Phenobarbital, rifampicin, and cimetidine increase propranolol clearance.

Amiodarone, calcium channel blockers, dipyridamole, disopyramide, phosphodiesterase-5-inhibitors, prostacyclins, and quinindine increase the level of propranolol.

Sotalol

Sotalol is primarily used as an antiarrhythmic drug and is discussed in the section on antiarrhythmics.

Atenolol[6]

Mechanism of Action

It selectively blocks β1 receptors.

Indications

Marfan syndrome (dilated aorta), aortopathy from other causes (bicommissural aortic valve with aortic root dilation), and selected supraventricular (**Table 2**).

Pharmacokinetics

- *Beta-blocking effect*: Onset: Oral: 1 hour; peak effect: Oral: 2–4 hours
- *Absorption*: Oral: 50%; Half-life: Children and adolescents (5–16 years of age): 4.6 hours; prolonged with renal impairment; End-stage renal disease: 15–35 hours
- *Excretion*: Feces (50%); urine (40% as unchanged drug). Clearance reduced in renal impairment

Important Adverse Effects

Bradycardia and hypotension. At higher doses, β1 is lost and bronchospasm may occur.

Specific Precautions

Abrupt withdrawal can cause acute tachycardia, hypertension, and/or ischemia.

Monitoring of therapy is by measuring blood pressure and heart rate.

Key Interactions

Amiodarone may enhance the bradycardic effect of beta-blockers. Beta-blockers may enhance the hypoglycemic effect of insulin. Aspirin (analgesic dose) will decrease antihypertensive effect of atenolol.

Metoprolol

It is useful in acute management of tachyarrhythmias and cyanotic spells. It can be used whenever IV beta-blockers are desirable as an alternative to propranolol.

Oral metoprolol is a reasonable choice for long-term beta-blockade. Metoprolol is discussed in further detail under antiarrhythmic medications.

Esmolol

Esmolol is a short-acting beta-blocker that is exclusively for acute settings and only administered intravenously. IV metoprolol is a reasonable substitute.

Bisoprolol

Bisoprolol has the highest β1 selectivity among available beta-blockers. It has the distinct advantage of once daily dosing because of a half-life of 12–14 hours and therefore thus has a long duration of action beyond 24 hours. Bisoprolol is 50% lipophilic, metabolized by the liver and 50% hydrophilic, excreted by the kidneys. Bisoprolol is increasingly popular in children requiring oral beta-blockade.

Third Generation (Vasodilatory Beta-blockers, Nonselective)

Carvedilol[3-5,7-9]

Mechanism of action: Carvedilol is a nonselective β-adrenergic blocking agent with alpha 1-blocking activity. Carvedilol is a racemic mixture where the S(–) enantiomer is a beta-adrenoceptor blocker and the R(+) enantiomer is both a beta- and alpha-I adrenoceptor blocker. Carvedilol's action on alpha-1 adrenergic receptors relaxes smooth muscle in vasculature, leading to reduced peripheral vascular resistance and an overall reduction in blood pressure. At higher doses, calcium channel blocking and antioxidant activity can be seen. The antioxidant activity of carvedilol prevents oxidation of low-density lipoprotein and its uptake into coronary circulation.

Indications: Dilated cardiomyopathy and CHF.

Pharmacokinetics: Onset of action for alpha-blockade is within 30 minutes and beta-blockade is within 1 hour. The oral bioavailability is 25–35% due to significant first-pass metabolism in the liver. It is metabolized through aromatic ring oxidation and glucuronidation in the liver. Elimination half-life is significantly shorter in children (2.2 hours and children and adolescents is 3.6 hours). R(+)-carvedilol has a shorter half-life of 5–9 hours as against S(–) carvedilol (7–11 hours). Excretion is via the gut and urine. Renal function impairment may result in higher plasma concentrations (40–50% in moderate-to-severe renal impairment). Severe hepatic impairment patients have a four- to sevenfold increase in concentrations.

Important adverse effects: Hypotension, bradycardia, and reactive airway disease.

Monitoring: Heart rate, blood pressure, and renal and liver function need to be monitored.

Key interactions: Concomitant use of digoxin and carvedilol reduces the digoxin clearance from the body and hence it is recommended that the digoxin dose be reduced by 25%.

β-blockers in Chronic Heart Failure

The primary mechanism of action is to prevent and reverse adrenergically mediated myocardial dysfunction and remodeling. Other effects are upregulation of beta-adrenergic receptors. It was previously contraindicated due to negative inotropic properties, especially in acute phase of heart failure but its role in reversing adverse neurohormonal activation in chronic heart failure results in improved left ventricular functional and relief from heart failure symptoms. Other beneficial effects include antiarrhythmic effects, coronary vasodilation, antioxidant effects, and improved cardiac energetics. Beta-blockers was found to improve symptoms, survival, and ventricular remodeling in adults with mild-to-moderate heart failure with reduced ejection fraction (HFrEF). Carvedilol has demonstrated improved survival over metoprolol due to broader actions (beta-1, 2, and alpha-1 receptor blockade). However, more recent registry analyses have failed to demonstrate any benefits in adults. After these studies in adults, selected small reports found metoprolol and carvedilol were beneficial in children with heart failure with systemic ventricular dysfunction.[7,8] However, the only multicenter prospective, randomized, double-blind trial of carvedilol in children with HFrEF failed to detect a beneficial role.[9] In children with systemic left ventricle, it improves symptoms and echocardiographic indices of ventricular function. In patients with systemic right ventricle or single ventricle, current data do not support the use of carvedilol for managing heart failure.

It is necessary to be mindful of the following facts about carvedilol:

- The half-life of carvedilol in children is shorter than in adults and hence, higher doses are needed to produce a beneficial effect.
- Carvedilol increases the levels of digoxin, so one must monitor its use and decrease the dose of digoxin. Careful monitoring and documentation of vitals (especially heart rate and blood pressure) is important as carvedilol may cause hypotension and/or symptomatic bradycardia.

Labetalol

Labetalol is also a vasodilatory beta-blocker that has been available several years before carvedilol was introduced. It is primarily used for the management of pheochromocytoma and hypertensive emergencies.

Mechanism of action: Dose-related decrease in blood pressure through *β1, β2, and alpha* blockade without causing significant reflex tachycardia or a decrease in the heart rate.

Indication: Hypertensive emergency.

Pharmacokinetics

Peak effect: Oral: 1–4 hours; IV: 5–15 minutes. Metabolized in the liver by glucuronidation. Oral labetalol has a bioavailability of only 25% because of extensive first-pass effect.

Important adverse effects: Orthostatic hypotension, bronchospasm, nasal congestion, CHF, bradycardia, myopathy, rash, and AV block.

Specific precautions: Chronic labetalol therapy should not be discontinued abruptly; taper it over 1–2 weeks. It is contraindicated particularly in bronchial asthma, incompatible with sodium bicarbonate.

Monitoring: Labetalol should be initiated cautiously with careful monitoring of blood pressure, heart rate, and electrocardiogram, and use the lowest effective dose.

ANTIARRHYTHMIC DRUGS

Antiarrhythmic drugs are classified on the basis of the cellular site of action. **Table 4** enlists the modified classification of antiarrhythmic drugs.

TABLE 4: Revised classification of antiarrhythmic medication.[13]

Class	*Subclass*	*Pharmacological targets*	*Drugs*	*Major clinical applications*	*Therapeutic mechanism*
Class 0: Hyperpolarization-activated cyclic nucleotide-gated (HCN) channel blockers					
		HCN channel-mediated pacemaker current (If) block	Ivabradine	Congenital and postoperative junctional ectopic tachycardia; ectopic atrial tachycardia, dilated cardiomyopathy, inappropriate sinus tachycardia	Reduction in SA node automaticity
Class 1: Voltage-gated Na$^+$ channel blockers					
	Ia	Nav1.5 open state	Quinidine disopyramide	Brugada syndrome, SVT, and VT	Reduction in ectopic ventricular/atrial automaticity. Reduction in accessory pathway conduction
	Ib	Nav1.5 open state	Lidocaine and mexiletine	Ventricular tachyarrhythmias, type III long QT syndrome	• Reduction in ectopic ventricular automaticity • Reduction in DAD-induced triggered activity • Reduced re-entrant tendency by converting unidirectional to bidirectional block, particularly in ischemic, partially depolarized myocardium
	Ic	Nav1.5 inactivated state	Propafenone and flecainide	Permanent junctional reciprocating tachycardia (PJRT), multifocal atrial tachycardia, SVT, catecholaminergic polymorphic ventricular tachycardia	• Reduction in ectopic ventricular/atrial automaticity • Reduction in DAD-induced triggered activity. Reduced re-entrant tendency by converting unidirectional to bidirectional block Slowed conduction and reduced excitability, particularly at rapid heart rates blocking re-entrant pathways showing depressed conduction
Class 2: Beta-blockers autonomic inhibitors and activators)					
	IIa	Nonselective β and selective β1-adrenergic receptor inhibitors	• *Nonselective β inhibitors*: Carvedilol, propranolol • *Selective β1 adrenergic receptor inhibitors*: atenolol, esmolol, and metoprolol	• Supraventricular (atrial fibrillation, atrial flutter, and atrial tachycardia), arrhythmias • Rate control of atrial fibrillation and ventricular tachyarrhythmias (ventricular tachycardia, premature ventricular contraction) • *Note*: atenolol, propranolol, and nadolol are also used in LQTS; nadolol is used in catecholaminergic polymorphic ventricular tachycardia	• Reduction in SAN automaticity • Reduction in AVN automaticity • Reduction in ectopic, ventricular/atrial automaticity. Reduction in EAD-/DAD-induced triggered activity Reduced SAN re-entry. Reduction in AVN conduction terminating re-entry
	IIb	Nonselective β-adrenergic receptor activators	Isoproterenol	Accelerating rates of ventricular escape rhythm in cases of complete atrioventricular block before definitive pacemaker implantation	Increased escape ventricular automaticity. Suppression of bradycardia-dependent EAD-related triggered activity
	IIc	Muscarinic M2 receptor inhibitors	Atropine	Mild or moderate symptomatic sinus bradycardia	Increase in SAN automaticity. Increase in AVN conduction

Contd...

Contd...

Class	*Subclass*	*Pharmacological targets*	*Drugs*	*Major clinical applications*	*Therapeutic mechanism*
	IId	Muscarinic M2 receptor activators	Digoxin	Supraventricular tachyarrhythmias	Reduction in SAN automaticity. Reduced SAN re-entry. Reduction in AVN conduction, terminating re-entry
	IIe	Adenosine A1 receptor activators	Adenosine	Acute termination of AVN tachycardia and cAMP-mediated triggered VTs. Differentiation of sinus from atrial tachycardia	Reduction in SAN automaticity. Reduction in AVN conduction, terminating re-entry. Reduction in EAD-/DAD-induced triggered activity
Class III: K^+ channel blockers and openers					
Voltage dependent K^+ channel blockers	IIIa	• Nonselective K^+ channel blockers	• Amiodarone	• Ventricular tachycardia in patients without structural heart disease or with remote myocardial infarction; tachyarrhythmias with Wolff–Parkinson–White syndrome; atrial fibrillation with atrioventricular conduction via accessory pathway. Ventricular fibrillation and premature ventricular contraction; tachyarrhythmias associated with supraventricular arrhythmias and atrial fibrillation	• Increase in AP recovery time. Increase in refractory period, with decreased re-entrant tendency • *Note*: Amiodarone also slows sinus node rate and atrioventricular conduction
		• Kv11.1 (HERG) channel-mediated rapid K^+ current (IKr) blockers	• Sotalol	• Fetal atrial flutter, resistant AVRT, ectopic atrial nonselective tachycardia, neonatal refractory SVT. Atrial has two isomers tachyarrhythmia in the setting of congenital heart disease	• Nonselective beta-blocker. It has two isomers (D- and L-), both with K^+ channel blocking activity, while the L-isomer provides the majority of the beta-adrenergic blocking activity. Sotalol has a dose-related mechanism of action at lower doses the beta-adrenergic effects predominate, whereas the K^+ channel effects predominate at higher doses
Class IV: Ca_2^+ handling modulators					
	IVa	Block of Ca_2^+ current (ICa resulting in inhibition of SAN pacing, inhibition of AVN conduction, prolonged ERP, increased AP recovery time, increased refractory period, diminished repolarization reserve, and suppression of intracellular Ca_2^+ signaling; increased PR intervals)	Verapamil and diltiazem	Verapamil-sensitive ventricular tachycardia (Belhassen ventricular tachycardia)	Reduction in AVN conduction, terminating Re-entry Reduction in EAD-/DAD-induced triggered activity
Intracellular Ca_2^+ channel blocker	IVb	SR RyR2-Ca_2^+ channel blockers; reduced SR Ca_2^+ release: reduced cytosolic and SR (Ca_2^+)	Flecainide and propafenone	Catecholaminergic polymorphic ventricular tachycardia and PJRT	Reduction in DAD-induced triggered activity

(AP: action potential; AVN: atrioventricular node; AVRT: atrioventricular reciprocating tachycardia; cAMP: cyclic adenosine monophosphate; DAD: delayed afterdepolarization; EAD: early afterdepolarization; ERP: effective refractory period; LQTS: long QT syndrome; SA: sinoatrial; SAN: sinoatrial node; SR: sarcoplasmic reticulum; SVT: supraventricular tachycardia; VT: ventricular tachycardia)

SELECTED ANTIARRHYTHMIC DRUGS USED IN PEDIATRIC PRACTICE

Ivabradine

Ivabradine is a selective inhibitor of the hyperpolarization-activated cyclic nucleotide-gated (HCN4) channels involved in the funny current-related depolarization. Increased automaticity is the underlying mechanism of several pediatric tachyarrhythmias including junctional ectopic tachycardia (JET) and ectopic atrial tachycardia. By inhibition of the funny current and reduction of automaticity, ivabradine represents a plausible potential therapy for these conditions. Ivabradine demonstrates use dependence, resulting in a greater effect at higher heart rates. It has a hemodynamically neutral profile, in contrast to many alternative antiarrhythmic agents. This offers a distinct advantage in failing hearts. It has recently been reported to be successful in infants with congenital and postoperative JET.[14]

The recommended dose for congestive/postoperative JET is 0.05–0.15 mg/kg 12 hours oral (adult 2.5–7.5 mg).

Ivabradine in Pediatric Chronic Heart Failure[14]

It is an effective heart rate-reducing agent, lowers incidence of cardiovascular death and hospitalization for worsening heart failure in adult patients and is therefore recommended for the treatment of chronic heart failure in adults with an elevated heart rate and in sinus rhythm. Ivabradine safely reduced the resting heart rate of children with chronic heart failure and dilated cardiomyopathy. Ivabradine's effect on heart rate was variable, highlighting the importance of dose titration. Ivabradine treatment improves left ventricular ejection fraction, the clinical status and quality of life.

The starting dose of Ivabradine in pediatric patients with dilated cardiomyopathy is 0.02 mg/kg twice daily for children aged 6–12 months and 0.05 mg/kg twice daily for children aged >1–18 years. A starting dose of 2.5 mg twice daily is given for children weighing >40 kg. The doses can be adjusted every 2 weeks (increased or decreased). The duration of titration period is governed by the magnitude of heart rate reduction and could last up to 8 weeks or until the patient has >20% reduction in heart rate without bradycardia or symptoms of bradycardia. Titration involves a maximum of four steps. Patients who are initiated on 0.02 mg/kg twice daily can be up-titrated to 0.05, 0.10, 0.15, and 0.20 mg/kg twice daily, while those initiated on 0.05 mg/kg twice daily can be up-titrated to 0.10, 0.15, 0.20, and 0.30 mg/kg twice daily. Patients weighing >40 kg, who are started on 2.5 mg twice daily, can be up-titrated to 5, 7.5, 10, and 15 mg twice daily. The titration period should be followed by a 2-week maintenance period. Thereafter, the patients are monitored for at least 12 months (on treatment) with monthly visits up to 3 months and then every 3 months. Monitoring of N-terminal pro-B-type natriuretic peptide levels can be done for effectiveness of treatment.

Lidocaine

Mechanism of Action

It blocks the fast sodium channel and decreases the rate of phase 4 depolarization in ventricular myocardium.

Indications

Ventricular ectopy, tachycardia, and fibrillation; local anesthetic.

Pharmacokinetics

The onset of action is 45–90 seconds. The half-life is 2–3 hours. Therapeutic levels of lidocaine are in the range of 2–5 μg/mL. Lidocaine is eliminated in the urine.

Important Adverse Effects

The most prominent effects are in the central nervous system (CNS) and include lethargy, agitation, slurred speech, seizures, anxiety, euphoria, and hallucinations. They occur with over-dosage or accidental IV injection during local anesthesia. The listed cardiovascular adverse effects include bradycardia, hypotension, heart block, arrhythmias, and cardiovascular collapse.

Dose

IV: 1% solution 0.1 mL/kg (1 mg/kg) over 2 min, then 0.09–0.3 mL/kg/hr (15–50 μg/kg/min); or 30 mg/kg in 50 mL at 50 mL/hr for 2 min, then 1.5–5 mL/hr (15–50 μg/kg/min).

Specific Precautions

Use with caution in patients with hepatic disease, heart failure, hypotension, or shock.

Monitoring

Electrocardiogram (ECG) should be continuously monitored. It is necessary to monitor the IV site, because local thrombophlebitis is well described with prolonged infusions.

Key Interactions

β-blockers may increase lidocaine serum levels. Class I antiarrhythmics and amiodarone may increase adverse effects.

Mexiletine

Mechanism of Action

Mexiletine is a class IB lipid soluble antiarrhythmic drug. It inhibits the fast sodium channel with greater effects at faster heart rates. Effects are exaggerated in diseased tissue, dependent on potassium concentration. Mexiletine suppresses early after depolarizations.

Indications

Mexiletine has a specific pediatric application in long QT type III.[15]

Pharmacokinetics

Undergoes hepatic metabolism. The half-life of mexiletine is 10–14 hours. Mexiletine is eliminated in the urine.

Important Adverse Effects

Palpitations, bradycardia, chest pain, syncope, hypotension, atrial or ventricular arrhythmias, dizziness, confusion, ataxia, agranulocytosis, hepatitis, tremors, diplopia, and tinnitus.

Dose

Oral dose is 8 mg/kg as the first dose and this is followed by 4–8 mg/kg 8 hours starting 2 hours after stat dose (maximum 400 mg); IV infusion: 2–5 mg/kg over 15 minutes (maximum 250 mg), then 5–20 µg/kg/min (maximum 250 mg/hour).

Specific Precautions

Mexiletine is to be used with caution in patients with seizure disorders, severe heart failure, hypotension, or hepatic dysfunction. Blood dyscrasias have been reported.

Monitoring

Liver enzymes, complete blood count (CBC), ECG and, heart rate should be monitored.

Key Interactions

Phenobarbital, phenytoin, rifampicin, and other hepatic enzyme inducers may lower mexiletine plasma levels.

Flecainide

Mechanism of Action

Flecainide is a class IC lipid soluble antiarrhythmic drug. It has three major electrophysiological effects—(1) inhibitor of the fast sodium channel (and slow calcium channels at higher doses), (2) prolongs action potential duration, and (3) inhibitor of rapid repolarizing current.

Indications

They include supraventricular tachycardia in children that do not respond to beta-blockers, permanent junctional re-entrant tachycardia, multifocal atrial tachycardia, and selected cases of catecholaminergic polymorphic ventricular tachycardia.

Pharmacokinetics

Most of the antiarrhythmic drugs increase action potential during slow heart rates and attenuate it during high hits, a property known as "reverse use dependence." However, flecainide binds to target channels more effectively when the channel is stimulated at a fast rate, a property known as "use-dependent kinetics." It occurs due to sodium channel blockade, which results in reduced sodium loading and Na^+, K^+ adenosine triphosphatase (ATPase) stimulation during tachycardia. Hence, flecainide is proarrhythmic and should be avoided in structural heart disease.

In view of these properties, the drug should be started under strict observation. Doses should be gradually increased till steady state (five times the half-life of the drug) is achieved. The QRS duration should be monitored while increasing the drug dose. The half-life (T1/2) of flecainide is age-dependent (neonates 29 hours, infants 11–12 hours, and children 8 hours). It has a narrow therapeutic index, greater oral bioavailability (>90%), and is eliminated through renal (33%) and hepatic (66%) metabolism. Oral absorption of flecainide is decreased by milk products.

Important Adverse Effects

Prolongation of PR interval, QRS duration, bradyarrhythmias, depression of LV function due to negative inotropic effect, and neurological manifestation including obtundation and seizures. Other adverse effects include rash, blood dyscrasias, increased liver enzymes, tremor, and blurred vision.

Dose

2–3 mg/kg 12 hours oral (maximum 100 mg), may increase over 2 weeks to 7 mg/kg (maximum 200 mg) 8–12 hours.

Specific Precautions

Drug preparation (especially in newborns and infants), avoid in structural heart disease and ventricular dysfunction.

Monitoring

Electrocardiogram, blood pressure, and heart rate.

Key Interactions

It interacts with drugs that are metabolized or inhibit/induce the cytochrome P4502D6 enzyme, include amiodarone and acetazolamide. Flecainide can also potentiate the effect of digoxin. Concomitant administration with medications that prolong QT interval should be avoided.

Amiodarone

Mechanism of Action

Amiodarone inhibits adrenergic stimulation; prolongs the action potential and refractory period of both atrial and ventricular myocardium; and decreases AV and sinus nodal function.

Indications

Drug-resistant arrhythmias, congenital postoperative JET; amiodarone is commonly used as first line therapy to manage JET and other supraventricular arrhythmias, particularly in patients with structural cardiac abnormalities or decreased cardiac output.[12,16] Amiodarone in children and young adults with critical, drug-resistant arrhythmias had an efficacy rate of 84% in early postoperative tachyarrhythmias, 91% in atrial tachyarrhythmias, 93% in JET.

Pharmacokinetics

The oral absorption ranges from 35 to 65%. It is metabolized in the liver and the GI tract via the cytochrome P450 system, primarily via cytochrome 3A4, and has an active metabolite desethyl amiodarone. Amiodarone is highly bound to plasma proteins (>96%).The metabolites are eliminated by biliary excretion and enterohepatic circulation. The half-life has not been well described in children. However, it is very long in adults (15–142 days, median 58 days, following a single dose and 40–55 days in adults receiving chronic therapy).

Important Adverse Effects

Bradycardia, heart block, sinus arrest, hypotension, heart failure, and myocardial depression. Administering smaller and slower doses decreases the frequency of hemodynamic adverse effects of amiodarone. Although amiodarone prolongs the QT-interval, there is low risk of torsades de pointes because amiodarone blocks all channels. Chronic oral administration of amiodarone is associated with numerous adverse effects including rash, headache, nausea, peripheral neuropathy, corneal microdeposits, pulmonary fibrosis, and hypo/hyperthyroidism. These adverse effects occur rarely in children younger than 10 years of age.

Hypotension can be potentially fatal with IV use; skin discoloration and subcutaneous fat necrosis if administered intravenously through peripheral line due to extravasation, photosensitivity, rash, and pruritus.

Specific Precautions

Severe sinus node dysfunction and second- or third-degree AV block are contraindications. Some IV amiodarone preparations contain benzyl alcohol, which has been associated with the potentially fatal "gasping" syndrome in neonates (metabolic acidosis, respiratory distress, gasping respirations, CNS dysfunction, hypotension, and cardiovascular collapse). It is mandatory to always administer IV amiodarone through central venous line due to risk of subcutaneous fat necrosis if administered through peripheral line due to extravasation, especially in neonates and infants.

Dose

- *IV*: 15 mg/kg in 50 mL 5% D at 5 mL/hr (25 µg/kg/min) for 4 hours, then 1–3 mL/hour (5–15 µg/kg/min, maximum 1.2 g day)
- *Oral*: 4 mg/kg (maximum 200 mg) 8 hours 1 week, 12 hours 1 week, then 12–24H; after starting tablets, taper IV infusion over 5 days.
- *Pulseless ventricular fibrillation (VF) or ventricular tachycardia (VT)*: 5 mg/kg IV over 3–5 minutes.

Monitoring

For hypotension, bradycardia, and AV block.

Key Interactions

Although it is primarily metabolized via the cytochrome P450 3A4 pathway, amiodarone is a substrate of multiple additional pathways of the cytochrome P450 system (1A2, 2C8, 2C19, and 2D6). It is an inhibitor of many cytochrome P450 pathways (1A2, 2A6, 2136, 2C9, 2C19, 2D6, and 3A4) and p-glycoprotein and hence, has many drug interactions. These interactions can either affect the metabolism of amiodarone or, more commonly, amiodarone affects the metabolism of the concomitant medication. Amiodarone increases serum concentrations of digoxin (by approximately 50%), class 1A antiarrhythmic drugs, beta-blockers, lidocaine, and flecainide. Antiarrhythmics which increase the serum concentrations of amiodarone include nondihydropyridine calcium channel blockers (verapamil and diltiazem). It is important to be checked for potential interactions before initiating by amiodarone or any concomitant medications.

Sotalol

Sotalol is fast emerging as a drug of choice for many pediatric supraventricular tachycardias because of its excellent safety profile and high effectiveness.[17]

Mechanism of Action

- Nonselective beta-blocker. It has two isomers (D and L), both with K^+ channel blocking activity, while L-isomer provides beta-adrenergic blocking activity.
- *It has dose related mechanism of action*: At lower doses, beta blocker and at high dose K^+ channel blocker.

Indications

Fetal atrial flutter, resistant re-entrant supraventricular tachycardia (AV and AV nodal), and etopic atrial tachycardia with conversation rates 85–89%.

Pharmacokinetics

It has excellent oral bioavailability (90–100%). It is renally eliminated. Half-life for neonates, infants, and children are 8.4, 7.4, and 9 hours, respectively.

Important Adverse Effects

- *Proarrhythmic effects*: QT prolongation, bradycardia, torsades de pointes
- *Monitoring*: ECG—for arrhythmia.

Key Interactions

Digoxin, lidocaine, amiodarone, sildenafil, propafenone, and quinidine all interact with sotalol. Concomitant usage needs careful monitoring of heart rate, blood pressure and ECG.

Metoprolol

Mechanism of Action

Metoprolol is a second-generation, cardioselective inhibitor of β1-adrenergic receptors. It is classified as a class II antiarrhythmic agent. It has no intrinsic sympathomimetic activity and a weak membrane stabilizing activity.

Indications

Tachyarrhythmias, hypertension, and acute management of hypercyanotic spell.

Pharmacokinetics

- *Onset of action*: Immediate release metoprolol has an onset of action as an antihypertensive in 15 minutes and causes full β-blockade within 1 hour.
- *Duration of action*: The β-blocking activity after a single immediate release oral dose is 3–6 hours, with longer duration observed with higher doses.

Absorption

Almost completely absorbed when administered orally.

Bioavailability

Ranges between 50 and 70% due to extensive first-pass metabolism.

Half-life: Neonates 5–10 hours and adults 3–7 hours.

Metabolism

Hepatic metabolism of metoprolol varies significantly in individual patients based upon the existence of the debrisoquine genetic polymorphism. Extensive hydroxylators may require several doses of the drug daily, whereas poor hydroxylators may do well with a single daily dose.

Important Adverse Effects

Bradycardia, worsening of AV block, hypotension, heart failure, and reduced peripheral circulation.

Specific Precautions

Metoprolol can exacerbate CHF and asthma.

Monitoring

Monitor heart rate and blood pressure.

Key Interactions

Nonsteroidal anti-inflammatory drugs (NSAIDs) may decrease the antihypertensive effect. When β-blockers and digoxin are given concomitantly, AV block and potential digoxin toxicity are possible. Diltiazem may cause hypotension, bradycardia, and AV conduction disturbances. Metoprolol toxicity (bradycardia, fatigue, and bronchospasm) may be seen when given with diphenhydramine due to inhibition of cytochrome P450 metabolism.

■ CALCIUM CHANNEL BLOCKERS

Calcium channel blockers are useful in selected supraventricular arrhythmias beyond infancy and for re-entrant idiopathic fascicular ventricular tachycardia that has a characteristic right bundle branch block with left axis deviation.

Verapamil

Mechanism of Action

Verapamil blocks calcium channels in vascular smooth muscle and myocardium during depolarization. Verapamil has the greatest influence on cells in the SA and AV nodes. Calcium channel blockade becomes more apparent at faster rates. Verapamil is effective in depressing-enhanced automaticity.

Indications

Verapamil-sensitive ventricular tachycardia (Belhassen ventricular tachycardia); selected supraventricular tachycardias beyond infancy.

Pharmacokinetics

Peak effect is seen in 1–2 hours for the oral, immediate release form and within minutes of the IV form. The duration is 6–8 hours for oral and 10–20 minutes of the IV form. It is metabolized in the liver with a half-life of 4–7 hours in infants/children and 4–12 hours in adults. Elimination is in the urine.

Important Adverse Effects

Cardiovascular: Severe hypotension resulting in asystole and cardiovascular collapse has been reported in infants with IV use. Verapamil may also cause bradycardia, heart block, and worsening of CHF nervous system: dizziness, fatigue, seizures, headache, gingival hyperplasia, constipation, and nausea.

Specific Precautions

Verapamil is not recommended for those younger than 1 year of age. Administer verapamil with continuous ECG monitoring and IV calcium at bedside. Avoid IV use in neonates and young infants because of the risk of cardiovascular collapse. Have IV calcium chloride 10 mg/kg available at the bedside to treat hypotension. Use verapamil with caution in patients with severe left ventricle dysfunction, sick sinus syndrome, hepatic or renal impairment, and hypertrophic cardiomyopathy. Verapamil administration may worsen myasthenia gravis and may decrease neuromuscular transmission in patients with Duchenne muscular dystrophy.

Dose

IV: 0.1–0.2 mg/kg over 10 minutes (adult 5–10 mg), then 5 μg/kg/min. Oral: 1–3 mg/kg 8–12 hours (adult 80–120 mg).

Monitoring

Electrocardiogram and blood pressure should be monitored. Follow hepatic enzymes with long-term use.

Key Interactions

Verapamil can result in serious cardiovascular effects when combined with beta-blocking agents, digoxin, quinidine, and disopyramide. Verapamil may increase serum concentrations of digoxin, quinidine, cyclosporine, and carbamazepine. Phenobarbital and rifampicin may decrease verapamil serum concentrations. Erythromycin may increase serum concentration of verapamil. Concomitant aspirin use may prolong bleeding times. Verapamil may prolong the recovery from vecuronium.

Diltiazem

Mechanism of Action

Diltiazem blocks inward calcium channels, with effects on the sinoatrial (SA) and AV nodes.

Indications

Same as in verapamil. Diltiazem is a useful alternative in infants.

Pharmacokinetics

Diltiazem has an extensive first-pass effect and is metabolized in the liver. It has a half-life of 3–4.5 hours and is not dialyzable.

Important Adverse Effects

Bradycardia, hypotension, AV block, tachycardia, flushing, peripheral edema, dizziness, headache, rash, nausea, constipation, dyspepsia, and elevation of liver enzymes.

Specific Precautions

Diltiazem should be avoided in neonates. Use of diltiazem with β-blockers or digoxin can result in conduction abnormalities. Use with caution in left ventricular dysfunction and with hepatic and renal dysfunction. It is contraindicated in hypotension, sinus node dysfunction, or heart block.

Dose

Oral 1 mg/kg Q 8 hours (adult 60 mg); increase if required to maximum 3 mg/kg (adult 180 mg); IV bolus 0.15–0.45 mg/kg.

Monitoring

Liver function tests, blood pressure, and ECG.

Key Interactions

The risk of bradycardia or heart block is increased with beta-blocker or digoxin use. Diltiazem may decrease metabolism of cyclosporine, carbamazepine, digoxin, lovastatin, midazolam, and quinidine. Diltiazem use may increase the effect of digoxin and fentanyl. Rifampicin may decrease diltiazem serum concentration. Cardiac effects of anesthetics may be potentiated by diltiazem.

Digoxin

Digoxin is one of the oldest cardiovascular medications with fairly extensive use in pediatric practice. It has been used for heart failure and for selected tachyarrhythmias. However, in recent times, its importance has diminished considerably with the advent of safer alternatives.

Mechanism of Action

Digoxin is a cardiac glycoside with cholinergic and antiadrenergic effects which serve to slow the sinus rate and AV node conduction by prolonging the effective refractory period. It also has direct effects on the atrial muscle to shorten the refractory period of atrial myocytes and accelerate conduction. Digoxin has a minor effect on ventricular muscle to increase repolarization. It also blocks Na^+/K^+ATP and increases intracellular calcium, which is responsible for its inotropic properties, but may also contribute to its proarrhythmic effects. The electrocardiographic effects of digoxin include decreased heart rate, prolonged PR, shortened QT, and ST-T wave depression.

Indications

Digoxin is used as first-line therapy for fetal supraventricular tachycardia (SVT) in the absence of hydrops and is associated with the least risk to mother and fetus. Flecainide and digoxin were more effective at conversion of fetal SVT to normal sinus rhythm than treatment with sotalol. Digoxin can be employed in rate control strategies for arrhythmias that originate in the atrium including EAT, atrial fibrillation, and atrial flutter. Digoxin is also utilized in re-entrant SVT when the re-entry circuit includes the AV node. Its use in heart failure from a variety of causes has declined lately. However, the positive inotropic effects do enable some degree of symptom relief in patients with heart failure.

Pharmacokinetics

Digoxin has a narrow therapeutic index. The oral bioavailability is approximately 75%. Infants require larger doses per unit body weight than adults and older children due to increased clearance and a larger volume of distribution. The half-life is shorter in infants (18–33 hours) than in children (37 hours), thus maintenance therapy should be divided into twice daily doses in infants but can be given as a single dose in children. Elimination is primarily renal and dosages need to be decreased with renal compromise. The dosages commonly used for digoxin is shown in **Table 5**.

Important Adverse Effects

Sinus bradycardia, AV block, sinus block, atrial ectopic beats, bi- and trigeminy, atrial tachycardia with AV block,

TABLE 5: Digoxin dosing.

	Oral		Intravenous	
Age group	*Loading dose*	*Maintenance dose*	*Loading dose*	*Maintenance dose*
Preterm	20 μg/kg	5–8 μg/kg/day	15 μg/kg	3–4 μg/kg/day
Term	30 μg/kg	6–10 μg/kg/day	20 μg/kg	5–8 μg/kg/day
1 month to 2 years	40–60 μg/kg	10–12 μg/kg/day	30–40 μg/kg	7.5–12 μg/kg/day
2–5 years	30–40 μg/kg	7.5–10 μg/kg/day	20–30 μg/kg	6–9 μg/kg/day
5–10 years	20–30 μg/kg	5–10 μg/kg/day	15–30 μg/kg	4–8 μg/kg/day
>10 years	10–15 μg/kg	2.5–5 μg/kg/day	6–12 μg/kg	2–3 μg/kg/day

ventricular arrhythmias, vomiting, and hyperkalemia are associated with toxicity.

Specific Precautions

Digoxin should not be used in children with pre-excitation as it can accelerate conduction along the accessory pathway leading to life-threatening ventricular arrhythmias in the setting of atrial flutter or fibrillation. Because of renal excretion, it has to be avoided or used in reduced doses in children with renal dysfunction.

Monitoring

Symptoms of digitalis toxicity include fatigue, nausea, vomiting, diarrhea, headache, and blurred vision. Proarrhythmic effects include AV node block, profound sinus bradycardia or SA block, atrial or nodal ectopy, and ventricular arrhythmia.

Key Interactions

Digoxin has serious drug interactions with multiple drugs including calcium channel blockers, carvedilol, propafenone, amiodarone, quinidine, erythromycin, tetracycline, nonsteroidal anti-inflammatories, and azole antifungals, which increase digoxin levels; β-blockers and calcium channel blockers can potentiate bradycardia and heart block; diuretics can exacerbate hypokalemia; and spironolactone interferes with digoxin assays.

Adenosine

Adenosine is invaluable in the diagnosis and acute management of tachyarrhythmias.

Mechanism of Action

Adenosine is an endogenous purinergic agent that blocks conduction through the AV node by increasing potassium channel conductance and depressing slow, inward calcium current. Adenosine also causes peripheral vasodilation.

Indications

Adenosine is indicated for termination of paroxysmal SVT (specifically AV nodal or AV re-entrant tachycardia). More importantly, the information recorded during termination of tachyarrhythmias is valuable from a diagnostic standpoint because it often unravels the underlying mechanism.

Pharmacokinetics

Adenosine is metabolized by erythrocytes (cellular uptake) with a half-life of <10 seconds.

Important Adverse Effects

Flushing, arrhythmias (atrial fibrillation, bradycardia, and heart block), hypotension, light-headedness, headache, apprehension, and blurred vision.

Specific Precautions

Bronchospasm may occur with adenosine use in asthmatics. Use adenosine with caution in patients with underling SA or AV nodal dysfunction or obstructive lung disease. The initial dose of adenosine should be decreased in patients receiving dipyridamole.

Dose

0.05–0.1 mg/kg stat by rapid IV push (adult 3 mg), increase by 0.1 mg/kg (adult 3 mg) every 2 minimum to maximum 0.5 mg/kg (adult 18 mg). Use the two-syringe technique for administration of the drug, immediately followed by a normal saline flush into a proximal IV access.

Monitoring

Continuous ECG, blood pressure, and respiratory rate. ECG should be recorded in all patients to document the mechanism of termination.

Key Interactions

Dipyridamole potentiates the effect of adenosine. Theophylline and caffeine antagonize the effect of adenosine. Concomitant use of carbamazepine increases the risk of heart block.

PULMONARY VASODILATORS

The outlook of pulmonary hypertension may have improved after the introduction of drugs that specifically result in pulmonary vasodilation. These drugs target different pathways that contribute to increased pulmonary vascular resistance.

- *Drugs that stimulate*: Nitric oxide (NO)-cyclic guanosine monophosphate (GMP) system: Sildenafil and tadalafil
- *Soluble guanylate* cyclase *stimulators*: Riociguat
- *Endothelium receptor blockers*: Bosentan, ambrisentan, and macitentan
- *Prostanoids*: Epoprostenol, treprostinil, iloprost, and beraprost.

While Chapter 18 describes the indications and use of these medications in some detail, this chapter describes the pharmacology of this important class of drugs. Essential details are summarized here in **Table 6**.

Inhaled Nitric Oxide

Mechanism of Action

Nitric oxide is produced endogenously from 1-arginine by NO synthases. Inhaled NO diffuses rapidly across the alveolar-capillary membrane into the pulmonary smooth muscle. The pathophysiological effects of NO are mediated through the increased intracellular concentrations of cyclic guanylate monophosphate (cGMP), leading to smooth muscle relaxation.

Adverse Effects

Methemoglobinemia may occur with sustained high concentrations of inhaled NO (80 ppm). Inhaled NO combines with hemoglobin and is rapidly oxidized to methemoglobin, leading to tissue hypoxia without cyanosis. The acute withdrawal of inhaled NO therapy may precipitate rebound pulmonary arterial hypertension (PAH), which may be ameliorated with the use of phosphodiesterase 5 (PDE-5) inhibitors.

Monitoring

Patients receiving inhaled NO should be monitored for formation of nitrogen dioxide (NO_2) and methemoglobinemia.

TABLE 6: Pulmonary vasodilators in children.

Pharmacologic pathway	*Medication class*	*Mechanism of action vasodilation and inhibition of vascular remodeling*	*Therapeutic agents*	*Route of administration*	*Adverse effects*
cGMP augmentation	· Inhaled nitric oxide (iNO)	· Via diffusion across the alveolar capillary membrane →↑cyclic GMP in pulmonary smooth muscle cells (SMC) → SMC relaxation	· iNO	Inhaled	· Methemoglobin formation of NO_2
	· Phospho-diesterase (PDE-5) inhibitors	· Via PDE-5 inhibition→↑ cGMP in pulmonary arteriolar smooth muscle cell→ pulmonary vasodilation and inhibition of vascular remodeling	· Sildenafil and tadalafil	· Oral and IV	· Headache, flushing, dizziness, hypotension, and priapism
	· Soluble guanylate cyclades (sGC) stimulator	· Via sGC (independent of NO, but also increases sGC sensitivity to NO) →↑cGMP→ pulmonary vasodilation	· Riociguat	· Oral	· Headache, dyspepsia, hypotension, and teratogenicity
cGMP augmentation	Prostaglandin	Via cell-surface G-protein receptors on pulmonary endothelial cells, or platelets →↑cAMP → Pulmonary and systemic vasodilation, inhibition of vascular, remodeling and inhibition of platelet aggregation	Epoprostenol treprostinil, iloprost beraprost	IV, inhaled, subcutaneous and oral	Flushing Headache Hypotension Jaw Pain thrombocytopenia
	PDE-3 inhibitors	Via PDE-3 inhibition →↑cAMP in arterial SMCs and cardiac myocytes→ pulmonary and systemic vasodilation and inotropy	Milrinone	IV	Hypotension thrombocytopenia
· ET receptor blockade	· ET-1 antagonists	· Via specific competitive dual ET-A and ET-B receptor blockade → pulmonary vasodilation and inhibition of vascular remodeling	· Bosentan	· Oral	· Liver toxicity · Anemia · Headache · Flushing nasal-congestion · Peripheral edema
	· ET-A antagonists	· Via selective ET-A receptor blockade, pulmonary vasodilation, antiproli-feration, and ET-1 clearance	· Ambrisen-tan	· Oral	· Extremity pain, teratogenicity

(AMP: adenosine monophosphate; cAMP: cyclic adenosine monophosphate, cGMP: cyclic guanylate monophosphate; ET: endothelin, NO: nitric oxide)

NO_2 is easily converted to nitric acid that is highly toxic to the respiratory tract.

Dose

1–40 ppm (up to 80 ppm); 0.1 L/min of 1,000 ppm added to 10 L/min gives 10 ppm.

(NO) = Cylinder (NO) × [1 – (Patient FiO_2/Supply FiO_2)]. (NO) = Cylinder (NO) × NO flow/Total flow.

Key Interactions

No known interactions.

Specific Challenges

Many hospitals do not possess the facility of NO administration because it is expensive and cumbersome. Oral and IV sildenafil achieves equivalent actions in most circumstances.

Clinical Uses

Selected cases of persistent pulmonary hypertension in the newborn, acute pulmonary hypertensive crisis in the postoperative period are the most common reasons to administer iNO.

Sildenafil[18,19]

Mechanism of Action

Sildenafil is a potent PDE-5 inhibitor that increases cGMP in the smooth muscle of pulmonary vasculature.

Pharmacokinetics

Oral sildenafil citrate is absorbed rapidly after administration during fasting. The mean absolute bioavailability is 40%. Maximum plasma concentrations are achieved 60 minutes after administration, with a half-life of approximately 4 hours in adults. When taken with food, the rate of absorption is slowed, with time to Cmax delayed by 1 hour. Metabolism of sildenafil occurs primarily by hepatic cytochrome P450 (CYP) enzymes such as CYP3A4 and CYP2C9. CYP3A4 inducers and medications, such as bosentan, decrease the levels of sildenafil, hence monitoring may be advisable with coadministration with CYP3A4 inducers. Alternatively, CYP3A4 inhibitors increase serum concentrations of sildenafil. N-desmethyl sildenafil is an active metabolite of sildenafil and is believed to account for 20% of its pharmacological effects. Sildenafil and its metabolites are 96% bound to plasma proteins.

Adverse Effects

The most frequent adverse events include headache, agitation, flushing, rhinitis, dizziness, hypotension, peripheral edema, dyspepsia, diarrhea, myalgia, back pain, and visual disturbances. Serious adverse effects requiring drug discontinuation occur infrequently. Inhibition of PDE-5 at therapeutic sildenafil levels produce dose-related ocular effects including blurred vision, changes in light perception, and transient blue-green visual abnormalities. Sildenafil has also been associated with hearing loss. The association between use of high-dose sildenafil and late death in children on sildenafil monotherapy is being explored.

Specific Precautions

Patients with a creatinine clearance <30 mL/min, hepatic cirrhosis, or concomitant use of CYP3A4 inhibitors may require a reduction in their sildenafil dose. Sildenafil should not be used concomitantly with systemic nitrates.

Monitoring

Oral sildenafil has less systemic effects and has been started in the outpatient setting. Eye screening and hearing assessment in extremely premature infants should be considered.

Dose

It is reasonable to start with an oral dose of 0.3 mg/kg/dose and increase every 3–6 hours until effective. It is perhaps not useful to increase the dose beyond 1 mg/kg/dose. The standard adult dose is 20 mg thrice daily.

Key Interactions

Coadministration of sildenafil with bosentan leads to decreased sildenafil plasma concentrations and increased bosentan concentrations. Bosentan decreases the maximum plasma concentration (Cmax) of sildenafil by 55.4% and the area under the plasma concentration versus time curve over a dosing interval (area under curve—AUC) by 62.6%, whereas sildenafil increases the Cmax of bosentan by 42.0% and AUC by 49.8%. The recommendations of dose adjustment are not available, but caution is advised. There is no significant pharmacokinetic interaction between sildenafil and warfarin.

Tadalafil[20]

Mechanism of Action

Tadalafil is a potent inhibitor of PDE-5 and increases the concentration of cGMP, which results in pulmonary vasodilation.

Pharmacokinetics

After a 20 mg tablet was administered in healthy adult subjects, tadalafil was absorbed rapidly with the median time to maximal concentration of 4 hours and a half-life of 35 hours. Steady-state plasma concentrations are achieved within 5 days of initiation of tadalafil at 20 mg or 40 mg daily. Unlike sildenafil, there does not seem to be any effect from food intake. The hepatic CYP3A4 pathway metabolizes tadalafil.

Adverse Effects

Headache, flushing, nasal congestion, dyspepsia, nausea, and myalgia.

Specific Precautions

Coadministration of PDE-5 inhibitors with other vasodilators may lead to hypotension. Concomitant use of potent inducers or inhibitors of CYP3A is not recommended. The dose should be reduced in patients with mild-to-moderate renal or hepatic impairment. Tadalafil is not recommended in patients with severe renal or hepatic disease and should not be used in patients taking nitrates. Use in neonates is contraindicated due to lack of maturation of glucuronidation pathway.

Monitoring

Tadalafil has less systemic effects and has been started in the outpatient setting. Use in children <4 years has not been described.

Dose

20 mg daily oral, increase every 4 weeks to 40 mg daily.

Key Interactions

Tadalafil exposure is decreased with concomitant bosentan by 41.5% in healthy adult volunteers, though no pharmacokinetic drug interactions have been noted between tadalafil and ambrisentan.

Riociguat[21]

Mechanism of Action

Riociguat stimulates soluble guanylate cyclase (sGC) independently of NO and increases the sensitivity of sGC to NO, resulting in increased cGMP levels.

Pharmacokinetics

Riociguat is rapidly absorbed and maximum plasma concentration is reached between 0.5 and 1.5 hours. The mean elimination half-life is 5–10 hours.

Indications

Riociguat significantly improves exercise capacity and pulmonary vascular resistance in patients with chronic thromboembolic pulmonary hypertension.[21]

Adverse Effects

In the PATENT-1 study, the most common serious adverse event in the 2.5 mg—maximum group was syncope. In the CHEST-1 study, the most common serious adverse events were right ventricular failure and syncope. Common side effects observed in patients treated with riociguat include headache, dizziness, indigestion, peripheral edema, nausea, diarrhea, and vomiting.

Specific Precautions

Riociguat carries a boxed warning alerting patients and healthcare professionals that the drug should not be used in pregnant women because it can harm the developing fetus. Patients should not take riociguat with any nitrates or PDE-5 inhibitors as this combination may lead to severe hypotension. Riociguat alters the regulation of bone homeostasis in juvenile rats and the riociguat-related bone findings are of concern with respect to potential pediatric use, especially in infants and younger children. It is also avoided in dialysis patients.

Dose

Dosing in adults starts at 0.5–1.0 mg three times daily with increases of 0.5 mg three times a day every 2 weeks to a maximum of 2.5 mg three times daily both for PAH and chronic thromboembolic pulmonary hypertension.

Key Interactions

Riociguat (2.5 mg three times daily) has no pharmacodynamics interaction with warfarin.

Epoprostenol[22]

Mechanism of Action

Epoprostenol is a prostacyclin analogue with anti-proliferative, anti-platelet, and vasodilatory effects on the pulmonary and systemic vascular beds.

Pharmacokinetics

Epoprostenol has a rapid onset of action, reaching plasma steady-state concentrations within 15 minutes. Epoprostenol is obligated to a continuous IV therapy due to ultra-short elimination half-life of 2–3 minutes. In human blood, epoprostenol is rapidly hydrolyzed and metabolized to 6-keto-PGF1 alpha. This metabolite is biologically inactive and eliminated in the urine.

Adverse Effects

Side effects are generally related to vasodilation and are dose-dependent. The most common side effects include flushing, headache, nausea, diarrhea, jaw discomfort while eating, foot-pain, rash, and thrombocytopenia.

Specific Precautions

Severe adverse events such as bradycardia, systemic hypotension, and thrombocytopenia resulting from insufficient or excessive dosage of epoprostenol may occur. Patients with pulmonary veno-occlusive disease or pulmonary vein disease may develop life-threatening pulmonary edema. Patients with pneumonia or other parenchymal lung disease may develop worsening ventilation-perfusion mismatch.

Monitoring

Systemic blood pressure, heart rate, and side effects should be monitored at initiation of administration.

Dose

Dilute to 2–10 μg/mL, new syringe every 8 hours. <8 kg: 12 μg/10 mL diluted at 0.25–0.75 mL/hr (5–15 ng/kg/min); >8 kg: 500 μg in 50 mL diluent at 0.03–0.09 mL/kg/hr (5–15 ng/kg/min). Chronic pulmonary hypertension: 2 ng/kg/min IV, increase to 20–40 ng/kg/min. T1/2 is 1 minute.

Key Interactions

Epoprostenol inhibits platelet aggregation and has anti-hypertensive effects. Therefore, coadministration epoprostenol with anticoagulants or platelet inhibitors may exacerbate bleeding and use with other vasodilators may worsen hypotension.

Bosentan[6,22-24]

Mechanism of Action

The endothelin (ET)-A receptor and ET-B receptor on vascular smooth muscle mediates vasoconstriction and cell proliferation in pulmonary vascular smooth muscle cells. The ET-B receptor on endothelial cells mediates vasodilation, antiproliferation, and ET-1 clearance. Bosentan is a highly specific, competitive, dual ET-1 receptor antagonist which binds to ET-A and ET-B receptors.

Pharmacokinetics

Bosentan is rapidly absorbed after oral administration and is unaffected by food intake. In the prospective pharmacokinetic study (FUTURE-1 trial), bosentan pharmacokinetics were studied after multiple dosages (2 or 4 mg/kg) twice daily in pediatric patients with PAH. The median time to maximum plasma concentration was 3.0 hour for both dosing regimens. The mean maximum plasma concentration was 583 and 649 ng/mL in patients receiving 2 or 4 mg/kg twice daily, respectively. In the BREATHE-3 trial, the mean maximum plasma concentrations were 685, 1,136, and 1,200 ng/mL in children receiving bosentan doses of 31.25 mg, 62.5 mg, or 125 mg twice daily, respectively. The corresponding values for median time to maximum plasma concentration were 2.5, 1.0, and 1.8 hours, respectively. Bosentan is metabolized in the liver by CYP2C9 and CYP3A4.

Adverse Effects

Bosentan is generally well-tolerated in the pediatric population. In the FUTURE-1 trial, the most frequent adverse events include abdominal pain, vomiting, chest pain, extremity pain, fatigue, flushing, headache, and nasal congestion. In BREATHE-3, the most common adverse events were flushing, edema, and headache. Bosentan has a potential risk of dose-dependent increases in aminotransaminase levels [>3 times the upper limit of normal (ULN) in 11–14% and >8 times in 2–7% of adults]. In pediatric studies, the incidence of elevated aminotransaminase levels (>3× ULN) were 3% in extended FUTURE-2 trial and 16% in the BREATHE-3 trial.

Specific Precautions

Bosentan is not recommended in patients with moderate or severe hepatic impairment. Teratogenicity is a significant concern in pregnant women. Decreases in sperm count have been observed in patients taking endothelin receptor antagonists (ERAs). Bosentan may decrease the effectiveness of oral contraceptive agents. It may also cause anemia.

Monitoring

Liver function tests should be monitored monthly. As bosentan is teratogenic, pregnancy should be tested regularly in women in reproductive age group.[6]

Dose

1 mg/kg 12 hours oral for 1–4 weeks (adult 62.5 mg), then 2 mg/kg 12 hours (adult 125 mg).

Key Interactions

Concomitant use of bosentan with inhibitors of CYP2C9 or CYP3A4 should be cautioned. The pharmacokinetics of bosentan was not affected by coadministration with warfarin. Because sildenafil inhibits CYP3A4 activity, the concomitant use of sildenafil leads to an increase in bosentan concentrations. Likewise, bosentan reduces the concentration of sildenafil.

Ambrisentan[25]

Mechanism of Action

Affinity for the ET-A receptor by ambrisentan is 4,000-fold greater than its affinity for the ET-B receptor. The possible impact of higher selectivity for the ET-A receptor includes greater vasodilation and preserved ET-1 clearance.

Pharmacokinetics

Ambrisentan is rapidly absorbed after oral administration to maximal concentrations within 1.7–3.3 hours. The pharmacokinetics of ambrisentan is not affected by food intake. Steady state is achieved after 3–4 days of therapy. Half-life: Approximately 15 hours for the 5 mg once daily dosing in adult patients. Metabolism: The primary metabolic pathway of ambrisentan is hepatic glucuronidation. Ambrisentan is also metabolized by CYP3A4 and CYP2C19 isozymes. A current pediatric study evaluated exposure to ambrisentan at doses from 2.5–10 mg; the mean Cmax was 737.7 ± 451.5 ng/mL, mean time to peak plasma concentration was 3.2 ± 2.1 hours and mean AUC was 6,656.8 ± 4,245.5 ng/mL, which were similar to those in adult studies.

Adverse Effects

Ambrisentan was generally well tolerated in most clinical studies. In the ARIES study, the most frequent adverse events included peripheral edema, nasal congestion, upper respiratory tract infection, headache, flushing, and nausea. Side effects were not dose-dependent. In the pediatric study, 5 of 38 patients (13%) discontinued ambrisentan due to severe headache, lack of clinical efficacy, or near syncope.

Specific Precautions

Ambrisentan is not recommended in patients with moderate or severe hepatic impairment. No pharmacokinetic change in ambrisentan levels was found in mild or moderate renal impairment (creatinine clearance of 20–150 mL/min). There is no information in patients with severely reduced renal function with creatinine clearance of <20. Teratogenicity is another effect of ERAs. The effects of ambrisentan on embryo-fetal abnormalities were observed in animal models but have not been evaluated or published in pregnant women. Ambrisentan is contraindicated in women who are or may become pregnant.

Monitoring

The incidence of elevated hepatic aminotransferase levels was 2.8 % in the ARIES study and was similar to the placebo group. Monthly liver function testing for ambrisentan is no longer on the Food and Drug Administration (FDA) label, but most pediatric centers still perform routine monitoring, every 3–4 months. Pregnancy test should be carried out regularly in female patients on ambrisentan.

Dose

5 mg daily oral (maximum 10 mg).

Key Interactions

Ambrisentan is partially metabolized by CYP3A4 and CYP2C19 and caution should be exercised with concomitant use of medications that are strong inhibitors of either or both of these. Administration of ambrisentan with warfarin does not have any significant drug interaction. There are also no drug-to-drug interactions between ambrisentan and sildenafil.

Macitentan

Mechanism of Action

Macitentan is an orally active, non-peptide dual endothelin ET-A and ET-B receptor antagonist for the treatment of PAH.

Pharmacokinetics

The dose-proportionality coefficient beta for Cmax [95% confidence interval (CI)] was 0.83 (0.79, 0.87) indicating less than dose-proportional pharmacokinetics of macitentan. A pharmacologically active oxidative depropyl metabolite, ACT-132577 was present in the plasma, whereas two minor metabolites were detected in the urine. The pharmacokinetics of macitentan are dose proportionate over a range from 1 to 30 mg after once daily administration.

Adverse Effects

Adverse events more frequently associated with macitentan than with placebo were headache, nasopharyngitis, anemia, and bronchitis.

Specific Precautions

ERAs are contraindicated in pregnancy. It is necessary to obtain baseline liver enzymes and monitor as clinically indicated. ERAs can also cause anemia. Decreases in sperm count have also been observed in patients taking ERAs. There are currently no studies in children with macitentan.

Dose

10 mg once daily oral; <5 years introduce over 10 days.

Key Interactions

Strong CYP3A4 inducers (rifampicin) reduce exposure to macitentan and should be avoided. Strong CYP3A4 inhibitors (ketoconazole and ritonavir) increase exposure to macitentan and should be avoided. Macitentan does not cause clinically relevant changes in sildenafil or warfarin exposure.

DIURETICS[26]

Diuretics are perhaps the most extensively used of all the medications listed in this chapter. They are almost always the first line of therapy for heart failure and are of great value in perioperative intensive care. Long-term oral diuretics are valuable adjuncts to other medication in ambulant management of heart failure. This section describes commonly used diuretics in pediatric cardiac practice.

Loop Diuretics

Loop diuretics are the most commonly used among all the diuretics because its efficacy.

Furosemide

Mechanism of Action

Furosemide acts through inhibition of $Na^+/K^+/2Cl^-$ cotransporter in ascending loop of Henle.

Indications

It is the first line of therapy for management of volume overload in CHF and following cardiac surgery.

Pharmacokinetics

The onset of action of loop diuretics is 30–60 minutes after oral administration. The peak effects occur within 1–2 hours and the duration of action is 6–8 hours. After an IV injection, the diuresis begins in 5 minutes and typically lasts for 2 hours. The hepatic metabolism of the drug is minimal, and the half-life is approximately 30 minutes.

Adverse Effects

Adverse effects of furosemide use include serious depletion of total body Na^+ manifesting in hyponatremia or extracellular fluid volume depletion associated with hypotension, reduced glomerular filtration rate (GFR), or circulatory collapse. It can cause extracellular fluid volume depletion associated with hypotension. Electrolyte imbalances including hypokalemia, hyponatremia, hypomagnesemia, and hypocalcemia are common. Also reported are dizziness, urticaria, nausea, pancreatitis, headaches, photosensitivity, diarrhea, dehydration, and anemia. Ototoxicity is known to occur from high doses of furosemide. Other effects may include hypochloremia, metabolic alkalosis, hypercalciuria, agranulocytosis, thrombocytopenia, nephrocalcinosis, prerenal azotemia, hyperuricemia, and interstitial nephritis. Oral solutions contain sorbitol, which may cause diarrhea.

Specific Precautions

Loop diuretics are potent agents. Excess amounts may lead to profound diuresis with fluid and electrolyte loss. Close medical supervision and dose evaluation is required. Initiating angiotensin-converting-enzyme (ACE) inhibitors during active diuresis may precipitate hypotension.

Monitoring

Serum sodium, potassium, chloride and bicarbonate, renal function [blood urea nitrogen (BUN) and creatinine (Cr)], blood pressure are all to be monitored. Long standing use may require tests for monitoring ototoxicity.

Dose

0.5–1 mg/kg 6–24 hours (oral, IV).

Key Interactions

Nonsteroidal anti-inflammatory drugs decrease the effect of furosemide. There is increased ototoxicity with aminoglycosides and ethacrynic acid; and drugs affected by potassium depletion such as digoxin. There is increased anticoagulation by warfarin when patients are on concomitant furosemide therapy.

Thiazide Diuretics

Hydrochlorothiazides

These are often used to supplement the effects of loop diuretics especially when there is refractoriness to the effects of loop diuretics. They are used as sole agents when mild diuresis is adequate. They are also useful adjuncts is antihypertensive therapy.

Mechanism of action: Thiazides act by inhibition of Na^+/Cl^- co-transporter in distal convoluted tubule.

Indications: Thiazide and thiazide-like diuretics are used for the treatment of mild-to-moderate hypertension. Additionally, they are used for the treatment of edema caused by heart failure, bronchopulmonary dysplasia, nephrotic syndrome, or after cardiac surgery.

Pharmacokinetics: Hydrochlorothiazide has an onset of action within 2 hours of oral administration, with duration of action of 6–12 hours. The oral absorption in the GI tract is approximately 60–80%. The half-life of hydrochlorothiazide is 5–15 hours and is eliminated almost completely via the kidneys as unchanged drug.

Adverse effects: Caution is advised for patients with severe renal disease, reduced hepatic function, diabetes mellitus, systemic lupus erythematosus, and gout. Adverse side effects of hydrochlorothiazide may include drowsiness, paresthesia, hypokalemia, hyponatremia, hypochloremic metabolic alkalosis, hyperglycemia, nausea, vomiting, anorexia, pancreatitis, cholestasis, hypotension, agranulocytosis, thrombocytopenia, leukopenia, prerenal azotemia, polyuria, and photosensitivity.

Monitoring: Serum electrolytes, renal function (BUN and Cr), blood glucose, triglycerides, uric acid, blood pressure, and fluid balance should all be monitored.

Dose: 1–1.5 mg/kg every 12–24 hours in children; (adult dose: 25–50 mg).

Key interactions: There is a decreased antihypertensive effect with NSAIDs. There is evidence of increased potassium losses when given concomitantly with steroids and amphotericin B; and increased hypersensitivity reactions to allopurinol. Increased hyperglycemia has been noted with diazoxide along with decreased effectiveness of antidiabetic agents. Incidence of hypotension is increased if given with ACE inhibitors. Renal toxicity has been commonly noted with concomitant use of cyclosporine.

Metolazone

Metolazone is essentially a thiazide-like diuretic that is especially used to supplement the effects of loop diuretics especially when there is refractoriness to the effects of loop diuretics.

Mechanism of action: Metolazone acts through inhibition of Na^+/Cl^- cotransporter in distal convoluted tubule.

Pharmacokinetics: Metolazone has an onset of action of approximately 1 hour and duration of action of 12–24 hours.

Oral absorption of the drug is dependent on the preparation used, and protein binding is 95%. The half-life is 6–20 hours and 70–95% of the drug is eliminated unchanged in the wine.

Adverse effects: Cautious use is recommended in patients with severe renal disease, reduced hepatic function, diabetes mellitus, systemic lupus erythematosus, gout, and in patients with high triglyceride or cholesterol levels. Common adverse reactions include palpitations, chest pain, hypotension, headaches, drowsiness, rash, and GI irritation. Hypokalemia, hyponatremia, hypochloremia, metabolic alkalosis, hyperglycemia, thrombocytopenia, leukopenia, aplastic anemia, and hyperuricemia have also been reported.

Monitoring: Serum electrolytes, renal function (BUN and Cr), blood glucose, triglycerides, uric acid, blood pressure, and fluid balance should be monitored.

Dose: 0.1–0.2 mg/kg daily orally (adult 5–10 mg).

Key interactions: There are also increased potassium losses with steroids and amphotericin B; and increased hypersensitivity reactions to allopurinol. Digoxin toxicity may be caused by metolazone-induced hypokalemia and hypomagnesemia.

Potassium-sparing Diuretics

The simultaneous use of potassium-sparing diuretics along with loop diuretics mitigates the significant side effect of hypokalemia. Whenever loop diuretics are to be used in twice daily doses or more, it is a good idea to combine with potassium-sparing diuretics.

Spironolactone[27]

Mechanism of action: Spironolactone is a potassium-sparing diuretic that competes with aldosterone for binding to receptor sites in the distal tubule of the kidneys. It increases the excretion of sodium, chloride, and water, preventing the excretion of potassium and hydrogen. The effect of aldosterone on arteriolar smooth muscle may also be blocked.

Indications: Potassium-sparing diuretics are commonly used to prevent potassium loss caused by the usage of loop and thiazide-like diuretics for the management of edema. Spironolactone is more commonly used and has been shown to increase success in the treatment of patients with CHF in animal models. It is used in the management of neonatal chronic lung disease. Potassium-sparing diuretics are also used to treat edema associated with hepatic cirrhosis and nephrotic syndrome as well as hypertension, hypokalemia, and primary aldosteronism.

Pharmacokinetics: Spironolactone is well absorbed after oral administration, with bioavailability at approximately 90%. The protein binding of the drug is greater than 90% with hepatic metabolism to multiple metabolites, including the active agent, canrenone. The half-life of spironolactone is 1.4 hours and that of canrenone is 13–24 hours. The duration of action of spironolactone is 2–3 days.

Adverse effects: Severe hyperkalemia may result when used with ACE inhibitors, potassium supplements, and NSAIDs. Use with caution in patients with decreased renal function, hyponatremia, dehydration, or reduced hepatic function. Adverse reactions associated with spironolactone include hyperkalemia, dehydration, hyponatremia, hyperchloremic metabolic alkalosis, headache, fever, diarrhea, vomiting, nausea, lethargy, rash, anorexia, agranulocytosis, coughing, and decreased renal function.

Monitoring: Serum potassium, blood pressure, renal function (BUN and Cr), and fluid balance.

Dose: Oral: 0–10 kg: 6.25 mg 12 hours, 11–20 kg: 12.5 mg 12 hours, 21–40 kg 25 mg 12 hours, >40 kg 25 mg 8 hours.

Key interactions: Potassium-sparing diuretics increases serum potassium when used with potassium supplements, ACE inhibitors, angiotensin receptor blockers, arginine, tacrolimus, sotalol, and cyclosporine. Amiloride decreases digoxin and lithium clearance. NSAIDs decrease the effects of amiloride. Spironolactone use may decrease the clearance of digoxin, may cause a decreased response to norepinephrine, and decrease the effects of oral anticoagulant.

ANGIOTENSIN-CONVERTING ENZYME INHIBITORS

As a class of drug, ACE inhibitors are now widely accepted for the management of heart failure and selected cases of hypertension in children. The afterload reduction that follows administration of this class of drugs makes it suited for the management of left ventricular dysfunction from any cause, large left-to-right shunts, and selected patients with aortic or mitral regurgitation. For the same reason, it is contraindicated in patients with outflow tract obstruction where any vasodilation can potentially result in hypotension.

Enalapril[28]

Mechanism of Action

Enalapril is a competitive inhibitor of angiotensin-converting enzyme and blocks the conversion of angiotensin I to angiotensin II. Angiotensin II is a potent vasoconstrictor, so reducing its blood level leads to less vasoconstriction.

Indications

They include systemic hypertension, CHF, left ventricular dysfunction, and proteinuria in steroid-resistant, mitral and aortic valve regurgitation.

Pharmacokinetics

The onset of action after oral administration is within 1 hour and after IV administration, it is within 15 minutes. Oral absorption is 60% in prodrug (enalapril) form (maximum effect, Oral: 4–8 hours; IV: 1–4 hours). Protein binding: 50–60% enalapril is a prodrug (inactive) that is transformed in the liver to enalaprilat (active). The time to peak serum concentration for enalapril is 0.5–1.5 hours; it is excreted mainly (60–80%) in urine. The half-life of enalapril in neonates is 10.3 hours (4.2–13.4 hours) and infants or children is 2.7 hours (1.3–6.3 hours), and for adults (healthy), it is 2 hours and for with CHF, it is 3.4–5.8 hours.

Adverse Effects

Hypotension, tachycardia, syncope, cough, dyspnea, diminished renal function, hyperkalemia, and eosinophilic pneumonitis. An isolated, dry cough has been reported in 17% (7/42) pediatric patients receiving ACE inhibitors and angioedema.

Specific Precautions

Hypersensitivity to enalapril or other ACE inhibitors. Also, patients with idiopathic or hereditary angioedema or a history of angioedema with administration of ACE inhibitors should not receive these drugs. ACE inhibitors should be used with extreme caution in neonates because of risk of renal failure. Administration during active diuresis can result in severe hypotension.

Monitoring

Blood pressure, BUN, creatinine, white blood cell (WBC), serum potassium, serum glucose. Monitoring for blood pressure effect should focus on the period 1–3 hours (enalapril) or 15–60 minutes enalaprilat (the active metabolite of enalapril) after dosing.

Dose

Initial or "test" dose 0.01 mg/kg/dose every 8–12 hours and titrate dose for response. 0.1 mg/kg (adult 2.5 mg) daily oral, increase over 2 weeks if required to maximum 0.5 mg/kg (adult 5–20 mg) 12 hours.

Key Interactions

In patients who are also receiving potassium supplements or a potassium-sparing diuretic (e.g., spironolactone), an additive hyperkalemic effect may occur.

ANGIOTENSIN II RECEPTOR ANTAGONISTS

Angiotensin II receptor antagonists have a theoretical advantages over ACE inhibitors based on the mechanism of action.

Losartan[29]

Mechanism of Action

Losartan (and its principal active metabolite E-3174) selectively blocks the binding of the potent vasoconstrictor angiotensin II to the AT-1 receptor. By inhibiting angiotensin II binding to these receptors, losartan reduces vasoconstriction and aldosterone secretion, which lowers systemic blood pressure. Angiotensin II receptor antagonists may be more inhibitory than ACE inhibitors on the renin-angiotensin system, and in addition, they do not affect the vascular response to bradykinin (a potent vasodilator) or induce as much cough or angioedema as ACE inhibitors. Losartan is also natriuretic and kaliuretic, which increases urine output.

Indications

Hypertension, aortic root dilation (Marfan syndrome and bicommissural aortic valve), heart failure, and ventricular dysfunction in children when ACE inhibitors are not tolerated because of cough.

Pharmacokinetics

The onset of action is in 6 hours; it is well absorbed with a bioavailability of 25–33%. It is metabolized in liver (14%) via cytochrome P450 isoenzyme CYP2C9 and 3A4 to active metabolite (E-3174) with extensive first-pass effect.

Adverse Effects

- *Cardiovascular*: Chest pain, hypotension, orthostatic hypotension, and tachycardia
- *Respiratory*: Cough, bronchitis, upper respiratory infection, nasal congestion, and sinusitis
- *Endocrine/metabolic*: Hypoglycemia and hyperkalemia
- *Hematologic*: Anemia and thrombocytopenia
- *Cutaneous/peripheral*: Cellulitis (patients with diabetic nephropathy)
- *Others*: Fever, flu-like syndrome, and angioedema.

Specific Precautions

Drugs that affect the angiotensin system in humans can cause injury or death to a fetus during the 2nd or 3rd trimester; therefore, losartan should be discontinued as soon as pregnancy is detected. Avoid use in nursing mothers since excretion in breast milk occurs. Because losartan can cause hypotension, especially with the initial dose, particular care should be used in those with low intravascular volume. It should be used with caution in patients who have baseline hepatic or renal dysfunction. It is often worth considering discontinuing potassium supplementation or potassium-sparing diuretics because of risk of hyperkalemia. Patients with unilateral renal artery stenosis or significant aortic or mitral stenosis are at risk for reduced systemic blood flow.

Monitoring

Blood pressure monitoring, serum electrolytes, BUN, serum creatinine, CBC, and urinalysis should be done regularly while on therapy.

Dose

0.5–2 mg/kg daily oral (adult 25–100 mg).

Key Interactions

Because losartan is metabolized in the liver by the cytochrome P450 system as a substrate of isoenzymes CYP3A4 and CYP2C9, it has multiple interactions with other drugs. The most significant interactions reported are as follows:

- Losartan and E-3174 levels are decreased by concomitant administration of phenobarbital and rifampicin
- Fluconazole decreases E3174 levels but increases losartan levels
- Losartan may increase the levels or effects of CYP2C8 (e.g., amiodarone) and CYP2C9 substrates (e.g., warfarin, phenytoin, and fluoxetine) substrates and lithium
- NSAIDs may reduce the effectiveness of losartan.

ANTITHROMBOTIC AGENTS

Antithrombotic therapy remains the initial management in children at risk or with thromboembolism. Here IV unfractionated heparin, low molecular weight heparin (LMWH), or warfarin with or without the addition of antiplatelet agents are used. Most critical circumstances with established clots resulting in vascular compromise may require the use of a thrombolytic agent, typically tissue plasminogen activator (tPA), for vascular recanalization and thrombus resolution.[30]

Tissue Plasminogen Activator (Alteplase)

Mechanism of Action

It binds to fibrin within a thrombus and converts plasminogen to plasmin, the enzyme that provides thrombus dissolution by degrading fibrin and fibrinogen into fragments.

Indications

Acute myocardial infarction (MI), acute ischemic stroke, acute massive pulmonary embolism, prosthetic valve thrombosis, and occluded central venous catheters. Alteplase has also been used in pediatric patients with systemic thrombosis or parapneumonic effusion (via chest tube instillation).

Pharmacokinetics

- *Onset of action*: For acute MI, the initial response is seen in 20–40 minutes
- *Volume of distribution*: Approximates plasma volume
- *Metabolism*: Liver
- *Half-life in adults*: 25–45 minutes following a 90-minute infusion
- *Elimination*: >50% of drug is cleared within 5 minutes after the infusion and 80% is cleared within 10 minutes. It must be given by continuous infusion to maintain thrombolytic activity.

Adverse Effects

Bleeding may occur at any site including GI hemorrhage, genitourinary hemorrhage, ecchymosis, retroperitoneal hemorrhage, epistaxis, gingival hemorrhage, intracranial hemorrhage, pericardial hemorrhage, and catheter insertion sites. The other adverse events include: hypotension, nausea, vomiting, fever, and allergic reactions.

Note: Doses used for catheter clearance have lower risk of adverse bleeding events.

Specific Precautions

Concurrent use of unfractionated heparin, LMWH, or oral anticoagulants may increase bleeding; arterial and venous punctures should be minimized; avoid intramuscular injections; risk of bleeding increases in cases of any recent major surgery/trauma/recent genitourinary or GI bleeding. Pregnancy, cerebrovascular disease, hypertension, patients with left heart thrombus, acute pericarditis, and subacute bacterial endocarditis are also risk factors for increased bleeding while on alteplase. Hemostatic defects, significant hepatic or renal dysfunction, hypertension, septic thrombophlebitis, or occluded IV cannula at an infected site also have an increased bleeding risk. Risks of alteplase therapy may be increased in patients with major early signs of infarct on computed tomographic (CT) scan and in those with severe neurological deficit at presentation.

Monitoring

Pre-treatment laboratories for systemic use should include prothrombin time/partial thromboplastin time (PT/PTT), platelet count, fibrinogen, fibrin degradation products, plasminogen, antithrombin, protein-C, and protein-S. Monitor for signs and symptoms of bleeding, renal and hepatic function, CBC with platelet count, reticulocytes, PT, activated partial thromboplastin time (aPTT), fibrinogen, fibrin degradation products, d-dimer, plasminogen, antithrombin, and protein C levels during infusion.

Dose

The initial dose is 0.1 mg/kg/hour IV for 6 hours while monitoring for bleeding and measuring fibrinogen levels. If sufficient response is not reached within 6 hours, the dose should be increased by 0.1 mg/kg/hour at 6-hour intervals, to a maximum of 0.5 mg/kg/hour. It is essential to maintain fibrinogen levels greater than 100 mg/dL. Duration of therapy is based on clinical response.

Arterial Thrombosis after Cardiac Catheterization

0.1 mg/kg bolus followed by an infusion of 0.5 mg/kg/hour for 2 hours followed by a heparin infusion.[21]

Venous Thrombosis

The initial dose is lower; 0.03 mg/kg/hour (0.06 mg/kg/hour in neonates) IV which is then adjusted based on clinical response.[22]

Key Interactions

Anticoagulants (unfractionated heparin, LMWH, direct thrombin inhibitors, and factor Xa inhibitors) and drugs that affect platelet function (aspirin, NSAIDs, and clopidogrel) may increase the risk of bleeding. Safety of concurrent use of aspirin or heparin with alteplase within the first 24 hours after the onset of symptoms is unknown and should be considered with caution. Antifibrinolytic agents may decrease effectiveness. Nitroglycerin may increase the hepatic clearance of alteplase.

Heparin (Unfractionated)

Mechanism of Action

Anticoagulation by heparin is mediated by antithrombin III, which primarily inactivates thrombin. In addition, heparin also inactivates activated coagulation factors IX, X, XI, XII, and plasmin. It also prevents the conversion of fibrinogen to fibrin.

Indications

Cardiac catheterization, prophylaxis, and treatment of thromboembolic disorders.

Pharmacokinetics

The absorption of drug when heparin is administered subcutaneously or intramuscular is erratic. Peak concentration is reached 2–4 hours after subcutaneous administration. The onset of action when heparin is administered IV is immediate and is 20–30 minutes when administered subcutaneously. It does not cross the placenta and does not appear in breast milk. It is largely protein bound (95%) and metabolism is via the liver and through the reticuloendothelial system. The mean half-life is 90 minutes (range of 1–2 hours). Factors that can prolong the half-life include obesity, renal dysfunction, hepatic dysfunction, malignancy, infection, and the presence of pulmonary embolism.

Adverse Effects

Adverse effects include hemorrhage, thrombocytopenia, epistaxis, hematuria, anaphylaxis, hematomas, erythema and pain at the injection site, heparin-induced thrombocytopenia, and thrombosis.

Specific Precautions

Preservative-free heparin should be used in neonates to prevent neonatal gasping syndrome caused by the preservative benzyl alcohol. Consider reduced heparin dosage if the child is therapeutically anticoagulated or on antiplatelet medications; has mild-to-moderate bleeding diathesis; uncontrolled hypertension; platelets <100,000 or 50% decrease from baseline; high risk or suspicion of bleeding at the time of initiation of heparin therapy (recent surgery within the past 2 days), recent trauma, arterial ischemic stroke, or cerebral sinus venous thrombosis, end-stage liver disease, renal failure, aneurysm (aortic or cerebral), GI/genitourinary hemorrhage bleeding within the past 14 days; thrombolytic therapy in the previous 12 hours; elevated baseline aPTT or international normalized ratio (INR); malnourished or with bacterial endocarditis.

Monitoring

Baseline laboratories prior to starting heparin therapy should include CBC with platelets, PT/INR, aPTT, and fibrinogen. After starting heparin: Cr should be obtained 4 hours after starting infusion, 4 hours after each rate change, followed by once a day (for therapeutic range); CBC with platelets and stool occult blood should be monitored daily.

Dose

The initial dose is 100 U/kg of heparin at the beginning of the catheterization. Check activated clotting time (ACT) before and after heparin administration. The goal is to keep ACT between 275 and 300 seconds. For infusion, the recommended dose typically ranges from 10 to 15 units/kg/hour.

Key Interactions

Anticoagulants, thrombolytic agents (alteplase, streptokinase, and urokinase), platelet inhibitors (aspirin, salicylates, NSAIDs, dipyridamole e, and clopidogrel), selective serotonin reuptake inhibitors (SSRIs), serotonin and norepinephrine reuptake inhibitor (SNRIs), and prostaglandin may increase the risk of bleeding. IV nitroglycerin may decrease the anticoagulant effect of heparin.

Low Molecular Weight Heparin: Enoxaparin[31]

Mechanism of Action

Enoxaparin is a LMWH that potentiates the activity of antithrombin III which primarily inactivates coagulation Factor Xa. Factor IIa (thrombin) activity is also inhibited, but to a much lesser degree than with unfractionated heparin.

Indications

Enoxaparin is used for the treatment of thromboembolic disorders including deep vein thrombosis and venous thromboembolism.

Pharmacokinetics

Based on antifactor Xa, enoxaparin is 100% bioavailable after subcutaneous injection. The peak activity is at 3–5 hours and the duration of action is approximately 12 hours. It does not cross the placental barrier and does not bind to most heparin-binding proteins. It is metabolized in the liver via desulfation and depolymerization.

Adverse Effects

Adverse effects include thrombocytopenia and bleeding.

Monitoring

Baseline investigations prior to starting enoxaparin therapy should include CBC with platelets, PT/INR, aPTT, creatinine, and fibrinogen. After starting enoxaparin Antifactor Xa (4 hours after second dose, 4 hours after each dose change) can be monitored. Thereafter, it is assessed weekly for inpatients and monthly for outpatients. CBC with platelets should also be monitored every 1–2 weeks. It is perhaps reasonable to consider monitoring bone density in infants and children on long-term use.

Dose

This is given in **Table 7**.

Key Interactions

Anticoagulants, thrombolytic agents (alteplase, streptokinase, and urokinase), and platelet inhibitors (aspirin, salicylates, NSAIDs, dipyridamole, and clopidogrel) may increase the risk of bleeding.

Warfarin

Warfarin still remains the most commonly used oral anticoagulant in children. There are a number of specific circumstances where it is indicated.

Mechanism of Action

Warfarin inhibits the synthesis of vitamin K-dependent clotting factors (II, VII, IX, and X) and the anticoagulants protein-C and protein-S by blocking the regeneration of vitamin K1 epoxide by vitamin K epoxide reductase complex.

Indications

Prophylaxis and treatment of thromboembolic disorders.

Pharmacokinetics

- *Bioavailability*: Rapidly and completely absorbed, with peak concentrations in 4 hours
- *Onset of action*: 24–72 hours, with the peak effect in 5–7 days
- *Duration*: The effects from a single dose last for 2–5 days
- *Protein binding*: Highly protein bound (99%)
- *Metabolism*: In the liver via CYP2C9
- *Half-life*: Approximately 40 hours; highly variable among individuals (range 20–60 hours) due to genetic variations in proteins CYP2C9 and VKORC I
- *Elimination*: 92% of the drug is excreted renally (mainly as metabolites) with the remaining excreted through the biliary tract.

Adverse Effects

Hemorrhage at a number of potential sites.

Specific Precautions

Contraindications to warfarin use are hypersensitivity to warfarin or any component, severe renal or hepatic impairment, hemorrhagic tendencies, cerebral or dissecting aortic aneurysms, active ulceration or bleeding, malignant hypertension, bacterial endocarditis, pericarditis and pericardial effusions, recent or potential surgery of CNS or eye, spinal punctures or lumbar block, pregnancy (serious birth defects have been associated with fetal exposure), and patients with a high potential for noncompliance with medications or monitoring.

Monitoring

Baseline investigations prior to starting therapy with warfarin should include CBC (for hemoglobin and hematocrit) with platelets, PT/INR, and fibrinogen. After starting warfarin, obtain PT/INR daily until therapeutic range is established (two times 24 hours apart, then every 72 hours thereafter while inpatient). It is also useful to monitor occult blood daily and CBC with platelets twice weekly during the first 2 weeks, then every 2–4 weeks thereafter. Target therapeutic INR for most pediatric indications is 2–3. Target range for mechanical prosthetic valves is usually higher (2.5–3.5). The prophylactic target INR range is 1.5–1.9.

Dose

Day 1 loading dose (if baseline INR is 1–1.3): 0.2 mg/kg (maximum dose of 10 mg); 0.1 mg/kg if patient has

TABLE 7: Dose of low-molecular-weight heparin in children.[14]

	Therapeutic dose (subcutaneous)	*Prophylactic dose (subcutaneous)*
Enoxaparin		
≤2 months of age	1.5 mg/kg twice daily	1.5 mg/kg once daily
>2 months of age	1 mg/kg twice daily	1 mg/kg once daily

TABLE 8: Recommended starting and maintenance doses of warfarin.[32]

International normalized ratio	*Action*
Initiation	
Day 1: Baseline 1–1.3	Give 0.1–0.2 mg/kg orally (maximum 10 mg)
Day 2–4: · 1.1–1.3 · 1.4–1.9 · 2–3 · 3.1–3.5 · >3.5	· Repeat initial loading dose · 50% of initial loading dose · 50% of initial loading dose · 25% of initial loading dose · Hold until INR <3.5 then restart at 50% of initial loading dose
Maintenance	
· 1.1–1.4 · 1.5–1.9 · 2–3 · 3.1–3.5 · >3.5	· Increase dose by 20% · Increase dose by 10% · No change · Decrease dose by 10% · Hold until INR <3.5 then restart at 20% of initial loading dose

(INR: international normalized ratio)

liver dysfunction. Days 2–4: loading dose is dependent on patient's INR. Aim to maintain an INR between 2 and 3. For mitral valve replacement, maintain an INR between 2.5 and 3.5. For aortic valve replacement, maintain an INR between 2 and 3 (**Table 8**).

Key Interactions

Warfarin has many drug-to-drug interactions. Only drugs that have significant/major interactions have been listed here. It is essential to consult a detailed reference for complete listing. Drugs that can increase the effects/toxicities of warfarin include: alcohol, allopurinol, aspirin, salicylates, NSAIDs, gemfibrozil, phenytoin, sulfonylureas, statins, amiodarone, fluconazole, ketoconazole, miconazole, voriconazole, metronidazole, omeprazole, amoxicillin, piperacillin, chloral hydrate, chloramphenicol, cimetidine, clopidogrel, fluorouracil, fosphenytoin, levofloxacin, moxifloxacin, phenobarbital, prednisone, SSRIs, streptokinase, sulfamethoxazole and trimethoprim, urokinase, delavirdine, nicardipine, testosterone, and ginkgo biloba.

Breast milk has decreased levels of vitamin K and therefore breastfed infants may be more sensitive to warfarin. Drugs that can decrease the effects of warfarin include: St. John's Wort, cyclosporine, bosentan, nevirapine, nafcillin, rifampicin, carbamazepine, cholestyramine, mesalamine, coenzyme Q10, phenobarbital, oral contraceptives, sucralfate, phytonadione, and foods containing vitamin K.

ANTIPLATELET AGENTS

Antiplatelet agents are widely used in a number of situations in pediatric cardiovascular disease.

Aspirin

Mechanism of Action

Aspirin is a salicylic acid derivative that inhibits both prostaglandin synthesis and platelet aggregation through inactivation of cyclo-oxygenase enzymes. Aspirin acts on the hypothalamus heat-regulating center to reduce fever.

Indications

Aspirin is used to treat pain, inflammation, fever, and for prevention of thromboembolism in a variety of situations. Anti-inflammatory doses are used in acute rheumatic fever and early phase of Kawasaki disease. It is prescribed in patients after palliation with a Blalock-Taussig shunt, bidirectional Glenn or Fontan procedure, and following ASD device closure to prevent thrombosis. Low-dose aspirin is used on a long-term basis in patients with Kawasaki disease who have associated coronary involvement.

Pharmacokinetics

- *Bioavailability*: Absorption is from the stomach and small intestine. Immediate-release formulation is completely absorbed, whereas the enteric-coated form is erratically absorbed.
- *Peak concentration*: The time to peak serum concentration is 1–2 hours (this may be delayed with controlled or timed-release preparations).
- *Duration*: The duration of analgesic/antipyretic effects is 4–6 hours.
- *Distribution*: It is widely distributed.
- *Metabolism*: It is metabolized in the liver.
- *Half-life*: The half-life of the active drug is 6 hours.
- *Elimination*: The elimination is through the kidneys (50–100% dialyzable).

Adverse Effects

- *CNS*: Tinnitus, headache, dizziness, confusion, and hyperpyrexia occur at high doses.
- *Skin*: Rash, urticaria, and angioedema are all described.
- *GI*: Nausea, vomiting, dyspepsia, epigastric discomfort, GI bleeding, and occult bleeding are all common side effects and can occur with low doses.
- *Hematologic*: Prolongation of prothrombin time, anemia, and thrombocytopenia are all well described.
- Others include bronchospasm and metabolic acidosis.

Specific Precautions

Contraindications to aspirin use are hypersensitivity to salicylates or other NSAIDs, bleeding disorders, hepatic failure, and children with chickenpox or flu symptoms because of the risk of Reye's syndrome.

Monitoring

Monitor salicylate levels when using high doses for anti-inflammatory effect.

Dose

Anti-inflammatory 80–100 mg/kg/day, antiplatelet 3–5 mg/kg/day.

Key Interactions

Anticoagulants can potentiate bleeding. Antiplatelet drugs including clopidogrel, dipyridamole, prasugrel, and ticlopidine increase the risk of bleeding. Aspirin may enhance the adverse GI effects (ulceration or bleeding) of systemic corticosteroids, whereas antacids may increase the excretion of salicylates. Salicylates may enhance the adverse and toxic effect of varicella virus-containing vaccines causing Reye's syndrome.

Clopidogrel[33]

This is the most commonly used alternative to aspirin. Occasionally, it is combined with aspirin to maximize antiplatelet effects.

Mechanism of Action

Clopidogrel is converted to an active metabolite which prevents binding of adenosine diphosphate (ADP) to platelet P2Y12 receptors. This irreversibly inhibits platelet aggregation for the entire lifespan of the platelets (7–10 days).

Indications

It is used for prevention of thrombosis. Common indications include Kawasaki disease with coronary involvement (especially in giant aneurysm) along with aspirin.

Pharmacokinetics

It is well absorbed, with a time-to-peak concentration of 1 hour and at least 50% bioavailability. Inhibition of platelet aggregation occurs 2 hours after an oral dose is administered and is dose-dependent. Peak response of 40–60% platelet inhibition occurs in 3–7 days. Complete recovery of platelet function occurs approximately 5–7 days after the last oral dose, when new platelets replace those affected by clopidogrel. Protein binding 98% is protein bound. It is metabolized extensively though the liver via oxidation by the cytochrome P450 system to an inactive metabolite that is then metabolized to the active thiol metabolite. It is 6 hours for the parent drug and 30 minutes for the active metabolite. 50% is excreted via kidneys and 46% is excreted via the GI system.

Adverse Effects

Gastrointestinal hemorrhage and epistaxis, and thrombotic thrombocytopenic purpura.

Specific Precautions

Clopidogrel should be used with caution in patients who may be at increased risk of bleeding. Clopidogrel should be discontinued 5 days before elective surgery. Risk of bleeding increases when clopidogrel is used concurrently with other antiplatelet drugs.

Monitoring

For signs of bleeding, periodic hemoglobin and hematocrit should be monitored. For efficacy determination it may be necessary to consider a platelet aggregation test.

Dose

The pediatric dose is 0.2 mg/kg once daily orally and the typical adult dose is 75 mg once daily.

Key Interactions

It is necessary to avoid use with omeprazole or esomeprazole as they inhibit the conversion to the active metabolite; lansoprazole and pantoprazole may have less effect on the active metabolite formation. Azole antifungals such as fluconazole and voriconazole should also be avoided due to the same reason. Anticoagulants (i.e., warfarin, heparin, enoxaparin, dabigatran, and rivaroxaban) or other antiplatelet agents (aspirin and dipyridamole) may increase the risk of bleeding. Concurrent use of NSAIDs may increase the risk of GI blood loss. Rifampicin may increase the effects of clopidogrel. Thrombolytics and concurrent use of SSRI and SNRIs may also result in an increased bleeding risk.

MEDICATIONS FOR ACUTE CARE SETTINGS

A detailed description on clinical uses of medications in acute care settings are described in the chapter on intensive care (Chapter 13). The following section will provide essential pharmacological information of the individual drugs.

Dopamine

Mechanism of Action

Dopamine is a precursor of norepinephrine that directly stimulates adrenergic and dopaminergic receptors and causes release of norepinephrine from nerve terminals. It is a sympathomimetic agent and the clinical effects have been found to be dose-dependent. At low doses, it exerts an effect on the dopaminergic receptors which produces renal, cerebral, coronary, and mesenteric vasodilation. At intermediate doses, it stimulates β1-adrenergic receptors that increase the heart rate and cardiac output and also stimulate indirect release of norepinephrine. At high doses, it activates alpha-adrenergic receptors inducing systemic and pulmonary vasoconstriction, increased heart rate, and increased blood pressure.

Indications

Treatment of low cardiac output, heart failure, and cardiogenic or septic shock.

Pharmacokinetics

- *Onset of action*: 5 minutes
- *Duration of action*: <10 minutes
- *Half-life*: 2 minutes.

Metabolism

About 75% in plasma, kidneys, and liver (to inactive metabolites by monoamine oxidase and catechol-ortho-methyltransferase) and 25% in sympathetic nerve-endings (transformed to norepinephrine).

Adverse Effects

They include sinus tachycardia, ectopic beats, peripheral or pulmonary vasoconstriction, widened QRS complexes, ventricular arrhythmias, systemic hypertension (contra-indicated in patients with pheochromocytoma), and palpitations.

Specific Precautions

Dopamine is to be infused diluted in dextrose with a maximal concentration of 3.2 mg/mL. It must be administered into a large vein, preferably a central venous catheter, with an infusion device allowing proper and reliable titration.

Dose

The dose has to be titrated to the desired effect as indicated below 5 μg/kg/min (low dosage): increased renal and mesenteric blood flow; increased urine output 5–15 μg/kg/min (intermediate dosage): increased renal blood flow, heart rate, cardiac contractility, and cardiac output >15 μg/kg/min (high dosage): systemic vasoconstriction and increased blood pressure.

Key Interactions

Drugs that antagonize the effect of dopamine include beta- and alpha-adrenergic blocking agents.

Dobutamine

Mechanism of Action

Dobutamine is a synthetic adrenergic agonist or sympathomimetic agent, indicated for the treatment of low cardiac output and heart failure.

Indications

Dobutamine stimulates adrenergic receptors causing increased contractility and some increase in the heart rate. It has less activity and minimal effects. The cardiovascular effects of dobutamine are mediated by direct β-adrenergic activity without norepinephrine release. Dobutamine also lowers central venous pressure and pulmonary capillary wedge pressure, but has no selective effect on pulmonary vascular resistance. Dobutamine may improve diastolic function and when used with adequate fluid replacement, it often increases urine output secondary to increased cardiac output and renal perfusion.

Pharmacokinetics

- *Onset of action*: 1–10 minutes
- *Maximum effect*: 10-20 minutes
- *Metabolism*: It is metabolized in tissues and the liver to inactive metabolites by catechol-ortho-methyltransferase followed by glucuronidation
- *Half-life*: 2 minutes.

Adverse Effects

Sinus tachycardia, ectopic beats, palpitations, hypertension, chest pain, premature ventricular contractions, and ventricular arrhythmias.

Specific Precautions

Dobutamine is a stable product in various solutions unless alkaline for 24 hours. It is recommended to dilute it with normal saline or dextrose with a maximal concentration of 5 mg/mL. It should be administered into a central vein, except for transient and/or urgent scenarios and should be administered using an infusion device allowing proper and reliable titration. Avoid the use of same IV access for administration of drugs such as sodium bicarbonate, heparin, loop diuretics, and some antibiotics such as cephalosporins and penicillin.

Dose

2–20 μg/kg/min.

Key Interactions

Beta-adrenergic blocking agents and calcium products may diminish the therapeutic effects of dobutamine.

Adrenaline

Mechanism of Action

Epinephrine, the end product of endogenous catecholamine synthesis, is a potent stimulator of alpha-1, beta-1 and beta-2-adrenergic receptors resulting in relaxation of smooth muscle of the bronchial tree, cardiac stimulation, and dilatation of skeletal muscle vasculature. Its effects are dose-dependent: at low doses, it causes vasodilatation (beta-2 receptors); at high doses, it may however produce vasoconstriction (alpha receptors) of skeletal and vascular smooth muscle with a subsequent increase of myocardial oxygen consumption. Moreover, it has marked metabolic effects particularly in the glucose homeostasis (hyperglycemia) and it may induce leukocytosis.

Indications

Sympathomimetic, bronchodilator, nasal decongestant, and antidote for hypersensitivity reactions. It is used in the treatment of hemodynamic compromise including decreased cardiac contractility and chronotropy (low cardiac output syndrome, severe hypotension and bradycardia, and myocardial dysfunction) and during cardiopulmonary resuscitation.

Pharmacokinetics

- *Onset of action*: IV: <1 minute
- *Inhalation*: Within 1 minute
- *Subcutaneous*: Within 20–40 minutes with varying levels of absorption
- *IM*: Within 5–10 minutes, more complete and rapid absorption if injected into the anterolateral thigh (vastus lateralis)
- *Absorption*: Active concentrations are not achieved by oral ingestion
- *Duration*: Very short, requiring a continuous infusion
- *Metabolism*: Hepatic (extensive) and renal (to a lesser degree) metabolism by the enzymes catechol-ortho-methyltransferase and monoamine oxidase
- *Half-life*: 2–3 minutes
- *Elimination*: Renal (after metabolization by hepatic glucuronidation and sulfation).

Adverse Effects

- *Cardiovascular*: Sinus tachycardia, hypertension, cardiac arrhythmias, angina, and sudden death. Use cautiously in cases of myocardial ischemia, since it may increase myocardial oxygen consumption.
- *Respiratory*: Rebound broncho- or laryngospasm and nasal congestion.

Specific Precautions

Epinephrine should be protected from light and air. Oxidation turns the drug pink and then a brown color. It is incompatible with alkaline solutions and may be administered with other vasoactive drugs and muscle relaxants. It must be administered into a central vein, except (transiently) in urgent scenarios, with an infusion device allowing proper and reliable titration. It should not be used if solution is discolored or if it contains precipitants. Storage is between 15–25°C (68–86°F) and it is not to be refrigerated.

Dose

Continuous IV infusion: 0.01 µg/kg/min, CPR dosage through different routes -IV or intracardiac (0.1 mL/kg of 1/10,000), endotracheal tube (0.1 mL/kg of 1/1,000).

Key Interactions

Drugs that may enhance vasopressor and cardiac effects of epinephrine include beta-blocking agents (propranolol, atenolol, and esmolol), alpha-blocking agents (phentolamine, phenoxybenzamine, and some phenothiazines), alpha and beta-blocking agents (labetalol), tricyclic antidepressants, and halogenated anesthetic gases.

Vasopressors

Vasopressors are indicated for septic shock and for hypotension in presence of outflow tract obstruction.

Noradrenaline

Mechanism of Action

Norepinephrine, a precursor of epinephrine, stimulates alpha-adrenergic (strong action) and beta-1 (mild action) receptors inducing a strong systemic vasoconstriction, which might increase systemic arterial pressure and thus coronary perfusion. Alpha effects predominate over beta effects, with more intense vasoconstriction than inotropic or chronotropic action, which explains a mild effect on cardiac contractility and heart rate (cardiac output).

Indications

Norepinephrine or noradrenaline is an adrenergic-agonist agent with potent alpha-adrenergic and weaker sympathomimetic (beta-1) action. Norepinephrine has long been used in sepsis as a treatment for vasodilatory shock.

Pharmacokinetics

- *Onset of action*: Almost immediate
- *Duration*: Very short, requiring a continuous infusion
- *Metabolism*: Rapidly metabolized by catechol-ortho-methyltransferase and monoamine oxidase
- *Half-life*: 1–2 minutes
- *Elimination*: By renal excretion (80–95% as inactive epinephrine metabolites).

Adverse Effects

Palpitations, sinus tachycardia, reflex bradycardia, cardiac arrhythmias, hypertension, chest pain, and dyspnea.

Specific Precautions

Norepinephrine is unstable in alkaline solutions and should therefore be diluted in dextrose or at least in saline solution (D5W/NS) with a maximal concentration between 4 and 16 mg/mL (in case of severe fluid restriction). It must be administered into a central vein, except and transiently in urgent scenarios, with an infusion device allowing proper and reliable titration.

Dose

0.05–2 µg/kg/min.

Key Interactions

Drugs that may enhance the effects of norepinephrine—atropine sulfate.

Phenylephrine

Mechanism of Action

Phenylephrine is a potent alpha-agonist (alpha-adrenergic stimulator) with very little beta-adrenergic activity. Therefore, it produces a selective systemic arterial vasoconstriction, causes vasoconstriction of the nasal and conjunctival arterioles, and stimulates the dilator muscle of the pupil producing mydriasis.

Indications

It is used as a pure vasoconstrictor drug to treat hypotension and vascular failure in distributive shock, and is particularly useful for the treatment of tetralogy of Fallot's hypoxic spells unresponsive to sedation, volume load, and beta-blocking or whenever it is required to increase peripheral vascular resistance.

Pharmacokinetics

- *Metabolism*: In the liver and the intestines by monoamine oxidase
- *Half-life*: 2.5 hours.

Adverse Effects

Cardiovascular: Hypertension, angina, severe reflex sinus bradycardia, arrhythmias, severe peripheral vasoconstriction. Phenylephrine is contraindicated in case of severe hypertension, pheochromocytoma, ventricular arrhythmias, and myocardial disease.

Specific Precautions

Phenylephrine is compatible with normal saline, dextrose solutions, and Ringer's lactate. For IV boluses: dilute 1 mg/mL (add 1–9 mL of diluting solution); recommended continuous infusion concentrations are 20–60 μg/mL. It should be administered into a central vein, except and transiently in urgent scenarios, with an infusion device allowing proper and reliable titration.

Dose

- *IM/SC*: 0.1 mg/kg/dose (maximum 5 mg) every 1–2 hours as required
- *IV bolus*: 5–20 μg/kg/dose every 15–20 minutes as required
- *IV continuous infusion*: 0.5–5 μg/kg/min titrated to effect.

Vasodilators

Vasodilators are specifically indicated when afterload reduction is desired as in ventricular dysfunction, large left-to-right shunts, and regurgitation of left-sided valves.

Milrinone[34]

Mechanism of Action

Milrinone is an analog of inamrinone that inhibits phosphodiesterase III, thus increasing cyclic adenosine monophosphate (cAMP) which potentiates the delivery of calcium to myocardial contractile units resulting in a positive inotropic effect. Milrinone has been demonstrated to improve cardiac index and to lower filling pressures, systemic and pulmonary arterial pressures, and resistances in the neonatal population. It induces an increase in cardiac output and it seems to preserve normal myocardial oxygen consumption. It may also produce diastolic relaxation (lusitropic effect) and reduce ventricular preload. Most importantly, it results in relaxation of vascular smooth muscle (predominantly systemic) producing vasodilatation.

Indications

Short-term treatment of acute cardiac failure and post-operative low cardiac output syndrome. It may also be indicated as a co-therapy for PAH.

Pharmacokinetics

- *Onset of action*: 5–15 minutes
- *Maximum effect*: Within 20 minutes
- *Half-life*: 3 hours; Duration: 30 minutes to 2 hours (dose-dependent)
- *Distribution*: Neonates: Unknown; Infants: 0.9 ± 0.4 L/kg (after cardiac surgery); Children: 0.7 ± 0.2 L/kg (after cardiac surgery); Adults: 0.3 ± 0.1 L/kg
- *Protein-binding*: 70%
- *Metabolism*: Milrinone is excreted unchanged
- *Half-life (prolonged in case of renal impairment)*: Infants: 3.1 ± 2 hours (after cardiac surgery); Children: 1.86 ± 2 hours (after cardiac surgery); Adults: 1.69 ± 0.18 hours (after cardiac surgery).

Adverse Effects

Ventricular and supraventricular arrhythmias, thrombocytopenia, and hypotension.

Specific Precautions

Milrinone is compatible with normal saline, half-saline plus dextrose solutions, with a maximum recommended concentration of 200 μg/mL. It should be administered with an infusion device allowing proper and reliable titration.

Dose

IV loading dose of 50 μg/kg over a period of 15 minutes, followed by a continuous maintenance dose of 0.25–1 μg/kg/min. In specific circumstances, the loading dose may be skipped to avoid the risk of hypotension.

Key Interactions

Milrinone interacts with furosemide producing a precipitate.

Levosimendan[35]

Mechanism of Action

Levosimendan is a pyridazinone-dinitrate that belongs to a new class of drugs, the calcium sensitizers. In contrast with other inotropic agents, this medication increases the sensitivity of the heart to calcium, thereby increasing cardiac contractility without a rise in intracellular calcium. It acts by binding to myocardial troponin-C by a calcium-dependent manner causing a configuration change in tropomyosin that exposes actin and myosin elements, allowing a more efficient contraction. It offers the advantage of increasing systolic force without compromising coronary perfusion. Moreover, levosimendan opens adenosine triphosphate (ATP)-sensitive potassium channels in vascular smooth muscles causing vascular relaxation (vasodilatory effect), coronary artery dilatation, and myocyte mitochondria activation. The drug is also believed to exert a cardioprotective effect by opening the mitochondrial (ATP) sensitive potassium channels in cardiomyocytes.

Indications

Levosimendan is a new inodilator used in the treatment of decompensated cardiac failure and as an elective drug in patients with perioperative risk of ventricular failure. It is a useful alternative to milrinone.

Pharmacokinetics

It has a very rapid (in a dose-proportional manner) onset of action, with a half-life of 1 hour. The duration of action is 2–4 hours. Protein-binding: 97–98%; metabolism: reduced in the gut into an amine metabolite; elimination: 296–368 mL/min; 70% of the unchanged drug is excreted by the urine (30%) and feces (40%).

Adverse Effects

Palpitations, flushing, and hypotension.

Specific Precautions

Levosimendan may be diluted in normal saline or in dextrose solutions and administered ideally in a reliable central line, except in an emergency situation. It should be administered under comprehensive hemodynamic monitoring.

Dose

Loading dose of 12 μg/kg over 1 hour, followed by a continuous infusion of 0.1–0.2 μg/kg/min.

Prostaglandin E1

Mechanism of Action

Prostaglandin E1 causes vasodilation by exerting direct effects on vascular and ductus arteriosus smooth muscle.

Indications

Prostaglandin E1 is used for the temporary maintenance of patency of the ductus arteriosus in neonates with ductal-dependent congenital heart disease.

Pharmacokinetics

- *Onset of action*: Rapid; dilation of ductus arteriosus typically occurs within 30 minutes of IV infusion.
- *Duration*: Ductus arteriosus will begin to close within 1–2 hours after infusion is discontinued.
- *Maximum effect*: In acyanotic congenital heart disease, the maximal effect is seen in 1.5–3 hours, with a range of 15 minute – 11 hours. In cyanotic congenital heart disease, the usual maximal effect is seen within 30 minutes.
- *Half-life*: The half-life is 5–10 minutes, therefore, prostaglandin E1 must be administered by continuous infusion.
- *Metabolism*: About 70–80% of prostaglandin E1 is metabolized by oxidation during one pass through the lungs. One active metabolite (13–14 dihydro-PGE1) has been identified in neonates.
- *Elimination*: 90% of prostaglandin E1 is excreted in the urine as metabolites within 24 hours.

Adverse Effects

Fever, flushing, bradycardia, systemic hypotension, tachycardia, and edema. Apnea may occur in about 10% of neonates, with greater risk in those weighing <2 kg at birth; usually occurs during the first hour of the infusion.

Dose

Always by continuous infusion: 0.05–0.2 μg/kg/min IV usually started at a higher dose until the duct patency is established and then titrated to lower levels. In duct-dependent systemic circulation started at a higher dose until the duct patency and maintain infusion at the same dose and it is not advisable to taper.

Reference for all the drug doses are from Frank Shann drug doses pocket book.[36]

REFERENCES

1. Packer M, Bristow MR, Cohn JN, Colucci WS, Fowler MB, Gilbert EM, et al. The effect of carvedilol on morbidity and mortality in patients with chronic heart failure. US Carvedilol Heart Failure Study Group. N Engl J Med. 1996;334(21):1349-55.
2. Munoz R, da Cruz EM, Vetterly CG, Cooper DS, Berry D. Handbook of Pediatric Cardiovascular Drugs, 2nd edition. London: Springer; 2014.
3. Bristow MR. What type of beta-blocker should be used to treat chronic heart failure? Circulation. 2000;102:484-6.
4. Fröhlich H, Zhao J, Täger T, Cebola R, Schellberg D, Katus HA, et al. Carvedilol compared with metoprolol succinate in the treatment and prognosis of patients with stable chronic heart

failure: carvedilol or metoprolol evaluation study. Circ Heart Fail. 2015;8(5):887-96.

5. Poole-Wilson PA, Swedberg K, Cleland JG, Di Lenarda A, Hanrath P, Komajda M, et al. Carvedilol Or Metoprolol European Trial Investigators. Comparison of carvedilol and metoprolol on clinical outcomes in patients with chronic heart failure in the Carvedilol or Metoprolol European Trial (COMET): randomised controlled trial. Lancet. 2003; 362(9377):7-13.
6. Berger RMF, Gehin M, Beghetti M, Ivy D, Kusic-Pajic A, Cornelisse P, et al. A bosentan pharmacokinetic study to investigate dosing regimens in paediatric patients with pulmonary arterial hypertension: FUTURE-3. Br J Clin Pharmacol. 2017;83(8): 1734-44.
7. Shaddy RE, Tani LY, Gidding SS, Pahl E, Orsmond GS, Gilbert EM, et al. Beta-blocker treatment of dilated cardiomyopathy with congestive heart failure in children: a multi-institutional experience. J Heart Lung Transplant. 1999;18(3):269-74.
8. Läer S, Mir TS, Behn F, Eiselt M, Scholz H, Venzke A, et al. Carvedilol therapy in pediatric patients with congestive heart failure: a study investigating clinical and pharmacokinetic parameters. Am Heart J. 2002;143(5):916-22.
9. Shaddy RE, Boucek MM, Hsu DT, Boucek RJ, Canter CE, Mahony L, et al. Pediatric Carvedilol Study Group. Carvedilol for children and adolescents with heart failure: a randomized controlled trial. JAMA. 2007;298(10):1171-9.
10. Storch CH, Hoeger PH. Propranolol for infantile haemangiomas: insights into the molecular mechanisms of action. Br J Dermatol. 2010;163(2):269-74.
11. Hogeling M, Adams S, Wargon O. A randomized controlled trial of propranolol for infantile hemangiomas. Pediatrics. 2011;128(2):e259-66.
12. Polymerou I, Ojala T, Bonou P, Martelius L, Tzifa A. Successful treatment of cardiac haeman-giomas with oral propranolol: a case series of two patients. Eur Heart J Case Rep. 2019;3(2): pii: ytz093.
13. Lei M, Wu L, Terrar DA, Huang CL. Modernized classification of cardiac antiarrhythmic drugs. Circulation. 2018;138(17):1879-96.
14. Bonnet D, Berger F, Jokinen E, Kantor PF, Daubeney PEF. Ivabradine in children with dilated cardiomyopathy and symptomatic chronic heart failure. J Am Coll Cardiol. 2017; 70(10):1262-72.
15. Zhu W, Mazzanti A, Voelker TL, Hou P, Moreno JD, Angsutararux P, et al. Predicting patient response to the antiarrhythmic mexiletine based on genetic variation. Circ Res. 2019;124(4): 539-52.
16. Hill AC, Silka MJ, Bar-Cohen Y. A comparison of oral flecainide and amiodarone for the treatment of recurrent supraventricular tachycardia in children. Pacing Clin Electrophysiol. 2019;42(6):670-7.
17. Celiker A, Ayabakan C, Ozer S, Ozme S. Sotalol in treatment of pediatric cardiac arrhythmias. Pediatr Int. 2001;43(6):624-30.
18. Humpl T, Reyes JT, Holtby H, Stephens D, Adatia I. Beneficial effect of oral sildenafil therapy on childhood pulmonary arterial hypertension: twelve-month clinical trial of a single-drug, open-label, pilot study. Circulation. 2005;111(24):3274-80.
19. Barst RJ, Ivy DD, Gaitan G, Szatmari A, Rudzinski A, Garcia AE, et al. A randomized, double-blind, placebo-controlled, dose-ranging study of oral sildenafil citrate in treatment-naive children with pulmonary arterial hypertension. Circulation. 2012;125(2):324-34.
20. Takatsuki S, Calderbank M, Ivy DD. Initial experience with tadalafil in pediatric pulmonary arterial hypertension. Pediatr Cardiol. 2012;33(5):683-8.
21. Ghofrani HA, D'Armini AM, Grimminger F, Hoeper MM, Jansa P, Kim NH, et al. Riociguat for the treatment of chronic thromboembolic pulmonary hypertension. N Engl J Med. 2013;369(4):319-29.
22. Humbert M, Barst RJ, Robbins IM, Channick RN, Galiè N, Boonstra A, et al. Combination of bosentan with epoprostenol in pulmonary arterial hypertension: BREATHE-2. Eur Respir J. 2004;24(3):353-9.
23. Ivy DD, Rosenzweig EB, Lemarié JC, Brand M, Rosenberg D, Barst RJ. Long-term outcomes in children with pulmonary arterial hypertension treated with bosentan in real-world clinical settings. Am J Cardiol. 2010;106(9):1332-8.
24. Carter NJ, Keating GM. Bosentan: in pediatric patients with pulmonary arterial hypertension. Paediatr Drugs. 2010;12(1): 63-73.
25. Takatsuki S, Rosenzweig EB, Zuckerman W, Brady D, Calderbank M, Ivy DD. Clinical safety, pharmacokinetics, and efficacy of ambrisentan therapy in children with pulmonary arterial hypertension. Pediatr Pulmonol. 2013;48(1):27-34.
26. Lowrie L. Diuretic therapy of heart failure in infants and children. Prog Pediatr Cardiol. 2000;12(1):45-55.
27. Jacob MS, Tang WH. Aldosterone-receptor antagonists in heart failure: insights after EMPHASIS-HF. Curr Heart Fail Rep. 2011;8(1): 7-13.
28. Hsu DT, Zak V, Mahony L, Sleeper LA, Atz AM, Levine JC, et al. Enalapril in infants with single ventricle: results of a multicenter randomized trial. Circulation. 2010;122(4):333-40.
29. Lacro RV, Dietz HC, Sleeper LA, Yetman AT, Bradley TJ, Colan SD, et al. Atenolol versus losartan in children and young adults with Marfan's syndrome. N Engl J Med. 2014; 371(22):2061-71.
30. Monagle P, Chan A, Massicotte P, Chalmers E, Michelson AD. Antithrombotic therapy in children: the Seventh ACCP Conference on Antithrombotic and Thrombolytic Therapy. Chest. 2004;126(3 Suppl):645S-87S.
31. Ignjatovic V, Najid S, Newall F, Summerhayes R, Monagle P. Dosing and monitoring of enoxaparin (Low molecular weight heparin) therapy in children. Br J Haematol. 2010;149(5): 734-8.
32. Krishna MR, Kunde MF, Kumar RK, Balaji S. Ivabradine in post-operative junctional ectopic tachycardia (JET): breaking new ground. Pediatr Cardiol. 2019;40(6):1284-8.
33. Wessel DL, Berger F, Li JS, Dähnert I, Rakhit A, Fontecave S, et al. Clopidogrel in infants with systemic-to-pulmonary-artery shunts. N Engl J Med. 2013;368(25):2377-84.
34. Hoffman TM, Wernovsky G, Atz AM, Kulik TJ, Nelson DP, Chang AC, et al. Efficacy and safety of milrinone in preventing low cardiac output syndrome in infants and children after corrective surgery for congenital heart disease. Circulation. 2003;107(7):996-1002.
35. Namachivayam P, Crossland DS, Butt WW, Shekerdemian LS. Early experience with levosimendan in children with ventricular dysfunction. Pediatr Crit Care Med. 2006; 7(5):445-8.
36. Shann F. Drug Doses, 17th edition. Mount Pleasant VIC: JR Medical Books; 2017.

13

CHAPTER

Pediatric Cardiac Intensive Care

Vishal Singh

INTRODUCTION

Pediatric cardiac intensive care is a rapidly evolving specialty for the perioperative management of the critically ill children after complex congenital heart disease (CHD). Dedicated pediatric cardiac intensive care units (PCICUs) manned by intensive care physicians with basic training as pediatricians, anesthesiologists, or pediatric intensive care and coordinating a multidisciplinary approach is associated with better outcomes.[1] As we enter into the third decade, a few major centers in India have set a template for a dedicated cardiac intensive care unit (ICU) with outcome very close to international standards though the data shared is still in the nascent stage. Rakhi et al. collated retrospective data from a combined adult and PCICU and compared it with prospective data of 634 children in a dedicated PCICU, and reported better outcomes in terms of earlier extubation, deintensification, and discharge from the ICU.[2] The challenge is to ensure that pockets of excellence are not incidental, and while mortality is reduced significantly, morbidity is still a challenge and protocol-based care with stress on pre-emption, reduced morbidity, and complications is the way to go for encouraging and retaining this rare breed of dedicated intensive care physicians. A template to improve quality of care in this arena cannot be fathomed without ensuring retention and motivation of the dedicated ICU team members including doctors, nurses, respiratory therapist, and paramedical aids.

The purpose of this document is to give a brief overview with conceptual understanding related to perioperative management of CHD in PCICU. PCICU caters not only to the pre- and postoperative CHD scenarios, but also critical catheterization interventions in neonates and infants. This is an endeavor to outline the broad principles of preoperative stabilization of a sick neonate, infant with CHD and other acute presentations with myocardial dysfunction, with an aim to optimize cardiopulmonary dynamics and end-organ perfusion and a detailed understanding of postoperative intensive care management after surgery and catheterization laboratory intervention for complex CHD.

PREOPERATIVE INTENSIVE CARE UNIT CARE

Successful critical care management and stabilization of preoperative sick CHD patients involve a quick preoperative assessment based on history and physical assessment not only related to the cardiac and respiratory scenarios, but also directed to the extent of cardiopulmonary impairment, airway abnormalities, and associated extracardiac anomalies. Besides addressing the immediate circulation, airway, and breathing (CAB) to stabilize hemodynamics and gas exchange, it is also relevant to prevent further end-organ damage, while the patient is optimized for surgical intervention.

A neonate or infant with heart disease typically presents with one of the following: heart failure or cardiogenic shock, hypoxia, and arrhythmias.[3] Associated comorbidities such as pneumonia and bloodstream infections often complicate the initial presentation. Interaction with the referring neonatologist, pediatrician, and other frontline healthcare workers is necessary in our aim to improve outlook for CHD children.[4]

Congenital heart defects are complex and can be difficult to categorize. Rather than trying to outline management for each individual defect in a critical presentation, a physiologic approach trying to get answers for the following questions in a scenario makes sense[5] (**Table 1**).

- How does the systemic venous return reach the systemic arterial circulation to maintain cardiac output (CO)? Whether intracardiac mixing, shunting, or outflow obstruction exist?
- Is the circulation in series or parallel?
- Is the pulmonary blood flow (PBF) increased or decreased?
- Is there a volume load or pressure load on the ventricle?

The chapter on neonatal heart disease (*see* Chapter 48) as well as the introductory chapter on CHD (*see* Chapter 20) elaborates the principles of physiology of specific congenital heart defects and lays a foundation for their management.

TABLE 1: Symptom based approach to congenital heart disease.[3]

Physiologic category	Conditions
Duct-dependent systemic blood flow	Hypoplastic left heart syndrome, critical coarctation, interruption of aortic arch, and critical aortic stenosis
Duct-dependent pulmonary blood flow	Pulmonary atresia, critical pulmonary stenosis, and Ebstein anomaly
Obstruction of pulmonary venous return	Obstructed total anomalous pulmonary venous return, mitral atresia with a restrictive patent foramen ovale
Parallel circulation with poor mixing	D transposition with intact ventricular septum
Increased pulmonary blood flow; pretricuspid shunt	Anomalous pulmonary venous drainage (unobstructed)
Increased pulmonary blood flow; post-tricuspid shunt	Unrestrictive ventricular septal defect, patent arterial duct and aortopulmonary window, and persistent truncus arteriosus

Severe Hypoxemia

This is an important category that merits immediate and precise ascertainment of the underlying heart diagnosis.

Ductal Dependent Pulmonary Circulation

The cyanotic forms of CHD present in the ICU and emergency with severe hypoxemia in the neonatal period with or without respiratory distress. Optimal stabilization is based on template of pediatric advanced life support (PALS) guidelines.

Circulation

Fluid boluses10–20 mL/kg over half an hour to 1 hour is often administered for stabilization in the event if baby is acutely ill.

Airway and Breathing

Noninvasive or invasive ventilation targeting oxygen saturation 70–75% is sometimes necessary if the baby appears distressed. It is reasonable to allow for mild metabolic alkalosis, with mild hyperventilation.

Prostaglandin (PGE_1) Infusion

Initiating prostaglandin E1 (PGE_1) infusion in the dosage range of 0.01–0.05 μg/kg/min in patients with decreased blood flow maintains or reestablishes blood flow through the ductus arteriosus. By increasing the PBF, PGE_1 also improves mixing of venous and arterial blood at the atrial level especially in patients with transposition of great arteries, with adequate atrial communication, allowing time to stabilize rather than rushing in for surgical correction. An exception to this is obstructed total anomalous pulmonary venous connection (TAPVC), where the patient presents with severe hypoxemia with respiratory distress, congested lungs, and circulatory collapse and do not benefit from PGE_1, necessitating immediate surgery.[5]

While the neonate is optimized, neurological evaluation and analysis of blood for renal, hepatic, and hematologic profile besides ruling out sepsis is imperative to assess the effects of hypoxia on end-organ profile.

The common side effects of PGE_1 infusion such as apnea, hypotension, and fever are aggravated if the dosage range is breached, but intermittent apnea occasionally necessitates noninvasive ventilation or intubation preoperatively. If the patient has to be transported with PGE_1 infusion, it is often worthwhile to intubate a neonate pre-emptively or provide reliable noninvasive ventilation support. However, it is important to ensure that hyperoxia is avoided to prevent excessive pulmonary vasodilation and systemic hypoperfusion.

Prostaglandin E1 infusion improves oxygenation singularly in patients with decreased pulmonary perfusion such as critical pulmonary stenosis or atresia by sustaining ductal dependent pulmonary circulation, with improvement in end-organ oxygen delivery (DO_2) and correction of lactic acidosis.

Neonates with transposition of great arteries, with intact ventricular septum (IVS), need adequate mixing of oxygenated and deoxygenated blood at the atrial level. A restrictive atrial communication may require balloon atrial septostomy that can be accomplished in the ICU, under echocardiographic guidance. In a few infants with hypoplastic left heart syndrome (HLHS), due to mitral valve hypoplasia and restrictive atrial septal defect, there is profound pulmonary venous congestion with desaturation, and this may require atrial septostomy or stenting of the atrial septum.[6]

Besides a quick clinical examination, a chest X-ray, an electrocardiogram, and a comprehensive echocardiography with color Doppler evaluation assist in confirming the diagnosis in neonate, though in complex univentricular situations or delayed presentations, a cardiac magnetic resonance imaging (cMRI) and cardiac catheterization to assess shunt fraction, pulmonary artery wedge pressure, pulmonary artery pressures, aortopulmonary and major aortopulmonary collateral arteries (APCA and MAPCA) are relevant.

Decreased PBF in preoperative patients with parallel circulation (single ventricle physiology) is reflected with hypoxemia with oxygen saturation <75%. Preoperatively, this may be due to a closing ductus arteriosus, increased pulmonary vascular resistance (PVR) secondary to parenchymal lung disease, or increased pulmonary venous pressure secondary to obstructed pulmonary venous drainage or restrictive atrial septal defect. If PVR elevated sedation, paralysis and controlled hyperventilation with mild respiratory alkalosis usually helps. However, in extreme scenarios, inhaled nitric oxide (iNO) and intravenous (IV) pulmonary vasodilators are also required to improve PBF.

It is essential to optimize systemic DO_2 and inotropes are occasionally required to augment CO.

In low- and middle-income country (LMIC) scenarios, quite a few times the patient with tetralogy physiology presents to the hospital with severe cyanosis, gasping respiration, excessive crying, and irritability. This conundrum of symptoms is referred to as mentioned here.

Hypercyanotic Spell

This is usually triggered with excessive crying, dehydration, and fever.

The baby on presentation may appear dusky with hyperpnea (rapid deep breathing) with significant decrease in oxygen saturation. On examination, the outflow tract murmur may be absent or soft and short. In severe spells, the baby may present with loss of consciousness (LOS) with poor systemic perfusion. There are multiple theories for the underlying mechanism precipitating cyanotic spells. While Woods et al.[7] reported that hypoxemic spell are due to spasm of infundibulum of the right ventricle (RV), with progressive right-to-left shunt and metabolic acidosis, the catecholamine surge further exacerbates the spasm due to tachycardia and increased myocardial contractility. Guntheroth et al.[8] reported that episodes of paroxysmal hyperpnoea are the cause rather than effect, as it increases systemic venous return with increased right-to-left shunting and increased work of breathing. Kothari et al.[9] contested the views mentioned above and emphasized the stimulation of mechanoreceptors in RV as the underlying mechanism. Catecholamine-induced tachycardia and increased contractility compounded with decreased RV volumes can trigger a reflex mediated by the mechanoreceptors resulting in peripheral vasodilatation which precipitates a spell by diverting systemic venous return to the aorta.

The management centers upon stabilization of vitals as per PALS protocol (ABCDE approach).[10]

- Provision of oxygen 100%, while the infant is made comfortable in mother's lap with knee chest position.
- Initiate IV fluids (balanced salt solutions/normal saline/ Ringer lactate) 10 mL/kg/dose over half an hour, to be repeated as per the hemodynamics and then continue fluids at requisite maintenance 100 mL/kg/day.
- Morphine 0.1 mg/kg bolus or pethidine 1 mg/kg/ bolus slowly. Can be given IV, and if no venous access, subcutaneously or intramuscular route preferred.
- Injection metoprolol bolus 0.1 mg/kg/dose can be repeated three times every 5 minutes, followed by infusion of 1–5 µg/kg/min or injection propranolol 0.1 mg/kg followed by infusion. Injection esmolol 0.5 mg/kg/dose followed by infusion at 50 µg/kg/min can also be used to reduce the heart rate and allow infundibular relaxation. Monitor for bradycardia.
- Increase systemic vascular resistance (SVR) with phenylephrine 5–20 µg/kg/dose followed by infusion 0.1–0.5 µg/kg/min. If phenylephrine is not available, methoxamine and norepinephrine should be considered.
- Correct metabolic acidosis with sodium bicarbonate 1 mEq/kg/dose, based on venous blood gas assessment, if pH < 7.3 with metabolic acidosis.
- It is prudent not to rush and intubate these patients as the sudden fall in SVR with sedation and paralysis worsens their condition. It is always wise to manage them with noninvasive continuous positive airway pressure (CPAP) delivered in a comfortable position (mother's lap) if necessary.

Congestive Heart Failure (*See* Chapters 17 and 48)

Congenital heart disease with increased PBF usually presents with symptoms suggestive of congestive heart failure (CHF), frequently aggravated by respiratory infection. Heart failure or cardiogenic shock in the first and second week of life is usually a manifestation of left heart obstructive lesions such as critical aortic stenosis, HLHS, coarctation of aorta with *duct-dependent systemic circulation*. The left-to-right shunts with CHF usually manifest after 3–4 weeks once PVR falls.

The characteristic features of heart failure are tachypnea with increased work of breathing, intercostal and subcostal retractions:

- Tachycardia
- Hepatomegaly
- Failure to thrive, interrupted feeding, increased sweating, irritability, and drowsiness
- Pallor and prolonged capillary refill time (CRT).

The manifestations mimic sepsis and occasionally aspiration related to gastroesophageal reflux and community-acquired respiratory sepsis may further compound issues. In preterm infants, occasionally a symptomatic patent ductus arteriosus (PDA) with CHF manifests as difficulty to wean off ventilator with congested lung fields and hepatomegaly.

While sepsis can be a frequent comorbid factor with neonatal presentation of CHD, the importance of checking saturation in all the four limbs and blood pressure recording in all four limbs, with a high index of suspicion, is the first step toward timely intervention, diagnosis, and minimizing end-organ damage.

The cardiac defects with ductal dependent systemic circulation, such as left-sided obstructive lesions (coarctation of aorta, critical aortic stenosis, HLHS, and interrupted aortic arch), present with rapidly progressive cardiogenic shock precipitated by ductal closure.

Stabilization

The initial stabilization involves resuscitation as per PALS protocol.

Circulation

Measured fluid boluses (10 mL/kg over half an hour/1 hour, once or twice while assessing for s/o fluid overload).

Prostaglandin E1 infusion = 0.01–0.05 μg/kg/min, titrated based on frequent duct patency assessment on two-dimensional (2D) echo with color Doppler.

Avoid excessive vasoconstriction. A balance of inodilators (dobutamine/milrinone with low-dose adrenaline) to maintain inotropy with decreased systemic afterload.

Airway and Breathing

Noninvasive/invasive ventilation targeting oxygen saturation 80–85%, [low FiO_2, controlled positive end-expiratory pressure (PEEP) based on presence of pulmonary edema] and mild hypercarbia (PCO_2 > 55–60 mm Hg) with mild respiratory acidosis (pH 7.30–7.35) to titrate PVR to improve systemic blood flow. If the work of breathing is not excessive and systemic perfusion is maintained with no metabolic acidosis, especially in a patient delivered with antenatal diagnosis and in neonatal intensive care unit (NICU) care, it is not essential to intubate and ventilate. Spontaneous ventilation is occasionally better to achieve an adequate systemic perfusion and balance of Qp and Qs. $Qp/Qs = (SaO_2 - ScVO_2)/(SpvO_2 - SpaO_2)$ and assuming normal oxygen extraction (O_2ER) of 25–30%, an SaO_2 of 70–75% and an $ScVO_2$ of 40–50% suggest appropriately balanced systemic and pulmonary circulation with Qp/Qs = 1.

In situations with excessive PBF with left-to-right shunts with pulmonary edema, diuretics would be a part of treatment strategy for decongestion. The strategy is again titrated with the aim of reducing Qp and optimizing Qs. If systemic perfusion is compromised, with suspected sepsis, these patients may require add-on inodilators and invasive or noninvasive ventilation support with the aim of titrating oxygen saturation below 90%, with hypercarbia (controlled hypoventilation at room air) and restricting shunt fraction with mildly increased PVR. Due to limited oxygen reserve, occasionally, these children may desaturate suddenly with aggravating factors such as pain and airway secretions have to be monitored stringently. Occasionally, dilated cardiomyopathy and myocarditis patients may present with similar symptoms, and the diagnosis is clinched with the help of antecedent history, electrocardiogram (ECG), chest X-ray, and echocardiography. The management guidelines are essentially similar in acute scenario, though there may be a case for levosimendan intermittent infusion weekly as a salvage therapy for scenarios awaiting heart transplant. Due to its longer half-life with no increase in myocardial oxygen demand, levosimendan, a calcium sensitizer with improved inotropy and afterload reduction, is a promising add-on to the arsenal. Calcium infusion as an inotrope is relevant in neonates and early infants and in LMIC hypocalcemia as a reversible cause of dilated cardiomyopathy is frequently observed.

It is important that the basics of neonatal and infant care including temperature regulation (prevent hypothermia), glucose and calcium homeostasis are optimized, and metabolic acidosis (pH < 7.30) corrected during resuscitation once ventilation is adjusted.

Monitoring

Besides the hemodynamic monitoring involving electrocardiogram, noninvasive blood pressure in right upper limb, right lower limb especially in ductal dependent systemic circulation, oxygen saturation, it may be worthwhile to monitor end-tidal CO_2 in ventilated patients (to assess improvement in pulmonary circulation in ductal dependent pulmonary circulation). End-tidal CO_2 values will increase and be close to normal range once pulmonary circulation is restored.

Additionally, mixed venous oxygen saturation checked with central venous blood gas, and serial plasma lactate assessment are good surrogates for improvement in systemic circulation and end-organ perfusion. Strategies to shorten the waiting time for surgical intervention and to prevent high plasma lactate levels before surgery have a direct connect with long-term neurocognitive outcome.[11]

The goal of resuscitation is to ensure optimization of clinical status with end-organ protection to ensure better postoperative outcomes. Renal dysfunction and necrotizing enterocolitis (NEC) are occasionally precipitated consequent to compromised end-organ oxygenation and the patients have to be strictly monitored for the same for timely intervention.

Arrhythmia (*See* Chapter 52)

Arrhythmias often present in neonates without structural heart defects, e.g., atrial flutter, congenital atrioventricular (AV) block. They can present with hemodynamic compromise and require stabilization based on the PALS guidelines. Congenital AV block may also occur in association with corrected transposition or heterotaxy syndromes, besides as a manifestation of maternal lupus and after initial stabilization the patient is taken for an emergency permanent pacemaker implantation. Chapter 52 discusses the common rhythm disorders seen in neonates, infants, and children in detail.

POSTOPERATIVE CARDIAC INTENSIVE CARE

One of the main requirements for providing good quality of care in a PCICU is to understand that the job of intensive care physician starts much before the operated child is admitted to the PCICU. Detailed information on the case of the child is required in advance before the day of admission. It is imperative to understand the preoperative anatomy and hemodynamics of the cardiac defect (detailed echo, catheterization data) associated comorbidities, nutritional status, surgical plan, and the possible perioperative and postoperative complications.

Every intensive care physician should be familiar with the intraoperative course and it works well to be familiar with the entire process of anesthesia induction, surgical techniques, cardiopulmonary bypass (CPB), and myocardial protection.

Pediatric Cardiac Intensive Care Unit Workflow

Before the patient is transferred to the PCICU, a careful and standardized preparation of the bed must be completed to avoid glitches and streamline the admission process. A checklist approach involving nursing requisites, monitoring tools, ventilation and resuscitation equipment, standard medication plans (sedation, pain therapy, antibiotics, inotropes and vasopressors, vasodilators, diuretics, fluid therapy, and infusions), and investigation check lists.

Postoperative Transfer of the Patient and Handover

This is a critical first step in postoperative management. Well-rehearsed protocol needs to be followed here. **Box 1** describes the PCICU handover protocol.

BOX 1: Pediatric cardiac intensive care unit handover protocol.

Surgical aspects:
- Intraoperative course, complications, and surprises
- Drains (pleural and mediastinal)
- Pacing wires
- Intraoperative epicardial/transesophageal echo assessment (residual gradient, valve insufficiency, residual shunt, and myocardial function)
- RV/PA step up especially relevant in multiple VSD, large VSD
- Any intraoperative arrhythmias, and how were they managed
- Intraoperative bleeding and how it was managed

Anesthesiology aspects:
- Endotracheal tube size (cuffed or uncuffed)
- Airway concerns
- *Central venous catheter*: Site of insertion and size
- *Arterial access*: Site and size
- Ventilation setting (mode, FiO_2, tidal volume, rate, peak pressure, and PEEP)
- Endotracheal secretions, any evidence of pulmonary hemorrhage
- LA, RA, PA monitoring lines and indications
- Anesthesia medications, inotropes, pressors, and vasodilators
- Heparinization and real-time coagulation status including activated clotting time
- Use of blood products (packed red blood cells, fresh frozen plasma, and platelet concentrates)
- Last arterial blood gas analysis
- Cerebral NIRS (SvO_2)
- Surgical prophylaxis

Cardiopulmonary bypass:
- Bypass time
- Aortic cross clamp time
- Total circulatory arrest time (if applicable)
- Cardioplegia and myocardial protection strategy
- Hemofiltration (modified or conventional ultrafiltration)

(LA: left atrium; NIRS: near-infrared spectroscopy; PA: pulmonary artery; PEEP: positive end-expiratory pressure; RA: right atrium; RV: right ventricle; VSD: ventricular septal defect)

Cardiopulmonary Bypass: Basic Principles (*See* Chapter 15)

Basic components of a CPB circuit include two venous cannulae that drain systemic venous blood from the superior and inferior vena cava (IVC) (or one venous cannula from the right atrium), a cardiotomy reservoir, a heat exchanger, a membrane oxygenator, a roller pump, and an arterial filter. An arterial cannula returns oxygenated blood to the aorta, although occasionally the innominate, axillary or femoral artery is used for the same. Occasionally, a second arterial cannula is used, such as during repair of an interrupted aortic arch, when one cannula is placed in the ascending and a second in the descending aorta to perfuse the lower body to allow selective antegrade and retrograde perfusion while repair is underway.

Before initiation of CPB, the circuit is primed with standardized quantities of crystalloid solution, glucose, buffer [sodium bicarbonate or tris-hydroxymethyl amino-methane (THAM)], heparin, calcium, and either whole blood or packed red blood cells (RBCs) and albumin. The tubing length is minimized but the priming volume can exceed the normal blood volume of neonates by 300%, resulting in hemodilution. This reduces hematocrit and alters plasma and coagulation homeostasis, with significant intraoperative and postoperative hazards including interstitial edema from decreased oncotic pressure, increased propensity for bleeding, etc. Heparin is administered at 1–3 mg/kg based on the baseline activated clotting time (ACT).

Induced hypothermia by adjusting the heat exchanger not only facilitates reduction of metabolic needs and oxygen requirement, but also facilitates surgical repair by allowing flow rate to be decreased. It allows greater interval between cardioplegia redosing, and end-organ protection especially when deep hypothermic circulatory arrest (DHCA) is induced for complex arch and pulmonary veins repair. Hemodilution is desirable during moderate-to-deep hypothermic CPB as hypothermia induces increased viscosity and RBC rigidity. Recent trials suggest a nadir of 25% hematocrit is associated with favorable acute- and long-term neurological outcome[12] but most perfusion strategies target a hematocrit of 30–36%. DHCA < 40 minutes is usually well-tolerated.[13] Regional perfusion techniques to counter the adverse outcomes of DHCA have been evolving, but their efficacy in altering neurodevelopmental outcome still needs to be proven.

Hypothermia induces alkalosis, and using an alpha stat strategy the pH is maintained at 7.40, irrespective of temperature. With the pH stat strategy, CO_2 is added to the circuit to maintain a temperature corrected pH of 7.40 and pH stat strategy has favorable effect based on early outcomes,[14] but no major impact on long-term neurological outcome. Hypothermia induces inflammation and capillary leak altering postoperative course.

Cardiopulmonary Bypass-induced Inflammation and Effect on Postoperative Physiology

The exposure of plasma proteases to the nonendothelial lining of CPB circuit with activation of *systemic inflammatory response syndrome (SIRS)* with deranged coagulation and *ischemia reperfusion injury* with release of proinflammatory reactive oxygen species, cytokines with complement activation, and resultant parenchymal injury especially pulmonary and myocardial are two mechanisms influencing post-CPB end-organ injury.

A uniformly adopted strategy of intraoperative steroids, modified ultrafiltration (MUF), and heparin-coated circuits is used in most adequately resourced environments to circumvent the inflammatory CPB response and end-organ dysfunction.[15,16]

Ultrafiltration removes water, reverses hemodilution, and eliminates low molecular weight inflammatory mediators. Heparin-bonded circuits have been associated with reduced intraoperative incidence of microthrombi as well as reduction in inflammatory response with diminished complement activation.

Initial Evaluation and Basic Patient Monitoring

Immediately after receiving from operation theater (OT) or catheterization laboratory, the essential clinical parameters must be assessed by the on-service intensivist to confirm that the patient is clinically stable, while the monitor variables are being recorded.

Respiration

Assess if the chest excursion is adequate, symmetrical, and the desired tidal volume is being delivered, besides a quick assessment of air entry and adventitious sounds. If patient is extubated on arrival, special attention should be given to proximal airway and presence/absence of stridor should be recorded, while the patient is positioned appropriately with DO_2 by nasal prongs or mask, or noninvasive ventilation as a transient support if chest excursion is shallow or severe airway reactivity is detected.

Circulation

Palpation of the central and peripheral pulsations provides vital information on volume, rate, and regularity of pulse, and pulse volume reflects the pulse pressure. Capillary filling assessment (normal CRT < 2 seconds) is a surrogate of peripheral microvascular perfusion and provides an indirect estimate of CO and peripheral vascular resistance. This should be checked with the limb slightly elevated to determine arterial perfusion rather than venous stasis and the child should be in a neutral thermic environment. A very prolonged CRT > 6 seconds has strong correlation with compromised stroke volume (SV).[17]

Auscultation for shunt murmur, e.g., with modified Blalock–Taussig–Thomas shunt at the endotracheal (ET) tube and infraclavicular zone, precordial auscultation for heart sounds, valve clicks, and assessment of murmur that suggests residual shunts or lesions are important. Assessment of essential vitals on monitor [heart rate, arterial blood pressure (ABP), central venous pressure (CVP), left atrial pressure (LAP), oxygen saturation, skin, and rectal or esophageal temperature] should be done simultaneously. The core peripheral temperature gradient improves as the patient rewarms and circulation improves, but it does not predict circulatory collapse nor consistently correlate well with hemodynamic parameters.[17]

Diuresis

Urine color and volume should be noted. An altered color of urine in the early postoperative period may suggest hemolysis.

Bleeding

The following items need to be noted: mediastinal and pleural drainage, color of drainage (bright red, dark red, and serosanguinous). If sternum is open, it is necessary to assess for pericardial collection and adequacy of suction applied to drainage.

Neurological Assessment

Sensorium should be assessed if already extubated. If ventilated and electively sedated, or under effect of anesthesia, it is necessary to note what are the drugs being administered as infusion or bolus for sedation, analgesia, or paralysis. It is vital to evaluate pupils and look for evidence of spontaneous limb movements and spontaneous breathing beyond supportive ventilation, especially with sedation holiday once every day. If sedation is wearing off, it is important to assess need for restraints.

Assessment of Catheters, Lines, and Site Examination

This is an integral part of the initial assessment.

Endotracheal tube fixation and ET cuff pressure must be checked on arrival.

Initial Tests

In parallel, the first blood samples are taken and include an arterial and central venous blood gas analysis, an ACT, a chest X-ray is ordered and a baseline end-organ assessment biochemistry profile is evaluated. A standard 12-lead ECG is recorded. A screening 2D echocardiogram with color Doppler to assess for residual lesions, myocardial contractility, pleural and pericardial collection, and assessment of pulmonary arterial hypertension (PAH) is prudent if intraoperative imaging not documented.

Blood Gas Analysis

Besides the usual parameters for adequacy of gas exchange and metabolic parameters including blood glucose, it is important to record mixed venous saturation (SvO_2) as an index of circulation besides plasma lactate. Also, baseline hemoglobin, serum electrolytes with serum calcium are relevant component of these records.

Hemodynamic Monitoring: Correlation with Clinical Data

The goals of postoperative hemodynamic monitoring are to establish an objective assessment of patient clinical status, predict potential adverse events, and guide proactive management. It is imperative to have a continuous ECG monitoring, invasive blood pressure, respiratory monitoring (pulse oximetry capnography), rectal or esophageal and skin temperature monitoring, and CVP. LAP monitoring and pulmonary artery pressure are monitored in specific scenarios. Near-infrared spectroscopy (NIRS) and central mixed venous oxygen saturation ($ScVO_2$) are gaining significance as a marker of adequacy of circulation and DO_2, over dynamic variables.[18] In isolation, the relevance of these parameters as markers to predict outcome and pre-empt a sentinel event is beyond the scope of this document, but every variable has its own relevance when examined in conjunction with clinical context.

Electrocardiogram

A 12-lead ECG identifies heart rate abnormalities, ischemic changes, and rhythm disturbances. Associated changes in blood pressure or atrial pressure tracings can lend additional weight to identification of rhythm disturbances. Tachycardia and limited monitor fidelity may conceal P waves and blur QRS morphology and careful attention to CVP or left atrial (LA) trace with arterial pulse contours may help unmask the underlying rhythm, besides atrial wire ECG which is an important adjunct in diagnosis of junctional rhythm variants.

A reduction in size of the QRS complex is significant and may be the first sign of pericardial collection or myocarditis. ECG abnormalities should be promptly and thoroughly analyzed as they may be the first sign of impending circulatory dysfunction.

Arterial Blood Pressure

Invasive blood pressure provides a continuous display of the arterial waveform. The slope of the upstroke is indirectly proportional to the myocardial contractility (**Fig. 1**). A slow rising upstroke is indicative of poor myocardial contractility,

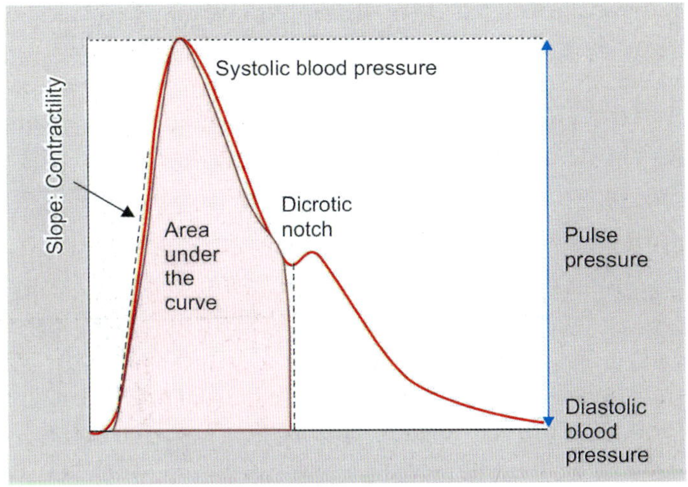

Fig. 1: Information that can be gathered from the arterial pressure contour. The area under the curve often gives a good idea of the stroke volume.[19]

but also observed with aortic stenosis or left ventricular outflow tract (LVOT) obstruction and elevations in SVR. The area under the systolic waveform is proportional to the SV. A low pulse pressure may reflect a low SV or elevated SVR, while a widened pulse pressure due to elevated systolic and depressed diastolic pressures is seen in low SVR states (warm shock), aorta to pulmonary run off, and patients with aortic regurgitation. Mean arterial pressure [systolic BP + 2(Diastolic BP)/3] monitoring goals based on underlying cardiac physiology and myocardial status make more clinical sense in ICU to titrate vasoactive therapy.

Central Venous Pressure

The CVP is the mean right atrial (RA) pressure, which approximates the right ventricular end-diastolic pressure, when right ventricular compliance and tricuspid valve function are normal. Rather than the numerical value, it is the CVP or RA pressure trace which is more informative. CVP is definitely not an absolute guide to fluid responsiveness but a high CVP definitely indicates myocardial dysfunction warranting inotropy rather than fluids. In the immediate postoperative period, a high CVP indicates the need to rule out cardiac tamponade. The atrial pressure waveform normally demonstrates three positive and two negative waves in coordination with cardiac cycle (**Fig. 2**).

When ventricular function and compliance is diminished, atrial systole generates an end-diastolic pressure that is higher (prominent a wave) than baseline. Cannon "a" waves result when atrial systole coincides with a closed tricuspid valve (AV dissociation). Prominent v waves are observed with tricuspid insufficiency, while prominent x and y descents are associated with pericardial restrictive disease.

Left Atrial Pressure

In the presence of underlying cardiopulmonary disease, there is no correlation between RA and LA pressures. LAP is

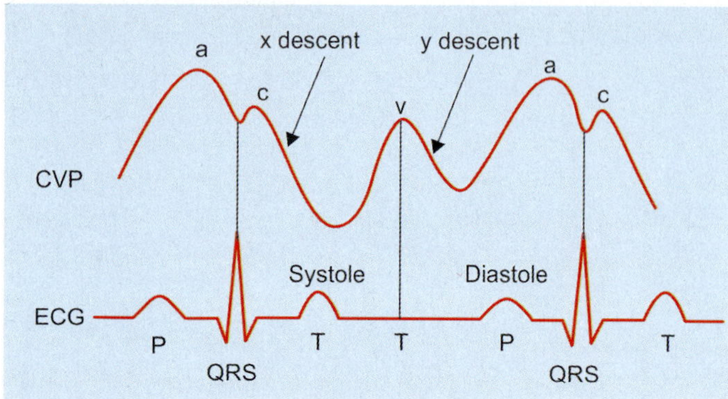

Fig. 2: The timing of individual right atrial or central venous pressure waves in relation to the ECG and cardiac cycle.[19]
(CVP: central venous pressure; ECG: electrocardiography)

a surrogate of left ventricular end-diastolic pressure. The LA line should be handled very carefully when used to avoid air embolus in the systemic circulation.

Left atrial pressure monitoring is relevant in very selected cases of left ventricular dysfunction [ALCAPA, regressed LV with delayed arterial switch in transposition of the great arteries (TGA) IVS], tetralogy of Fallot (TOF) with small left ventricular configuration with increased LA return on pump due to collaterals, and AV valve regurgitation in single ventricle physiology or AV septal defect repair.

Near-infrared Spectroscopy and Mixed Venous Oxygenation

Measurement of central venous oximetry allows for assessment of the relationship between oxygen demand and delivery (oxygen transport balance). While plasma lactate also reflects adequacy of tissue perfusion and oxygenation, O_2ER increases and becomes critical well before lactate production exceeds its clearance.[19]

The relationship between CO and O_2ER is curvilinear and only when the low cardiac output state (LCOS) becomes decompensated the O_2ER becomes critical (**Box 2**). Central mixed venous oxygen saturation ($ScVO_2$) estimation at pulmonary artery origin is ideal in the absence of shunt. Splanchnic O_2ER (IVC) increases first when CO falls, while superior vena cava (SVC) and jugular bulb oximetry value is variable as changes in PCO_2 alters cerebral O_2ER as cerebral blood flow is uncoupled with cerebral metabolism.

$$VO_2/DO_2 = O_2ER = SaO_2 - SvO_2/SaO_2$$

The body is able to preserve constant oxygen consumption (VO_2) over a wide range of DO_2 by adjusting O_2ER ratio (supply independent VO_2). But below a critical DO_2, the increased O_2ER fails to support consumption (supply dependent VO_2). The critical DO_2 remains same and correspondingly the critical O_2ER values also hover between 50 and 60% irrespective of the cause of failure to deliver oxygen to tissues.

Vincent and De Backer[20] analyzed the VO_2/DO_2 relation in sepsis and acute respiratory distress syndrome (ARDS) and observed that supply dependent VO_2 may be observed at a higher DO_2 and hence O_2ER (interpreted with SVO_2) should be closely monitored in critically ill patients as a guide to adequacy of circulation to titrate therapy to ensure O_2ER is restored in normal range.

> **BOX 2:** Oxygen extraction ratio.[18]
>
> *Oxygen extraction ratio (O_2 ER)*: $SaO_2 - SvO_2/SaO_2$ (SaO_2: Arterial O_2 saturation; SvO_2: Mixed venous O_2 saturation (usually from SVC)
> - *25%*: Normal
> - *30–40%*: Increased
> - *40–50%*: Impending shock
> - *>50–60%*: Shock with lactic acidosis
>
> (SVC: superior vena cava)

Near infrared spectroscopy relies on the relative transparency of biological tissue such as skin and bone to near infrared light, where oxy- and deoxyhemoglobin have differing absorption spectra. The equipment algorithm can evaluate nonpulsatile signal of the microcirculation where 75% of blood is venous and the derived oxygen saturation is a surrogate of tissue venous oxygen saturation, correlating well with SVC and jugular venous saturation in case of cerebral NIRS. Mesenteric and renal NIRS are important components of multisite NIRS and mesenteric NIRS values correlate well with decreased perfusion and impending LCOS as splanchnic circulation decreases due to autoregulation and O_2ER increases.

Near-infrared spectroscopy and cerebral oximetry is implemented as a surrogate for cerebral venous oxygen saturation, but with a caveat that cerebral circulation is usually preserved, due to autoregulation in patients with compromised circulation and hence is a relatively late indicator of deteriorating CO and perfusion.

The debate favoring intermittent versus continuous invasive $ScVO_2$ monitoring in pediatric patients with sepsis is still ongoing. Sankar et al.[21] favored continuous monitoring, with 36% patients in continuous monitoring versus 19% in intermittent meeting the primary end point of reversal of shock at 6 hours. But adoption of continuous monitoring as a standard of care in LMIC countries needs stronger evidence.

Lactate

Lactate measurement may not conform to the ideals of hemodynamic monitoring with its intermittent availability through invasive access as a late marker of tissue hypoxia, but is an essential tool as an index of adequacy of perfusion and a reliable downstream surrogate of oxygen supply and demand. An elevated lactate can be an index of tissue hypoxia and anaerobic metabolism (type A) or aerobic metabolism (type B) as in hepatic and renal dysfunction in isolation or acting in combination. Occasionally, it is a tissue adaptive response to hypoxia to preserve crucial substrates while preserving the redox state. Hence, lactate should never be seen in unison, but in correlation with presence or absence of associated signs of tissue hypoxia. A rising or persistent level is a poor prognostic sign. Recently, it has been shown that lactate can act as a biomarker, with higher mortality rates in presumed sepsis, even with no evidence of organ dysfunction.[22]

Echocardiography

Two-dimensional echocardiography is an essential diagnostic tool to assess myocardial contractility, residual defects, pericardial and pleural collection, and a hemodynamic tool to assess fluid responsiveness in PCICU especially in postoperative ICUs.

While left ventricular systolic function can be assessed by determining fractional shortening (FS = end-diastolic dimension- end-systolic dimension/end-diastolic dimension) (FS = 0.28 – 0.40) in unidimensional M mode, calculation of the ejection fraction (EF) is based on the 2D imaging of the left ventricular systolic function by quantifying changes in ventricular volume (EF = end-diastolic volume – end-systolic volume/end-diastolic volume) [left ventricular ejection fraction (LVEF) = 0.68 ± 0.09)]. Right ventricular systolic function is most often qualitative and based on the inward motion of right ventricular free wall (eye balling) toward interventricular septum, though tricuspid annular plane systolic excursion (TAPSE) is emerging as a reliable quantitative variable for the same. Similarly, ventricular wall thickness and volumes can be assessed providing a glimpse into diastolic function and operating volumes.

Inferior vena cava collapsibility on spontaneous breathing and distensibility on positive pressure besides LVOT velocity time integral (VTi) variability with respiration are important surrogates of fluid responsiveness in low output states and in conjunction with other variables assist streamlining fluid strategy for individual case scenarios.

Low Cardiac Output State

Postoperative myocardial dysfunction secondary to CPB-induced reperfusion injury is especially common after prolonged cross clamp times and is further exacerbated by deep hypothermic circulatory arrest (DHCA). The adverse effects of CPB are enhanced in neonates due to limited reserve, as cardiomyocytes are predominantly composed of noncontractile elements. Besides calcium stores in immature myocardium are lesser, compounded by an immature sarcoplasmic reticulum. Also, the neonatal myocardium is exposed to a higher oxygen demand per unit mass necessitating a relatively greater CO and minute ventilation. The infant myocardium is less compliant and less responsive to fluids and inotropes and more susceptible to increased ventricular afterload[23] due to vascular dysfunction with pulmonary and systemic endothelial injury and enhanced reactivity. The surgical approach and preexisting ventricular dysfunction based on underlying pathology only exacerbates the postoperative myocardial dysfunction (**Fig. 3**).

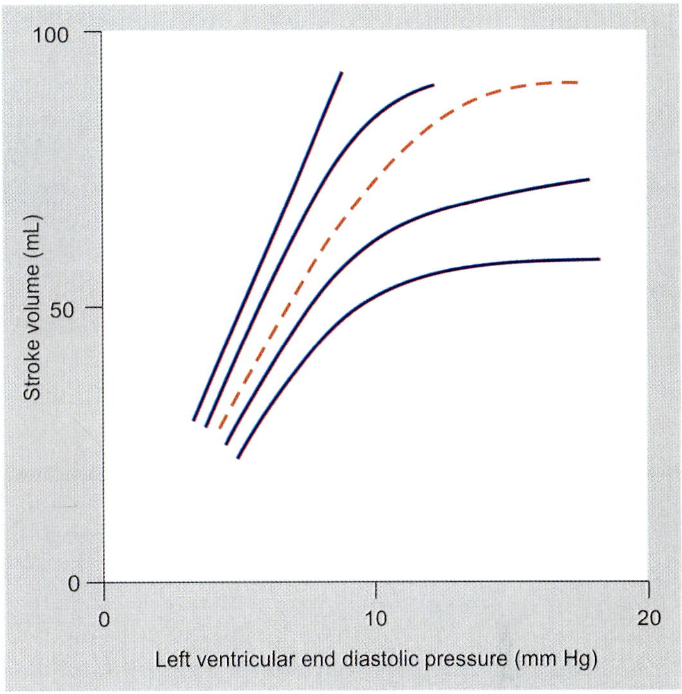

Fig. 3: Frank-Starling Curves—the ability of the heart to change its force of contraction and therefore stroke volume in response to changes in venous return. Each heart operates on a family of curves, based on its contractility and afterload. An increased afterload and decreased contractility shifts it to the right of baseline and a decreased afterload with normal or improved contractility shifts it to the left for a given left ventricular end-diastolic pressure.

In the immediate postoperative period, besides primary myocardial dysfunction, pericardial tamponade (rapid accumulation of fluid, air, or blood in the pericardial space) with decreased venous return as the transmural pressure is decreased, precipitate an acute catastrophe with hypotension and arrest.

Tachycardia, rising venous pressures with poor peripheral perfusion with IVC distension are the initial signs, with RA and right ventricular compression in diastole on echocardiography. Pulsus paradoxus is the most sensitive sign, with >10 mm Hg difference in systolic pressure during inspiration. Emergency pericardiocentesis is the corrective management.

Low CO state is basically a scenario of inadequate DO_2 relative to demand with impaired oxygen transport balance. It manifests as tachycardia, poor peripheral perfusion with increased core-peripheral temperature gradient, oliguria, and rising lactate trend with or without metabolic acidosis on blood gas analysis. Low CO state is the most common determinant of impaired DO_2 and this may be due to inadequate venous return and preload, excessive afterload, myocardial dysfunction, arrhythmias, and significant residual defects which should be addressed systematically.

Several factors are responsible for increasing the oxygen demand, including the systemic inflammatory response to bypass, fever, endogenous and exogenous catecholamines, stress response, wakefulness, and agitation besides work of spontaneous breathing. Optimization of oxygen transport balance involves reduction of oxygen demand with optimization of supply.

Mechanical ventilation with resultant lesser load on respiratory muscle diverts 50% of CO to vital organs. In extreme scenarios *mechanical ventilation as a therapeutic tool* is relevant, especially in severe ventricular dysfunction.

Similarly avoiding hyperthermia, sedation and analgesia impact oxygen reserves spontaneously.

Inadequate preload often results from an aggressive strategy to decrease total body water, with CPB ultrafiltration exacerbated with peritoneal drainage and diuresis in postoperative period. Besides vascular dysfunction with capillary leak decreases intravascular volume. Diastolic dysfunction with its restrictive physiology demands elevated filling pressure and adds on to the deficit. Assessment of fluid responsiveness based on IVC distensibility in a ventilated patient and IVC collapsibility in a spontaneously breathing patient often enables optimize fluid supplementation[24] without inducing overload. Lack of response to fluid with elevated filling pressures is a guide to optimize the inotrope and pressors. Diastolic and systolic ventricular dysfunction can both result in low CO state.

Diastolic dysfunction refers to a reduction in diastolic distensibility, filling, or relaxation of the ventricle due to restrictive physiology as in TOF or ischemic ventricle. The low output state results from inadequate ventricular filling against an elevated ventricular pressure due to inadequate relaxation.

Therapy for diastolic dysfunction entails maintaining adequate ventricular preload at a higher filling pressure, ensuring optimal heart rate and rhythm (ensuring AV synchrony and adequate time for ventricular filling in diastole), minimizing intrathoracic pressure (ITP) by encouraging spontaneous breathing and restrict positive-pressure ventilation (PPV) where feasible.

Inodilators such as milrinone may have a beneficial role, but vasoactive agents that lead to venodilation, compromise venous return and inotropes with chronotropic effect further exacerbate diastolic dysfunction. The ideal inodilator is one which improves myocardial contractility, with improved relaxation (lusitropy) without increase in heart rate and myocardial oxygen demand.

Systolic dysfunction is the intrinsic ability of heart muscle to shorten and generate force independent of changes in volume loading conditions. In systolic dysfunction, the EF and SV are reduced and ventricular end-diastolic pressure is elevated. In contrast to the left ventricle (LV), the RV has diminished contractile elements. A significant portion of thin-walled highly compliant right ventricular pressure and volume outflow is modified by LV contractility, termed as *systolic ventricular interdependence*. With either ventricle, the systolic dysfunction hampers the ventricular response to volume and exacerbates afterload sensitivity.

Therapy for systolic dysfunction, begins with:

- Optimize ventricular loading conditions.
- Reduce ventricular preload and afterload decreasing ventricular wall stress and myocardial oxygen demand.
- Ventricular diastolic volume and pressure may be reduced by increasing venous capacitance with venodilators or decreasing intravascular volume with diuretics.
- Reduced afterload also enhances ventricular ejection and may be accomplished with medications and utilizing PPV as a therapeutic tool.

Pharmacological Approach to LCOS

The rationale for selecting vasoactive agents is based on the presence of right and left ventricular systolic and diastolic dysfunction as well as the function of venous capacitance and pulmonary and systemic arterial resistance vessels.

Vasoactive agents that selectively induce venodilatation (nitroglycerin) decrease systemic venous return and ventricular diastolic volume and pressure with no effect on afterload.

Vasoactive agents that selectively dilate arterial resistance vessels (sodium nitroprusside) decrease afterload and enhance ventricular ejection.

Vasopressors increase SVR, with no effect on myocardial contractility (vasopressin) or mild improvement in contractility (norepinephrine). Vasopressors may have utility in vasoplegic state post-CPB.[25] Vasopressin becomes relevant especially in small-for-gestational age neonates and early infants with preoperative stress and myocardial dysfunction with higher incidence of catecholamine resistance exacerbated by low cortisol levels.[26] Besides, in low doses, vasopressin acts upon the oxytocin receptors and this may help reduce pulmonary vascular resistance and mitigate the LCOS in selected neonates and young infants. However, NEC can manifest occasionally from intense splanchnic vasospasm.

Inotropic agents (dopamine, dobutamine, and epinephrine) improve EF and SV with improvement in myocardial contractility and dose-dependent tachycardia. Ventricular filling pressure remains same unless venous capacitance is increased. Myocardial VO_2 invariably increases as a result of enhanced contractile function and elevated heart rate.

Inodilators (milrinone and levosimendan) may improve diastolic function with improved lusitropy and decrease in afterload with no increase in heart rate and improved myocardial oxygen transport balance. **Table 2** summarizes information on commonly used inotropes and vasopressor agents.

The hallmark of successful management of LCOS involves careful anticipation and aggressive cardiopulmonary management. It is imperative to rule out residual lesions after surgery by a detailed postoperative echocardiography assessment. The management strategy involves the following:

TABLE 2: Vasoactive medicines used in pediatric cardiac intensive care.[27]

Medication and dose	*Target receptors*	*Effect on heart rate and ventricular contractility*	*Effect on systemic vascular resistance*	*Effect on cardiac output*	*Effect on blood pressure*	*Effect on pulmonary vascular resistance*	*Main uses*	*Safe for peripheral use?*
Inodilators								
Dobutamine 2–20 µg/kg/min	αββββ	↑↑↑	↓	↑↑↑	Variable	↓	Low cardiac output	Yes
Milrinone 0.375–0.75 µg/kg/min	cAMP	↑↑	↓↓	↑↑↑	Variable	↓	Low cardiac output	Yes
Isoproterenol 2–10 µg/min	ββββ	↑↑↑↑↑	↓	↑↑↑	Variable		Bradycardia	Yes
Pure vasopressors								
Vasopressin 0.001–0.0008 U/kg/min	V1 and V2	↓	↑↑↑	↔/↓	↑↑↑	↓	Vasoplegic shock, sepsis	No
Phenylephrine 40–180 µg/min	Aααα	↓	↑↑↑	Variable	↑↑↑	↑↑	Vasoplegic shock, cyanotic spell	Yes, use with caution
Inotropes-pressors								
Epinephrine 0.01–2 µg/kg/min	αβββ	↑↑↑	↑	↑↑↑	↑↑		Bradycardia, cardiogenic shock, sepsis, and anaphylaxis	Use with extreme caution and for short periods
Dopamine, low 1–4 µg/kg/min	Dopaminergic receptor (D)	↔	↓	↑	↓		Low cardiac output state as an alternative to epinephrine	Probably not
Dopamine, medium 4–10 µg/kg/min	αβββD	↑	Variable	↑↑	Variable			
Dopamine, high 10–20 µg/kg/min	αααβD	↑↑	↑↑	↑	↑↑↑	↑		

- Improving circulation while reducing oxygen demand
- Normothermia and volume optimization
- Selection of inotropes, inodilators, and vasoactive agents based on individual disease scenario
- Titrating doses—avoid tachycardia
- Reducing pulmonary vascular reactivity in biventricular repair
- Utilizing PPV as a therapeutic tool based on underlying surgical intervention.

Cardiopulmonary Interactions: Ventilation as a Therapeutic Tool

In an era where early extubation is considered as a major factor affecting ICU length of stay and health economics, it is prudent that selection of cases for the same is linked to basic understanding of postoperative physiology of the underlying CHD. Ventilation is a valuable tool in pediatric intensive care and is far more effective in improving circulatory physiology when implemented judiciously.

Positive-pressure ventilation has a beneficial effect in systolic dysfunction (especially in postoperative arterial switch operation for transposition with regressed LV, anomalous coronary artery from pulmonary artery, complex biventricular repair for double outlet RV) as it reduces right ventricular preload and left ventricular afterload by reducing exaggerated negative pressure breathing and decreasing LV systolic transmural pressure (Ptm) with a positive ITP (Ppl) (Ptm = Intravascular systolic pressure– Ppl). This impacts myocardial oxygen demand positively as the exaggerated work of breathing in compromised states diverts a significant amount of CO to respiratory work with considerable increase in oxygen demand.

Noninvasive ventilation postextubation as a preemptive measure works well with the background of systolic dysfunction. In patients operated for univentricular physiology, the key to limiting morbidity and improving survival with functional univentricular circulation is to maintain a balanced ratio of pulmonary-to-systemic blood flow with adequate systemic DO_2 by titrating ventricular loading and vascular resistance of pulmonary and systemic vascular beds. A low CO state if it ensues after a Fontan operation is likely due to diastolic dysfunction stressing the

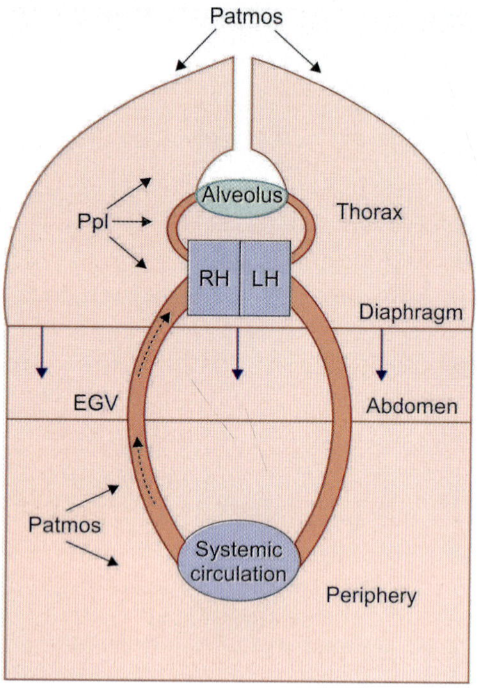

Fig. 4: Simplifying cardiopulmonary interaction:[28] Model of the circulation, showing factors that influence systemic venous drainage. The right heart (RH) and intrathoracic great veins are subjected to pleural pressure (Ppl), which varies throughout the respiratory cycle. Intra-abdominal pressure increases with inspiratory diaphragmatic descent, and normalizes to atmospheric (Patmos) with expiration. Peripheral venous pressure is unaffected by respiration and so remains at atmospheric pressure throughout the respiratory cycle. Systemic venous drainage (broken arrow) depends on a driving pressure gradient between extra-thoracic great veins (EGV) and the right atrium, and so during spontaneous respiration is maximized during inspiration as the pleural and right atrial pressure falls and the intra-abdominal pressure (and EGV) pressure rises.[28]

role of optimizing ventricular filling. Minor changes in ITP exert significant influences on PBF and CO. Spontaneous ventilation and negative ITP with inspiration significantly improves PBF and CO[28,29] with univentricular physiology.

In patients postbidirectional cavopulmonary shunt, PBF is sensitive to cerebral vascular resistance, ITP, and PVR and optimal ventilation is targeted at improving cerebral vasodilatation and pulmonary arterial flow. Early extubation and spontaneous ventilation with mild hypercarbia works best (**Fig. 4**), but if hypoxia and decreased PBF compromise CO, minute ventilation should be titrated to reduce PVR and improve cerebral blood flow. Mild hypercarbia with improvement in cerebral blood flow uncoupled with cerebral tissue metabolism improves PBF, bypassing effects of mild respiratory acidosis on PVR.

Postoperative diastolic dysfunction exacerbating pre-existing restrictive myocardial pathology invariably benefits from spontaneous breathing with improved ventricular filling.[30] This is particularly relevant in TOF with severe RV diastolic dysfunction due to delayed intervention in LMIC. Spontaneous breathing improves the antegrade pulmonary artery flow in diastole with improved CO and limits pulmonary regurgitation after repair.[31] But, if LCOS ensues post-TOF repair with systolic dysfunction aggravating poor circulation, it may be worthwhile to reduce work of breathing and improve tissue oxygen transport balance. As a principle, it is wise to minimize airway pressure during PPV and wean once circulation improves.[32]

Postoperative Arrhythmias

Postoperative arrhythmias, after surgery for complex CHD, can be benign as premature ventricular or atrial beats and fulminant as in with ventricular tachycardia (VT) or ventricle fibrillation. The reported incidence may vary between 15 and 50%. Junctional ectopic tachycardia, supraventricular reentrant tachycardia (accessory pathway), ectopic atrial tachycardia, and VT are the most common arrhythmias. They all require careful assessment and in many instances intervention as they can precipitate LCOS, prolonged mechanical ventilation, and increased risk of cardiac arrest. Risk factors for the development of tachyarrhythmias include younger age, prolonged CPB, and cross-clamp duration, or DHCA.[33] Delayed interventions with chronic hemodynamic stress, atrial stretch, electrolyte, and acid base imbalance with vasoactive drugs at high-dosage range can further exacerbate tachyarrhythmia.

Ventricular tachycardia is associated with rapid progression to hemodynamic compromise. It is rarely observed in current practice with improvement in surgical expertise and better myocardial protection. A wide QRS complex tachycardia with hemodynamic instability should be approached as VT pending diagnosis. If pulseless or with hemodynamic instability, PALS tachyarrhythmia approach is recommended.[34] A detailed discussion on tachyarrhythmias is presented in Chapter 52.

Accurate diagnosis of arrhythmias is the key to timely intervention. Narrow complex tachycardia is classified as automatic or reentrant rhythm. Re-entrant rhythms are usually sudden onset and respond to adenosine or synchronized cardioversion with abrupt termination. They also may respond to overdrive pacing (twice the heart rate) that is feasible via the pacing wires that are often placed at the time of surgery.

The automatic tachyarrhythmias [junctional ectopic tachycardia (JET)] and atrial ectopic tachycardia (AET) have a slow rise and slow decline in heart rate (warm up and cool down phenomena). They are usually catecholamine responsive, and do not respond to cardioversion or overdrive pacing. A 12-lead ECG or rhythm strip is essential to make the diagnosis and in some scenarios, atrial wire ECG can help identify the presence or absence of P waves, especially in JET. Tachycardia induces increased myocardial VO_2 with decreased diastolic coronary filling, and alters the balance between DO_2 and consumption with decreased SvO_2 and elevated lactate.

Management of JET involves volume optimization, core cooling (34.5–36°C), maintaining normal magnesium levels and normokalemia, minimizing sympathetic overdrive (control fever, pain, and optimize or reduce dosing of inotrope and pressors). Dexmedetomidine has emerged as a promising agent especially with sympatholytic effects and reduction in heart rate, and judicious use of neuromuscular blockade are imperative in halting worsening of JET.[35] Overdrive atrial pacing especially if it is a junctional slow rhythm helps restore hemodynamic balance, but if hemodynamically worsening with fast rate, amiodarone is the first line for JET. The dose as per PALS protocol is 5 mg/kg as bolus given over half an hour to 1 hour followed by infusion at 10 µg/kg/min.[36] Beta-blockers, especially if myocardial contractility is acceptable, can be an option for JET in a few scenarios with stable hemodynamics. Oral ivabradine at a dosage of 0.1 mg/kg/day in two divided doses to a maximum of 0.3 mg/kg/day is emerging as an additional option.[37] For ectopic atrial tachycardia (EAT), beta-blockers (esmolol) are usually effective. Similarly, in reentrant postoperative tachyarrhythmias, when hemodynamically stable beta-blockers (esmolol infusion or intermittent metaprolol dose administration) exert beneficial rate control effect (*see* Chapter 52).

Bradyarrhythmias observed in the postoperative period include sinus bradycardia as in sick sinus syndrome and varying degrees of AV dissociation. While atrial pacing with temporary pacing wires usually works well for sinus bradycardia, AV sequential pacing is preferred for AV dissociation. Permanent pacemaker installation (PPI) may be required for complete heart block in case it does not reverse by the end of second week after surgical intervention.

Postoperative Pulmonary Hypertension

Pulmonary hypertension manifesting as increased pulmonary vascular reactivity after cardiac surgery is observed after open heart surgery for TAPVC repair, truncus arteriosus, complete AV canal defect, large VSD with delayed intervention, Taussig–Bing anomaly, etc. This is further exacerbated with presence of preoperative ventilation or sepsis, besides comorbid associations as Down syndrome. The vasoconstriction may be triggered by reduced endogenous nitric oxide production with impaired pulmonary artery relaxation and alterations of the endothelin-1 pathways exacerbated by post-CPB inflammatory response with ischemia reperfusion injury.[38]

Postoperatively there may be a rapid and critical increase in PVR with pain, fever, agitation, and tracheal suction. This results in rapid increase in PVR [pulmonary hypertensive crisis (PHC)] with decreased PBF with RA and RV acute dilatation with drop in systemic CO and poor coronary perfusion with impending cardiac arrest.[39]

Prevention of PHC is crucial when dealing with postoperative care of above disease spectrum, neonatal heart surgery, and in patients with pulmonary venous hypertension.

PULMONARY HYPERTENSIVE CRISIS

Do's

- Rule out residual anatomic lesions
- Leave right-to-left shunt (pop-off) in borderline high-risk scenarios at atrial or ventricular level
- Optimal sedation—anesthesia:
  - Intermittent neuromuscular blockade with extremely labile PVR
  - Opioids/alpha-blockers in combination. Avoid benzodiazepines.
- Moderate hyperventilation
- Moderate alkalosis
- Adequate inspired oxygen (oxygen saturation above 95% in complete corrections and above 80% in univentricular physiology)
- Titrate PEEP to optimize normal lung volumes and oxygenation. Avoid overdistension
- Optimize hematocrit (30–35%).

INOTROPIC SUPPORT

To counter severe RV failure and counteract right-to-left interventricular septal shift resulting in LV compromise, inotropic support in the form of inodilators (milrinone/levosimendan/dobutamine) may be required along with vasopressors to counter low SVR with pulmonary vasodilators and improve systemic perfusion. Vasopressin due to its interaction with lung oxytocin receptors resulted in low PVR in a limited patient cohort.[40]

Milrinone and levosimendan unlike dobutamine improve myocardial contractility with no increase in myocardial VO_2 by preventing tachycardia.

PULMONARY VASODILATORS

(See Chapter 10 for a detailed description)

Inhaled nitric oxide may be considered for treatment of postoperative PAH in mechanically ventilated patients to improve oxygenation and reduce risk of PHC.[39] iNO works by activating cyclic guanosine monophosphate (cGMP) dependent signaling pathways in pulmonary vascular smooth muscle cells, resulting in selective pulmonary vasodilation. Miller et al.[41] analyzed infants with CHD receiving iNO postoperatively and this group had reduced incidence of PAH crisis with shorter postoperative stay. The authors recommended iNo at dose of 10 ppm when infants are operated for scenarios with high risk for PHC. Journois et al.[42] also reported lower mortality with use of iNO in AV canal defects with reduction of PHC postoperatively. Though a detailed Cochrane database review by Bizarro et al.[43] questioned the effectiveness of iNO on survival and hemodynamic secondary end points. In quite a few low resource settings, the availability and cost of iNO is a hindering factor and a combination of vasodilators and other strategies have sustained good outcomes. Though far from ideal, iNO still has a pivotal role in preventing PHC. Therapeutic trial entails administration at 20 ppm, with maximum dosage 80 ppm postoperatively for 48–72 hours before weaning it off gradually to avoid rebound PH under sildenafil cover. Methemoglobinemia is a potential risk with prolonged usage with dosage exceeding 40 ppm.

Concomitant sildenafil citrate (IV or oral) should be administered to prevent rebound PAH in patients who have evidence of worsening PAH on withdrawal of iNO, despite gradual weaning[44] or in combination with other vasodilators in those with poor response to iNO.[40] Sildenafil and tadalafil exert phosphodiesterase (PDE)-5 inhibitor activity with improved cGMP levels with superior NO dependent pathway signaling and vasodilatation.[45]

Mourani et al.[46] recommended a dose of 0.5 mg/kg/day to a maximum of 2 mg/kg/day. IV sildenafil is also available and can be used as an infusion at 0.03–0.07 mg/kg/hour, after a bolus dose of 0.4 mg/kg stat over 3 hours. Sildenafil should be avoided in pulmonary hemorrhage and with parenchymal injury due to potential risk of increasing ventilation perfusion (VQ) mismatch.

Endothelin receptor antagonists (ERAS): Bosentan can also be used in exceptional circumstances in acute settings. Beghetti et al.[47] meta-analysis revealed that Bosentan in a dose range 2 mg/kg/day is safe effective and well tolerated therapy in children. Ambrisentan with its once daily administration and reduced adverse effects is also promising.

Inhaled prostaglandin (iloprost) may be effective in postoperative PAH.[39] They have been found to be effective in cases with failed iNO therapy and have a potential utility for reducing PVR in postoperative acute scenarios.

MANAGEMENT OF POSTOPERATIVE PULMONARY HYPERTENSION

Avoid

- Agitation/pain
- Respiratory and metabolic acidosis
- Alveolar hypoxia
- Atelectasis or overdistension
- Excessive hematocrit
- Low output and coronary perfusion
- Increased afterload.

Acute Pulmonary Hypertensive Crisis

Acute PHC is a life-threatening emergency requiring aggressive management as risk of circulatory collapse is high. Cardiopulmonary resuscitation with aim to optimize ventilation and normalize CO_2 with bag to tube ventilation, bolus of norepinephrine/epinephrine, sedation, and neuromuscular relaxation when indicated usually restore circulation in majority of patients. Inotropes and inodilators with resultant decrease in RV afterload while improving RV contractility and sustaining adequate coronary perfusion pressure with preserved LV output and DO_2 are recommended, while balancing out with pulmonary vasodilators. Extracorporeal support may have to be considered early when ventilator and pharmacological initiatives fail.

Pulmonary Hypertension Concerns in Univentricular Physiology with Partial (Glenn Procedure) and Total Cavopulmonary Anastomosis (Fontan Procedure)[39]

Enhanced vascular reactivity exacerbated by preoperative hypoxia occasionally precipitates PHC in Glenn patients with cessation of SVC flow and risk of shunt thrombosis. This presents as deep cyanosis with compromised DO_2. Management involves optimization of ventilation (mild hypercarbia, avoid high PEEP), iNO and inotropy and fluid titration with vasopressors to optimize systemic CO. Extracorporeal membrane oxygenation (ECMO) should be kept as an option standby if the circulation and oxygenation does not improve with these measures.

In patients with total cavopulmonary correction low PVR (transpulmonary gradient <5 mm Hg) is a prerequisite for adequate ventricular filling. In borderline cases, titration of PVR with iNO in combination with pulmonary vasodilators, milrinone, and short duration support ventilation (mild hypercarbia with low mean airway pressure) with transition to spontaneous breathing once parameters optimize, is the way ahead.

Postoperative Respiratory Management and Respiratory Dysfunction

Positive-pressure ventilation is closely interlinked with myocardial recovery and hemodynamics after surgery for CHD. Patients most affected are those with significantly impaired myocardial contractility, pulmonary vascular disease, and passive PBF after univentricular palliation. The key to optimal mechanical ventilation is to adopt strategies that improve hemodynamics and gas exchange, while patient recovers from the post-CPB inflammatory cardiopulmonary dysfunction.

As regards postoperative respiratory management, the approach is moving toward early extubation.[48] Advantages of early extubation include minimizing the need for postoperative sedation, reducing ICU length of stay, and improving patient and family interaction. Early extubation protocol evolves positively only when the anesthesiologist, intensivist, and cardiac surgeon are on the same page to ensure that weaning criteria is adequately fulfilled. This includes:

- Hemodynamically stable patient with good myocardial contractility and no residual deficits on intraoperative echocardiography and minimal inotropic support

- Awake and alert patient with adequate pain relief
- Adequate gas exchange with no metabolic acidosis and plasma lactate (adequacy of microcirculation) in normal range
- No active bleeding
- The CPB time should not be very prolonged (<150 minutes) and no DHCA
- Urine output is adequate and mixed venous oxygen saturation and peripheral temperature corroborate optimal circulation and DO_2.

Most patients require supplemental oxygen via standard nasal cannula, but a few patients may be candidates for noninvasive ventilation through high-flow nasal cannula (HFNC) or nasal CPAP based on their cardiopulmonary behavior.

The algorithm works for most of the elective cardiac scenarios with (risk-associated congenital heart surgery) RACHS score <4, but in complex scenarios and neonatal interventions, respiratory dysfunction is a major determinant of morbidity.

In neonates, the functional residual capacity is reduced due to the high chest wall to lung compliance ratio, and they are predisposed to atelectasis and VQ mismatch. Besides the respiratory work postextubation is enhanced due to significant energy being consumed to expand the rib cage rather than generating tidal volume. The diaphragm also has less contractile reserve with increased arterial venous oxygen content difference. This diverts 25–50% of CO to sustain work of breathing in extreme situations, especially with decreased lung compliance due to post-CPB inflammatory stress with capillary leak phenomenon and surfactant deficiency. An increased respiratory load coupled with a limited CO state is a common convergence in patients after surgery for CHD and increases the propensity to develop ventilator failure.[49] Neonates and early infants with complex scenarios are hence candidates for extended ventilation beyond 48 hours postoperatively in specific situations with myocardial compromise and invariably require noninvasive support postextubation to sustain adequate gas exchange with no significant increase in work of breathing.

There are several factors that impair ventilatory (CO_2 handling) function postcardiac surgery. Ventilatory function is the result of the interplay between neuromuscular competency which includes the central and peripheral nervous system and respiratory musculature, respiratory muscle DO_2 versus demand, and respiratory load which is affected by lung compliance, airway resistance, and minute ventilation. Neuromuscular competence may be compromised as a result of central nervous system depression due to sedatives, diaphragmatic paresis or paralysis, compromised further by disuse atrophy of the respiratory musculature. This worsens further with malnutrition and excessive use of muscle relaxants.

Dead space ventilation accentuates ventilation perfusion mismatch with increased arterial-end tidal CO_2 gradient which further gets exacerbated by PPV. These factors along with preoperative ventilation and malnutrition contribute significantly to weaning failure and occasionally prolonged ventilation with extubation failures with recurrent reintubation in infants, especially after delayed interventions in LMICs. This necessitates gradual ventilatory de-escalation with respiratory rehabilitation occasionally aided by tracheostomy[50] to ensure successful weaning in a few scenarios.

Airway resistance may be elevated due to several factors. Upper airway obstruction may result from postextubation croup. In neonates and infants, the cross section of the subglottic region is smaller compared to older children. Postoperative recurrent laryngeal nerve injury and vocal cord paralysis can further exacerbate the problem. Lower airway obstruction can be due to external vascular compression as in vascular rings or abnormal aortopulmonary collaterals and occasionally due to interstitial edema with compression of small airways. If significant, can result in hyperinflation with flattened diaphragms with reduced ventilation capacity. These issues are addressed with a balance of airway positioning, ET tubes with microcuff, adequate pain relief avoiding patient agitation, and occasionally steroids and bronchodilators.

Pulmonary hemorrhage secondary to reperfusion injury, small multiple collaterals due to delayed intervention in TOF physiology or pulmonary edema due to LV dysfunction require titration of PEEP while on ventilation to sustain adequate oxygenation and later gradual weaning with extubation aided by noninvasive ventilation to ensure alveolar recruitment.

Phrenic nerve injury resulting in diaphragmatic paresis can be due to topical application of ice during surgery (reversible), redo operations, and difficult dissection and surgeries involving aortic arch, pulmonary arteries, or SVC. Diaphragm paresis is suspected during failed weaning or difficult weaning with hypercarbia, increased work of breathing, and elevated hemidiaphragm on chest X-ray. Confirmation is with ultrasound or fluoroscopy during spontaneous breathing. It is now often a requirement in PCICU to assess diaphragm thickness and movement before extubation to pre-empt noninvasive ventilation and ensure work of breathing is not a deterrent postextubation. While in a few cases, noninvasive ventilation can tide over paresis but paralysis with paradoxical hemidiaphragm movement may necessitate plication of affected diaphragm.

Chylothorax is a complication of congenital heart surgery and can result due to thoracic duct injury or occasionally with complex biventricular repair or univentricular palliation with higher systemic venous pressures. It can present with respiratory distress, worsening oxygenation, and persistent drainage from postoperative chest tube. If the infant has been fed, the pleural effusion appears creamy and the diagnosis is confirmed with pleural fluid triglyceride level >110 mg/dL and total cell count >1,000 cells/mm^3 with lymphocytosis. The management strategy involves total parenteral nutrition (PN) with NPO though this can be detrimental with pre-existing malnutrition and hence enteral nutrition (EN) with medium chain triglycerides based diet with adequate protein supplement (2–3 g/kg/day) and supplementation of essential fatty acids, diuretics, and IV somatostatin at 10 µg/kg/dose 8-hourly for 3–5 days often corrects the course. Thoracic duct plication is the last reprieve in resistant cases.

Renal Concerns

Acute kidney injury (AKI) is invariably a high-risk association with complex congenital heart intervention. Fluid titration based on clinical assessment confirmed with echocardiography parameters such as IVC distensibility on ventilation (>20% variation) and collapsibility (>50% variation) with inspiration on spontaneous breathing besides VTi across LVOT (>10% variation with inspiration), eyeballing of ventricular volumes and filling pressures, helps avoid fluid overload.[24] As a protocol, IV fluids should be restricted to 50–60% maintenance for weight in open heart procedures and approximately 70% for closed heart interventions, but this is just a rough guide and modifiable based on preoperative morbidity, intraoperative third spacing, and postoperative drainage and hemodynamics. Once postoperative drainage is under control, cumulative isotonic fluid supplementation (maintenance plus inotrope n sedation dilution) needs strict justification targeting normal electrolyte balance besides adequate glycemic control (RBS 100–150 mg/dL). Blood loss should be replaced with blood products as is the norm in such situations.

Urine output is a relevant surrogate of CO, circulation, and renal function and as per the kidney diseases improving global outcome (KDIGO) criteria, it is an important parameter besides serum creatinine to assess AKI[51] (**Table 3**).

As a baseline urine output of 2 mL/kg/hour after cardiac surgery is minimum to ensure adequate fluid balance. These patients most often have a combination of prerenal cardiac failure (LCOS, capillary leak, and volume deficit) besides renal injury due to CPB-induced SIRS. In cases with third spacing and ascites, high intra-abdominal pressure (compartment syndrome) precipitates low renal perfusion pressure and oliguria. Also, pre-existing obstructive or renal parenchymal pathology aggravated by drug-induced toxicity, e.g., amino-glycosides add on to the risk spectrum.

MANAGEMENT/PREVENTION OF ACUTE KIDNEY INJURY PROGRESSION

- *Strict input/output, electrolytes monitoring*: Cumulative fluid overload status: Fluid overload and AKI are an example of bidirectional risk. Fluid overload exceeding 10% is a red herring and delay in renal replacement therapy increases risk of mortality.
- Review nephrotoxic medications.
- Diuretics—furosemide bolus or infusion. If there is no response to furosemide then consider other class of diuretics (metolazone and chlorothiazide). Furosemide nonresponsiveness is considered if urine output <1 mL/kg/hour at 2 and 6 hours with a furosemide dose of 0.8–1.2 mg/kg/dose and is predictive of worsening AKI.[52] Currently none of the biomarkers have yet been proven as a consistent predictive tool, except urine neutrophil gelatinase association lipocalcin (NGAL) as a predictive tool for initiating and withdrawing dialysis in noncardiac patients with sepsis.[53]
- Avoid flogging with drugs and address optimization of volume and perfusion pressure.
- In neonates with asphyxia adenosine receptor antagonist (theophylline), by inhibiting adenosine-induced vasoconstriction improves renal blood flow and diuresis.
- Theophylline or aminophylline—recommended as a single dose for AKI prevention with birth asphyxia—anti-inflammatory role and vasodilatory effect due to PDE inhibition with increased cyclic adenosine monophosphate (AMP).
- Therapeutic levels—4–8 µg/mL and should be monitored to avoid toxicity. Cardiac surgery associated AKI no perceived significant benefit with xanthine derivatives is reported as of 2021.[52]

TABLE 3: Neonatal kidney diseases improving global outcome acute kidney injury classification.[51]

Stage	*Serum creatinine (SCr)*	*Urine output*
0	No change rise of <0.3 mg/dL	≥0.5 mL/kg/hour
1	SCr rise ≥0.3 mg/dL within 48 hours or SCr rise >1.5–1.9 × reference SCr within 7 days	<0.5 mL/kg/hour for 6–12 hours
2	SCr rise >2.0–2.9 × reference SCr	<0.5 mL/kg/hour for ≥12 hours
3	SCr rise >3 × reference SCr; SCr >2.5 mg/dL or receipt of dialysis	<0.3 mL/kg/hour for ≥24 hours or anuria

Reference serum creatinine value is the available previous value
S. creatinine >2.5 mg/dL correlates with estimated glomerular filtration rate 10 mL/min/1.73 m^2

Renal replacement therapy is indicated

Oliguria with resultant fluid overload resulting in:

- Hypertension
- Pulmonary compromise and pulmonary edema
- Abdominal compartment syndrome—peritoneal drainage is occasionally good enough to reverse AKI progression[52]
- Hyperkalemia
- Metabolic acidosis
- Hyponatremia
- Uremia
- Hypocalcemia
- Hyperphosphatemia
- Intermittent hemodialysis is more appropriate for patients >10 kg and hemodynamically stable
- Peritoneal dialysis is most appropriate for patients <10 kg, hemodynamically stable, especially after surgery for CHD
- No major abdominal deterrents (except with abdominal wall defects, gastroschisis, abdominal surgery, and NEC)
- Continuous renal replacement therapy (CRRT) most appropriate for patients who are hemodynamically unstable of any size. Fluid and caloric intake can be modified liberally with CRRT.

Neurological Issues

Patients with CHD may have congenital brain abnormalities linked to genetic or syndromic diagnoses. In fetus with left heart obstructive lesion or transposition physiology, cerebral development may be impaired as a consequence of diminished cerebral blood flow and oxygenation.[54] Nearly 20% of full-term neonates with CHD display evidence of periventricular leukomalacia on magnetic resonance imaging (MRI). Preoperative management strategies are crucial and timing of intervention is a key to optimize out comes. The degree of lactate elevation and severity of hypoxia with delay in intervention potentially contributes to significant neurological compromise.[55]

Operative strategies based on age, complexity of repair with prolonged intervention are associated with worse outcomes. CPB and circulatory arrest impair cerebral vascular autoregulation. NIRS monitoring during and immediately following surgery is a good indicator of cerebral flow and oxygenation and low NIRS values have been correlated with seizures corroborated with 24-hour electroencephalogram (EEG) monitoring and cerebral dysfunction with MRI abnormalities.[56]

Low cerebral and mixed venous oxygen saturation is linked to greater incidence of adverse events such as cardiac arrest in ICU. Cardiac arrest occurs in 1–3.5% of PCICU admissions, and has a significant deleterious effect on developmental outcome of children with heart disease. Cardiac arrest and LCOS states unresponsive to resuscitation require initiation of extracorporeal life support (ECLS). Approximately 50% of ECLS survivors have been found to have range of disabilities on formal neurodevelopmental evaluation.[57] The rate of normalization of plasma lactate postresuscitation is directly correlated with better neurodevelopment outcome. Meanwhile hyperthermia and hyperglycemia are also relevant postoperative factors adversely affecting neurological outcome if poorly controlled.

Therapeutic hypothermia after pediatric cardiac arrest (THAPCA) trial did not show a significant benefit to cooling (32–34°C) versus normothermia (36–37.5°C). But cooling works for neonates, adults, and in animal models, by effectively reducing metabolic oxygen demand. Either way fever is bad and should be prevented with continuous core temperature measurement. For kids who are persistently comatose after arrest, it is reasonable to choose targeted temperature management (TTM) to 32–34°C for 2 days followed by 36–37.5°C for 3 days.[58]

Sedation and Analgesia, and Neuromuscular Blockade

Postoperative analgesia, sedation, and reduction of anxiety are an essential part of care in PCICU. Opioids, alpha-blockers (dexmedetomidine), and benzodiazepines are used in varied combination as per individual unit protocol. The patients on mechanical ventilation and with open sternum occasionally require neuromuscular blockade. Excessive usage of these drugs for prolonged duration can precipitate critical care induced myopathy, especially when the ICU stay is extended. Hence, it is imperative to rationalize and limit usage and give periodic sedation holiday to assess the ability of patient to move and comprehend.

The *ABCDEF* approach is designed to facilitate better outcomes and mobility with shorter ICU LOS, by making it an essential tool for daily evaluation while planning patient management:

- *A*ssess, prevent and manage pain
- *B*oth spontaneous awakening trial (SAT) and spontaneous breathing trial (SBT)
- *C*hoice of analgesia and sedation
- *D*elirium—assess prevent and manage
- *E*arly mobility and exercise
- *F*amily engagement and empowerment.

Sedatives and analgesics that act by altering synaptic transmission at gamma-amino butyrate type A (benzodiazepines, propofol, and chloral hydrate) and N-methyl D aspartate NMDA receptors (ketamine) interfere with normal brain development and hence the frequency of dosage has to be calibrated. Opioids on prolonged usage also can hamper developmental outcomes and it is prudent to ensure the choice and duration of these agents is reviewed daily to minimize the neurological side effects.

Nutrition

Poor nutritional status and failure to thrive are frequent associations in children with heart disease. The contributing factors being gastroesophageal reflux disease (GERD), interrupted feeding due to tachypnea, and altered suck swallow coordination. This is compounded with high-energy expenditure due to high metabolic rate and reduced splanchnic blood flow especially in L-R shunts and bowel wall edema with right heart failure. In LMICs, recurrent respiratory infections worsen the nutritional status further. Surgical intervention cannot be delayed in view of poor nutrition and nutritional rehabilitation postoperatively is an important parameter determining length of stay and outcome.[59,60]

Postoperatively, CPB-induced stress induces metabolic dysregulation with increased energy expenditure and negative protein balance. Indirect calorimetry is the ideal method to ensure estimation of resting energy expenditure and plan nutrition strategy.[61] The average resting energy expenditure is 55–60 kcal/kg/day for 3–5 days after surgery with variations based on complexity and nutritional energy goals should be defined accordingly with protein intake 1–2 g/kg/day (**Table 4**). Between 6 and 10 days with attenuation of inflammatory response and C-reactive protein (CRP) normalization, it is desirable to increase nutritional supplements to catch up with the normal metabolic response to 100–120 kcal/kg/day with protein intake 3 g/kg/day for term and 3.5–4 g/kg/day in preterm intervention.[62]

Energy repletion with adequate EN is associated with shorter duration of mechanical ventilation and shorter feeding interruptions avoiding PN. A daily review of supplementation of micronutrients, vitamins, and electrolytes is extremely relevant to optimize holistic outcomes.

Postoperative feeding concerns involve abdominal distension with feeding intolerance and increased NG aspirates exacerbated by sepsis, spontaneous breathing with noncuffed tubes and electrolyte disturbances. Prokinetic and antireflux measures, transpyloric continuous feeds may help in tiding over the nutritional delays besides addressing the primary etiology. Continuous EN may allow for increased nutrient intake and assimilation because it minimizes myocardial VO_2 and decreased aspiration and osmotic load.[63,64] Gastrointestinal (GI) bleeding can be secondary to operative stress, coagulopathy, thrombocytopenia, and can be an early sign of NEC. NEC is an inflammatory bowel disease associated with prematurity, prostaglandin usage and LCOS, septic shock with prolonged and high-dose vasopressors. NEC can be associated with any critical heart disease but the association is stronger with HLHS and truncus arteriosus. The diagnosis of NEC involves clinical, laboratory, and radiological findings of pneumatosis intestinalis with or without peritonitis. The treatment consists of IV broad-spectrum antibiotics and bowel rest with total PN and surgical intervention if necessary for bowel necrosis or perforation. GI bleed due to other issues involves conservative management with cold saline washes, antacids, and addressing coagulopathy issues if any.

Gastroesophageal reflux disease is commonly associated with CHD and is more frequent in syndromic babies. The mainstay of therapy involves antacids and prokinetics, individualized for specific case scenarios, with surgical intervention such as fundoplication or prolonged transpyloric feeding reserved for severe cases.

One has to be vigilant for associated GI defects such as malrotation in heterotaxy syndrome, esophageal atresia in CHARGE syndrome, hind-gut atresia in VACTERL syndrome while managing postoperative care of CHD patients.

Hematological Issues

Immediately following CPB, bleeding secondary to hypofibrinogenemia, thrombocytopenia, residual heparinization, and poor clot formation is a challenge especially in neonates and delayed interventions with deep cyanosis. Whole blood is ideal but where not feasible, blood product

TABLE 4: Determination of nutritional requirements for infants with congenital heart disease.[62]

	Critical care	*Step-down/acute care*
Energy	• Determine by indirect calorimetry, if available • Provider REE (55–60 kcal/kg) in the first 3–5 days after surgery or until CRP is <2 mg/dL	120–150 kcal/kg; 140–200 kcal/kg for catch-up growth equation (kcal/kg): Kcal/kg for weight age X ideal body weight/current weight
Protein	Term: 3–3.5 g/kg Preterm or LBW: 3–4 g/kg	
Fluid	As per critical care fluid restriction (generally 50–80% MIVF with liberalization after medication wean and sternal closure)	• <3 kg: 120 mL/ kg • >3 kg: 100 mL/kg • Consider + 10–15% to compensate for increased losses with tachypnea, diarrhea, emesis, and diuresis
Micro-nutrients	• *Potassium*: 2–5 mEq/kg • *Sodium*: At least 2–3 mEq/kg even it sodium restriction is required • Supplement iron and vitamin D in breastfed infants and those with low formula intakes	

(CRP: C-reactive protein; LBW: low birth weight; MIVF: maintenance intravenous fluids; REE: resting energy expenditure)

transfusion and supplementation of specific blood products or factors based on thromboelastography (TEG–ROTEM) studies serve as a good template to rationalize therapy based on specific coagulation zone identification. Antifibrinolytics [epsilon aminocaproic acid (EACA) and tranexamic acid (TA)] are occasionally useful in reducing bleeding especially in redo interventions.

Once drainage is controlled, restrictive blood cell transfusion strategy is reasonable for patients with acyanotic heart disease, while cyanotic patients (palliated cyanotic heart disease) require a slightly higher hematocrit to optimize DO_2. Fresh frozen plasma is not recommended as colloidal volume or protein supplement. In case colloid supplementation is required 5% or 20% albumin based on serum albumin levels, patient volume and clinical status may be considered.[65]

Postoperative anticoagulation is important when dealing with systemic-to-pulmonary artery shunts, low flow venous grafts (Fontan procedure), and prosthetic valve replacements. IV unfractionated heparin (antithrombin III inhibitor) is the first line and anticoagulation is further sustained with coumadin derivatives in case of prosthetic valves and Fontan grafts. In children predisposed to recurrent thrombosis daily subcutaneous low molecular weight heparin may have to be considered, while antiplatelet agents such as aspirin/clopidogrel are preferable in cases with shunts made of synthetic material (such as polytetrafluoroethylene or Gore-Tex) and cannulae of ventricular assist devices.

Tissue plasminogen activator (tPA) is important in cases with thrombosis to lyse clots and is more helpful in treating rather than preventing thrombosis but this cannot be used for several weeks in the postoperative period because of the prospect of refractory bleeding.

Endocrine Dysfunction

Transient postoperative hyperglycemia is an adaptive neuroendocrine response to operative stress and frequently observed in critically ill children with congenital heart surgery. This is a metabolic response with acute relative resistance to insulin and breakdown of reserves exacerbated by glucocorticoids supplemented during CPB. While tight glycemic control (120–140 mg/dL) has been debated, in practice we intend to target random blood sugar (RBS) between 100 and 150 mg/dL, but sustained severe hyperglycemia (above 180–270 mg/dL) warrants insulin therapy.

Transient adrenal insufficiency is occasionally observed after intervention in complex CHD with severe myocardial dysfunction and also in malnourished infants with preoperative morbidity with an incidence rate of 19%.[66] It manifests as catecholamine-resistant hypotension resistant to fluids and inotropes. In low resource environments, it is more of a clinical diagnosis as the serum cortisol reports have a minimum turnaround time of around 3 hours. Failure to generate increase in serum cortisol after adrenocorticotropin hormone (ACTH) challenge is diagnostic but in real time it is more often a clinical diagnosis warranting IV steroids supplementation (IV hydrocortisone/IV methylprednisolone) for short duration (24–48 hours) with the hemodynamic status determining the duration of therapy in real time.

The sick euthyroid syndrome is observed after complex surgical intervention. It is diagnosed with declining thyroid stimulating hormone (TSH), total T3 and T4 levels with reduction in rT3 and elevated T3 uptake. Altered thyroid axis can exacerbate increased inotrope scores and altered vascular autoregulation. A few cases with syndromic association or with severe malnourished status invariably manifest hypothyroidism with low T3 levels and elevated TSH. These cases do require thyroid supplementation in the preoperative and immediate postoperative period especially when associated with LCOS or postoperative AV dissociation. As a protocol, preoperative thyroid profile screening can help in identifying patients which may require supplementation.

Infection Issues

Healthcare-associated infections (HAIs) after pediatric cardiac surgery are linked to younger age, preoperative morbidity, malnutrition, preoperative ventilation, greater operative complexity with open sternum, and CPB related SIRS with immunosuppression. Also, redo interventions with multiple blood transfusions, exacerbated by syndromic associations such as 22q11 deletion, impair immune responsiveness.

The rate of HAI is an index of ICU morbidity and is rightly a parameter for quality improvement initiatives. HAI and long ICU stay are mutually coexistent, besides an increase in mortality risk and healthcare costs. Modifiable risk factors for HAI are best addressed with the bundle approach whereby all aspects of device insertion, ongoing device handling, injection practices, site dressings, and other patient related concerns are addressed with an idea to prevent infection. The most common incriminating HAIs are hospital associated bloodstream infections (HABSIs), ventilator associated pneumonia (VAP), and surgical site infection (SSI). Sepsis exacerbations usually manifest as vasopressor-resistant hypotension or hypoxic respiratory failure with pulmonary hypertension and rapidly progressive multiorgan dysfunction. Sepsis screen includes complete blood count with differential and band cell count, and sepsis biomarkers CRP, procalcitonin (PCT) besides blood, tracheal, urine, and cerebrospinal fluid (CSF) cultures. PCT as a marker for sepsis in acute postoperative phase supercedes CRP with its sensitivity and specificity still debated, but a negative PCT definitely has got a high predictive value for absence of bacterial and fungal sepsis. Li et al.[67] evaluated 238 patients and concurred that PCT values in the first 72 hours are high based on the duration of CPB, and after 72 hours persistent elevation or increase is suggestive of postoperative sepsis especially in the first week after surgery. The dynamic or serial evaluation of PCT is more important than the absolute value to predict postoperative infection. Rodriguez et al.[68] alluded to a combination of PCT trends and white blood cell (WBC) count with band forms as a tool to predict postoperative sepsis, while Surti et al.[69] in a prospective analysis of a cohort of Indian patients reported that worsening thrombocytopenia was the strongest predictor of sepsis after pediatric cardiac surgery.

The antimicrobial therapy and escalation is entirely based on the local bacterial milieu and sensitivity patterns. Based on the existential flora, the antibiotic policy is programmed yearly in consult with infection control department, with adequate stress on antimicrobial stewardship in order to curtail antimicrobial resistance (AMR). Nursing education and reinforcement on infection control practice and hand hygiene for all healthcare professionals is the key to reduce the incidence of HAI. The hemodynamic stabilization involves judicious use of volume, inotropes, ventilation, and vasopressors. If no improvement is observed with optimal medical management, ECLS support is recommended especially in hypoxic respiratory failure with oxygenation index >40 for >4 hours with 100% FiO_2.[70]

Exposure to broad-spectrum antimicrobials entails prophylactic antifungal therapy specifically in immunocompromised hosts with syndromic and comorbid associations.[65]

EXTRACORPOREAL LIFE SUPPORT

Extracorporeal membrane oxygentation (ECMO) is approved essential therapeutic intervention for salvaging neonates, infants with severe postoperative heart failure, myocarditis, or as a bridge to transplantation in cardiomyopathy substrates.[71]

Extracorporeal membrane oxygenation is implemented for pre- and postoperative patients with CHD with cardiogenic shock or failure to come off CPB and in substrates with myocarditis, refractory arrhythmias, and cardiomyopathy. It is also an important salvage tool in resistant hypoxic respiratory failure as alluded to earlier induced by sepsis, acute lung injury post-CPB, or pulmonary hemorrhage, and also in septic shock with vasopressor-resistant hypotension with rapidly evolving multiorgan dysfunction.

The aim of ECMO is to offer the failing myocardium a chance to recover while the body is provided with adequate circulation and oxygenation through ECMO device with oxygenator.

In neonates with CHD, ECMO can be utilized for preoperative stabilization (e.g., D-TGA with pulmonary hypertension), failure to wean from CPB, or LCOS postoperatively. Cardiac arrest as an indication for ECMO is referred as extracorporeal cardiopulmonary resuscitation (ECPR) and in PCICU, it is now imperative to be prepared with ECPR drills and resources.[72] The ECMO survival to discharge hovers around 50% according to STS database study.[73] In a data analysis to be published from our institution, the ECMO survival rate overall is around 53% (**Box 3**).

The outcome varies significantly based on the underlying anatomy with high mortality with Ross-Konno, Truncus repair (approximately 70%) versus 14% mortality with ALCAPA. Our organization reported 25% mortality for D-TGA, IVS with regressed LV (late presentation) after ECMO (**Box 4**). Chauhan et al. also reported a 29% mortality after ECMO in the D-TGA, IVS substrate, and regressed LV.[74]

Extracorporeal membrane oxygenation can be initiated in the operating room with failure to come off bypass or in ICU with resistant LCOS with worsening circulation, increasing plasma lactate and tissue hypoxia.[75] It is always better to intervene and initiate ECMO before cardiac arrest in high-risk substrates. Norwood procedure is one such scenario where the outcomes are better when intervention

BOX 3: Indications for extracorporeal membrane oxygenation.[71]

Use of extracorporeal life support for cardiac failure should be considered for patient with evidence of inadequate and organ perfusion and oxygen delivery resulting from inadequate systemic cardiac output.

- Hypotension despite maximum doses of two inotropic or vasopressor medications
- Low cardiac output with evidence of end-organ malperfusion despite medical support as described above: persistent oliguria, diminished peripheral pulses
- Low cardiac output with mixed venous, or superior caval central venous (for single ventricle patients) oxygen saturation <50% despite maximal medical support
- Low cardiac output with persistent lactate >4.0% mmol/L and persistent upward trend despite optimization of volume status and maximal medical management

BOX 4: Contraindications for extracorporeal membrane oxygenation.[71]

- Use of extracorporeal life support (ECLS) is not recommended under certain circumstances, particularly if there is strong evidence for lack of capacity to recover or be treated
- Cardiopulmonary extracorporeal life support is inappropriate if
- The condition is irreversible and/or
- There is no timely, reasonable therapeutic option and/or
- High likelihood of poor neurological outcome
- Absolute contraindications: ECLS is not recommended in the following circumstances
- Extremes of prematurity or low birth weight (<30 weeks gestational age or <1 kg)
- Lethal chromosomal abnormalities (e.g., trisomy 13 or 18)
- Uncontrollable hemorrhage
- Irreversible brain damage
- Relative contraindications
- Intracranial hemorrhage
- Less extreme prematurity or low birth weight in neonates (<34 week gestational age or <2.0 kg)
- Irreversible organ failure in a patient ineligible for transplantation
- Prolonged intubation and mechanical ventilation (>2 week) prior to ECLS

is timed before severe metabolic acidosis and elevated lactate levels manifest as markers of prolonged end-organ compromise, as the long-term neurological outcome is likely to be compromised with delay. Providing adequate systemic blood flow and optimizing circulation with normalizing lactate is an immediate goal of ECLS support and if any significant residual lesions, it should be corrected once on ECMO.

The ECMO is VA (venoarterial) ECMO with central cannulation in most situations except for myocarditis/cardiomyopathy in older children where femoral or neck cannulation may be done. This entails the venous drainage cannula in the right atrium or SVC/IVC and arterial cannula in ascending aorta. In specific situations with LV distension (compromising coronary circulation) and LA hypertension, LA vent cannula is required to unload the left heart and prevent pulmonary edema/hemorrhage. Anticoagulation targeting ACT between 180 and 220 seconds, with heparin infusion and if heparin resistance, bivalirudin infusion (APTT target twice normal values) is imperative with extracorporeal circulation. Inotropes are kept at a minimum and optimized once weaning initiated with myocardial recovery. The goal of mechanical ventilation on ECMO is to optimize lung volumes with minimal lung injury. Most often low ventilation pressures with tidal volumes 4–6 mL/kg and PEEP (8–10 cmH_2O) with FiO_2 at room air is ideal on ECMO and ventilation is optimized to physiology once ECMO is weaned based on 2D echocardiography with color Doppler assessment for improvement in myocardial contractility, pulsatile arterial trace, improving $ETCO_2$ trends suggestive of improved forward PBF aided by improving urine output, reduced third spacing, normal lactate, and improved circulation. It is imperative that EN with partial parenteral nutrition is sustained during ECMO runs besides micronutrient supplementation relevant to myocardial optimization.

Extracorporeal cardiopulmonary resuscitation for refractory cardiopulmonary arrest can be applied for the purpose of supporting a patient for cerebral cardiopulmonary resuscitation (cerebral–CPR) or for the purpose of supporting organs for donation.[72] Newborns, infants, and children after complex cardiac surgical intervention have a 10-fold higher risk for in-hospital cardiac arrest and their survival to discharge following ECPR has been reported at higher than 50%. In our institution, the survival to discharge is around 45% though ECMO is weaned successfully in approximately 60%. Successful outcome is dependent on type of underlying cardiac disease, with fulminant myocarditis having a better outcome vis-à-vis single ventricle palliations. ECPR cannot be a replacement for high-quality CPR and in adequately manned PCICU ECPR best outcomes are associated with process initiation 10 minutes from CPR onset in witnessed arrest and completion of ECPR with restoration of circulation within 30 minutes.

PEDIATRIC CARDIAC INTENSIVE CARE UNIT: WAY FORWARD

Pediatric cardiac intensive care unit with its inherent nature of work is a quaternary ICU with ready access for 24-hour EEG monitoring, extensive hemodynamic monitoring and availability of ECLS, advanced support such as renal replacement therapy, and heart transplants care protocols and manpower.[76] In today's day and age, sustaining the unit is a much bigger challenge than a regular pediatric ICU. Besides avoiding community acquired infections is essential in a PCICU and hence it is not a good idea to merge it with general PICU. The cost constraints in LMIC warrants judicious use of resources and hence monitoring assets such as NIRS monitor and 24-hour EEG monitor are in limited numbers and have to be sustained based on patient triaging on a day-to-day basis.

The PCICU entails a system and proactive impetus collaboratively provided by the senior pediatric intensivist, pediatric cardiothoracic and vascular surgeon, pediatric cardiologist, nurse-in-charge, and respiratory therapist to ensure that essence of team work is not lost while quality centric care is optimized. The role of pediatric cardiac intensivist as a coordinator for all limbs to ensure that holistic care plans are not disjointed is paramount. The intensive care team can be a mix of trained and certified cardiac intensive care fellows with a background pediatric or anesthesiology training. Sustaining the team involves a regular feature of academic reviews in house with research initiatives and data collaboration to enhance outcomes.[77]

Nursing ratios and nursing education with quality improvement initiatives and monitoring go a long way in improving care while maintaining employee growth, satisfaction, and dedication.

The role of respiratory therapists, occupational therapist has become even more important with focus on early mobilization to ensure patient well-being and morale. Besides a team of nutrition rehabilitation specialists and pharmacists with a daily cover complete the essence of multidisciplinary overview to improve outcomes in the critical subset of patients.

The pediatric cardiac intensive care physician has to drive a daily work plan-based culture at all levels to ensure that minor details are not missed in the overall complexity of scenarios. We have evolved a thought process at our center listed below to streamline work patterns on a daily basis.

FRICHMAN-R is the acronym that summarizes the individual elements here: Fluids and electrolytes, nutrition, imput, output, insensible losses, volume and appearance of drains and, urine color. Diuresis optimization with electrolyte screen is based on renal profile.

Daily assessment of nutritional goals and nutrition supplementation titrated with feeding tolerance.

Serum albumin monitored intermittently besides RBS.

Respiratory care: Assessment of need for ventilation invasive and noninvasive, SAT and SBT based on hemodynamic status.

Daily review—ventilation and oxygenation goals.

Troubleshooting—solutions for weaning and extubation failures with a checklist approach.

Infection profile: Sepsis screen, biomarkers, follow-up on culture reports, de-escalation/escalation/antifungal prophylaxis.

Cardiac status and circulation: Hemodynamic status review—define hemodynamic goals, arrhythmias, de-escalating/escalating inotropes, and pressors. Afterload reduction.

Initiation of pulmonary vasodilators in pulmonary hypertension.

Screening echocardiography to rule out residual lesions and assess myocardial function. It may be necessary occasionally to consider cardiac catheterization or CT scan in selected cases.

Need for anticoagulations when prosthetic shunts and valves in place. Assess lower limb pulsations (post-catheterization intervention).

Hematology: Assess need for blood and blood products. If pancytopenia or neutropenia, involve hematoncology consultant and assess need for targeted therapy. Reserved blood product status review in conjunction with blood bank services.

Multiorgan review: Hepatic and renal monitoring, besides RBS. Endocrine profile (thyroid and adrenal axis evaluation) based on case scenario and preoperative status. Investigations and management related to syndromic associations and pre-existing comorbid disease review.

Abdomen: Abdominal girth monitoring, distension, presence/absence of bowel sounds, stool passed/not passed. Requirement for imaging and involving pediatric surgeon for specialty review.

Ascites, third spacing with evidence of compartment syndrome and appropriate management strategy.

Hepatomegaly as sign of congestive cardiac failure (CCF), splenomegaly in sepsis, and associated hematological disorders.

Neurological status: Awake status, sedation holiday, pupillary reaction, movement, and reflexes of all limbs. Pain assessment, need for conversation, and family presence. Positive reinforcement and reassurance while rounding to allay anxiety.

Referrals: Multispecialty referrals for specific concerns. Coordinate with ancillary management limbs such as pharmacy, nutritional rehabilitation, respiratory therapist, and occupational rehabilitation.

It is important to evolve clinical early warning screen such as cardiac hospital early warning scores for nurses and attending alike to ensure intervention before significant cardiopulmonary compromise ensues (**Table 5**).

TABLE 5: Cardiac-Children's hospital early warning signs.[78]

	0	*1*	*2*	*3*	*Score*
Behavior/ Neuro	· Playing/sleeping appropriately · Alert, at patient's baseline	Sleepy somnolent when not disturbed	Irritable, difficult to console, increase in patient's baseline seizure activity	· Lethargic, confused, floppy · Reduced response to pain · Prolonged or frequent seizures · Pupils asymmetric or sluggish	
Cardio-vascular	· Skin tone appropriate for patient · Capillary refill ≤2 seconds	· Pale · Capillary refill 3–4 seconds · Mild tachycardia · Intermittent ectopy or irregular HR (not new)	· Gray · Capillary refill 4–5 seconds · Moderate tachypnea	· Gray and mottled · Capillary refill >5 seconds · Severe tachycardia · New onset bradycardia · New onset/increase in ectopy, irregular HR or heart block	
Respiratory	· Within normal parameters · No retractions	· Mild tachypnea/ increased WOB (flaring, retracting) · Up to 40% supplemental oxygen · Up to 1 L NC > patient's baseline need · Mild desaturations < patient's baseline · Intermittent apnea self-resolving	· Moderate tachypnea/ increased WOB (flaring, retracting, grunting, and use of accessory muscles) · 40–60% oxygen via mask · 1–2 L NC > patient's baseline need · Nebs Q 1–2 hours · Moderate desaturations < patient's baseline · Apnea requiring repositioning or stimulation	· Severe tachypnea · RR < normal for age · Severe increased WOB (i.e., head bobbing and paradoxical breathing) · >60% oxygen via mask · >2 L NC > patient's baseline need · Nebs q 30 minutes—1 hour · Severe desaturations < patient's baseline · Apnea requiring interventions other than repositioning or stimulation	
Staff concern		Concerned			
Family concern		Concerned or absent			
		Mild	*Moderate*	*Severe*	
Infant		≥10%↑For age	≥10%↑For age	≥10%↑For age	
Toddler and older		≥10%↑For age	≥10%↑For age	≥10%↑For age	

(HR: heart rate; NC: nasal cannula; WOB: work of breathing)

CONCLUSION

The very strength of our present and growing abilities to diagnose and treat anatomic cardiovascular defects in critical care setting highlights the need and potential for development of new models of care. The novel care paradigm would involve artificial intelligence, data review synced with clinical examination with point-of-care tests, to align, synchronize, and improve outcome with good neurocognitive and quality of life outcome.

Informatics and big data will increasingly be used to establish reproducible standards of care, and provide collaborative platforms to enhance real-time learning and rapid hypothesis testing.[79] Adequately protected data on clinical practice and outcome will be shared in comprehensive and open registries to enhance outcome with shared learnings.[77]

Shared knowledge and experience base will go a long way in optimizing cost-effective critical care with no quality compromise in LMICS and improve holistic outcomes.

REFERENCES

1. Pronovost PJ, Angus DC, Dorman T, Robinson KA, Dremsizov TT, Young TL. Physician staffing patterns and clinical outcomes in critically ill patients: a systematic review. JAMA. 2002; 288(17):2151-62.
2. Balachandran R, Nair SG, Gopalraj SS, Vaidyanathan B, Kumar RK. Dedicated pediatric cardiac intensive care unit in a developing country: does it improve the outcome? Ann Pediatr Cardiol. 2011;4(2):122-6.
3. Marwali EM, Heineking B, Haas NA. (2017). Pre and Postoperative management of Pediatric patients with congenital heart disease. Intech Open science open minds. [online] Available from: https://www.intechopen.com/books/pediatric-and-neonatal-surgery/pre-and-postoperative-management-of-pediatric-patients-with-congenital-heart-diseases. [Last accessed March 2021].
4. Saxena A. Pediatric cardiac care in India: current status and the way forward. Future Cardiol. 2010;14(1):1-4.
5. Schuette JJ, Fraisse A, Wessel DL. Preoperative care of the pediatric cardiac surgical patient. Roger's Textbook of Pediatrics, 5th edition. Delhi: Lippincott Williams and Wilkins; 2016.
6. Gossett JG, Rocchini AP, Lloyd TR, Graziano JN. Catheter based decompression of the left atrium in patients with hypoplastic left heart syndrome and restrictive atrial septum is safe and effective. Catheter Cardiovasc Interv. 2006;67(4):619-24.
7. Wood P. Attack of deeper cyanosis and loss of consciousness (syncope) in Fallots tetralogy. Br Heart Journal. 1958;20(2):282-6.
8. Yates MC, Rao PS. Pediatric cardiac emergencies. Emerg Med. 2013;3:6.
9. Kothari SS. Mechanism of cyanotic spells in tetralogy of Fallot – the missing link? Int J Cardiol. 1992;37(1):1-5.
10. Taksande A, Gautami V, Bakshi K. Hypercyanotic spells. JMGIMS. 2009;14(ii):7-9.
11. Ricci MF, Anderson JC, Joffe AR, Watt MJ, Moez EK, Robertson CMT, et al. Chronic neuromotor disability after complex cardiac surgery in early life. Pediatrics. 2015;136(4):e922.
12. Wypij D, Jonas RA, Bellinger DC, Del Nido PJ, Mayer JE Jr, Bacha EA, et al. The effect of hematocrit during hypothermic cardiopulmonary bypass in infant heart surgery. Results from the combined Boston hematocrit trials. J Thorac Cardiovasc Surg. 2008;135(2): 355-60.
13. Wypij D, Newburger JW, Rappaport LA, du Plessis AJ, Jonas RA, Wernovsky G, et al. The effect of duration of deep hypothermic circulatory arrest in infant heart surgery on late neurodevelopment. The Boston Circulatory Arrest Trial. J Thorac Cardiovasc Surg. 2003; 126(5):1397-403.
14. Bellinger DC, Wypij D, du Plessis AJ, Rappaport LA, Riviello J, Jonas RA, et al. Development and neurological effects of alpha stat versus pH stat strategies for deep hypothermic cardiopulmonary bypass in infants. J Thorac Cardiovasc Surg. 2001;121(2):374-83.
15. Allen M, Sundarajan S, Pathan N, Burmester M, Macrae D. Anti-inflammatory modalities: their current use in pediatric cardiac surgery in the United Kingdom and Ireland. Pediatr Crit Care Med. 2009;10(3):341-5.
16. Checchia PA, Bronicki RA, Costello JM, Nelson DP. Steroid use before pediatric cardiac operations using cardiopulmonary bypass: An international survey of 36 centres. Pediatr Crit Care Med. 2005;6(4):441-4.
17. Amanfo GO, Cheifetz MI. Pediatric postoperative care. Critical Care Clinics: Pediatric critical care. 2013;29(2):185-212.
18. Bronicki RA, Chang AC. Management of the postoperative pediatric cardiac surgical patient. Crit Care Med. 2011;39(8): 1974-84.
19. Bronicki RA, Spenceley NC. Hemodynamic monitoring. Rogers Textbook of Pediatric Intensive Care, 5th edition. Delhi: Lippincott Williams and Wilkins; 2016. pp. 1120-36.
20. Vincent JL, De backer D. Oxygen transport–the oxygen delivery controversy. Intensive Care Med. 2004;30(11):1990-6.
21. Sankar J, Singh M, Kumar K, Sankar MJ, Kabra SK, Lodha R. Intermittent versus Continuous monitoring in children with septic shock: a randomized, non-inferiority trial. Intensive Care Med. 2020;46(1):82-92.
22. Levy B. Lactate and shock stat: The metabolic view. Curr Opin Crit Care. 2006;12(4):315-21.
23. Romero TE, Freidman WF. Limited left ventricular response to volume overload in the neonatal period. A comparative study with the adult animal. Pediatr Res. 1979;13(8):910-15.
24. Singh Y, Tissot C, De Luca D, Fraga MV, Yousef N, Cortes RG, et al. International evidence based guidelines on point of care ultrasound (POCUS) for critically ill neonates and children issued by the POCUS working group of the European Society of Paediatric and Neonatal Intensive Care (ESPNIC). Critical Care. 2020;24(1):65.
25. Polito A, Parisini E, Ricci Z, Picardo S, Annane D. Vasopressin for treatment of vasodilatory shock: an ESICM systematic review and meta-analysis. Intensive Care Med. 2012;38(1):9-19.
26. Singh VK, Sharma R, Varma A. Vasopressin in the pediatric cardiac intensive care unit: myth or reality. Ann Pediatr Cardiol. 2009;2(1):65-73.
27. Farkas J. Vasopressors EMCrit Project. The Internet book of critical care. 2020.
28. Shekerdemian L, Bohn D. Cardiovascular effects of mechanical ventilation. Arch Dis Child. 1999;80(5):475-80.
29. Penny DJ, Redington AN. Doppler echocardiographic evaluation of pulmonary blood flow after the Fontan operation. The role of the lungs. Br Heart J. 1991;66(5):372-4.
30. Shekerdemian LS, Bush A, Shore DF, Lincoln C, Redington AN. Cardiorespiratory responses to negative pressure ventilation after tetralogy of Fallot repair. A hemodynamic tool for patients with low output state. J Am Coll Cardiol. 1999;33(2):549-55.
31. Cullen S, Shore D, Redington A. Characterization of right ventricular diastolic performance after complete repair

of tetralogy of Fallot. Restrictive physiology predicts slow postoperative recovery. Circulation. 1995;91(6):1782-9.
32. Walsh MA, Merat M, La Rotta G, Joshi P, Joshi V, Tran T, et al. Airway pressure release ventilation improves pulmonary blood flow in infants after cardiac surgery. Crit Care Med. 2011;39(12): 2599-604.
33. Delaney JW, Moltedo JM, Dziura JD, Kopf GS, Snyder CS. Early postoperative arrhythmias after pediatric cardiac surgery. J Thorac Cardiovasc Surg. 2006;131(6):1296-300.
34. Kleinman ME, Chameides L, Schexnayder SM, Samson RA, Hazinski MF, Zaritsky AL, et al. Part 14: Pediatric advanced life support: 2010 American Heart Association guidelines for cardiopulmonary resuscitation and emergency cardiovascular care. Circulation. 2010;122(18 Suppl 3):S876-S908.
35. El Amrousy DM, Elshmaa SN, EL-Feky W, Hassan S, Elsanosy M, Hablas N, et al. Efficacy of prophylactic dexmeditomidine in preventing postoperative junctional ectopic tachycardia after pediatric cardiac surgery. J Am Heart Assoc. 2017;6(3):e004780.
36. Cools E, Missant C. Junctional ectopic tachycardia after congenital heart surgery. Acta Anaesthesiol Belg. 2014;65(1):1-8.
37. Krishna MR, Kumar RK, Kumar RK, Balaji S. Ivabradine in post-operative junctional ectopic tachycardia (JET): Breaking new ground. Pediatr Cardiol. 2019;40(6):1284-88.
38. Celermajer DS, Cullen S, Deanfield JE. Impairment of endothelium-dependent pulmonary artery relaxation in children with congenital heart disease and abnormal pulmonary hemodynamics. Circulation. 1993;87:440-6.
39. Kaestner M, Schranz D, Miera O, Warnecke G, Apitz C, Hansmann G. Pulmonary hypertension in the intensive care unit. Expert consensus statement on the diagnosis and treatment of paediatric pulmonary hypertension. The European Paediatric Pulmonary Vascular Disease Network endorsed by ISHLT and DGPK. Heart. 2016;102(Suppl 2):i57-66.
40. Brunner N, De Jesus Perez VA, Richter A, Haddad F, Denault A, Liao X, et al. Perioperative pharmacological management of pulmonary hypertensive crisis during congenital heart surgery. Pulm Circ. 2014;4(1):10-24.
41. Miller OI, Tang SF, Keech A, Pigott NB, Beller E, Celermajer DS. Inhaled nitric oxide and prevention of pulmonary hypertension after congenital heart surgery: a randomized double blind study. Lancet. 2000;356(9240):1464-9.
42. Journois D, Baufreton C, Mauriat P, Pouard P, Vouhé P, Safran D. Effects of inhaled nitric oxide administration on early postoperative mortality in patients operated for correction of atrioventricular canal defects. Chest. 2005; 128(5):3537-44.
43. Bizzarro M, Gross I, Barbosa FT. Inhaled nitric oxide for the postoperative management of pulmonary hypertension in infants and children with congenital heart disease. Cochrane database Syst Rev. 2014;(7):CD005055.
44. Miller OI, Tang SF, Keech A, Celermajer DS. Rebound pulmonary hypertension on withdrawal from inhaled nitric oxide. Lancet. 1995;346(8966):51-2.
45. Stocker C, Penny DJ, Brizard CP, Cochrane AD, Soto R, Shekerdemian LS. Intravenous sildenafil and inhaled Nitric oxide: a randomized trial in infants after cardiac surgery. Intensive Care Med. 2003;29(11):1996-2003.
46. Mourani PM, Sontag MK, Ivy DD, Abman SH. Effects of long term sildenafil treatment for pulmonary hypertension in infants with chronic lung disease. J Pediatr. 2009;154(3): 379-84.e1-2.
47. Beghetti M. Bosentan in pediatric patients with pulmonary arterial hypertension. Curr Vasc Pharmacol. 2009;7(2):225-33.
48. Mittnacht AJ, Thanjam M, Srivastava S, Joashi U, Bodian C, Hossain S, et al. Extubation in the operating room after congenital heart surgery in children. J Thorac Cardiovasc Surg. 2008;136(1):88-93.
49. Field S, Kelly SM, Macklem PT. The oxygen cost of breathing in patients with cardiorespiratory disease. Am Rev Respir Dis. 1982;126(1):9-13.
50. Watters FK. Tracheostomy in infants and children. Respir Care. 2017;62(6):799-825.
51. Selewski TD, Charlton JR, Kent LA, Jetton JG, Guillet R, Mhanna MJ, et al. Neonatal acute kidney injury. Pediatrics. 2015;136(2): e463-9.
52. Carlisle M, Soranno D, Basu R, Gist KM. Acute kidney injury and fluid overload in pediatric cardiac surgery. Curr Treat Options Pediatr. 2019;5(4):326-42.
53. Varnell CD, Goldstein SL, Devarajan P, Basu RK. Impact of near real time urine neutrophil gelatinase associated lipocalcin assessment on clinical practice. Kidney Int Rep. 2017;2(6): 1243-9.
54. Limperopoulus C, Majnemer A, Shevell MI, Rosenblatt B, Rohlicek C, Tchervenkov C. Neurological status of newborns with congenital heart defects before open-heart surgery. Pediatrics. 1999;103(2):402-8.
55. Ricci MF, Andersen JC, Robertson CM, Joffe AR, Watt MJ, Moez EK, et al. Chronic neuromotor disability after complex cardiac surgery in early life. Pediatrics. 2015;136(4):e922-33.
56. Kussman BD, Wypij D, Laussen PC, Soul JS, Bellinger DC, DiNardo JA, et al. Relationship of intraoperative cerebral oxygen saturation to neurodevelopmental outcome and brain magnetic resonance imaging at 1 year of age in infants undergoing biventricular repair. Circulation. 2010;122(3):245-54.
57. Lequier L, Joffe AR, Robertson CM, Dinu IA, Wongswadiwat Y, Anton NR, et al. Two-year survival, mental and motor outcomes after cardiac extracorporeal life support at less than 5 years of age. J Thorac Cardiovasc Surg. 2008;136(4):976e3-83e3.
58. Duff JP, Topilan AA, Berg MD, Chan M, Hazinski MF, Atkins DL, et al. 2019 American Heart Association focused update on pediatric advanced life support: an update to the American heart guidelines for cardiopulmonary resuscitation and emergency cardiovascular care. Circulation. 2019;140(24):e904-14.
59. Vaidyanathan B, Roth SJ, Gauvreau K, Shivaprakasha K, Rao SG, Kumar RK. Somatic growth after ventricular septal defect repair in malnourished infants. J Pediatr. 2006;149(2): 205-9.
60. Vaidyanathan B, Nair SB, Sundaram KR, Babu UK, Shivaprakasha K, Kumar RK, et al. Malnutrition in children with congenital heart disease (CHD). Determinants and short-term impact of corrective intervention. Indian Pediatr. 2008;45(7):541-6.
61. Leong AY, Field CJ, Larsen BM. Nutrition support of the postoperative cardiac surgery child. Nutr Clin Pract. 2013; 28(5):572-9.
62. Roman B. Nourishing little hearts: Nutritional implications for congenital heart defects. Nutr Issues Gastroenterol. 2011;35(8): 11-34.
63. Forchielli ML, McColl R, Walker WA, Lo C. Children with congenital heart disease: a nutrition challenge. Nutr Rev. 1994;52(10): 348-53.
64. Hagau N, Culcitchi C. Nutritional support in children with congenital heart disease. Nutr Ther Metab. 2010;28(4):172-84.
65. Weiss SL, Peters MJ, Wong HR, Zimmerman JJ, Kissoon N, Tissieres P. Surviving sepsis campaign international guidelines for the management of septic shock and sepsis associated organ dysfunction in children. Intensive Care Med. 2020;46(Suppl 1):510-67.

66. Menon K, Ward RE, Lawson M, Gaboury I, Hutchison JS, Hébert PC, et al. A prospective multicenter study of adrenal function in critically ill children. Am J Respir Crit Care Med. 2010;182(2):246-51.
67. Li X, Wang X, Li S, Yan J, Li D. Diagnostic value of procalcitonin on early postoperative infection after pediatric cardiac surgery. Pediatr Crit Care Med. 2017;18(5):420-8.
68. Rodriguez H, Munguira BJ, Lorenzo M, Gómez-Sánchez E, Álvarez FJ, Tamayo E, et al. Procalcitonin and white blood cells, combined predictors of infection in cardiac surgery patients. J Surg Res. 2017;212:187-94.
69. Surti J, Jain I, Mishra A, Shah K, Kandre Y, Tripathi P, et al. Predictive efficacy of procalcitonin, platelets and white blood cells for sepsis in pediatric patients undergoing cardiac surgeries who are admitted to intensive care units: single center experience. Ann Pediatr Card. 2018;11(2):137-42.
70. Butt WW, Chiletti R. ECMO for neonatal sepsis in 2019. Front Pediatr. 2020;8:Article 50.
71. Roeleveld PP, Mendonca M. Neonatal cardiac ECMO in 2019 and beyond. Front Pediatr. 2019;7:Article 327.
72. Laussen PC, Geurguerian AM. Establishing and sustaining an ECPR program. Front Pediatr. 2018;6:Article 152.
73. Mascio CE, Austin EH, Jacobs JP, Jacobs ML, Wallace AS, He X, et al. Perioperative mechanical circulatory support in children; an analysis of the Society of Thoracic Surgeons Congenital Heart Surgery Database. J Thorac Cardiovasc Surg. 2014;147(2):658-64.
74. Chauhan S, Malik M, Malik V, Chauhan Y, Kiran U, Bisoi AK. Extra corporeal membrane oxygenation after pediatric cardiac surgery: a 10-year experience. Ann Card Anaesth. 2011; 14(1):19-24.
75. Jung C. Assessment of microcirculation in cardiogenic shock. Curr Opin Crit Care. 2019; 25(4):410-6.
76. Frankel LR, Hsu BS, Mysore MR, Conway EE Jr. Criteria for critical care infants and children: PICU admission, discharge, and triage practice statement and levels of care guidance. Ped Crit Care Med. 2019;20(9):847-82.
77. Gaies M, Pasquali SK, Charpie JR. Improvement in pediatric cardiac surgical outcomes through interhospital collaboration. JACC. 2019;74(22): 2786-95.
78. McLellan MC, Connor JA. The Cardiac Children's Hospital Early Warning Score (C-CHEWS). J Pediatr Nurs. 2013;28(2):171-8.
79. Treidman JK, Newburger JW. Trends in congenital heart disease the next decade. Circulation. 2016;133:2716-33.

14

CHAPTER

Catheter-based Interventions

Shreepal Jain

INTRODUCTION

Pediatric cardiac interventions started in mid- 1960s, when balloon atrial septostomy (BAS) was performed by William Rashkind to palliate newborns and infants with transposition of the great arteries (TGA).[1] Following the footsteps of coronary interventions, pediatric cardiac interventions have made a remarkable progress in the last couple of decades. Currently, cardiac catheterization is done mainly for therapeutic interventions rather than for diagnostic purposes. Transcatheter interventions are mainly performed to dilate narrow valves or vessels, close abnormal communications, and to create or maintain patency of communications to improve oxygenation. More recently, valves are being replaced with transcatheter techniques. Most of these procedures are being performed in our country with great degree of safety and efficacy. Some of these interventions can palliate or cure the defect by themselves, while the others are being used in conjunction with the surgical procedures for more effective and sometimes less morbid palliation.[2] Catheter interventions play a complementary role in the management of pediatric heart disease and should be part of comprehensive services that include imaging, intensive care, and pediatric cardiac surgery. While a growing proportion of children with heart disease are taken care of in the catheterization laboratory, it is important to understand that surgery is the primary mode of therapy for majority of pediatric heart disease. Performing catheter interventions require specialized training and expertise. Catheter interventions should only be undertaken in institutions that have a surgical program because selected complications (e.g., device embolization) require emergency surgery as a bail out procedure.

ATRIAL SEPTOSTOMY PROCEDURES

Balloon Atrial Septostomy

Balloon atrial septostomy is one of the earliest interventional cardiac procedures to have been performed. Rashkind and Miller first performed it in 1966 on a neonate with transposition of the great vessels and severe desaturation.

Balloon atrial septostomy is a life-saving procedure in infants with TGA with intact interventricular septum, especially younger than 1 month of age who cannot be immediately scheduled for surgical correction. Because of septal thickening with age, BAS is not very effective in older infants (>1–2 months of age).[2] It is also indicated for palliating newborns in whom all systemic, pulmonary, or mixed venous blood must traverse a restrictive interatrial communication to return to the active circulation. These include a small minority of patients with tricuspid atresia, mitral atresia, and some instances of total anomalous pulmonary venous connection. The procedure is usually performed from the femoral vein, although it can be accomplished easily via the umbilical vein.[3] It is most often done under fluoroscopic guidance, although it can be carried out at the bedside using echocardiographic guidance.[3,4] The balloon is inflated in the left atrium and then "jerked" across the interatrial septum, the entire procedure being repeated until there is no resistance to the movement of the balloon (**Figs. 1A and B**). The success of the procedure is indicated by increase in the oxygen saturation and by increase in the size of the interatrial communication on echo. "Fracture" of the septum primum with excessive movement is also an indicator of a good and lasting septostomy.

The role of BAS has declined somewhat with the advent of early neonatal arterial switch operation. Selected pediatric cardiac programs are able to offer surgery in the first few days of life, thereby avoiding the need for BAS as an interim palliation.

Indications[5]

- Low saturations despite prostaglandin E1 (PGE1) infusion and when the atrial septal defect (ASD) is restrictive and when arterial switch procedure is not immediately feasible.
- Patients with restrictive ASD, not "fit" for immediate surgery because of a co-morbid condition (e.g., having sepsis or respiratory infection).
- *Restrictive ASD in TGA patients with large ventricular septal defect (VSD) or patent ductus arteriosus (PDA)*: To decrease left atrial pressure and pulmonary venous

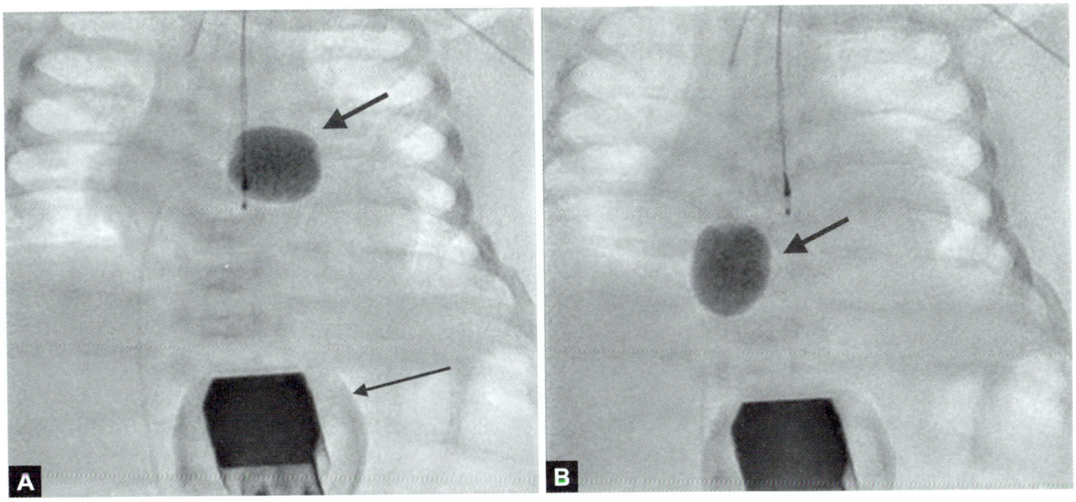

Figs. 1A and B: Balloon atrial septostomy procedure being done under fluoroscopic and transthoracic echo guidance (thin arrow). (A) Balloon (bold arrow) passed from the inferior vena cava (IVC) across the foramen ovale into the left atrium (toward the left of spine); (B) The balloon is pulled into the right atrium (to the right of the spine) with a jerky movement to tear open the interatrial septal communication.

hypertension. This indication is now less frequent reason to do balloon atrial septostomy because early arterial switch operation is often undertaken in TGA-VSD as well.

Atrial septostomy may be considered for selected conditions other than transposition where a restrictive atrial communication is responsible for reduced cardiac output (e.g., tricuspid atresia with restrictive atrial communication; pulmonary atresia with intact ventricular septum and restrictive atrial communication; total anomalous pulmonary venous connection with restrictive atrial communication) or severe pulmonary venous hypertension with pulmonary edema [mitral atresia and hypoplastic left heart syndrome (HLHS)].

Complications

They include atrial arrhythmias (often transient), injury to inferior vena cava, tricuspid valve [from inadvertent entry of balloon into right ventricle (RV)] and vascular access-related problems. However, with increasing experience, echo guidance and improved hardware, these have become very rare. The incidence of strokes from air or thrombus in the venous circuit that preferentially embolize to the aorta, and then to the brain are shown to be common with BAS, and this is one of the reasons why some units prefer to avoid it and do an arterial switch early instead.

Blade and Static Balloon Dilatation Atrial Septostomy

Blade atrial septostomy is an adjunct to BAS that was first described by Park and colleagues in 1978.[6] This procedure is indicated in select babies beyond 1 month of age who require an atrial septostomy for palliation but their atrial septum is too thick or tough for a simple BAS to tear. The blade is introduced through a long sheath and withdrawn slowly across the IAS in a controlled fashion. This action is repeated a few times with the blade being opened in different directions until there is no resistance to the withdrawal of the fully opened blade. This is usually followed by static balloon dilatation using standard balloons. In most cases, an adequate and permanent ASD is created, palliating the patient until a more definitive solution is available. Stenting of the IAS has been performed in some of these cases to ensure a lasting opening.[2]

BALLOON DILATATIONS

Balloon dilatation procedures are mainly used for dilatation of valves or vascular structures. The valves commonly undergoing dilatation in pediatric age group include the semilunar valves (pulmonary and aortic). Vascular structures include aorta, branch pulmonary arteries, and systemic and pulmonary veins.

Balloon Valve Dilatations (Valvuloplasty)

Significant pulmonary and aortic valve stenoses account for almost 10% of all congenital heart diseases (CHDs).[7]

Pulmonary Valve Dilatation

Severe pulmonic stenosis (PS) can present at any age, even in adulthood. Data obtained from a sequential follow-up study suggest that patients with PS with a gradient across the stenotic valve of >50 mm Hg had a better outcome at 20 years' follow-up when treated with surgery as compared with no intervention.[8] This forms the basis of the commonly used threshold for balloon pulmonary valvuloplasty (BPV). First reported in 1982, balloon valvuloplasty remains the treatment of choice for valvar pulmonary stenosis in patients of all ages.[9] The procedure is performed under sedation or general anesthesia. Patients are usually observed in hospital overnight and then discharged home the following day. Postprocedural care is minimal, with activity limitation for about 48–72 hours to allow healing of catheter entry sites.

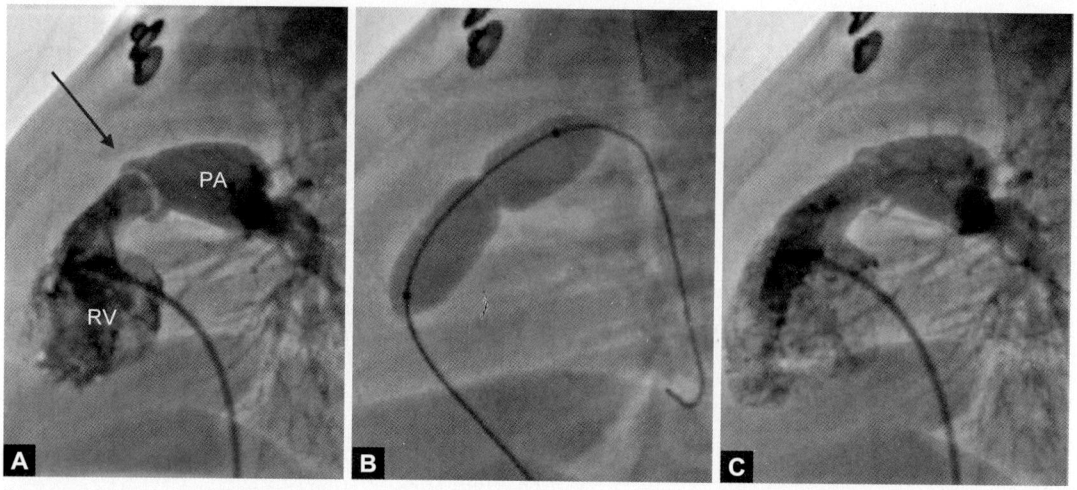

Figs. 2A to C: Balloon pulmonary valvotomy procedure being performed in the lateral view on fluoroscopy. (A) Right ventricular (RV) angiogram showing a thin doming pulmonary valve (arrow) along with a dilated main pulmonary artery (PA); (B) Balloon positioned across the pulmonary valve and inflated. Waist visualized on the balloon at the level of valve; (C) RV angiogram after balloon dilatation showing improved flow across the valve.

In PS, balloon dilation is effective in most patients (**Figs. 2A to C**). The main exception is the subset of patients with so-called "dysplastic pulmonary valve" (common in Noonan syndrome), where the valve is thick and adhered to the wall of the main pulmonary artery (PA) in part. It is often associated with supravalvar narrowing. Measurement of the annulus size on echocardiography and on angiography is extremely important to determine the balloon size needed for adequate dilatation. The balloon diameter chosen is equal to 1.2–1.4 times the diameter of the pulmonary annulus but for dysplastic valves one may go up to 1.5 times the annular diameter. To avoid marked drop in systemic blood pressure (common while using large balloons when annulus size is >20 mm) and to reduce the trauma to the veins at the site of entry, a double balloon technique is occasionally used.[2] When using this technique, the combined diameters of the two balloons should equal 1.5–1.7 times the measured diameter of the valve annulus. With pure stenosis, the gradient across the valve should reduce to <20 mm Hg. In some cases, relief of valvar obstruction unmasks an infundibular obstruction resulting in a persistent residual right ventricular outflow gradient. Experience has shown that this infundibular obstruction is usually dynamic and regresses with time. Follow-up for pulmonary valve balloon dilatation now extends to nearly 25 years. Efficacy is long-lasting in most cases, although about 8% of individuals require repeat dilatation for restenosis.[10] Although dilation results in mild-to-moderate valvular regurgitation, the physiologic consequences of the insufficiency are rarely significant in childhood and adolescence since it is a low pressure regurgitation. Thus, the main long-term issues are the need for observation for the relatively rare cases of restenosis, the continued need for endocarditis prophylaxis, and the unknown long-term (e.g., 30–60 years) effects of the pulmonary regurgitation (PR).

Critical PS in the newborn: Critical stenosis of pulmonary valve presents in the newborn with cyanosis, cardiac failure, or occasionally with sudden cardiovascular collapse following ductal closure. Very little blood can flow across the valve and majority of the systemic venous return to the heart shunts from right to left across the foramen ovale. Left-to-right shunting at the level of the ductus arteriosus maintains pulmonary blood flow and is life-saving. As the normal constriction of the ductus arteriosus occurs, the infant becomes progressively and severely hypoxemic and acidotic. These neonates need to be stabilized in the intensive care unit (ICU) with intravenous (IV) fluids, PGE1 infusion to maintain ductal patency, correction of acidosis and electrolyte imbalance, and positive inotropes to maintain perfusion. In this group of patients, the procedure is technically more demanding than in older children. In early series, technical failures and serious complications were common.[11] Refinements in technique and technology (such as use of coronary angioplasty wires and very low profile balloons for those with pin-hole critical stenosis) have resulted in progressively improved outcome. In current practice, technical success (i.e., successful dilation of the valve) is achieved in almost all cases. Clinical success, which is defined as relief of significant hypoxemia with no more than mild residual valvular obstruction, occurs in 94% of patients.[12] Overall, the prognosis of patients with isolated critical PS with normally developed RV (i.e., nonhypoplastic) is excellent through childhood, however, long-term sequelae need further follow-up. Those with hypoplastic RV may need additional procedure in the form of ductal stenting or a Blalock–Taussig (BT) shunt to maintain reliable pulmonary blood flow.

Indications[5]

- Immediate intervention required for:
  - Newborns with severe PS who are duct-dependent
  - Infants, children, or adults with right ventricular dysfunction due to severe PS, regardless of the valve gradient.

- Elective balloon dilation for:
  - Asymptomatic or symptomatic patients with valvular PS having peak instantaneous gradient by echo Doppler of >64 mm Hg.
  - Neonates and infants with any degree of PS who have mild hypoxia due to mild hypoplasia of RV, even if right ventricular function is normal.
  - Patients with valvular PS due to dysplastic valve, who meet the above criteria.

Complications

- Transient bradycardia, premature beats, and systemic hypotension during balloon inflation
- Development of subvalvar obstruction secondary to infundibular muscle spasm
- Damage to tricuspid valve apparatus
- RV or PA perforation
- Reperfusion pulmonary edema after relief of stenosis.

Aortic Valve Dilatation

Severe aortic stenosis (AS) presents with shock, syncope, angina, or cardiac failure. Balloon aortic valvotomy (BAV) is an acceptable palliative procedure that relieves obstruction either by separating fused leaflets or by creating small tears that increase the size of the valve orifice.[13] It is common for the procedure to result in some degree of aortic regurgitation (AR). The size of the balloon should preferably not exceed 90% of the size of the annulus and certainly should never perhaps be more than the aortic annulus. Attempts to alleviate obstruction completely with the use of larger balloons (exceeding annular diameter) result in an unacceptable amount of regurgitation defeating the very purpose of nonsurgical dilatation. Hence, a reduction in the gradient by 60–70% or a residual gradient of <40 mm Hg is considered acceptable. This can usually be accomplished without inducing significant AR. Despite using a conservative approach and a stepwise dilatation, significant residual obstruction or aortic insufficiency occurs in about 10% of patients.[14-16] During the early years of BAV, a significant number of patients did not get effective dilatation due to "ping-pong" effect (i.e., inability of the balloon to stabilize itself across the aortic valve during inflation). This is more commonly seen in those with normal left ventricular contractility. With the advent of long balloons (5–6 cm in length) and with the use of rapid ventricular pacing during dilatation, this difficulty has been overcome in majority of the patients. The benefit achieved after aortic valve dilation is for variable duration of time. Intervention-free survival is reported to be 50–60% at 10 years after dilation.[17] The need for subsequent intervention or surgery may result from the development of recurrent obstruction, aortic valve insufficiency, or both. In the first case, repeat valve dilation is an option, however, when aortic insufficiency becomes severe, surgery is the only modality of treatment. Thus, follow-up care of patients after intervention for aortic valve disease is quite important. Depending on the severity of residual stenosis and insufficiency, patients may be limited from competitive and contact sports. It is mandatory to evaluate them at regular intervals for assessing their symptomatic status and hemodynamics by echocardiography and color flow mapping. All of them need lifelong infective endocarditis prophylaxis.

Critical AS in the newborn: Critical AS encompasses a spectrum with hypoplastic mitral annulus and/or left ventricle and/or ascending aorta at one end, while the other end comprises of those patients with normal sized mitral valve, left ventricle, and the ascending aorta. Most of the patients with former anatomical subset have what is essentially a hypoplastic left heart syndrome (HLHS) and will need treatment on those lines. For those belonging to the latter subset, balloon aortic valvuloplasty is a preferred option, although some centers practice surgical aortic valvuloplasty.[18] In this group of patients, there is a variable reduction of left ventricular contractility. Although the LV function tends to recover in the majority after balloon dilation, in a few of them there is such severe myocyte injury that the ventricle does not recover even after successful relief of the narrowing.[18]

The efficacy of balloon valvotomy in newborn critical AS is comparable to that of surgical valvotomy and thus has largely replaced the surgical procedure. Mechanical ventilation, inotropic support, and PGE1 infusion are administered to the patient depending on the clinical situation. After BAV, some infants need several days of continued intensive care with inotropic support to allow recovery of left ventricular performance. Aortic valve is commonly approached by the "retrograde approach" from the femoral artery. The "antegrade" approach from the femoral vein across the interatrial septum into the left atrium and then crossing the aortic valve antegradely is another strategy. This procedure, however, has a higher incidence of failure in delivering the balloons and a significant incidence of damage to the mitral valve apparatus. Also, this approach is more prone to ventricular arrhythmias which are ill tolerated by some with poor LV contractility. Another option is a transcarotid approach which gives a direct access to the aortic valve requiring less catheter manipulation, less procedural time, and a very minimal complication rate.[18]

Reported early survival of newborns after balloon dilation of critical AS is close to 90% in patients without significant left ventricular hypoplasia. Most deaths were procedure related. Subsequent mortality was negligible when followed for up to 8 years.[19] Nowadays, with more experience, the procedural mortality is around 4%, but subsequent intervention remains quiet prevalent. The actuarial freedom from reintervention is only 32% at 15 years.[20] If reintervention is necessary in childhood, it is likely to be necessary in the first year of life. Recurrent AS, severe aortic insufficiency, or both necessitate reintervention. Patients with isolated restenosis may benefit from repeat balloon dilation, but many of these patients with predominantly regurgitant lesion will undergo autograft root replacement (Ross procedure) or aortic valve repair.

To summarize, aortic valve disease is a lifelong disease, and patients who require dilation of aortic stenosis as newborns are likely to have significant residual disease and on-going cardiovascular concerns. Although all patients with AS require cardiac follow-up, newborns with critical AS require frequent evaluation during growth and are virtually certain to need subsequent aortic valve interventions during infancy, childhood, and possibly throughout adulthood. With appropriate follow-up management, however, the majority of these children remain asymptomatic.

Indications[5]

- Immediate intervention required for:
  - Newborns with severe AS who are duct-dependent (balloon dilation or surgical valvotomy)
  - Infants or children with left ventricular dysfunction due to severe AS, regardless of the valve gradient
- Elective balloon dilation for:
  - Asymptomatic or symptomatic patients with AS having >64 mm Hg peak instantaneous gradient or >40 mm Hg mean gradient by echo-Doppler or peak-to-peak gradient of ≥50 mm Hg, measured invasively at cardiac catheterization
  - Patients with symptoms due to AS (angina and exercise intolerance) or electrocardiogram (ECG) showing ST-segment changes at rest or during exercise: balloon dilation may be considered for lower gradients (invasively measured) of ≥40 mm Hg
  - Selected asymptomatic child or adolescent with a peak-to-peak gradient (invasively measured) of ≥40 mm Hg, but without ST-T wave changes, if the patient wants to participate in strenuous competitive sports. This participation will be contingent to near elimination of gradient without development of significant AR and, ideally, regression of the left ventricular hypertrophy.

Complications

- Femoral arterial injury with pulse loss and late complications such as reduction of limb size in comparison with contralateral limb
- Thromboembolic stroke
- Significant aortic valve regurgitation; this may necessitate emergency aortic valve repair or replacement or the Ross operation
- Injury to the mitral valve apparatus; this is particularly a concern with the antegrade approach
- Myocardial perforation, especially in newborns. This is a very rare event and almost unheard of with modern hardware.

Mitral Valve Dilatation

Rheumatic mitral valve stenosis (MS) is still a common lesion in children in India. The pliable leaflets, fusion of commissures, and absence of calcification make these valves most suitable for a dilation procedure, which has been demonstrated to be effective in children. Most of the patients with juvenile MS have small left atria and severe pulmonary hypertension (PHT). Hence, they are unable to tolerate acute mitral regurgitation if it were to occur following the balloon mitral valvotomy (BMV). Hence, it is better to accept a mild residual MS rather than producing acute mitral regurgitation in an effort to achieve complete relief of the stenotic element. The anatomy of congenital mitral stenosis is quite variable and is generally not suitable for balloon dilation, although the procedure has occasionally been effective for this lesion.

The procedure can be performed by using standard valvuloplasty balloon catheters. In older children, the specially designed Inoue balloon is found to be safe, simple, and effective.[21] The decision to proceed with balloon valvuloplasty for congenital mitral stenosis should be based on a comprehensive echocardiographic assessment of mitral valve anatomy. The procedure is less likely to be effective when there is a single papillary muscle or severe shortening or virtual absence of the chordal apparatus (the "arcade-type" mitral valve). In view of suboptimum results either with surgery or with balloon dilatation for congenital MS, our threshold for any form of intervention in congenital MS is quite high unless the patient is symptomatic despite medical treatment or has progressive worsening of PHT.

Indications[22]

- Transcatheter balloon valvuloplasty is indicated for symptomatic patients with moderate-to-severe isolated rheumatic mitral stenosis or asymptomatic patients with moderate-to-severe rheumatic MS/restenosis associated with PHT.
- Transcatheter balloon valvuloplasty is reasonable for the treatment of symptomatic children >5 years of age with congenital mitral stenosis or restenosis who have mitral valvemorphologythatisfavorableforballoonvalvuloplasty (i.e., thickened leaflets and fused commissure).

Complications

- Iatrogenic mitral regurgitation as a result of injury to leaflet (often in the form of tear)
- Cardiac tamponade during trans-septal perforation to enable entry of the balloon assembly into the left atrium
- Atrial or ventricular perforation (rare)
- Transient rhythm abnormalities
- Stroke from an unrecognized left atrial clot that is displaced during the procedure
- Femoral venous trauma from the large caliber of the balloon dilation assembly.

Dilatation of Vascular Structures

Coarctation of the Aorta

Coarctation of the aorta (CoA) occurs in 0.04% of individuals and accounts for 5% of heart defects.[6] Like AS, critical coarctation presents in the newborn period with severe heart failure or shock when the ductus arteriosus closes. Older patients are most often asymptomatic but sometimes present with hypertension or complication of hypertension pertaining to cerebrovascular or cardiovascular systems. They can come to attention due to a murmur produced by an associated bicommissural aortic valve or by presence of intercostal collaterals. All patients with significant coarctation require treatment. Balloon dilation has been used as a treatment for coarctation since the 1980s. It was first used to successfully dilate postsurgical recurrent CoA. The dense scar tissue surrounding the recurrent coarctation makes repeat surgery difficult and provides some insurance against aortic rupture during balloon dilatation, hence, this mode of treatment has become the preferred approach for tackling recoarctation. As regards native coarctation, however, there is still substantial variation in practice. Surgery is the benchmark against which interventional catheter treatment must be judged. In newborns, the preferred treatment is surgical because there is a high rate of recurrent obstruction after balloon dilation. In infants and older children with coarctation, balloon angioplasty is widely used as the primary form of therapy, but opinion is divided, and surgery continues to remain a common option. The controversy surrounding these options relates to the varying reported rates of recurrence and aneurysm formation at the site of balloon dilatation. For example, the incidence of aneurysm formation (the most worrisome complication of this procedure) has been variously reported as ranging from <2 to 40% of cases.[23-25] Revised Indian guidelines on mode of intervention for coarctation based on the age and weight of the patient were published recently.[5]

In newborns with coarctation presenting with shock or cardiovascular collapse secondary to severe left ventricular dysfunction, balloon dilatation is often the preferred procedure as a salvage therapy. Transcatheter balloon dilatation procedure has been made easier by the use of axillary arterial approach.[26] The use of a femoral arterial access has a high risk of significant vessel damage, particularly in a premature neonate suffering from aortic coarctation with impaired flow to the lower part of the body. The advantage of using axillary arterial access is that it is not an end-artery and the arm continues to be perfused by the second intercostal artery as well as by the acromial artery. Moreover, the axillary artery is better felt in neonates, especially in those with coarctation with low cardiac output and nonpalpable femoral pulses (**Figs. 3A to C**).

In patients who present after adolescence and into adulthood, stenting of the coarctation at catheterization is now considered as the first-line therapy. Stents result in effective and predictable relief of the obstruction in the majority of cases. The complications with this procedure are relatively infrequent. At follow-up, recurrent coarctation and aneurysm formation are relatively uncommon[27-29] (**Figs. 4A to C**).

Indications[5]

- Patients with resting CoA gradient ≥20 mm Hg
- Patients of CoA presenting with left ventricular dysfunction, even though the gradient across is <20 mm Hg, where left ventricular dysfunction is considered to be due to tight CoA
- Patients with gradient <20 mm Hg, but having upper limb hypertension, left ventricular hypertrophy, or significant collateral formation
- Patients with hypertension who have >50% narrowing at the site of CoA, relative to aortic diameter at diaphragm on computed tomography angiography (CTA)/cardiac

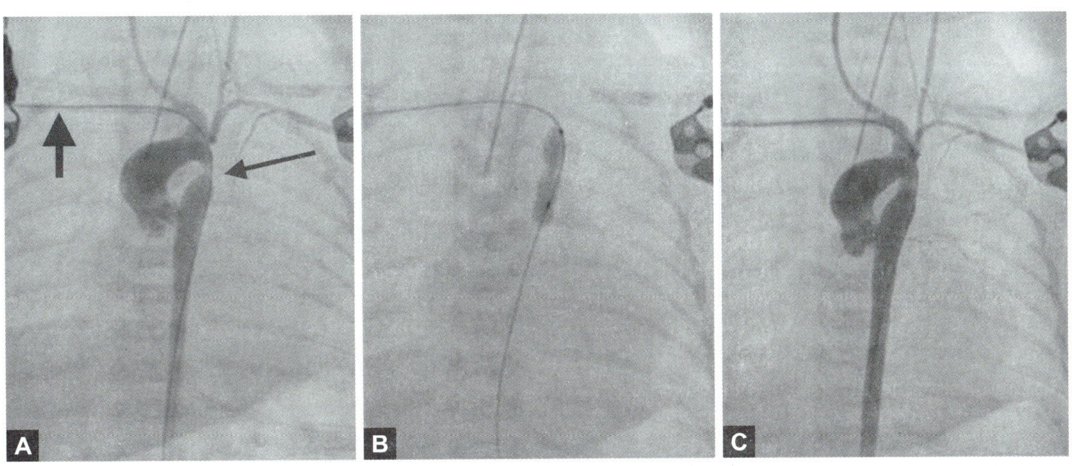

Figs. 3A to C: Balloon dilatation of critical coarctation in a neonate via the axillary artery approach (bold arrow). (A) Aortogram via a sheath placed in the right axillary artery shows a discrete coarctation of the postsubclavian aorta; (B) Balloon dilatation of coarctation; (C) Postdilatation angiogram showing a well-opened aortic segment.

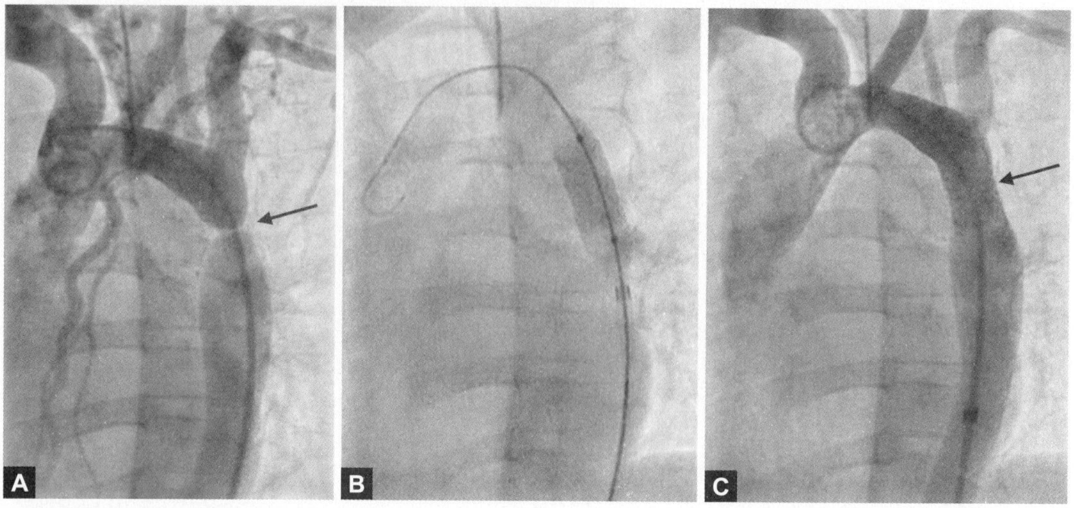

Figs. 4A to C: Stenting of coarctation of aorta. (A) Aortogram in lateral anterior oblique (LAO) view showing a discrete postsubclavian coarctation of aorta (arrow); (B) Balloon mounted stent being inflated across the coarctation segment; (C) Poststenting aortogram showing well-positioned stent (arrow) with unobstructed flow across the segment.

magnetic resonance imaging (cMRI)/angiography, irrespective of pressure gradient

- Intervention is not indicated if Doppler gradient across coarctation segment is <20 mm Hg with normal left ventricular function and no upper-limb hypertension.

Mode of intervention:[5]

- *Neonatal presentation*: Surgery is preferred. Aortic arch hypoplasia, if associated, should also be repaired.
- Critically ill neonates who are considered high risk for surgery (shock-like syndrome and severe left ventricular dysfunction): Balloon angioplasty may be considered to tide over the crisis.
- *Infants with native coarctation*: Surgery is perhaps the best approach but balloon angioplasty may also be considered.
- *Infants with re-coarctation*: Balloon angioplasty is the procedure of choice.
- *Children <25 kg with native coarctation*: Balloon angioplasty or surgery, both are reasonable options.
- *Children <25 kg with re-coarctation*: Either balloon angioplasty or stenting of the coarctation site may be considered.
- *Children >25 kg and adults with native coarctation or recoarctation*: Catheter-based stenting is generally preferred because it offers a more complete relief of the narrowing, and there is a lower likelihood of aortic injury with stenting.
- Elective endovascular stenting of aorta is generally avoided in children <10 years of age because of limitations in the vessel size as well as the challenges related to growth requiring redilation in the future.

Complications

- Femoral artery injury from the balloon catheter or stent assembly
- Dissection at the site of dilation of the aorta
- Aneurysm formation at the site of angioplasty
- Restenosis of the dilated segment; this is common in neonates
- Stent malposition or migration
- In-stent restenosis with a reduction in lumen that necessitates redilation in 10–15% of cases
- Persistent hypertension; this is inevitable in older patients. Even after successful management of coarctation, there is life-long risk of systemic hypertension meriting lifelong follow-up. Additionally, vascular complications such as late aortic dissection and berry aneurysm formation in the cerebral vessels are unaffected by relief of coarctation.

Branch Pulmonary Artery Stenosis

The dilation of all varieties of branch pulmonary artery stenosis is a widely accepted procedure, in large part because most of these lesions (especially those beyond the hilum) are not easily amenable to surgical repair. Results are inconsistent and relief is often partial, i.e., some percentage reduction of the gradient or percentage improvement in the measured stenosis rather than actually abolishing the gradient or producing a vessel of normal diameter. The technique for dilation of these stenoses is similar to that for pulmonary valve dilation. The balloon size must be equal to or slightly larger than the "normal" vessel on each side of the stenosis or three to four times the diameter of the actual narrowing (**Figs. 5A to C**). There is a suggestion that the use of high pressure balloon in these lesions will improve the results in selected cases. However, the data from VACA registry for dilation of branch pulmonary arteries does not show significant difference with high pressure balloons.[2]

Presence of branch pulmonary artery stenosis in the presence of PR [especially seen after surgical repair of tetralogy of Fallot (TOF)] can further increase the PR

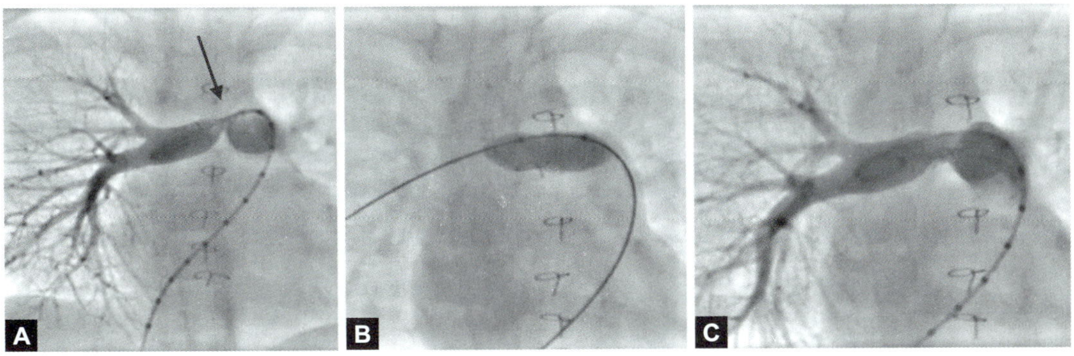

Figs. 5A to C: Balloon dilatation of the right pulmonary artery (RPA) in an operated case of tetralogy of Fallot. (A) Right pulmonary artery angiogram showing discrete stenosis of the proximal RPA (arrow); (B) Balloon dilatation of the RPA; (C) Postdilatation angiogram showing an opened up segment.

leading to progressive right ventricular dilation and reduced function. These patients are at increased risk of decreased exercise tolerance, arrhythmias, and sudden cardiac death. Studies have shown that relief of branch PA stenosis reduces insufficiency and improves right ventricular systolic function.[30]

Although the short-term results are quite gratifying, there is a high incidence of restenosis over a period of time. Less than 20% of these dilated vessels are maintained at near normal diameter with insignificant gradient during the follow-up.[2] There is a definite morbidity and rarely mortality related to the procedure. Since there are no predictors of success, balloon dilation is performed as a therapeutic trial. More recently, cutting balloons have been used with more encouraging results.[31]

Due to suboptimum results with balloon dilatation, stents are being increasingly used to dilate these obstructions. Since their introduction, intravascular stents have become the primary mode of therapy for branch pulmonary artery stenosis in children beyond 5 years of age. The experience with stents in these lesions has significantly changed the approach to branch pulmonary artery stenosis. The results are excellent and they virtually eliminate any gradient and open the vessel to achieve a normal end diameter. The initial results have been sustained over years. In addition, it has been demonstrated that if the appropriate stents are implanted initially, these stents can be dilated further up to the adult diameter of the vessel. Balloon dilation alone of branch pulmonary stenosis is presently recommended only for patients who urgently require some therapy for their lesion but who are too small for implanting an intravascular stent that can be dilated to adult size at a later date. Recently, there have been isolated reports of biodegradable stents being successfully used in neonates with significant branch PA stenosis.[32]

Indications[5]*:* Percutaneous interventional therapy (balloon dilatation ± stenting) is the treatment of choice for focal branch and/or peripheral PA stenosis with >50% diameter narrowing, an elevated RV systolic pressure >50 mm Hg (or >50% of systemic pressure), difference in perfusion of both lungs of >20% (on lung perfusion scan), and/or symptoms.

Complications

- Pulmonary artery injury/perforation
- Stent malpositioning/migration
- "Jailing" of side branches.

Systemic Vein Stenosis

Dilation of stenosed systemic veins, particularly postsurgical, is acutely successful and carries little risk. The surgical alternative for these lesions is poor. These are usually seen in the venous baffles following Senning or Mustard operation for transposition. The other common postoperative venous stenosis is seen in the superior vena cava (SVC) following repair of sinus venosus ASD or at the site of SVC cannulation for various open heart procedures. Stenoses can also develop from indwelling lines in the veins or from external compression. Like pulmonary branch stenosis, the results are not uniform or predictable. As with balloon dilation of other vessels, there is immediate hemodynamic, anatomic, and symptomatic improvement, however, recurrence of the stenosis is almost a rule. The balloon diameter chosen should be equivalent or slightly larger than that of the adjacent normal segment of the vessel or baffle.

Due to high rates of restenosis, primary therapy for these venous lesions has become implantation of intravascular stents. The venous stent delivery procedure is similar to any other intravascular stents. For stent delivery, a single balloon of a diameter not less than that of the adjacent nearest normal vein is used. The results of implantation of stents within systemic veins have been excellent.[33] Some in-stent restenosis in the venous location has occurred when the stents were dilated to a diameter significantly larger than the adjacent vessel at the time of implant. In these instances, the lumen within the stent "remodels" with neointima to the size of the normal adjacent vessel.

Indications[22]

- Venous balloon angioplasty is reasonable to consider for the management of peripheral venous obstruction or "complex" venous stenosis in cases in which no viable alternative therapy exists.

- Venous balloon angioplasty may be reasonable in the management of central venous obstruction, but its usefulness as a definitive therapy has not been established.

Complications

- Vascular perforation
- Restenosis
- Thrombus formation
- Stent migration or embolization.

Pulmonary Vein Stenosis

Pulmonary vein stenosis can present as an isolated congenital lesion or in association with other cardiac defects. It can also be acquired after corrective surgery for various anomalous pulmonary venous connections or after lung transplantation. More rare causes include external compression from tumors, sarcoidosis, and mediastinitis. This lesion is often progressive and fatal if it occurs bilaterally. Treatment modalities include surgery, balloon angioplasty, cutting balloon angioplasty, and venous stenting. However, to date, there is not a single procedure that produces a high rate of patency consistently and does not require reintervention. Pulmonary vein balloon dilation provides only transient relief. The procedure is acutely successfully in most cases; however, restenosis has been observed in all attempted cases. Attempted dilation of these lesions may be recommended in an infant or child who is severely symptomatic. High pressure balloons and cutting balloons too have been used in an attempt to improve immediate and long-term results.[34] The experience with intravascular stents in pulmonary vein stenosis to date has had no better results than dilation alone and has been associated with a high percentage of complications. In highly select situations where the vessel size is 7 mm or greater, sustained benefit can be expected.[22] Stents have been placed in pulmonary veins surgically under direct vision with limited short-term success.

Indications[22]

- Pulmonary venous angioplasty and stenting are indicated for the management of acquired pulmonary vein stenosis after lung transplantation or for external compression due to tumors in older children and adolescents.
- Pulmonary venous angioplasty is reasonable to consider in the management of pulmonary vein stenosis after surgical repair for anomalous pulmonary vein connections.
- Pulmonary venous angioplasty and stenting may be considered in the management of isolated congenital pulmonary vein stenosis.
- Pulmonary venous angioplasty and stenting may be considered for the management of acquired pulmonary vein stenosis after lung transplantation or for external compression due to tumors in infants and young children.
- Pulmonary venous stenting may be considered for the management of postoperative pulmonary vein stenosis after surgical repair for anomalous pulmonary vein connections.

Complications

- Vessel dissection
- Pulmonary hemorrhage
- Stent malposition
- Stent embolization—can have devastating consequences since the procedure is performed in the left atrium.

TRANSCATHETER CLOSURE OF INTRACARDIAC SHUNTS

Earliest successful experience with transcatheter closure of PDA lead to further experimentation with closure of other defects such as ASD. Gradually, the techniques were extended to closure of VSD and other defects such as aortopulmonary window and rupture of sinus of Valsalva.

Atrial Septal Defect

Atrial septal defects are among the more common defects and account for about 10% of all CHDs.[1] Most of the children are asymptomatic and are incidentally detected due to murmur. Some may present with repeated respiratory tract infections and failure to thrive usually beyond infancy. A very small minority (<5%) will present with cardiac failure during infancy. All ASDs of consequence (either symptomatic or producing right ventricular volume overload on echo) need to be closed. Since the impact of ASD is evident only after first few decades of life, the timing of closure is elective unless the child is significantly symptomatic. In our practice, most children are advised to undergo closure between 3 and 5 years of age (preschool going) or at the time of diagnosis if this occurs later. Mills and King were the first to describe transcatheter closure of secundum ASD in 1976. They successfully treated 5 patients with defects as large as 26 mm using a "double umbrella device."[35] Device technology matured in the 1980s and 1990s. Now most secundum ASDs are closed by placement of a transcatheter device. Patients with ASD are screened by echocardiography to determine whether they are candidates for transcatheter approach. Closure using a device is possible only for secundum defects, not sinus venosus or atrioventricular canal-type ("primum ASD") ASDs. The defect must have adequate surrounding margins and must be of a size that permits placement of the device. Although devices to close very large defects (up to 40 mm in diameter) are available, the larger devices fit only in the heart of an adult.[36] In general, device closure is not advised if there are deficient rims (<5 mm), if weight of the patient is <10–15 kg or if the defect size is >20 mm/m^2.[5] There are various devices currently in use for closure of ASD. Majority of them have double disks of fine nitinol wire mesh

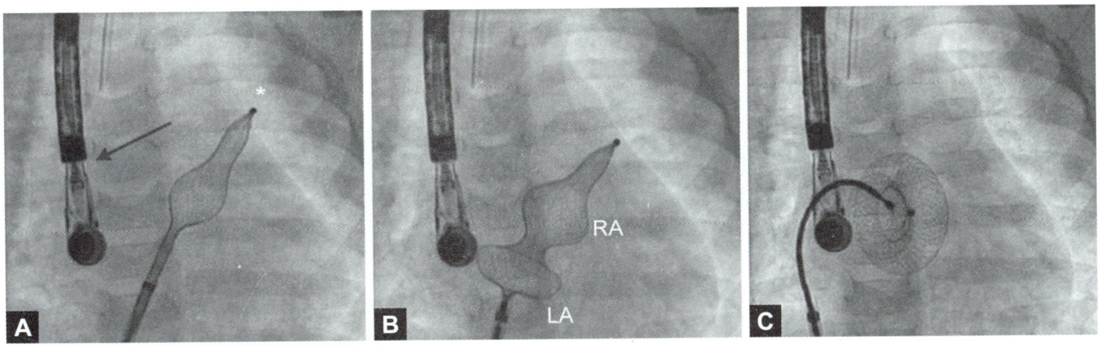

Figs. 6A to C: Fluoroscopic images of deployment of septal occluder device for closure of ostium secundum atrial septal defect (ASD) with the left superior pulmonary vein (LSPV) technique under transesophageal echocardiographic (TEE) guidance (arrow). (A) The left atrial disk of the occluder device being opened in the LSPV (*); (B) Rest of the occluder device being deployed by withdrawing the sheath. The left atrial disk is still fixed in the LSPV; (C) Left atrial disk completely opened after pushing the delivery cable resulting in deployment of the device.

filled with polyester fibers. The two disks are fixed on either sides of the ASD by a central "hub" of the same material—the diameter of the hub corresponding to the size of the ASD. The device is delivered through a 7–12 French sheath and is removable without damaging the device or the patient even after full deployment until it is released (**Figs. 6A to C**).

Patients usually undergo ASD closure with one day's hospitalization. Some centers which perform ASD closure with intracardiac echocardiography do it even as a day-care procedure. Device placement is performed under a combination of fluoroscopic and transesophageal or intracardiac echocardiographic guidance. In younger children, a general anesthetic is administered to permit transesophageal echocardiography. In selected patients, general anesthesia is not needed because it is possible to guide- device placement using transthoracic echocardiography alone. Patients typically remain supine for several hours after the procedure but may ambulate normally by the time they leave hospital. Subsequently care is straightforward, with avoidance of contact sports for about 3 months. Thereafter, they are allowed resumption of all normal activities without restriction. Patients receive low-dose aspirin and adhere to bacterial endocarditis prophylaxis precautions for 6 months. At that time, a follow-up echocardiography examination is performed to document effective and complete ASD occlusion, after which prophylaxis is no longer needed. The follow-up echo also includes evaluation of surrounding structures such as the systemic and pulmonary veins, the ventricular inflows, the atrioventricular valves, right ventricular size and shape, biventricular function, presence of a thrombus on the device, and any evidence of pericardial effusion.

Several studies have documented the efficacy and safety of ASD closure using a device in comparison to surgery. In general, these studies shows no or little difference in efficacy rates between the two strategies (95–98%), with longer hospital stay and higher rate of complications after surgical closure.[37,38] While all ASDs can be closed surgically, the same is not true for device closure. Appropriate patient selection improves results and reduces complications. Many techniques have been described to improve success rates of closing large ASDs and size of defect has almost ceased to become a contraindication to ASD closure.[39] The risk of major complications is low after both surgical or device closure, therefore statistical comparisons of major complications are not very meaningful. The main difference in complication rate is attributable to the morbidity of surgery related to bleeding, infection, pain, and pericardial effusion (postpericardiotomy syndrome), which do not happen after device closure. Device integrity has not been an issue with the newer generations of devices, and other problems, such as formation of subacute thrombus on the device, have been rare.[40]

Indications[5]

- *In an asymptomatic child*: Elective closure between 3 and 5 years.
- *Symptomatic ASD in infancy (congestive heart failure and PA hypertension)*: Seen in about 8–10% of cases. Early closure is recommended after ruling out associated lesions (e.g., total anomalous pulmonary venous drainage, left ventricular inflow obstruction, and aortopulmonary window).
- *If presenting beyond ideal age*: Elective closure irrespective of age as long as there is left-to-right shunt with right heart volume overload and pulmonary vascular resistance (PVR) is not significantly elevated.

Complications

These are generally rare in today's times and include:

- Device migration, malposition, or embolization requiring surgical retrieval and surgical closure of the ASD.
- Cardiac erosion or perforation leading to tamponade from pericardial accumulation of blood. This is potentially fatal but fortunately rare and affects 1 in 2–3,000 device implants. It can happen several months after implantation which is why long-term follow-up is important.

- Heart block; varying degree of atrioventricular (AV) dissociation can happen especially when relatively large devices are used in small children.
- Air embolism is an avoidable acute complication that is largely prevented by attention to details during the implantation process.
- Stroke from embolization of thrombotic material on the device surface is a rare complication and is avoided by administration of antiplatelet therapy for 6 months after the procedure.
- *Migraine*: Episodes of headache suggestive of migraine are relatively common for the first few months after implant and are perhaps related to platelet activation on the device surface and release of vasoactive substances. They often subside with dual antiplatelet agents (aspirin plus clopidogrel).
- Nickel allergy has been previously reported but is exceedingly rare with current devices that have a coating of inert material such as ceramic.

Ventricular Septal Defect

Ventricular septal defect is the single most common heart defect, accounting for almost 40% of all defects.[6] Patients with large VSDs present with overt congestive heart failure in infancy. Moderate defects may have more subtle manifestations of heart failure, such as failure to thrive, and patients with smaller defects are typically asymptomatic.[41] VSD closure is indicated in infants with heart failure, PHT, or failure to thrive. In the absence of these manifestations, indications for closure are less clear, but most concur that closure is appropriate when the shunt through the defect exceeds 2:1, i.e., when the pulmonary blood flow is at least twice as much as the systemic cardiac output.

In contrast to ASDs, surgical closure remains the mainstay of treatment for VSD. In selected cases, device closure is being performed with increasing frequency with improvement in technique and technology. Like ASD, device closure of VSD is performed under both fluoroscopic and ultrasound guidance. The procedure is much more complex than that for ASD. The need to manipulate relatively large and stiff catheters through the heart increases the risk of this procedure, especially in very small infants. Another option for small infants with muscular VSDs is a combined surgical-catheter (hybrid) approach. In this method, a midline sternotomy is performed, the heart is exposed [without the need for cardiopulmonary bypass (CPB)], and the device-delivery catheter is advanced under echocardiographic guidance. The major advantage of this technique is the ability to close VSDs that are in portions of the heart that are difficult to reach by standard open surgical technique (e.g., apical VSDs). Also, in the absence of use of CPB, the pulmonary, cerebral, and renal complications are perhaps less commonly seen with the potential of reduced hospital stay.[42] However, with parallel improvement is bypass technology, an exposure to CPB is no longer associated with much morbidity.

The main selection criterion for device closure of VSD is the type and location of the VSD and the size of the patient. Muscular defects, especially those situated in the midportion of the septum, are ideally suited for this procedure and the first-generation devices for VSD closure were developed to close these defects. Patients who are of sufficient size (>8 kg) to permit placement of the delivery catheter and in whom location of the VSD allows device placement without valve impingement are candidates for the procedure. Although the devices were originally designed for muscular VSDs, the most common, hemodynamically significant VSDs are perimembranous ventricular septal defects (pmVSDs). The proximity of these VSDs to the aortic valve precluded device closure. However, with the advent of various newer devices, the success rate of transcatheter closure of pmVSD has increased significantly, whereas complications, such as aortic or tricuspid regurgitation and device embolization, have reduced considerably.[43] Several reports have demonstrated that the procedure is efficacious, reporting success rate from 86 to 100%. These reports include patients with postoperative residual VSDs and some who were considered poor surgical candidates.[44-48] However, the incidence of heart blocks after closure of pmVSD has merited concern, with complete atrioventricular block (AVB) being the most malignant. Incidence of complete AVB has ranged from 1.1 to 5.7% in various reports.[45] In addition, other types of postprocedure heart blocks (PPHB), including right bundle branch block (RBBB), left bundle branch block (LBBB), and first-degree AVB, could progress to high-degree AVB. Yang et al. documented that compared with the patients without PPHB, the patients suffering PPHBs were characterized by a significantly longer distance between the aortic valve and the defect, a shorter distance from the lower rim of the defect to the septal leaflet of the tricuspid valve, and a larger diameter difference between the occluder and VSD.[45]

Devices other than the membranous VSD occluder have been used to close pmVSD like the Amplatzer Duct Occluder (ADO) I and II (Abbott, Abbott Park, Illinois, USA), which were designed for closure of PDA. ADO I has the advantage that it does not have two disks like the other devices, and hence does not impinge onto the conduction tissue due to clamp force (**Figs. 7A to C**). Also compared to other devices, it is relatively cheaper. ADO II has the advantage that it requires smaller sheath size and can be deployed from the arterial side thus avoiding the need to form an arteriovenous loop. However, since it is available in sizes up to 6 mm, pmVSD measuring >5.5 mm cannot be closed with this device. KONAR-MF (Lifetech, Shenzhen, China) is a new occluder device with a hybrid

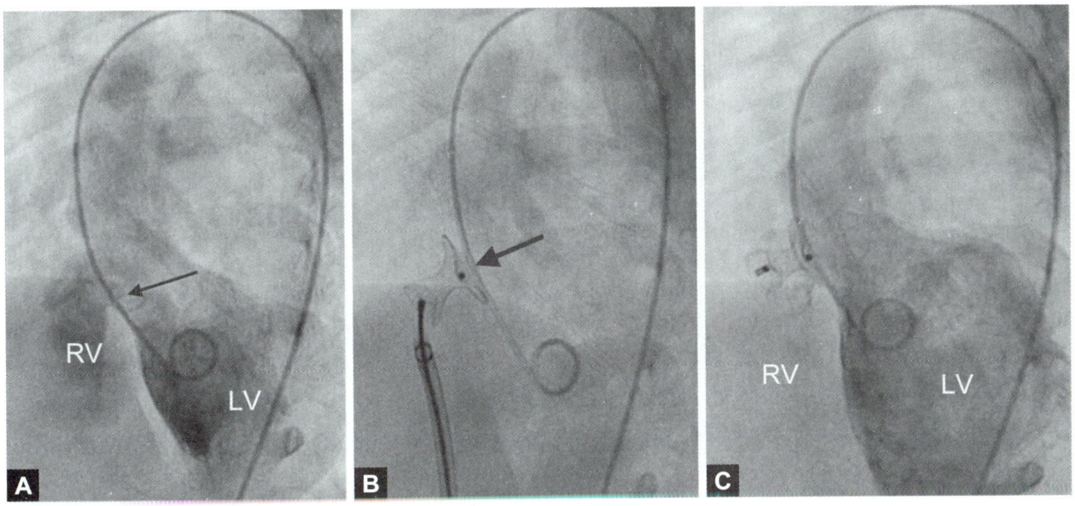

Figs. 7A to C: Transcatheter closure of a perimembranous ventricular septal defect (VSD) with an Amplatzer ductal occluder device (ADO I). (A) Left ventricular (LV) angiogram showing a moderate-sized perimembranous VSD (arrow) with contrast entering the right ventricle (RV); (B) ADO I device (bold arrow) being deployed from the venous side; (C) LV angiogram after device deployment showing resolution of the shunt.

design between single disk and double disk occluders with the advantage of low profile allowing delivery through relatively smaller sheaths, softer material producing reduced chances of AVB, and double-sided screws allowing antegrade as well as retrograde deployment across the VSD.[49] Follow-up care of children after device occlusion of VSD is essentially the same as after ASD closure.

Indications[5]

- Mid-muscular VSD, anterior muscular VSD, and postoperative residual VSD
- Perimembranous VSD with at least 4 mm distance from the aortic valve.

Contraindications

- VSD with pulmonary vascular obstructive disease
- Pre-existing left bundle branch block or conduction abnormalities
- Any AR
- Associated lesions requiring surgery
- Inlet and subpulmonic VSD.

Device should not be deployed if any of the following findings develop at the time of procedure:

- Any degree of AR
- *Conduction defect*: Complete heart block (CHB)/left bundle branch block
- Mitral or tricuspid regurgitation.

Complications

- Device migration/embolization
- Tricuspid and mitral valve regurgitation
- Hemolysis from residual flows
- Transient ischemic attack/stroke
- Ventricular tachycardia
- Atrioventricular heart block.

Patent Ductus Arteriosus

Patent ductus arteriosus accounts for 10% of CHD. Larger PDAs may lead to congestive heart failure or pulmonary vascular disease. Those with moderate-sized shunts may present with failure to thrive. Most often children with a PDA have a small left-to-right shunt, are asymptomatic, and present with a continuous murmur.

Transcatheter closure of PDA has been extensively studied. Smaller PDAs (<3 mm) can be safely and completely closed with coils. A European registry series reported an overall efficacy of 95% in >1,200 procedures performed between 1994 and 2001.[50] In this series, successful occlusion was less likely in larger PDAs. Since that large European report, the ADO I device has proven efficacious, with a closure rate of 100% in one report,[51] and is particularly useful in the closure of larger PDAs (**Figs. 8A to C**). Some investigators in an attempt to decrease cost (especially in developing countries) have used ingenious techniques to deliver multiple coils in an attempt to close large PDAs.[52] These coils are either delivered using a bioptome or a balloon occlusion technique. The incidence of residual shunts is somewhat higher with coils when compared to occlusive devices but the cost benefits are considerable. The second-generation PDA device, ADO II, is a versatile device for closure of ducts of various shapes, lengths, and diameters up to 5.5 mm.[53] It requires a smaller delivery sheath size and can also be delivered from the arterial side.

Recently, many operators have started closing PDAs in extremely low birth weight (ELBW) neonates by transcatheter route using a variety of devices and with encouraging results.[54] However, in view of a very steep learning curve and high chances of complications in inexperienced hands, this modality is presently not the standard of recommendation for preterm PDA closure.

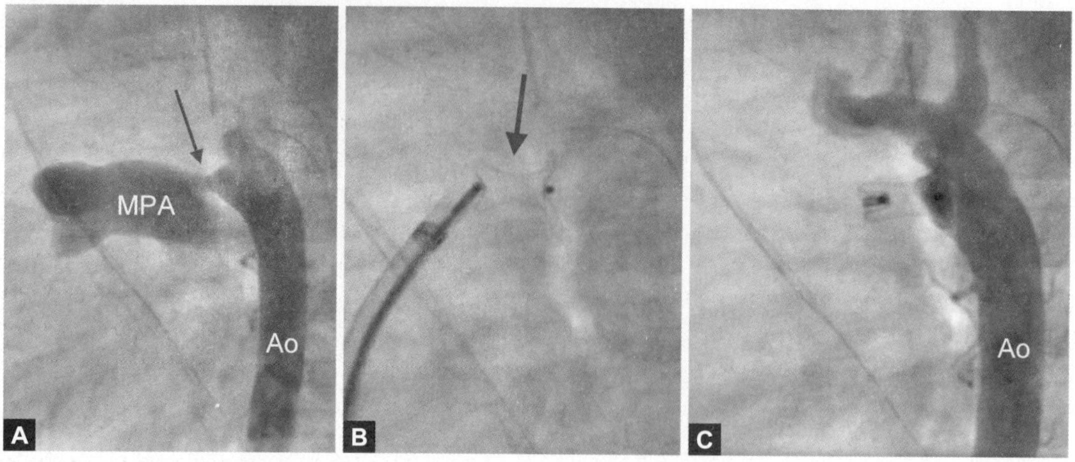

Figs. 8A to C: Patent ductus arteriosus (PDA) closure by Amplatzer duct occluder (ADO I) device. (A) Aortogram (Ao) demonstrating a moderate-sized PDA (arrow) with contrast entering the main pulmonary artery (MPA); (B) ADO I device being deployed across the PDA from the PA side; (C) Aortogram showing complete occlusion of the PDA.

Indications[22]

- Transcatheter PDA occlusion is indicated for the treatment of a moderate-sized or large PDA with left-to-right shunt that results in any of the following: Congestive heart failure, failure to thrive, pulmonary overcirculation (with or without PHT), or an enlarged left atrium or left ventricle, provided the anatomy and patient size are suitable.
- Transcatheter PDA occlusion is reasonable in the presence of a small left-to-right shunt with normal-sized heart chambers when the PDA is audible by standard auscultation techniques.

Complications

- Inadvertent device embolization into the pulmonary and systemic circulation
- Device obstruction to aortic (creating an iatrogenic coarctation) or pulmonary flow, especially in small infants
- Transient left ventricular systolic dysfunction
- Residual flow producing hemolysis
- Recanalization.

CARDIAC INTERVENTIONS IN COMPLEX CONGENITAL HEART DISEASE

Pulmonary Atresia with Intact Interventricular Septum

Newborns with pulmonary valve atresia present like those with critical pulmonary stenosis, and the initial medical management is identical. The subsequent management of these patients varies enormously because the disorder is very heterogeneous. Some patients are born with a well-developed RV, whereas others are born with severe right heart hypoplasia but patent tricuspid valve and may also have communications between the cavity of the RV and the coronary arteries (coronary cameral fistulae). These fistulae are often associated with coronary artery stenosis and the coronary artery flow depends on maintaining a high pressure in the RV. A variety of treatment approaches are used to deal with the heterogeneity of this disorder. When the right heart is well-developed, the treatment may be much like the treatment for pulmonary stenosis, but surgical management is required when there is significant underdevelopment of any of the right heart structures. Surgery may be directed at achieving a biventricular repair or toward single ventricle palliation, depending on the severity of anatomic abnormalities.

Cardiac catheterization is performed in almost all patients with pulmonary atresia. The first goal of the procedure is to complete the diagnostic assessment: Angiography is the only way to determine the extent of coronary artery involvement. Patients with a well-developed right heart are candidates for transcatheter treatment. Innovative strategies have been developed that allow the interventionist to perforate the atretic valve plate safely using radiofrequency energy.[55,56] Thereafter, sequential balloon dilation of the valve can be performed. In developing countries where cost considerations play a major role in decision-making, perforation of the pulmonary valve with the widely available hard end of the coronary guide-wire is used as an effective and cheaper alternative.[57] Patient selection is the most important factor determining success of both the techniques. Pericardial tamponade arising from inadvertent perforation of the right ventricular outflow tract remains a major concern with both techniques. Despite adequate relief of outflow obstruction, it is not uncommon for patients to require surgical BT shunt/PDA stent for having a predictable and augmented pulmonary blood flow.[55,57,58]

Follow-up concerns in infants with pulmonary atresia vary depending on initial anatomy and the type of intervention performed. After transcatheter perforation and dilation, oxygen saturation is assessed for evidence of atrial right-to-left shunting and degree of pulmonary blood flow. Echocardiography is performed to quantify residual obstruction as well as the direction of the atrial shunt so as to know how well the RV hypertrophy and restriction is involuting following relief of obstruction. In patients without significant residual hypoxemia (SaO_2 >90% on room air), the prognosis through childhood tends to be quite good, although some will require repeat intervention for restenosis. As is true for almost all therapies for CHD, the truly long-term (decades) outcomes are not well-known and will require on-going study.

Stenting of the PDA in Duct-dependent Circulations

Ductal stenting is now emerging as a less invasive alternative to systemic-pulmonary shunt for palliating duct-dependent circulations. Compared with surgical alternatives, ductal stenting can avoid complications such as chylothorax, phrenic, or recurrent laryngeal nerve injury or PA distortion, which are well described after placement of a surgical aortopulmonary shunt. Pulmonary atresia with intact ventricular septum, TOF with pulmonary atresia, and tricuspid atresia with pulmonary atresia are some of the indications for ductal stenting. The procedure is usually performed under general anesthesia with endotracheal intubation. Intravenous prostaglandin is stopped about 4–6 hours prior to the stent delivery so as to let the duct constrict a little. This prevents migration of the stent during and immediately after the delivery. Most of the children remain on small-dose aspirin till such time the presence of the stented duct is required. The stenting can be performed from the arterial or the venous side; each having its merits and demerits. Local vascular injury, PA obstruction, ductal spasm, stent migration, acute or subacute stent thrombosis, excessive pulmonary blood flow through the stented ductus, and in-stent restenosis are some of the complications reported with this procedure. Early restenosis is common in the stented ductus, and consequently, the palliation provided by this procedure is less reliable and often of shorter duration than can be expected from a surgical aortopulmonary shunt. In a study of 51 infants with cyanotic CHD who underwent ductal stenting, Alwi and colleagues reported a freedom from reintervention rate of 89% at 6 months, which decreased to 55% at 12 months.[59] Restenosis can be due to in-stent tissue growth or due to constriction of the aortic or pulmonary end of the ductus if left uncovered by the stent.

Hypoplastic Left Heart Syndrome

Neonates with HLHS have hypoplastic left ventricle and ascending aorta secondary to various combinations of mitral and aortic valve atresia/stenosis. This results in systemic outflow obstruction and subsequent duct-dependent systemic, cerebral, and coronary circulations. It is a highly fatal disease with approximately 90% patients dying within the first month of life without any intervention. The objective of stage I palliation for HLHS or any single-ventricle physiology is to provide an unobstructed systemic outflow tract, unrestrictive interatrial communication, a controlled source of pulmonary blood flow, and a reliable source of coronary blood flow. These objectives were met with the surgical procedure described by Norwood in 1981 and by the Sano modification of the Norwood procedure described in 2001.

The first hybrid palliative approach to HLHS was reported in 1993 with surgical banding of the branch PAs, percutaneous stenting of the arterial duct and atrial septostomy or septectomy with the goal of achieving distal PA pressure <50% of the systemic pressure and a reduction in systemic oxygen saturation to approximately 80%.[60] Survival of 82% till stage II, palliation has been documented.

The complications and risks of the hybrid palliation include stent embolization, development of retrograde coarctation, and development of proximal stenosis of uncovered ductus. PA banding may result in pulmonary arterial distortion and need for angioplasty at the time of the second palliation. Balloon atrial septostomy (BAS) in these patients may result in inadequate decompression or need for repeat BAS. Postoperative management of such patients in the ICU can be quite challenging and requires a deep understanding of factors influencing systemic and PVRs.

Stenting of the Right Ventricular Outflow Tract

In selected young infants with TOF who are not candidates for corrective surgery stenting of the right ventricular outflow tract can buy time until corrective surgery can be accomplished. This is increasingly used in infants with small branch pulmonary arteries and coronary artery crossing the outflow tract as an alternative to the BT shunt. The procedure improves saturation for 4–6 months and enables growth of the pulmonary arteries.

CLOSURE OF ABNORMAL VASCULAR COMMUNICATIONS: EMBOLIZATION THERAPY

Embolization of abnormal or persistent arterial or AV structures has been available for >30 years. The embolization techniques were developed and perfected primarily by the vascular radiologists working in the abdominal viscera, gastrointestinal areas, and central nervous system, particularly in "end artery" vessels. Many materials and devices, including the patients' own clotted blood, Gelfoam, colloidal plugs, "glues", detached balloons, and coil occlusion devices, have been used for these peripheral occlusion.

The Gianturco (Cook, Inc.) coils are the most commonly used of all these occlusion devices for patients with congenital cardiac defects. These coils are made of spring wire with polyester fibers enmeshed in the coils, which are available in several sizes and multiple diameters and lengths. The coil is introduced into the delivery catheter through a straight metal "loader" as a straight wire. When it is delivered by extrusion out of the distal end of the catheter, it coils like a small "pigtail." Once delivery with this particular coil has been started, there is no way of withdrawing the coil back into the catheter. The Gianturco coil occludes the vessel by the creation of a mass of fabric and wire in which a thrombus is formed. The coil occlusion device usually is delivered into a vessel with a discrete distal narrowing, where it will fix in place and not migrate further through the vessel. Often, several coils are placed in a single vessel to achieve complete occlusion. In the absence of a distal narrowing, some other type of device for fixation such as the Amplatzer vascular plug is used. The coils are only usable in tubular structures with a distended diameter up to 7–8 mm. For larger vessels or vessels without an area of discrete stenosis, coils can be used in conjunction with other intravascular occlusion devices to complete the occlusion of the vessel. Recently, Amplatzer vascular plug is being used to occlude these abnormal communications. It has a smaller and maneuverable delivery system. In addition, the control over the plug is far superior than the coils.

Many abnormal collateral vessels or persistent surgically created systemic to pulmonary artery shunts are associated with the more complex lesions. These vessels need occlusion when systemic flow competes with normal pulmonary flow, particularly when the major defect is corrected, e.g., TOF with pulmonary atresia. These communications traditionally required surgical division during the corrective procedure or as a separate procedure. However, the same can be achieved now in the catheterization laboratory. Other lesions in which these devices may be useful are AV fistulae, including systemic, coronary-cameral, and peripheral as well as pulmonary AV fistulae. In these lesions, it is critical to identify the stenotic or "end" vessel into which the device can be fixed in order to reduce the dangers of migration to vital structure.

ROLE OF INTRAVASCULAR STENTS IN CONGENITAL HEART DISEASE

As discussed under the individual lesions, the major problems with vascular dilation procedures relate to the need for overdilation of the vessel and to restenosis of the lesions, either acutely with vessel recoil or over the long term. The use of intravascular stents has provided a definitive solution to this problem. There has been extensive favorable experience and >10 years' follow-up in patients with PA branch stenosis and systemic vein stenosis. In the single-center series of Mullins et al. at Texas Children's Hospital, >655 stents were implanted in 340 patients with PA and systemic veins stenosis. Further dilation of these stents has been successful for as long as 4 years after implant.[2] To be used in the growing patients, the stent that is used initially must be capable of being dilated to a full adult-vessel diameter.

The largest group of patients in this series had lesions involving the central pulmonary arteries in postoperative patients and postoperative central systemic vein or systemic venous baffle stenosis. Many of these stenotic veins had a totally occluded initial lumen; some of the venous channels were purposely perforated with a wire or long needle. The mean vessel diameter increased from 5 to 12 mm (with an increase in area from 20 to 113 mm^2). The success was lasting, with fewer than 0.5% showing restenosis during the period of follow-up. The number of complications from the procedure or the stents themselves was minimal. Intravascular stents in the branch pulmonary arteries and systemic veins have been demonstrated to provide definitive therapy for these lesions and offer an entirely new outlook for these previously inoperable patients.[4]

The intravascular stents are now used in many other areas such as the aorta and other intravascular stenosis. There are new developments in the area of split, "open ring" stents and biodegradable stents that would make these forms of therapy possible for the infants and small children. "Covered" stents have been used in the adult catheterization laboratories for the treatment of ruptured vessels, including aortic aneurysms. In addition, this type of covered stent has been used for transcatheter completion of a lateral tunnel Fontan procedure.[61]

PERCUTANEOUS PULMONARY VALVE IMPLANTATION

Over the last couple of decades, a great deal of experience has been gathered in percutaneous transcatheter replacement of pulmonary valves. Various valves (Medtronic, Edward-Sapien) are being used for this purpose. These are stent mounted valves delivered through the femoral vein or internal jugular vein using long sheaths. The procedure is being done mainly for those patients with RV-PA conduits who have a free PR or PS with PR due to valve degeneration. In those with a significant PS, the narrowing is relieved by balloon dilation prior to implantation of the valve.[62] This procedure is being performed in adolescents and adults who have almost completed their growth. Complications include device instability/dislodgement, coronary compression due to stent placement, branch PA obstruction, homograft rupture, stent fracture, and local vascular injury due to the large sheaths required for valve delivery (22–24 Fr). Percutaneous pulmonary valve implantation (PPVI) is associated with a significantly decreased mortality, a shorter length of hospital stay, a lower rate of 30-day readmission, and recurrent PR as compared to surgical pulmonary valve implantation (SPVI) throughout the follow-up duration.

SPVI results in a significantly lower rate of postprocedural infective endocarditis than PPVI.[63] Newer valves such as the Venus-P valve are designed to suit those with surgically corrected TOF with free PR in whom RV-PA conduit was not used and are more likely to have wider RV outflow tracts.

TRANSCATHETER REPLACEMENT OF OTHER VALVES

Transcatheter valve implantation in positions other than pulmonary valve have also been reported, although mainly in adults.[64] Presently, these systems have a larger profile making them unsuitable for pediatric patients. These valves are implanted over failed bioprosthetic valves, and hence provide the patient with a favorable less invasive alternative.

HYBRID PROCEDURES

A hybrid approach combines the best of both surgical and transcatheter therapy into a single procedure. The best example of a hybrid approach is the management of HLHS with a hybrid Norwood procedure. Other examples include device closure of muscular VSD in small infants via a midline sternotomy approach (perventricular VSD device closure), intraoperative stent implantation on branch pulmonary arteries, etc. Major advantages of hybrid approach include precise deployment of device/stent, preventing vascular injury, and avoiding adverse effects of CPB.

REFERENCES

1. Rashkind WJ, Miller W. Creation of an atrial septal defect without thoracotomy: palliative approach to complete transposition of the great arteries. JAMA. 1966;196(11):991-2.
2. Bridges ND, O'Laughlin MP, Mullins CE, Freed MD. From Moss and Adams' Heart Disease in Infants, Children and Adolescents, 6th edition. Philadelphia: Lippincott Williams and Wilkins; 2001. pp. 26-324.
3. Ashfaq M, Houston AB, Gnanapragasam JP, Lilley S, Murtagh EP. Balloon atrial septostomy under echocardiographic control: six years' experience and evaluation of the practicability of cannulation via the umbilical vein. Br Heart J. 1991;65(3):148-51.
4. Kakadekar AP, Hayes A, Rosenthal E, Huggon IC, Baker EJ, Qureshi SA, et al. Ballloon atrial septostomy in the intensive care unit under echocardiographic control: nine years' experience. Cardiol Young. 1992;2(2):175-8.
5. Saxena A, Relan J, Agarwal R, Awasthy N, Azad S, Chakrabarty M, et al. Indian guidelines for indications and timing of intervention for common congenital heart diseases: revised and updated consensus statement of the Working group on management of congenital heart diseases. Ann Pediatr Card. 2019;12(3):254-86.
6. Park SC, Neches WH, Zuberbuhler JR, Lenox CC, Mathews RA, Fricker FJ, et al. Clinical use of blade atrial septostomy. Circulation. 1978;58(4):600-06.
7. Hoffman JI, Kaplan S. The incidence of congenital heart disease. J Am Coll Cardiol. 2002; 39(12):1890-900.
8. Nugent EW, Freedom RM, Nora JJ, Ellison RC, Rowe RD, Nadas AS. Clinical course of pulmonary stenosis. Circulation. 1977;56(1): 36-71.
9. Kan JS, White RI Jr, Mitchell SE, Gardner TJ. Percutaneous balloon valvuloplasty: a new method for treating congenital pulmonary-valve stenosis. N Engl J Med. 1982;307(9):540-2.
10. McCrindle BW. Independent predictors of long-term results after balloon pulmonary valvuloplasty. Valvuloplasty and Angioplasty of Congenital Anomalies (VACA) Registry Investigators. Circulation. 1994;89(4):1751-59.
11. Zeevi B, Keane JF, Fellows KE, Lock JE. Balloon dilation of critical pulmonary stenosis in the first week of life. J Am Coll Cardiol. 1988;11(4):821-24.
12. Gournay V, Piechaud JF, Delogu A, Sidi D, Kachaner J. Balloon valvotomy for critical stenosis or atresia of pulmonary valve in newborns. J Am Coll Cardiol. 1995;26(7):1725-31.
13. Helgason H, Keane JF, Fellows KE, Kulik TJ. Balloon dilation of the aortic valve: studies in normal lambs and in children with aortic stenosis. J Am Coll Cadiol. 1987;9(4):816-22.
14. Scoller GF, Keane JF, Perry SB, Sanders SP, Lock JE. Balloon dilation of the congenital aortic valve stenosis: results and influence of technical and morphological features on outcome. Circulation. 1988;78(2):351-60.
15. Shaddy RE, Boueek MM, Sturtevant JE, Ruttenburg HD, Orsmond HS. Gradient reduction, aortic valve regurgitation and prolapse after balloon aortic valvoplasty in 32 consecutive patients with congenital aortic stenosis. J Am Coll Cardiol. 1990;16(2):451-56.
16. O'Connor BK, Beekman RH, Rocchini AP, Rosenathal A. Intermediate-term effectiveness of balloon valvuloplasty for congenital aortic stenosis: a prospective follow-up study. Circulation. 1991;84(2):732-38.
17. Reich O, Tax P, Marek J, Rázek V, Gilík J, Tomek V, et al. Long-term results of percutaneous balloon valvoplasty of congenital aortic stenosis: independent predictors of outcome. Heart. 2004:90(1):70-76.
18. Justino H, Petit CJ. Percutaneous common carotid artery access for pediatric interventional cardiac catheterization. Circ Cardiovasc Interv. 2016;9(4):e003003.
19. Egito ES, Moore P, O'Sullivan J, Colan S, Perry SB, Lock JE, et al. Transvascular balloon dilation for neonatal critical aortic stenosis: early and midterm results. J Am Coll Cardiol. 1997;29(2):442-7.
20. Sullivan PM, Rubio AE, Johnston TA, Jones TK. Long-term outcomes and re-interventions following balloon aortic valvuloplasty in pediatric patients with congenital aortic stenosis: a single-center study. Catheter Cardiovasc Interv. 2016;89(2): 288-96.
21. Joseph PK, Bhat A, Francis B, Sivasankaran S, Kumar A, Pillai VR, et al. Percutaneous transvenous mitral commissurotomy using an Inoue balloon in children with rheumatic mitral stenosis. Int J Cardiol. 1997;62(1):19-22.
22. Feltes TF, Bacha E, Beekman RH 3rd, Cheatham JP, Feinstein JA, Gomes AS, et al. On behalf of the American Heart Association Congenital Cardiac Defects Committee of the Council on Cardiovascular Disease in the Young, Council on Clinical Cardiology, and Council on Cardiovascular Radiology and Intervention. Indications for cardiac catheterization and intervention in pediatric cardiac disease: a scientific statement from the American Heart Association. Circulation. 2011;123(22):2607-52.
23. Heggon IC, Qureshi SA, Baker EJ, Tynan M. Effect of introducing balloon dilation of native aortic coarctation on overall outcome in infants and children. Am J Cardiol. 1994;73(11): 799-807.
24. Shaddy RE, Boueck MM, Sturtevant JE, Ruttenberg HD, Jaffe RB, Tani LY, et al. Comparison of angioplasty and surgery for unoperated coarctation of the aorta. Circulation. 1993;87(3): 793-99.
25. Tynan M, Finley JP, Fontes V, Hess J, Kan J. Balloon angioplasty for the treatment of native coarctation: results of valvuloplasty and angioplasty of congenital anomalies registry. Am J Cardiol. 1990;65(11):790-92.
26. Michel-Behnke I, Schranz D. Axillary artery access for cardiac interventions in newborns. Ann Pediatr Card. 2008;1(2):126-30.

27. Thanopoulos BD, Hadjinikolaou L, Konstadopoulon GN, Tsaousis GS, Tripokiadis F, Spirou P. Stent treatment for coarctation of the aorta intermediate term follow-up and technical considerations. Heart. 2000;84(1):65-70.
28. Marshall AC, Perry SB, Keane JF, Lock JE. Early results and medium-term follow-up of stent implantation for mild residual or recurrent aortic coarctation. Am Heart J. 2000;139(6): 1054-60.
29. Tyagi S, Singh S, Mukhopadhyay S, Kaul UA. Self and balloon-expandable stent implantation for severe native coarctation of aorta in adults. Am Heart J. 2003;146(5):920-8.
30. Petit CJ, Gillespie MJ, Harris MA, Seymour TL, Liu TY, Khan A, et al. Relief of branch pulmonary artery stenosis reduces pulmonary valve insufficiency in a swine model. J Thorac Cardiovasc Surg. 2009;138(2):382-9.
31. Bergersen LJ, Perry SB, Lock JE. Effect of cutting balloon angioplasty on resistant pulmonary artery stenosis. Am J Cardiol. 2003;91(2):185-9.
32. Peters B, Ewert P, Berger F. The role of stents in the treatment of congenital heart disease: current status and future perspectives. Ann Pediatr Cardiol. 2009;2(1):3-23.
33. Frazer JR, Ing FF. Stenting of stenotic or occluded iliofemoral veins, superior and inferior vena cavae in children with congenital heart disease: acute results and intermediate follow up. Catheter Cardiovasc Interv. 2009;73(2):181-8.
34. Cook AL, Prieto LR, Delaney JW, Rhodes JF. Usefulness of cutting balloon angioplasty for pulmonary vein in-stent stenosis. Am J Cardiol. 2006;98(3):407-10.
35. Mills NL, King TD. Nonoperative closure of left-to-right shunts. J Thorac Cardiovasc Surg. 1976;72(3):371-8.
36. Lopez K, Dalvi BV, Balzer D, Bass JL, Momenah T, Cao Q, et al. Transcatheter closure of large secundum atrial septal defects using the 40-mm Amplatzer septal occluder: results of an international registry. Catheter Cardiovasc Interv. 2005;66(4): 580-4.
37. Du ZD, Hijazi ZM, Kleinman CS, Silverman NH, Larntz K, Amplatzer L. Comparison between transcatheter and surgical closure of secundum atrial septal defect in children and adults: results of a multicentre nonrandomized trial. J Am Coll Cardiol. 2002;39(11):1836-44.
38. Formigari R, Di Donato RM, Mazzera E, Carotti A, Rinelli G, Parisi F, et al. Minimally invasive or interventional repair of atrial septal defects in children: experience in 171 cases and comparasion with conventional strategies. J Am Coll Cardiol. 2001,37(6): 1707-12.
39. Dalvi BL, Jain SA. Atrial septal defect: step-by-step catheter closure. J Struct Heart Dis. 2016;2(1):15-32.
40. Krumsdorf U, Keppeler P, Horvth K, Zadan E, Schrader R, Sievert H. Catheter closure of atrial septal defects and patent foramen ovale in patients with an atrial septal aneurysm using different devices. J Interv Cardiol. 2001;14(1):49-55.
41. Weidman WH, Blount Jr SG, DuShane JW, Gersony WM, Hayes CJ, Nadas AS. Clinical course in ventricular septal defect. Circulation. 1977;56(1S):156-69.
42. Bacha EA, Hijazi ZM, Cao QL, Abdulla R, Starr JP, Quinones J, et al. Hybrid pediatric cardiac surgery. Pediatr Cardiol. 2005;26(4): 315-22.
43. Morray BH. Ventricular septal defect closure devices, techniques, and outcomes. Intervent Cardiol Clin. 2019;8(1):1-10.
44. Thanopolus BD, Tsaousis GS, Konstadopoulon GN, Zarayelyan AG. Transcatheter closure of muscular ventricular septal defects with Amplatzer ventricular septal defect occluder: initial clinical applications in children. J Am Coll Cardiol. 1999;33(5):1395-459.
45. Yang R, Kong XQ, Sheng YH, Zhou L, Xu D, Yong YH, et al. Risk factors and outcomes of post-procedure heart blocks after transcatheter device closure of perimembranous ventricular septal defect. J Am Coll Cardiol Interv. 2012; 5(4):422-7.
46. Holzer R, Balzer D, Lock K, Hijazi ZM. Device closure of muscular ventricular septal defects using Amplatzer muscular ventricular septal defect occluder: immediate and midterm results of a US registry. J Am Coll Cardiol. 2004; 43(7):1257-63.
47. Bridges ND, Perry SB, Keane JF, Goldstein SA, Mandell V, Mayer Jr JE, et al. Preoperative transcatheter closure of congenital muscular ventricular septal defects. N Engl J Med. 1991; 324(19):1312-17.
48. Arora R, Trehan V, Thakur AK, Mehta V, Sengupta PP, Nigam M. Transcatheter closure of congenital muscular ventricular septal defect. J Interv Cardiol. 2002;17(2):109-15.
49. Haddad RN, Daou LS, Saliba ZS. Percutaneous closure of restrictive-type perimembranous ventricular septal defect using the new KONAR multifunctional occluder: mid-term outcomes of the first middle-eastern experience. Catheter Cardiovasc Interv. 2020;96(3):E295-302.
50. Magee AG, Huggon IC, Seed PT, Qureshi SA, Tynan M. Transcatheter coil occlusion of the arterial duct: results of the European Registry. Eur Heart J. 2001;22(19):1817-21.
51. Ebeid MR, Masura J, Hijazi ZM. Early experience with the Amplatzer ductal occluder for closure of the persistently patent ductus arteriosus. J Interv Cardiol. 2001;14(1):33-6.
52. Kumar RK, Anil SR, Kannan BR, Philip A, Sivakumar K. Bioptome assisted coil occlusion of moderate-large patent ductus arteriosus in infants and small children. Catheter Cardiovasc Interv. 2004;62(2):266-71.
53. Bhole V, Miller P, Mehta C, Stumper O, Reinhardt Z, De Giovanni JV. Clinical evaluation of the new Amplatzer duct occluder II for patent arterial duct occlusion. Catheter Cardiovasc Interv. 2009;74(5):762-9.
54. Almeida-Jones M, Tang NY, Reddy A, Zahn E. Overview of transcatheter patent ductus arteriosus closure in preterm infants. Congenit Heart Dis. 2019;14:60-64.
55. Humpl T, Soderberg B, MeCrindle BW, Nykanen DG, Freedom RM, Williams WG, et al. Percutaneous balloon valvotomy in pulmonary atresia with intact ventricular septum: impact on patient care. Circulation. 2003;108(7):826-32.
56. Justo RN, Nykanen DG, Williams WG, Freedom RM, Benson LN. Transcatheter perforation of the right ventricular outflow tract as initial therapy for pulmonary valve atresia and intact ventricular septum in the newborn. Cathet Cardiovasc Diagn. 1997;40(4): 408-13.
57. Pinto RJ, Dalvi BV. Transcatheter guidrewire perforation of the pulmonary valve as a pallative procedure in pulmonary atresia with intact interventricular septum. Indian Heart J. 2004;56(6):661-3.
58. Ovaert C, Qureshi SA, Rosenthal E, Baker EJ, Tynan M. Growth of the right ventricle after successful transcatheter pulmonary valvotomy in neonates and infants with pulmonary atresia and intact ventricular septum. J Thorac Cardiovasc Surg. 1998;115(5):1055-62.
59. Alwi M. Stenting the ductus arteriosus: case selection, technique and possible complications. Ann Pediatr Card. 2008;1(1):38-45.
60. Gibbs JL, Wren C, Watterson KG, Hunter S, Hamilton JR. Stenting of the arterial duct combined with banding of the pulmonary arteries and atrial septectomy or septostomy: a new approach to palliation for the hypoplastic left heart syndrome. Br Heart J. 1993;69(6): 551-5.
61. Metton O, Calvaruso D, Stos B, Ali WB, Boudjemline Y. A new surgical technique for transcatheter Fontan completion. Eur J Cardiothorac Surg. 2011;39(1):81-5.
62. Giugno L, Faccini A, Carminati M. Percutaneous pulmonary valve implantation. Korean Circ J. 2020;50(4):302-16.
63. Zhou Y, Xiong T, Bai P, Chu C, Dong N. Clinical outcomes of transcatheter versus surgical pulmonary valve replacement: a meta-analysis. J Thorac Dis. 2019;11(12):5343-51.
64. Webb JG, Wood DA, Ye J, Gurvitch R, Masson JB, Rodés-Cabau J, et al. Transcatheter valve-in-valve implantation for failed bioprosthetic heart valves. Circulation. 2010;121(16):1848-57.

15 CHAPTER

Principles of Pediatric Cardiac Surgery

Biswa Panda, Balaji Srimurugan

INTRODUCTION

Congenital heart surgery, now in its eighth decade of evolution, has seen tremendous progress in diagnostic precision, technical and infrastructure improvisation, skill modifications, and postoperative care. There has been a continuous growth in knowledge in these fields in the last 30–40 years with dramatic improvements in outcome. The cohesiveness of the team of caregivers has seen a direct impact on the patient outcome and efficiency of the system.

In developing countries, congenital heart diseases (CHDs) are a major cause of mortality and morbidity. Most congenital heart defects are amenable to surgical or catheter-based correction or palliation. In experienced centers, the current era mortality after common congenital heart defects is <3%. Hence, heart surgery when indicated, should be recommended without hesitation.

HISTORICAL ASPECTS

Surgery on heart was a dreaded thought less than a century ago and was known for professional death of the surgeon. In 1937, Robert Gross successfully performed the first patent ductus arteriosus (PDA) ligation in a 7-year-old child. Alfred Blalock, with the help from Helen Taussig, in 1944, performed the first Blalock–Taussig (BT) shunt (Blue Baby Surgery) which generated the great interest among medical fraternity. Performance of the first successful open-heart surgery using a heart lung machine in 1953 changed the earlier misconceptions and perceptions, and interest towards the treatment of heart defects grew leaps and bounds resulting in rapid evolution of surgical techniques.

COMMON CONGENITAL HEART DISEASES IN CLINICAL PRACTICE

For ease of understanding, a surgical classification and incidence of the defects is compiled and listed in **Table 1**.

ROLE OF PREOPERATIVE CARE AND OPTIMIZATION IN THE IMPROVEMENT OF SURGICAL OUTCOME

In the current era, weight and age are no more a limitation for heart surgery. Newborn babies safely undergo complex open-heart surgeries with good outcome. However, in smaller babies, a higher morbidity and abundant resource consumption is expected. The experience and skill of the treating team and the support system are important modulators of outcome (**Fig. 1**).

A better outcome is expected in a stable child, without inotropes, without active infection, and with the satisfactory organ functions. Hence, when a baby comes with multiple comorbidities, it is important to stabilize the baby before exposing to a major stress of surgery and cardiopulmonary bypass (CPB). Inotropes such as dobutamine help in balancing the hemodynamics and ensuring adequate tissue perfusion. In neonates with closing ducts, prostaglandin E1 helps in patency of the PDA and stabilizing patients with duct dependent systemic and pulmonary circulation.

Any suspicion of sepsis must be confirmed by culture and sensitivity tests and appropriate antibiotics must be instituted. Unless emergency, surgery should be deferred for 2–3 weeks after infective episode. During this period, the inflammatory response of the organs get normalized preventing a flare up following a CPB run. Occult infections of the urinary tract, otitis media, and dental caries should be ruled out. During waiting period, a nutritional rehabilitation plan should be considered.

In certain situations, emergency surgery needs to be done in spite of risk factors [e.g., obstructed total anomalous pulmonary venous connection (TAPVC), pulmonary atresia/stenosis with uncontrolled spells, prostaglandin nonresponsive PDA in severe coarctation of aorta (CoA) or interrupted arch, etc.]. In such patients, a stormy postoperative course is anticipated.

TABLE 1: Surgical classification of congenital heart defects.

	Primary physiology	*Cardiac defect*	*Approximate incidence*
Acyanotic	Left-to-right shunts	Ventricular septal defect (VSD)	20%
		Atrial septal defect	10–12%
		Patent ductus arteriosus	10–12%
		Atrioventricular (AV) septal defect	2–3%
		Aortopulmonary window	0.5–1%
	Left-sided obstructive lesions	Coarctation of aorta	8–10%
		Congenital aortic stenosis	10%
		Congenital mitral stenosis	1%
		Interrupted aortic arch	1%
Cyanotic (two ventricle repair feasible)	Reduced pulmonary blood flow	Tetralogy of Fallot and variants*	10%
		Severe pulmonic stenosis (PS) with atrial communication	5–8%
		Pulmonary atresia with intact ventricular septum	5%
		Ebstein anomaly	0.5%
	Increased pulmonary blood flow	Transposition	5%
		Total anomalous pulmonary venous return	2%
		Persistent truncus arteriosus	1%
Cyanotic: Single ventricle physiology	Reduced pulmonary blood flow	• Single ventricle (double-inlet left or right ventricle) with pulmonic stenosis or atresia • Tricuspid atresia with restrictive VSD or severe PS	<5%
	Increased pulmonary blood flow	• Single ventricle with no PS • Hypoplastic left heart syndrome	<3%

*TOF variants include tetralogy of Fallot with pulmonary atresia, double-outlet right ventricle, corrected transposition with VSD and PS, AV septal defect with PS.

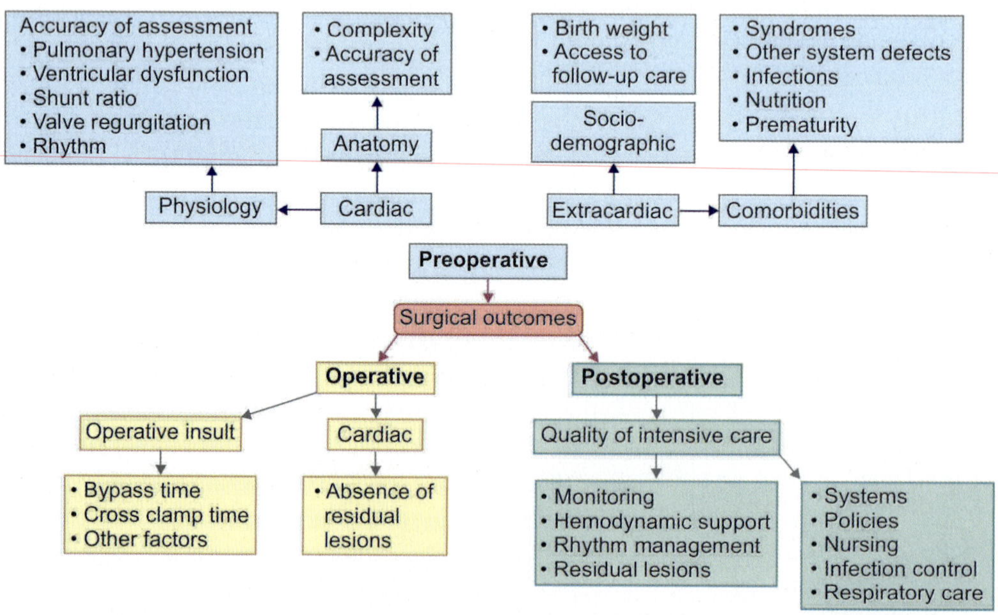

Fig. 1: The figure demonstrates that pediatric heart surgery is a complex endeavor and results are often determined by a number of preoperative, operative, and postoperative factors. Optimization of each of these elements is needed to ensure a good outcome.

Immunization and Heart Surgery

Children with CHD should receive immunization as per schedule. Cardiac surgery need not be deferred if a child has recent history of immunization. Patients with asplenia undergoing elective surgeries need immunization against Gram-positive cocci. Following heart surgery, usually an interval of 3–4 weeks is considered for immunization.

ROLE OF COHESIVE MULTIDISCIPLINARY TEAM APPROACH IN IMPROVING OUTCOME AFTER CARDIAC SURGERY

The optimal care of pediatric patients with complex CHD requires collaboration and a multidisciplinary team approach from surgery, cardiology, anesthesiology, critical care, and other medical subspecialties (**Flowchart 1**). It is essential that an effectively functioning cardiac team be established in the care of complex CHD patients to reduce their morbidity and mortality. The vital components of a highly effective team not only include clinical excellence throughout all disciplines but must include excellence in leadership, trust, accountability, respect, and a shared mental model of the heart center's mission and values. If these components are maximized, the quality of patient care excels, optimizing the lives of children with CHD.

OPEN HEART SURGERY VERSUS CLOSED HEART SURGERY

Cardiac surgeries are broadly classified into two divisions, open and closed heart surgeries. Any cardiac or extracardiac procedure that requires the help of CPB is called open heart surgery and if CPB is not utilized, it is known as closed-heart surgery. This is in contrast to the popular myth that heart chambers must be opened in order to be categorized as open-heart surgery. Common open-heart surgeries are atrial septal defect (ASD) closure, ventricular septal defect (VSD) closure, tetralogy of Fallot (TOF) repair, TAPVC repair, etc. and common closed heart surgeries are PDA ligation, coarctation repair, pulmonary artery (PA) banding, etc. Few surgeries can be either open heart or closed heart as per the clinical situation, example BT shunt, bidirectional Glenn shunt, etc.

SURGICAL APPROACHES FOR HEART SURGERY

Median sternotomy through a vertical incision form the suprasternal notch to the xiphisternum is the most common route to access the heart. It provides good exposure of the heart as well as great vessels and is very convenient for instituting the CPB. Left posterolateral thoracotomy is routinely used for accessing the distal arch, proximal descending aorta, or the left PA (PDA ligation, CoA repair, BT shunt, or Potts shunt). Left anterolateral thoracotomy gives access to left ventricular (LV), right ventricular (RV) surface, and the PA (PA band and pacemaker insertion). Right thoracotomy helps for minimally invasive surgeries [ASD closure and mitral valve replacement (MVR)] and surgeries involving right PA (BT shunt). Limited sternotomies are useful in selected surgeries. **Figures 2A to C** show the common surgical approaches for cardiac surgery.

ROLE OF CARDIOPULMONARY BYPASS IN CARDIAC SURGERY

Cardiopulmonary bypass is a technique by which a mechanical device (heart–lung machine) temporarily takes over the function of heart and lungs, so that, that defect in the heart can be repaired without affecting the cardiac output or oxygenation. The components of the CPB system are (1) heart–lung machine which runs the various components of the circuit, (2) oxygenator which performs gas exchange, (3) circuit tubing which receive blood from the patient and delivers back, (4) venous reservoir which maintains the minimum level in the process, (5) hemoconcentrator which removes the extra fluid, (6) filters which remove the air and particulate materials, (7) hemotherm which helps in temperature regulation, and (8) cardioplegia delivery system (**Fig. 3**).

Flowchart 1: Elements and personnel that constitute a comprehensive pediatric cardiac program. Not all elements may be present in every center and adaptations are necessary.

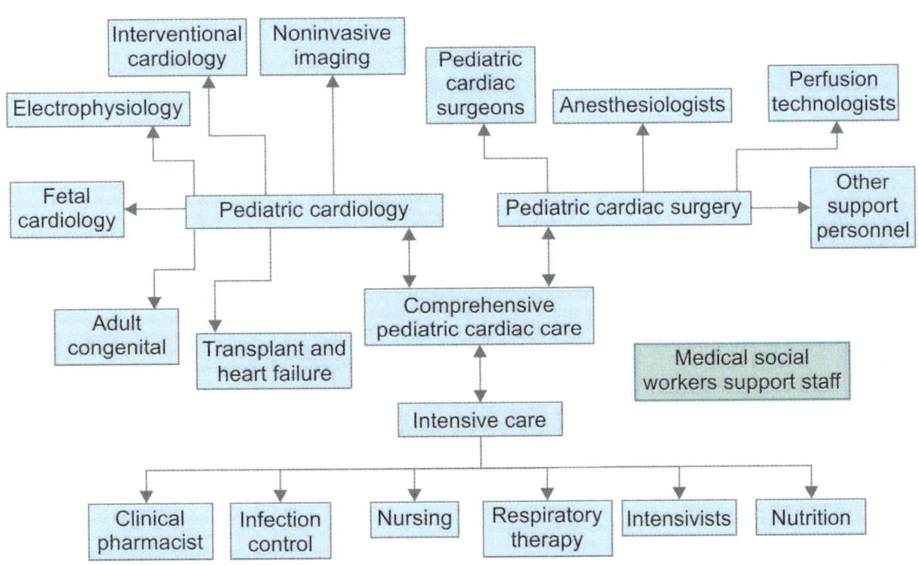

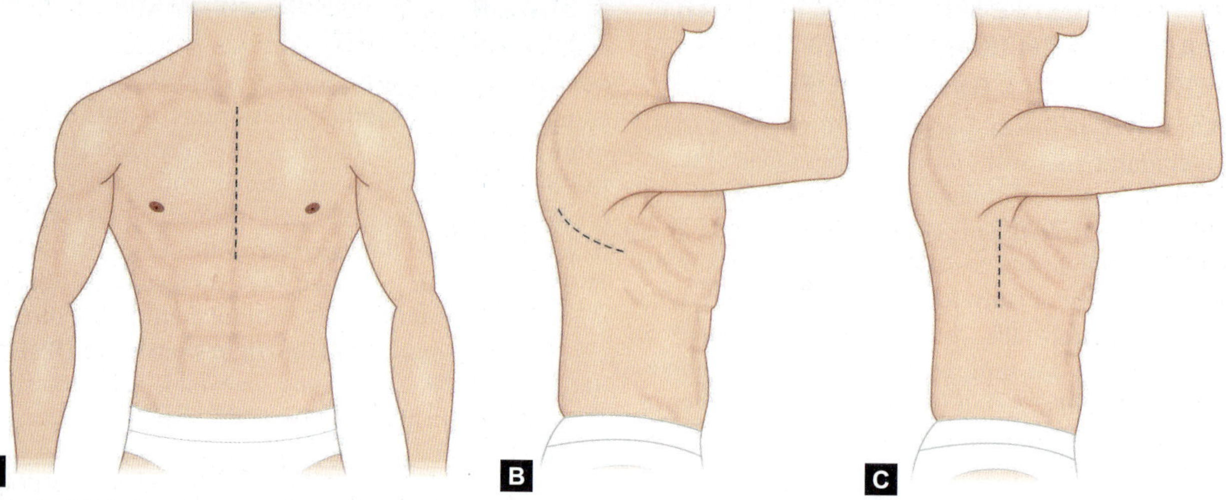

Figs. 2A to C: (A) Median sternotomy (most commonly used approach); (B) Posterolateral thoracotomy; (C) Axillary thoracotomy (minimally invasive).

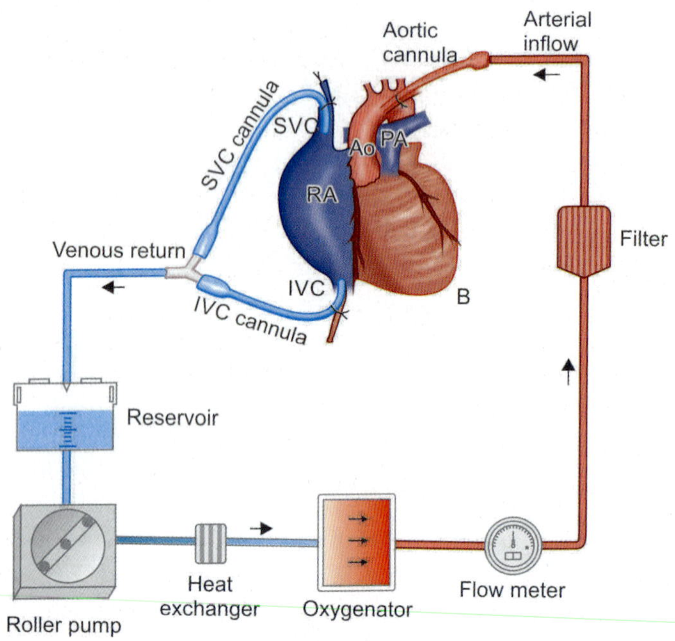

Fig. 3: Schematic diagram of a simplified cardiopulmonary bypass circuit.

During CPB, the venous cannulas and tubing siphon the deoxygenated blood, which collects in the venous reservoir. A roller or centrifugal pump sends this blood to the oxygenator for gas exchange after which the arterial tubing and cannulas return the blood back to the aorta. A minimum amount of fluid (mixture of blood and/or crystalloid solution and electrolytes) need to be maintained in the CPB circuit and is called priming fluid. The cardioplegia is a potassium-rich solution, when injected into the coronary arteries through the aortic root, produces diastolic cardiac arrest. Cessation of cardiac activity gives an access to the interior of the heart for repair of the defects. Suction tubing called vents are used to keep the bloodless field for good visibility as well as for avoiding distension of cardiac chambers. Preservation of cardiac function, also known as "myocardial protection" is an important key to a good outcome. Hypothermia, cessation of electrical activity by periodic administration of cardioplegia, and avoidance of distension of heart during surgery are as equally important as a flawless surgical repair of the defect.

Cardiopulmonary bypass, though an integral part of open-heart surgery, has many adverse effects on the body. The exposure of the blood particles to the extracorporeal, nonendothelized surface of the CPB circuit exacerbates a systemic inflammatory response syndrome (SIRS) with capillary leak. The neonates and low-weight infants, with long CPB time, this response can lead to multiorgan dysfunction. Neurological dysfunction (air embolism), acute respiratory distress syndrome (ARDS), sepsis, and coagulation disorders are common complications of CPB. Over the last two decades, the safety with CPB has significantly improved.

DEEP HYPOTHERMIA AND CIRCULATORY ARREST

Hypothermia is an essential tool for reducing the metabolic demand of the body, thus improving the organ safety. As per the temperature range, hypothermia is categorized as mild (32–35°C), moderate (28–32°C) and profound (<32°C). With a deep hypothermia, the circulation can be reduced (low flow perfusion) or stopped for few minutes [deep hypothermic circulatory arrest (DHCA)] to perform aortic arch surgery or complex intracardiac repair in neonate or infant. The impact of hypoperfusion on the brain is dependent on the degree of hypothermia and duration of circulatory arrest. In selected surgeries involving the aortic arch, the blood flow to the brain is maintained, but the body circulation is stopped (selective antegrade cerebral perfusion). This allows a longer time of safety for executing complex procedure without causing brain damage.

PALLIATIVE VERSUS CORRECTIVE SURGERY

A surgical technique, which achieves the anatomic continuity and physiologic correction of the circulation, is known as a corrective procedure (e.g., PDA ligation and VSD closure). In a palliative procedure, neither anatomic nor physiologic normalcy is achieved, but the surgery targets to improve the hemodynamic and prepares the child for the next stage definitive repair (e.g., BT shunt and PA banding). Palliative surgery is performed in a child if the anatomy, age, or weight does not allow a single stage corrective surgery. Most palliative surgeries are performed in patients with single ventricle physiology. In certain situations, the surgery achieves normal physiology, but the anatomy remains abnormal. Such operations are called physiologic correction [e.g., Senning operation, simple closure of the VSD in a patient with corrected transposition of the great arteries (CTGA) and VSD].

WHY SURGICAL TIMING IS IMPORTANT FOR OPTIMUM RESULTS?

In children with increased pulmonary blood flow, delay in surgery leads to repeated life-threatening chest infections and failure to thrive. With time, the pulmonary vascular disease becomes established and the child becomes inoperable. In cyanotic children, there can be life-threatening hypoxia and the survivors face hypoxic organ damage.

Surgery before the recommended age unduly exposes the child to CPB. The small size of the chest cavity and heart creates a challenge for surgical access and exposure. Also, there is a need for a heightened expertise for anaesthetic and intensive care and management of smaller children, than older children with the same defect. In certain diseases, if operated early, frequent reoperations are needed as the child quickly outgrows small-sized prosthetic materials that were used in the first surgery.

Table 2 lists the preferred age of surgery for common congenital heart defects.

SURGICAL STRATEGIES OF COMMON ACYANOTIC HEART DISEASES

Atrial Septal Defect

Patent foramen ovales (PFOs) and small ASDs, which do not cause RV volume overload, do not require any intervention. Asymptomatic unoperated patients usually develop symptoms of mild functional impairment or arrhythmias in the second or third decade of life. **Figures 4A to C** demonstrate individual types of ASD. For ostium secundum defects,

TABLE 2: Preferred age for surgery in common congenital heart diseases.

Atrial septal defect closure	2–4 years
Ventricular septal defect closure	3–6 months
Partial anomalous pulmonary venous communication repair	2–4 years
Ligation of the patent arterial duct	3–6 months; earlier if indicated; preterm babies require early surgery
Coarctation repair	• Infants and children—on diagnosis • Neonatal—emergency surgery
Tetralogy of Fallot repair	5–9 months
Repair of the atrioventricular septal defect	3–6 months
Transposition with intact ventricular septum	• Arterial switch operation—0–4 weeks • Senning operation—4–6 months
Transposition with ventricular septal defect	Arterial switch + VSD closure—2–8 weeks
Transposition with ventricular septal defect and pulmonic stenosis	Rastelli/Réparation à l'Etage Ventriculaire (REV)/Nikaidoh procedure—1–2 years
Bidirectional Glenn shunt	6–9 months
Fontan operation	4–6 years
Truncus and aortopulmonary (AP) window repair	1–3 months; AP window may dictate earlier operation
Pulmonary artery banding	4–8 weeks
Blalock–Taussig shunt	Emergency as per situation
Total anomalous pulmonary venous return	• Obstructed—emergency upon diagnosis • Nonobstructed—1–2 months

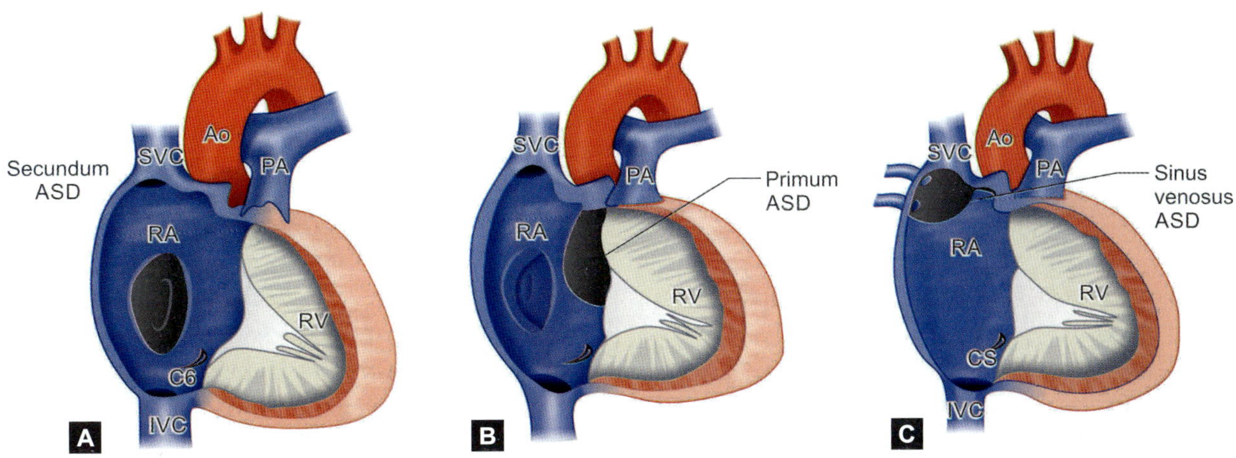

Figs. 4A to C: Illustration depicting the types of atrial septal defects: (A) Ostium secundum ASD; (B) Ostium primum ASD; (C) Sinus venosus ASD. (Ao: aorta; CS: coronary sinus; IVC: inferior vena cava; PA: pulmonary artery; RA: right atrium; RV: right ventricle; SVC: superior vena cava)

ASD device closure is preferred whenever the size and the location of the defect is appropriate for this technique. In small children and larger defects with absent rims, surgical ASD closure is recommended. Autologous pericardium is the patch material of choice. Sinus venosus defects with anomalous pulmonary venous drainage require surgical patch closure and rechanneling of the pulmonary veins to the left atrium. Ostium primum ASDs are managed by patch closure of the defect and repair of associated mitral or tricuspid leaflet defects.

Atrial septal defect closure is usually performed though a standard median sternotomy and CPB. Heart is stopped with cardioplegia and right atrium opened to suture the patch to the ASD margin. Cosmetic approaches such as ministernotomy, limited posterolateral thoracotomy (LPT), right anterolateral thoracotomy, right axillary approach, and port access surgery are feasible in suitable candidates.

Atrial septal defect closure is a low-risk surgery with very low operative mortality (<0.5%) and morbidity. Closure of an ostium primum septal defect carries with it a small risk of heart block. Recurrent pericardial effusion can be a challenge in few children.

Ventricular Septal Defect

The decision and optimal timing of VSD closure is based on the size of the defect, age of the patient, symptoms, and location of the defect. The VSDs are classified as small, moderate, and large on the basis of the size and resultant pulmonary blood flow. The complete anatomical information about the size and the location of the defect (perimembranous, subaortic, subpulmonic, and muscular) is mandatory prior to surgery (**Fig. 5**). This helps in the management of CPB strategy, chamber approach to access the VSD, and planning of the surgical technique. Information about presence of multiple VSDs is helpful in avoiding residual intracardiac shunts and thus improving surgical outcome.

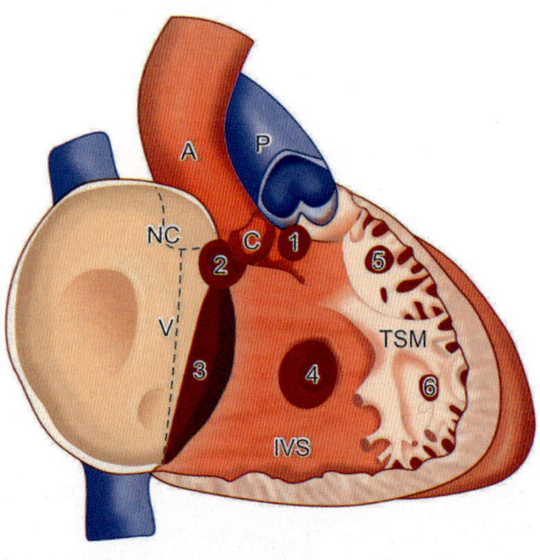

Fig. 5: Schematic representation of the position of ventricular septal defects (VSD) as seen from the right ventricular side. (1) Subpulmonic VSD, also known as doubly committed or juxta-arterial VSD; (2) perimembranous/conoventricular VSD; (3) inlet septal VSD; (4) posterior muscular; (5) outlet muscular; (6) apical muscular.

The standard approach is through median sternotomy and CPB. After cardiac arrest, the VSD can be approached in different ways as per the location. The most common type, perimembranous VSDs, are approached by opening the right atrium and retracting the tricuspid valve. The commonly used patch materials for VSD closure are polytetrafluoroethylene (PTFE), dacron, pericardium, and bovine pericardium. The patch material is sewed to the VSD margin with polypropylene sutures using either continuous or interrupted stitches. Attention is needed in the posteroinferior margin to avoid injury to the conduction bundle and the superior margin to protect the aortic valve. The midmuscular, posterior muscular, and inlet muscular defects can be easily accessed and closed through the tricuspid valve approach. Apical muscular VSDs are sometimes difficult to approach from the tricuspid valve and may require a limited right ventriculotomy for visualization. Subpulmonic VSDs are easily closed through the PA. Subaortic VSDs can be accessed from the tricuspid valve or the aorta or both depending on the extent of the VSD.

Operative mortality for the VSD closure is <1%. However, presence of multiple comorbidities, long-term preoperative ventilation and hospital stay, infections, and airways problems affect the outcome significantly. Heart block is a potential risk and is seen in 1% of cases. Inlet VSDs are at risk of heart block due to close proximity of the bundle to the VSD patch.

Children presenting late with elevated pulmonary vascular resistance and borderline operability, benefit from a small shunt between the left and right chambers of the heart in the form of VSD fenestration or VSD flap valve or PFO. This serves as a "pop-off" for the hypertensive right ventricle, which can be life-saving during episodes of pulmonary hypertensive crisis. Modern pulmonary vasodilators such as sildenafil, milrinone, and inhaled nitric oxide are the helpful in the postoperative management in selected patients.

In children with subarterial VSDs, the aortic cusp prolapse into the VSD results in cusp deformity and aortic regurgitation. Even if the left-to-right shunt is not significant, these children need early surgery to avoid progressive aortic valve damage. In the presence of moderate-to-severe aortic regurgitation, the aortic valve is repaired or replaced at the time of VSD closure. In patients with small VSDs, the risk of infective endocarditis is no longer an indication for VSD closure.

Patent Ductus Arteriosus

In infants, surgery is advised for hemodynamically significant PDAs if catheter intervention is not possible. In neonates with large PDA, surgery (PDA ligation) is the treatment of choice. The approach is through the left posterolateral thoracotomy by opening the fourth intercostal space. The lung is retracted and PDA isolated. PDA can be ligated, clipped or divided as per the surgical team's preference. PDA ligation, though carries 1–2% risk of residual patency, avoids the possibility of catastrophic hemorrhage associated with PDA division and suturing.

In children, where PDA is associated with other cardiac defects such as VSD and atrioventricular (AV) canal defect, the approach is through the median sternotomy and PDA is ligated during the correction of the associated major intracardiac anomaly. Aortic arch assessment is mandatory before decision for PDA ligation. Sometimes, the PDA can be extremely large and does not have a stump and is called "window ductus." These PDAs are closed from the sternotomy approach and with the help of CPB.

Patent ductus arteriosus interruption is a relatively low-risk procedure and mortality risk is <1%. PDA ligation in preterm babies and neonates carries a higher mortality and morbidity risk due to associated comorbidities and the proneness to infection in such candidates.

"Park and Ride concept of PDA ligation" is a term used when the surgical team does the PDA ligation in the neonatal intensive care unit (NICU) itself. In preterm, premature babies with low body weight, merely the transfer of the baby to the operation theater (OT) and back can precipitate life-threatening instability. In such situations, the surgery is done bedside itself without much mobilization of the baby.

Atrioventricular Septal Defect

The surgery for AV septal defect is planned as per the anatomical type. The principles of surgery aim to eliminate the intracardiac shunting (VSD and ASD) and repair of the AV valves.

- *Complete AV septal defect*: The ideal age for surgery in these patients is between 3 and 6 months. However, with Down syndrome, surgery is planned around 3 months of age, before the pulmonary vascular changes progress. AV septal defects can sometimes be quite complex and may not allow easy correction. These complex forms are often associated with heterotaxy and situs ambiguous. Standard approach is through midline sternotomy and CPB and cardioplegic arrest. The right atrium is opened and anatomy inspected for planning for the most suitable positioning of the VSD and ASD patch. The commonly used two-patch repair involves closure of the VSD with a Gore-Tex or Dacron patch and then ASD closure with autologous pericardium (**Fig. 6**). The positioning of the VSD patch is the most critical step of this operation as it decides the orifice sizes of the mitral and tricuspid components. The AV node is located posteroinferior to the AV canal and can be injured by the posteroinferior sutures of the VSD and ASD patch. The mitral and the tricuspid valves are repaired to optimize valve function. The other techniques used are "modified single patch repair" and "single patch repair."

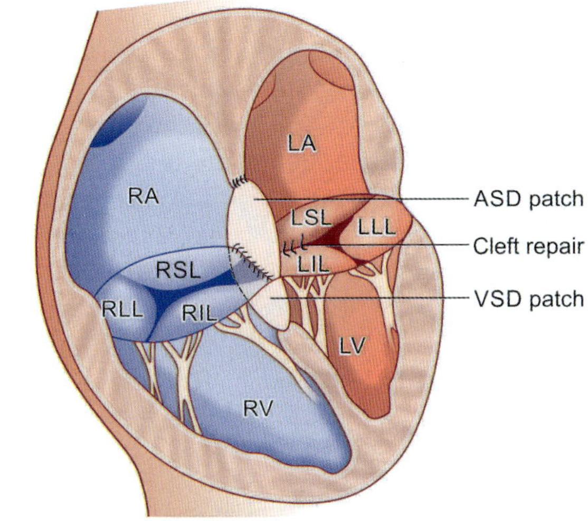

Fig. 6: Schematic illustration showing a surgically corrected complete atrioventricular septal defect.
(ASD: atrial septal defect; LA: left atrium; LIL: left inferior leaflet; LLL: left lateral leaflet; LSL: left superior leaflet; LV: left ventricle; RA: right atrium; RIL: right inferior leaflet; RLL; right lateral leaflet; RSL: right superior leaflet; RV: right ventricle; VSD: ventricular septal defect)

- *Intermediate AV septal defect*: The ideal age for surgery is between 1 and 2 years. Children with severe mitral regurgitation become symptomatic, needing early surgery. In this anomaly, the VSD component is small and is partially closed by the chordae of the bridging leaflets. The surgical technique involves the use of an autologous pericardial patch to close the VSD as well as the large ASD. Interrupted sutures in the supraventricular crest (VSD margin) eliminate the incidence of residual shunts. The cleft in the anterior mitral leaflet is repaired by interrupted or continuous sutures to achieve competency.
- *Partial AV septal defect*: These patients clinically behave like ostium secundum ASDs and operated around 2–3 years of age. The large ostium primum ASD is closed with autologous pericardial patch. The inferior margin is formed by the supraventricular crest and contains chordae from the mitral and tricuspid components as well as the conduction bundle and needs special attention to avoid heart block. The cleft in the anterior mitral leaflet is closed to achieve competency.

The surgical mortality is <5% following complete AV canal repair and <2% for partial and intermediate AV canal repair. The incidence of postoperative complete heart block following AV canal repair is around 2%. Children with complete AV canal can have pulmonary hypertensive crisis resulting in stormy postoperative recovery.

Strict follow-up is advised in these patients as progressive left AV valve regurgitation requiring reoperation (repair/replacement) is seen in a significant number of patients. Children presenting late and with borderline operability can show progressive pulmonary hypertensive disease even after a successful surgery.

Aortopulmonary Window

The left-to-right shunt resulting from AP window leads to excessive pulmonary blood flow and pulmonary arterial hypertension. These children present in early infancy with features of congestive heart failure and failure to thrive. In larger defects, as the pulmonary bed is exposed to systemic pressure, the pulmonary vascular resistance progresses and the child becomes inoperable toward the later part of infancy. The ideal age for AP window repair is between 1 and 3 months of age.

The standard approach is through the median sternotomy and CPB. Once the heart is arrested with cardioplegia, the communication between the aorta and PA is divided and the resultant defects are closed with two separate patches, thus separating the systemic from pulmonary circulation (two-patch technique). Sandwich technique is an alternative method where only the anterior part of the communication is opened, the patch is sutured to the posterior, superior, and anterior margin of the window. The anterior margin of the patch is incorporated in the anterior suture line thus completing the septation. In children with small communication, a surgical ligation can be attempted. During patch implantation, the origin of the left coronary artery should be protected.

Current era surgical mortality ranges between 1 and 2%. Postoperative pulmonary hypertension can be a concern during recovery. Reoperation is rare after AP window repair.

SURGICAL STRATEGIES OF COMMON CYANOTIC HEART DISEASES

Tetralogy of Fallot

Diagnosis of TOF is an indication of surgery and surgical time is planned on the basis of age of the patient, symptoms, and the PA anatomy. The ideal age for TOF repair (total correction) is around 6–9 months of age. In very symptomatic patients with frequent spells, surgery can be done as early as 3 months. Although TOF repair can be performed in the neonatal period or early infancy, it is not routinely favored as this can be resource consuming and may not give equivalent outcome. In such high-risk cyanotic patients, a palliative BT shunt helps in improving oxygenation and salvaging the child. An elective TOF repair is planned after the child becomes 6–9 months of age.

The goal of TOF repair is (1) closure of the VSD, (2) relief of right ventricular outflow tract (RVOT) obstruction, (3) preservation of the competence of pulmonary and tricuspid valve, and (4) protection of the myocardial function (**Figs. 7A and B**). The surgery is performed through midline sternotomy and hypothermic CPB. After cardioplegic arrest, the right atrium is opened to expose the VSD through the tricuspid valve. The VSD is closed with a polytetrafluoroethylene (PTFE) (Gore-Tex), Dacron patch or pericardium with special attention to avoid damage to the conduction bundle and the aortic valve. The orientation of the VSD patch routes the LV to the aorta eliminating the aortic override. The hypertrophied septal and parietal bands in the infundibular region are divided either from the tricuspid valve approach or by a right ventriculotomy incision. If only pulmonary valvar stenosis is the culprit, a simple commissurotomy form the infundibular or PA incision relieves the obstruction preserving the valve competency. However, hypoplastic pulmonary annulus requires interruption and reconstruction with a transannular patch. Extensive incision in the RVOT creates a good outflow, but creates a profound pulmonary regurgitation affecting early and postoperative outcomes. Hence, a limited incision in the RVOT is advised and small residual gradient is accepted. In suitable anatomy, attempt is made to create a competent pulmonary valve using monocusp technique or anterior

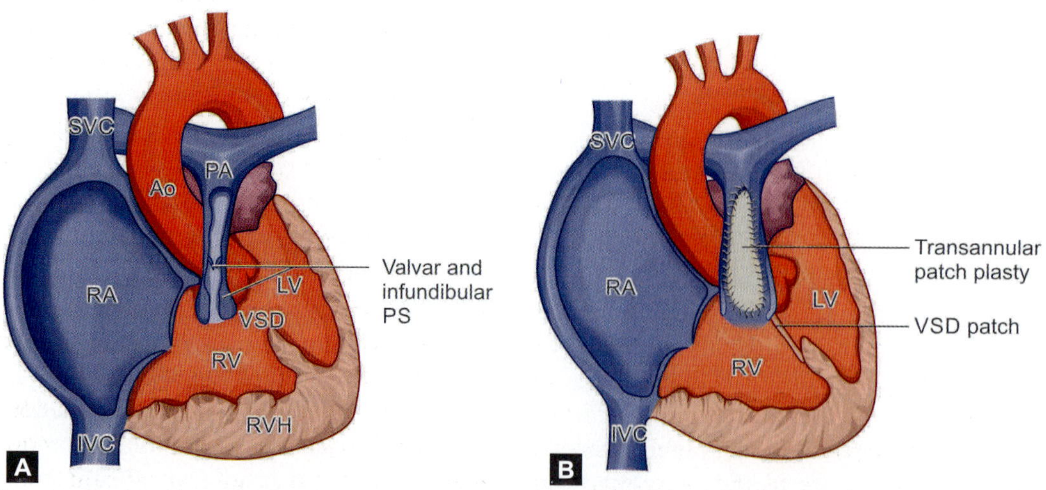

Figs. 7A and B: (A) Uncorrected tetralogy of Fallot; (B) Surgically corrected tetralogy of Fallot; depicting closure of the ventricular septal defect, relief of right ventricular outflow obstruction with infundibular muscle resection and transannular patch plasty.
(Ao: aorta; IVC: inferior vena cava; PA: pulmonary artery; PS: pulmonary stenosis; RA: right atrium; RV: right ventricle; RVH: right ventricular hypertrophy; SVC: superior vena cava; VSD: ventricular septal defect)

leaflet augmentation (Sung technique). Patch materials such as autologous pericardium, PTFE membrane, and bovine pericardium are used for the valve reconstruction. Associated problems such as multiple VSDs, PDA, and branch PA stenosis are addressed during the repair. In patients with prior BT shunt, the shunt divided and ends sutured in the beginning of the procedure, once the CPB is established.

Intraoperative transesophageal echocardiography helps in defining the adequacy of repair and presence of residual defect. Direct pressure measurement (by a needle connected to pressure monitoring line) of the aorta (LV pressure), RV cavity, augmented RVOT, and distal PAs guide us in localizing the residual obstruction, if any. In general, the P RV/LV ratio (Kirklin index) less than 0.7 denotes a satisfactory repair. Any residual intracardiac shunt or significant RVOT gradient must be addressed immediately.

The operative mortality following TOF repair in the current era is between 1 and 2%. The hypertrophied right ventricle aggravates the diastolic dysfunction following surgery. In patients with right ventriculotomy and severe pulmonary regurgitation due to transannular patch, the RV dysfunction leads to stormy postoperative course with increased mortality and morbidity. Incidence of heart block after TOF repair is 1%. In older polycythemic patients, the associated coagulopathy results in excessive postoperative bleeding and needs special attention. Arrhythmia, especially junctional ectopic tachycardia (JET), can be life-threatening in the postoperative period. With the modified surgical techniques, improved myocardial protection, and aggressive intensive care, the incidence of JET is now rare.

The children with repaired tetralogy require long-term follow. Although the pulmonary regurgitation is generally well tolerated, the RV dilates with time. In some children, gradually the right ventricle becomes dysfunctional with reduction in exercise capacity. Pulmonary valve replacement is indicated in such patients. Some children present with arrhythmia decades after surgery. Older age at surgery is a known risk factor for this long-term complication.

Tetralogy of Fallot with Absent Pulmonary Valve Syndrome

In these patients, the tethered diminutive pulmonary valve is also regurgitant. The main PA and the branch pulmonary arteries are aneurysmally dilated leading to compression on the airways. The preferred age for surgery is between 1 and 2 years of age. The surgery is similar to TOF repair, but special attention is given to create a competent pulmonary valve, either in the form of a monocusp or valved RV to PA conduit. The dilated pulmonary arteries need plication or reduction to eliminate the compression effect on the bronchi. Patients with severe obstruction of airways become symptomatic in early infancy and need early intervention.

Tetralogy of Fallot with Pulmonary Artesia

As the correction involves a conduit implantation, the surgery is deferred till the child is 1–2 years of age, so that a reasonably large conduit can be placed. The surgery is performed through the midline sternotomy and CPB. VSD is closed with a prosthetic patch. A valved conduit (either a bovine internal jugular vein conduit, or aortic or pulmonary homograft or a handmade valved conduit with PTFE or bovine pericardium) is used to establish the continuity between RV and PA. The surgical mortality is <5%. The child needs reoperation at a later age (usually after 5–10 years) for the conduit change. Symptomatic patients presenting with significant desaturation in the neonatal or early infancy period require a palliative BT shunt or PDA stenting as a temporary measure.

Children with hypoplastic and nonconfluent pulmonary arteries with major aortopulmonary collateral artery (MAPCA)-dependent circulation require multistage fashion. Staging is done for (1) centralization of the pulmonary arteries by attaching PA branches to create a confluence and implantation of the large MAPCAs to them (unifocalization procedure), (2) augmentation of the blood flow to the pulmonary system by creation of unilateral or bilateral BT shunts, or a central shunt, and (3) once the pulmonary arteries are of good size, the final stage surgery done with VSD closure and implantation if an RV to PA conduit.

Management of Double Outlet Right Ventricle

Management of double-outlet right ventricle (DORV) is planned as per (1) size and location of the VSD, (2) presence or absence of the pulmonary stenosis, (3) age and weight of the patient, and (4) relation of the great arteries (**Table 3**). The surgery aims at creation of a wide connection from LV to aorta, and relief of left ventricular outflow tract (LVOT) or RVOT obstruction, if present (**Figs. 8A to D**).

If the VSD is subaortic in location, it is tunneled to the aorta with a large patch. Any associated infundibular or valvar pulmonary stenosis if present are relieved as in TOF repair. In DORV with subpulmonic VSD, the VSD cannot be routed to the aorta avoiding LV and RV outflow obstruction. Hence, the LV is easily routed to the pulmonary valve to create a transposition and then arterial switch operation is performed. In patients with remote VSDs, the LV to aorta path becomes long tunnel and with time invariably results in LVOT obstruction. Hence, they are treated in the single ventricle pathway.

Patients with excessive pulmonary blood flow present in early infancy with features of CCF. If the VSD tunneling cannot be done in a small baby, a palliative PA banding helps to allow growth of the child for an elective DORV repair at a later age. Children with severe pulmonary stenosis presenting in early life benefit from a BT shunt or PDA stenting.

TABLE 3: Surgical approach to double outlet right ventricle (DORV) as dictated by specific type.

Type of DORV	*Physiology*	*Management plan*
DORV with subaortic VSD	VSD type	VSD routing to aorta
DORV with subaortic VSD and PS	TOF type	DORV tunneling and RVOTO relief
DORV with subpulmonic VSD	TGA type	VSD routing to PA and arterial switch operation
DORV with noncommitted VSD	Large nonroutable VSD	Single ventricle pathway (PA banding → BDGS → Fontan)
DORV with AVSD + heterotaxy ± PS	As VSD or TOF as per pulmonary stenosis	DORV tunneling + AV canal repair+ RVOTO relief
DORV with CTGA ± situs abnormalities ± PS	As VSD or TOF as per pulmonary stenosis	Complex biventricular repair/single ventricle approach

(AVSD: atrioventricular septal defect; BDGS: bidirectional Glenn procedure; CTGA: corrected transposition of great arteries; PA: pulmonary artery; PS: pulmonic stenosis; RVOTO: right ventricular outflow tract obstruction; TOF: tetralogy of Fallot; TGA: transposition of great arteries; VSD: ventricular septal defect).

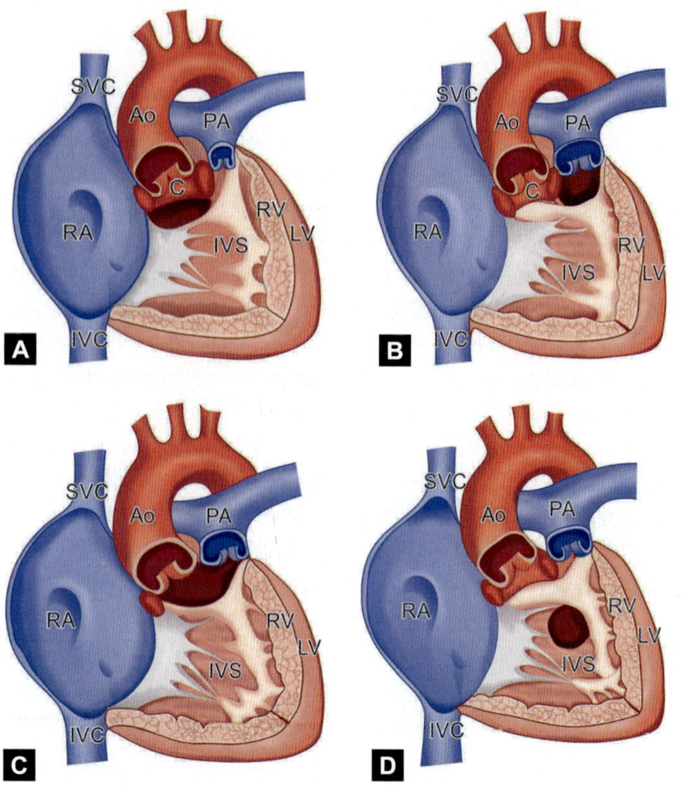

Figs. 8A to D: Types of double outlet right ventricle (DORV). (A) DORV with subaortic VSD; (B) DORV with subpulmonic VSD; (C) DORV with doubly committed VSD; (D) DORV with remote VSD.

(Ao: aorta; C: conal septum; IVC: inferior vena cava; IVS: interventricular septum; PA: pulmonary artery; RA: right atrium; RV: right ventricle, SVC: superior vena cava; VSD: ventricular septal defect)

This prepares the baby for a corrective surgery with conduits at a later age.

Surgical Strategies for Transposition in its Full Spectrum

Transposition of the great arteries (TGA) complex is broadly classified into three groups as per morphology and management plans.

1. TGA with intact ventricular septum
2. TGA with VSD
3. TGA with VSD and PS.

Transposition of the Great Arteries with Intact Ventricular Septum

Neonatal arterial switch operation is the ideal treatment. The preoperative optimization may require prostaglandin infusion to maintain the ductal patency and a balloon atrial septostomy to improve the interatrial mixing. Beyond 4 weeks of age, the left ventricle starts regressing and becomes unsuitable for taking the load of systemic cardiac output. With the improved cardiac intensive care support and new generation inodilators, the arterial switch operation can be performed up to the age of 3 months, though some of the babies need extracorporeal membrane oxygenation (ECMO) support in the early postoperative period to support the regressed left ventricle.

The arterial switch operation is an anatomic correction and targets to connect the left ventricle to the aorta, the right ventricle to the PA, and the coronary arteries to the base of the new aorta. A thorough understanding of the coronary artery anatomy is necessary for a successful outcome. With median sternotomy, the heart and great vessels are exposed. Hypothermic CPB utilized to support the heart and lungs during surgery. PDA or ductal ligament is divided. With cardioplegia heart is arrested. Then aorta and pulmonary arteries are transected above the level of sinus of Valsalva. The coronary arteries are harvested from the aorta. Two openings are made in the neoaorta and the coronaries are reimplanted. This is the most critical part of the operation as any error would result in myocardial ischemia and mortality. The distal aorta is moved posterior to the transected PA by LeCompte maneuver and then anastomosed to the PA (neoaortic) root and distal main PA is brought anteriorly and is connected to the aortic (neopulmonary) root (**Figs. 9A and B**). Any associated ASD or PFO is closed through the right atrium.

The current mortality for arterial switch operation is <5%. This surgery has significant learning curve in operative as well as postoperative management; hence, a higher mortality and morbidity can be expected in a low volume pediatric center. Early mortality can be related to coronary transfer problem or LV failure. Being a corrective surgery,

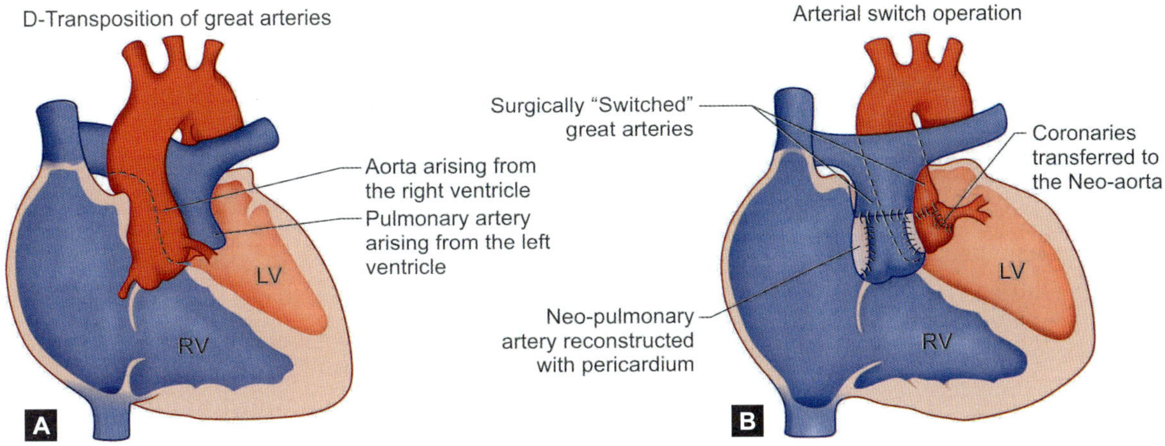

Figs. 9A and B: (A) Transposition of great arteries showing ventriculo-arterial discordance; (B) The arterial switch operation showing the "switched" great arteries along with coronary translocation.

arterial switch operation gives excellent long-term survival and quality of life. Late complications such as supravalvar pulmonary stenosis, supravalvar aortic stenosis, aortic root dilatation, and aortic regurgitation require reoperation.

Some children present late with a regressed left ventricle and are unsuitable for arterial switch operation. A staged approach of preparing the left ventricle and then performing arterial switch is beneficial. In the first stage, a BT shunt is created to increase the saturation and volume overload of the heart, and the PA is banded to increase the afterload of the left ventricle. This results in LV hypertrophy and increase in LV muscle mass which is followed up with serial echocardiography. Once the LV is prepared (usually 3–4 weeks), the arterial switch is performed and BT shunt and PA band are removed (two-stage switch operation).

In the developing world, many children present late and the resources, expertise, and economy restrict a two-stage arterial switch operation. In such patients with regressed left ventricle, atrial switch or Senning operation is the procedure of choice. Usual age for surgery is between 4 and 6 months of life. The surgery is performed via median sternotomy and CPB. The heart is arrested with cardioplegia. The SVC, IVC, and coronary sinus are directed to the mitral valve and left ventricle, which is connected to the pulmonary circulation. The pulmonary veins are channeled through a baffle to the tricuspid valve and right ventricle, which is connected to the systemic circulation. Inability of the RV to cope up as a systemic ventricle (RV dysfunction), baffle leak, and baffle obstruction are the common complications following a Senning operation. The mortality after Senning operation is around 2–3%. The main concerns after a Senning operation related to long-term complications such as RV failure, which is almost inevitable after 20–30 years and atrial arrhythmias.

Transposition of the Great Arteries with Ventricular Septal Defect

In children with TGA and VSD, the right-to-left shunting of blood across the VSD, the lungs keep the oxygen saturation at a higher level, and the volume overload of the left ventricle prevents the regression. Hence, the switch operation can be performed till 3 months of age. However, the ideal age of surgery for TGA-VSD is between 3 and 6 weeks as the prolonged exposure to excessive pulmonary blood flow results in the dilatation of the PA leading to increased surgical risk and also the elevated pulmonary vascular resistance results in a stormy postoperative course. Beyond 4–6 months of age, the pulmonary vascular bed develops static changes resulting in early Eisenmengerization.

Surgery is performed with median sternotomy and hypothermic CPB and cardioplegic arrest. Depending on the location of the VSD, either subpulmonic or perimembranous or inlet or muscular, the VSD is closed and then the arterial switch operation is performed. The relative mismatch between the sizes of the aorta and the PA can be a technical challenge and results in coronary compromise and early mortality. Hence, early surgery is advocated.

The surgical mortality rate is <5% in a high-volume specialist pediatric center. With timely surgery, the LV dysfunction is unusual unless associated with a coronary problem. Delayed surgery precipitates the risk of postoperative pulmonary hypertensive crises. Postoperative heart block rate approaches 2% in patients with TGA and VSD. Due to the disproportion that generally exists between aortic root and pulmonary root, there is a chance of neoaortic dilatation resulting in aortic regurgitation in the long-term follow-up.

Transposition of the Great Arteries, Ventricular Septal Defect, and Pulmonary Stenosis

This category of patients presents with a TOF like physiology and usually present beyond neonatal period. The spectrum of corrective procedures for these defects are customized as per the age of presentation, location of VSD, size of the conal septum, and the coronary anatomy, the details of which are beyond the scope of this discussion. The common procedures contemplated during a surgical planning are as follows:

- *Rastelli procedure*: The LV is routed to the aorta through the VSD by an intracardiac tunnel. The native stenotic PA is transected and is connected to the RV infundibulum with valved conduit (either Contegra or handmade Gore-Tex/Bovine pericardial conduit).
- *Réparation à l'Etage Ventriculaire (REV) procedure*: This procedure involves the excision of the native PA and closure of the pulmonary valve. The LV is routed to the aorta using the intracardiac tunnel to close the VSD. With LeCompte maneuver, the transected PA is brought anterior to the aorta and the RVOT is reconstructed either directly by a transannular patch with monocusp or with a conduit.
- *Nikaidoh procedure*: This involves the excision of the aortic root from the RV outflow and transposing it posteriorly to the pulmonary root and then reconstructing the pulmonary outflow anteriorly with a conduit.

In view of the complexity and requirement of artificial conduits, these surgeries are planned beyond 1 year of age and are delayed if the clinical conditions allow. The larger baby allows a bigger size patch for tunneling, thus reducing the incidence of LVOT obstruction, and a bigger conduit, thus reducing reoperations for conduit change. The current era mortality for these complex surgeries are between 5 and 10%.

If the child is very symptomatic in the neonatal or early infancy period, a palliative BT shunt or PDA stenting can help in improving the saturation and preparing the baby for the corrective surgery.

Total Anomalous Pulmonary Venous Connection Repair

Total anomalous pulmonary venous connection (TAPVC) includes distinct anatomic subtypes that are based on the site of drainage of the pulmonary veins (**Figs. 10A to C**). The goal of the TAPVC repair is to establish a direct connection between the common pulmonary venous chamber and the left atrium, and to close the ASD. Obstruction of the pulmonary venous drainage either at the level of vertical vein or the ASD warrants emergency surgery. Patients with severe form of the disease need neonatal TAPVC repair. Infradiaphragmatic TAPVC are most often obstructed because of the complex path the oxygenated blood takes to reach the right atrium. In the unobstructed TAPVC, elective surgery is planned around 1–2 months of age.

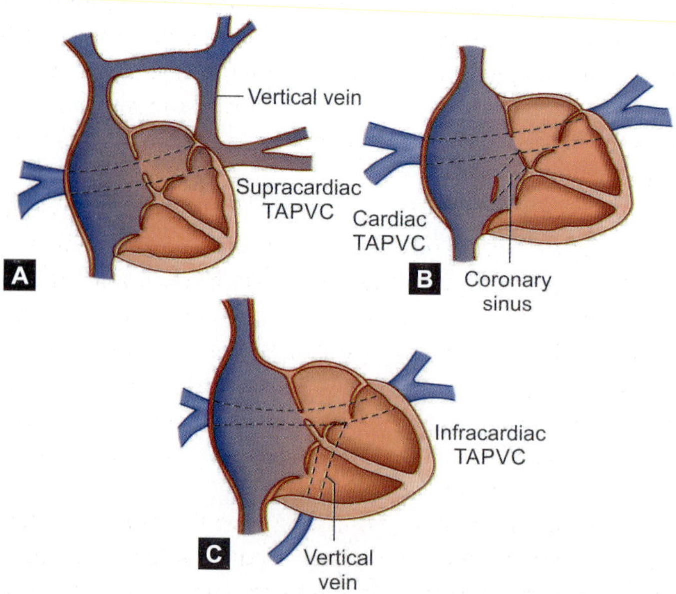

Figs. 10A to C: Types of total anomalous pulmonary venous connection (TAPVC) classified based on the anatomical pattern of venous drainage. (A) Supracardiac TAPVC; (B) Cardiac TAPVC; (C) Infracardiac TAPVC.

The standard approach is through a midline sternotomy and hypothermic CPB with cardioplegic arrest. In supracardiac and infracardiac TAPVC, the common pulmonary venous chamber is anastomosed to the back wall of the left atrium. The approach can be from the right side approach behind interatrial groove (Schumaker technique), the left side approach by lifting the heart (Doty technique), superior (caval approach), or transatrial. The ASD is closed, usually with a fenestrated patch. The vertical vein is usually ligated, unless a suprasystemic pulmonary pressure causes hemodynamic instability.

In coronary sinus type of cardiac TAPVC, the roof of the coronary sinus is unroofed till the mitral valve to create a spacious route for the flow of pulmonary venous blood. A generous pericardial patch is used to close the ASD along with the coronary sinus orifice, thus diverting the coronary sinus blood to the left atrium. Similarly, the right atrial TPAVC needs unroofing of the wall between left atrium and the common pulmonary venous chamber, and patch closure of the ASD.

The surgical mortality of TAPVC repair varies from 1 to 3%. Infants with unobstructed TAPVC usually have a good recovery. On the other extreme, in neonates with poor pulmonary venous anatomy, ventilated, septic, in multiorgan failure, and with preoperative cardiopulmonary resuscitation, the mortality can be as high as 30–40%. In the postoperative period, the pulmonary arterial hypertension can result in a slow recovery. Pulmonary vasodilators such as sildenafil, milrinone, and inhaled nitric oxide are useful in managing pulmonary hypertensive crises. The relatively small size of the underfilled LA and LV may need some time to adapt to the load of systemic circulation.

Recurrence is seen in nearly 10% patients after TAPVC repair. Progressive pulmonary venous obstruction is a life-threatening condition. Mixed TAPVC, poor pulmonary venous anatomy, and preoperative pulmonary venous obstruction are known risk factors for recurrence. Reoperation can give a satisfying result only in selected patients with suitable anatomy.

Truncus Arteriosus

In persistent truncus arteriosus, the children become symptomatic by the end of the first month of life and congestive cardiac failure with failure to thrive ensues. The preferred time for surgery is between 1 and 3 months of life, before the onset of advanced pulmonary vascular disease. Some neonates with uncontrolled failure and ventilator dependence need surgery as early as the second week of life. A preoperative testing of the DiGeorge syndrome guides in modulating the intraoperative and postoperative management plans.

The surgery is performed under hypothermic CPB and cardioplegic arrest through a midline sternotomy. Though the technical approach varies as per the type of truncus, the essential steps are: (1) separation of the pulmonary trunk or confluence containing both the branch pulmonary arteries from the truncal root, (2) repair of the truncal valve if warranted, (3) closure of the defect in the aortic trunk either directly or with a patch, (4) creation of an opening in the RV outflow tract, (5) closure of the VSD, and (6) establishment of the continuity between the right atrium (RA) and PA confluence using a valved conduit.

The valved conduit pathway in the RVOT avoids the pulmonary regurgitation and thus helps in faster recovery. However, several other approaches such as Barbero-Marcial techniques and nonvalved conduit reconstruction are also adopted by various surgical teams with comparable long-term results.

The surgical mortality following truncus repair under 10%. The postoperative pulmonary hypertensive episodes and coexisting noncardiac morbidities usually prolong recovery following neonatal truncus surgery. Children with borderline operability, benefit from a planned fenestration in VSD patch/valved patch or PFO. The postoperative pulmonary hypertensive surges decompress into the left side of the heart and maintains the cardiac output during the crisis period.

These children require reoperation for conduit change once they outgrow the conduit, depending on the rate of weight gain by the child and the conduit degeneration. The aortic regurgitation can progress requiring repair or replacement of aortic valve.

COARCTATION OF AORTA

In neonates and young infants with aortic coarctation, surgical repair is ideal as recurrence after balloon dilatation is common. The diagnosis of a significant narrowing is an indication of early surgery. In neonates with critical coarctation, prostaglandin helps in establishing the PDA flow and maintenance of distal circulation. This allows preoperative optimization of the child for surgery. If the PDA is nonresponsive to prostaglandin, balloon dilatation is advised in critically-ill babies with LV dysfunction and multiorgan failure. This helps in salvaging the patient. Elective surgery can be done at a later age when the coarctation recurs.

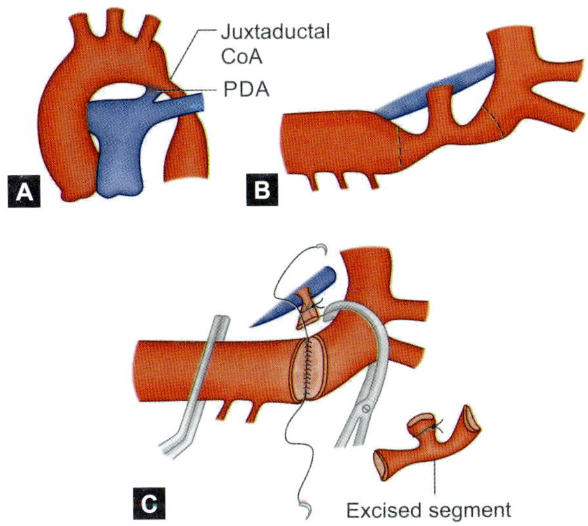

Figs. 11A to C: (A) Depicts the coarctation in relation to the patent ductus arteriosus and the aortic arch vessels; (B) Dotted lines show the site of incision; (C) Following the application of the proximal and the distal clamps, the coarcted segment along with the ligated ductal tissue is excised and end-to-end anastomosis is performed.

(CoA: coarctation of aorta; PDA: patent ductus arteriosus)

The standard approach is through the left posterolateral thoracotomy through the third intercostal space. The narrow segment with the proximal and distal normal aorta is dissected (**Figs. 11A to C**). The coarctation area is excised between aortic clamps. The healthy descending aorta is anastomosed to the distal aortic arch (end-to-end anastomosis). In children with hypoplasia of distal aortic arch, the incision extended to the undersurface of the narrow arch and the distal aorta is anastomosed (extended end-to-end anastomosis). Long segment coarctation can be managed by utilizing the proximal part of the subclavian artery as a flap to establish the aortic continuity (subclavian flap technique). In bigger children where mobilization is a challenge, patch augmentation of the coarcted segment is advocated. In patients with long segment coarctation, where direct anastomosis is not feasible, a prosthetic interposition tube graft helps in bypassing the obstruction and maintains the distal circulation.

The operative mortality for coarctation repair is 1–2%. In neonates, the associated comorbidities might adversely affect the outcome. Postoperative chylothorax and recurrent laryngeal nerve palsy can be seen. Paraplegia is a very rare complication and can be avoided by preserving collaterals, inducing mild hypothermia (34°C), and shortening the clamp time. Recurrence following coarctation repair is seen in 10–20% of children and balloon dilatation is the treatment of choice for recurrent coarctation.

Presence of associated major intracardiac defects such as VSD, TGA, or TAPVC requires simultaneous correction of all the defects through the midline sternotomy and CPB. These are complex procedures and carry a mortality risk related to the primary intracardiac procedure.

TABLE 4: Staged approach to single ventricle physiology.

Stage	*Operation*	*Timing*
Stage 1	Pulmonary artery banding	4–6 weeks of life, once the neonatal PVR drops
	Blalock–Taussig shunt	Neonatal or early infancy; emergency if low saturation
Stage 2	Bidirectional Glenn shunt	6–9 months after sufficient growth of pulmonary arteries and decline in pulmonary vascular resistance
Stage 3	Fontan completion	4 years or later after near complete development of the pulmonary vascular bed

(PVR: pulmonary vascular resistance)

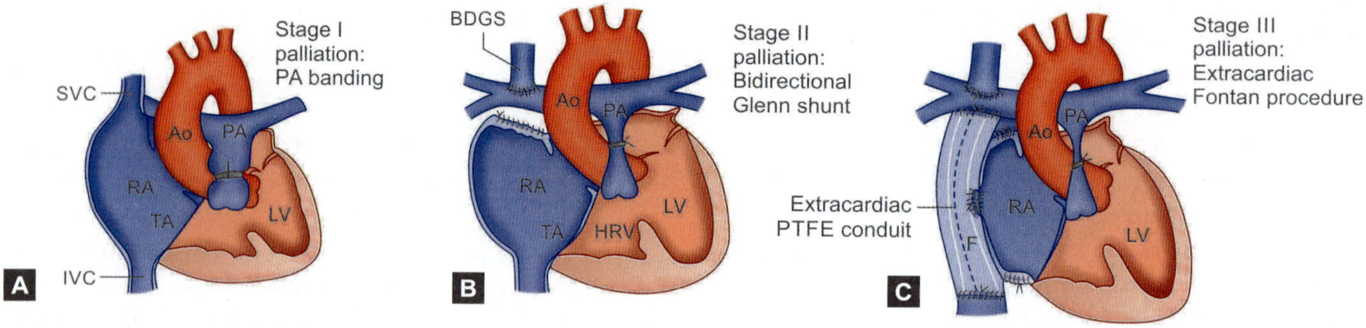

Figs. 12A to C: Stages of single ventricle palliation (Figures A, B, and C depict a heart with single ventricle physiology-tricuspid atresia with increased pulmonary blood flow. (A) Stage I palliation—pulmonary artery banding; (B) Stage II palliation—bidirectional Glenn shunt (superior cavopulmonary connection); (C) Stage III palliation—Fontan procedure (total cavopulmonary connection).

(Ao: aorta; IVC: inferior vena cava; PA: pulmonary artery; RA: right atrium; SVC: superior vena cava; IVC: inferior vena cava; TA: tricuspid atresia; HRV: hypoplastic right ventricle; BDGS: bidirectional Glenn shunt; F: Fontan connection)

SURGICAL MANAGEMENT SINGLE VENTRICLE PHYSIOLOGY: THE STAGED APPROACH

Cardiac anomalies, which cannot be anatomically and/or functionally separated to systemic or pulmonary circulations, are considered under single ventricle palliation. The defects might be in the ventricular level and/or valve levels (inflow/outflow). The common anomalies needing single ventricle palliation are tricuspid atresia, mitral atresia, double inlet left ventricle, hypoplastic left heart syndrome (HLHS), hypoplastic right heart syndrome, unbalanced AV canal defects, nonroutable DORV, few heterotaxy syndromes, etc.

As there is only one functional ventricle, this takes the role of systemic ventricle (LV). The systemic venous return (deoxygenated blood) is routed directly to the lungs without entering the right atrium or right ventricle. This concept is called Fontan circulation. For a successful Fontan physiology, few prerequisites must be met. In the earlier era, these were known as "Ten Commandments." The current understanding is that, for a successful Fontan operation, the basic requirements are (1) good sized pulmonary arteries, (2) normal or low pulmonary vascular resistance, (3) no obstruction to pulmonary venous return, or systemic outflow, (4) normal ventricular function, (5) sinus rhythm, and (6) normal function of AV valves and aortic valve.

The patients with single ventricle anatomy need a staged approach (**Table 4**).

The preparation of single ventricle palliation starts in the newborn period itself and strategy to achieve a good Fontan circulation is worked out. Children with pulmonary stenosis or atresia present with desaturation and need a BT shunt for survival. However, if there is no pulmonary stenosis, the excessive pulmonary blood flow results in elevated PVR. Hence, a PA band is necessary in these children to control the heart failure and protect the pulmonary vascular bed (**Figs. 12A to C**). Both the BT shunt and PA band are nonreliable circulations for optimum pulmonary blood flow and the clinical condition depends on the variations in the systemic and pulmonary vascular resistance. As the child gets older, the second stage surgery (Glenn shunt) is considered (**Figs. 12A to C**).

The goal of a bidirectional Glenn shunt is to (1) reduce the volume overload off the single ventricle allowing optimization of the ventricular function and (2) optimization of the pulmonary blood flow with adequate oxygenation with no risk of pulmonary vascular disease. The bidirectional Glenn shunt can be performed as open-heart surgery or a closed-heart surgery (off pump). With a median sternotomy, the SVC is transected from the right atrium and is anastomosed to the superior surface of RPA resulting in direct flow of the venous blood to the lungs. The main PA is ligated and BT shunt divided (if any present) to eliminate the antegrade blood flow, making the SVC as the sole source for the lungs. The aim is to keep the PA pressure low, so as to facilitate the passive flow of blood to the pulmonary arteries.

As the child grows, there is progressive fall in the relative flow in superior vena cava not being able to fulfill the oxygen requirement. This results in worsening cyanosis after 3–4 years of age, necessitating the Fontan operation. In patients with no antegrade pulmonary blood flow to the lungs, the lack of hepatic factor in lungs predisposes to the development of progressive pulmonary arteriovenous malformation, which resolves after Fontan operation. The "One and a half ventricle repair" technique involves keeping antegrade blood flow through the PA to avoid the AV malformations. However, the antegrade blood flow can elevate the pulmonary vascular pressure leading to Glenn dysfunction. Some children develop cyanosis few years after Glenn operation due to the development of collaterals between SVC and IVC circulation.

The Fontan operation aims to divert the IVC blood into the pulmonary circulation directly. This can be achieved by interposing a PTFE graft between inferior vena cava and PA (extracardiac conduit Fontan) or creation of a tunnel in the lateral wall of the right atrium (lateral tunnel Fontan). The flow of blood in the lungs is passive and is aided by negative intrathoracic pressure. Activity related pumping of lower limb muscles acts as peripheral heart aiding to the blood flow to the lungs. In children with elevated PA pressure or borderline narrow branch pulmonary arteries, a small fenestration is created between the Fontan circuit and the left atrium (fenestrated Fontan operation). This helps as a pop off for the elevated pressure in the Fontan circuit and maintains the cardiac output, thus allowing easy acceptance of the new circulation.

Being a nonpulsatile circulation, a higher Fontan pressure is needed for passive flow into the PA and the left heart. Lower ventricular end-diastolic pressure (EDP) helps in forward flow at a lower Fontan pressure. A high pressure in the Fontan circuit results in seepage of fluid into the extravascular space leading to recurrent pleural effusion and ascites. With time, the tissues get adjusted to this elevated systemic venous pressure and the Fontan circulation gets established. In most of the children, it takes a 2–4 weeks' time to get used to this new circulation. However, if the anatomy is unfavorable or the preoperative assessment is inadequate, the Fontan circulation worsens with time resulting in recurrent massive pleural effusions, chylothorax, ascites, generalized edema, plastic bronchitis, and hemodynamic compromise. This Fontan failure needs to be addressed early with catheterization to establish a diagnosis and creation of a good-sized fenestration if was not made earlier. For some children not responding to the conservative management, the Fontan is taken down and converted back to the Glenn circulation.

It is increasingly apparent that life after a Fontan is challenging after the initial 20 years. Long-term complications relate to liver damage, rhythm problems, and specific complications such as protein losing enteropathy and plastic bronchitis. The basis for these complications is the chronic exposure to elevated central venous pressure. Liver injury is evident through elevation of gamma-glutamyl transferase (GGT) and abnormal degree of fibrosis that is detectable through transient elastography (Fibroscan) and later through ultrasound. There is a higher than normal incidence of liver cancer 30 years after Fontan operation.

In single ventricle candidates presenting late, a single-stage Fontan operation can be considered if the anatomy is suitable.

ROLE OF SYSTEMIC TO PULMONARY ARTERY SHUNTS

Patients with low oxygen saturation and history of spells benefit from a systemic to pulmonary shunt. The target of these procedures is to establish a connection between a systemic artery and PA and augment the pulmonary blood flow to (1) improve oxygenation of the child, (2) augment growth of branch pulmonary arteries, and (3) prepare the baby for the next stage surgery.

Modified BT shunt is the most common systemic to PA shunt preferred. This can be performed through a median sternotomy or a posterolateral thoracotomy. Surgery involves placement of an interposition graft between subclavian or innominate artery and the branch PA of the same side. Expanded PTFE (Gore-Tex) tube graft is the commonly used material. The diameter of the graft is decided according to the weight of the child and the size of the target PA. A suitable BT shunt maintains saturation between 80 and 85%. Anatomical reasons resulting in smaller grafts provide inadequate saturation and carry a risk of premature blockage. Overcirculation due to a large size shunt results in excessive steal from the aorta resulting in stormy postoperative course with systemic malperfusion and congestive cardiac failure. Usually, this surgery is done as a closed heart procedure. However, associated procedures (such as atrial septectomy, PA plasty) or hemodynamic instability mandates CPB use.

Classical BT shunt was the original technique where the transected subclavian artery was directly anastomosed to the ipsilateral right PA. The complications related to limb vascularity and technical complexity in shunt division at the time of next stage surgery have made this technique unpopular. A central shunt involves the implantation of the graft in the main PA to allow uniform flow in both the branches. Various modifications such as Waterston's and Pott's shunt are no longer used.

The BT shunt surgery carries a mortality risk of 5–8% in a specialized pediatric unit and higher in low volume centers. A thorough understanding to achieve a balance between systemic and pulmonary vascular resistance and a multidisciplinary team approach is needed to achieve good outcome. Shunt revisions and stormy postoperative course can be expected following BT shunt surgery. Outcomes are also influenced by the age, weight, preoperative conditions, and associated comorbidities.

ROLE OF PULMONARY ARTERY BANDING IN SINGLE VENTRICLE AS WELL AS TWO VENTRICLE SITUATIONS

Pulmonary artery banding is a palliative procedure used to control the excessive pulmonary blood flow when a corrective or definitive procedure cannot be performed at a younger age. The ideal age for a PA banding is between 4 and 6 weeks of life. In the current era, main indications are: (1) multiple muscular VSDs (Swiss cheese septum), (2) single ventricle physiology with increased pulmonary blood flow, and (3) preparation of the left ventricle for arterial switch operation in the babies with TGA and intact septum who present late.

Pulmonary artery banding can be a part of a complex open-heart procedure. However, isolated PA banding is a closed-heart procedure. The approach for the surgery is via midline sternotomy. The thymus is preserved and pericardium opened only in front of the great arteries to avoid excessive adhesion of the heart during the next stage surgery. Main PA is isolated and a Mersilene tape is passed around it and fixed at the desired level. Traditionally, Trusler's rule is followed for planning the band circumference, and hemodynamic as well as ABG guided adjustments help in good balance between systemic and pulmonary blood flow. Minimally invasive approaches such as ministernotomy, left anterolateral thoracotomy, and left posterolateral thoracotomy can be attempted in selective children.

Though a relatively less complex procedure, PA banding carries a mortality risk of nearly 3–5%. The lability of the pulmonary vascular resistance takes time to settle and can result in a stormy postoperative course. The expected saturation after a PA band for multiple VSDs is around 85–95% and for complex single ventricle physiology is around 75–85%.

MANAGEMENT OF CORONARY ARTERY ANOMALIES

Although coronary artery anomalies are not rare, only few of them which are functionally significant need a surgical repair.

- Anomalous origin of left coronary artery from pulmonary artery (ALCAPA) becomes obvious in the 3rd to 4th week of life once the coronary steal becomes prominent after the fall in the pulmonary vascular resistance. As the left coronary artery territory is supplied by collaterals from the right coronary system and there is continuous steal of coronary blood to the low-pressure PA, these children develop LV dysfunction and endocardial and papillary muscle fibrosis resulting in mitral regurgitation. The ventricular dysfunction worsens with time warranting early surgery. In few children, the intercoronary collateral develops early maintaining myocardial perfusion, and the symptoms are delayed. Children with VSD or PDA with elevated pulmonary pressure, the coronary steal is limited and the symptoms appear late resulting in a masking of diagnosis.
- The ideal surgery aims to establish a two-coronary system by removing the left coronary ostium from the PA and implanting on the aorta (coronary transfer technique; **Figs. 13A and B**). In the earlier era, creation of a coronary baffle to the proximal aorta in the supravalvar pulmonary area (Takeuchi technique) was used. In older patients with unfavorable anatomy left internal mammary grafting of the left anterior descending coronary artery is adopted. In small children, moderate-to-severe mitral

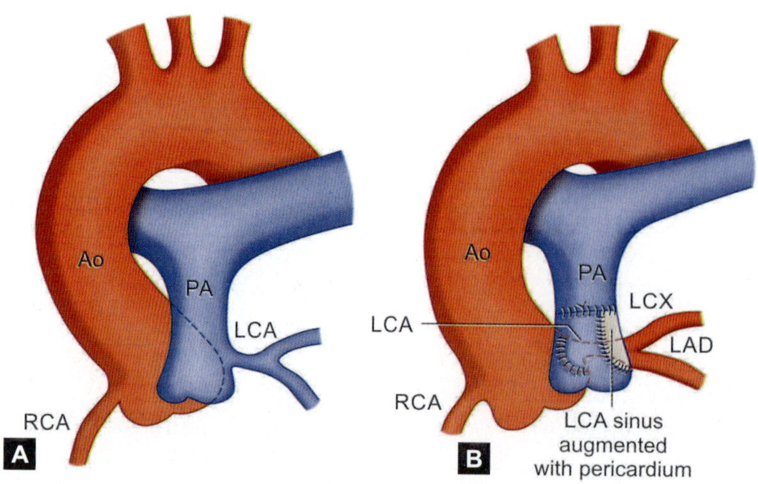

Figs. 13A and B: (A) Anomalous origin of left coronary artery from pulmonary artery; (B) Coronary translocation: Rerouting of left coronary defect to the aorta and closing the pulmonary artery defect with a patch of autologous pericardium.
(Ao: aorta; LAD: left anterior descending artery; LCA: left coronary artery; LCx: left circumflex artery; PA: pulmonary artery; RCA: right coronary artery)

regurgitation usually recovers to some degree. However, in bigger patients and profound mitral regurgitation, mitral valve repair or replacement becomes necessary.

- The surgical mortality ranges between 10 and 20% depending on the extent of ventricular dysfunction, valve regurgitation, and preoperative morbidity. These subsets of patients are known for long-term ventilation and ICU stay with frequent requirement of mechanical LV support in the form of ECMO or left ventricular assist device (LVAD).
- Anomalous aortic origin of coronary artery is a rare anomaly and a known cause of sudden death in young adults and athletes. Coronary ostioplasty and repositioning is the commonly preferred approach. Bigger children benefit from left internal mammary grafting of the left anterior descending coronary artery.
- Coronary aneurysms and fistulas to various cardiac chambers are usually managed by catheter or device closure. Larger coronary aneurysms need surgical exclusion of the segment and bypass grafting of the distal coronary artery. Hemodynamically significant coronary cavernous fistula requires patch closure of both ends of the fistula under CPB.

HYPOPLASTIC LEFT HEART SYNDROME

The HLHS patients need a three-stage palliation to achieve a stable circulation. The first stage surgery Norwood operation is done in the first 2–4 weeks of life. The aorta and PA are joined to create the systemic outflow (Damus–Kaye–Stansel procedure) and the hypoplastic aortic arch is repaired (**Figs. 14A and B**). The pulmonary blood flow is established by a modified BT shunt or RV to PA conduit (Sano shunt).

The delicate balance between systemic and pulmonary blood flow is imperative to maintain a good cardiac output and cardiac function. The current era mortality after Norwood operation ranges from 10 to 30% in specialized pediatric centers. The second stage surgery Glenn shunt is performed at 4–6 months of age to establish a stable circulation.

MANAGEMENT OF PEDIATRIC VALVE DISEASES

Catheter-based therapy is now offered to most congenital stenotic lesions of the pulmonary and aortic valve as well as for isolated rheumatic mitral valve stenosis. Surgery is primary more of therapy for regurgitant lesions and congenital mitral stenosis.

Surgery for Mitral Valve Diseases

Congenital mitral valve lesions are common, presenting either as stenosis in the supravalvar, valvar, or subvalvar region or as mitral regurgitation. Supravalvar mitral stenosis in the form of cor triatriatum or supramitral membrane (ring) has excellent outcome with excision. Congenital stenosis of the mitral valve needs commissurotomy and chordae release. The most common subvalvar obstruction in the form of parachute mitral valve, requires release of subvalvar apparatus to create a spacious mitral outflow. In these anatomies, recurrent obstructions are common needing reoperations. Children with anatomy unsuitable for repair need MVR.

Cleft in the mitral leaflets is the most common cause of congenital mitral regurgitation and closure of the clefts usually gives a good result. Chordal rupture is another cause of mitral valve regurgitation in infants needing repair in the form of creation of neochordae. Mitral regurgitation due to annular dilatation is usually secondary to LV dilatation. Correction of the primary pathology usually resolves this issue. Symptomatic children benefit from annular plication to control the regurgitation.

For mitral valve lesions in infants and young children, repair is the primary goal unless the anatomy is totally unsuitable. MVR is extremely challenging in view of the small

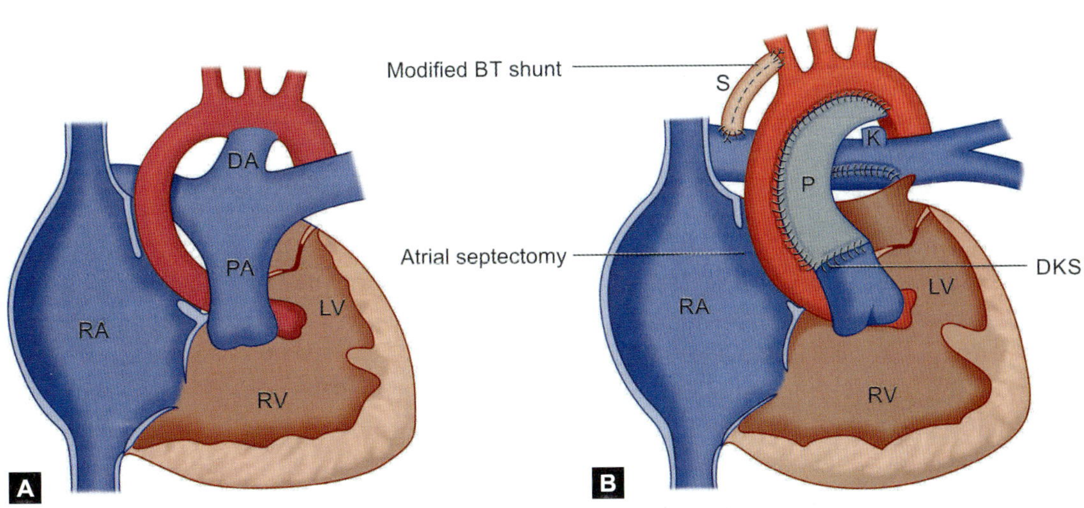

Figs. 14A and B: (A) Hypoplastic left heart syndrome (HLHS); (B) Stage I Norwood palliation for HLHS.
(Ao: aorta, DKS- Damus–Kaye–Stanzel anastomosis; LV: left ventricle; PA: pulmonary artery; RA: right atrium; RV: right ventricle)

size of the annulus and no availability of such small valves. In extremely small children, a supra-annular placement of mitral valve can be considered. Reoperation to replace the valve is needed once the child grows.

Ebstein Anomaly of Tricuspid Valve

The primary pathology is apical displacement of tricuspid valve leaflets and annular dilatation leading to tricuspid regurgitation. The surgery aims to restore the tricuspid valve competency and right ventricle size. The "cone technique" involves release of the tricuspid leaflets from the RV wall and then attaching to the new annulus created by plication of the dilated atrialized right ventricle. This new orientation gives a cone shape to the valve outflow and prevents regurgitation. In bigger children and adults with severely damaged and regurgitant valve leaflets, tricuspid valve replacement is the treatment of choice. Newborns with severe form of disease, where two-ventricle repair is not feasible, are managed by "Starnes approach." The tricuspid valve is closed with a pericardial patch, atrial septectomy created for the systemic venous outflow, and a systemic to pulmonary arterial shunt implanted to establish pulmonary blood flow. These children are staged to Glenn and Fontan operation at a later age.

COSMETIC PEDIATRIC CARDIAC SURGERY

Cosmetic pediatric surgery aims to achieve a small and good-looking scar without compromising any surgical outcome. Usually simple surgeries are performed through the cosmetic approach as they limit access to many areas of heart and can compromise safety. Ministernotomy (partial sternotomy) is useful in surgeries such as ASD closure, VSD closure (subpulmonic), and PA band. A limited right thoracotomy is preferred in selected candidates for ASD closure and MVR. The CPB is to be established with peripheral cannulation using femoral, neck, or axillary vessels. In suitable patients, a small anterolateral thoracotomy can be used for PA banding or pacemaker insertion.

Limited incisions are usually avoided in small babies, where the visibility is as such compromised due to size. The cosmetic approaches are avoided for staged surgeries as the next stage surgery being a redo procedure, inevitably requires median sternotomy.

ROLE OF HYBRID APPROACH IN PEDIATRIC CARDIAC DISEASES

During intervention for certain congenital heart defects, the combined technical expertise of pediatric cardiac surgeon and interventional pediatric cardiologist yields a better result. The goals of hybrid approach are: (1) to reduce the cumulative impact of multiple interventions required to treat complex congenital heart defects, (2) to deliver the most efficient and cost-effective care, (3) to reduce morbidity and mortality, and (4) to improve the quality of life.

In small children with symptomatic secundum ASDs, hybrid approach with limited sternotomy and ASD device placement through a controlled access via right atrium helps in avoiding open-heart surgery. Device deployment in a muscular VSD can be achieved by a controlled access from the RV surface via a subxiphoid incision. In complex HLHS scenario, hybrid procedure is extremely helpful. Through a median sternotomy, the cardiac surgeon performs bilateral PA banding. The interventional cardiologist creates a balloon atrial septostomy via a purse string-controlled approach in the right atrium and then implants the PDA stent via a direct access in the main PA. In complex redo-surgeries, intraoperative stent placements in the inaccessible areas of branch pulmonary arteries are becoming popular.

This combined cardiac team procedure normally gives the best result when performed in a hybrid operating suite. In selected hybrid surgeries, use of CPB can be easily avoided. A postprocedural angiography confirms the adequacy of the repair.

IMPLANTS USED IN CONGENITAL HEART SURGERY

As the reconstruction of a compatible anatomical pathway involves closure of defects, construction of tunneled pathways, creation of functional valves and implantation of conduits, and prosthetic materials form an integral part of congenital heart surgery. The patches can be autograft (autologous pericardium, right atrial tissue, and PA patch), homograft (pericardium, PA, or aortic patch), xenograft (bovine or equine pericardial patch), or synthetic (PTFE and Dacron patch). Routinely used prosthetic tube grafts are synthetic (Gore-Tex and Dacron tube grafts).

The commonly used valved conduits are Contegra (bovine jugular vein xenograft) and aortic or pulmonary homograft. The homografts are harvested form human cadavers, sterilized and stored in liquid nitrogen. Xenograft conduits are harvested from porcine or bovine sources, processed in glutaraldehyde to make them nonantigenic and then stored. After implantation, both the homografts and xenografts degenerate with time, get calcified and become stenotic. Implantation of valved conduit at a young age commits the patient to reoperation for a conduit change. Hence, elective surgeries requiring conduit placement are planned at a later age to accommodate a larger conduit to reduce the number of reoperations.

ROLE OF PEDIATRIC AND NEONATAL EXTRACORPOREAL LIFE SUPPORT

Even with the maximum medical management, some children with CHD will persist with a severe refractory low cardiac output and require extracorporeal life support for survival. Currently available mechanical circulatory supports are (1) ECMO, (2) ventricular assist device (VAD), and (3) intra-aortic balloon pump (IABP) (rarely used). The optimal candidates are patients with cardiac or respiratory dysfunction refractory to medical management.

Extracorporeal Membrane Oxygenation

In the past decades, ECMO has established itself as the therapeutic mainstay for pediatric short-term mechanical circulatory support. It is flexible in its ability to provide support even for the smallest patients and can be instituted by peripheral cannulation. The indications are categorized into (1) preoperative optimization, (2) postoperative refractory cardiorespiratory dysfunction, (3) nonsurgical candidates with temporary instability (sepsis), and (4) as a bridge to LVAD insertion or as a bridge to heart, lung, or heart–lung transplant.

Ventricular Assist Device

In children with end-stage heart failure, LVAD can be used as a bridge to heart transplantation or as a destination therapy. With time, the VAD system has seen a continuous improvement in cannulation techniques, circuit miniaturization, flow dynamics, and centrifugal pump efficiency. Various hardware models are available in market (e.g., Berlin heart, Syncardia, Heart-mate, Heart-ware, and Jarvik heart). They aim at minimizing the complications such as thrombosis and hemorrhage-related neurological complications, ambulation of the patient to a near normal life and maintaining an event-free effective circulatory system for long duration. In children with reversible myocardial pathology, the VAD is explanted once the ventricular function completely recovers.

Intra-aortic Balloon Pump

Intra-aortic balloon pump is commonly used in adult practice for augmentation of cardiac output. However, smaller femoral vessels, greater elasticity of the aorta, and inability of the device to track high heart rate commonly seen in pediatric practice limit its use.

SCOPE OF PEDIATRIC HEART TRANSPLANTATION

Cardiomyopathy and complex congenital heart defects are the most common indications for pediatric heart transplantation. Children with repaired congenital heart defects who do not fare well after surgery are usually selected for transplantation. The candidate evaluation is very important from medical as well as social and financial standpoint for a successful long-term survival. Suitable donor availability can be a challenge to match recipient's heart size and intrathoracic space. Proximity of donor and recipient's hospital and a good logistic networking is important in limiting the time between organ harvest and implantation. A longer cold ischemia time (>4 hours) is associated to higher mortality and morbidity. Orthotopic heart transplantation is the procedure of choice. Standard approach through median sternotomy and a bicaval technique is the preferred technique. Postoperative extracorporeal life support is required in 30–40% patients to tide over the recipient's pulmonary hypertension-related donor heart failure.

In the current era, the 1-year survival following pediatric heart transplantation is 80–90%. After transplantation, the children require lifelong immunosuppression and are at dangers such as graft rejection, cardiac allograft vasculopathy, infections, and malignancy. Children with cardiac allograft vasculopathy develop accelerated atherosclerosis and graft failure needing retransplantation. Heart transplantation for children remains the safest and most efficient therapy for children with end-stage heart failure. It is also the only viable option for all single ventricles palliated in the Fontan pathway, who eventually succumb to end stage heart and circulatory failure.

CONCLUSION

We have attempted to provide concise information about common congenital heart surgeries that would help pediatricians in understanding the available medical and surgical treatment modalities of common congenital heart defects, which helps in counseling and providing the right advise to the parents. As an elaborate description is beyond the scope of this book, readers are advised to refer the following publications for a detailed information.

SUGGESTED READING

1. Kouchoukos NT, Blackstone EH, Hanley FL, Kirklin JK. Kirklin/Barret-Boyes. Cardiac Surgery, 4th edition. Amsterdam: Elsevier Science; 2012.
2. Mavroudis C, Backer CL. Pediatric Cardiac Surgery, 4th edition. Hoboken: Wiley Blackwell; 2013.
3. Shllke F, del Nido P, Swanson S. Sabiston and Spencer Surgery of the Chest, 9th edition. Amsterdam: Elsevier Science; 2015.

16

CHAPTER

Counseling Families of Children with Heart Disease

Sangeetha Viswanathan

INTRODUCTION

Being told that your child may have a heart defect is understandably a very stressful experience for any parent and as physicians we play a crucial role in helping the family deal with what is often an unexpected and life-changing experience. Parents undergo a range of emotions when confronted with the news that their child has a heart defect including shock, grief, guilt, anger, and depression which translate into heightened anxiety and stress.[1,2] This can impede the ability of the family to care for the child with congenital heart disease (CHD).[3]

As children with CHD often have a long and sometimes complicated medical journey ahead of them, it is crucial that the family are co-opted as equal partners along with the healthcare team in the decision-making and management process. Establishing a strong, trusting relationship with the family right at the outset allows for free and honest discussion and unbiased decision-making with the interests of the child and the family at its core.

Although we are all well-trained practitioners who can "reel off" differential diagnoses at the tip of our tongues when we graduate, we often find ourselves unprepared to effectively deal with the emotional and psychological needs of families in real life. This aspect of patient care is unfortunately not emphasized in our curriculum as medical trainees and we end up having to "learn on the job" in order to fulfill this very important role as a "healer" of wounds not only physical but also emotional and psychological.[2]

In this chapter, we will touch upon the general approach to counseling parents and children with chronic disease and also specific aspects that are unique to CHD by journeying together with a typical family as they confront the news that their newborn daughter has CHD. Salient tips regarding ideal counseling practices will be highlighted alongside their story.

THE FIRST ENCOUNTER

The family gather anxiously outside the ICU waiting for the specialist to tell them what is wrong with their perfectly formed little girl who seemed completely well after being discharged from their local hospital at 24 hours of age after an uneventful pregnancy and normal vaginal delivery. Suddenly at 2 days of age they noticed that she was lethargic, pale, and breathing rapidly and brought her to the emergency department. An echocardiogram has revealed a tight coarctation and the appropriate management has been initiated with clinical improvement. Now the medical team are faced with the task of speaking to the family and appraising them about the diagnosis and management plan.

A Suitable Setting and Team Approach

A suitable environment for counseling should include a room with adequate seating for the family and healthcare staff, stationery so that illustrative drawings can be drawn to clearly communicate the structural problem and proposed treatment to the family and some tissues and a bottle of water for the family members. It is often helpful for the physician to have a nurse present to provide additional support to the family. This also ensures that there is seamless and uniform messaging by all members of the team. "Counseling in the corridor" at this critical juncture should be strongly avoided and discouraged. Team leaders should set an example to their team members by their behavior and set the scene for further communication with the patient's family.

The family is taken into the counseling room outside the ICU with the parents, grandfather, and uncle being present for the session. The physician and nurse introduce themselves by name and designation. The physician summarizes the events since birth addressing the child by name whenever possible. She then updates the family regarding the current status of the child saying "Jothi was very sick when she was brought to the emergency department and required immediate care. You did a great job bringing her to the hospital at the right time. We have placed a drip to give medications and fluids and performed tests to find out the reason for her sickness and she is now much better.

Usually when babies present in this fashion, one of the most common causes is infection but all the blood tests pertaining to infection are negative. The next thing that we usually look for is a possible heart problem and that was why I was involved in her care. We have done a heart scan and it does show a heart problem." The physician then pauses for the information to sink in.

Giving Time and Avoiding Blame

It is critical that the physician appears unrushed and able to give all the time required by the family. If the chief consultant has other tasks at hand, an able deputy should take up the task of counseling the family. It is highly unsatisfactory for the family to have a rushed counseling session leaving them with unanswered questions and heightened anxiety.

Reassurance to the family that the child is being stabilized and that the clinical condition is improving sets their mind at rest and they are then able to take in the more technical discussions regarding the diagnosis and planned treatment strategy. It is also useful to address any guilt that the parents may carry and appreciate their prompt action in seeking medical attention at the right time. Care should be taken to avoid blaming the parents for delay in presentation or less than perfect care of the patient.

Often parents have questions on their minds like "Will my child survive?," "What is the long-term outlook for the condition?," "Can she have a normal life? Go to school, play with other children, etc." It is often helpful to address some of these questions pre-emptively during the course of the counseling session. Parents should also be given an opportunity to ask questions either during or at the end of the session.

The family appears distraught and the mother starts to cry. Tissues are handed to her to wipe her tears. The physician then continues...

"Let me explain exactly what the problem is so that you can understand the exact nature of the defect and the treatment plan."

She then draws an illustration of the normal heart and explains the chambers and blood vessels (tubes) taking care to use nontechnical layman terminology. Next she draws an illustration of the baby's condition—in this case coarctation of the aorta.

She explains, "The reason that the baby looked well with no problems initially was due to the presence of an additional blood tube that was supplying the lower half of the body which is present in all newborns. This blood tube usually closes in 1–2 days after birth and then the blood supply to the lower body is affected resulting in the baby becoming pale, cold, lethargic, and breathless.

We have now started a medicine to keep this blood tube open and this seems to be working well. The baby now looks much better. In fact you will be able to see her shortly.

Sometimes young babies when given this medication may develop slow breathing and if this happens we may need to support the baby's breathing with a machine. But right now she is breathing well on her own. Even if we need to support her breathing it will only be temporary as long as the baby requires it. Once she starts breathing well on her own we can take her off the machine. This machine support may not be needed but I am just explaining this to you so that you do not get worried if we need to use it later."

By now the mother appears more settled and the family seem to have accepted that there is a problem but reassured that things are stable at the present. The physician takes this opportunity to enquire further about the family background; parents occupation, whether they have other children, extended family support, etc.

Communicating Effectively and Understanding the Family Circumstances

During counseling, it is very important to use simple language and illustrative aids to help the family understand underlying structural defects easily. The physician should be prepared to do this multiple times if required. The illustrations can be given to parents and some of them may request that the name of the diagnosis be written down to enable them to learn more about the condition or communicate to other family members. A well-informed parent is an asset in patient care and although we have all faced situations where parents come to us with information from "Dr Google," which might not be entirely contextual, we should appreciate the parent's initiative to be involved and informed. We would perhaps do the same in their shoes...

Also, it is important to understand the family circumstances; their education level, occupation, and financial ability as this will inform the style and content of our counseling.[4] Unfortunately, families in our part of the world have to grapple not only with the diagnosis and management but also with how they will fund this entirely unexpected medical expenditure.

After the initial shock of the diagnosis, Jothi's family are now anxious and want to be reassured that all will be well.

Dad asks; "Now that she has improved with this medication will she be okay?"

The physician responds, "The medication is only a short-term solution to the problem. We cannot keep her on the medication forever. Something more permanent has to be done to relieve the problem and that involves an operation."

The room falls silent. The mother speaks up hesitantly "But she is such a small baby, will it not be risky?"

The physician responds, "Whenever we undertake surgery in children with heart defects, we have to weigh the risks and benefits. We should not undertake procedures that are unnecessary but where necessary we have to understand that although there may be risks involved, the benefits of treatment outweigh the risks. Of course, any surgery related to the heart does carry a small risk but the chances of a successful outcome are more than 95% in these children." She clarifies, "If 100 children undergo this operation more than 95 of them will have a successful operation without any serious side effects.[5]

Unfortunately there is no natural cure for this condition and no long-term medical treatment that will cure the condition. If surgery is not carried out in this condition, the child will not be able to survive."

Communicating Risk

It is important to address parents' concerns regarding risks associated with treatment. One should not falsely claim that there is no risk associated with the treatment proposed. The risk should be placed in a context that can be easily understood and the parents should be convinced that the risk is unavoidable or that the benefits outweigh the risks. In situations where the benefit is uncertain, this should be clearly explained and the parents should be invited to make a decision with the help and support of the medical team.

It is not uncommon for parents to ask 'What would you do if this were your child?' Some physicians may choose not to answer this question and simply respond that these are individual decisions and that it would be unwise to superimpose their personal views to influence the family's decision. Others may choose to say that they would choose a particular mode of treatment in the hypothetical scenario that they were in the parents' shoes but reinforce that whatever the family decides will be respected and supported by the medical team. This is particularly important in the context of fetal diagnosis and decision-making regarding continuation of pregnancy.

Jothi's parents seem convinced that surgery is unavoidable. They are both teachers on a meagre income and the cost of cardiac surgery will be quite a burden on them but Jothi is precious to them and they are determined to do whatever is necessary to ensure that she survives and is given a fighting chance.

They do however have further questions regarding the long-term outlook and ask "Once the operation is done successfully will she have a normal life?"

The physician sets out to explain as follows. "Most children with this condition who have a successful operation go on to lead a normal life. They go to school, play with their friends, and can have families themselves when they grow up. However, a small percentage of them may need further treatment either in the form of repeat surgery or a keyhole type of procedure if there is a recurrence in the problem. In our center, I would say 2 in 10 children require repeat procedures but 8 out of 10 children are completely well.[5]

We do need to see them regularly and monitor their blood pressure as some of these children can develop high blood pressure but usually this can be managed well with medications if required."

Implications of the Diagnosis and the Likely Roadmap

A proportion of children with CHD require repeat procedures in later life. This is particularly the case in children with single ventricle physiology where a staged approach is needed, children with conduits which will need to be replaced in later life and children with conditions where residual hemodynamic problems are anticipated such as tetralogy of Fallot (TOF) with pulmonary regurgitation. Families need to be made aware of the entire journey that a child with CHD needs to make into adulthood. For most simple heart lesions which thankfully form the major proportion of the CHD burden in our part of the world, this will only involve regular outpatient visits and surveillance. However, for patients with moderately complex or highly complex cardiac problems, the story is quite different and may involve repeated interventions both surgical and transcatheter. A clear roadmap should be drawn so that the family are mentally and financially prepared to undertake this journey. Having a child with complex CHD can take a toll on the family; affecting the relationship between the parents and also impacting siblings who may not receive adequate parental attention in the changed circumstances.

Following their conversations with the medical team, the family is ready to proceed with treatment but confess that they may not be able to bear the financial burden completely. Pediatric cardiac programs are often heavily subsidized by parent hospitals and nongovernmental organization (NGOs) and usually supplementary funding can be obtained through alternative sources. The physician assures the family that help is at hand and in a happy ending to this family's story, the child undergoes successful surgery with a good hemodynamic result and is discharged home on no medications with normal blood pressure readings. The family are deeply grateful and happy and will be attending outpatient review in 2 months.

SPECIFIC COUNSELING CONUNDRUMS

Fetal Counseling

Case Example 1

A 24-year-old primigravid woman presents for a fetal echocardiogram at 18 weeks' gestation due to suspicion of a ventricular septal defect (VSD) on routine anomaly screening. A fetal echocardiogram confirms a moderate sized VSD and the family is counseled. As there is only an isolated VSD, the fetal cardiologist explains that the outlook is good and that the defect may restrict spontaneously or may require surgery if it remains moderate sized within 6 months of life. The overall survival is expected to be >95% as mortality for VSD surgery is around 5% in good pediatric cardiac centers.[6] The mother can have a normal vaginal delivery and the baby can be reassessed postnatally to make further decisions regarding need for intervention. The lady and her family are unhappy with the fetus having a cardiac problem and opt to terminate the pregnancy despite the overall good outlook for the cardiac lesion.

Case Example 2

A 31-year-old primigravid woman who has undergone treatment for infertility presents for a routine fetal echocardiogram at 17 weeks' gestation. Fetal echocardiogram reveals that the fetus has hypoplastic left heart syndrome. The fetal cardiologist explains the diagnosis and the need for staged surgery which can only be palliative. The overall survival at 10 years is quoted at around 70% with a high risk for the first-stage procedure, the Norwood.[7,8] It is explained that there is likely to be a significant need for repeated interventions to deal with the pulmonary arteries and the aorta. Also, long-term complications such as protein losing enteropathy and cardiac dysfunction are outlined. For this mother however this is a precious pregnancy and she has conceived after many years of IVF treatment. She decides to continue with the pregnancy and prepares for a long journey with complex CHD.

These two cases illustrate the high degree of variability in patients' perception of CHD and the individual circumstances that influence decision-making.

Avoiding Personal Bias

One of the most difficult aspects of good counseling is to avoid being directive. Decision-making needs to be patient led rather than physician led and there is a huge variability in individual reactions to the diagnosis of CHD that is dependent on individual value systems, religious faith, and personal circumstances. The clinician must take care to remain unbiased and willing to support the patient and their family in whatever decision they may arrive at. After all it is their life and their decision and the role of the physician is to actualize the patient's or parents' decision regarding their or their family's health.

Recurrence Risk and Future Pregnancies

The risk of recurrence of CHD is an important concern for families and specific counseling is required to address this issue. Having a previous child with CHD increases the risk of CHD by 3–4% in the next pregnancy.[9] There is still a >96% chance of having a child with a normal heart. There are however specific lesions such as left-sided obstructive lesions which seem to recur at higher rates and the nature of the lesion should inform the tone of counseling. However, overall there is a very good chance of having an unaffected child and families wishing to have another child should be supported and encouraged in this process. Fetal echocardiography can be carried out electively in early pregnancy to rule out CHD in these pregnancies.

Transitional Counseling

Case Example

A 15-year-old boy with a Fontan circulation who has been under pediatric cardiac care since birth attends clinic with his parents. He has been doing very well from a clinical point of view and his cardiac status is optimal. His parents however are unhappy that he has stopped taking his aspirin therapy over the past 3 months. He is aggressive and angry at home and does not want to go to school. Although he had been a good student in the past he is now failing examinations and falling behind. It is a difficult consultation with the parents blaming the child and each other. The boy sits silently looking at the floor waiting to get out of the consulting room.

The physician asks the parents to leave the room and speaks to the boy on his own. It becomes obvious that he is being bullied and made fun off in school due to his scar and his inability to participate on par with his peers in sports. He does not want to change in a common changing room with the other boys and is being teased and called a "girl" by his peers.

Empowering the Young Person

Counseling patients who are transitioning from being children to young adults can be very tricky. The child sees the physician as another adult, an establishment figure and winning their trust can take a long time. The first step is to empower the young person in looking after their own health, perhaps explaining to them the long journey that they have undertaken so far will help. Reaffirming that the obstacles that they have faced and overcome are a testament to their strength and that there is nothing that they cannot achieve if they set their mind. Assuring them that you will always be there when they need a friendly ear while explaining to the parents that it is important for the young person to gain independence gradually and to take responsibility for their own well-being may be useful. Sometimes additional resources including a psychologist may be required. Meeting other children with CHD can make them realize that they are not alone and may allow them to learn coping strategies from other survivors of CHD. Ideally patients should be seen in transitional clinics along with an adult congenital heart disease (ACHD) specialist to enable smooth transfer of care into adulthood.

Reproductive Counseling

Case Example 1

A 24-year-old lady comes to clinic accompanied by her husband and parents-in-law. She has been "recently" diagnosed to have Eisenmenger syndrome and has been advised not to get pregnant. Her husband is the only son of his parents and they are keen to "see their grandchildren before they die." They have come for specialist advice and management.

An echocardiogram reveals a large patent ductus arteriosus with clear clinical and echo signs of Eisenmengerization. The lady has established pulmonary vascular disease and clearly should not get pregnant.

This is not an uncommon scenario in our society where huge importance is placed on role of marriage and child birth in a woman's life. Ideally this lady, her parents, and her partner should have been counseled prior to marriage and the situation clearly explained. The presence of Eisenmenger syndrome is not a contraindication to marriage but her partner should have been made aware that it would not be possible for her to safely get pregnant as pregnancy in these patients carries a very high mortality of nearly 40–50%.[10]

In this case, the husband was a very understanding and compassionate man and understood the circumstances that led to the current situation. The couple were given advice regarding contraception and pregnancy avoidance. She underwent tubal ligation and the family are considering adopting a child.

Case Example 2

A 20-year-old visits clinic with her partner of many years. They have been together since school as the girl journeyed through life with complex CHD having undergone an atrial switch operation in early life. She currently has good ventricular function and is clinically well with no arrhythmia. The couple are planning to get married and want to know if they can safely start a family.

Patients who have undergone the atrial switch operation have the right ventricle (RV) supporting systemic circulation. In the long term, the systemic RV tends to fail and usually this occurs in the third or fourth decade of life. Currently this patient can successfully undergo pregnancy and she is advised to not delay having children but to have them early when her cardiac function is maintained. They come back a month later with a wedding invitation.

Some subsets of patients like those with the RV in systemic position, patients with a good Fontan circulation, those with moderate valve disease may be better off getting pregnant early as their disease is expected to progress with time and should be counseled accordingly.

Confidentiality

Reproductive counseling is a very important and often neglected area of CHD care. Patients are often lost to follow-up as they transition into adulthood and turn up to clinic already pregnant. Ideally counseling should be carried out preconception and care delivery should be planned ahead of time with clear plans in place for antepartum, intrapartum, and postpartum management.

Reproductive counseling in our country is often a "family affair" with not only the couple but also extended families being involved. This can lead to particular problems for the counseling physician but it is important to give the woman a choice to be counseled privately or with just her partner. One should also bear in mind that the woman's health and welfare is the physician's paramount priority and all other considerations only secondary.

Communicating Uncertainties

This is one of the most difficult situations confronting a clinician while counseling a patient or family. "Honesty" they say is the best policy and in this scenario this is the only approach that will work. It is important for the clinician to communicate clearly the uncertainties in diagnosis or treatment and fully involve the patient/family in the decision-making process. Existing literature should be discussed and the merits and demerits of the proposed plan explained in detail. Acknowledging that this is not an easy decision to make and assuring the patient and family that they will have the full support of the medical team irrespective of their decision is important. When the outcome of the procedure cannot be guaranteed or when despite a good procedural outcome clinical relief of symptoms cannot be guaranteed, this should be clearly communicated to the patient and family.

Lesion-specific Counseling

Benign/Relatively Insignificant Conditions

This includes small atrial septal defect (ASD), ventricular septal defect (VSD), patent ductus arteriosus (PDA), mild valve lesions such as mitral valve prolapse with trivial to mild mitral regurgitation, etc. The emphasis of counseling should be to reassure the family and to empower them to treat the child as normal with no activity restrictions. In lesions that have a risk of endocarditis, this risk should be highlighted with an emphasis on good dental hygiene.

Innocent Murmurs

The emphasis of counseling in this setting is to explain to the family that an innocent murmur which is very common in children occurring in 7 out of 10 children at some point during childhood is a benign phenomenon related to flow of blood through a normal heart. The thin body habitus and hyperdynamic circulation seen in children produce a noise much like "water running through a tap." Once a normal heart structure has been demonstrated on an echocardiogram, there is absolutely no cause for concern. It should be highlighted that innocent murmurs are likely to be heard during acute illnesses such as respiratory infections. The patient and family should be advised an unrestricted life and given tips regarding healthy living including a balanced diet and regular exercise.

Heart Disease Needing Corrective Surgery

This includes lesions such as moderate-to-large VSD, ASD, PDA, and total anomalous pulmonary venous connection which can be completely corrected by surgery. Once corrective surgery has been performed, these children have essentially normal hearts and only need infrequent follow-up. Once the shunt lesions have been completely abolished and endothelialization has occurred over the prosthetic patch, there is no increase in the risk of endocarditis compared to a normal heart. These children can be advised unrestricted activity including competitive sport. Procedure specific complications related to surgery including bleeding, thromboembolic episodes including stroke, wound infections, etc., should be discussed whilst obtaining consent prior to the procedure. The risk to life although small should be mentioned but placed in the context of risk benefit analysis.

Heart Disease Needing Corrective Intervention

This includes lesions such as moderate-to-large ASD, PDA, and VSD, which are device suitable and also valve stenosis (particularly pulmonary stenosis) which is balloon dilated. These corrective interventions when performed at the right time usually result in restoration of normal hemodynamics and normalization of cardiac structure and dimensions over a period of time. Device endothelialization occurs within 6 months and antiplatelet medication if any can be stopped at this point. There is no increased risk of endocarditis following endothelialization and complete abolition of the shunt. Patients who undergo device closures particularly with large intracardiac devices or in positions vulnerable to conduction system damage (e.g., perimembranous VSD closure) do require long-term rhythm surveillance and this should be highlighted prior to device closure. Procedure-specific complication such as bleeding, thromboembolic episodes including the risk of stroke, and device embolization should be discussed whilst obtaining consent prior to the procedure. The risk to life although small should be mentioned but placed in the context of risk–benefit analysis.

Defects Requiring Correction with Future Reoperations

This includes conditions such as truncus arteriosus, TOF with absent pulmonary valve syndrome, TOF requiring a transannular patch, atrioventricular septal defect (AVSD) with residual mitral regurgitation (MR), etc. The possibility of residual lesions and need for future intervention/surgery should be discussed. Operations that require conduit placement in early infancy invariably require revision and perhaps multiple reoperations during childhood and early adult life. This should be highlighted to the family. The possibility of future transcatheter revision avoiding redo sternotomy may also be mentioned.

Single Ventricle Physiology

The emphasis in this subset of patients is to explain the need for multiple surgeries in a preplanned staged manner at appropriate ages. The complications of single ventricle palliation including protein losing enteropathy, plastic bronchitis, ventricular dysfunction, valve leakage, and arrhythmia should be highlighted. The need for close lifelong follow-up and possible need for lifelong medical therapy should be mentioned. The possibility of needing cardiac transplantation if the patient develops complications may also be mentioned.

Syndromic Children/Chromosomal Anomalies with Heart Disease

The possibility of genetic diagnoses associated with CHD, especially in syndromic children, should be explained. Certain lesions may be associated with specific genetic/chromosomal abnormalities, e.g., AVSD with Down syndrome, truncus arteriosus or TOF with DiGeorge syndrome. The implications of the suspected genetic diagnosis should be explained and specialist genetic consultation should be sought.

UNIQUE CHALLENGES IN THE INDIAN CONTEXT

Financial Cost of Pediatric Cardiac Care

In addition to dealing with the psychological impact of having a child with CHD, parents in our part of the world have to deal with the financial stress that this brings with it. Physicians will often need to factor in the likely cost of any procedure or hospitalization required and explore the financial ability of the patient's family. This might influence decision-making regarding the management of a patient. For example, surgical pulmonary valve replacement is only 1/10th the cost of transcatheter valve replacement and is often preferred even in patients who have anatomy suitable for transcatheter therapy due to its forbidding cost.

Fortunately many parent hospitals subsidize pediatric cardiac programs and in addition nongovernmental organization (NGOs) and private donors help to make it possible for patients from low-income families to undergo cardiac surgery and go on to lead productive lives.

Lack of Robust Patient Support Groups and Resources

Although the concept of support groups is well established in the west, it is yet to gain steam in our part of the world. Support groups are an invaluable resource for patients providing useful information, guidance, and support to parents and patients to help them navigate the difficult journey through CHD. Online resources are however widely available which can be easily accessed from any part of the world and can help clinicians caring for patients with CHD and their families.

CONCLUSION

In conclusion, counseling is a critical step in the management pathway of patients with CHD and warrants increased focus in the training of future clinicians involved in caring for children with CHD and their families. Establishing a trusting relationship with patients and their families facilitates ease of treatment and ensures patient compliance with therapies. In addition, it goes a long way to help mitigate the risk of litigation that physicians encounter in modern medical practice.

REFERENCES

1. Lumsden MR, Smith DM, Wittkowski A. Coping in parents of children with congenital heart disease: a systematic review and meta-synthesis. Lumsden MR, Smith DM, Wittkowski A. J Child Fam Stud. 2019;28(3):1736-53.
2. Vainberg LD, Vardi A, Jacoby R. The experiences of parents of children undergoing surgery for congenital heart defects: a holistic model of care. Front Psychol. 2019;10:2666.
3. Uzark K, Jones K. Parenting stress and children with heart disease. J Pediatr Health Care. 2003; 17(4):163-8.
4. Lisanti AJ. Parental stress and resilience in congenital heart disease: a new frontier for health disparities research. Cardiol Young. 2018;28(9):1142-50.
5. Sen S, Garg S, Rao S, Kulkarni S. Native aortic coarctation in neonates and infants: immediate and midterm outcomes with balloon angioplasty and surgery. Ann Pediatr Cardiol. 2018; 11(3):261-6.
6. Vaidyanathan B, Roth SJ, Rao S, Gauvreau K, Shivaprakasha K, KrishnaKumar R. Outcome of ventricular septal defect repair in a developing country. J Pediatr. 2002;140(6):736-41.
7. Kane JM, Canar J, Kalinowski V, Johnson TJ, Hoehn S. Management options and outcomes for neonatal hypoplastic left heart syndrome in the early twenty-first century. Pediatr Cardiol. 2016;37(2):419-25.
8. Javed R, Cetta F, Said SM, Olson TM, O' Leary PW, Qureshi MW. Hypoplastic left heart syndrome: an overview for primary care providers. Pediatr Rev. 2019;40(7):344-53.
9. Fesslova V, Brankovic J, Lalatta F, Villa L, Meli V, Piazza L, Ricci C. Recurrence of congenital heart disease in cases with familial risk screened prenatally by echocardiography. J Pregnancy. 2011;2011:368067.
10. Duan R, Xu X, Wang X, Yu H, You Y, Liu X, et al. Pregnancy outcome in women with Eisenmenger's syndrome: a case series from west China. BMC Pregnancy Childbirth. 2016;16(1):356.

Pediatric Cardiovascular Disease

2 PART

17
CHAPTER

Heart Failure in Children

Sumitra Venkatesh, R Krishna Kumar

INTRODUCTION

Heart failure is a clinical syndrome that results from a wide variety of causes in children.[1] It is important for the pediatrician to be familiar with the nuances of recent advances in diagnosis and management of various causes of heart failure which have translated into a vastly improved outlook. The prognosis of heart failure in children is critically dependent on identifying the precise etiology quickly and treating the exact cause. Acute care of severely compromised children has vastly improved, and most children can be salvaged through good intensive care. This is somewhat different from adults with heart failure where the list of potential causes, especially treatable causes, is much smaller.

There is considerable diversity in the clinical presentation and etiology of heart failure depending on the age of the child. Neonates, infants, toddlers, older children, and adolescents all have important differences in clinical manifestation and etiology.

Additionally, there are important considerations in the Indian context. A few causes are unique to the Indian context. These include rheumatic fever and rheumatic heart disease and aortoarteritis in older children and adolescents, calcium and vitamin D deficiency and Beriberi in infants and young children; and scorpion sting-related ventricular dysfunction and diphtheritic myocarditis in very specific settings.[2,3] The management of heart failure is often challenged by resource limitations in many Indian healthcare settings.

The purpose of this chapter is to lay a robust framework for the pediatrician to enable accurate diagnosis of heart failure in various age groups and to enunciate the principles of diagnostic workup so that the cause of heart failure is correctly identified in the overwhelming majority. The recent advances in therapy of heart failure will be discussed in some detail. The evidence from clinical trials of the commonly used drugs in pediatric heart failure will be presented. Additionally, the principles of acute care of critically ill children with severe cardiovascular compromise will also be presented. These principles are vital to caregivers who are involved in stabilizing these children prior to referral for definitive management.

DEFINITION

Heart failure is generally understood as a progressive clinical and pathophysiological syndrome occurring due to a complex interplay of molecular, circulatory, and neuro-hormonal derangements that result from inability of the heart to meet the metabolic demands of the body either at rest or during activity. The presence of typical signs and symptoms of respiratory distress, growth failure, and exercise intolerance together with features of elevated filling pressures in the form of liver enlargement, venous engorgement, and edema are typical clinical manifestations.

A simple definition of heart failure would be the inability of the heart to function adequately to meet the metabolic demands of the body. This definition also includes situations where cardiac output is reduced at rest or during activity and situations where the cardiac output is maintained at the cost of elevated filling pressures. It is often not intuitively obvious that the definition of heart failure actually includes conditions in children where a heart disease is responsible for relatively subtle manifestations such as failure to thrive alone. Therefore, for example, a 5 year old child with an atrial septal defect (ASD) with failure to thrive as the only manifestation that gets corrected after closure of the defect would be classified as having heart failure. In strictest terms, the definition of heart failure should also include situations where heart disease is only manifest on formal testing through measurement of oxygen consumption at peak exercise.

A broad and inclusive definition of heart failure serves to identify the need to treat children with heart disease prior to development of changes that may have a potential for long-term consequences. For example, in a child with aortic or mitral valve regurgitation, waiting for overt clinical manifestations may result in irreversible damage to the heart muscle. Such a definition also allows for fine-tuning drug treatment strategies. Most clinical trials on medications for heart failure in children include poor weight gain as an inclusion-criteria.[4]

EPIDEMIOLOGY

There are almost 5 million adults with heart failure in India alone with an annual incidence ranging between 0.5 and 2 million, but there is no comprehensive pediatric database regarding the incidence or prevalence of heart failure in our country.[5] Literature suggests around 12,000–35,000 pediatric cases of heart failure-related hospitalizations in the United States (US) alone annually, with congenital heart disease (CHD) and cardiomyopathies being the leading causes of failure in the current era.[6] According to a few European studies, cardiac failure in children accounts for 10–33% of all cardiac admissions with >50% of them being due to structural CHD and about 20% due to cardiomyopathies.[7] Though incidence of heart failure in children with CHD accounts for 6–24% in a few European studies, the US database shows almost 60% of the hospital discharges in children with heart failure had a presence of an underlying CHD. The incidence of CHD in adults admitted with heart failure was <1% in both.[8] No such data is available from the Indian subcontinent. There is perhaps a need to establish large multicenter registries to understand the profile of heart failure among children in the Indian context. The true incidence and prevalence of pediatric heart failure would be much more difficult to ascertain as this would require a community-based surveillance. Given the relative rarity, such a study would be almost impossible to conduct at the community level. However, a multicenter pediatric heart failure registry would help estimate the overall disease burden.

ETIOLOGY

It is vital to recognize that heart failure is the end result of a wide range of conditions. The two unique features of heart failure in children are that there are a large number of possible causes and that the majority of these causes can be addressed through specific treatments. For this reason the most important step in managing heart failure in a child is to determine the exact cause. Interestingly, even in some of the situations where the exact cause is not identified, the child may recover completely after aggressive supportive treatment (for example, acute myocarditis). This situation is quite different from adults where the outlook is not as favorable and where the majority of the heart failure results from a limited set of causes such as ischemic heart disease.

The causes of heart failure in children vary in different age groups and there are important regional differences as well. **Figure 1** presents a convenient classification of causes of heart failure in children based on the underlying mechanism. Many of these conditions are structural defects that can be corrected through surgery or occasionally through catheter-based intervention. The other major category is myocardial disease that manifests as ventricular dysfunction. It is important to recognize that heart failure from ventricular dysfunction in children has diverse causes, many of which are treatable (**Flowchart 1**). A number of these conditions are mislabeled as idiopathic cardiomyopathies.

The etiology of heart failure is different in different age groups (**Fig. 2**). This is useful information because it enables us to limit the possible causes to a relatively smaller list of conditions.

Regional and sociocultural differences in the etiology result from the higher frequency of specific conditions in certain areas. In India, rheumatic fever and rheumatic heart disease is prevalent in many parts and is a common cause of heart failure in school-going children and adolescents. Beriberi is still prevalent in specific pockets of the country

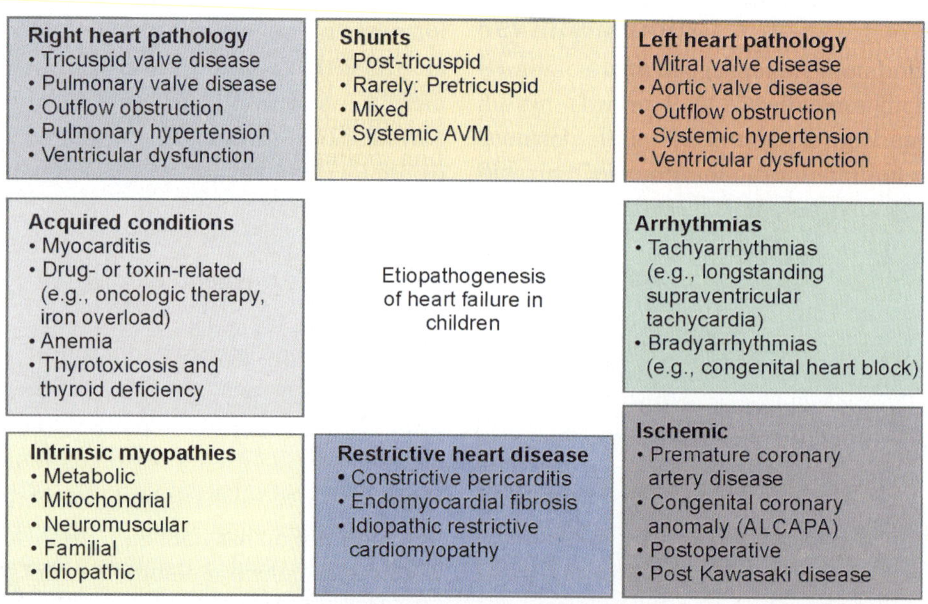

Fig. 1: A convenient classification of causes of heart failure in children as determined by underlying mechanism. ALCAPA: anomalous left coronary artery from pulmonary artery. This is not meant to be a comprehensive list of conditions but serves as a general guide. (AVM: arteriovenous malformation)

Flowchart 1: Classification of systolic ventricular dysfunction in children.

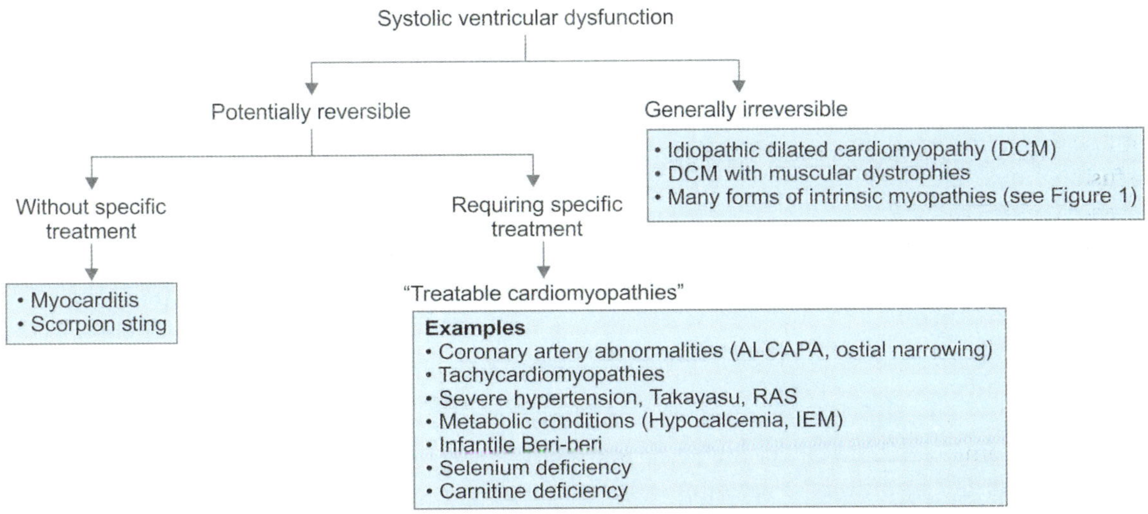

(ALPACA: anomalous left coronary artery from pulmonary artery; IEM: inborn errors of metabolism; RAS: renal artery stenosis)

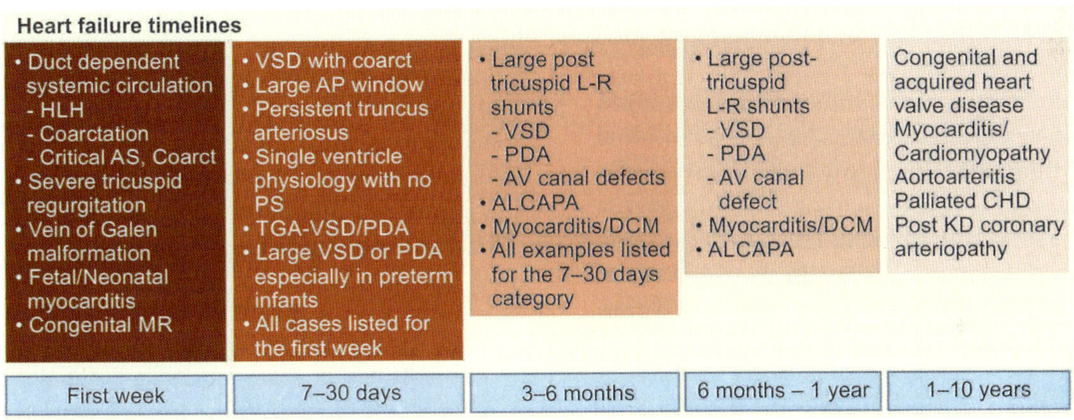

Fig. 2: Age-related possible etiology of heart failure.
(ALCAPA: anomalous left coronary artery from pulmonary artery; AP: aortopulmonary; AS: aortic stenosis; AV: atrioventricular; CHD: congenital heart disease; DCM: dilated cardiomyopathy; HLH: hypoplastic left heart; KD: Kawasaki disease; MR: mitral regurgitation; VSD: ventricular septal defect; PS: pulmonary stenosis; TGA: transposition of the great arteries; PDA; patent ductus arteriosus)

with very specific dietary practices in breastfeeding mothers that result in severe thiamine deficiency.[7] Similarly, severe calcium and vitamin D deficiency can present as heart failure with ventricular dysfunction in breastfed infants of mothers with severe vitamin deficiency.[9]

Heart failure may also occur transiently in certain acute care settings. Examples include severe sepsis in pediatric intensive care settings and in the postoperative period following cardiopulmonary bypass during palliative or corrective cardiac surgeries. More recently during the COVID pandemic, heart failure has been seen after exposure to the virus. This is often a part of the multi-system inflammatory syndrome (MISC) in children and adolescents with myocarditis. As with any other illness, the context of heart failure is of paramount importance.[10]

PATHOPHYSIOLOGY

Developmentally, heart is the first organ to be completely formed during embryogenesis. It begins beating as a heart tube at around 3 weeks of gestation and is completed by 9–10 weeks after a complex process of looping, septation, formation of valves, coronaries, and conduction system. Any insult during the process of cardiogenesis may cause structural, functional, or conduction abnormalities in the heart. Though fetal heart structurally resembles an adult heart, it functions in a parallel circuit, rather than the normal circulation in series. This implies that the left ventricle (LV) pumps into the head and upper part of the body and the right ventricle (RV) pumps to the ductus arteriosus, placenta, and lower part of the body. During failure or obstruction of either of the ventricles, the other ventricle compensates well in terms of function. Due to this very reason, many CHDs are well tolerated in fetal life and manifest clinically only after birth. The myocardium, on the other hand, continues to develop for a few months beyond fetal life albeit with smaller and lesser number of myocytes. The neonatal myocardium has decreased intracellular calcium and certain specific structural proteins such as titin and troponin I. These factors make the fetal/neonatal myocardium relatively stiff. Hence, the compensatory mechanism varies from those in adults and makes the fetal heart more prone to heart failure in conditions such as arrhythmias, cardiomyopathies, restrictive foramen ovale or arterial duct (causing venous hypertension in fetus), and high output states such as twin-to-twin transfusion. Thus, age is an important determinant of pediatric heart failure with >50% of the cases occurring in infancy (especially in the first 3 months of age). Most western literature mention that close to 70% of heart failure in children occurs during infancy and that almost 50% of these infantile cases have primary myocardial disease as the cause.[1]

After birth, there are changes in myocytes and an increase in ventricular compliance. The pulmonary vascular resistance also begins to fall in the first 3 months of life. This is also the period of transition from fetal to neonatal circulation. In cases of large left-to-right shunts such as ventricular septal defect or patent arterial duct, there is an extra volume of blood entering the pulmonary circulation. The LV contracts more forcefully to maintain the systemic cardiac output and compensate for the blood that is shunted into the pulmonary vasculature. This leads to the symptoms of congestive cardiac failure inspite of the normal ventricular systolic function.

The fundamental physiologic concepts required to understand the intricate relationship between preload, afterload, and contractility as well as the Frank–Starling's principle are discussed in Chapter 4.

Pathophysiology in Pressure Overload Conditions

The classic example here is that of severe aortic stenosis in neonates. There is an obstruction to the outflow from the LV in systole which reduces the LV output. In animal research, the obstruction has shown to cause myocyte hyperplasia (increase number of cells) and myocardial hypertrophy (increased contractile elements per cell) and a decreased LV cavity in fetal life. As mentioned earlier, due to the parallel circulation in utero, the RV compensates for the decreased cardiac output from LV, most of the times except in most severe cases. This mechanism changes after birth as the circulation transitions from parallel to a circulation in series. The RV is then unable to maintain the necessary cardiac output leading to poor perfusion, metabolic acidemia culminating in cardiogenic shock.

Pathophysiology in Volume Overload Conditions

The fundamental mechanisms of volume overload include large left-to-right shunts, valve regurgitations, and the high output state. The pathophysiology of heart failure from shunt lesions is discussed in chapters relating to individual CHDs (*see* Chapters 20 to 25). The LV is volume loaded in large post-tricuspid shunts. The LV decompensates from having to deal with a significantly higher volume of blood returning from the pulmonary veins as a result of the shunt between ventricles or the great vessels. Generally large pretricuspid shunts, such as ASD, are better tolerated and do not result in overt heart failure because the volume overload affects the RV that is better adapted to deal with larger volumes. However, even the RV may be overwhelmed in extremely large shunts as in total anomalous pulmonary venous return.

Heart failure develops in acute severe valve regurgitations or after compensatory mechanisms fail in chronic valve regurgitation. Regurgitation of right-sided heart valves are generally clinically less obvious for a long period of time. The best example is chronic pulmonary regurgitation after repair of tetralogy of Fallot. These patients remain relatively symptom free for decades until decompensation sets in. On the other hand, aortic and mitral regurgitation tend to have a relatively shorter period of compensation and overt heart failure tends to set in earlier.

In high output states, there is an excessive demand imposed because of specific extracardiac conditions such as anemia, thyotoxicosis, and beriberi. Decompensation results after a variable period when the heart is subject to excessive overload.

Direct Myocardial Injury

A wide variety of insults can directly impair ventricular function. These diverse conditions include genetic factors, viral infections, drugs and toxins, metabolic and electrolyte abnormalities, ischemia, chronic hypoxia, and immunologic insults. The list is very long and discussed in greater detail in Chapters 43 and 45. Many of these factors are partially or completely reversible. Compensatory mechanisms involve hyperplasia and hypertrophy of unaffected myocytes. Myocardial dysfunction leads to ventricular dilation that enables the heart to function at higher volumes for a variable period of time until clinically manifest decompensation sets in.

COMPENSATORY RESPONSE

A variety of compensatory mechanisms are activated by the body that is very useful in the short term (**Flowchart 2**). However, over time, they lead to adverse consequences that further reduce the efficiency of the heart muscle pump.[11]

Cardiac failure leads to an increased release and a decreased uptake of norepinephrine causing peripheral vasoconstriction. This in turn increases the systemic vascular resistance (SVR) and boosts the mean arterial pressure leading to improved perfusion of selected vital organs. The increased sympathetic activity also stimulates β-receptors, thereby increasing the heart rate to subsequently augment cardiac output (which is directly proportional heart rate and stroke volume).

Flowchart 2: Compensatory mechanisms in heart failure.

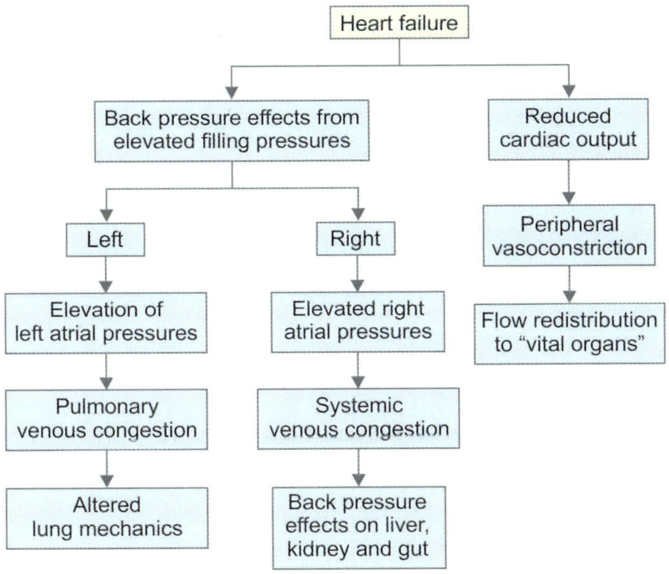

Heart failure also stimulates the renin–angiotensin–aldosterone system (RAAS) that increases the circulating levels of renin, angiotensin II, and aldosterone. Renin leads to breakdown of angiotensinogen to angiotensin I which is converted to angiotensin II in the presence of angiotensin-converting enzyme (ACE). Angiotensin II plays multiple roles in cardiac failure. It is a potent vasoconstrictor that helps in maintaining end-organ perfusion and causes sodium retention at the proximal tubules directly. It additionally stimulates the thirst center of the brain, stimulating release of arginine vasopressin hormone (AVP), which is known to be inappropriately elevated in patients with heart failure. This results in retention of water, peripheral vasoconstriction, hyponatremia, and an increased production of endothelin which is a powerful vasoconstrictor. Also, angiotensin II [illegible] aldosterone. Aldosterone causes sodium resorption in the distal tubules, causing salt and water retention leading to an increased cardiac preload and thus an increased cardiac output in the initial stages. In a normal heart, atrial natriuretic peptide and the brain natriuretic peptide (BNP) are two important hormones that are secreted to counter-regulate the RAAS activation. These are secreted due to stretching of the atrium or myocardium. The natriuretic peptides cause increased production of cyclic guanosine monophosphate (cGMP), whereas in those with heart failure, there is a peripheral resistance to the natriuretic peptides causing vasoconstriction and volume overload.

Both the above neurohormonal mechanisms eventually cause cardiomyocyte injury with fibrosis and apoptosis of cardiac cells leading to progressive heart failure, thus offering only a temporary stability to the circulatory system. Most contemporary pharmacotherapy used in treating heart failure (especially in adults) target these compensatory mechanisms.

EFFECT OF HEART FAILURE ON ORGAN SYSTEMS AND THEIR CLINICAL IMPLICATIONS IN CHILDREN

Nutrition and Growth

Malnutrition and growth disturbance are highly prevalent in pediatric heart failure. The magnitude of the problem is directly related to the severity of the cardiac lesion and the hemodynamic effects. Malnutrition during the period of rapid growth in infancy also results in permanent physical or developmental impairment. Birth weight of babies with CHD is often normal or near normal for gestational age; failure to grow occurs as energy is diverted away from growth and healing toward other critical functions.[12] The mechanism for growth failure in children with heart disease is still not completely understood; growth essentially occurs in an anabolic state, when exogenous caloric intake exceeds energy expenditure. Increased metabolic rate, insufficient calorie intake, inflammation, and malabsorption of ingested calories are the various potential reasons for failure to grow in this population. Additionally, fatigue on feeding, anorexia, vomiting, and fluid restriction contribute to malnutrition in these babies.[13] Excessive loss of proteins (protein losing enteropathy) and steatorrhea were seen to be commonly associated in children with heart failure. Also, hepatomegaly and gut edema associated with heart failure decrease the gastric volume (leading to deficient intake) and causes dysmotility with malabsorption of nutrients respectively. Indirect evidence of inadequate calorie intake has been proven by studies that have shown short-term gain in growth (weight and height) while on measured enteral feeds. The high resting energy expenditure with the increased metabolic demand in children with heart failure adds to the above burden leading to significant growth failure.[14,15]

Weight is more affected than height in acyanotic congenital heart lesions that may cause pulmonary hypertension (PH), whereas both height and weight are equally affected in those with cyanotic heart diseases such as transposition of the great arteries (TGA). Patients with isolated obstructive lesions such as pulmonary stenosis or coarctation of the aorta (CoA) have also shown reduced linear growth, albeit to a smaller extent. Studies have shown that close to a quarter of patients with DCM and almost 50% of those listed for heart transplant or ventricular assist device (VAD) implantation are malnourished.[16] Assist devices support facilitates nutritional rehabilitation by reducing symptoms of heart failure and improving hemodynamics allowing concomitant increase in dietary intake and decreased metabolic demand. Most studies have also noted that the weight is often more affected than height. Though cardiac surgery in malnourished patients poses additional risk, many centers worldwide no longer wait for the ideal weight prior to surgery as early surgical correction of the underlying cardiac lesion will eliminate heart failure and hypoxemia, leading to catch-up growth in infancy.[17,18]

Delay in skeletal maturity is directly related to the severity of hypoxemia. There may be an endocrine involvement that causes delayed puberty in adolescents with severely cyanotic CHD, which often does not begin until a height age of 12–13 years has been achieved.[19]

Neurocognitive Development

The spectrum of neurodevelopmental delay in children with chronic heart failure and complex CHD includes one or more of the following possibilities—mild developmental delay, motor deficit, cognitive impairments, attention deficit and hyperactivity, delay in language and communication skills, and poor social interaction. These may persist well into school age and beyond. There are reports showing moderate-to-severe impairment in at least one area of neurodevelopment in children who required cardiac surgery in infancy. These children are also known to have special needs at school; with learning disabilities and speech impairment. This subset of children must be monitored continuously to determine the need for early intervention and individualized education plan. Usually a multidisciplinary team intervention is required in most of these cases, which includes a developmental pediatrician, neurologist, psychologist, physiotherapist, occupational therapist, and speech therapist in addition to the pediatric cardiologist.

Liver

The liver receives almost 25% of the total cardiac output from dual sources, the hepatic artery and portal vein. Blood then flows through the sinusoids and reaches the hepatic veins, which carry the blood to inferior vena cava (IVC) to eventually drain into the right atrium.[19] This dual blood supply is quite beneficial as liver continues to function even if one source fails. Heart and liver are in close relation to each other and hence any impairment in cardiac function may lead to associated hepatic dysfunction. Hepatic dysfunction is noted in 20–30% of cases with cardiac failure.[20] In cases of CHD leading to left or right heart failure, hepatic dysfunction ensues due to the primary cardiac defect or postpalliative surgery such as Fontan (especially in single ventricle pathology).

The mechanism causing the liver affliction may be multifactorial ranging from passive liver congestion, chronic hypoxia, volume overload to low cardiac output state (hypoperfusion of the liver).[21] Over time, congestive hepatopathy and hepatic ischemia may lead to hepatic cirrhosis, fibrosis, and portal hypertension.

Passive liver congestion is seen in as high as 65% cases of severe heart failure. Congestive hepatopathy resulting from elevated right atrial pressure is seen in a wide variety of conditions that include ASDs with PH, Eisenmenger syndrome, Ebstein anomaly, single ventricle physiology (after Fontan procedure), d-TGA (after atrial switch surgery), late after tetralogy of Fallot repair with chronic pulmonary regurgitation and right ventricular failure.

Though details of Fontan surgery is covered in a separate chapter (*see* Chapter 39), post-Fontan hepatopathy needs a special mention in heart failure as it is one of the most common sequelae of the procedure and also one of the most common causes of hepatic injury in children with heart failure. Post-Fontan hepatopathy occurs mainly due to passive congestion and hypoxia due to ventricular dysfunction. Chronic elevation of central venous pressure is seen due to the continuous, nonpulsatile backpressure on the liver in the absence of a subpulmonic pump. Failure of the single, systemic functional ventricle causes a decreased cardiac output. All of these cause significant structural and functional alteration of the liver parenchyma leading to hepatic fibrosis followed by cirrhosis. These complications are often only incidentally detected on follow-up when specifically looked for and may even progress to hepatocellular carcinoma in a few cases.

Apart from clinical signs of right heart failure, laboratory investigations reveal elevated indirect bilirubin level, liver enzymes, especially gamma-glutamyl transaminase, deficiency of liver coagulation factors, and elevated lactate dehydrogenase levels. Evidence of hepatic fibrosis is identified early through specific tests that include elastography and later they are apparent on routine ultrasound and computed tomography (CT) scans.

Kidneys

Kidneys are known to be affected in 10–25% of children with heart failure. Acute kidney injury (AKI) is an abrupt and sustained change in renal function frequently encountered in children with heart disease. It is an important independent risk factor for increased morbidity and mortality in these cases. Repeated episodes of AKI lead to chronic kidney disease (CKD) eventually. Since long, clinicians have noted the bidirectional and concomitant nature of heart and renal dysfunction in children diagnosed with CHD and heart failure. The diagnosis of AKI varies in different studies as some studies are based on serum creatinine levels whereas others based on urine output. Oliguria is quite a sensitive prognostic marker in children with AKI. In adult population, even small increments in creatinine values have shown detrimental effects in terms of morbidity and mortality.

Cardiorenal syndrome (CRS) is the term used to define the coexistence of cardiac and renal dysfunction in children with heart failure. The cause here is multifactorial involving volume status, inflammation, neurohormonal interactions, and use of pharmacological agents, with the pathophysiology simply being poor renal perfusion. Reduction in cardiac output and renal artery flow is perceived by the kidneys as hypoperfusion; this stimulates the compensatory neurohormonal, up-regulatory mechanisms that cause sodium and water reabsorption along with the activation of RAAS pathway in an attempt to increase cardiac output and renal perfusion.[22] A systemic venous congestion occurs due to reabsorption of sodium and water, which impedes the forward flow of blood through renal vasculature leading to decreased glomerular filtration and increased protein excretion. This leads to oliguria which subsequently increases volume overload, symptomatically worsening cardiac failure. Though the pediatric data on CRS is scarce, most studies have noted an increasing need for mechanical circulatory support and mortality in children with heart failure with worsening renal functions.

Children undergoing corrective cardiac surgeries are exposed to cardiopulmonary bypass, aortic cross-clamping, hypothermic circulatory arrest, and a low cardiac output with multiple nephrotoxic pharmacological agents in the postoperative period.[23] All these may lead to or worsen renal failure in these children with an increased need for renal replacement therapy and duration of hospital stay. Risk of AKI and mortality increases with younger age at surgery, longer cross-clamp time, higher preoperative creatinine values, need for prolonged postoperative support (ventilation and inotropes), requirement of nitric oxide, cyanosis, and complexity of the surgery (additional details in Chapter 13).

Lungs

Lung is one of the most affected organs and the pulmonary vascular tone is one of the most important determinants of heart failure. Pulmonary hypertension (PH) occurs due to chronic pulmonary venous congestion with elevated filling pressures as seen in cases of systolic and diastolic ventricular dysfunction (secondary to left ventricular disease).[24] This additionally leads to an impaired gas exchange in the fluid filled alveoli due to pulmonary edema. Presence of PH is a predictor of poor prognosis and worse outcome in many subsets of pediatric heart failure. Reversibility of PH with pharmacotherapy or interventions denotes better survival and an improved outcome in children with cardiac failure. Additional details on PH are provided in Chapter 18.

CLINICAL FEATURES AND RECOGNITION OF HEART FAILURE

The clinical features of pediatric heart failure reflect hemodynamic derangements and the neurohormonal compensation that occurs subsequently. Hence, a good knowledge of the mechanism causing the mismatch between the metabolic demand and cardiac output is essential for clinical recognition of the condition (*see* **Flowchart 2**).

These hemodynamic changes may occur at different times and therefore the clinical manifestations also vary between patients.[25]

Symptoms are mainly age and pathophysiology dependent. The common symptoms seen in all cases of heart failure irrespective of the cause are poor growth, respiratory distress, and exercise intolerance. Age-adjusted scores of cardiac failure that are used to quantify the symptoms are a poor predictor of worsening clinical outcomes.

Neonates

The first few days after birth is a period of transition away from fetal circulation and is marked by a number of metabolic changes that occur during the birth process. The SVR increases and so does the oxygen demand. Neonatal heart is less compliant than the adult heart and hence more prone to failing.[26] This is especially true for the preterm or small for gestation babies where the myocardial fibers have limited cardiac energy stores and fewer contractile elements per cell.

The common reasons for cardiac failure on the first day of life include birth asphyxia, metabolic derangements (hypocalcemia and hypoglycemia), severe anemia, fetal distress, arrhythmias, neonatal myocarditis, and sepsis, in addition to severe structural CHD. Left heart failure results in pulmonary venous congestion consistently manifesting as tachypnea (RR >60 breaths per minute). Neonates may not have visible subcostal, intercostal and suprasternal retractions, nasal flaring, and grunting. Auscultation of the respiratory system is generally unhelpful and reveals more wheeze than rales in early neonatal age. Sinus tachycardia (heart rate >150 bpm) is a consistent early feature of a failing heart. Any resting heart rate of >220–230 bpm would point to primary arrhythmia as the cause of heart failure. Neonates with complete heart block may have a heart rate of less than 55 bpm and those with severe hypoxic ischemic encephalopathy can present with a relative bradycardia with heart rate ranging between 90 and 100 bpm. A bounding pulse is suggestive of high-output failure or shunting at the great artery level in the form of a large patent arterial duct, aortopulmonary window, or persistent truncus arteriosus.

Prolonged capillary refill time with cold and mottled extremities are pointers to low cardiac output and poor perfusion. Often the neonate with reduced cardiac output acquires an ashen pale appearance. Presence of an enlarged liver is an additional important feature of heart failure.

Physical examination of the heart offers some clues to the presence of underlying heart disease, but findings are often of limited sensitivity and specificity (*see* Chapter 48).

Infants

Lesions causing heart failure beyond the first week of life until early infancy are those with increased left-to-right shunting of the blood due to the fall in pulmonary vascular resistance. Most common amongst these are ventricular septal defects, atrioventricular septal defects, persistent truncus arteriosus, total anomalous pulmonary venous drainage, and aortopulmonary window. Babies with multiple shunts (in number or levels) present earlier than those with a single lesion. Other rare lesions such as anomalous left coronary artery from pulmonary artery may also present with heart failure at this age with symptoms of excessive irritability, which may be the only clue to the underlying infantile angina (*see* **Fig. 2**).

In infants, heart failure seriously affects feeding and this contributes to poor weight gain. Suck-rest-suck cycle is quite pathognomonic of heart failure and is similar to exercise intolerance in older patients. Sucking is an energy-consuming activity and is an exercise mimic for a baby. Heart failure causes frequent interruption during feeds, allowing the infant to rest and continuing to feed thereafter. This increases the feeding time and decreases the quantity of feed taken by these infants leading to poor weight gain. The respiratory pattern in these infants gives an important clue to the presence of cardiac failure in most cases. Silent tachypnea without much work of breathing is usually seen in CHD with mild-to-moderate pulmonary overcirculation. As the severity of pulmonary edema increases, these babies present with all the signs of respiratory distress and air hunger in the form of subcostal and intercostal retractions and alae nasal flaring. Respiratory distress with tachypnea and dyspnea is often the first evidence of cardiac failure in infants.

Older Children and Adolescents

The most common symptoms in older children with heart failure are decreased exercise capacity, shortness of breath, and easy fatigability. Though many children may not admit to having these complaints directly, they do increase their rest or sleep times, thereby giving a clue to worsening of symptoms. Few may even avoid strenuous activity entirely. Weight loss may occur due to chronic anorexia and nausea caused by gut edema and also due to the medications prescribed for medical management of heart failure. A sudden increase in weight on follow-up suggests development of edema, which is usually accompanied by abdominal pain and distension from hepatic congestion and ascites. Excessive sweating and paroxysmal nocturnal dyspnea are commonly seen in older children. Pedal edema may go unnoticed in the pediatric age, but periorbital edema on awakening is a well-recognized symptom in these children.

Classification of Functional Status in Heart Failure

Classification of functional status in heart failure in pediatric population is very challenging due to the variation in normal respiratory rates and heart rates across various age groups; different levels of exercise capacities at different stages of development and the varied etiology of heart failure (metabolic, congenital structural cardiac abnormality, myocardial dysfunction).

BOX 1: Modified Ross classification of heart failure in infants.

- *Class I*: No symptoms/limitations
- *Class II*: Mild tachypnea/sweating during feeds in infants/dyspnea on exertion in older children but no growth failure
- *Class III*: Significant tachypnea or sweating during feeds/marked dyspnea on exertion/prolonged feeding time with growth failure
- *Class IV*: Symptoms (tachypnea, retractions, grunting, and sweating) even at rest with growth failure

The Ross Heart Failure Classification was developed to provide a global assessment of heart failure severity in infants and later modified to be applicable to all pediatric ages (**Box 1**).[27] This scoring system is based on volume consumed per feed, time taken per feed, pattern of respiration, respiratory rate, heart rate, peripheral perfusion, hepatomegaly, and presence of third heart sound or diastolic rumble. The modified Ross classification is comparable to the New York Heart Association (NYHA) classification for adults.

There are various scoring systems for pediatric heart failure which include only clinical parameters like the one devised by Reithmann and colleagues called the Pediatric Clinical Heart Failure score.[28] This uses data like time taken for feeding, volume of feed apart from the vital parameters on physical examination to derive the score and is mainly used for clinical research purposes. Another by Connolly and team considers the signs, symptoms, echocardiography findings, and the presence of single ventricle physiology along with the outcomes in terms of ventricular function on therapy, degree of functional capacity, and presence of ventricular arrhythmias in the New York University Pediatric Heart Failure Index.[29] But, none of these are as popular and useful as the modified Ross classification for classification of heart failure in children mentioned earlier.

COMMON DIAGNOSTIC TESTS AND THEIR INDICATIONS

Laboratory Investigations

The following laboratory tests are generally indicated:

- *Complete blood count* to rule out anemia (can cause/aggravate heart failure), leukocytosis for underlying infection.
- *Renal function tests*: Elevated blood urea nitrogen (BUN) and creatinine are seen in decompensated heart failure.
- *Liver function tests*: Congestive hepatomegaly elevates the liver enzymes [serum glutamic pyruvic transaminase/serum glutamic oxaloacetic transaminase (SGPT/SGOT and lactic dehydrogenase (LDH)] and causes prolongation of partial thromboplastin time (PTT). Hyperbilirubinemia (direct and indirect) is seen in hepatic venous congestion associated with severe right

heart failure. Hypoalbuminemia is also seen in chronic heart failure due to poor nutrition and liver dysfunction.

- *Serum electrolytes*: Hyponatremia occurs due to expansion of extracellular fluid volume (dilutional) with a normal total body sodium, while hypokalemia and hypochloremia occur commonly due to prolonged use of diuretics. Hyperkalemia is seen in some cases due to impaired tissue perfusion causing release of intracellular potassium and due to poor renal perfusion causing reduced glomerular filtration rate.
- *Thyroid function tests*: While both severe hypothyroidism and hyperthyroidism can lead to heart failure, they may also contribute to worsening in select cases.
- Specific viral panels to identify viruses that can cause myocarditis (e.g., BioFire Film array) may be considered in very specific circumstances (*see* Chapter 43).
- *Arterial blood gas*: Mild-to-moderate heart failure shows mild hypoxemia on blood gas analysis. Severe hypoxemia is seen in severe heart failure. Ventilation-perfusion mismatch causes hypocapnia in early pulmonary edema, later progressing to hypercapnia and respiratory acidosis due to reduced vital capacity and poor ventilation.
- *Natriuretic peptides*: BNP/N-terminal pro-BNP levels correlate well with Ross heart failure/NYHA classification of severity of heart failure in children.[30] These are useful markers to differentiate between respiratory and cardiac cause in cases of respiratory distress. BNP values of >300 pg/mL suggests a poorer prognosis.
- Cardiac enzymes [troponin I/T, creatine phosphokinase-MB (CPK-MB)] are useful in selected instances of suspected myocarditis and cardiomyopathy (*see* Chapters 43 and 45).
- *Lactates*: Elevated levels indicate dcreased tissue perfusion or decreased metabolism due to liver dysfunction in decompensated heart failure and are useful to monitor response to therapy in acute settings.

Chest Radiography

The chest X-ray yields vital information regarding the cardiac shape and size, pulmonary blood flow (plethora or oligemia), presence of pulmonary edema or venous congestion, pulmonary artery dilation, and pleural effusion.

Electrocardiogram

Sinus tachycardia is common although heart rates consistently beyond what is normal age should raise suspicion of tachyarrhythmia. A number of specific diagnostic clues are offered by the electrocardiogram (ECG). They include evidence of ischemia or infarction [ALCAPA (anomalous coronary artery from pulmonary artery) or coronary occlusion from any cause], hypocalcemia (suggested by long QT interval), tachyarrhythmia, bundle branch block pattern, and ventricular hypertrophy patterns.

Echocardiography

Echocardiography provides real-time and instant information regarding cardiac structure, systolic and diastolic function, chamber volumes, presence of structural abnormalities and septal defects, aortopulmonary level shunts, venous (systemic and pulmonary) and great artery anatomy, atrioventricular valve status, coronaries, outflow tracts, aortic arch, shape and size of ventricles, wall thickness, pulmonary pressures, and presence of pericardial effusion. This data aids in accurate diagnosis and helps in offering appropriate and optimal treatment (*see* Chapter 9).

Advanced Cardiac Imaging (*see* Chapter 10)

Cardiac Computed Tomography Scan

Cardiac CT with angiography helps in better delineation of the vascular structures in complex CHD. It is particularly useful in lesions with multiple aortopulmonary collaterals or anomalous venous connections that lead to pulmonary overcirculation leading to heart failure.

Cardiac Magnetic Resonance Imaging

Cardiac magnetic resonance imaging (cMRI) helps in finer diagnosis in complex CHD and offers better tissue characterization. It permits calculation of the actual ventricular volume and function with other hemodynamic parameters which cannot be accurately done with two-dimensional (2D)-echocardiography. The myocardial changes in cardiomyopathy and myocarditis and the severity of cardiac involvement, as assessed from cMRI, are useful to differentiate between the two conditions and also help to plan further therapy.

Cardiac Catheterization

Cardiac catheterization is seldom needed for diagnostic purposes (*see* Chapter 11) today; it is largely used to perform therapeutic interventions to manage specific lesions (*see* Chapter 14).

Exercise Testing and the 6-minute Walk Test

Exercise testing and 6-minute walk distance estimation is particularly useful to accurately determine the functional status of affected patients and can be used to monitor response to therapy.

Endomyocardial Biopsy

Endomyocardial biopsy is an invasive procedure with some risk and so it is reserved for specific diagnosis of myocarditis (viral/giant cell myocarditis) and in post-transplant work up.

DIFFERENTIAL DIAGNOSES

Many diseases present with heart failure due to an increased metabolic demand or impaired cardiac function. Common noncardiac causes that increase preload (volume overload conditions), increase afterload (hypertension), reduce oxygen-carrying capacity of blood (anemia), or increase metabolic demand (sepsis) can ultimately lead to heart failure. Lymphatic obstruction and venous obstruction syndromes (e.g., Budd–Chiari) also present with signs that resemble right heart failure. Often, right heart failure can present with vague abdominal symptoms such as nausea, vomiting, right-sided abdominal pain, anorexia, and weight loss. Pulmonary edema due to damage to the alveolar-capillary membrane is one of the most common conditions that mimics heart failure and may occur due to noncardiac causes such as in respiratory infections, acute respiratory distress syndrome, sepsis, hemorrhagic shock, and poisoning. Apart from respiratory conditions [such as acute respiratory distress syndrome (ARDS), pneumonia, pulmonary edema, emphysema, pulmonary embolism, and pulmonary fibrosis], acute kidney failure, nephrotic syndrome, and cirrhosis of liver may also present with symptoms and signs resembling that of heart failure.

It could be a clinical challenge to identify heart failure in children in the presence of other conditions like the above-mentioned respiratory diseases. Even a simple viral bronchiolitis in early infancy may appear ominous in some. Failure to thrive due to any other cause such as renal tubular acidosis or other metabolic conditions may also have signs such as tachypnea (due to acidosis) with tachycardia and hepatosplenomegaly that can be confused with heart failure. Neuromuscular diseases such as Duchenne muscular dystrophy and Friedreich's ataxia can also affect heart leading to heart failure and patients must undergo cardiac evaluation periodically as a standard of care. Genetic syndromes and chromosomal anomalies are frequently associated with cardiac disease causing heart failure.

All of these need a complete and thorough cardiovascular evaluation to enable early recognition and treatment of heart failure. An acutely sick child with poor perfusion, irrespective of the cause (e.g., sepsis) will show all signs of heart failure that include poorly felt pulses, mottled skin, cold extremities, cyanosis (due to sluggish circulation and impaired gas exchange), tachycardia, tachypnea, and hypotension mimicking cardiac failure.

Lack of history for progressive heart failure or CHD, with absence of a gallop rhythm or nonelevated jugular venous pressure (JVP) on examination may suggest a noncardiac cause. Investigations such as chest X-ray, ECG, echocardiography, measurement of pulmonary capillary wedge pressure on catheterization, and serum BNP usually help in clearly distinguishing a purely cardiac cause for heart failure from a noncardiac one.

MANAGEMENT OF HEART FAILURE IN CHILDREN

Management Goals

As stated previously, diagnostic work-up should be toward identifying the precise etiology because the vast majority of causes of heart failure in children are correctable. Even in situations where it is not possible to correct the underlying cause, it is important to characterize the underlying mechanism to enable therapy that is tailored to the physiological derangement. For example, heart failure from systolic ventricular dysfunction requires the administration of vasodilators while heart failure from restrictive physiology requires careful usage of diuretics and vasodilators are unlikely to help. At all times, it is essential to be mindful of physiology while planning medications in children with heart failure.

Over the years, there have been significant advances in management of heart failure in adults, whereas management is not so established in children. Though the etiology of heart failure is more varied and significantly different in children, the goals of therapy for both the populations remain the same. The main goals of heart failure therapy are to correct the underlying cause, reduce associated morbidity and mortality, improve functional status, and help improve quality of life.

Perhaps the most important goal of management is to identify the precise etiology of cardiac failure, so as to enable treatment of the root cause. This is particularly important as the most common reason for heart failure in children is structural CHD, which can be corrected in most cases, thanks to the substantial advances in pediatric cardiac surgery and interventional cardiology. In cases where no successful strategy is available, the aim is to modify the neurohormonal responses to heart failure and their pathophysiological consequences in order to stimulate endogenous repair mechanisms.

For the sake of therapy, heart failure can be considered to be in four stages (as in adult heart failure management strategies). Stage A is where there is a risk for heart failure (exposure to anthracyclines and presence of dystrophinopathies) and mainly requires observation with periodic evaluation to detect signs of heart failure and administration of medications to prevent/delay the onset of heart failure. Stage B includes those cases with asymptomatic structural abnormality. Stage C is when there is an underlying structural abnormality [like reduced LV ejection fraction (EF)] along with symptoms of heart failure.[31] Pediatric heart failure guidelines does suggest use of ACE inhibitors, beta-blockers, or aldosterone antagonists for therapy in stages B and C, though most randomized controlled trials (RCTs) do not show clear positive results. Stage D requires inotropic or mechanical circulatory support with mixed outcomes in chronic cases. Another unique challenge of treating pediatric heart failure with drugs approved from the adult armamentarium is difficulty in identifying the most optimal dosing pattern due to substantial variation in pharmacokinetics and pharmacodynamics in children which depends significantly on age and developmental maturity.[32]

General Measures

Supportive management helps prevent rapid deterioration of cardiac status and acute events, allowing the physicians some buffer time until definitive and potentially curative therapy is instituted.

Important among these are:

- *Fluid management*: Restriction of fluid in take is generally recommended especially when edema or lung congestion is unresponsive to diuretic therapy or in the presence of hyponatremia. Fluid administration is indicated less commonly when there is an absolute or relative volume depletion. Typically, these are situations where the ventricle is stiff and needs a higher "preload" to generate the required cardiac output. Examples include the stiff RV early after repair of tetralogy of Fallot and hypertrophic cardiomyopathy. Strict monitoring and balance of blood pressure and perfusion parameters is helpful while hydrating a child in heart failure.
- *Rest and activity recommendations*: This is a frequently overlooked part of therapy that helps significantly by reducing the load on a compromised myocardium and prevents worsening of symptoms during acute heart failure. In infants, "rest" translates into expressed/tube feeds and avoiding direct breastfeeding. Recent studies have shown that regular physical activity shows small, but sustained increment in cardiac functions even in children with complex CHD (as a part of cardiac rehabilitation program).
- *Measures to increase the oxygen-carrying capacity of blood*: Anemia is one of the most common cause of high-output cardiac failure and anemia also increases the metabolic demand of the already compromised heart. Hence, building-up or maintaining optimal hemoglobin level becomes even more imperative. This is achieved by iron supplementation to maintain hemoglobin as close to normal as possible. Blood transfusion is usually reserved for patients with severe anemia (hemoglobin of 7 or lesser)
- *Oxygen*: Supplementary oxygen is sometimes necessary in children with heart failure, especially in the presence of pulmonary congestion or coexisting lung infections.
- *Diet*: Nutritional support is as important as medical therapy in cases of children with cardiac condition associated with growth failure. The standard recommendation is to provide adequate calories and proteins with the principle of increasing the calorie density and retaining the normal volume of feeds. This is normally achieved by adding medium chain triglycerides or sugar to the diet. The nutritional requirement in infants must provide around 150 kcal/kg/day to promote rapid growth and is usually better tolerated and achieved by providing small and frequent feeds. In older children and adolescents, 30 kcals/kg/day is a reasonable target. The three major macronutrients in diet should be in a balanced proportion with carbohydrates not exceeding 6 g/kg/day, proteins around 1.5–2 g/kg/day, and lipids of 2.5 g/kg/day. Addition of essential amino acids is necessary in critically ill children. Calcium and vitamin D supplementation as well as standard micronutrient supplementation must be recommended in infants as well as in older children unable to eat their regular meals.
- Sodium restriction is not strictly recommended in young children with heart failure (unlike in adults) as it is often impractical and interferes with nutritional intake. Also, most available feeding formulae are hypo-osmolar that control sodium intake. Sodium restriction is probably beneficial only in those cases with severe edema unresponsive to diuretic therapy.
- *Monitoring progress*: It is vitally essential to objectively monitor the effects of therapy through regular evaluation of body weight, intake versus output, clinical signs such as jugular venous pressure, liver size, respiratory rate, heart rate, and blood pressure (supine and sitting/standing). Chronic therapy is often guided by objective measurement of exercise capacity through the 6-minute walk test and measurement of anaerobic thresholds. In infants, the growth, appetite, and activity are useful surrogates of heart failure status. Additionally formal assessment of quality of life through questionnaires is sometimes useful in patients with chronic conditions.

Pharmacotherapy of Heart Failure

There is limited systematic evidence to support most of the heart failure medication in children. RCTs for heart failure are often are not practical in children. The challenges include significant diversity resulting from different etiologies and age groups, smaller number of patients available to recruit, low event rates requiring large numbers, and problems relating to doing RCTs in children in general. As a result much of what we practice in children is extrapolated from adult data. The broad principles and main goals are as follows:

- Increase cardiac output with improved end-organ perfusion with better myocardial synchrony.
- Decrease vascular resistance without decreasing tissue perfusion whenever physiologically appropriate. For instance, a reduction in SVR is not safe when there is dynamic or fixed left ventricular outflow obstruction.
- Optimize the preload without intra-arterial volume depletion.
- Potentially delay disease progression by establishing endogenous and exogenous repair mechanisms.

The four main groups of drugs to achieve these goals include diuretics, vasodilators, inotropes, and beta-blockers. There are a few newer antifailure agents available now with anecdotal experiences in pediatric heart failure management. All of these drugs are discussed in detail in the chapter

Flowchart 3: Management of acutely ill child with heart failure.

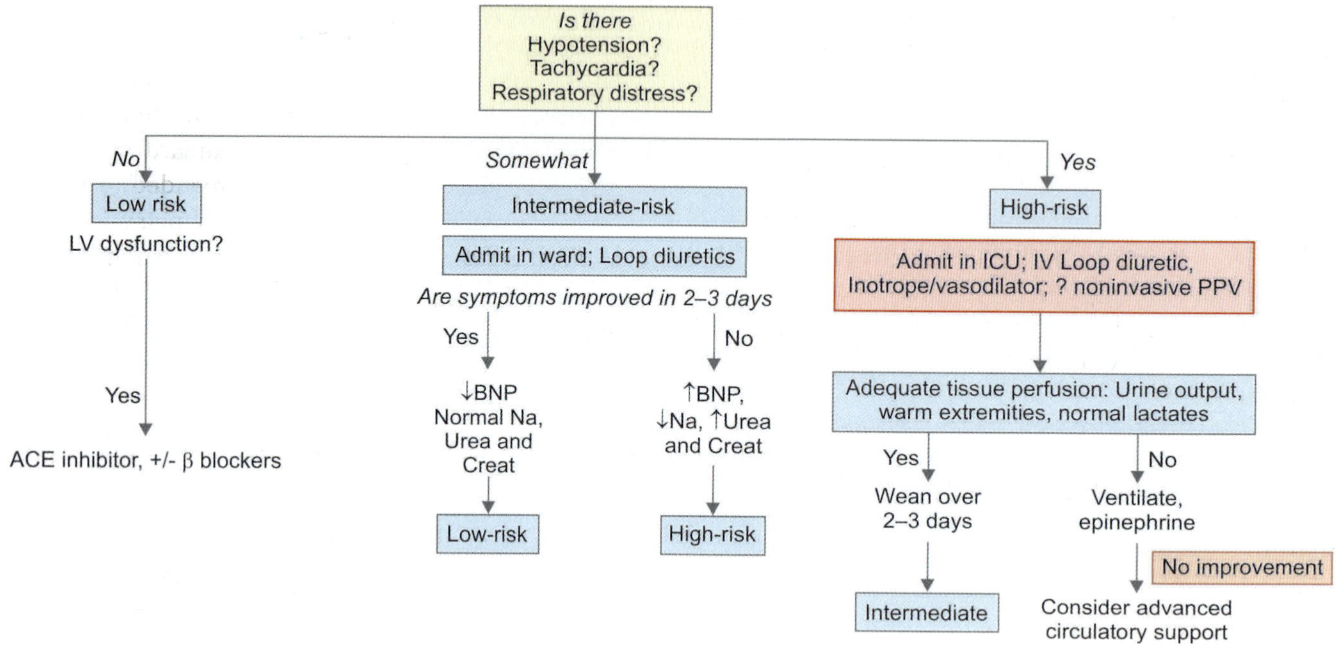

(ACE: angiotensin-converting enzyme; BNP: brain natriuretic peptide; Creat: creatinine; ICU: intensive care unit; IV: intravenous; LV: left ventricle)

on Pharmacology (*see* Chapter 12) and hence are briefly mentioned here. Additionally, we present a practical strategy for institution of heart failure therapy and hospitalization (**Flowchart 3**).

Diuretics

Diuretics form the mainstay therapy in almost all forms of heart failure by reducing the systemic and pulmonary congestion. Furosemide is the usual diuretic of choice in heart failure, given at an oral dose of 1–2 mg/kg q6–12 hours. In acute heart failure, dose of furosemide is 0.5–2 mg/kg q6–12 hours given as bolus intravenously and the dose for infusion is 1–3 mg/kg/day. For patients who have not previously received furosemide, it is often reasonable to start with low doses (~0.5 mg/kg/dose). These patients are generally quite sensitive and respond to low doses. Multiple doses results in some degree of progressive refractoriness that can be overcome by combining with thiazide diuretics such as metolazone.

Aldosterone antagonists (aldactone/spironolactone) decrease potassium loss and may prevent myocardial fibrosis. Spironolactone is used in a dosage of 0.5–1.5 mg/kg q 12 hours. Neonates may require higher dosage due to the higher levels of aldosterone in their circulation.

Hypovolemia and hypotension, hypokalemia and hyponatremia, and metabolic alkalosis are common with loop diuretics and electrolytes need to be monitored in acute settings. Additionally, renal failure may result from acute reduction in renal perfusion and this is more likely to happen when diuretics are combined with ACE inhibitors. Ototoxicity can result from prolonged administration of high doses.

Vasodilators

Vasodilators are to be administered in heart failure only when the altered physiology is likely to benefit from a reduction in vascular resistance. There are specific medications for the systemic and for the pulmonary circuit (*see* Chapters 12 and 18). In this section, we will discuss selected systemic vasodilators that are used to manage systemic (usually left) ventricular dysfunction. Systemic vasodilation is also reasonable as interim treatment of shunt lesions such as ventricular septal defect or patent arterial duct because there is a sound physiological basis. Reduction in SVR will divert blood toward the systemic circuit and thereby reduces the quantum of left-to-right shunt and pulmonary blood flow. Similarly in mitral or aortic regurgitation, there could be some benefit from improving forward flow into the aorta. However, systemic vasodilation could be catastrophic in conditions where there is obstruction to blood in the left side of the heart. Examples include mitral stenosis, subvalvar, valvar, or supravalvar aortic stenosis, dynamic LV outflow obstruction as in hypertrophic cardiomyopathy. Selected examples of vasodilators are discussed here.

ACE inhibitors: ACE inhibitors are now the most widely accepted oral vasodilators for management of heart failure in children. This is despite the fact that we do not have any RCTs in the pediatric age group. The afterload reduction that follows administration of this class of drugs makes it suited for the management of left ventricular dysfunction from any cause, large left-to-right shunts and selected patients with aortic or mitral regurgitation. They are commonly prescribed in outpatient setting in children with cardiomyopathy and children recovering from myocarditis, and in selected patients following cardiac surgery where there is residual LV dysfunction or valve regurgitation. The most commonly used ACE inhibitor in children in India is enalapril. The dose ranges from 0.1 to 0.5 mg/kg/day. It is strongly recommended to start at a lower dose and up-titrate to reach the maximum levels. Captopril has a shorter half-life. It is currently unavailable in India. Other ACE inhibitors available in India are long-acting. They include lisinopril and ramipril. Blood pressure must be recorded after the first dose. Serum electrolytes and renal functions must be monitored in specific settings. Neonates and young infants are particularly prone to renal failure after ACE inhibitors and considerable caution is warranted. Chronic cough is a common reason patients discontinue therapy with ACE inhibitors and switch to angiotensin receptor blockers (ARBs).

Angiotensin receptor blockers (ARBs): There is limited evidence to support the use of ARB in children. Currently, losartan at a dose of 0.75–1.4 mg/kg/day is used under supervision and only in those patients who do not tolerate ACE inhibitor.

Nitroglycerin/Nitroprusside: These medications are used in acute care settings where significant afterload reduction is desired. A good example is in the early postoperative intensive care unit (ICU) setting.

Inotropes

Digoxin: It is a cardiac glycoside and the only oral inotrope that has been used since many years in children with heart failure. The dose is 10 μg/kg/day orally with serum levels to be maintained between 0.5 and 0.9 nmol/L. It acts by blocking the Na-K adenosine triphosphatase (ATPase) pump causing an increase in intracellular sodium, which causes an influx of calcium into myocardial cells, thereby increasing the contractility. Other actions of digoxin include reducing sympathetic overactivity. It also improves systolic function due to neurohormonal modulating effect and is beneficial in patients with low EF, cardiomegaly, and with NYHA III/IV.[33] It has a narrow therapeutic index, complicated by age-dependent dose requirement and cannot be easily measured and hence must be used with caution in children with renal failure. The use of digoxin as a drug for management of heart failure has declined with the increasing availability of ACE inhibitors and specific therapy. However, in selected cases, there is symptom benefit and the resultant improvement in the quality of life may often be valued to warrant its continued use.

The management of heart failure in the acute care setting as well as various agents are discussed in detail in Chapter 12 (Essential Cardiac Pharmacology) and Chapter 13 (Pediatric Cardiac Intensive Care). These medications include intravenous inotropes and vasopressors, phosphodiesterase type III inhibitors such as milrinone, and calcium sensitizers (levosimendan).

Beta-blockers

In acute settings, beta-blockers are very useful in tachyarrhythmia-related heart failure or in selected high output states such as in thyrotoxicosis. They are also useful when ventricular filling may be worsened by tachycardia such as in mitral stenosis or reduction in contractility reduces outflow tract obstruction (hypertrophic obstructive cardiomyopathy). The rationale for beta-blockers in heart failure is counterintuitive in ventricular dysfunction and is discussed in detail in Chapter 12.

Newer Drugs in Pediatric Heart Failure

- *Nesiritide*: This is a B-type natriuretic peptide indicated in the management of acute, decompensated congestive cardiac failure and is associated with improved diuresis, decreased thirst, and improved functional status.[34] It also significantly decreases the pulmonary wedge pressure, mean pulmonary artery pressure, systolic blood pressure, SVR, central venous pressure, and cardiac index.
- *Ivabradine*: Acts on the sinus node with a beneficial effect in cases of systolic heart failure.[35] This has been noted to be especially useful in cases of cardiomyopathy induced by tachyarrhythmias.
- *Eplerenone*: This is a mineralocorticoid/aldosterone antagonist used in the treatment of systolic heart failure in adults.[36] It has also been proven to be well tolerated in children and is useful in decreasing blood pressure in cases of hypertension.
- *Combination of neprilysin inhibitor (sacubitril) and valsartan*: Inhibition of neprilysin decreases vaso-constriction, remodeling of the ventricles, and sodium retention. This in combination with an ARB is widely used in adults and studies are on-going in children for the treatment of heart failure. Few established pediatric cardiac centers use this combination while the child is awaiting a cardiac transplant.

Principles of Management of an Acutely Ill Child with Heart Failure (*see* Flowchart 3)

Management of a child in acute heart failure varies in terms of the medications used, as the armamentarium for drugs in pediatrics remain limited with poor availability of RCTs and inadequately validated extrapolation of adult studies to children. Any acutely ill child with heart failure must be managed in an intensive care setting for an optimal outcome (*see* Chapter 13).

In addition to routine drugs such as diuretics and ACE inhibitor, inotropes form the mainstay of therapy in an acutely ill child, whatever be the cause and type of heart failure. Inotropes in an acute care setting has to be appropriate and in alignment with the physiology of heart failure, with the main aim being to ensure end-organ perfusion (**Table 1**). Hence, a robust knowledge regarding the underlying pathophysiology and periodic assessments in the ICU will help in titration/addition/manipulation of antifailure therapy.

Apart from measures of providing supplementary oxygen in those with lung congestion, keeping the child propped-up (to decrease venous return) and use of intravenous bolus/infusion of diuretics (to decrease preload); choice of the right inotropic support is crucial to the management of acute heart failure.

Digoxin is the main oral inotropic drug used in selected symptomatic children with right or left ventricular dysfunction. Intravenous inotropes are reserved for cases of decompensated and hypotensive heart failure. It is prudent to be aware that though inotropy increases cardiac output and blood pressure, the final outcome is an increased demand and consumption of oxygen due to the limited contractile reserve of the failing myocardium.

Dobutamine, dopamine, and epinephrine are common choices of inotropes, with milrinone and levosimendan used as inodilators. A combination of these is used in conditions with LV dysfunction or acute mitral regurgitation leading to heart failure. Dopamine and dobutamine do increase the cardiac output with decrease in pulmonary and systemic vascular resistance, but also lead to tachycardia and tachyarrhythmia.

Milrinone is a phosphodiesterase-III inhibitor with vasodilatory and inotropic action that improves diastolic relaxation of the ventricles. This is generally the drug of choice in case of low cardiac output state seen in postoperative settings with proven efficacy. Presence of hypotension with severe ventricular dysfunction like in cases of outflow tract obstruction warrants use of vasoconstrictors, namely norepinephrine and vasopressin. Adrenaline is used as a pure inotrope in advanced ventricular dysfunction with hypotension.

In neonates with critical aortic stenosis or pulmonary stenosis (duct-dependent circulations), acute LV or RV failure may set in during early infancy and needs urgent management with prostaglandin infusion to keep up the circulation and an urgent balloon valvuloplasty.

TABLE 1: Physiological basis of heart failure therapy.*

Physiological category with examples	*Examples*	*Desired hemodynamic effect*	*Possible medications (physiologically appropriate)*
Left-to-right shunts	VSD, aortopulmonary window, CHD with increased pulmonary blood flow	Reduction of pulmonary blood flow and improved systemic blood flow	Systemic vasodilators
Valve regurgitation	Mitral and aortic regurgitation	Reduction of regurgitation fraction	Systemic vasodilators**
Systolic ventricular dysfunction	Myocarditis, cardiomyopathy and numerous other conditions	Improved cardiac output through reduced afterload and increased contractility	Systemic vasodilators, inotropes
Dynamic LV outflow obstruction	Hypertrophic obstructive cardiomyopathy	Reduction of gradient through reduction of contractility	Beta-blockers, cardioinhibitory calcium channel blockers (verapamil)
Fixed LV outflow obstruction	Discrete subaortic stenosis, valvar aortic stenosis	Improved cardiac output	Medications are generally ineffective, inotropes may help in short term, vasodilation contraindicated, vasopressors may help for short periods in maintaining perfusion
Diastolic dysfunction with preserved ejection fraction	Hypertrophic cardiomyopathy, systemic hypertension	Improved ventricular relaxation	Beta-blockers, cardioinhibitory calcium channel blockers (verapamil)
LV inflow obstruction	Mitral stenosis, supramitral ring	Improved ventricular filling	Diuretics
Elevated pulmonary artery pressures	The wide variety of conditions associated with pulmonary hypertension (*see* Chapter 18)	Improved RV function	Selective pulmonary vasodilators Inotropes
Isolated or predominant right ventricular systolic dysfunction	RV cardiomyopathy, late postoperative TOF	Improved RV function	Inotropes
Isolated or predominant right ventricular diastolic dysfunction	Early postoperative TOF	Improved RV filling	Medications are generally minimally effective
Tricuspid valve disease	Ebstein anomaly	Systemic venous congestion	Diuretics

(CHD: congenital heart disease; LV: left ventricle; RV: right ventricle; TOF: tetralogy of Fallot; VSD: ventricular septal defect)

*Diuretics are generally used in all of the above situations to help reduce pulmonary and systemic venous congestion

**Systemic vasodilators have a limited role in compensated chronic mitral and aortic regurgitation with normal ventricular function but may be quite useful in acute settings

Treatment of Advanced Pediatric Heart Failure and End-stage Heart Disease

Cardiac catheter interventions, palliative and total corrective surgeries are the ideal therapy for most structural heart diseases causing heart failure. Yet, there are a significant number of children with disease progression and refractory failure with complications as catastrophic as sudden cardiac death. Children with postoperative arrhythmias, ventricular tachycardia causing hemodynamic instability, symptomatic bradycardia, atrioventricular dyssynchrony, unexplained syncope, tachyarrhythmias, and severe LV systolic dysfunction are potential candidates for device therapy as per the expert consensus guidelines from American Heart Association.[37]

The main devices used in children are pacemakers, implantable cardioverter defibrillators (ICD), and cardiac resynchronization therapy (CRT). Observational studies have shown that there is a functional improvement in children with CRT, though there are no long-term trials to prove efficacy.[38]

Ventricular Assist Devices

Mechanical circulatory support is used in children who are refractory to medical therapy in terms of unloading the failing ventricle and maintaining end-organ perfusion. Children in cardiogenic shock or acute heart failure with underperfusion may be transiently stabilized with extracorporeal membrane oxygenation (ECMO) or extracorporeal life support. A permanent ventricular assist device can be implanted in chronic refractory cases as a destination therapy or bridge to cardiac transplantation. However, the prohibitive costs essentially eliminate consideration in the vast majority of Indian children.

Heart Transplantation

Cardiac transplantation is the therapy of choice for children in end-stage heart failure, refractory to medical and surgical therapy. Heart transplant significantly increases the functional capacity, survival, and quality of life with improving outcomes in the recent years. The most recent data from International Society for Heart and Lung Transplantation (ISHLT) shows a median survival of as high as 19 years in infants and 12 years in older children/adolescents.[39] ABO incompatible cardiac transplant is a novel approach to expand the donor pool in young infants as their immature immune systems do not produce relevant antibodies.[40]

The paucity of donors for pediatric hearts and absence of established systems for organ retrieval, transport, and coordinated efforts to ensure timely provision of hearts limit the use of pediatric heart transplants to very few centers. However, results from few Indian centers are quite encouraging.[41]

Future Directions in Pediatric Heart Failure Therapy

A major step toward this direction will be to conduct more randomized, controlled, and well-designed trials for antiheart failure drugs in children to obtain strong data to recommend their use. Continuous improvement in surgical techniques and cardiac interventions will help dealing with structural heart diseases in a more refined manner and reduce the incidence of heart failure. Advances in genetics and genomics of heart disease may enable better risk stratification and informed treatment of these conditions.[42] Most importantly, comprehensive heart failure programs that follow a multidisciplinary team approach are a must in centers offering pediatric cardiac care for an optimal management of heart failure in children.

Family Support and Psychosocial Support in Chronically Ill Children

Children with CHD are twice as likely to have psychological and behavioral problems when compared to the healthy population. As discussed earlier, these children may also have neurodevelopmental and intellectual impairments that can further challenge their educational and occupational status. Parental anxiety and stress are independent to the severity of illness and play a crucial role in the psychological well-being of these children. Lesser participation in outdoor activities as compared to peers and siblings, including sports (owing to decreased exercise capacity), frequent hospitalizations, and overall suboptimal health also significantly lower the quality of life.

In a country like India, the healthcare expenditure is usually "out-of-pocket," rather than government/public or insurance-based. The health-seeking behavior also varies greatly due to the disparity and diversity in economic and literacy status of the population. Many centers catering to children with heart disease are concentrated in the bigger cities and hence most patients have to commute and/or stay away from their own hometowns for prolonged periods of time. Multiple trips to a medical facility, prolonged admissions during procedures (interventions/surgery), arranging finances for management (drugs, device, surgery), and adherence to medications are the main concerns for the family. Frequent absenteeism from school (for the child) and work (for the parents) changes the family dynamics to a great extent, contributing negatively to the overall quality of life for the entire family.[43] Most of these issues can be tackled by support from pediatric psychologists offering counseling, behavior modification therapies, parent training, patient information booklets, etc. A combination of patient and family-centered work is very important to sustain the benefits of treatment and ensuring continuing care in these children. This clearly underscores the importance of comprehensive pediatric heart failure programs that include patient and family education, dietary-exercise-medicine counseling, and social services consultations.

CONCLUSION

Heart failure in children is a complex syndrome with varied etiology and therefore results in considerable diversity in clinical presentation. The most common etiology still remains structural heart disease that is often amenable to corrective procedures and may require short-term medical therapy. The significant lack of RCTs and well-designed, scientific studies in children forces us to adopt modified treatment strategies from adult literature as well as extrapolations from our understanding of physiological alterations. A holistic approach with integration of multiple pediatric specialties and a comprehensive pediatric care plan that includes supportive measures such as patient–family education, diet, immunization, exercise, compliance to medication, and timely follow-up is needed in providing optimal care to these children.

REFERENCES

1. Shaddy RE, George AT, Jaecklin T, Lochlainn EN, Thakur L, Agrawal R, et al. Systematic literature review on the incidence and prevalence of heart failure in children and adolescents. Pediatr Cardiol. 2018;39(3):415-36.
2. Sastry UMK, Kumar RK, Ghosh S, Bharath AP, Subramanian A, et al. Thiamine-responsive acute severe pulmonary hypertension in exclusively breastfeeding infants: a prospective observational study. Arch Dis Child. 2021; 106(3):241-6.
3. Hinton RB, Ware SM. Heart failure in pediatric patients with congenital heart disease. Circ Res. 2017;120:978-94.
4. Shaddy RE, Boucek MM, Hsu DT, Boucek RJ, Canter CE, Mahony L, et al. Carvedilol for children and adolescents with heart failure: a randomized controlled trial. JAMA. 2007; 298(10):1171-9.
5. Harikrishnan S, Sanjay G, Anees T, Viswanathan S, Vijayaraghavan G, Bahuleyan CG, et al. Clinical presentation, management, in-hospital and 90-day outcomes of heart failure patients in Trivandrum, Kerala, India: the Trivandrum Heart Failure Registry. Eur J Heart Fail. 2015; 17(8):794-800.
6. Hsu DT, Pearson GD. Heart failure in children: part I: history, etiology, and pathophysiology. Circ Heart Fail. 2009;2(1):63-70.
7. Massin MM, Astadicko I, Dessy H. Epidemiology of heart failure in a tertiary pediatric center. Clin Cardiol. 2008;31(8):388-91.
8. Webster G, Zhang J, Rosenthal D. Comparison of the epidemiology and co-morbidities of heart failure in the pediatric and adult populations: a retrospective, cross-sectional study. BMC Cardiovasc Disord. 2006;6:23.
9. Bansal B, Bansal M, Bajpai P, Garewal HK. Hypocalcemic cardiomyopathy-different mechanisms in adult and pediatric cases. J Clin Endocrinol Metab. 2014;99(8):2627-32.
10. Sperotto F, Friedman KG, Son MBF, Vander-Pluym CJ, Newburger JW, Dionne A. Cardiac manifestations in SARS-CoV-2-associated multisystem inflammatory syndrome in children: a comprehensive review and proposed clinical approach. Eur J Pediatr. 2021;180(2): 307-22.
11. Knudson JD, Cabrera AG. The pathophysiology of heart failure in children: the basics. Curr Cardiol Rev. 2016;12(2):99-103.
12. Leitch CA. Growth, nutrition and energy expenditure in pediatric heart failure. Prog Pediatr Cardiol. 2000;11(3):195-202.
13. Hansen SR, Dørup I. Energy and nutrient intakes in congenital heart disease. Acta Paediatr. 1993;82(2):166-72.
14. Menon G, Poskitt EM. Why does congenital heart disease cause failure to thrive? Arch Dis Child. 1985;60(12):1134-9.
15. Cameron JW, Rosenthal A, Olson AD. Malnutrition in hospitalized children with congenital heart disease. Arch Pediatr Adolesc Med. 1995;149(10):1098-102.
16. Hollander SA, Addonizio LJ, Chin C, Lamour JM, Hsu DT, Bernstein D, et al. Abdominal complaints as a common first presentation of heart failure in adolescents with dilated cardiomyopathy. Am J Emerg Med. 2013;31(4): 684-6.
17. Vaidyanathan B, Nair SB, Sundaram KR, Babu UK, Shivaprakasha K, Rao SG, Kumar RK. Malnutrition in children with congenital heart disease (CHD) determinants and short term impact of corrective intervention. Indian Pediatr. 2008;45(7):541-6.
18. Reddy NS, Kappanayil M, Balachandran R, Jenkins KJ, Sudhakar A, Sunil GS, et al. Preoperative determinants of outcomes of infant heart surgery in a limited-resource setting. Semin Thorac Cardiovasc Surg. 2015; 27(3):331-8.
19. White RI Jr, Jordan CE, Fischer KC, Dorst JP, Nagy JM, Garn SM, et al. Delayed skeletal growth and maturation in adolescent congenital heart disease. Invest Radiol. 1971;6(5):326-32.
20. Shah SC, Sass DA. "Cardiac Hepatopathy": a review of liver dysfunction in heart failure. Liver Res. 2015;1:1-10.
21. Asrani SK, Asrani NS, Freese DK, Phillips SD, Warnes CA, Heimbach J, et al. Congenital heart disease and the liver. Hepatology. 2012; 56(3):1160-9.
22. Udani SM, Koyner JL. The effects of heart failure on renal function. Cardiol Clin. 2010;28(3):453-65.
23. Riley A, Gebhard DJ, Akcan-Arikan A. Acute kidney injury in pediatric heart failure. Curr Cardiol Rev. 2016;12(2):121-31.
24. Shin JT, Semigran MJ. Heart failure and pulmonary hypertension. Heart Fail Clin. 2010; 6(2):215-22.
25. Masarone D, Valente F, Rubino M, Vastarella R, Gravino R, Rea A, et al. Pediatric heart failure: a practical guide to diagnosis and management. Pediatr Neonatol. 2017;58(4):303-12.
26. Chang AC, Towbin JA. Heart failure in children and young adults. Philadelphia: Saunders Elsevier; 2006.
27. Ross RD, Bollinger RO, Pinsky WW. Grading the severity of congestive heart failure in infants. Pediatr Cardiol. 1992;13(2): 72-5.
28. Reithmann C, Reber D, Kozlik-Feldmann R, Netz H, Pilz G, Welz A, et al. A post-receptor defect of adenylyl cyclase in severely failing myocardium from children with congenital heart disease. Eur J Pharmacol. 1997;330(1):79-86.
29. Connolly D, Rutkowski M, Auslender M, Artman M. The New York University Pediatric Heart Failure Index: a new method of quantifying chronic heart failure severity in children. J Pediatr. 2001;138(5):644-8.
30. Tissieres P, Aggoun Y, da Cruz E, Sierra J, Mensi N, Kalangos A, et al. Comparison of classifications for heart failure in children undergoing valvular surgery. J Pediatrics, 2006;149(2):210-5.
31. Rossano JW, Shaddy RE. Heart failure in children: etiology and treatment. J Pediatr. 2014;165(2):228-33.
32. Hsu DT, Pearson GD. Heart failure in children: part II: diagnosis, treatment, and future directions. Circ Heart Fail. 2009;2(5):490-8.
33. Jain S, Vaidyanathan B. Digoxin in management of heart failure in children: should it be continued or relegated to the history books? Ann Pediatr Cardiol. 2009;2(2):149-52.
34. Behera SK, Zuccaro JC, Wetzel GT, Alejos JC. Nesiritide improves hemodynamics in children with dilated cardiomyopathy: a pilot study. Pediatr Cardiol. 2009;30(1):26-34.

35. Romeo E, Grimaldi N, Sarubbi B, D'Alto M, Santarpia G, Scognamiglio G, et al. A pediatric case of cardiomyopathy induced by inappropriate sinus tachycardia: efficacy of ivabradine. Pediatr Cardiol. 2011;32(6):842-5.
36. Li JS, Flynn JT, Portman R, Davis I, Ogawa M, Shi H, et al. The efficacy and safety of the novel aldosterone antagonist eplerenone in children with hypertension: a randomized, double-blind, dose-response study. J Pediatr. 2010 Aug;157(2):282-7.
37. Epstein AE, DiMarco JP, Ellenbogen KA, Estes NA III, Freedman RA, Gettes LS, et al. ACC/AHA/HRS 2008 Guidelines for Device-Based Therapy of Cardiac Rhythm Abnormalities: a report of the American College of Cardiology/American Heart Association Task Force on Practice Guidelines (Writing Committee to Revise the ACC/AHA/NASPE 2002 Guideline Update for Implantation of Cardiac Pacemakers and Antiarrhythmia Devices): developed in collaboration with the American Association for Thoracic Surgery and Society of Thoracic Surgeons. Circulation. 2008;117(21): e350-408.
38. Cecchin F, Frangini PA, Brown DW, Fynn-Thompson F, Alexander ME, Triedman JK, et al. Cardiac resynchronization therapy (and multisite pacing) in pediatrics and congenital heart disease: five years experience in a single institution. J Cardiovasc Electrophysiol. 2009; 20(1):58-65.
39. Dipchand AI, Kirk R, Edwards LB, Kucheryavaya AY, Benden C, Christie JD, et al. The Registry of the International Society for Heart and Lung Transplantation: Sixteenth Official Pediatric Heart Transplantation Report-2013; focus theme: age. J Heart Lung Transplant 2013; 32(10):979e88.
40. West LJ, Pollock-Barziv SM, Dipchand AI, Lee KJ, Cardella CJ, Benson LN, et al. ABO-incompatible heart transplantation in infants. N Engl J Med. 2001;344(11):793-800.
41. Balakrishnan KR, Rao KG, Subramaniam GK, Tanguturu MK, Arvind A, Ramanan V, et al. Clinical profiles and risk factors for early and medium-term mortality following heart transplantation in a pediatric population: a single-center experience. Ann Pediatr Card 2021;14(1):42-52.
42. Pillekamp F, Khalil M, Emmel M, Brockmeier K, Hescheler J. Stem cells in pediatric heart failure. Minerva Cardioangiol. 2008;56(3):335-48.
43. Rohan JM, Verma T. Psychological considerations in pediatric chronic illness: case examples. Int J Environ Res Public Health. 2020;17(5):1644.

18 CHAPTER

Pulmonary Hypertension in Children

Shine Kumar KH

INTRODUCTION

Pulmonary hypertension (PH) in children is a rare disease of diverse etiology affecting all age groups from newborns to adolescents. The annual incidence and point prevalence of idiopathic pulmonary arterial hypertension (IPAH, previously known as primary PH) in pediatric population is estimated to be between 0.48–0.7 and 2.07–4.4 cases per million[1-3] compared to adult data of 1–3.3 and 5.6–25 cases per million, respectively.[4-6] In contrast, there is a higher prevalence of PH associated with congenital heart disease (CHD) in children compared to adults (10.1–15.6 vs. 3 cases per million).[1,2] The management principles are often adapted from adult data, but are limited by wide spectrum of etiologies and physiologic states unique to pediatric population.[7]

DEFINITIONS

Pulmonary hypertension refers to a mean pulmonary arterial pressure (mPAP) ≥25 mm Hg in children >3 months of age at sea level.[8] The term pulmonary arterial hypertension (PAH) is specifically used when mPAP is ≥25 mm Hg with pulmonary capillary wedge pressure (PCWP) <15 mm Hg and pulmonary vascular resistance index (PVRI) >3 Wood Units.m^2 (WU.m^2). This term is used to indicate elevation in pulmonary artery pressure as a result of elevation in pulmonary vascular resistance.

Pulmonary venous hypertension (PVH) refers to a PCWP or a pulmonary venous pressure >15 mm Hg.

In infants <3 months and neonates, no definite criteria exist regarding cut off value for defining PH. Recently following the 6th World Symposium on Pulmonary Hypertension (WSPH) held in Nice, 2018, the cut off for diagnosis of PH in children >3 months has been revised to mPAP >20 mm Hg based on adult data.[9]

CLASSIFICATION

The current classification of PH is based on guidelines from 6th World Symposium of Pulmonary Hypertension, held at Nice, 2018[9] (**Fig. 1**). Further, PAH due to CHD has been grouped into four categories viz Eisenmenger syndrome, left-to-right shunts (correctable and noncorrectable), PAH with coincidental CHD (PAH with small defects which per se does not contribute to elevated PVR) and postoperative PAH (PAH persisting or appearing after correction of CHD in absence of hemodynamically significant residual lesions).[10]

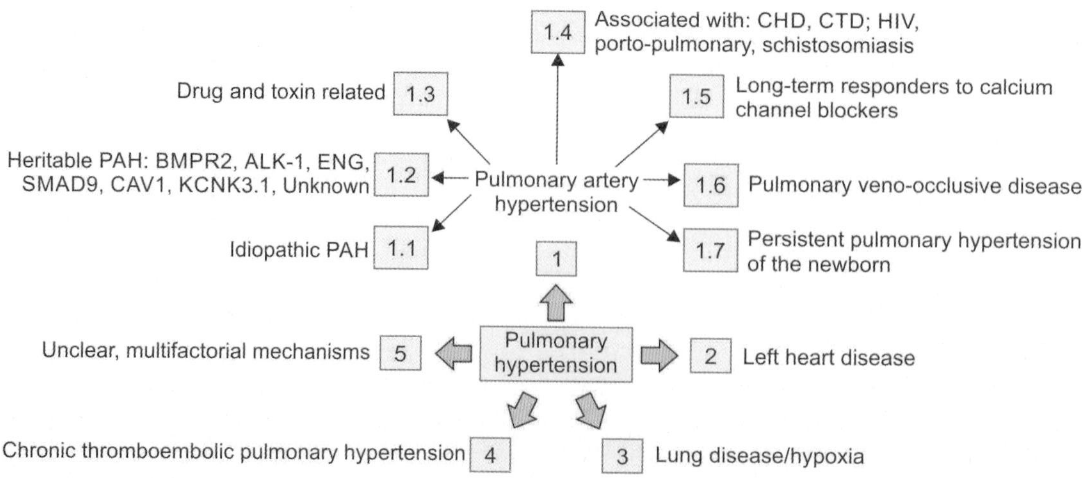

Fig. 1: Nice classification of pulmonary hypertension.
(CHD: congenital heart disease; CTD: connective tissue disease; HIV: human immunodeficiency virus; PAH: pulmonary arterial hypertension)

CLINICAL PRESENTATION

The clinical presentation in children are highly variable and, often, nonspecific. The symptoms essentially reflect an inability to augment cardiac output in the face of increased demand. Therefore, they often present with shortness of breath with exertion, fatigue, chest discomfort, syncope, or seizure mimics.[2,11] The symptoms may be subtle and as disease advances, children with PH may present with right heart failure with symptoms at rest. In children with CHD, especially large post-tricuspid left-to-right shunt, improvement in symptom status and failure to thrive may hint development of pulmonary vascular disease. At times a chest X-ray or an electrocardiogram (ECG) done for other indications may reveal finding suggestive of PH.

Because of a large variety of possible causes, PH is often incidentally identified during evaluation of a number of conditions that include congenital and acquired heart disease, lung and airway disease, severe spinal deformities with respiratory compromise, liver disease, inflammatory conditions of connective tissue and, hematological conditions. Exceptionally, chronic hypoventilation from underlying neuromuscular conditions can also result in PH. A family history should be carefully recorded because a small proportion of patients clinically labeled as IPAH may have first-degree relatives who are affected.

TABLE 1: World Health Organization (WHO) classification of functional status in pulmonary hypertension (PH).

Class I	• Patients with PH but without resulting limitation of physical activity • Ordinary physical activity does not cause undue dyspnea or fatigue, chest pain, or near syncope
Class II	• Patients with PH resulting in slight limitation of physical activity • They are comfortable at rest. Ordinary physical activity causes undue dyspnea or fatigue, chest pain, or near syncope
Class III	• Patients with PH resulting in marked limitation of physical activity • They are comfortable at rest. Less than ordinary activity causes undue dyspnea or fatigue, chest pain, or near syncope
Class IV	• Patients with PH with inability to carry out any physical activity without symptoms These patients manifest signs of right heart failure. Dyspnea and/or fatigue may even be present at rest • Discomfort is increased by any physical activity

EVALUATION

Clinical Examination

This includes the assessment of growth and development and immunization status (especially vaccination against pneumonia and influenza). Failure to thrive is a poor prognostic sign in children with PH. Pulse oximetry should be recorded in upper and lower limbs to rule out hypoxia from Eisenmenger syndrome, primary lung parenchymal and upper airway diseases. Systemic desaturation in a large left-to-right shunt may indicate early reversal of shunt with onset of pulmonary vascular disease. Clubbing suggests Eisenmenger physiology or lung disease or chronic liver disease (associated with portopulmonary hypertension) and pallor for anemia, which may worsen symptomatic status. Jaundice can occur in chronic liver disease. General physical examination should also include a search for cutaneous telangiectasia that may point to a specific disorder like hereditary hemorrhagic telangiectasia. Clinically a prominent left parasternal impulse or heave may be noted. The pulmonary component of second heart sound (S2) is loud, often palpable. The palpable P2 often follows just after a prominent systolic pulsation of the pulmonary artery in the left second interspace. The physiological splitting of S2 may be lost and is often single. Tricuspid or pulmonary regurgitation murmurs due to PH may be audible. The shunt murmurs and flow murmurs are usually absent with the development of PH. Raised jugular venous pressure, pedal edema, hepatomegaly, and ascites occur with failing right ventricular function. Splenomegaly may indicate portal hypertension. In general examination, look for any features of dysmorphism suggestive of chromosomal or genetic disorders such as Down syndrome which may predispose to the development of PH.

Assessment of Functional Status

In older children, especially in school-going age group, functional status is assessed by World Health Organization (WHO) functional classification (class I to IV) for PH.[12] This is similar to New York Heart Association (NYHA) except that the symptoms are being assessed in patient with PH (**Table 1**). An alternate functional classification system for children—Panama functional classification system—has been proposed, though not yet validated.[13] The aim was to overcome the limitations of WHO functional classification when used in younger children. This classification includes five classes (I, II, IIIa, IIIb, and IV) for children from newborn to 16 years. Each functional class is further divided into five age groups (0–6 months, 6 months–1 year, 1–2 years, 2–5 years, and 5–16 years) incorporating physical activity and developmental milestones unique to each age group.

Baseline Investigations

The chest X-ray typically shows dilated main pulmonary artery and branch pulmonary arteries (**Fig. 2**). PAH secondary to CHD shows absence of pulmonary plethora, proximally dilated branch pulmonary arteries with abrupt distal tapering, and absent vascularity toward lung periphery (**Fig. 3**). Chest X-ray helps in identifying any primary lung parenchymal diseases or spine and thoracic cage abnormalities contributing to PH. PVH is characterized by pulmonary edema, prominent upper lobe vessels (cephalization), and interlobar edema (**Fig. 4**).

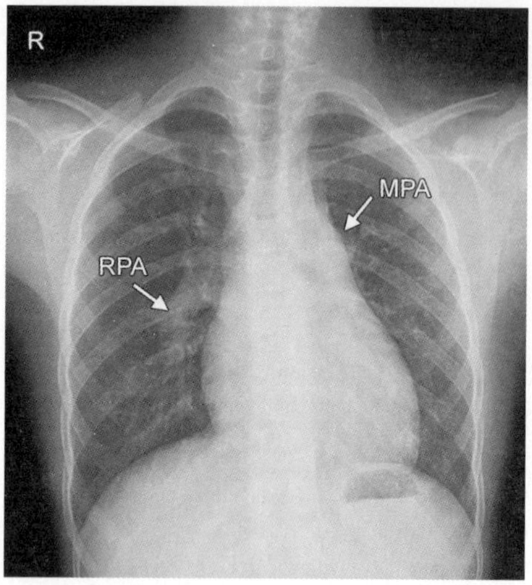

Fig. 2: Chest X-ray shows dilated main pulmonary artery (MPA) and right lower lobe branch (RPA) in a patient with idiopathic pulmonary arterial hypertension.

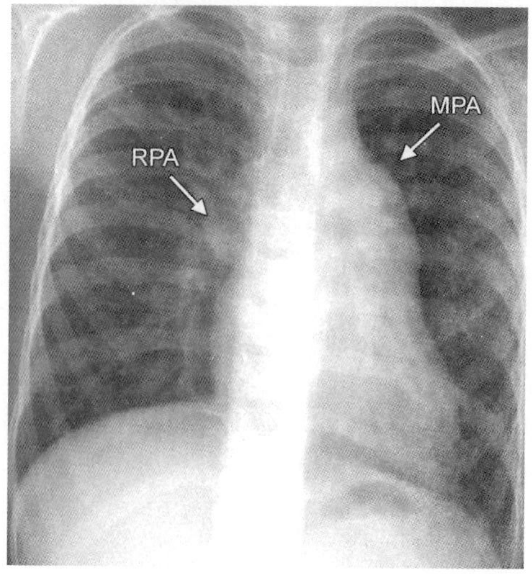

Fig. 3: Chest X-ray from a patient with Eisenmenger syndrome. Note the relatively dark peripheral lung fields with large hilar pulmonary arteries (arrows).

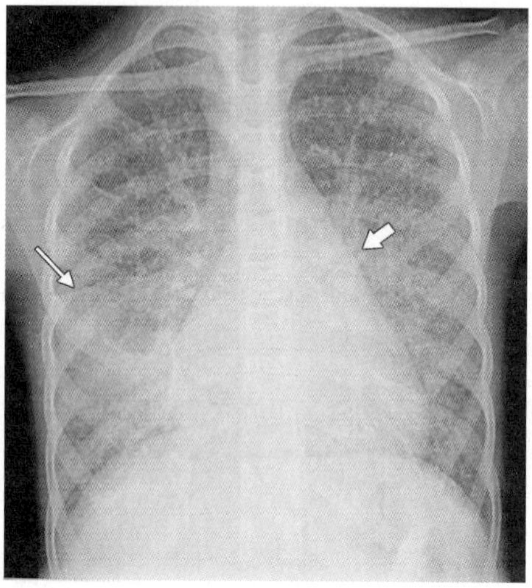

Fig. 4: Pulmonary venous hypertension as a cause of pulmonary hypertension in an adolescent with juvenile mitral stenosis. The straight left heart border is because of combined effects of enlarged main pulmonary artery and left atrial appendage (block arrow); Note the features of pulmonary venous hypertension as suggested by prominence of interlobar fissure (thin arrow).

The ECG usually shows right atrial enlargement and right ventricular hypertrophy with or without strain pattern depending on the severity of disease (**Fig. 5**). Right atrial enlargement is relatively less sensitive and tends to happen later in the disease process. Typical right axis deviation of QRS axis is helpful in older children, may not be helpful in younger children and newborns where it is the norm. Arrhythmias are rare and seen in advanced stage of disease.

Echocardiography is the primary tool for confirmation of diagnosis of PH. In addition, echocardiography helps in assessment severity of PH, evaluation of ventricular function, to rule out structural heart disease, and look for pericardial effusion, an important prognostic marker. Echocardiography should be carefully undertaken because there is potential for a number of specific conditions that can be missed and mislabeled as idiopathic PAH (**Table 2**). Some of these conditions are readily treatable.

Ultrasound Scan of Abdomen

The primary purpose of ultrasound scan (USS) abdomen is to rule out congenital portosystemic shunt (Abernethy malformations), a rare but potentially curable and often underdiagnosed cause for PH in children. In addition, any evidence of portal hypertension, hepatic, and renal malformations also can be evaluated (**Fig. 6**).

Six-minute Walk Test

Six-minute walk test is primarily used to assess physical activity in PH patient. This can be easily done in cooperative children who can follow the required instructions. The distance walked aid in monitoring progress of disease and management strategies. A six-minute walk distance of >300 meters is usually considered normal in children with PH. Advanced methods of cardiopulmonary exercise testing measuring oxygen consumption has significant logistic limitations in low resource setting.

Laboratory Blood Investigations

Table 3 lists routine and additional blood tests and rationale for evaluation of PH in children. There are no diagnostic tests and these are supplementary to other tests in arriving at etiological diagnosis for PH. The additional tests are done depending on the clinical suspicion of PH etiology.

Cardiac Catheterization

Cardiac catheterization remains the gold standard in confirming PH. An exact assessment of the mean pulmonary

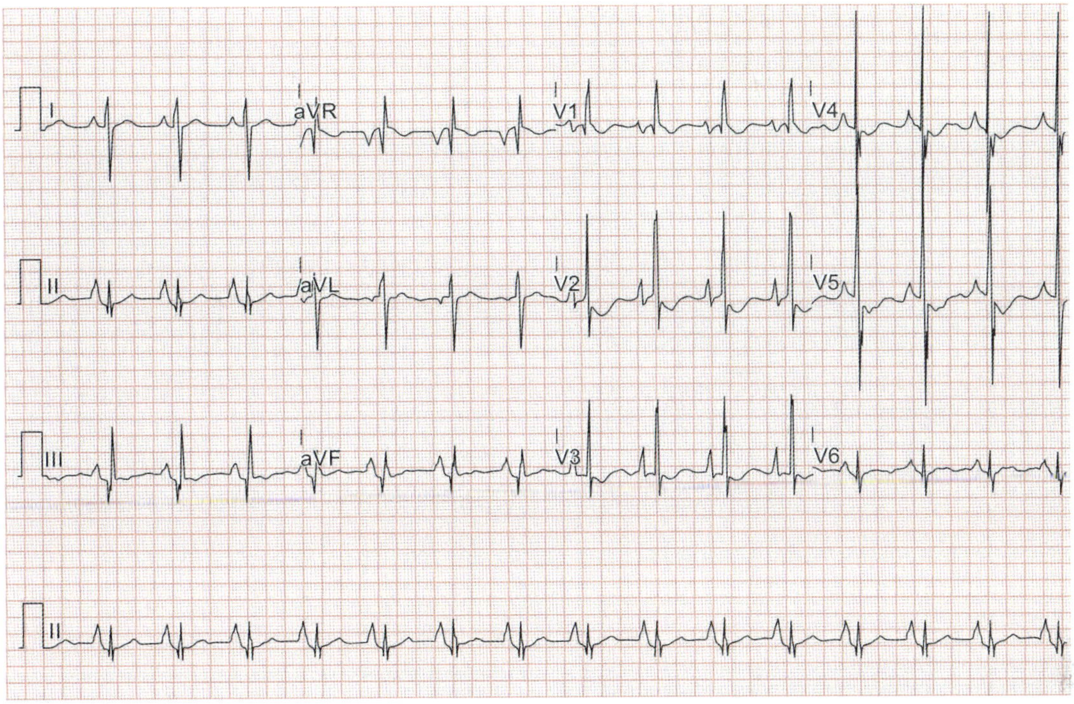

Fig. 5: Electrocardiogram (ECG) shows sinus rhythm with right atrial enlargement (peaked P waves in lead II), right axis deviation of QRS vector +150 (equiphasic QRS complex in lead aVR), right ventricular hypertrophy (R/S ratio in V1 11/2), and strain (ST depression and T inversion in leads V1-V3).

TABLE 2: Echocardiographic mimics of pulmonary hypertension.

Condition	*Details*
Large patent ductus arteriosus (PDA)	The flow across a large PDA tends to be low velocity (laminar) and may not be picked up. Indirect clues (left atrial and left ventricular enlargement and flow reversal in descending thoracic aorta) may point toward the diagnosis. The PDA itself can then be imaged
Aortopulmonary window	• Like in the case of patent ductus arteriosus, aortopulmonary window is suggested by flow reversal in descending aorta (suggesting aortic runoff) and left atrial and left ventricular enlargement • The ascending aorta is also enlarged and once suspected, AP window can be easily identified through careful imaging
Apical muscular ventricular septal defect	A large defect in the apical muscular septum may sometimes be missed unless carefully looked for
Hemitruncus (one pulmonary artery from aorta)	This is a rare anomaly that often gets labeled as idiopathic PAH. The right pulmonary artery is usually involved and comes off the ascending aorta
Obstructed total anomalous pulmonary venous connection (TAPVC)	Neonates with obstructed TAPVC are often incorrectly labeled as persistent pulmonary hypertension of the newborn. Careful imaging of the pulmonary veins and identification of the anomalously draining vertical vein enables the diagnosis
Pulmonary vein obstruction	Isolated pulmonary venous obstruction is rare. It can involve some of the veins or all pulmonary veins (Cor triatriatum)
Scimitar syndrome	Scimitar syndrome is often associated with pulmonary hypertension in infants. Associated anomalies (anomalous pulmonary venous drainage with or without obstruction and hypoplastic right lung with bronchopulmonary sequestration) enable the diagnosis
Vein of Galen malformation	A well-known cause of unexplained pulmonary hypertension in the newborn. This is identified by the vigorous flows in the superior vena cava
Coarctation of aorta in the neonate	Isolated coarctation often presents with severe pulmonary artery hypertension in the neonate
Absence of one pulmonary artery	Congenital absence of the right or left pulmonary artery may manifest as severe pulmonary hypertension
Abernethy malformation	Increasingly recognized as a potentially treatable cause for pulmonary hypertension. This requires careful imaging of the inferior vena cava and portal vein

(PAH: pulmonary arterial hypertension)

artery pressure can only be obtained invasively. The aim of catheterization is to confirm and assess severity and type of PH, evaluation of hemodynamics including oximetry, pulmonary and systemic output and vascular resistances, and assessment of responsiveness to selective pulmonary vasodilators (acute vasodilator test). The distinction between

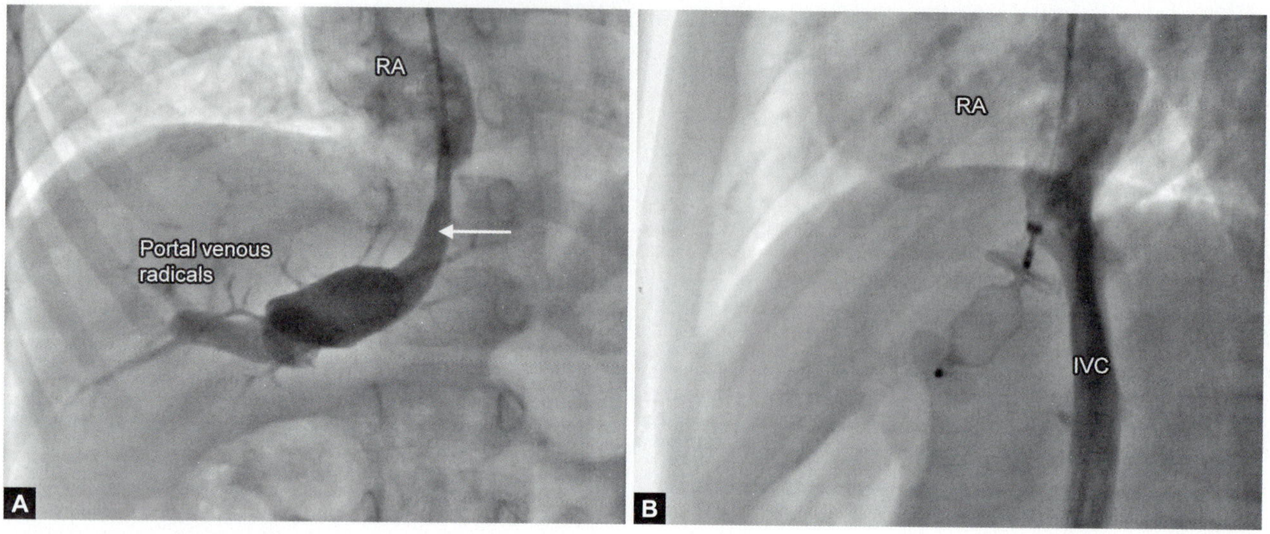

Figs. 6A and B: Angiogram obtained before and closure of Abernethy malformation (arrow). (IVC: inferior vena cava; RA: right atrium)

TABLE 3: Laboratory investigations in pulmonary hypertension in children.

Investigations	*Rationale*
Routine	
Hb and complete blood count	Anemia and polycythemia
ESR, CRP	CTD
Liver function tests	
Renal function tests	
Electrolytes—Na, K, Ca	
Thyroid function test	
APTT, PT/INR	Coagulation abnormalities
BNP	Myocardial strain
Specific tests	
Arterial blood gas	Lung and airway pathologies
ANA screen	Rheumatological disorders
Serology for hepatitis, HIV	If clinically suspected
Genetic screening	Heritable PH, IPAH

(ANA: antinuclear antibody; APTT: activated partial thromboplastin time; BNP: brain natriuretic peptide; CRP: C reactive protein; CTD: connective tissue disorder; ESR: erythrocyte sedimentation rate; Hb: hemoglobin; HIV: human immunodeficiency virus; INR: international normalized ratio; IPAH: idiopathic pulmonary arterial hypertension; PH: pulmonary hypertension; PT: prothrombin time)

precapillary PH (PAH) and postcapillary PH (PVH) is based on PCWP which can be only determined with certainty by catheterization. Catheterization is recommended in all patients at the time of diagnosis and is a safe procedure in expert hands.[14] A hemodynamically unstable patient presenting in heart failure or in presence of other significant comorbidities, catheterization may be deferred until stabilization with appropriate medical treatment.

Acute Vasodilator Test

This is done to identify acute responders to pulmonary vasodilators in cases of IPAH, familial PH and drug-induced PH, and to assess operability in borderline cases of CHD with severe PH. The recommended agent is inhaled nitric oxide (20 parts per million).[15] Testing with oxygen alone is no longer recommended unless there is associated hypoxia.[16] In children, the acute responder is defined as fall in mean pulmonary artery pressure by 20% or more from baseline with sustained or increased cardiac output and unchanged or improving ratio of pulmonary to systemic vascular resistance.[17,18] This criterion was first suggested by Robyn Barst and is known as the modified Barst criteria. A more rigid criteria defines acute responder as those with fall in PVRI to <5 WU.m^2 with normal or high cardiac output.[3] Acute responder tends to have better overall hemodynamics and long-term outcomes and respond well to Ca channel blockers as initial therapy. The percentage of acute responders ranges from 10 to 50% in different registries depending on defining criteria. Over time, responders tend to lose responsiveness and often require escalation of therapy. For assessment of operability in CHD (left-to-right shunts), a fall in PVRI to <4 WU.m^2 and or ratio of PVRI: systemic vascular resistance index (SVRI) <0.3 with vasodilator testing may indicate that shunt closure can be considered[19] after careful comprehensive clinical assessment, other relevant investigations and the baseline resting data in the catheterization laboratory.

Computed Tomography Scan of the Chest

A high-resolution computed tomography (CT) chest is done in cases of primary parenchymal lung disease and evaluation of airways. CT pulmonary angiography is done when pulmonary thromboembolism is suspected and to evaluate cardiac structures, especially pulmonary veins.

Magnetic Resonance Imaging

Magnetic resonance imaging (MRI) is the gold standard in evaluation of right ventricular function, though echocardiography remains the preferred imaging modality because of cost, convenience, and availability. In addition to anatomical details, ventricular volumes and cardiac output can be estimated. Specific utility in pediatric PH is limited and is rarely used as tool for evaluation.

Pulmonary Function Tests/ Polysomnography

Pulmonary function tests are primarily indicated in evaluation of children with lung diseases, neuromuscular diseases, and chest wall abnormalities as possible contributory factor for PH. The tests need cooperation and hence can be done only in older children. A significant restrictive pattern may point toward interstitial lung disease, pulmonary veno-occlusive disease (PVOD), or pulmonary capillary hemangiomatosis were the management strategies differ drastically from usual therapy. Polysomnography is done in children with obstructive sleep apnea syndrome. An arterial blood gas should always be obtained when pulmonary causes are suspected and elevated PCO_2 and low PO_2 suggest that the PAH is secondary to respiratory causes.

Genetic Testing

Genetic basis for PH has been well established in children with IPAH and heritable PAH (HPAH). The most common gene studied is bone morphogenic protein receptor 2 mutation (BMPR2), autosomal dominant with variable penetrance. Other genes implicated are ALK1 (activin-like kinase type 1), CAV1 (caveolin 1), ENG (endoglin), KCNK3 (potassium channel subfamily K, member 3), NOTCH3 (neurogenic locus notch homologue protein 3), and SMAD9 (Smad family member 9). EIF2AK4 (eukaryotic translation initiation factor 2 alpha kinase 4) is the specific gene described in PVOD. Genetic testing helps in diagnosis, prognostication, and counseling of family members regarding the risk of transmission to future generations.

Risk Stratification

The following features are considered as adverse prognostic signs in children with PH:

- Symptoms and functional class (WHO functional class III/IV), rapid progression of symptoms, syncope, and failure to thrive are all ominous signs and merit serious attention.
- Clinical evidence of right heart failure in the form of congested liver, elevated jugular venous pressure is an adverse prognostic sign. The onset of right ventricular dysfunction is a consistent marker of adverse prognosis.
- Significantly elevated levels of brain natriuretic peptide (BNP)/N-terminal pro b-type natriuretic peptide (NT-proBNP) levels suggest right ventricular dysfunction.
- Severe enlargement or right atrium or right ventricle (RV) or dysfunction of RV and pericardial effusion are all adverse prognostic markers that are identified by echocardiography.
- During catheterization, a cardiac index <2.5 L/min/m^2, ratio of mean pulmonary artery to mean systemic arterial pressure >0.75, mean right atrial pressure >15 mm Hg, and PVRI >15 WU.m^2 suggest advanced disease.

Drug Therapy

The recent availability of drugs that specifically result in pulmonary vasodilation has helped to improve the outlook of patients with PH. These drugs target different pathways that contribute to increased pulmonary vascular resistance. This section presents a brief summary of the common selective pulmonary vasodilators that are used for children with PH.

Phosphodiesterase Type 5 Inhibitors

Phosphodiesterase type 5 inhibitor (PDE5i) acts by inhibiting PDE5 enzyme in smooth muscles causing accumulation of cyclic guanosine monophosphate (cGMP) and vascular smooth muscle relaxation with subsequent vasodilation. Sildenafil and tadalafil are commonly used examples.

Sildenafil: The dosage in children <1 year of age is 0.5–1 mg/kg/dose three to four times/day including neonates.[8] In specific subsets such as bronchopulmonary dysplasia with PH, vigilant up titration of dosage up to 2 mg/kg/dose up to three to four times per day has been suggested.[20] In older children ≥ 8–20 kg, 10 mg three times a day and >20–40 kg, 20 mg three times a day is recommended.[21]

Intravenous sildenafil is available, and usage data is limited to persistent pulmonary hypertension of newborns (PPHNs). The dose is 0.4 mg/kg bolus over 3 hours followed by 1.6 mg/kg/day continuous infusion.[22]

The concerning adverse effect is hypotension at onset of therapy. It is prudent to initiate therapy with half the recommended dosage, especially in neonates and infants. Reported side effects include visual disturbances and muscle aches (especially at onset of therapy). These are rare in children.

Tadalafil: It is a more selective PDE5 inhibitor with longer duration of action when compared to sildenafil. Dosage in older infants and children is 1 mg/kg/dose once daily up to a maximum of 40 mg.[23-26] The safety profile and side effects are like that of sildenafil.

Endothelin Receptor Antagonists

Endothelin 1 is a neurohormone, which acts upon endothelin receptors A (ET_A) and B (ET_B) in endothelium and vascular smooth muscles. Endothelin receptor antagonists (ERAs) block these receptors attenuating the vasoconstrictor effects of endothelin.

Bosentan is a nonselective endothelin receptor blocker acting on both receptors. The maintenance dose for <10 kg including neonates is 2 mg/kg/dose twice daily.[8] For children above 10 kg, maintenance dosage is twice daily dosage of 31.25 mg in 10–20 kg, 62.5 mg in 20–40 kg and 125 mg in >40 kg.[27] The initial dosage is half the maintenance dose and can be up titrated to full dose after 4 weeks. The major side effect, though rare and reversible, is elevation of hepatic transaminases which require regular monitoring during initiation, escalation to full dose, and on follow-up.[28] An elevation to more than three times the baseline value warrants drug withdrawal. Other common side effects include anemia and male infertility.

Ambrisentan is selective ET_A receptor antagonist. The current dosage for children (>2 years old) under 20 kg is an initial dose of 2.5 mg once daily titrated up to 5 mg once daily. For 20–40 kg, the initial dose is 2.5 mg or 5 mg once daily titrated up to 10 mg once daily and for those over 40 kg, 5 mg once daily titrated up to 10 mg once daily.[29] Unlike bosentan, elevation of hepatic transaminases is exceedingly rare and after successful titration to required dosage, routine monitoring of liver function tests is not recommended.

Calcium Channel Blockers

This group of drugs acts by inhibiting calcium influx causing smooth muscle relaxation. This is specifically indicated in children with IPAH who are acute responders.[17,30,31] The commonly used drugs include nifedipine (initial dose 0.6–0.9 mg/kg/day in three divided doses, maintenance 2–5 mg/kg/day, maximum 120–240 mg/day), diltiazem (initial dose 1.5–2 mg/kg/day in three divided dose, maintenance 3–5 mg/kg/day, maximum 240–720 mg/day) and amlodipine (initial dose 2.5–5 mg/day and maintenance 2.5–5 mg/day twice daily, maximum 20 mg/day).[8] Calcium channel blockers are contraindicated in children <1 year.[32]

Prostacyclin and its Analogs

Prostacyclin is naturally occurring arachidonic acid metabolites with potent pulmonary and systemic vasodilator effects mediated by cell surface G-protein receptors resulting in increased intracellular cyclic adenosine monophosphate (cAMP) and resultant activation of protein kinase A causing smooth muscle relaxation. This class of agents is not freely available in India (unlike the other categories of drugs).

Epoprostenol was the first drug ever to be approved for use in PH by FDA (Food and Drug Administration, USA). The dosage across all age groups in children is 1–3 nanogram (ng)/kg/min as continuous intravenous (IV) infusion initially up to a maintenance dose of 50–80 ng/kg/min or higher in accordance with disease severity.[31,33,34]

Treprostinil: Another prostacyclin analog administered IV, subcutaneously (SC), or by inhalation. The IV and SC doses in children are similar to epoprostenol.[35,36] The initial dosage for inhalation is three breaths (18 µg) four times a day and up to nine breaths (54 µg) four times a day.[37]

Iloprost: Inhaler prostacyclin analog with initial dosage of 2.5 µg per inhalation 6–9 times per day with maintenance up to 5 µg to a maximum of 9 times per day.[38]

Prostacyclins are the drug of choice in high-risk children with PH and have proven survival benefit. The adverse effects are due to vasodilatation such as hypotension, flushing, jaw pains, and diarrhea. The need for continuous infusion when in parental form due to short half-life (6 minutes to 4 hours) and complications related to subcutaneous injection site or central IV lines mandates close monitoring. Currently, the very high cost and nonavailability limits its use in India.

Inhaled Nitric Oxide

Inhaled nitric oxide (iNO) acts directly on vascular endothelium such as endogenous NO producing vasodilatation through cGMP-dependent pathway. iNO has been approved by FDA as drug of choice in PPHN. The recommended dosage is 20 parts per million (ppm).[39,40] In addition, iNO has been used in various acute care settings in managing sick children with PH. The common adverse event is development of methemoglobinemia.

Other Supportive Therapy

Anticoagulation: The only indication for anticoagulation in children is thromboembolic PAH. There is no indication for routine use of anticoagulation in children in any other forms of PH including Eisenmenger syndrome.

Digoxin and diuretics: The use of digoxin and or diuretics may be helpful in symptomatic improvement of right heart failure. It is necessary to be cautious with aggressive diuresis to avoid a sudden fall in cardiac output in these patients who are dependent somewhat on high right ventricular filling pressures (preload dependent).

Oxygen therapy: Oxygen therapy is beneficial in patients who have PH from chronic alveolar hypoxia (saturation <92% and/or pO_2 <60%) secondary to primary lung diseases like bronchopulmonary dysplasia. Routine use of oxygen in PH due to CHD is not recommended.

Vaccination: In addition to all routine vaccinations, children with PH being high-risk subsets should be administered pneumococcal and influenza vaccination.

Catheter-based and Surgical Interventions

Atrial Septostomy

Atrial septostomy is indicated in children with recurrent syncope with WHO functional class III/IV in right heart failure as a bridge to transplant or to increase cardiac output. This procedure involves creation of an atrial septal defect in the cardiac catheterization laboratory to deliberately allow right-to-left shunting. This helps maintain cardiac output at the cost of systemic desaturation.

Potts Shunt

The Potts shunt involves establishing an effective communication between left pulmonary artery and descending aorta to decompress the hypertensive RV and improve cardiac output. This is generally accomplished surgically but can also be done in the catheter laboratory. This is a palliative procedure done in worsening patients for symptomatic benefit or as bridge to heart-lung or lung transplant.

Transplantation

Lung transplantations are primarily indicated in PH due to primary lung disease such as PVOD and IPAH or hereditary PAH refractory to medical therapy. The 5-year survival rate for lung transplantation in IPAH patients is 61% in western centers.[41] Transplantation is generally not advised for PAH associated with CHD since the long-term survival is better than post-transplant patients.

Selection of Pulmonary Vasodilators

A modified treatment algorithm based on availability of pulmonary vasodilator therapy and interventions for PH in Indian children is given in **Flowchart 1**. The high-risk category is benefitted from upfront combination therapy. The favored combination is of tadalafil and ambrisentan based on adult clinical trials.[42]

Flowchart 1: Modified algorithm for pulmonary vasodilator therapy in children in India.

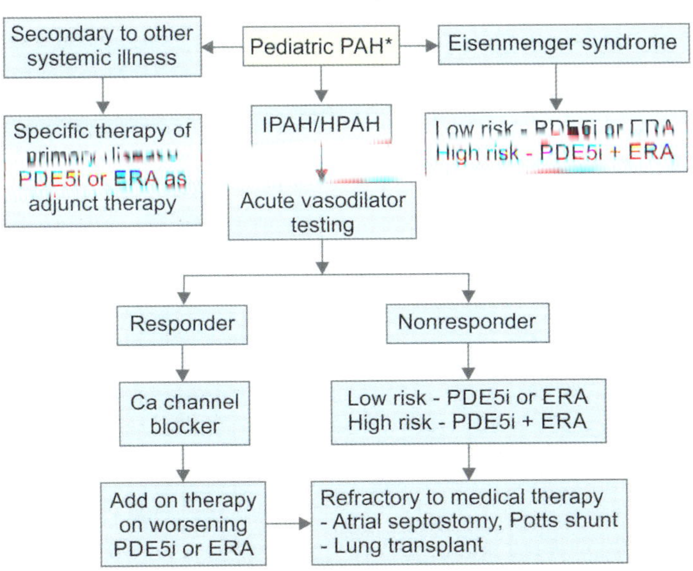

*Ideally in high risk patient in any category, the recommended drug of choice is prostacyclins. Since it is not available currently in India, the choice is based on available drugs.

(PDE5i: phosphodiesterase 5 inhibitor; ERA: endothelin receptor antagonist; IPAH: idiopathic pulmonary arterial hypertension; HPAH: hereditary PAH)

Source: Adapted from Abman et al. Pediatric pulmonary hypertension. Guidelines from AHA&ATS. Circulation. 2015;132.

Future Directions in Pulmonary Vasodilator Therapy in Children

The following are the next generation medications approved for use in adult population, yet to undergo clinical trials in children.

- *Macitentan*: Nonselective endothelin receptor antagonist
- *Riociguat*: Direct stimulator of soluble guanylate cyclase (sGC) receptors and sensitizes sGC to endogenous NO
- *Selexipag*: First oral prostacyclin analog, directly stimulating prostacyclin receptor.

OUTCOMES OF CHILDREN WITH PULMONARY HYPERTENSION

The outcomes of children with PH prior to advent of targeted therapy in last century were dismal with median survival of 10 months.[43] With introduction of prostacyclins and other targeted therapy in the first two decades of 21st century, the overall 5-year survival is 75–81%.[3,11] The outcome is best for Eisenmenger syndrome and worst for postoperative residual PAH in CHD with borderline operability.[1] The acute responders and those on combination therapy have better survival than nonresponders and those on monotherapy.

TREATABLE CAUSES OF PULMONARY HYPERTENSION IN CHILDREN

Pulmonary hypertension in children is characterized by a wide range of etiologies. There are certain subsets of children where the PH is curable, unlike adult population. The classical example of these are PPHN and PH associated with bronchopulmonary dysplasia. Rare but treatable conditions also include PH associated with massive adenotonsillar enlargement, congenital upper airway abnormalities, congenital portosystemic shunts (Abernethy malformations) and metabolic diseases such as wet beriberi prevalent in specific geographical populations in India.[44-46] Hence, though rare careful evaluation for curable causes is important in evaluation of PH in children.

CONCLUSION

The etiology of pulmonary hypertension in children is diverse and affects all age group from newborns to adolescents. The clinical presentation can be subtle, nonspecific, often presenting in advanced stage of disease. The advancement in pharmacological therapy, palliative interventions, early detection and timely intervention in CHD and increasing awareness have improved outcomes in children with PH. A thorough and systematic evaluation with focus on identifying treatable causes should be the norm in managing PH in children.

REFERENCES

1. Marín MJDC, Rotés AS, Ogando AR, Soto AM, Jiménez MQ, Camacho JLG, et al. Assessing pulmonary hypertensive vascular

disease in childhood. Data from the Spanish registry. Am J Respir Crit Care Med. 2014;190(12):1421-9.

2. van Loon RLE, Roofthooft MTR, Hillege HL, ten Harkel ADJ, van Osch-Gevers M, Delhaas T, et al. Pediatric pulmonary hypertension in the Netherlands: epidemiology and characterization during the period 1991 to 2005. Circulation. 2011;124(16):1755-64.
3. Moledina S, Hislop AA, Foster H, Schulze-Neick I, Haworth SG. Childhood idiopathic pulmonary arterial hypertension: a national cohort study. Heart. 2010;96(17):1401-6.
4. Escribano-Subias P, Blanco I, López-Meseguer M, Lopez-Guarch CJ, Roman A, Morales P, et al. Survival in pulmonary hypertension in Spain: insights from the Spanish registry. Eur Respir J. 2012;40(3):596-603.
5. Humbert M, Sitbon O, Chaouat A, Bertocchi M, Habib G, Gressin V, et al. Pulmonary arterial hypertension in France: results from a national registry. Am J Respir Crit Care Med. 2006;173(9):1023-30.
6. Peacock AJ, Murphy NF, McMurray JJV, Caballero L, Stewart S. An epidemiological study of pulmonary arterial hypertension. Eur Respir J. 2007;30(1):104-9.
7. Ivy DD, Abman SH, Barst RJ, Berger RMF, Bonnet D, Fleming TR, et al. Pediatric pulmonary hypertension. J Am Coll Cardiol. 2013;62(25 Suppl):D117-26.
8. Abman SH, Hansmann G, Archer SL, Ivy DD, Adatia I, Chung WK, et al. Pediatric Pulmonary Hypertension. Volume 132. Philadelphia: Lippincott Williams and Wilkins; 2015. p. 2037-99.
9. Hansmann G, Koestenberger M, Alastalo TP, Apitz C, Austin ED, Bonnet D, et al. 2019 updated consensus statement on the diagnosis and treatment of pediatric pulmonary hypertension: The European Pediatric Pulmonary Vascular Disease Network (EPPVDN), endorsed by AEPC, ESPR and ISHLT. J Heart Lung Transpl. 2019;38(9):879-901.
10. Simonneau G, Gatzoulis MA, Adatia I, Celermajer D, Denton C, Ghofrani A, et al. Updated clinical classification of pulmonary hypertension. J Am Coll Cardiol. 2013;62(25 Suppl):D34-41.
11. Zijlstra WMH, Douwes JM, Rosenzweig EB, Schokker S, Krishnan U, Roofthooft MTR, et al. Survival differences in pediatric pulmonary arterial hypertension: Clues to a better understanding of outcome and optimal treatment strategies. J Am Coll Cardiol. 2014;63(20):2159-69.
12. Lammers AE, Apitz C, Zartner P, Hager A, Dubowy KO, Hansmann G. Diagnostics, monitoring and outpatient care in children with suspected pulmonary hypertension/paediatric pulmonary hypertensive vascular disease. Expert consensus statement on the diagnosis and treatment of paediatric pulmonary hypertension. The European Paediatric Pulmonary Vascular Disease Network, endorsed by ISHLT and DGPK. Heart. 2016;102:ii1-13.
13. Lammers AE, Adatia I, Del Cerro MJ, Diaz G, Freudenthal AH, Freudenthal F, et al. Functional classification of pulmonary hypertension in children: report from the PVRI pediatric taskforce, Panama 2011. Pulmonary Circulation. 2011;1(2):280-5.
14. Bobhate P, Guo L, Jain S, Haugen R, Coe JY, Cave D, et al. Cardiac catheterization in children with pulmonary hypertensive vascular disease. Pediatr Cardiol. 2015;36(4):873-9.
15. Apitz C, Hansmann G, Schranz D. Hemodynamic assessment and acute pulmonary vasoreactivity testing in the evaluation of children with pulmonary vascular disease. Expert consensus statement on the diagnosis and treatment of paediatric pulmonary hypertension. The European Paediatric Pulmonary Vascular Disease Network, endorsed by ISHLT and DGPK. Heart. 2016;102 Suppl 2:ii23-9.
16. Guo L, Bobhate P, Kumar S, Vadlamudi K, Kaddoura T, Elgendi M, et al. Hyperoxia reduces oxygen consumption in children with pulmonary hypertension. Pediatr Cardiol. 2017;38(5):959-64.
17. Barst RJ. Pharmacologically induced pulmonary vasodilatation in children and young adults with primary pulmonary hypertension. Chest. 1986;89(4):497-503.
18. Yung D, Widlitz AC, Rosenzweig EB, Kerstein D, Maislin G, Barst RJ. Outcomes in children with idiopathic pulmonary arterial hypertension. Circulation. 2004;110(6):660-5.
19. del Cerro MJ, Moledina S, Haworth SG, Ivy D, Al Dabbagh M, Banjar H, et al. Cardiac catheterization in children with pulmonary hypertensive vascular disease: Consensus statement from the Pulmonary Vascular Research Institute, Pediatric and Congenital Heart Disease Task Forces. Pulm Circ. 2016;6(1):118-25.
20. Wardle AJ, Wardle R, Luyt K, Tulloh R. The utility of sildenafil in pulmonary hypertension: a focus on bronchopulmonary dysplasia. Arch Dis Child. 2013;98(8):613-7.
21. Barst RJ, Ivy DD, Gaitan G, Szatmari A, Rudzinski A, Garcia AE, et al. A randomized, double-blind, placebo-controlled, dose-ranging study of oral sildenafil citrate in treatment-naive children with pulmonary arterial hypertension. Circulation. 2012;125(2):324-34.
22. Steinhorn RH, Kinsella JP, Pierce C, Butrous G, Dilleen M, Oakes M, et al. Intravenous sildenafil in the treatment of neonates with persistent pulmonary hypertension. J Pediatr. 2009;155(6):841-7.
23. Takatsuki S, Calderbank M, Ivy DD. Initial experience with tadalafil in pediatric pulmonary arterial hypertension. Pediatr Cardiol. 2012;33(5):683-8.
24. Kohno H, Ichida F, Hirono K, Ozawa S, Yoshimura N, Nakamura T, et al. Plasma concentrations of tadalafil in children with pulmonary arterial hype tension. Ther Drug Monit. 2014;36(5):576-83.
25. Shiva A, Shiran M, Rafati M, Zamani H, Babazadeh K, Saeedi M, et al. Oral tadalafil in children with pulmonary arterial hypertension. Drug Res (Stuttg). 2015;66(1):7-10.
26. Small D, Ferguson-Sells L, Dahdah N, Bonnet D, Landry J, Li B. Pharmacokinetics and safety of tadalafil in a paediatric population with pulmonary arterial hypertension: a multiple ascending-dose study. Br J Clin Pharmacol. 2019;85(10):2302-9.
27. Rosenzweig EB, Ivy DD, Widlitz A, Doran A, Claussen LR, Yung D, et al. Effects of long-term Bosentan in children with pulmonary arterial hypertension. J Am Coll Cardiol. 2005;46(4):697-704.
28. Berger RMF, Gehin M, Beghetti M, Ivy D, Kusic-Pajic A, Cornelisse P, et al. A bosentan pharmacokinetic study to investigate dosing regimens in paediatric patients with pulmonary arterial hypertension: FUTURE-3. Br J Clin Pharmacol. 2017;83(8):1734-44.
29. Takatsuki S, Rosenzweig EB, Zuckerman W, Brady D, Calderbank M, Ivy DD. Clinical safety, pharmacokinetics, and efficacy of ambrisentan therapy in children with pulmonary arterial hypertension. Pediatr Pulmonol. 2013;48(1):27-34.
30. Sitbon O, Humbert M, Jaïs X, Ioos V, Hamid AM, Provencher S, et al. Long-term response to calcium channel blockers in idiopathic pulmonary arterial hypertension. Circulation. 2005;111(23):3105-11.
31. Barst RJ, Maislin G, Fishman AP. Vasodilator therapy for primary pulmonary hypertension in children. Circulation. 1999;99(9):1197–208.
32. Vorhies EE, Ivy DD. Drug treatment of pulmonary hypertension in children. Pediatric Drugs. 2014;16(1):43-65.
33. Rosenzweig EB, Kerstein D, Barst RJ. Long-term prostacyclin for pulmonary hypertension with associated congenital heart defects. Circulation. 1999;99(14):1858-65.
34. McIntyre CM, Hanna BD, Rintoul N, Ramsey EZ. Safety of epoprostenol and treprostinil in children less than 12 months of age. Pulm Circ. 2013;3(4):862-9.

35. Ivy DD, Claussen L, Doran A. Transition of stable pediatric patients with pulmonary arterial hypertension from intravenous epoprostenol to intravenous treprostinil. Am J Cardiol. 2007;99(5):696-8.
36. Levy M, Del Cerro MJ, Nadaud S, Vadlamudi K, Colgazier E, Fineman J, et al. Safety, efficacy and Management of subcutaneous treprostinil infusions in the treatment of severe pediatric pulmonary hypertension. Int J Cardiol. 2018; 264:153-7.
37. Krishnan U, Takatsuki S, Ivy DD, Kerstein J, Calderbank M, Coleman E, et al. Effectiveness and safety of inhaled treprostinil for the treatment of pulmonary arterial hypertension in children. Am J Cardiol. 2012;110(11):1704-9.
38. Ivy DD, Doran AK, Smith KJ, Mallory GB, Beghetti M, Barst RJ, et al. Short- and long-term effects of inhaled iloprost therapy in children with pulmonary arterial hypertension. J Am Coll Cardiol. 2008;51(2):161-9.
39. Roberts JD, Fineman JR, Morin FC, Shaul PW, Rimar S, Schreiber MD, et al. Inhaled nitric oxide and persistent pulmonary hypertension of the newborn. N Engl J Med. 1997;336(9):605-10.
40. Davidson D, Barefield ES, Kattwinkel J, Dudell G, Damask M, Straube R, et al. Inhaled nitric oxide for the early treatment of persistent pulmonary. Pediatrics. 1998;101(3):325-34.
41. Goldstein BS, Sweet SC, Mao J, Huddleston CB, Grady RM. Lung transplantation in children with idiopathic pulmonary arterial hypertension: An 18-year experience. J Hear Lung Transplant. 2011;30(10):1148-52.
42. Hoeper MM, McLaughlin VV, Barberá JA, Frost AE, Ghofrani HA, Peacock AJ, et al. Initial combination therapy with ambrisentan and tadalafil and mortality in patients with pulmonary arterial hypertension: a secondary analysis of the results from the randomised, controlled AMBITION study. Lancet Respir Med. 2016;4(11):894-901.
43. D'Alonzo GE, Barst RJ, Ayres SM, Bergofsky EH, Brundage BH, Detre KM, et al. Survival in patients with primary pulmonary hypertension: results from a national prospective registry. Ann Intern Med. 1991;115(5):343-9.
44. Bhat JI, Rather HA, Ahangar AA, Qureshi UA, Dar P, Ahmed QI, et al. Shoshin beriberi-thiamine responsive pulmonary hypertension in exclusively breastfed infants: a study from northern India. Indian Heart J. 2017;69(1):24-7.
45. Orji FT, Ujunwa FA, Umedum NG, Ukaegbe O. The impact of adenotonsillectomy on pulmonary arterial pressure in West African children with adenotonsillar hypertrophy. Int J Pediatr Otorhinolaryngol. 2017;92:151-5.
46. Uike K, Nagata H, Hirata Y, Yamamura K, Terashi E, Matsuura T, et al. Effective shunt closure for pulmonary hypertension and liver dysfunction in congenital portosystemic venous shunt. Pediatr Pulmonol. 2018;53(4):505-11.

19
CHAPTER

Syncope

Mani Ram Krishna

INTRODUCTION

The word syncope is a derivative of the Greek word "synkoptein" and translates roughly into "to cut short." It is defined as a transient loss of consciousness (LoC) with loss of tone due to cerebral hypoperfusion which is usually followed by a prompt recovery.[1] Syncope is a surprisingly common symptom in children with estimates suggesting that approximately 15% of the population would have experienced one episode of syncope during childhood.[2] The incidence peaks during the teenage years with girls more likely to experience it than boys. Although transient cerebral hypoperfusion is the final common pathway for LoC, the inciting events are varied. Accordingly the causes of syncope are classified into three major groups (**Flowchart 1**): (1) autonomic; (2) cardiovascular, and (3) neurological. Syncope, thus is an important clinical problem in childhood and pediatricians should adopt a structured approach toward its evaluation to ensure that the cause is correctly identified. In this chapter, we discuss autonomic syncope and present a clinical approach to syncope which can be easily practiced by a clinician in his outpatient clinic or the emergency room with good accuracy to identify the cause.

The majority of syncope in children are benign and can be attributed to autonomic instability (80–85%). However, a significant portion could experience symptoms secondary to a cardiovascular cause (5–10%). These causes have a potential to result in sudden cardiac death. It is possible to differentiate between the two causes in almost all cases through a detailed history and physical examination. An understanding of the pathophysiology will aid in understanding their clinical presentation.

AUTONOMIC SYNCOPE

Autonomic or reflex syncope is the most common cause of syncope in children. As the name suggests, this is a reflex response of the body to a sudden change which results in decreased cardiac output and LoC. Improvements in our understanding of this disease entity have permitted further subclassification of this disease entity.[3] Of these, the most clinically important is the neurocardiogenic syncope (NCS).

Flowchart 1: Causes of syncope in children.

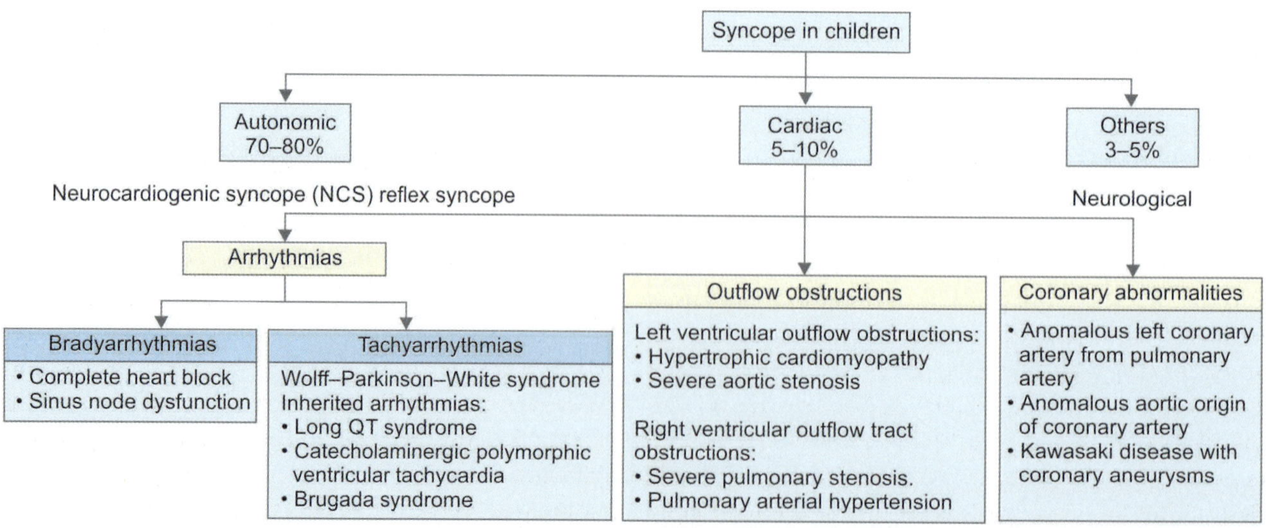

Source: Reproduced with permission from Krishna MK, Kunde MF. A clinical approach to syncope. Indian J Prac Pediatr. 2020;22(1):92-9.

Etiopathogenesis

The term vasovagal syncope (VVS) first coined by a British cardiologist, Dr Thomas Lewis, in the 1930s[4] still continues to be widely used although it has lost favor with specialists who prefer NCS. This is because NCS more appropriately explains the pathogenesis of the condition which is attributed to the Bezold-Jarisch (B-J) reflex.[5] The reflex was first described by van Bezold and later became popular after the animal studies conducted by Jarisch and his team in the last century. Any condition which results in a sudden decrease in the preload of the heart stimulates the cardiac mechanoreceptors in the ventricle (C-fibers) which pass the information on to the dorsal vagal nucleus in the medulla oblongata. Stimulation of the vagal center results in bradycardia and hypotension. Although meant to protect the heart and the circulation from the decreased preload, it paradoxically leads to LoC. Recently, the presence of C-receptors in the ventricle has been challenged by a few physiologists. Hence, the exact pathogenesis of NCS continues to be researched despite the condition being very common.

Clinical Features

A typical episode of NCS consists of a prodrome which is followed by LoC which then is followed by recovery.

Prodrome

This is usually abrupt. Most children will be able to recollect presyncopal symptoms when enquired after the recovery. Additionally the observation of onlookers provides clues regarding the condition of the child prior to LoC. The common symptoms described include dizziness, light-headedness, and the presence of visual aura. Some children describe nausea or a general feeling of unease. Onlookers describe the children typically as turning pale or more rarely to be hyperventilating.

Loss of Consciousness

The child loses consciousness for a brief period. During this phase, onlookers may notice some limb movements which may be described as convulsions. Incontinence is not typically a feature associated with autonomic syncope.

Recovery

Recovery from consciousness is usually within seconds to minutes. Postrecovery, the child may complain of fatigue. Full recovery usually happens within an hour.

A number of triggers and precipitants can be identified in almost every episode of NCS. Precipitants are remote events which tend to reduce the threshold for an episode while triggers precede the actual event. The common precipitants identified in children include inadequate sleep, emotional distress, dehydration, and viral illness while triggers include sudden change in posture (usually from supine to an upright posture), prolonged standing, or a noxious event.

On occasions, especially when episodes happen at school, children are not under the direct supervision of an adult and peer group children may not be able to accurately recollect the event. Hence, it is important to focus on the events preceding the LoC. This often provides the most valuable clue regarding the cause. Autonomic syncope almost exclusively occurs during an upright posture and syncope during a supine posture should alert the physician about a nonautonomic cause.

Often, there may be paroxysmal movements associated with syncope which can be misinterpreted as seizures. The term "convulsive syncope" has been used to describe these movements. They can usually be reliably differentiated from seizures using the following clues[6] as listed in **Table 1**.

TABLE 1: Distinguishing convulsive syncope from primary seizure.

Clinical parameter	*Convulsive syncope*	*Seizures*
Movements	Pleomorphic	Uniform and rhythmic
Prodrome	Almost always present	Unusual
Tongue biting	Rare and usually at the tip of the tongue	More likely at the sides of the tongue
Incontinence	Unusual	Frequent
Duration	Seconds	Much longer
Postictal phase	Fatigue is the dominant symptom	Confusion and weakness are more common

Investigations

A detailed history and a thorough physical examination are the only evaluation needed for a diagnosis of NCS. Recurrences are common and can occur in close to 60% of children. In children with recurrent syncope, investigations may be necessary to reassure the family. A common misdiagnosis is a seizure disorder. Convulsive syncope can be differentiated from true seizures based on certain clinical clues. When episodes are recurrent and when there is a strong suspicion of only a convulsive syncope, parents should be encouraged to record the episode on a video while someone arranges for medical attention. The only investigation which has diagnostic utility in autonomic syncope is the head up tilt table (HUTT) testing.[7] The HUTT test needs a specialized HUTT laboratory. A number of different protocols exist each claiming greater specificity than the other.[8] The testing is usually performed in the morning time. Some authorities recommend overnight fasting. It is important that resuscitation equipment and a physician or paramedic trained in cardiopulmonary resuscitation (CPR) are present during the study. The child is then placed supine for 10–20 minutes while his heart rate and blood pressure (BP) are monitored. The table is then slowly tilted to an almost upright position (70–80°) over a 10–20-minute period.[9] Three types of responses are possible[10]—vasodepressor response where the systolic BP drops by at least 20% or a cardioinhibitory type where the heart rate drops to <40 per minute without a significant drop in BP. A mixed response is also possible. An HUTT is reported to be positive when symptoms occur along with one of the hemodynamic responses. The child should then be immediately returned to the supine position and continued to be monitored. Intravenous fluids may be started. If initial testing is negative, the test can be repeated with a provocative agent. The commonly used agents are isoprenaline and nitrates.

Head up tilt table has a number of important disadvantages. Although it has been shown to have reasonable specificity (>80%), its sensitivity is very low. No single protocol has been shown to be consistently superior over others and the testing method varies greatly between HUTT laboratories.[8] The tests are not reproducible. The same person may experience varied results even with the same methodology. A positive HUTT also does not predict response to therapy. However, a major advantage of HUTT is its ability to clarify the diagnosis and allay fears about an alternate diagnosis for the family as well as the treating physician.

Treatment

The only treatment needed for autonomic syncope is reassurance and education about avoidance of triggers and precipitants.[11] Adequate consumption of water and maintenance of sleep hygiene helps prevent episodes. Addition of extra salt to the child's diet has been shown to be useful as well. If symptoms occur with sudden change of posture to upright, children can be encouraged to first move to a semirecumbent position before standing upright. Exercises to improve calf muscle tone have been shown to reduce frequency of symptoms.

In a small minority of patients symptoms persist despite lifestyle modifications. These patients may benefit from medications. The commonly used medications include:

- *Fludrocortisone*[12]: This is a mineralocorticoid. At a dose of 0.1 mg/day for adolescents, it aids in water and salt retention and helps maintain intravascular volume.
- *Beta-blockers*[13]: Beta-blockers are believed to mitigate the activation of the ventricular mechanoreceptors, thus preventing activation of the B-J reflex. A sustained release preparation of metoprolol at a dose of 0.5–1 mg per kg daily has been shown to reduce the number of episodes.
- Disopyramide at a dose of 1–4 mg/kg thrice daily has been found to be effective in a few studies. Its action is believed to be due to its anticholinergic activity.
- In exceptional circumstances, a pacemaker has been used in patients with severe symptoms.[14] This should be reserved for children with very frequent symptoms who have a sustained bradycardia or asystole on HUTT.

CARDIOVASCULAR SYNCOPE

The cardiovascular causes of syncope are shown in **Flowchart 1**. Most of these conditions result in syncope during exertion. They may be classified into three broad subsets. The individual disorders are discussed in detail in their respective sections.

Obstructive Lesions

These include obstruction to the left or right ventricle outflow tract. During normal activity, the cardiac output may be maintained. However, during exertion, the heart is usually unable to increase the cardiac output against a fixed resistance resulting in a drop in cardiac output and LoC.

Tachyarrhythmias

Any sympathetic overactivity decreases the threshold for arrhythmias. As discussed earlier in the chapter on arrhythmias, a number of inherited arrhythmia syndromes result in malignant ventricular arrhythmias during exercise.

Bradyarrhythmia

Both complete heart block (CHB) and sinus nodal dysfunction (SND) can result in syncope on exertion. An increase in heart rate is an integral response whenever an increase in cardiac output is warranted. Children with bradyarrhythmia cannot increase heart rate and thus cardiac output resulting in LoC.

Coronary Artery Disorders

Anomalous origin of the coronary arteries as well as coronary artery aneurysm and thrombosis due to Kawasaki disease can result in chest pain and syncope on exertion. This is due to a demand-supply mismatch similar to coronary artery disease in adults.

A CLINICAL APPROACH TO SYNCOPE

An often repeated quote is the only difference between syncope and sudden death is that the patient wakes up after a syncope. A patient presenting with syncope thus presents a valuable opportunity to prevent sudden death. Hence, although most episodes of syncope are benign, they should be evaluated thoroughly and systematically to ensure no serious cause is missed.

History

A detailed history is probably the most important diagnostic tool in syncope.[15] Often when episodes happen in school or when the child is not under parental supervision, an accurate description of the episode is difficult to obtain. Syncope is a dramatic event for a layman who may be flustered after witnessing it. The child may also be frightened because of the excessive attention. If we are able to win the confidence of the child, it is our experience that children can often accurately recollect events leading up to the LoC.

Leading questions may be necessary to identify potential precipitants and triggers. When we analyzed patients with NCS who presented to our outpatient clinic, we were able to identify a trigger or precipitant in every case who had presented to our unit over a 3-month period (unpublished data). An endeavor must be made to record five key elements in history for every child presents with syncope.

1. Time of the event.
2. *Activity leading to the event*: Cardiovascular syncope happens at the peak of exertion (mid-stride) while NCS almost exclusively happens at the completion of the activity.
3. *Posture at the time of syncope*: NCS occurs in the upright position.
4. *Associated symptoms*: The presence of chest pain, palpitation, and dyspnea on exertion are pointers toward a cardiac cause of syncope. Syncope without a prodrome and a history of palpitations has been shown to have a 100% specificity for cardiac syncope.[16]
5. *Family history*: Syncope, seizures, infant death, and sudden unexpected deaths in young adults.

Red flag signs for a cardiac syncope have been identified and the presence of any of them should prompt an immediate referral to a pediatric cardiologist. The red flag signs include the following:[17]

- Syncope on exertion
- Syncope without a prodrome
- Syncope in supine position
- Child with a known cardiac problem including Kawasaki disease
- Family history of cardiac disorders, sudden death[18], and drowning in multiple family members
- *Specific triggers for episodes*: Fever and auditory stimuli.

Physical Examination

All the vital signs should be carefully recorded including the pulse rate, BP, and oxygen saturation. It is recommended that orthostatic vital signs be recorded in each child with syncope. This implies measuring pulse rate and BP in the sitting and standing position (usually 2–5 minutes). This is often not possible in a busy outpatient or emergency room (ER) setting and are normal in a vast majority of children with NCS. However, should significant bradycardia or hypotension be documented, this may be diagnostic.

A thorough cardiovascular examination is mandatory in all children with syncope. The presence of cardiomegaly or a parasternal heave suggest obstruction to the left or right ventricular outflow respectively. A low volume pulse is present in severe aortic stenosis. The baseline heart rate is very low in CHB. An ejection systolic murmur at the base of the heart (2nd intercostal space) suggests outflow tract obstruction while a loud (and often palpable) pulmonary component of the second heart sound is diagnostic of severe pulmonary arterial hypertension (PAH).

A rapid neurological examination should also be performed with special attention for neurocutaneous markers and focal deficits.

Electrocardiogram

The electrocardiogram (ECG) is a cheap and readily available investigation and hence should be obtained whenever there is any uncertainty about the diagnosis of an autonomic syncope on history and physical examination. The ECG is probably the only investigation with any diagnostic utility in syncope. Significant outflow tract obstructions, severe PAH, CHB, hypertrophic cardiomyopathy (HCM), and the pre-excitation syndrome can be diagnosed or suspected based on a 12-lead ECG. The resting ECG is often normal in children with an inherited arrhythmia or a coronary artery abnormality.

Structured clinical evaluation has been part of recommendation for the evaluation of syncope for many decades. When Johnson and colleagues analyzed ER records in a tertiary care hospital over a 18-year period, retrospectively—a screening test using syncope on exertion, positive family history, abnormal cardiac examination, and abnormal ECG had a 100% sensitivity for diagnosing cardiac syncope.[19] Although extremely simple and practical, this is not practiced routinely even in large teaching hospitals. When the evaluation of syncope was reviewed in a large pediatric ER, an adequate history was not obtained in more than half the patients and investigations other than ECG which were ordered in almost all patients were not diagnostic in any.

REFERENCES

1. Shen WK, Sheldon RS, Benditt DG, Cohen MI, Forman DE, Goldberger ZD, et al. 2017 ACC/AHA/HRS Guideline for the Evaluation and Management of Patients With Syncope: Executive Summary, a Report of the American College of Cardiology/American Heart Association Task Force on Clinical Practice Guidelines and the Heart Rhythm Society. J Am Coll Cardiol. 2017;70(5):620-63.
2. McHarg ML, Shinnar S, Rascoff H, Walsh CA. Syncope in childhood. Pediatr Cardiol. 1997; 18(5):367-71.
3. Kanjwal K, Calkins H. Syncope in children and adolescents. Card Electrophysiol Clin. 2013;5(4):443-55.
4. Nahm F, Freeman R. Vasovagal syncope: the contributions of Sir William R. Gowers and Sir Thomas Lewis. Arch Neurol. 2001;58(3):509-11.
5. Grubb BP. Clinical practice. Neurocardiogenic syncope. N Engl J Med. 2005;352(10):1004-10.
6. Sheldon R. How to differentiate syncope from seizure. Card Electrophysiol Clin. 2013;5(4):423-31.
7. Kenny RA, Ingram A, Bayliss J, Sutton R. Head-up tilt: a useful test for investigating unexplained syncope. Lancet. 1986;1(8494):1352-5.
8. Buszko K, Kujawski S, Newton JL, Zalewski P. Hemodynamic response to the head-up tilt test in patients with syncope as a predictor of the test outcome: a meta-analysis approach. Front Physiol. 2019;10:184.

9. Benditt DG, Ferguson DW, Grubb BP, Kapoor WN, Kugler J, Lerman BB, et al. Tilt table testing for assessing syncope. American College of Cardiology. J Am Coll Cardiol. 1996;28(1):263-75.
10. Brignole M, Menozzi C, Del Rosso A, Costa S, Gaggioli G, Bottoni N, et al. New classification of haemodynamics of vasovagal syncope: beyond the VASIS classification. Analysis of the presyncopal phase of the tilt test without and with nitroglycerin challenge. Vasovagal Syncope International Study. Europace. 2000;2(1):66-76.
11. McLeod KA. Syncope in childhood. Arch Dis Child. 2003; 88(4):350-3.
12. Schleifer JW, Shen WK. Vasovagal syncope: an update on the latest pharmacological therapies. Expert Opin Pharmacother. 2015;16(4):501-13.
13. Sheldon R, Connolly S, Rose S, Klingenheben T, Krahn A, Morillo C, et al. Prevention of Syncope Trial (POST): a randomized, placebo-controlled study of metoprolol in the prevention of vasovagal syncope. Circulation. 2006;113(9):1164-70.
14. Brignole M, Menozzi C, Moya A, Andresen D, Blanc JJ, Krahn AD, et al. Pacemaker therapy in patients with neurally mediated syncope and documented asystole: Third International Study on Syncope of Uncertain Etiology (ISSUE-3): a randomized trial. Circulation. 2012;125(21):2566-71.
15. Strickberger SA, Benson DW, Biaggioni I, Callans DJ, Cohen MI, Ellenbogen KA, et al. AHA/ACCF Scientific Statement on the evaluation of syncope: from the American Heart Association Councils on Clinical Cardiology, Cardiovascular Nursing, Cardiovascular Disease in the Young, and Stroke, and the Quality of Care and Outcomes Research Interdisciplinary Working Group; and the American College of Cardiology Foundation: in collaboration with the Heart Rhythm Society: endorsed by the American Autonomic Society. Circulation. 2006;113(2):316-27.
16. Hurst D, Hirsh DA, Oster ME, Ehrlich A, Campbell R, Mahle WT, et al. Syncope in the pediatric emergency department - can we predict cardiac disease based on history alone? J Emerg Med. 2015;49(1):1-7.
17. Krishna MR, Kunde MF. A clinical approach to syncope. Indian J Pract Pediatr. 2020;22(1):92-9.
18. Colman N, Bakker A, Linzer M, Reitsma JB, Wieling W, Wilde AA. Value of history-taking in syncope patients: in whom to suspect long QT syndrome? Europace. 2009;11(7):937-43.
19. Johnson ER, Etheridge SP, Minich LL, Bardsley T, Heywood M, Menon SC. Practice variation and resource use in the evaluation of pediatric vasovagal syncope: are pediatric cardiologists over-testing? Pediatr Cardiol. 2014;35(5):753-8.

20
CHAPTER

Congenital Heart Disease

R Krishna Kumar, Anil Kumar Singhi

INTRODUCTION

A substantial portion of pediatric cardiac practice relates to congenital heart disease (CHD) because they are by far the most common cause of heart ailments in children.[1] There is tremendous diversity within the broad category of CHDs. The diversity is in anatomy, hemodynamics, associations, natural history, and complications. As a result, most pediatricians are somewhat intimidated. However, from the point of view of management, it is essential to be familiar with broad physiologic categories that often can be identified clinically as well. Additionally, it is also necessary to be aware of the natural history of common heart defects and how they can be altered by contemporary treatment options. This section will discuss, at first, key aspects of epidemiology, classification physiology, natural history, complications, and prevention from the broad overall perspective of CHD in general. Specific aspects of the above considerations relating to individual heart defects are discussed in detail in separate subchapters (*see* Chapters 21-40).

The following generalizations about CHD are worth stating at the outset:

- Heart defects are among the most common birth defects and are responsible for a significant proportion of infant mortality in many parts of the world including many parts of emerging economies such as India, China, Sri Lanka, Vietnam, and Indonesia. CHD ranks in the top 5 causes of infant mortality in most regions of the world including many parts of India.[2]
- In general, the most sinister and severe defects present early after birth. Indeed the earlier a defect presents, the more severe it is likely to be with a high likelihood of death without specific intervention.
- In spite a seemingly bewildering variety of individual defects, the broad physiologic categories of CHD are limited and they can be understood. This understanding is often adequate for the initial diagnosis and management of CHD in the primary care facility at the level of district hospital.
- Numerous advances in imaging, surgery, intensive care, and catheter interventions have vastly improved the outlook of patients with CHD in the past 3–4 decades. A number of Indian centers can now deliver comprehensive pediatric cardiac care and deliver outcomes that are comparable to international standards.[3]
- Timing of surgical or catheter intervention of CHD is an important decision. In general, there is a shift toward earlier intervention to enable the best long-term results for the heart, lung vasculature, and brain development as well as for the best general growth and development. However, there is also a need to exercise judgment in relatively mild lesions where the natural history may not be worse than results of interventions. Here, intervention is timed to ensure that the predicted outcomes are better than the anticipated natural history.
- While many heart defects are correctable through a single surgical or catheter procedures, many relatively complex defects require staged interventions. Many of the so-called corrections require continued follow-up. It is increasingly apparent that there are long-term concerns that surface later in life after "corrective" procedures. Some conditions, such as single ventricle physiology, can only be palliated and this generally accomplished in stages (**Flowchart 1**).

EPIDEMIOLOGY

Epidemiology of CHDs is covered extensively in the first chapter of this book and will not be repeated here. It is essential to recognize that the relative importance of CHD as a cause of infant mortality and morbidity progressively increases as overall infant mortality improves. Many parts of the world including most states in India are experiencing a progressive reduction in infant mortality rate (IMR) largely because common and easily preventable causes of infant mortality are declining. However, because of deaths, CHD is not being addressed particularly in infancy, the relative contribution of CHD of infant mortality progressively increases (**Fig. 1**).

Flowchart 1: A simplified working classification of congenital heart operations.

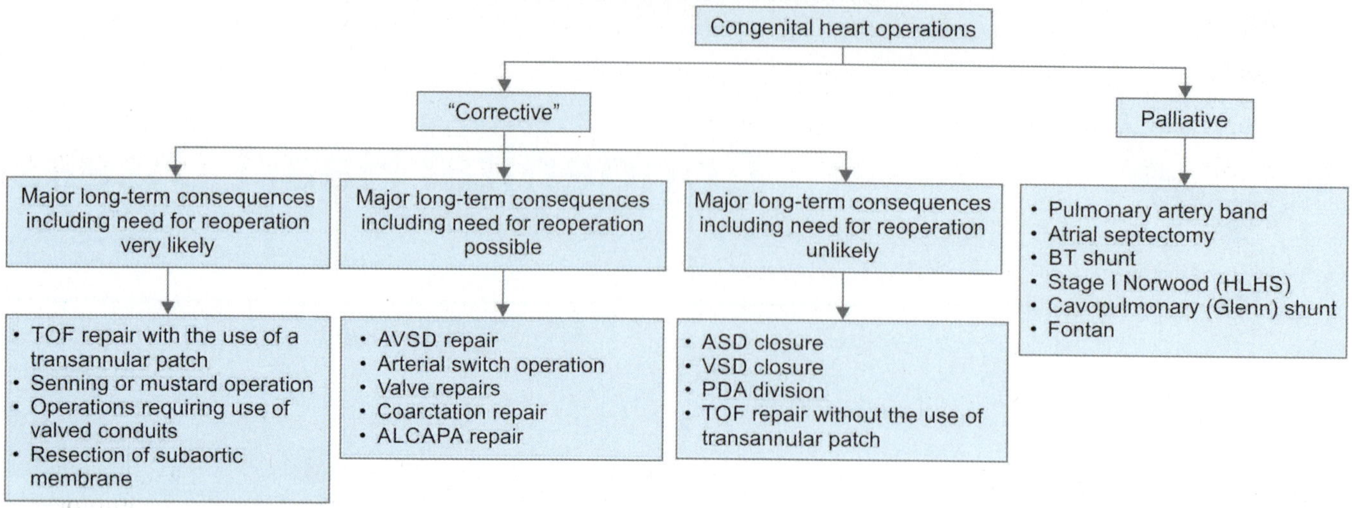

(ASD: atrial septal defect; ALCAPA: anomalous left coronary artery from pulmonary artery; AVSD: atrioventricular septal defect; BT: Blalock–Taussig; HLHS: hypoplastic left heart syndrome; PDA: patent ductus arteriosus; TOF: tetralogy of Fallot; VSD: ventricular septal defect).

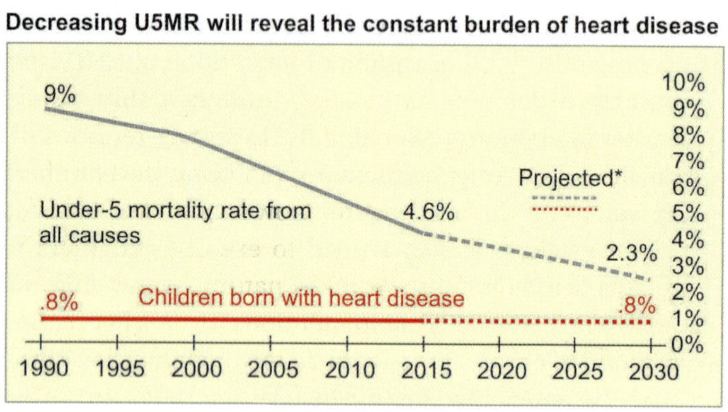

Fig. 1: This graph shows how congenital heart disease is "unmasked" as an important cause of infant mortality as infant mortality from other preventable causes decline.
Adapted with modification from: "A Case for the Invisible Child", Children's HeartLink. [online] Available from: http://theinvisiblechild.childrensheartlink.org/. [Last accessed October, 2020].

PHYSIOLOGICAL CATEGORIES OF CONGENITAL HEART DISEASE

It is often possible to identify the physiological category of CHD using history and physical examination supplemented by the chest X-ray and ECG (electrocardiogram). The rules required for this categorization are relatively simple and enable fairly accurate categorization.

The traditional and time-honored classification of CHD as acyanotic and cyanotic has significant shortcomings because there is considerable overlap (**Fig. 2**). Bedside assessment of cyanosis is seriously flawed and any desaturation (<95%) would classify a disease as cyanotic CHD. This classification still forms the basis for much of bedside teaching of pediatric cardiology. It is important to understand the limitations of this classification.

In the real world, a spectrum of oxygen saturations are encountered and there are conditions that are traditionally classified as cyanotic such as tetralogy of Fallot (TOF) can be quite "pink". Similarly patients with common left-to-right shunts develop cyanosis once there is a marked elevation in pulmonary vascular resistance (PVR). **Figure 2** attempts to display all congenital heart defects in the spectrum. While there are several conditions that are clearly cyanotic or acyanotic, the overlap is considerable.

The following physiologic categories are important from a conceptual standpoint:[4]

- Pretricuspid versus post-tricuspid shunts
- The ventricular septal defect-pulmonary stenosis (VSD-PS) physiology
- Single ventricle physiology
- Duct-dependent lesions
- Unfavorable streaming and parallel circulation.

Pretricuspid versus Post-tricuspid Shunts

Acyanotic heart disease with left-to-right shunts is traditionally classified as pretricuspid and post-tricuspid shunts. There are important differences in physiology that have an important bearing on clinical manifestations and natural history.

Left-to-right shunts at the level of the atria are known as pretricuspid shunts. They include atrial septal defects (ASDs) and partial anomalous pulmonary venous connection. The left-to-right shunt and the consequent excessive pulmonary blood flow are dictated by relative stiffness of the two ventricles. Since the right ventricle is relatively stiff (noncompliant) at birth and during early infancy, the shunt is small. Over the years, the right ventricle progressively enlarges to accommodate the excessive pulmonary blood flow. The pulmonary vasculature also becomes more capacious to gradually accommodate the excessive blood flow. This explains why ASDs typically do not manifest with symptoms of pulmonary overcirculation during infancy and childhood. The clinical signs are also easily explained by the physiology

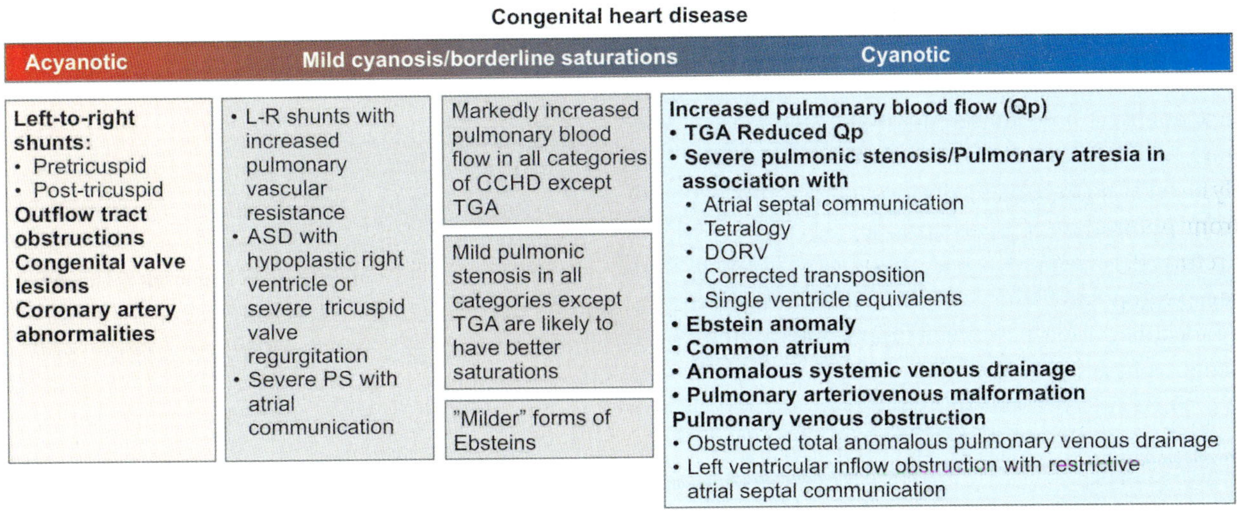

Fig. 2: The clinical spectrum of congenital heart disease. On the left are "pink conditions" and on right are "blue conditions." Between the two extremes are a number of conditions that can have some desaturation.
(ASD: atrial septal defect; CCHD: cyanotic congenital heart disease; DORV: double outlet right ventricle; PS: pulmonary stenosis; TGA: transposition of the great arteries)

of pretricuspid shunts. The diastolic flow murmur of ASD is across the much larger tricuspid valve and is therefore subtle or even inaudible. The second heart sound split is wide and fixed largely because of the prolonged "hang-out" interval resulting from increased capacitance of the pulmonary circulation. Additionally, the large communication at atrial level minimizes any differences in the impact of respiration on right versus left heart. Pulmonary arterial hypertension (PAH) is typically absent or at most mild. The presence of moderate or severe PAH in ASD is worrisome and may suggest the onset of irreversible changes in the pulmonary vasculature.

Post-tricuspid shunts are different in that there is direct transmission of pressure from the systemic to the pulmonary circuit at the ventricular level (VSD) or great arteries [patent ductus arteriosus (PDA) and aortopulmonary window]. For patients with large post-tricuspid shunts, symptoms begin in early infancy, typically after some regression of elevated pulmonary vasoconstriction in the newborn period together with progressive development of the pulmonary vascular tree. The excessive pulmonary blood flow returns to the left atrium and flows through the mitral valve resulting in the apical diastolic flow murmur that is a consistent marker of large post-tricuspid shunts. The left atrium and the ventricle are dilated as a result of this extra volume. Elevation in pulmonary artery pressures is an inevitable consequence of large (or unrestrictive) post-tricuspid shunts and is labeled as hyperkinetic PAH. This needs to be distinguished from elevation of PVR that results from sustained exposure to increased pulmonary blood flow.

Ventricular Septal Defect-Pulmonary Stenosis Physiology

This situation is characterized by a large communication at the ventricular level together with varying degrees of obstruction to pulmonary blood flow. Typically this is in the form of subvalvar (infundibular), valvar, annular (small valve annulus), and occasionally supravalvar stenosis. The free communication between the two ventricles results in equalization of pressures. Severity of PS dictates the volume of blood flowing through pulmonary arteries and therefore amount of oxygenated blood returning via pulmonary veins. Severe PS results in right-to-left shunt across the VSD with varying degrees of hypoxia and, consequently, cyanosis. Cyanosis is directly proportionate to the severity of PS. Because the right ventricle is readily decompressed by the large VSD, heart failure is unusual. The best example of VSD-PS physiology is TOF. In its least severe form, TOF is often not associated with cyanosis (pink TOF). Here, PS is significant enough to result in a large pressure gradient across the right ventricular outflow tract (RVOT), but not severe enough to result in a reduction in pulmonary blood flow. Pink TOF is typically associated with a loud ejection systolic murmur because of a reasonable volume of blood flowing across the RVOT. As the severity of PS increases, pulmonary blood flow declines and the intensity of murmur declines progressively. Other examples of VSD-PS physiology include double-outlet right ventricle (DORV) with subaortic VSD and PS, corrected transposition with PS, and atrioventricular septal defect with PS. These conditions are often indistinguishable from TOF at the bedside.

Single Ventricle Physiology

This refers to a group of conditions where there is complete mixing of pulmonary and systemic venous returns. In addition to single ventricle (double inlet ventricle), a variety of conditions come under the category of single ventricular physiology. Atresia of one of the atrioventricular (AV) valves, severe hypoplasia of one of the ventricles, severe straddling of one of the AV valves over a large VSD are all examples of situations where there is mixing of pulmonary and systemic venous returns. The clinical manifestations are dictated by whether or not there is PS. In absence of PS, there is excessive pulmonary blood flow especially in infants because of the relatively lower PVR. As a result, the proportion of oxygenated blood from pulmonary veins that mixes with the systemic venous return is high. As a result, cyanosis is minimal and measured oxygen saturation may be in the 90s. However, the price for this preserved oxygenation is heart failure and development of permanent elevation of PVR (pulmonary vascular obstructive disease or PVOD). Over time, if the child survives infancy, PVR progressively increases with increasing cyanosis.

Single ventricle and its physiologic variants can be associated with varying degrees of pulmonary stenosis. Here, the situation is quite similar to VSD-PS physiology except for relatively severe hypoxia because of free mixing systemic and pulmonary venous return.

Duct-dependent Lesions

An infant or a newborn with CHD that is dependent on the patency of the ductus arteriosus for survival can be termed as suffering from a duct-dependent lesion. Typically, these are newborns in which either the systemic blood supply is critically dependent on an open PDA [duct-dependent systemic circulation (DDSC)] or pulmonary blood flow is duct-dependent [duct-dependent pulmonary circulation (DDPC)].

Closure of the PDA in DDSC results in systemic hypoperfusion (often mislabeled as neonatal sepsis). Examples of DDSC include hypoplastic left heart syndrome where the entire systemic circulation is supported by the right ventricle through the PDA, interrupted aortic arch where the descending aortic flow is entirely through the PDA. Severe coarctation and critical aortic stenosis are also examples of DDSC.

Closure of PDA in DDPC results in severe hypoxia and cyanosis in the affected newborn. Examples of DDPC include all forms of pulmonary atresia (irrespective of underlying heart defect) where the PDA is the predominant source of pulmonary blood flow. There are examples of pulmonary atresia where pulmonary blood supply is from major aortopulmonary collaterals. These children may survive even after the PDA closes. Critical pulmonic stenosis ("nearly-atretic" pulmonary valve) can present as duct-dependent pulmonary blood flow.

Neonates with duct-dependent physiology require prostaglandin E1 (PGE1) for survival. Early recognition of a duct-dependent situation allows early initiation of PGE1 and stabilization until definitive procedure can be accomplished.

Unfavorable Streaming and Parallel Circulation

Unfavorable streaming refers to a situation where oxygen-rich pulmonary blood flow is directed toward the pulmonary valve and poorly oxygenated blood toward the aortic valve. An extreme form of unfavorable streaming is the parallel circulation in the transposition of great arteries (TGA) with intact ventricular septum. Here, survival is dependent of the presence of a communication (ideally at atrial level) that allows mixing of pulmonary and systemic venous return. The presence of a VSD may improve the situation in TGA but significant cyanosis is usually present unless the pulmonary blood flow is torrential.

DIAGNOSTIC APPROACH

The diagnostic approach is dictated by age at presentation (**Box 1**). The primary focus of the diagnostic approach in a newborn is to exclude critical and potentially lethal CHD. While clinical manifestations provide clues to the presence of CHD in neonates, the endeavor is to identify CHD even before the manifestations occur. This is because once clinical manifestations are apparent, there is often very little time to intervene. Therefore, the focus has shifted to systematic screening of all neonates within the first 24–48 hours after birth (*see* Chapter 6). Indeed, with the advent of routine prenatal cardiac evaluation, CHD is increasingly identified before birth allowing for delivery to be planned in advance at a tertiary center that has a comprehensive pediatric heart program well before any adverse consequences occur (*see* Chapter 47). Nonetheless, it is necessary for pediatricians to be familiar with how heart disease presents in the newborn as majority of neonates are still not screened in India and screening may still miss a small proportion of critical CHD and a significant proportion of noncritical defects that require close follow-up intervention later in life. Manifestations are often not specific for CHD and clinical evaluation often do not identify the underlying defect and, in many instances, the physiological category. The most important question here is "does the newborn have critical CHD?" Once serious heart disease is suspected, the focus is on rapidly arriving at a precise diagnosis through echocardiography, stabilizing the condition, and expeditiously transporting the baby to an appropriate tertiary care facility. The principles of evaluation of neonates with suspected CHD are enunciated in Chapter 48.

Selected heart defects manifest for the first time later during infancy. They constitute an important proportion of CHD and are often relatively easy to salvage through corrective surgery. These babies characteristically manifest with symptoms that provide important clues to the presence of underlying CHD and the likely physiology. Physical examination often provides useful clues to the underlying defect. Chest X-ray and ECG allow further refinement of the

BOX 1: Congenital heart diseases (CHDs) classified by natural history.

- Conditions that seldom permit survival beyond the neonatal period:
  - Critical obstruction to pulmonary blood flow (duct-dependent pulmonary circulation):
    - Pulmonary atresia with inadequate aortopulmonary collaterals (tetralogy of Fallot with pulmonary atresia, pulmonary atresia with intact ventricular septum, pulmonary atresia in association with any other cardiac malformation)
    - Critical pulmonic stenosis (isolated or in association with other forms of CHD)
    - Severe forms of Ebstein malformation of the tricuspid valve
  - Critical obstruction to systemic blood flow (duct-dependent systemic circulation):
    - Hypoplastic left heart syndrome
    - Critical aortic stenosis
    - Aortic atresia
    - Arch interruption
    - Coarctation
  - Transposition of great arteries with intact ventricular septum
  - Total anomalous pulmonary venous drainage
- Conditions that seldom permit survival or correction beyond early childhood:
  - Complex defects associated with increased pulmonary blood flow:
    - Single ventricle, double-outlet right ventricle, tricuspid atresia, transposition with ventricular septal defect, corrected transposition with ventricular septal defect, persistent truncus arteriosus, and common atrioventricular (AV) canal
  - Large post-tricuspid left-to-right shunts:
    - Large ventricular septal defects
    - Large patent ductus arteriosus
    - Aortopulmonary window
  - Severe left ventricular inflow obstructions (alone or in combination with other malformations:
    - Congenital pulmonary vein stenosis, Cor triatriatum, supramitral ring, mitral atresia, and congenital mitral stenosis
  - Severe left ventricular outflow obstruction:
    - Severe aortic stenosis in infancy
    - Severe coarctation in infancy
  - Anomalous origin of the left coronary artery from the pulmonary artery
  - Defects associated with severely reduced pulmonary blood flow**:
    - "Severe" tetralogy of Fallot, single ventricle with severe pulmonary stenosis (PS), double-outlet right ventricle with severe PS, corrected transposition with VSD and severe PS, tricuspid atresia with severe PS, transposition with ventricular septal defect and severe PS, pulmonary atresia in association with any of the above.
- Congenital heart defects that allow survival to adulthood:
  - Left-sided obstructive lesions:
    - Bicuspid aortic valve
    - Subaortic membrane
    - Coarctation
    - Supravalvar aortic stenosis
  - Right-sided obstructive lesions:
    - Valvar pulmonic stenosis
    - Double chamber right ventricle (infundibular stenosis)
  - Left-to-right shunts:
    - Atrial septal defects and other pretricuspid shunts
    - Patent ductus arteriosus**
    - Ventricular septal defects**
  - Conditions associated with reduced pulmonary blood flow:
    - "Less severe" forms of tetralogy of Fallot#, complex defects with "balanced circulation" (conditions in which the pulmonic stenosis is just severe enough to protect the lungs from excessive pulmonary blood flow: examples include, single ventricle, double-outlet right ventricle, tricuspid atresia, and corrected transposition)
    - Tetralogy of Fallot with pulmonary atresia and major aortopulmonary collaterals
    - Ebstein anomaly of the tricuspid valve
  - Eisenmenger syndrome (severe pulmonary artery hypertension with shunt reversal):
    - Large ventricular septal defects, patent ductus arteriosus, atrial septal defects, and other conditions associated with increased pulmonary blood flow
  - Cyanotic conditions with normal pulmonary blood flow:
    - Pulmonary arteriovenous malformation
    - Left superior vena cava to an unroofed coronary sinus
  - Cyanotic heart disease with increased pulmonary blood flow:
    - Unobstructed total anomalous pulmonary venous drainage
  - Others:
    - Ruptured or unruptured aneurysm of sinus of Valsalva
    - Coronary-cameral fistula
    - Uncomplicated corrected transposition of the great arteries

**Small ventricular septal defects and patent ductus arteriosus allow survival to adulthood. Patients with large ventricular septal defects and patent ductus arteriosus often develop irreversible changes in the lung vasculature (Eisenmenger syndrome) when they survive to adulthood.

#Patients with tetralogy of Fallot who survive to adulthood typically have mild resting cyanosis during infancy. Cyanosis increases with age and may eventually become severe.

assessment and echocardiography allows precise diagnosis and planning of the exact intervention.

Timely diagnosis of CHD in the neonates or infants and prompt treatment translate into saving a number of lives. Often these babies require just a single intervention and can expect to lead near normal lives. The focus worldwide has therefore shifted to early diagnosis. There is a global emphasis on sensitizing pediatricians toward newborn screening and developing centers with capability for neonatal and infant heart surgery.[5]

The relatively "milder" forms of CHDs are naturally selected to survive beyond infancy. Some of these defects are significant and merit surgery or catheter intervention later in life. Many other can be followed up at specific intervals to monitor for adverse consequences.

An accurate history together with a systematic and meticulous physical examination allows identification of the physiology of the majority of CHDs shown in **Figure 2**. The chest X-ray and ECG allow further refinement of this diagnosis. With the wide availability of echocardiography, there is a tendency to bypass the basic bedside evaluation. However, there is still considerable value to history, physical examination, ECG, and chest X-ray. A number of problems result when echocardiography is divorced from clinical context. For example, a small insignificant ASD or patent foramen ovale in an asymptomatic neonate becomes a source of anxiety to young parents who then obtain repeated echocardiograms. A large patent arterial duct with laminar flows can be missed if not carefully looked for in an infant in whom there is clinical evidence of pulmonary hypertension. The foundations of history and physical examination are given in Chapter 5. ECG and chest X-ray are discussed in Chapters 7 and 8, respectively.

NATURAL HISTORY OF CONGENITAL HEART DISEASE

Natural history covers a whole spectrum from benign conditions with near normal life expectancy to critical CHD that are mostly fatal in infancy (**Fig. 3**). Indeed variations in the natural history allow us a convenient way to classify CHD (*see* **Box 1**). This classification is useful in population based surveys of CHD. Sinister defects that present early in neonatal period and are generally fatal without prompt treatment are classified as critical.[6] Defects that allow survival beyond the first month of life but need attention in infancy are classified as "major." A number of CHDs present late or allow survival to adulthood. These are typically identified during school health screening programs. Some of these require intervention later in life. Finally, there are number of patients with "minor" lesions that do not generally impact longevity.

It is very important to have a good knowledge of natural history of individual CHDs in order to take the right management decisions. Surgical or catheter interventions should only be done if expected outcome after the procedure is superior to the predicted natural history. While it is clear that timely intervention has the ability to dramatically alter the natural history for critical CHD like transposition and total anomalous pulmonary venous return, the utility of intervening is a lot more controversial in conditions such as a small ventricular septal defect.

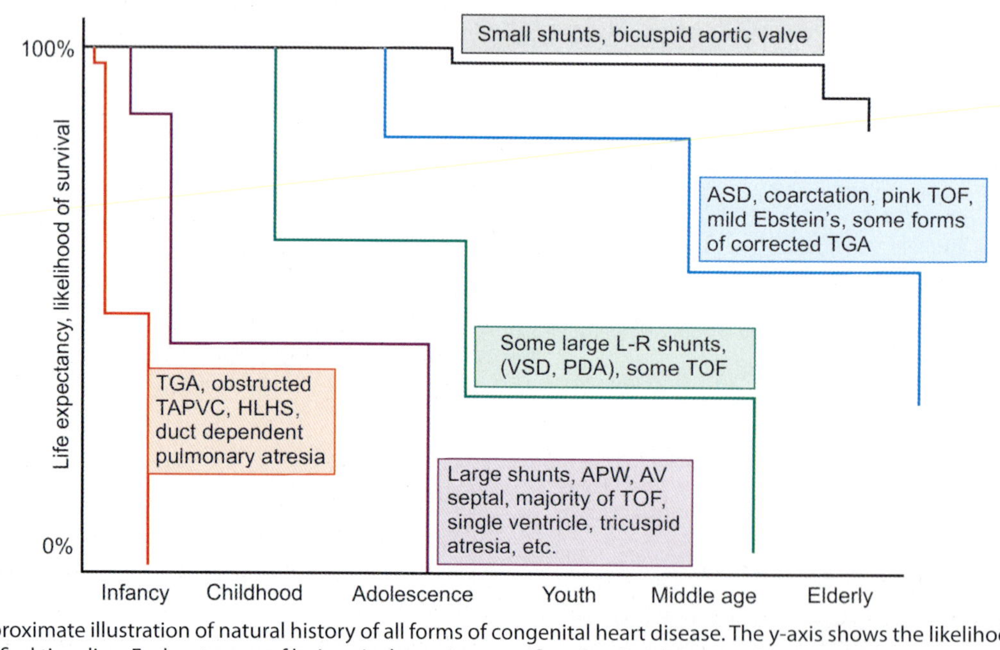

Fig. 3: This is an approximate illustration of natural history of all forms of congenital heart disease. The y-axis shows the likelihood of survival and the x-axis shows a simplified time line. Each category of lesions is shown in a specific color. Conditions such as bicuspid aortic valve and small defects can expect to have a near normal survival. On the other hand, very few babies with critical CHD can expect to survive beyond the first year of life.
(ASD: atrial septal defect; APW: aortopulmonary window; AV: atrioventricular; HLHS: hypoplastic left heart syndrome; PDA: patent ductus arteriosus, TAPVC: total anomalous pulmonary venous communication; TOF: tetralogy of Fallot; TGA: transposition of the great arteries; VSD: ventricular septal defect)

Natural history data is generated by long-term follow-up studies.[7] It is no longer possible to obtain this information on the most serious forms of CHD because it is unethical to follow them without intervention. However, landmark publications that examined the natural history of CHD at birth through meticulous follow-up have provided us with valuable data that informs our clinical decisions today. It is important to be conscious of the survivorship bias in CHD that results from encounters with exceptional survivors. All conditions will have examples of patients who live well beyond the predicted natural history and keep visiting healthcare facilities to create an erroneous impression (bias) of a good survival. For example, if we do encounter an occasional older child with total anomalous pulmonary venous communication in our clinic who seems to be doing rather well, it would be incorrect to assume that this disease has a good outlook when, in reality, nearly 90% babies with total anomalous pulmonary venous connection (TAPVC) do not survive beyond infancy.

Another important consideration in the natural history of CHD is the spontaneous closure of atrial and ventricular septal defects. In general, small defects that are seen at a young age have the highest likelihood of spontaneous closure. Additionally, the exact anatomy matters. Fossa ovalis ASDs are more likely to close when compared to primum or sinus venous ASDs and muscular and membranous VSDs are more likely to close when compared to inlet VSDs. Outlet VSDs are likely to close through prolapse of the right coronary cusp of the aortic valve with the potential for aortic regurgitation.

Finally, it is important to be aware of specific events that complicate the course of common CHDs during the lifetime of a patient. Bacterial endocarditis (*see* Chapter 41) is a possibility in many lesions and the most common source is from the oral cavity underscoring the need for attention to oral-dental hygiene throughout life. A host of complications result from chronic hypoxia that includes erythrocytosis and its effects, brain abscess, and cerebrovascular events. Pulmonary hypertension (*see* Chapter 18) accompanies a number of defects is a major determinant of outcome.

COMPLICATIONS AND COMORBIDITIES

A number of complications can potentially develop as a result of having a CHD (**Table 1**). These complications affect a variety of other organ systems and this can have a profound effect on overall health and longevity as well as quality of life.

Infections Associated with Congenital Heart Disease

Respiratory Infections

Lower respiratory infections are widely recognized as the number one cause of mortality children after the first month of life in most low- and middle-income countries.[8] Infants with large left-to-right shunts are at the risk of frequent respiratory infections that are often severe.[3,9] CHD is typically detected first at the time of a major respiratory infection. These are challenging and difficult. Specific strategies are discussed at the end of Chapter 22.

Endocarditis

See Chapter 41

Brain Abscess

Brain abscess is a significant cause of morbidity in patients with uncorrected or partially palliated congenital cyanotic heart disease (CCHD).[10] The incidence of brain abscess in the population with CHD varies from 5 to 18.7%. Mortality as a result of brain abscess was previously high (30% and 45% in some series), but has decreased dramatically over the last few decades. However, this is still a cause of significant morbidity. Risk factors include, severe hypoxia, increasing age (rare before the age of 2 years) and, severe erythrocytosis.

Pulmonary Vascular Obstructive Disease and Eisenmenger Syndrome

Delays in corrective treatment because of limitations in access result in a high prevalence of PVOD in CHDs that are associated with increased pulmonary blood flow and infants with large post-tricuspid shunts are especially vulnerable.[1] These delays are a result of economic challenges and limited awareness among caregivers on the need for timely correction. A clinical spectrum results from varying degrees elevation in PVR. At one end of this spectrum are children remain operable with mild degree if increase in PVR. At the other extreme are CHD patients with marked elevation in PVR and irreversible changes and right-to-left shunts (Eisenmenger syndrome). Within spectrum are also patients who are classified as "borderline" where it is often not easy to be sure about operability.[11] The available guidelines are largely based on expert consensus that is not yet substantiated by evidence from appropriately designed prospective studies.[12] There are no clearly defined thresholds for PVR, ratios of pulmonary and systemic vascular resistance, and response to selective pulmonary vasodilators that consistently separate the "operable" from "inoperable." This is because there are inherent limitations in accuracy of data obtained through cardiac catheterization. A comprehensive holistic approach that combines clinical examination, chest X-ray, ECG, echocardiography, and invasive data is the best way to decide on regarding operability in this challenging group of patients.[11]

Children with cyanotic heart disease and increased pulmonary blood flow, such as single ventricle without pulmonic stenosis truncus arteriosus, transposition with a large patent arterial duct or VSD, have a rapid onset of

TABLE 1: Common complications of congenital heart disease.

Lesion category	*Common complications*
• Duct-dependent systemic blood flow in the newborn: – Hypoplastic left heart syndrome – Critical coarctation – Interrupted aortic arch – Critical aortic stenosis	Systemic hypoperfusion with closure of the duct with resultant impairment of liver, kidney, and gut perfusion. Adverse neurologic and neurodevelopmental consequences result from cerebral hypoperfusion. Death is inevitable without specific interventions
• Duct-dependent pulmonary blood flow in the newborn: – Pulmonary atresia intact ventricular septum – Pulmonary atresia with other CHD conditions – Critical pulmonary stenosis – Severe Ebstein anomaly	Hypoxia occurs with closure of the ductus. This can result in serious neurologic and neurodevelopmental consequences if persistent and fatal if untreated
• Conditions associated with increased pulmonary blood flow: – Left-to-right shunts – Admixture lesions with increased pulmonary blood flow [transposition with ventricular septal defect (VSD), persistent truncus arteriosus, double-outlet right ventricle, tricuspid atresia with unrestricted pulmonary blood flow, single ventricle, etc.]	• Early: – Heart failure – Vulnerability to lower respiratory infections that are frequent prolonged and difficult to treat – Growth retardation • Late: – Pulmonary vascular obstructive disease and Eisenmenger syndrome – Development of valve dysfunction – Aortic regurgitation in VSD – Mitral regurgitation in atrial septal defect – Ventricular dysfunction from prolonged volume overload
• Conditions with reduced pulmonary blood flow and right to left shunting in the heart tetralogy of Fallot (TOF) • Other conditions with TOF (VSD with pulmonic stenosis) physiology	• Cyanotic spells • Ischemic Stroke • Brain abscess • Seizure disorders • A variety of adverse long-term neurodevelopmental consequences – Cognitive impairment – Lower intelligence quotient (IQ) – Learning disturbance • Consequences of erythrocytosis
• Obstructive lesions • Aortic and pulmonary valve stenosis • Subaortic obstruction • Supravalvar aortic stenosis • Isolated infundibular stenosis • Coarctation • Peripheral pulmonic stenosis	• Heart failure • Ventricular dysfunction • Sudden death • Dysrhythmias
Congenital valve regurgitation	• Heart failure • Ventricular dysfunction • Dysrhythmia

increase in PVR. They are often inoperable at an early age, sometimes during infancy itself.

Growth and Nutrition

Poor growth with underweight for age, decreased length/height for age, and underweight-for-height are all relatively common in children with CHD.[13] The underlying causes of this failure to thrive may be multifactorial, including innate growth potential, severity of cardiac disease, increased energy requirements, decreased nutritional intake, malabsorption, and poor utilization of absorbed nutrition.[14] These factors are particularly common and severe in low- and middle-income countries. Although nutrition should be carefully assessed in all patients, failure of growth is not a contraindication to surgical repair, and patients should receive surgical repair where indicated as soon as possible.[3,15] Close attention should be paid to nutritional support—primarily enteral feeding, with particular use of breast milk in infancy—in the perioperative period and in the pediatric intensive care unit (PICU). This nutritional support requires specific attention and allocation of resources, including appropriately skilled personnel. Thereafter, it is essential to monitor growth and development and to identify causes for failure to catch-up or grow appropriately.

Neurological and Neurodevelopmental Consequences of Congenital Heart Disease

Overt neurological problems that include occurrence of strokes and development of a substrate for long-standing seizures are particularly in patients with cyanotic congenital heart defects (*see* Chapter 51). However, covert neurological problems have become a source of major concern.

Neurodevelopmental disabilities are among the most common, and arguably the most damaging, sequelae of complicated childhood diseases including CHDs.[16] Previous studies have reported that children with CHD who under_ went corrective/palliative cardiac surgery in infancy have more problems related to reasoning, learning, executive function, inattention and impulsive behavior, language skills, and social skills when compared with their counterparts without CHD.[16-19] These studies also suggest that there is a distinctive pattern of neurodevelopmental delay in areas of intelligence, academic achievement, language, visual disturbance, attention disorders, fine motor skills, and psychosocial maladjustment. A prospective single-center study from India identified neurodevelopmental delay in 15% of infants with no prior identified neurological anomalies undergoing corrective heart surgery on 1-year follow-up.[20]

As these children who had cardiac surgery during infancy reach adulthood, the persistent neurodevelopmental disabilities can impair their overall educational achievements, scope of employability, insurability, and quality of life.[16]

The etiology of neurodevelopmental delay in children with CHD is multifactorial. A recent review has identified categories of pediatric patients with CHD at high risk for developmental disorders or disabilities.[21] The same is presented in **Table 2**.

Many factors are innate and nonmodifiable including presence of structural anomalies of the brain and associated genetic syndromes. Other factors pertinent to low-middle-income countries (LMICs) include late presentation due to delay in diagnosis, timely referral and lack of access to tertiary pediatric care, suboptimal preoperative clinical status, malnutrition, and infective complications.[3]

Prolonged hemodynamic insult due to long-standing cyanosis or heart failure can further compromise the neurological status. In addition, the perioperative period and strategies adopted for neuroprotection during cardiac surgery also can play a role. It is possible that the prevalence and severity of neurodevelopmental sequelae in children after CHD surgery are likely to be more in the context of lower middle income countries (LMICs) in view of the above factors.

Quality of Life and Psychosocial Consequences in Congenital Heart Disease

Systematic studies on the health-related quality of life (HRQOL) in all age groups of children with CHD have shown a substantial reduction across most domains.[22,23] The clinical severity of CHD appears to have minimal impact on overall HRQOL. A number of psychosocial challenges have been identified in patients with CHD and these come in the way of integration within the society, employability, and overall self-esteem.

TABLE 2: Categories of pediatric CHD patients at high risk for developmental disorders or disabilities*.

1.	Neonates or infants requiring open heart surgery (cyanotic and acyanotic types), for example, HLHS, IAA, PA/IVS, TA, TAPVC, TGA, TOF, tricuspid atresia
2.	Children with other cyanotic heart lesions not requiring open heart surgery during the neonatal or infant period, for example, TOF with PA and MAPCA(s), TOF with shunt without use of CPB, and Ebstein anomaly
3.	Any combination of CHD and the following comorbidities:
	3.1 Prematurity (37 weeks)
	3.2 Developmental delay recognized in infancy
	3.3 Suspected genetic abnormality or syndrome associated with developmental delay
	3.4 History of mechanical support (ECMO or VAD use)
	3.5 Heart transplantation
	3.6 Cardiopulmonary resuscitation at any point
	3.7 Prolonged hospitalization (postoperative LOS 2-week in the hospital)
	3.8 Perioperative seizures related to CHD surgery
	3.9 Significant abnormalities on neuroimaging or microcephaly*
4.	Other conditions determined at the discretion of the healthcare providers

(CHD: congenital heart disease; CPB: cardiopulmonary bypass; ECMO: extracorporeal membrane oxygenation; HLHS: hypoplastic left heart syndrome; IAA: interrupted aortic arch; LOS: length of stay; MAPCA: major aortopulmonary collateral artery; PA/IVS: pulmonary atresia with intact ventricular septum; TA: tricuspid atresia; TAPVC: total anomalous pulmonary venous connection; TGA: transposition of the great arteries; TOF: tetralogy of Fallot; VAD: ventricular assist device)

*Adapted from: Marino BS, Lipkin PH, Newburger JW, Peacock G, Gerdes M, Gaynor JW, et al. American Heart Association Congenital Heart Defects Committee, Council on Cardiovascular Disease in the Young, Council on Cardiovascular Nursing, and Stroke Council. Neurodevelopmental outcomes in children with congenital heart disease: evaluation and management: a scientific statement from the American Heart Association. Circulation. 2012;126(9):1143-72.[21]

PRINCIPLES OF MANAGEMENT: TIMING OF INTERVENTION IN CONGENITAL HEART DISEASE

The decision about when to intervene in CHD requires carefully balancing the results of the procedure with the expected natural history of the individual conditions. The extraordinary variety of conditions complicates the decision-making process. Further, during the last 30 years, there have been numerous advances in the field of pediatric cardiology and pediatric cardiac surgery. These advances have enabled improved results from operations and transcatheter interventions and have allowed the procedures to be performed early. In addition, we now have information on the natural history of many congenital heart conditions. An increasing number of studies are being published on the long-term results of operations and interventions for CHD.

Because of the wealth of information available to us, the decision about "when to intervene in CHD" now involves careful consideration of a number of variables that influence

Flowchart 2: The principle behind deciding on when to intervene.

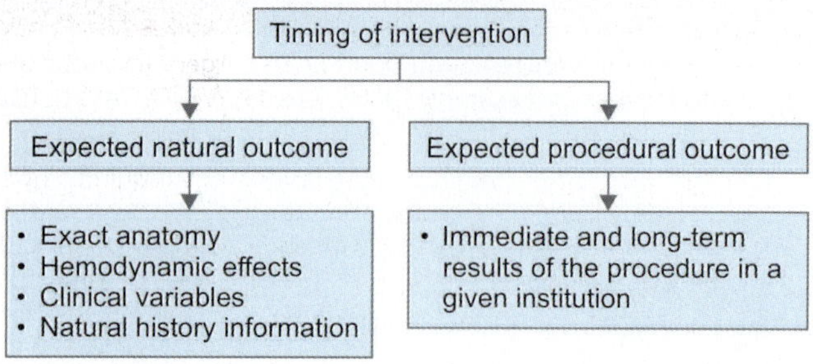

natural history and procedural outcome (**Flowchart 2**). *There are no simple rules for the numerous CHD conditions and the decision-making process has to be individualized for every patient.* At all times, there has to be a careful comparison of immediate and long-term procedural outcome with the natural history.

The enormous variety of CHD conditions encountered complicates attempts at predicting the natural history. It is important to gather complete information for every patient and the following requirements must be met:

- The precise anatomic diagnosis
- Accurate hemodynamic assessment
- Thorough clinical evaluation
- Natural history information.

Without obtaining complete information, it is hazardous to make a statement on the natural history. We have come across numerous examples of patients with Eisenmenger syndrome who were reassured after a clinical evaluation alone in early infancy that their defect would close on its own.

The enormous variety of CHD conditions encountered complicates attempts at predicting the natural history. It is important to gather complete information for every patient and the following requirements must be met:

- The precise anatomic diagnosis
- Accurate hemodynamic assessment
- Thorough clinical evaluation
- Natural history information.

Without obtaining complete information, it is hazardous to make a statement on the natural history. For example, reassuring an infant's family with a large VSD that the defect will close spontaneously without complete evaluation will be a serious error. A number of patients have developed Eisenmenger syndrome as a result of such false reassurances.

The section on individual CHDs outlines the various considerations and principles for each condition. However, the reader is also advised to read the recently published Indian guidelines that specifically look into timing of intervention of individual CHDs.[24]

PREVENTION OF CONGENITAL HEART DISEASE

The definite cause for CHD is not well known and presumed to be multifactorial in etiology in most instances. Detailed epidemiological studies showed that identifiable genetic or environmental cause can be noted in up to 20–30% of CHD. The genetic influences attributed to single gene disorder in 3–5% of cases, gross chromosomal anomaly or aneuploidy in 8–10% cases and copy number variation (CNV) in 3–25% of the cases. The de novo autosomal dominant and recessive cases are found in 8 and 2%, respectively. A possible environmental cause is linked in 2% cases of CHD. Avoidance of possible teratogenic exposure may be an approach to prevent CHD but its impact is likely to be quite limited. Similarly, avoiding the impact of specific genetic influences may also have a limited role overall.[25]While the risk of CHD in offspring or siblings of patients with CHD have been defined to some extent (*see* **Box 1**), they are of limited value in counseling because the risks are too low to avoid conception altogether.

Preconceptual and Periconceptual Prevention

Primary prevention is the best form of prevention because there is a prospect of preventing the possible cause of CHD even before the onset of the disease. Two possible causes of CHD such as genetic factors and exposure to teratogen are included in preconceptional prophylaxis.

Consanguinity and Association with Congenital Heart Disease

Consanguinity of marriage is reported to be associated with increased possibility of CHD.[26] Consanguinity is widely prevalent in many societies and declines as education and human development indices improve. However, there is a need to educate the population as a whole on the potential harmful impact of consanguinity on the prevalence of a number of genetic conditions.

Counseling for Specific Conditions

Diagnosis of CHD at any stage comes with great responsibility for the clinician and team. Antenatal diagnosis by fetal anomaly scan and fetal echocardiography requires a detailed counseling session. The parents and family members will be eager to know about the disease and its prognosis along with a management plan if the pregnancy is continued (*see* Chapter 47). A good counseling should include comprehensive communication of risks of recurrence of CHD in the next child (**Table 3**). This is a common source of anxiety in many families (*see* Chapter 16).[27,28] Continued support during pregnancy through regular counseling forms an integral part of management for antenatal diagnosis of CHD.[29]

Identifying Carrier State

Some genetic disorders such as catch-22 and Noonan syndrome are associated with increased risk of CHD. Noonan syndrome is commonly associated with pulmonary

TABLE 3: Risk of recurrence for common isolated congenital heart disease.[28]

Lesion	*Father affected (%)*	*Mother affected (%)*	*One sibling affected (%)*	*Two siblings affected (%)*
ASD	1.5–3.5	4.–6	2.5–3	8
AVSD	1–4.5	11.5–14	3–4	10
VSD	2–3.5	6.–10	3	10
AS	3.–4	8.–18	2	6
PS	2–3.5	4–6.5	2	6
TOF	1.5	2–2.5	2.5–3	8
CoA	2.–3	4–6.5	2	6
HLHS	21	21	2.–9	6
D-TGA	2	2	1.5	5

(AS: aortic stenosis; ASD: atrial septal defect; AVSD: atrioventricular septal defect; CoA: coarctation of the aorta; D-TGA: d-loop transposition of the great arteries; HLHS: hypoplastic left heart syndrome; PS: pulmonary stenosis; TOF: tetralogy of Fallot; VSD: ventricular septal defect).

TABLE 4: Medication in pregnancy and teratogenicity.[34]

Medication in pregnancy	*Possible cardiovascular toxicity*
Paroxetine	ASD, VSD, and ventricular outflow tract obstruction
Bupropion	Left outflow tract obstruction
Valproic acid	ASD, VSD, TOF, PA, HPRH
Lithium	Ebstein anomaly, mitral atresia, and CoA
Ibuprofen	TGV, VSD, and bicuspid aortic valve
Indomethacin	Premature closure of the ductus
Vitamin A	PS and outflow tract abnormalities
Nitrofurantoin	HLHS and ASD
Cephalosporins	ASD

(ASD: atrial septal defect; CoA: coarctation of the aorta; HLHS: hypoplastic left heart syndrome; HPRH: hypoplastic right heart; PA: pulmonary atresia; PS: pulmonary stenosis; TGV: transposition of the great vessels; TOF: tetralogy of Fallot; VSD: ventricular septal defect)

outflow obstruction and hypertrophic cardiomyopathy. Catch 22 syndrome has a range of cardiac anomalies, most common being conotruncal anomaly (*see* Chapter 53). The parents and siblings of these genetic syndromes can be carriers of the gene. Thereby, they are at a high risk of having a syndromic offspring with CHD. It is important to determine the carrier state of these genetic defects so that we can prevent occurrence of these syndromes.

MMR Vaccination

Congenital rubella syndrome is one of the very important causes of CHD caused by infection of pregnant lady in early pregnancy with rubella virus. Immunization of the girls in early age with MMR (measles, mumps, rubella) vaccination and later Rubella booster dose successfully can prevent the occurrence of Rubella infection of mother and can prevent congenital rubella syndrome.[30] Along with folic acid supplementation, MMR vaccination are two practical public health measures that can impact the incidence of CHD in a population.

Folic Acid Supplements

Folic acid deficiency has been linked with the development of CHD, such as malformation of great arteries and septal defects.[31] Folic acid also found to attenuate the toxic effect of arsenic on heart. Though some studies have not found significant association of folic acid deficiency linked with severe heart disease, majority of the literature is in favor of folic acid supplementation being beneficial in the prevention of CHD.[32,33]

Avoiding Specific Drugs and Teratogens

Multiple drugs have been linked with teratogenic effects causing CHD. Avoidance of such drugs found to be useful in the prevention of CHD (**Table 4**). Additionally there are specific environmental exposures that are associated with occurrence of CHD (**Table 5**).

TABLE 5: Toxic exposure in pregnancy.

Exposure in pregnancy	*Possible cardiovascular toxicity*
Diabetes mellitus (hyperglycemia)	TGV, VSD, AVSD, HPLHS, PDA, and CM
Fever (hyperthermia)	PDA, VSD, and pulmonary valve
Phenylketonuria	VSD, PDA, TOF, and single ventricle abnormalities
Organic solvents	Conotruncal defects, TOF, PS, HPLHS, TAPVR, and CoA

(ASD: atrial septal defect; AVSD: atrioventricular septal defect; CoA, coarctation of the aorta; CM: cardiomyopathy; HPLHS: hypoplastic left heart syndrome; HPRH: hypoplastic right heart; PDA: patent ductus arteriosus; PS: pulmonary stenosis; TAPVR: total anomalous pulmonary venous return; TGV: transposition of the great vessels; TOF: tetralogy of Fallot; VSD: ventricular septal defect)

Maternal disease and intake of medications for the same is also one of the reasons for development of CHD. Maternal hypertension and maternal diabetes are the two diseases, which will top the list. Pregnant ladies with hypertension irrespective of drug treatment are at higher risk for CHD? The risk possibility is 80% more than women without hypertension.[35] Similarly, diabetic mothers have 8.8% risk of babies having CHD, most commonly hypertrophic cardiomyopathy. High maternal vitamin E intake is also reportedly associated with risk for CHD in the baby.[36,37]

There are other factors, which are linked with heart disease in the fetus. Some of them are maternal smoking,[37] maternal occupational pesticide, herbicide, and fungicide exposure.[38] The insecticide use is found to be linked with development of septal defect, whereas herbicides and insecticides in combination in hypoplastic left heart syndrome, insecticide, and fungicide add to the risk of TOF.[25,38]

Antenatal Detection of Congenital Heart Disease: Screening and Fetal Echocardiography (*see* Chapter 47)

Screening for CHD can happen in early pregnancy. First trimester fetal scan detection can detect markers linked with suspicion of CHD which can be useful in prevention of CHD. Elevated nuchal translucency or edema more than 6 mm is found to be associated with elevated risk of CHD. When nuchal translucency is combined with abnormal ductus venosus flow, the risk of CHD increases multifold and these two indicators when abnormal warrant detail fetal echocardiography.[39]

Down syndrome is the most common disease which is detected in antenatal scan. It is screened by triple test and presence of other congenital defects such as duodenal atresia.

Down syndrome is associated with 40% possibility of CHD and a detailed fetal echocardiogram can help to detect CHD. Similarly is a suspected case of genetic anomaly in fetus detected by amniocentesis, a follow-up detail echocardiogram will greatly aid in detection of CHD and take appropriate measure.

Congenital heart disease detection is aided by these early scans. If the first trimester indicators are positive, a second trimester screening transabdominal echocardiogram can be done at 12–15 weeks of gestation. Transvaginal echocardiogram can be done even a little earlier by an expert cardiologist. In the second trimester, 16–18 weeks is the ideal time for a detailed cardiac evaluation. This allows a fairly detailed diagnosis and detailed counseling.

The decision to terminate pregnancy based on the results of the fetal echocardiogram should only happen after careful counseling with the family and a thorough discussion with obstetrician (*see* Chapter 47). The legal limit for termination is up to 20 weeks as per existing law in India. In specific cases, this can be extended to 24 weeks of gestation after careful review of expert opinion.

CONCLUSION

This chapter seeks to provide basic information on general aspects of congenital heart disease epidemiology, physiology, natural history, complications, broad principles of management and prevention. The details of specific defects are covered in the next 20 chapters (*see* Chapters 21-40).

REFERENCES

1. Kumar RK, Iyer P, Iyer KS, Hugo-Hamman C. Global burden of pediatric heart disease and pediatric cardiac care in low and middle-income countries. In: Wernovsky G, Anderson RH, Kumar K, Mussato K, Redington A, Tweddel J, Tretter J, (Eds). Anderson's Pediatric Cardiology, 4th edition. Philadelphia: Elsevier; 2019.
2. GBD 2017 Congenital Heart Disease Collaborators; Global, regional, and national burden of congenital heart disease, 1990–2017: a systematic analysis for the Global Burden of Disease Study 2017. Lancet. 2020;4(3):185-200.
3. Reddy SN, Kappanayil M, Balachandran R, Sudhakar A, Sunil GS, Raj BR, et al. Preoperative determinants of outcomes of infant heart surgery in a limited-resource setting. Semin Thorac Cardiovasc Surg. 2015;27(3):331-8.
4. Kumar RK. Congenital heart disease. In: Parthasarathy A, Menon PSN, Nair MKC, (Eds). IAP Textbook of Pediatrics, 7th edition, Section 7. New Delhi: Jaypee Brothers Medical Publishers; 2019. pp. 563-84.
5. Zheleva B, Atwood JB. The invisible child: childhood heart disease in global health. Lancet. 2017;389(10064):16-8.
6. Saxena A, Mehta A, Sharma M, Salhan S, Kalaivani M, Ramakrishnan S, et al. Birth prevalence of congenital heart disease: a cross-sectional observational study from North India. Ann Pediatr Cardiol. 2016;9(3):205-9.
7. Nadas AS. Report from the Joint Study on the Natural History of Congenital Heart Defects. I. General introduction. Circulation. 1977;56(1 Suppl):I3-4.
8. Liu L, Oza S, Hogan D, Perin J, Rudan I, Lawn JE, et al. Global, regional, and national causes of child mortality in 2000-13, with projections to inform post-2015 priorities: an updated systematic analysis. Lancet. 2015;385(9966):430-40.
9. Bhatt M, Roth S, Kumar RK, Gauvreau K, Chengode S, Nair SG, et al. Management of infants with large, unrepaired left-to-right shunts and respiratory infection requiring mechanical ventilation. J Thorac Cardiovasc Surg. 2004;127(5):1466-73.
10. Udayakumaran S, Onyia CU, Krishnakumar R. Forgotten? Not yet—Cardiogenic brain abscess in children—a case series based review. World Neurosurg. 2017;107:124-9.
11. Viswanathan S, Kumar RK. Assessment of operability in congenital cardiac shunts with increased pulmonary vascular resistance. Cathet Cardiovasc Interv. 2008;71(5):665-70.
12. Lopes AA, Barst RJ, Haworth SG, Rabinovitch M, Al Dabbagh M, Del Cerro MJ, et al. Repair of congenital heart disease with associated pulmonary hypertension in children: what are the minimal investigative procedures? Consensus statement from the Congenital Heart Disease and Pediatric Task Forces, Pulmonary Vascular Research Institute (PVRI). Pulm Circ. 2014;4(2):330-41.
13. Vaidyanathan B, Radhakrishnan R, Sarala DA, Sundaram KR, Kumar RK. What determines nutritional recovery in malnourished children after correction of congenital heart defects? Pediatrics. 2009;124(2):e294-9.
14. Argent AC, Balachandran R, Vaidyanathan B, Khan A, Kumar RK. Management of undernutrition and failure to thrive in children with congenital heart disease in low and middle income countries. 2017;27(S6):S22-S30.
15. Vaidyanathan B, Roth SJ, Rao SG, Gauvreau K, Shivaprakasha K, Kumar RK. Outcome of ventricular septal defect repair in a developing country. J Pediatr. 2002;140(6):736-41.
16. Gaynor JW, Stopp C, Wypij D, Andropoulos DB, Atallah J, Atz AM, et al. International Cardiac Collaborative on Neurodevelopment (ICCON) Investigators. Neurodevelopmental outcomes after cardiac surgery in infancy. Pediatrics. 2015;135(5):816-25.
17. Bellinger DC, Wypij D, Rivkin MJ, DeMaso DR, Robertson RL Jr, Dunbar-Masterson C, et al. Adolescents with d-transposition of the great arteries corrected with the arterial switch procedure: neuropsychological assessment and structural brain imaging. Circulation. 2011;124(12):1361-9.
18. Gaynor JW, Nord AS, Wernovsky G, Bernbaum J, Solot CB, Burnham N, et al. Apolipoprotein E genotype modifies the risk of behavior problems after infant cardiac surgery. Pediatrics. 2009;124(1):241-50.
19. Creighton DE, Robertson CM, Sauve RS, Moddemann DM, Alton GY, Nettel-Aguirre A, et al. Western Canadian Complex Pediatric Therapies Follow-up Group. Neurocognitive, functional, and health outcomes at 5 years of age for children after complex cardiac surgery at 6 weeks of age or younger. Pediatrics. 2007;120(3):e478-86.

20. Solomon RS, Sasi T, Sudhakar A, Kumar RK, Vaidyanathan B. Early neurodevelopmental outcomes after corrective cardiac surgery in Indian infants. Indian Paediatrics. 2018;55(5): 400-4.
21. Marino BS, Lipkin PH, Newburger JW, Peacock G, Gerdes M, Gaynor JW, et al. American Heart Association Congenital Heart Defects Committee, Council on Cardiovascular Disease in the Young, Council on Cardiovascular Nursing, and Stroke Council. Neurodevelopmental outcomes in children with congenital heart disease: evaluation and management: a scientific statement from the American Heart Association. Circulation. 2012;126(9): 1143-72.
22. Raj M, Sudhakar A, Roy R, Soman S, Antony L, Champaneri B, et al. Health-related quality of life in infants and toddlers with congenital heart disease: a cross-sectional survey from South India. Arch Dis Child. 2018;103(2):170-5.
23. Raj M, Sudhakar A, Roy R, Champaneri B, Sudevan R, Kabali C, et al. Health-related quality of life (HRQOL) in children and adolescents with congenital heart disease: a cross-sectional survey from South India. BMJ Paediatr Open. 2019;3(1):e000377.
24. Saxena A, Relan J, Agarwal R, Awasthy N, Azad S, Chakrabarty M, et.al. Indian guidelines for indications and timing of intervention for common congenital heart diseases: revised and updated consensus statement of the Working group on management of congenital heart diseases. Ann Pediatr Cardiol. 2019;12(3): 254-86.
25. Pierpont ME, Brueckner M, Chung WK, Garg V, Lacro RV, McGuire AL, et al. Genetic Basis for Congenital Heart Disease: Revisited: A Scientific Statement From the American Heart Association. American Heart Association Council on Cardiovascular Disease in the Young; Council on Cardiovascular and Stroke Nursing; and Council on Genomic and Precision Medicine. Circulation. 2018;138(21):e653-711.
26. Shieh JT, Bittles AH, Hudgins L. Consanguinity and the risk of congenital heart disease. Am J Med Genet A. 2012;158A(5): 1236-41.
27. Kovacevic A, Simmelbauer A, Starystach S, Elsässer M, Müller A, Bär S, et al. Counseling for prenatal congenital heart disease-recommendations based on empirical assessment of counseling success. Front Pediatr. 2020;8:26.
28. Nees SN, Chung WK. Genetic basis of human congenital heart disease. Cold Spring Harb Perspect Biol. 2019.
29. Kovacevic A, Bär S, Starystach S, Simmelbauer A, Elsässer M, Müller A, et al. Objective assessment of counselling for fetal heart defects: An Interdisciplinary Multicenter Study. J Clin Med. 2020;9(2):467.
30. Berger BE, Navar-Boggan AM, Omer SB. Congenital rubella syndrome and autism spectrum disorder prevented by rubella vaccination-United States, 2001-2010. BMC Public Health. 2011;11:340.
31. Mao B, Qiu J, Zhao N, Shao Y, Dai W, He X, et al. Maternal folic acid supplementation and dietary folate intake and congenital heart defects. PLoS One. 2017;12(11):e0187996.
32. Na L, Bai Q, Xiumei Z, Lingzi Z, Deqin H, Xuanxuan Z, et al. Research into the intervention effect of folic acid on arsenic-induced heart abnormalities in fetal rats during the periconception period. BMC Cardiovasc Disord. 2020;20:139.
33. Leirgul E, Gildestad T, Nilsen RM, Fomina T, Brodwall K, Greve G, et al. Periconceptional folic acid supplementation and infant risk of congenital heart defects in Norway 1999-2009. Paediatr Perinat Epidemiol. 2015;29:391-400.
34. Lynch TA, Abel DE. Teratogens and congenital heart disease. J Diagn Med Sonogr. 2015; 31(5):301-5.
35. Tabib A, Shirzad N, Sheikhbahaei S, Mohammadi S, Qorbani M, Haghpanah V, et al. Cardiac malformations in fetuses of gestational and pre gestational diabetic mothers. Iran J Pediatr. 2013;23:664-8.
36. Smedts HP, de Vries JH, Rakhshandehroo M, Wildhagen MF, Verkleij-Hagoort AC, Steegers EA, et al. High maternal vitamin E intake by diet or supplements is associated with congenital heart defects in the offspring. BJOG. 2009;116(3):416-23.
37. Feng Y, Yu D, Yang L, Da M, Wang Z, Lin Y, et al. Maternal lifestyle factors in pregnancy and congenital heart defects in offspring: review of the current evidence. Ital J Pediatr. 2014;40:85.
38. Rocheleau CM, Bertke SJ, Lawson CC, Romitti PA, Sanderson WT, Malik S, et al. Maternal occupational pesticide exposure and risk of congenital heart defects in the National Birth Defects Prevention Study. National Birth Defects Prevention Study. Birth Defects Res A Clin Mol Teratol. 2015;103(10):823-33.
39. Vigneswaran TV, Homfray T, Allan LD, Simpson JM, Zidere V. Persistently elevated nuchal translucency and the fetal heart. J Matern Fetal Neonatal Med. 2018;31(18):2376-80.

21
CHAPTER

Atrial Septal Defect

Sudeep Verma, Vejendla Gouthami

INTRODUCTION

An atrial septal defect (ASD) is referred as a hole of variable size in the atrial septum. Inter-atrial communications other than patent foramen ovale (PFO) accounts for 7–10% of all congenital heart disease (CHD).[1] Two-third of all these are secundum defects and they include fossa ovalis defects or sinus venous defect.[2] ASD occurs as a part of various congenital heart defects in 30–50% of the patients.[1]

EPIDEMIOLOGY AND GENETICS

The female to male ratio is 2:1 in patients with secundum ASD, while gender ratio is equal for sinus venosus and primum ASD.[3,4] ASD is a feature of two conditions that are inherited in autosomal dominant manner. The first one is with bony abnormality with prolonged PR interval known as Holt-Oram syndrome (HOS).[5] The other is syndrome of ASD without bony abnormality but associated with prolonged atrioventricular conduction.[6,7] Mutations in *NKX2.5* gene have been associated with familial ASD and progressive prolongation of atrioventricular conduction.[8] Familial clustering of ASD is well documented without any conduction abnormality. Mutations in TBX5 produce the HOS, associated with malformations of the upper limb and CHDs.[9] Other genetic conditions associated with ASD include the Noonan syndrome. Distinctive *PTPN11 SOS1* is identified to be related to Noonan syndrome.[10] Family relatives positive for gain of *TBX 20* mutations present with large secundum ASD.[11]

NATURAL HISTORY

Approximately one-third of secundum ASDs close spontaneously between 1 and 2 years of age.[12] Foramen ovale usually becomes anatomically closed within 2–3 years after birth but it may remain patent for longer time, and in 15–25% of the individuals, it persists into adult life.[13] ASD can close spontaneously, remain open, or may enlarge with time. Hemodynamically significant defects only occasionally close in the first year of life. It is unlikely for defect >8 mm to get closed spontaneously. For defect under 3 mm in size diagnosed during infancy, 100% spontaneous closure observed by one and half year of age.[1] Between 3 and 8 mm ASD, 80% patients reported to have spontaneous closure in early childhood.[1] Natural history studies suggest that repair of a hemodynamically significant ASD before 25 years of age should allow a normal life expectancy. Pulmonary vascular disease is less common when compared to other left-to-right shunts (such as ventricular septal defects). While it typically occurs usually after 20 years of age in 5–10% of patients with untreated ASD (mostly in females), a series from India documented early onset of pulmonary hypertension and shunt reversal from pulmonary vascular disease (Eisenmenger reaction) in first two decades of life in 10–20% of cases.[14]

EMBRYOLOGY[15]

The sequence of events leads to formation of atrial chamber occurs between 4 and 6 weeks of gestation. The chamber destined to become atria start separating from each other by growth of the septum from the posterosuperior wall of the common atrium. This growth known as septum primum grows toward the atrioventricular junction, where the developing endocardial cushion is separating atria from the ventricles. This septum primum fuses with the endocardial cushion, but before the complete closure of the septum primum, multiple openings appear in the midportion maintaining communication between the two atria. Another septum, known as septum secundum, develops from the posterosuperior portion of the atrial wall, just to the right of the origin of septum primum. This septum also grows inward toward the atrioventricular junction. This septum reached mid way to partly cover the central hole in septum primum, with its semilunar edge forming crista dividens of fetal heart (**Fig. 1**).

The ostium secundum ASD occurs in the region of fossa ovalis, anterior to the rims of crista dividens, as a result of excessive resorption in septum primum or due to inadequate development of septum secundum. Normally after birth, PFO closes due to fusion of its valve with the limbus of the fossa ovalis due to increase in left atrial (LA) pressure.

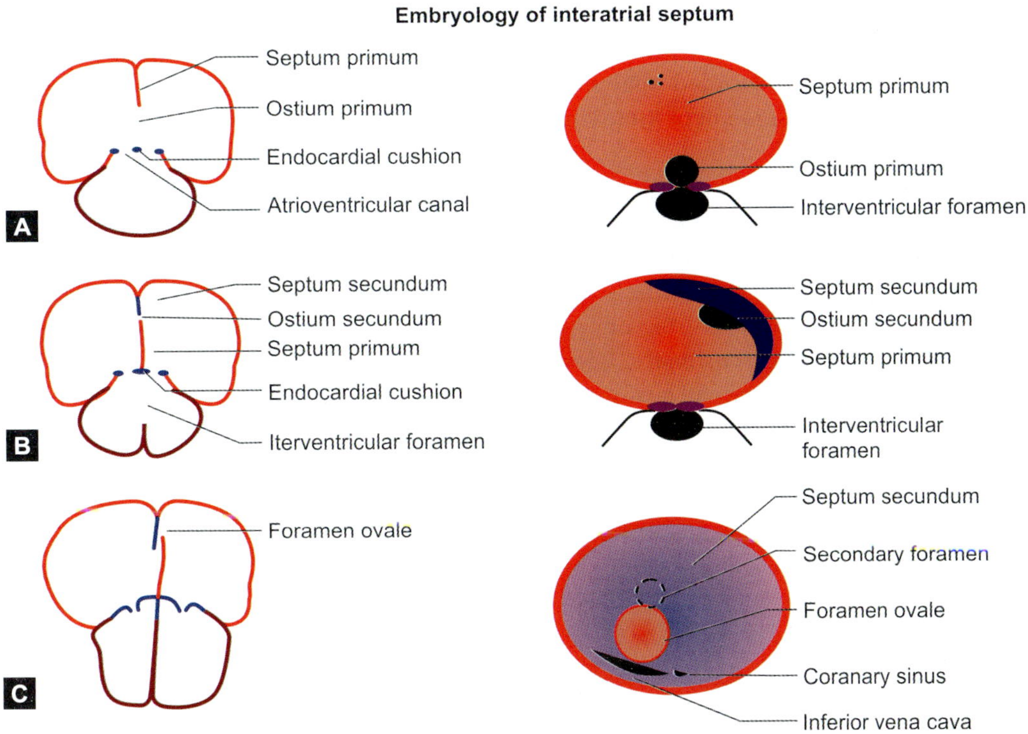

Figs. 1A to C: Embryogenesis of atrial septum.

This process takes a variable amount of time and may not happen altogether in about a third of the population.

Sinus venosus ASD is not related to abnormalities of septum secundum or primum and considered to represent a defect in the wall between the right upper pulmonary vein and posterior aspect of the superior vena cava (SVC).

Ostium primum ASD results from a deficiency in central lower portion of the atrial septum bordering tricuspid and mitral valve rings. This is often accompanied by cleft or separation in the anterior mitral leaflet.

TYPES OF ATRIAL SEPTAL DEFECTS (FIG. 2)

Ostium secundum (fossa ovalis) location is the most common type and accounts for 60–70% of all ASDs. It includes the central portion of the atrial septum at the position of foramen ovale.

Ostium primum defect is at the central lower end of septum bordering tricuspid and mitral valve annulus. As an isolated defect, it contributes to 15% of all ASD.

The sinus venous ASD exists outside the confines of fossa ovalis at the junction of SVC to the right atrium and is invariably associated with anomalous drainage of the right upper pulmonary vein. It accounts for 5–10% of all ASDs. ASDs adjacent to inferior vena cava are sometimes referred to as inferior sinus venous defects. They are often isolated defects with normal pulmonary venous drainage.

The coronary sinus type ASD is rare (<1%) and situated between the left atrium and the coronary sinus. It usually includes the ostium of the coronary sinus in the right atrium.

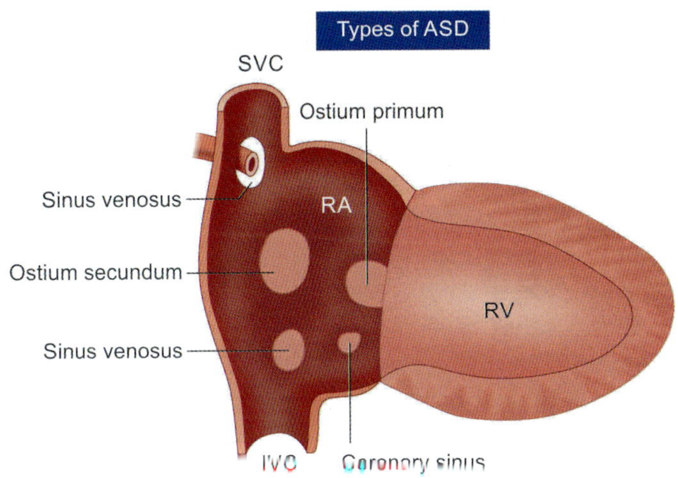

Fig. 2: Sketch showing types of atrial septal defect.
(IVC: inferior vena cava; RA: right atrium; RV: right ventricle; SVC: superior vena cava)

Common atrium refers to the absence of interatrial septal septum. It is associated with the Ellis–van Creveld syndrome. The presence of bilateral superior vena cavae with direct draining of left SVC to the left side of common atrium is a frequent association.

ASSOCIATED DEFECTS

Anomalous drainage of the pulmonary veins is almost invariably associated with the sinus venosus type of ASD.[16] They are uncommon in fossa ovalis type of ASDs. Anomalous systemic venous drainage (persistent left SVC to left atrium) is frequent in common atrium.

Pulmonary stenosis is a common association in patients with ASD who have the Noonan syndrome. The pulmonary valve is typically dysplastic. It must be noted that flow acceleration through a normal valve as a result of increased pulmonary blood flow can result in gradient being recorded across the valve by Doppler.[17]

Mitral valve prolapse (MVP) is identifiable in a significant proportion of the cases of secundum ASD. This is believed to result from the relative smallness of the left ventricle as a result of chronic right ventricle volume overload. Significant mitral regurgitation (MR) requiring surgical correction is less common. However, the mitral valve needs careful evaluation as MR may be underestimated and may become manifest after the ASD is closed.

Tricuspid regurgitation (TR) mainly results from annular dilatation from long-standing atrial shunt causing progressive TR and as a result of associate pulmonary hypertension.

PHYSIOLOGY AND HEMODYNAMICS OF ATRIAL SEPTAL DEFECT[18-20]

The shunt across the ASD depends mainly on the relative compliance (distensibility) of the ventricles. Soon after birth and during early infancy, the right ventricle is relatively stiff or noncompliant. As a result, the ASD does not result in significant left-to-right shunt. As the age advances, the pulmonary vascular resistance decreases and the physiological right ventricular hypertrophy regresses. This results in better right ventricular distensibility or compliance. The shunt across the ASD gradually increases. The right ventricle gradually dilated to accommodate the excessive blood flowing through it. The pulmonary vasculature also dilated to accommodate the flow. Over a period of time, significant shunt develops across the ASD. This results in progressive dilatation of the right atrium, the right ventricle, and the pulmonary arteries. The excessive flow across the tricuspid and pulmonary valve can be heard as diastolic and systolic flow murmurs, respectively.

During adulthood with increasing age, the left ventricle becomes stiffer (less compliant) with high left ventricular (LV) filing pressure. Hypertension or coronary artery disease contributes to this process, this increases the left-to-right shunt across the ASD. Additionally, progressive right atrial enlargement results in the development of atrial arrhythmia, particularly atrial flutter or fibrillation. The incidence of atrial arrhythmia increases with advancing age. It is as high as 13% at 40 years of age and 52% in those who are 60 years of age or older.

Cyanosis is rare in ASD. Its presence should alert the possibility of underlying pulmonary arterial hypertension. Other causes for cyanosis in the presence of ASD include common atrium, left SVC draining directly to left atrium, Eustachian valve, or Thebesian valve diverting blood from inferior vena cava (IVC) directly toward ASD.

Heart failure is rare with ASD. A small portion of infants with large ASD and excessive pulmonary blood flow (<5%) may be symptomatic with failure to thrive. Older children or adults can develop heart failure if they develop a significant mitral valve disease (severe MR or severe rheumatic mitral stenosis—the Lutembacher syndrome).

While isolated ASD does not result in above-mentioned manifestations, it is important to appreciate here that in selected congenital heart defects postnatal survival depends upon sizeable atrial communication in the form of a PFO or a large ASD. These include right heart obstructions such as pulmonary atresia-intact interventricular septum, critical pulmonary stenosis or tricuspid atresia, total anomalous pulmonary venous return, transposition and mitral atresia.

CLINICAL FEATURES

Most of the patients are asymptomatic and incidentally detected during routine evaluation. A small subset of ASD in infancy (<5%) can present with heart failure, poor growth, and recurrent respiratory tract infection. Older children with moderate shunt often are asymptomatic while those with large shunt may occasionally present with complaints of fatigue and dyspnea. Symptoms appear relatively early in common atrium and can be more pronounced. The onset of dyspnea on exertion in a patient with ASD may suggest the possibility of development of pulmonary hypertension.

Examination

The general physical examination may reveal facial dysmorphism and other features of Noonan syndrome. The distinctive appearance of the HOS, i.e., hypoplastic thumb with an accessory phalanx and difficult thumb opposition should be specifically looked for.

The cardiac physical findings depend upon the shunt ratio. Inspection and palpation are seldom remarkable. However, selected patients with large shunts have a hyperdynamic precordium in the left parasternal region. Those with a significant left-to-right shunt (Qp/Qs > 1.8) usually have wide and fixed splitting of second heart sound, a soft pulmonary midsystolic murmur at second and third intercostal space and a soft, mid-diastolic tricuspid valve flow murmur.

Wide split is the result of delay in pulmonary component due to increased ejection time together with increased hangout interval from increased pulmonary vascular capacitance. Wide split in inspiration remained unchanged in expiration. The fixed splitting of the second heart sound is more specific for ASD if it is also appreciated in the sitting position. During inspiration, inflow to the right atrium is increased with concomitant decrease in left-to-right shunt across the ASD; in expiration, the decrease in venous return is compensated by increase in left-to-right shunt across ASD, thus keeping the volume across right heart constant in both phases of respiration.[21,22] The pulmonary component of S2 is relatively loud even in the absence of pulmonary hypertension. However, a palpable P2 is usually indicative of significant PAH with elevation of pulmonary vascular resistance.

The pulmonary ejection midsystolic murmur in ASD begins just after the S1, is of grade 2/6 or 3/6 with maximum intensity in the second or third intercostal space; it is impure and superficial (due to proximity of the pulmonary artery to the chest wall) and peaks in early and midsystole. Any murmur louder than 3/6 in ASD is suggestive of coexisting pulmonary valve stenosis or associated mitral valve disease.

The diastolic flow murmur at tricuspid valve area is often subtle and may not be easily picked by the uninitiated trainee. It is brief, low-pitched, soft, and localized to the left lower parasternal region. When the ASD is relatively small, the diatonic murmur may not be present.

When significant pulmonary hypertension develops, the P2 becomes strikingly loud and often palpable. A parasternal heave is also often felt. The S2 continues to have a fixed split. The diastolic flow murmur disappears and the systolic murmur becomes softer and shorter. A systolic ejection click may result from the dilated pulmonary artery.

Cyanosis occurs in common atrium with increased pulmonary blood flow and in those with pulmonary hypertension. In infants in spite of large defect, typical auscultatory findings may be absent.

X-ray in Atrial Septal Defect[23] (Fig. 3)

The chest X-ray findings in ASD are discussed in the chapter on chest X-ray (*see* Chapter 8). In summary, the chest X-ray often becomes abnormal after infancy and the changes are related to the amount of left-to-right shunt, which is related to size of defect and age. The abnormalities include increased lung vascularity, right atrial enlargement, dilatation of main pulmonary artery, and its branches. In patients with pulmonary vascular obstructive disease, the pulmonary artery and its branches are very much enlarged with persistent cardiomegaly that may indicate the presence of underlying TR.

ECG in Atrial Septal Defect (Figs. 4 to 7)

The ECG has certain characteristic features in ASD and it is of potential diagnostic value. The various types of ASD have distinct features (**Table 1**) that are also of potential diagnostic value.

Atrioventricular conduction defects are relatively common in ASD. As discussed earlier, advanced first-degree heart block occurs commonly with familial ASD and less frequently in nonfamilial ASD.[5-7]

The QRS axis is usually deviated to right side with frontal vector of +90 to 180. In older children and adults, electrical axis may be in the +70 to 90 range particularly with small ASD. Left axis deviation is exceptional and can be seen with primum ASD or with Noonan syndrome.[24] The typical rsR' or rSR' in the right precordial leads in ASD results from volume overloading and dilatation of the right ventricle.[23,25]

Atrial fibrillation and flutter are more common in the fourth decade of life because of long-standing atrial enlargement.

Echocardiography (Figs. 8 to 12)

The preferred investigation of choice for confirming the presence of ASD is echocardiography.

The standard transthoracic echocardiogram is essentially adequate to confirm the diagnosis, identify the exact anatomic type and associated anomalies, define the physiology, and determine the suitability for transcatheter closure in the vast majority of cases. It is important to make the distinction between a PFO and small ASD on one hand and a significant defect that will need closure in the future. With the wide availability of echocardiography, atrial communications are commonly identified in neonates and small infants. Small defects invariably close and do not require repeated echocardiography to check their status.

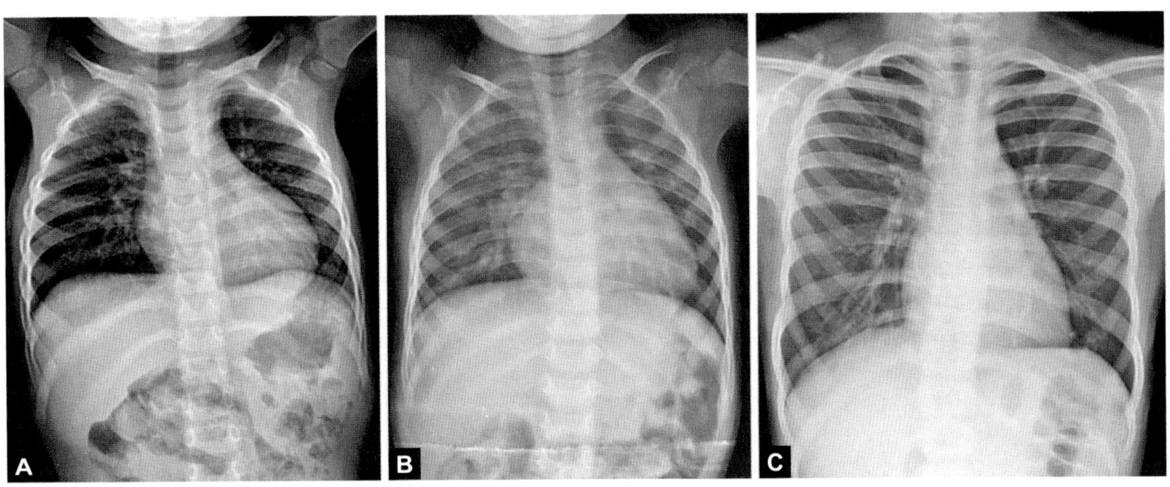

Figs. 3A to C: Chest X-ray in atrial septal defect showing right heart dilatation, prominent PA, and increased vascularity.

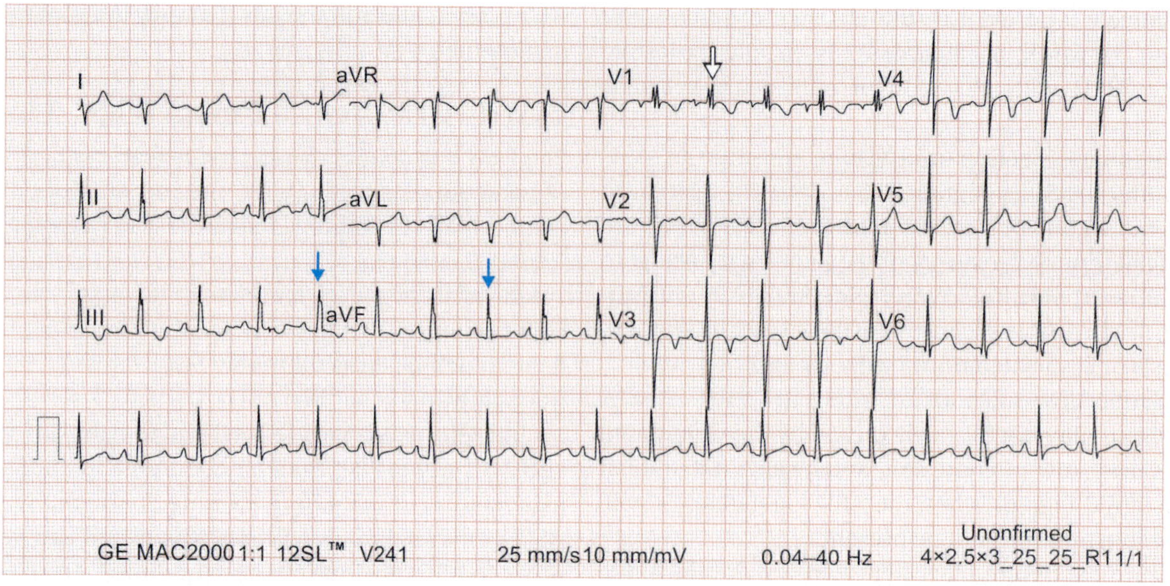

Fig. 4: Typical electrocardiogram (ECG) of ostium secundum atrial septal defect (ASD). Normal P axis, right axis deviation, rsR′ in V1 (white arrow), splintered QRS—crochetage in III, aVF (blue arrows).

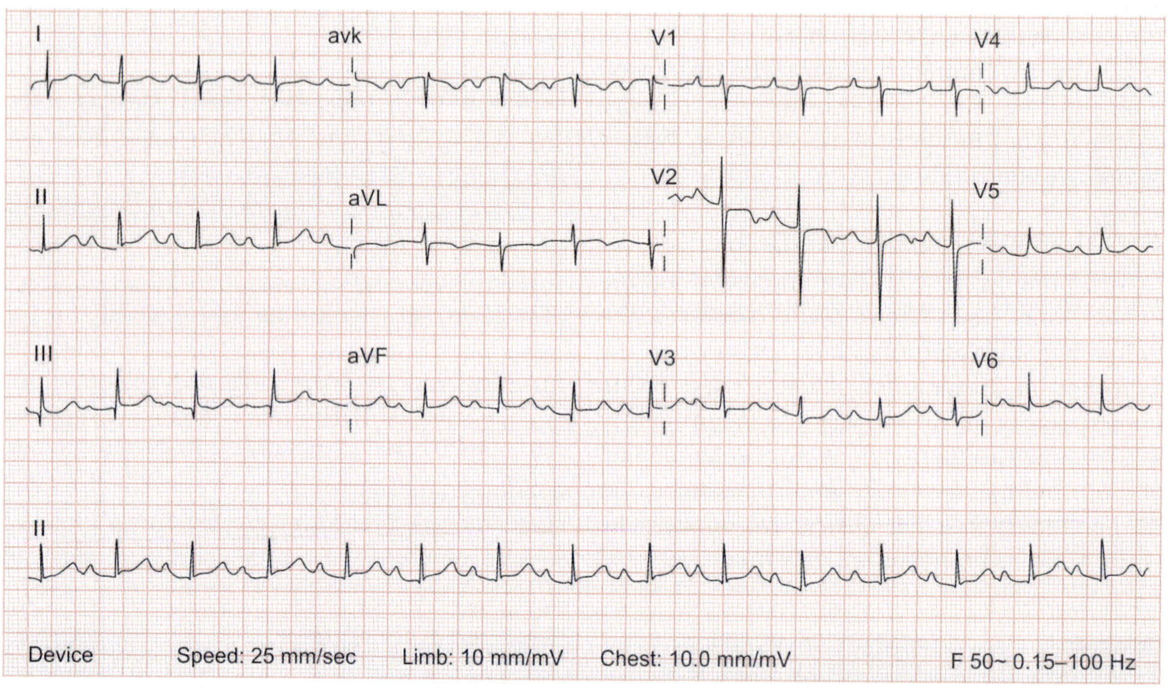

Fig. 5: Electrocardiogram (ECG) of atrial septal defect (ASD) with prolonged PR interval. HR: 100/min, normal P axis, PR interval of 200 ms, other typical signs of ASD not seen

Defects that are associated with volume overload of the right ventricle merit follow-up evaluations. Some of these may also close but it is less common.

Once an ASD is identified in the echocardiogram, systematic efforts are necessary to characterize it in detail. In those patients where a catheter-based closure is contemplated, the defect size should be accurately measured in multiple views and it is vital to ascertain whether the margins are adequate to hold the device. Associated abnormalities are common and therefore a thorough, systematic, and comprehensive study is warranted in all patients. The physiological consequences are nearly always accompanied by clinical manifestations. It is important to corroborate echocardiographic findings with clinical examination, ECG, and chest X-ray.

Transesophageal echocardiography (TEE) is reserved for those patients (often older and relatively obese) where the details of the ASD are not sufficiently delineated by transthoracic echocardiography. Additionally, TEE enables accurate guidance of transcatheter closure.

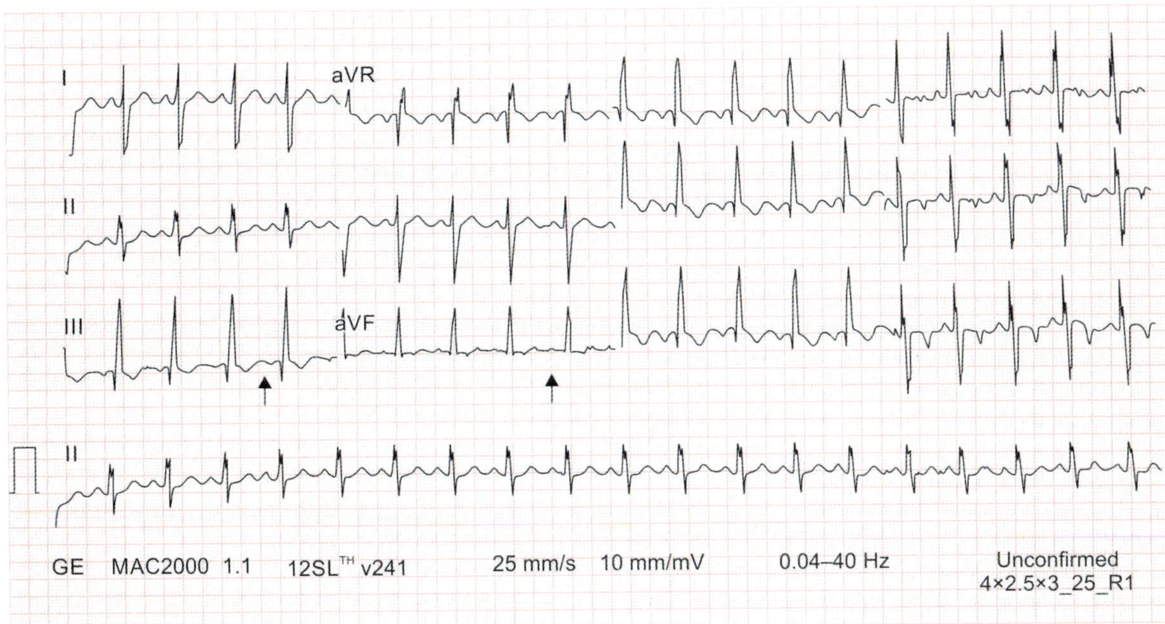

Fig. 6: Electrocardiogram (ECG) of sinus venosus atrial septal defect (ASD). Heart rate (HR): 125/min, P axis—abnormal (negative P in II, aVF)—black arrows, peaked P, QRS axis: right axis deviation, qR pattern in V1, prominent RV forces.

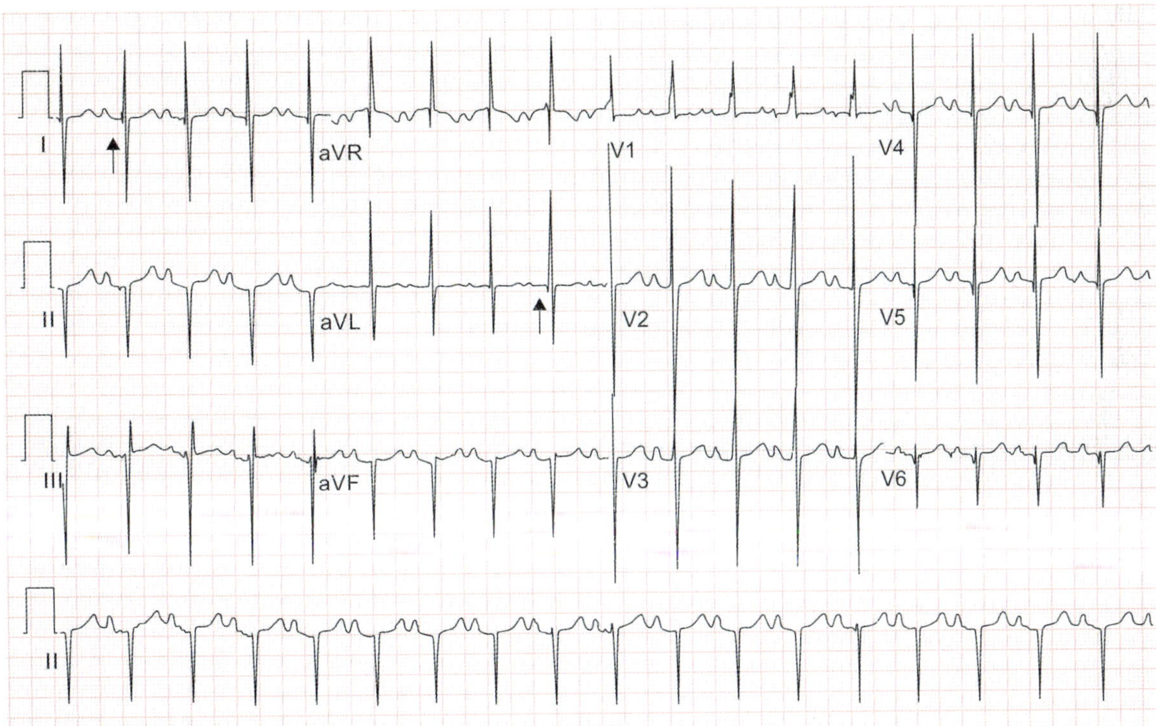

Fig. 7: Electrocardiogram (ECG) of ostium primum atrial septal defect (ASD). Heart rate (HR): 150/min, normal P axis, PR interval—160 ms, QRS axis: left axis deviation-superior axis, rR' in V1, q wave in I and aVL—counterclockwise loop—denoted by arrows.

Cardiac Catheterization

In ASDs, the most diagnostic information can be obtained noninvasively and cardiac catheterization is generally undertaken to perform catheter closure. In the present era, the main indication for diagnostic cardiac catheterization in ASD is to assess operability by measuring pulmonary vascular resistance in patients with associated pulmonary hypertension.

MANAGEMENT[19,20,28] (FIGS. 13A AND B)

A large ASD is one that is clinically manifested or associated with significant right atrial and right ventricular enlargement from volume overload. Often the size of these defects is equal or more than that of the mitral valve annulus which is the other outlet for the left atrium.[20] Symptoms are generally rare and the purpose of closing the ASD is to prevent complications from progressive enlargement of right atrium

TABLE 1: Electrocardiographic changes in atrial septal defects (ASDs).

Type of atrial septal defect (ASD)	*P axis P wave*	*QRS axis*	*Others*
Ostium secundum ASD **(Fig. 4)**	• Normal—left and inferior • Peaked pointed but not tall	• Vertical clockwise depolarization • Right axis deviation is seen in infants and with development of pulmonary hypertension	• rSR is seen in right precordial leads • PR interval prolongation is more commonly seen with familial secundum ASD **(Fig. 5)**
Sinus venosus ASD **(Fig. 6)**	• Abnormal P axis- leftward and superior • More than 30 degree • Shift between sinus rhythm to ectopic atrial rhythm can be seen	Same as secundum ASD	Same as secundum ASD
Ostium primum ASD **(Fig. 7)**[26]	Normal P axis	• Left axis deviation with counterclockwise depolarization • Splintering of S wave in inferior leads	PR interval prolongation seen in 50% cases
Common atrium[27]	• Abnormal—leftward and superior. Inverted P wave in the inferior leads • Occasional shift between sinus rhythm to ectopic atrial rhythm	• Left axis deviation with counterclockwise depolarization and • Splintering of S wave in inferior leads	Precordial leads like in secundum ASD

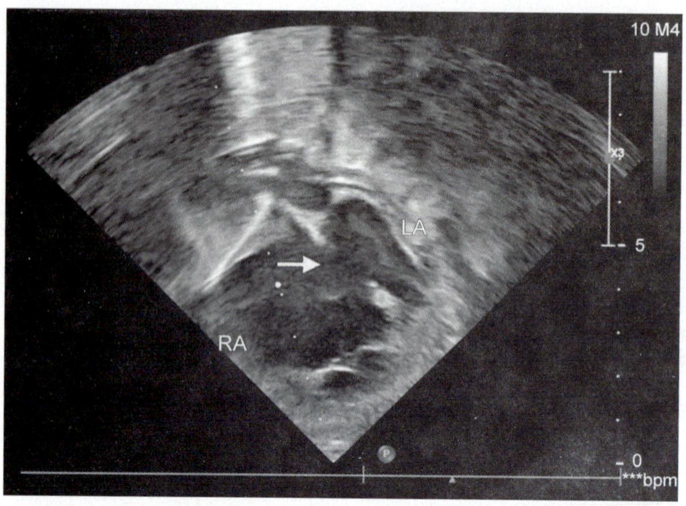

Fig. 8: Echocardiography subcostal view. Defect in atrial septum—typical ostium secundum atrial septal defect (ASD) with good margins (arrow).

and right ventricle (atrial arrhythmias) and perhaps to prevent the development of pulmonary hypertension. The relationship between the ASD and the future development of PAH is not clear since only a small percent develops this problem. The revised and updated consensus statement of the working group on management of CHD has recently described the indications and timing of ASD closure.[28]

SPECIAL CATEGORIES

Atrial Septal Defect in Infancy

A small percentage of ASD in infants (<5%) presents with symptoms usually in the form of failure to thrive and recurrent respiratory infections. Tachypnea is uncommon. The first step in here is to treat the secondary causes such as anemia and respiratory infection and maximize efforts to ensure adequate nutrition and rule out associated genetic conditions. Medical treatment in the form of diuretics may be tried. In truly refractory cases, the ASD may be closed and surgical closure is generally preferred here.

Atrial Septal Defect in Children and Adolescents

Large shunts in the children can be closed either by transcatheter method using occlusive devices or surgically. The surgical approach depends upon the expertise and experience of the surgeon. It can be done using the standard median sternotomy or through cosmetically appealing approaches such as the ministernotomy, limited posterior thoracotomy, or through the right axillary approach. Catheter closure has emerged as an attractive solution in the last two decades and nearly 70–80% of secundum defects in the fossa ovalis region are suited for closure using occlusive devices. The specific criteria include size of the defect and adequacy of the margins. It is important to exclude associated conditions such as MR or anomalous pulmonary venous drainage prior to catheter closure.

Primum ASDs cannot be closed in the catheter laboratory. Selected sinus venosus defects in adults are now being closed in the catheter laboratory by means of covered stents deployed in the SVC but this is largely experimental and presently not recommended for growing children. For coronary sinus defects also currently surgery is the treatment of choice.

POSTSURGICAL/DEVICE CLOSURE CARE (FIGS. 14 AND 15)

Long-term surgical results are excellent. After transcatheter closure of ASD antiplatelet therapy should be continued

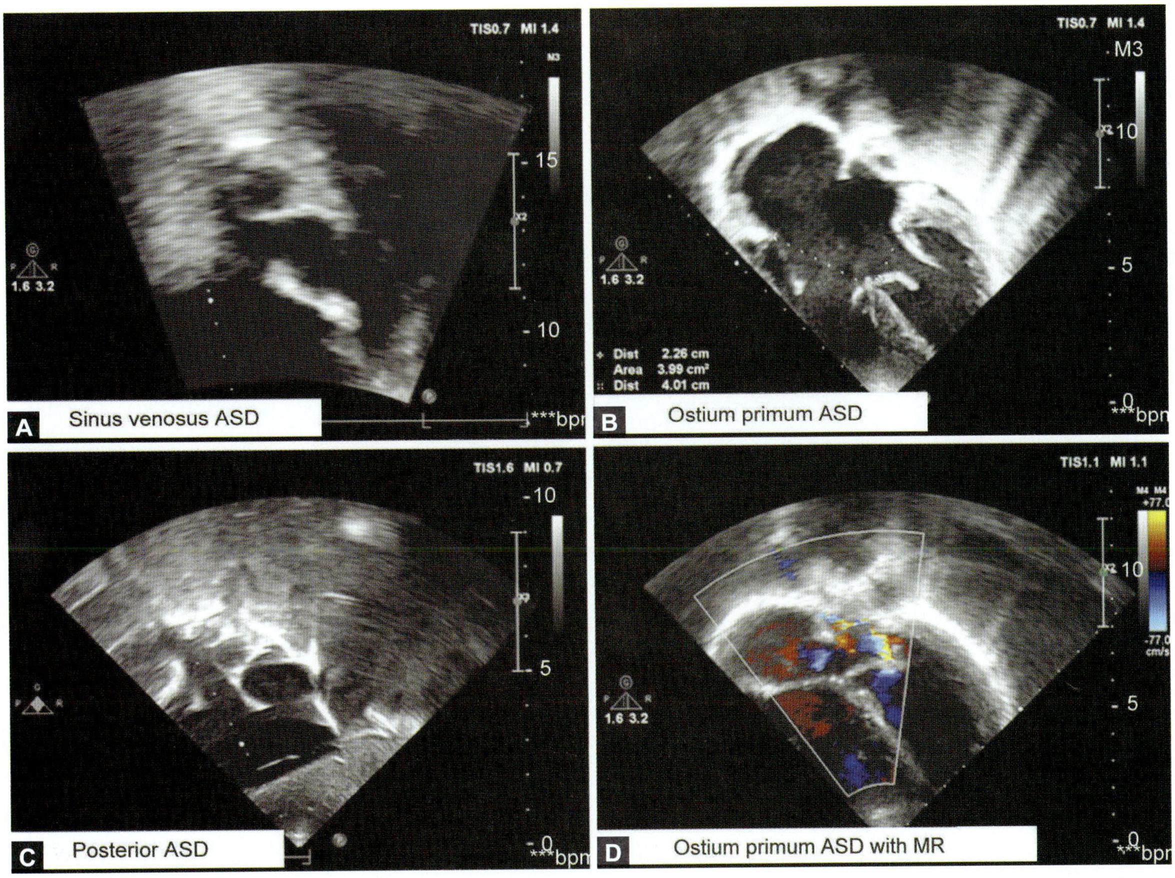

Figs. 9A to D: Types of atrial defects. (A) Sinus venosus atrial septal defect (ASD); (B) Ostium primum ASD; (C) ASD with deficient posterior inferior rim; (D) Ostium primum ASD with color interrogation showing mitral regurgitation (MR).

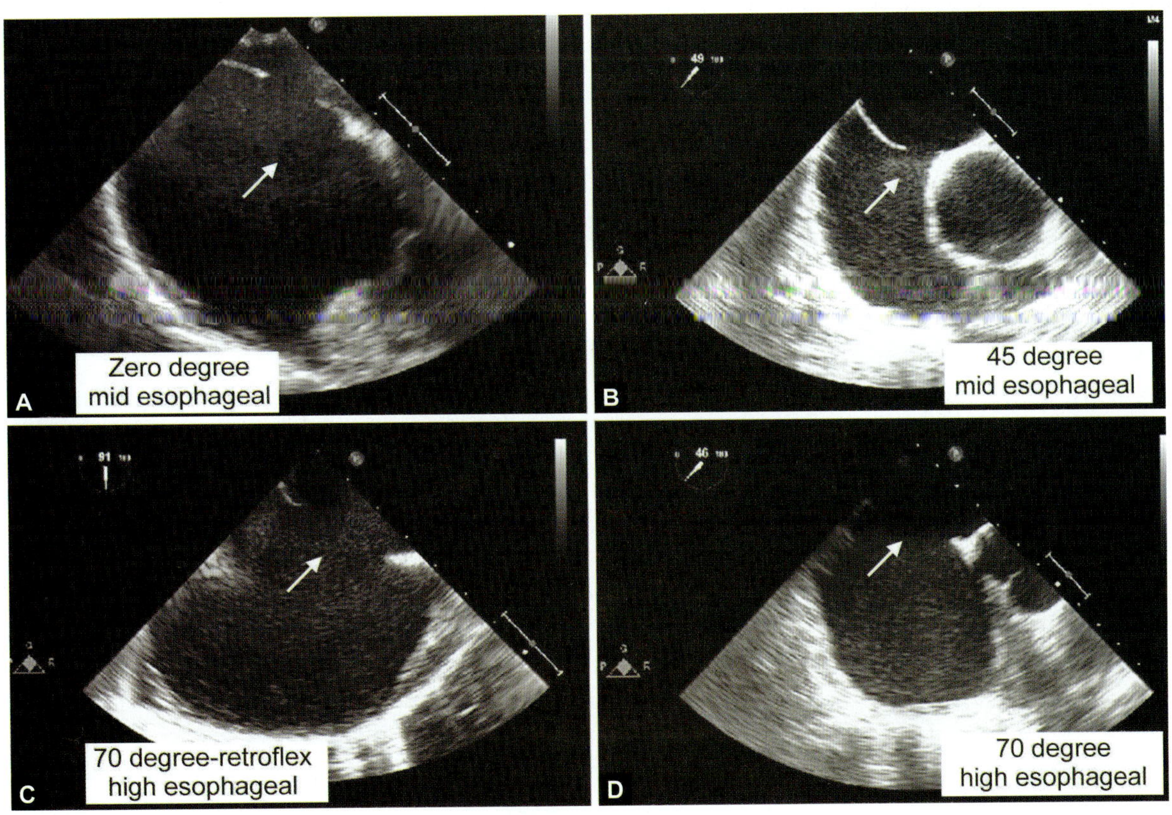

Figs. 10A to D: Transesophageal echocardiogram (TEE) for atrial septal defect (ASD) rims assessment. (A) 0° midesophageal view; (B) 45° midesophageal view; (C) 70° retroflexion showing inferior rim; (D) High esophageal 70° view.

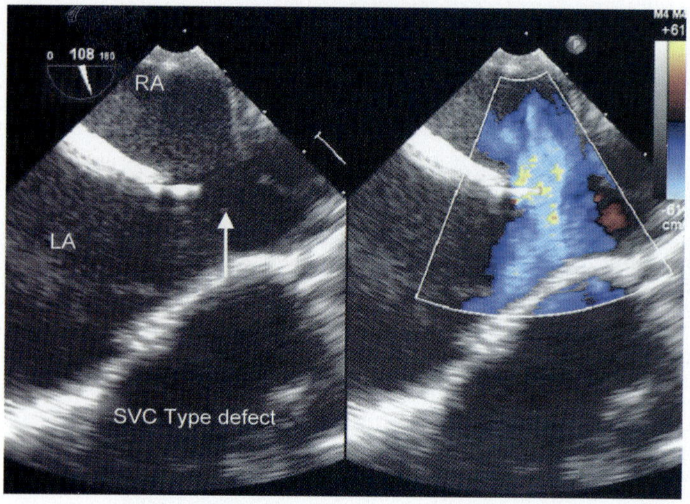

Fig. 11: Transesophageal echocardiogram (TEE) showing sinus venosus atrial septal defect (ASD).

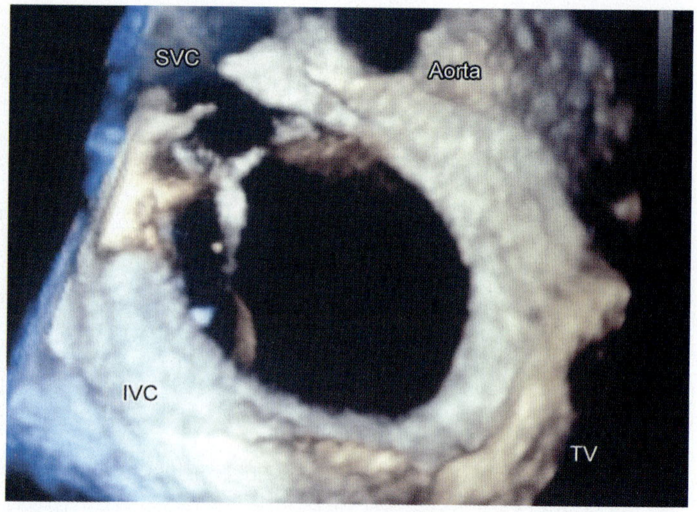

Fig. 12: Three-dimensional transesophageal echocardiogram showing atrial septal defect (ASD) profile with rims.
(IVC: inferior vena cava; SVC: superior vena cava; TV: tricuspid valve)

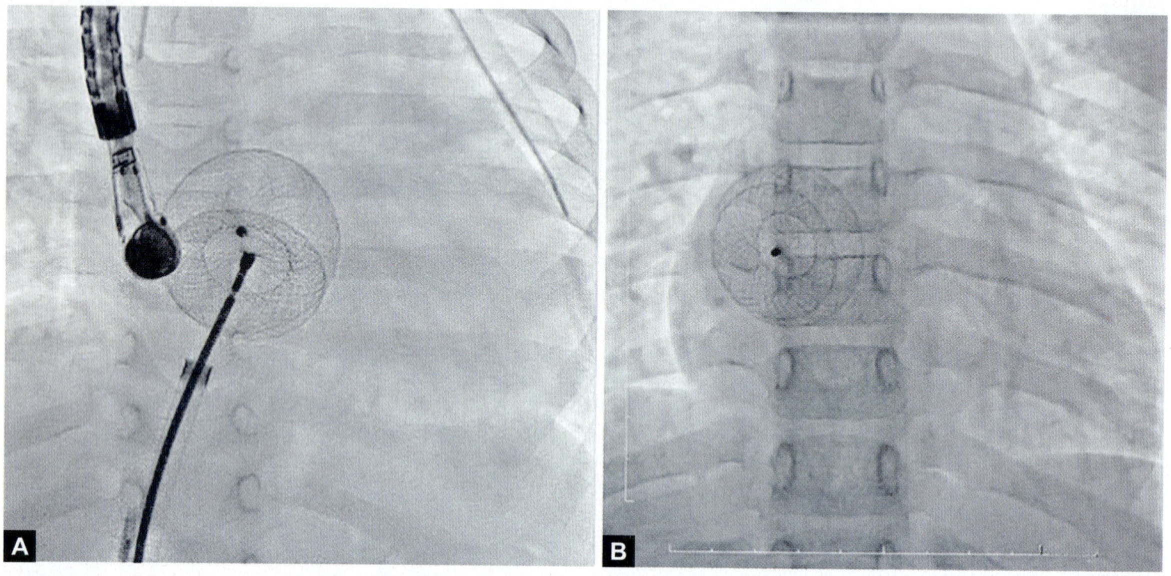

Figs. 13A and B: (A) Transcatheter closure of ASD using atrial septal occluder under transesophageal echocardiogram (TEE) and fluoroscopy guidance; (B) Device profile under fluoroscopy after release.

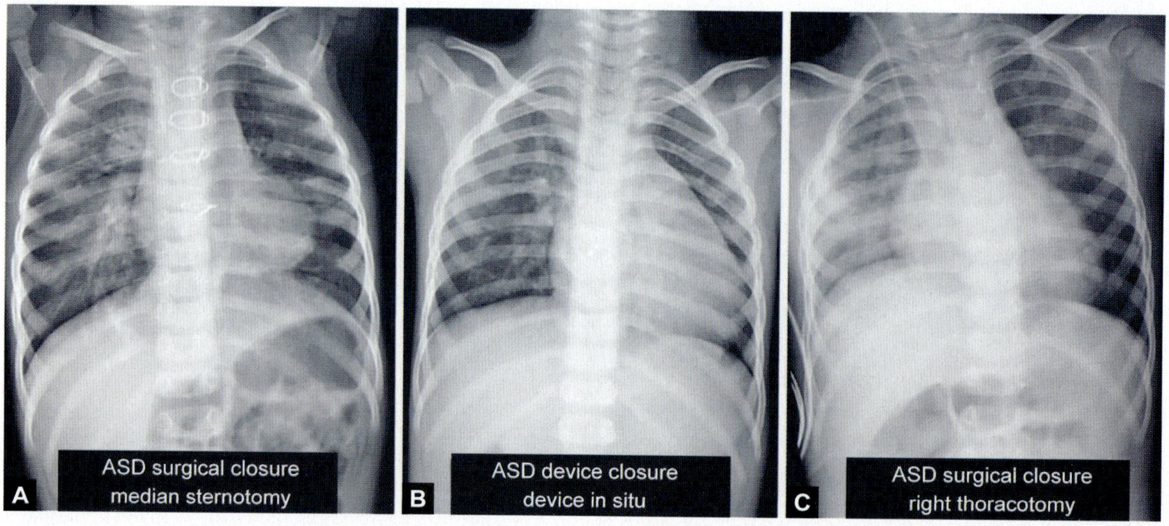

Figs. 14A to C: Chest X-ray after ASD closure. (A) Through median sternotomy—sternal wires seen; (B) Transcatheter device closure—device in situ; (C) Through right thoracotomy—central line from IJV, crowding of right ribs, right lung haziness.

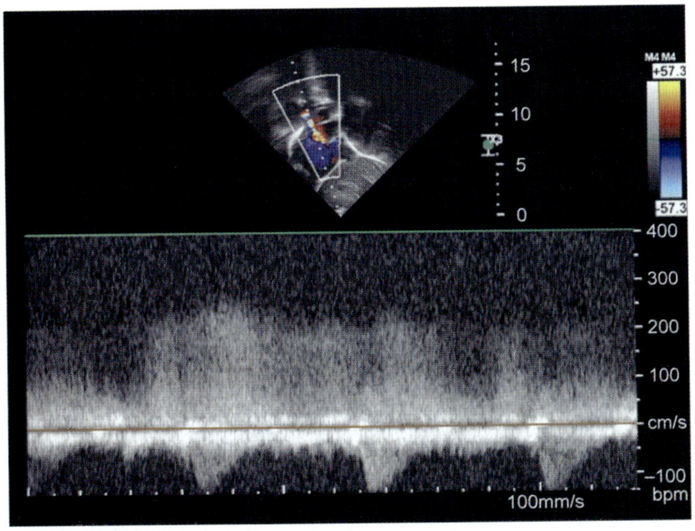

Fig. 15: Doppler across SVC to RA junction in a postoperative case of sinus venosus ASD during follow-up. Showing continuous wave pattern suggestive of obstruction.

for 6 months after device placement while awaiting endothelialization of the device. Complications such as device migration, heart block, device erosion are rare. After surgical closure, early complications include pericardial collections that can occasionally be substantial. Following sinus venosus ASD, SVC obstruction (*see* **Fig. 11**) and sinus node dysfunction may occur, atrial arrhythmias may occasionally occur after surgical or catheter ASD closure, particularly in older patients. Routine follow-up is needed until 1 year for ASD closed with surgery or with transcatheter method and longer follow-up is dictated by the specific condition. Infective endocarditis prophylaxis is generally recommended after device closure of ASD for a period of 6 months.

CONCLUSION

Atrial septal defect is a relatively common congenital defect that typically presents beyond infancy and early childhood. The exact anatomic type of ASD and the associate defects can potentially impact clinical features. The characteristic clinical finding for uncomplicated ASD is a wide and fixed split of the second heart sound. While the ECG may help in differentiating various types of ASD, echocardiography is the most useful investigation for diagnosis of ASD and its subtypes. Transesophageal echocardiography is sometimes needed to plan catheter based closure for ASD. The management of ASD includes either surgical closure through the median sternotomy or thoracotomy approach. Catheter-based closure is an option for defects in the fossa ovalis region with adequate rims.

REFERENCES

1. Park MK. Paediatric Cardiology for Practitioners, 5th edition. Missouri: Mosby Elseiver; 2007. pp. 161-5.
2. Hoffman JIE, Kaplan S. The incidence of congenital heart disease. J Am Coll Cardiol. 2002; 39(12):1890-900.
3. Flyer DC, Buckley LP, Hellenbrand WE. Report of the New England Regional Infant Cardia Program. Pediatrics. 1980;65(Suppl): 37-461.
4. Webb G, Gatzouilis MA. Atrial septal defects in the adult: recent progress and overview. Circulation. 2006;114(15):1645-53.
5. Silvermann ME, Copeland Jr AJ, Hurst JW. The Holt–Oram syndrome: the long and short of it. Am J Cardiolo.1970;25(1):11-7.
6. Bizarro RO, Callahan JA, Feldt RH, Kurland LT, Gordon H, Brandenberg RO. Familial atrial septal defect with prolonged atrioventricular conduction. A syndrome showing the autosomal dominant pattern of inheritance. Circulation. 1970;41(4):677-83.
7. Bjornstad PG. Secundum type of ASD with prolonged PR interval and autosomal dominant mode of inheritance. Br Heart J. 1974; 36(12):1149-54.
8. Bjornstad PG, Leren TP. Familial atrial septal defect in the oval fossa with progressive prolongation of the atrioventricular conjunction caused by mutations in the NKX2.5 gene. Cardiol Young. 2009;19(1):40-4.
9. Holt M, Oram S. Familial heart disease with skeletal malformations. Br Heart J. 1960;22(2): 236-42.
10. Marino B, Digilio MC, Toscano A, Giannotti A, Dallapiccola B. Congenital heart disease in children with Noonan syndrome: an expanded cardiac spectrum with high prevalence of atrioventricular canal. J Pediatr. 1999;135(6): 703-6.
11. Kirk EP, Sunde M, Costa MW, Rankin SA, Wolstein O, Castro ML, et al. Mutations in cardiac T-box factor gene TBX20 are associated with diverse cardiac pathologies, including defects of septation and valvulogenesis and cardiomyopathy. Am J Hum Genet. 2007;81(2): 280-91.
12. Cayler CG. Spontaneous functional closure of symptomatic atrial septal defects. N Engl J Med.1967;276(2):65-73.
13. Hagen PT, Scholz DG, Edwards WD. Incidence and size of patent foramen oval during the first 10 decades of life: an autopsy study of 965 normal hearts. Mayo Clin Proc. 1984;59(1):17-20.
14. Cherian G, Uthaman CB, Durairaj M, Sukumar IP, Krishnaswami S, Jairaj PS, et al. Pulmonary hypertension in isolated secundum atrial septal defects: high frequency in young patients. Am Heart J. 1983;105(6):952-7
15. Van Mierop LHS. Embryology of the atrioventricular canal region and pathogenises of endocardial cushion defects. In: Feldt RH, Mcgoon DC, Ongley PA, et al., (Eds). Atrioventricuar Canal Defects. Philadelphia: WB Saunders, 1976. pp. 1-12.
16. Ettedgui JA, Siewers RD, Anderson RH, Park SC, Pahl E, Zuberbuhler JR. Diagnostic echocardiographic features of the sinus venous defect. Br Heart J. 1990;64(5):329-31.
17. Eidem BE, Cetta F, O'Leary PW. Echocardiography in Paediatric and Adult Congenital Heart Disease, 1st edition. Philadelphia: Lippincott Williams and Wilkins, a Wolters Kluwer Business; 2010. p. 93.
18. Mainwaring Rd, Mirali-Akbar H, Lamberti JJ, Moore JW. Secundum type atrial septal defects with failure to thrive in the first year of life. J Cardiol Surg. 1996;11(2):116-20.
19. Allen HD, Driscoll DJ, Shaddy RE, Feltes TF. Moss and Adams' Heart Disease in Infants, Children and Adolescents: Including the Fetus and Young Adult, 7th edition. Philadelphia: Lippincott Williams and Wilkins, a Wolters Kluwer Business; 2008. p. 634.
20. Rudolph AM. Congenital Diseases of the Heart: Clinical-Physiological Considerations, 3rd edition. West Sussex: Wiley-Blackwell; 2009. pp. 182-8.
21. Kumar S, Luisada AA. The second heart sound in atrial septal defect. Am J Cardiol. 1971; 28(2):168-72.

22. O'Toole JD, Reddy PS, Curtiss EI, Shaver JA. The mechanism of splitting of the second heart sound in atrial septal defect. Circulation. 1977;56(6):1047-53.
23. Perloff JK, Marelli AJ. Clinical Recognition of Congenital Heart Disease, 6th edition. Philadelphia: Elsevier Saunders; 2012. pp. 219-31.
24. Harrison DC, Morrow AG. Electrocardiographic evidence of left axis deviation in patients with defects of the atrial septum of the secundum type. N Engl J Med. 1963;269:743-5.
25. Liebman J, Nadas AS. The vectorcardiogram in the differential diagnosis of atrial septal defect in children. Circulation. 1960;22:956-75.
26. Brandenburg RO, Burchell HB, Toscano-Barbosa E. Electrocardiographic studies of cases with intracardiac malformations of the atrioventricular canal. Proc Staff Meet Mayo Clin. 1956;31(19):513-23.
27. Hung JS, Ritter DG, Feldt RH, Kincaid OW. Electrocardiographic and angiographic features of common atrium. Chest. 1973;63(6):970-5.
28. Saxena A, Relan J, Agarwal R, Awasthy N, Azad S, Chakrabarty M, et al. Indian Guidelines for indications and timing of intervention in common congenital heart diseases: revised and updated consensus statement of the working group on management of congenital heart disease. Ann Pediatr Cardiol. 2019;12(3):254-86.

22 CHAPTER

Ventricular Septal Defect

Nageswara Rao Koneti

INTRODUCTION

Isolated ventricular septal defect (VSD) is the common congenital heart defect constitutes approximately 20% of all congenital heart defects.[1] The median incidence of VSD is 2,829/1,000,000 live births. The prevalence varies from 3 to 5/1,000 live births.[2] Multiple VSDs are seen in 20% of the cases. Supracristal VSD is more commonly seen in Asian population. In another 25% of cases with congenital heart disease such as tetralogy of Fallot, double outlet right ventricle, truncus arteriosus, tricuspid atresia, and interruption of aortic arch, VSD is obligatory.

GENETIC FACTORS

The etiology of VSD is multifactorial like any other congenital heart disease (CHD). Between 5 and 8% of CHD have chromosomal defects. Major chromosomal abnormalities such as Down syndrome, DiGeorge syndrome, and Turner syndrome are associated with CHD. Single-gene mutations such as *NKX2.5*, *TBX5*, and *GATA4* had been shown association with septal defects.[3] Maternal VSDs are associated with recurrence risk of 6–10% and in one offspring carries 2% risk in the subsequent child.[4]

EMBRYOLOGY OF INTERVENTRICULAR SEPTUM

The septum has both mesenchymal and muscular components. Conotruncal and endocardial cushions are the origin for the mesenchymal tissue. The muscular septum originates from a cluster of cells which produce primitive interventricular septum (IVS). Embryologically, IVS develops from three important structures: (1) atrioventricular (AV) cushions developing into membranous septum, (2) outflow tract ridges which form outlet septum, and (3) myocardium surrounding primary interventricular foramen toward greater curvature develops into muscular IVS proper (excluding outlet septum). The bifurcation of the AV conduction bundle is the landmark that separates these three parts of IVS.[5]

Muscular Septum

Two separate components together form muscular septum (1) anterior part develops from bulboventricular fold (circular constriction presents between developing right and left ventricles) and (2) the posterior part or caudal part is caudal extension of the trabecular part.[6]

At 5 weeks, muscular septum is identifiable between the trabecular portion of the both ventricles. Embryonic right and left ventricles balloon while the myocardium in the primary interventricular foramen (lining bulboventricular fold) remains as small circular tube. This wave of passive growth is followed by a second wave of symmetric active in-growth of left and right ventricular cardiomyocytes. This is followed by third waves of active proliferation of cardiomyocytes already present in IVS.[7]

Membranous Septum

Superior and inferior AV endocardial cushions form AV membranous septum at their site of fusion. The interventricular membranous septum forms after delamination of the medial leaflets of tricuspid valve.[5]

Outflow Septum

Outflow septum develops fusion of proximal portions of septal and parietal ridges at 7.5 weeks of gestation.[8] The portion of ridges below arterial valves forms a muscular partition between subpulmonary and subaortic vestibules. This outlet part of IVS is initially supported exclusively by developing right ventricle. The myocardial cuff surrounding the proximal outflow tracts develops differential regression, with predominant regression on the left side (resulting regression of myocardium separating aortic valve from mitral valve) and proliferation of right side (resulting in further separation of tricuspid and pulmonary valves). This differential myocardial regression aligns the aorta with developing left ventricle and outlet septum with the crest of the muscular ventricular septum.[9]

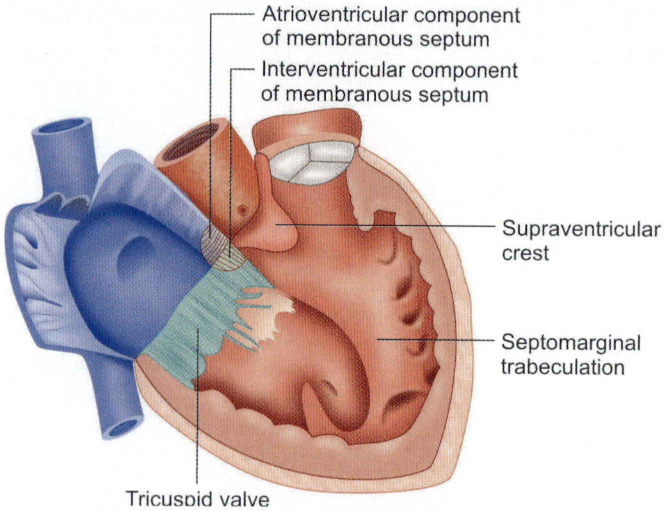

Fig. 1: Schematic diagram of interventricular septum from the right ventricular side showing membranous septum and its relationship to tricuspid valve and AV component. The red color-shaded portion is trabecular septum.

MORPHOLOGY

Ventricular septum is divided into membranous septum and muscular septum (**Fig. 1**). Perimembranous septum or membranous septum is the thinnest portion of the ventricular septum joining the inlet and outlet components of the muscular septum. The relationship of the membranous septum to the aortic valve and tricuspid valve is important. Membranous septum is below the noncoronary and right coronary cusps of the aortic valve. It is divided into pars atrioventricularis and pars interventricularis by the septal leaflet of tricuspid valve.[10] The muscular septum is divided into inlet, trabecular, and outlet septum. Largest part of the IVS constitutes trabecular portion extends from membranous septum to the apex and superiorly to the infundibular septum.[11] Muscular VSDs can be divided into anterior, posterior, mid, and apical muscular VSD. The right ventricular outlet has muscular infundibulum. This muscular trabecular septum separates the subarterial regions. Septomarginal trabeculae is a "y"-shaped septal band separates between right ventricular apical trabecular portion to conus. Perimembranous VSD can extend into inlet septum and outlet septum.

CLASSIFICATION OF VENTRICULAR SEPTAL DEFECT

Sotos classification: This is one of the earliest morphological classifications based on the location of the VSD.[10]

- Perimembranous VSD:
  - Inlet extension
  - Trabecular extension
  - Infundibular extension
- Muscular VSD:
  - Posterior (inlet)
  - Trabecular
  - Infundibular
- Subarterial infundibular (also known as subpulmonic/doubly committed/supracristal defects)
- Mixed defects.

However, classification by Congenital Heart Surgery Nomenclature and Database proposed a simplified version for the better understanding of location VSD on the right ventricular side from the surgical point of view.[12]

- *Type 1*: Subarterial, supracristal, conal VSD, and infundibular
  - A VSD that lies below the semilunar valve
- *Type 2*: Perimembranous, paramembranous, and conoventricular
  - A VSD that involves membranous septum and is bordered by an AV valve
- *Type 3*: Inlet and AV canal type
  - A VSD that involves the inlet of right ventricular septum immediately inferior to the AV valve apparatus
- *Type 4*: Muscular
  - A VSD completely surrounded by muscular septum
- *VSD Gerbode*: Left ventricle to right atrial shunt
  - The communication between left ventricle to right atrium through membranous septum.

The classification based on the size of the defect and amount of shunt is as follows:

- *Small VSD*: Diameter of VSD <1/3rd of aortic orifice. Shunt ratio (Qp/Qs) is <1.5:1. Normal pulmonary artery (PA) pressure
- *Moderate VSD*: Diameter of the VSD is between 1/3rd and 2/3rd of aortic orifice. Qp/Qs is >1.5:1. PA pressure varies from normal to elevated but subsystemic.
- *Large VSD*: Diameter of VSD is >2/3rd of the aortic orifice. Qp/Qs varies depends on pulmonary vascular resistance (PVR). PA systolic pressure is near systemic or systemic.

Perimembranous Ventricular Septal Defect

These defects are located in the membranous septum. The boundaries always involve fibrous continuity between AV valve (septal leaflet of tricuspid valve) and semilunar valves (noncoronary and right coronary sinuses of aortic valve). That is why the tissue of septal leaflet often covers perimembranous VSD in the natural process of spontaneous closure. Sometimes even the aortic sinuses may get prolapsed into perimembranous VSD.

Inlet Ventricular Septal Defect

The defect in the inlet location along with the tricuspid valve is called as inlet VSD. It can be an extension of perimembranous VSD. Inlet VSDs are also a part of many AV septal defects.

Muscular Ventricular Septal Defect

These are midmuscular (trabecular), apical muscular, anterior muscular, and posterior muscular types. Often, muscular

VSDs are multiple and sometimes "Swiss-cheese" with multiple openings in the right ventricular side of the IVS.

Outlet Ventricular Septal Defect

These are the defects in the outlet septum called as subarterial, infundibular, or doubly committed VSDs. There are no reports of spontaneous closure of these defects. The septum below the right coronary sinus is absent; this may lead to prolapse of the right coronary cusp and subsequently aortic regurgitation.

Conoventricular or Malaligned Ventricular Septal Defect

Defects in the conal septum with either anterior or posterior malalignment are called as conoventricular VSDs. These are commonly associated with other structural heart defects. Anterior malalignment is seen in tetralogy of Fallot, whereas posterior malalignment in aortic arch interruption.

PHYSIOLOGY AND HEMODYNAMICS

The shunt across the VSD is dependent on the size and relative resistance produced in the pulmonary and systemic vasculature. Fetal diagnosis of small VSDs is often difficult due to insignificant shunt in the presence of high PVR. The shunt across VSD depends on the pressure changes in the ventricles during cardiac cycle. The neonatal PVR in the immediate postnatal period is high; therefore, cardiac murmur due to VSD is generally inconspicuous. Cardiac murmurs and shunt across the defect appear once the PVR drops during neonatal period. It is delayed in these cases due to altered alveolar to arterial ratio in the lungs in the presence of VSD.[13] The magnitude of the shunt is based on the size of the VSD and PVR. Typically, infant will have respiratory distress and feeding difficulties between 6 weeks and 3 months of age where PVR falls significantly and net left-to-right shunts increase, i.e., pulmonary blood flow (Qp) versus systemic blood flow (Qs). They have high baseline PVR and infant may have more problems related to respiratory pathology rather left-to-right shunt. As the left-to-right shunt (Qp/Qs) increases, the pulmonary blood flow, pulmonary venous return, and volume of left atrium and left ventricle also proportionately increase. The dilated left ventricle due to high end-diastolic volume increases the end-diastolic pressure as per the Frank–Starling mechanism. This causes increase in left atrial filling pressure and subsequently pulmonary capillary wedge pressure. Therefore, infant presents with congestive heart failure (CHF) due to both increased pulmonary blood flow and increased left heart filling pressures.

Untreated long-standing cases with large or moderate VSDs develop pulmonary arterial changes due to injury to pulmonary capillary endothelium. The small- and medium-sized pulmonary arteries develop medial hypertrophy and smooth muscle cell proliferation. There are various irreversible pathological stages described in chronic left-to-right shunt. The PVR increases as the distal vascular bed capacity decreases due to musculature and hypertrophy. And finally, the shunt across the VSD will become right to left and this is referred to as Eisenmenger syndrome. The pulmonary arterial pressure and right ventricular pressure will be equal to the systemic pressure.

NATURAL HISTORY OF VENTRICULAR SEPTAL DEFECT

About 10% of patients with large VSDs die in 1st year due to CHF and lower respiratory infections.[14] Common causes of mortality among infant and young children with VSD are lower respiratory tract infection and congestive cardiac failure. Early surgery may reduce mortality and morbidity significantly. Among unoperated patients with all the types of VSDs combined, 27% die by 20 years and 53% by 40 years of age.[15] The natural history of VSD is influenced by multiple factors such as size, location, age at which the defect is recognized, number of VSD, and association with other malformations. The possible outcomes for a child with VSD can be any or multiple of the following paths:[16]

- Spontaneous diminution in size or closure
- Development of right ventricular outflow tract obstruction (RVOTO)
- Development of aortic regurgitation
- Development of left ventricular (LV) outflow tract obstruction
- Development of pulmonary vascular obstructive disease (PVOD)
- Infective endocarditis.

Spontaneous Closure

Spontaneous decrease in the size of VSD and closure are common outcomes in some of the children with VSD. The mechanisms of closure differ between perimembranous VSD and muscular. Most common mechanism responsible for the closure of perimembranous defects is progressive adherence of septal leaflet of tricuspid valve to the margins of VSD. Uncommonly, prolapse of aortic valve cusp may adhere to the subaortic margin. Muscular defects close by either proliferation of fibrous tissue or hypertrophied muscles in the right ventricle.[17,18] Krovetz et al. in their study of 692 children with VSD showed that up to 70% of VSD close spontaneously. An inverse relationship exists between the probability of the spontaneous closure and age at which the patient was first observed. Most defects destined to close do so within the first year of life, with 60% closing before 3 years of age, and 90% closing before 8 years of age.[19] Smaller defects (those <3 mm) are more likely to close.

Up to 85% small muscular VSDs do spontaneously close. Perimembranous VSD with left ventricle to right atrial shunt (Gerbode defect), malaligned VSD, subpulmonic VSD, and inlet VSD are less likely to close spontaneously.[20]

Right Ventricular Outflow Tract Obstruction

Progressive obstruction of right ventricular obstruction among children with VSD is usually due to hypertrophy of the right ventricular muscle bundles in outflow tract.[21] Incidence of RVOTO at various levels is seen in 13%. Right ventricular mid cavity or infundibular obstruction is called as Gasul phenomenon.[22-24] This acquired RVOTO occurs due to long-standing left-to-right shunt with a force into the right ventricle which stimulates the proliferation of infundibular muscles in a genetically predisposed individual.

Aortic Valve Regurgitation

Aortic cusp prolapse and aortic regurgitation are more common with subpulmonic VSD and perimembranous VSDs, which are in direct contact with the aortic valve. Right coronary cusp prolapses most frequently through VSD. Venturi effect, absence of structural support for the leaflets, and abnormal commissural separation are the main mechanisms for the development of aortic valve prolapse. Incidence of aortic cusp prolapse and subsequent regurgitation range from 2 to 7% in various studies.[22,25,26]

Infective endocarditis is a known risk in cases of restrictive perimembranous VSD. Incidence of infective endocarditis is <2% and it usually occurs after the age of 4–5 years.[27-29] The natural history in small perimembranous VSD is generally uneventful but the risk of infective endocarditis has to be kept in mind during the follow-up. Perimembranous VSD has jet effect on septal tricuspid valve causing the endothelial injury and hence it is a site of growth of vegetations. On rare situations, vegetations at the base of the septal tricuspid leaflet cause perforation and produce LV to right atrial shunt (acquired indirect Gerbode defect). Occasionally, the site of infective endocarditis can be on the aneurysm of the IVS.[30,31] Muscular defects have a low incidence of infective endocarditis because the jet is dissipated within the right ventricular cavity without striking the septal tricuspid leaflet.[31,32] Subpulmonic VSDs have a risk of endocarditis that can occur on the pulmonary valve. Dental hygiene remains the key for prevention of infective endocarditis.

CLINICAL FEATURES

The clinical spectrum of isolated VSD is wide and varies depending upon the size of defect and amount of shunt. It may range from being asymptomatic to severe heart failure. Clinical symptomatology and physical signs can be broadly divided into two groups on the basis of size of defect: (1) small VSD and (2) moderate-to-large VSD.

Small Ventricular Septal Defect

Patients are asymptomatic with normal growth and development. The clinical course is benign throughout the infancy even up to late adulthood, but they are at risk for infective endocarditis. Risk of infective endocarditis increases with dental caries and other conditions with bacteremia. Small perimembranous and muscular VSD have higher chances (40–80%) of spontaneous closure.[22] These patients are often referred to a cardiologist for a systolic murmur detected on routine examination or at the time of an incidental illness. The murmur can be audible as early as 2 weeks depending on the PVR. Normal precordial activity but a systolic thrill along the left sternal border can be felt. First and second heart sounds are normally heard. Presence of S3 suggests significant left-to-right shunt. Detailed description of murmurs in VSD is described separately.

Moderate-to-Large Ventricular Septal Defect

Infants with moderate-to-large VSDs present with symptoms due to CHF by 4–8 weeks, as the PVR decreases. The symptoms are predominantly due to significant left-to-right shunt leading to increased pulmonary vascularity and thus causing volume overload to left heart and CHF.[30] The following are the symptoms during infancy:[33]

- Increased respiratory rate (tachypnea), increase in the work of breathing due to decrease in lung compliance and chest retractions
- Feeding difficulties with suck-rest-suck cycle and easy fatigability due to decompensated heart failure
- Excessive sweating of forehead (diaphoresis) due to sympathetic overdrive as a compensatory phenomenon
- Failure to thrive due to hypercatabolic state and poor feeding
- Recurrent respiratory infections: (1) anatomical relationship between pulmonary arteries, left atrium to the tracheobronchial tree, (2) pulmonary over circulation leading to alveolar and peribronchial exudates, and (3) reduced ciliary motion in the terminal bronchioles
- Symptoms of wheezing, tachypnea, respiratory distress: engorgement of pulmonary circulation due to increased flow and pulmonary venous congestion leading to pulmonary edema and combination with compression of airways.

Congestive heart failure symptoms decrease as the amount of shunt decreases over the period due to the increase in PVR. These groups of patients will have asymptomatic period before the Eisenmenger reaction sets in. VSD with Eisenmenger disease presents with exercise intolerance and cyanosis in view of fixed cardiac output and shunt reversal.[34] They have higher risk of cerebral vascular accidents. Clinical approach should include assessment of general physical growth and achievement of milestones and also evaluation for syndromic features. Most of the syndromes are associated with significant VSD. Harrison's groove with precordial bulge can be noted in long-standing large left-to-right shunts. Pulse may be low volume in cases with significant left-to-right shunt with heart failure. In moderate-to-large VSDs, precordial pulsations are visible due to LV volume overload. The apical impulse is LV type, hyperdynamic, displaced downward and outward. LV S3 is audible. Precordial bulge and parasternal heave become obvious in cases with pulmonary hypertension. PA pulsations and palpable P2 are important clinical clues for the diagnosis of pulmonary hypertension. They will have right ventricular type apex; loud second heart sound with close split, and (P2 component—booming character) a diastolic tap is felt (corresponds to loud palpable P2). An ejection clicks (pulmonary, related to dilatation of PA) is present all over the precordium.[34] Presence of a systolic thrill usually suggests either restrictive VSD or associated with RVOTO.

Cardiac Murmurs

- Holosystolic or pansystolic murmurs are absent at birth due to high PVR but audible murmur appears as soon as PVR falls and shunt begins. Restrictive VSD produces pansystolic murmur. Shunt velocity across the defect determines the grade of the murmur, the higher the velocity in a restrictive VSD, the louder is the murmur. Pansystolic murmur is usually harsh in character compared to the murmur due to mitral regurgitation at apex which is soft and blowing in character. The site of the murmur gives subtle clues that are of limited specificity about the location of the defect. Murmur due to perimembranous VSD can be heard along the left lower sternal border. Harsh loud pansystolic murmur at 2nd and 3rd intercostal space usually suggests subpulmonic VSD. Muscular VSD can be heard along the sternal border based on the location. Larger defects have lesser grade murmur and may not be pansystolic in most of the cases. The murmur becomes soft as the restriction across the defect becomes less in the latter half of the ventricular systole. The systolic murmur due to large shunt becomes inconspicuous once the PVR increases to systemic level over the period of time.[35]

  A harsh loud systolic murmur of >4/6 grade needs exclusion of development of acquired RVOTO including double chambered right ventricle or infundibular obstruction.
- Early systolic murmur is a feature of small closing muscular VSD. The VSD will be obliterated during later part of cardiac systole leading to obliteration of the shunt results in early systolic murmur.
- Mitral diastolic murmur is commonly heard in a hemodynamically significant VSD with left-to-right shunt >2:1. The increased flow across the normal mitral valve produces relative turbulence is the basis for the short mid-diastolic murmur. This tends to be subtle and is often missed unless specifically sought. It is best heard with the bell of the stethoscope. Mitral mid-diastolic murmur associated with presystolic accentuation or associated thrill suggests the presence of congenital mitral valve abnormalities causing obstruction of mitral valve. Various congenital mitral valve abnormalities including supramitral ring, single papillary muscle (parachute valve), etc., may be associated with and needs to be looked for.
- A new early diastolic murmur may be audible over pulmonary area due to pulmonary regurgitation (Graham Steell murmur) in Eisenmenger patients. This murmur is usually high pitched and holodiastolic in nature.

DIAGNOSTIC EVALUATION

Chest X-ray

Radiological findings are useful to assess the vascularity, which indirectly gives idea about the amount of shunt. Plethora is seen in cases with significant left-to-right shunt. Cardiomegaly is seen in patients with heart failure. This is due to specific chamber enlargement including left ventricle, left atrium, and PA. Both plethora and pulmonary venous hypertension are noticed in large shunts. This is due to raised left atrial filling pressures due to large shunts leading to increased pulmonary capillary wedge pressures (**Fig. 2**).

Untreated patients or a subset of patients with persistent PVR show reduction in cardiothoracic ratio, dilated central pulmonary arteries, and peripheral pruning (**Fig. 3**).

Electrocardiogram

Various changes are seen based on the amount of the shunt and pulmonary hypertension. The electrocardiogram (ECG) findings in a small VSD with shunt (Qp/Qs <1.5:1) may

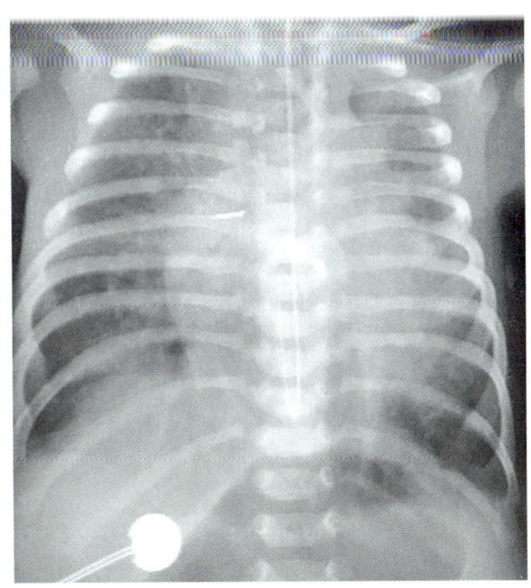

Fig. 2: Chest X-ray of an infant with refractory congestive heart failure due to large perimembranous ventricular septal defect (VSD) showing gross cardiomegaly and plethora (increased vascularity).

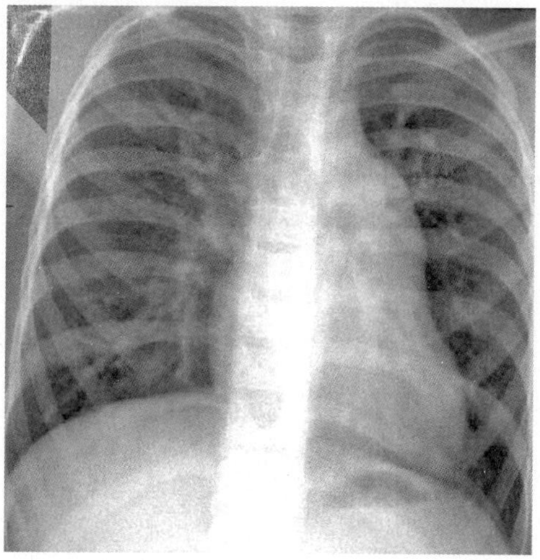

Fig. 3: Chest X-ray of a grown-up patient with unoperated large ventricular septal defect (VSD) presented with cyanosis due to Eisenmenger syndrome. Cardiothoracic ratio is normal (0.5), dilated main pulmonary arteries, and absent plethora.

have subtle findings including mild left atrial enlargement. Prominent "q" waves in V5 and V6 suggest the presence of significant left-to-right shunt leading to LV volume overload. Moderate defects show volume overload features including enlargement of the left atrium and the left ventricle and prominent "q" waves in the lateral leads. Large VSDs (Qp/Qs >2:1) typically have biventricular forces as evidenced by high voltages in the mid precordial leads (Katz-Wachtel phenomenon) (**Fig. 4**). The frontal plane QSR axis is usually rightward except in inlet VSD where left axis is a feature due to posterior-inferior course of the conduction system (**Fig. 5**). ECG changes such as monophasic "R" wave in V1 and deep S waves in V5 and V6 are common in patients with pulmonary hypertension (**Fig. 6**).

Echocardiogram

Transthoracic echocardiogram (TTE) is mandatory in all cases of clinically suspected VSD. TTE provides information

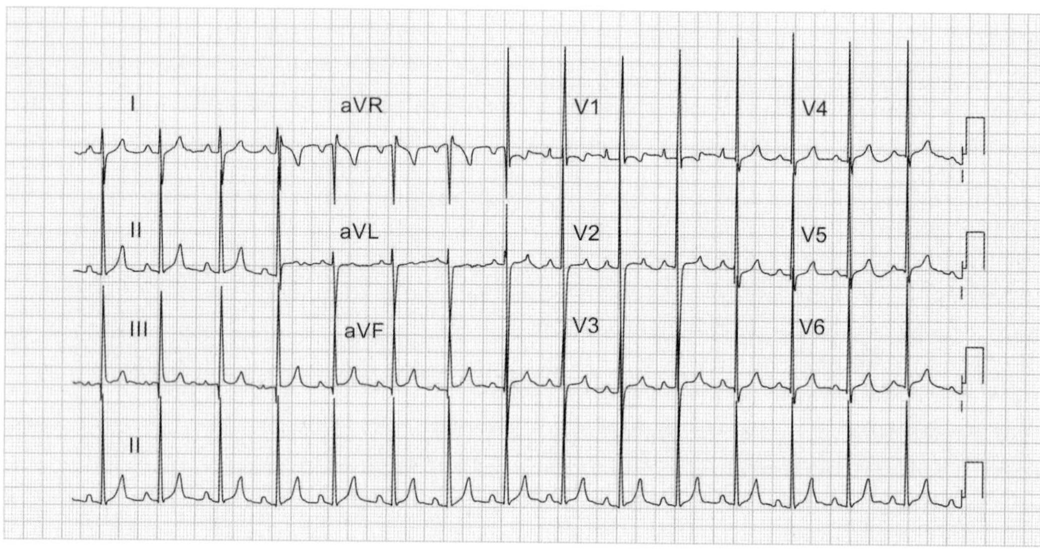

Fig. 4: A 12-lead electrocardiogram of a 3-year-old child with large perimembranous ventricular septal defect (VSD) showing normal sinus rhythm, rightward QRS axis (+105), presence of biventricular (both right and left) hypertrophy. The mid-precardial (V2-V4) voltages are high called as "Katz-Wachtel phenomenon."

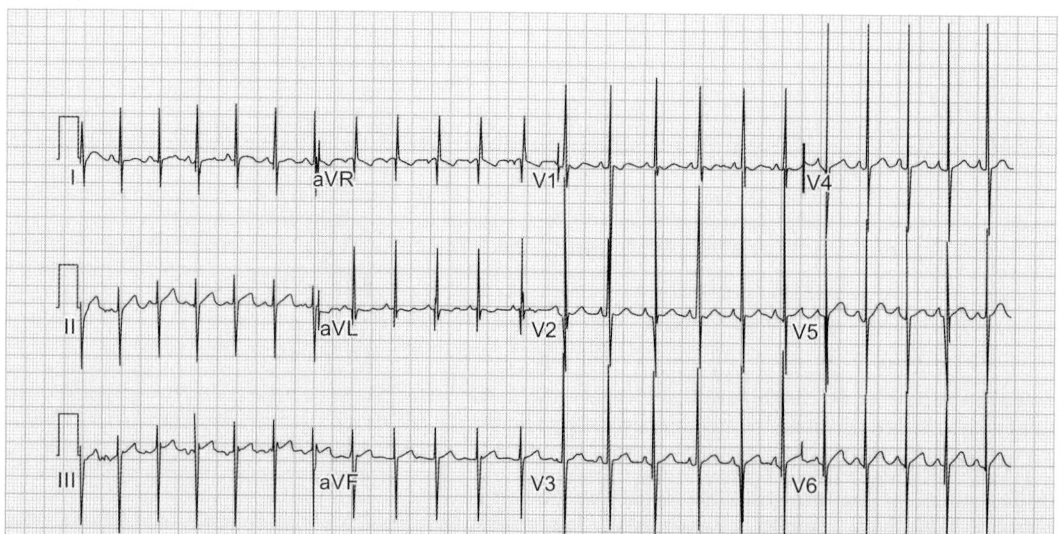

Fig. 5: A 12-lead electrocardiogram of an infant with large inlet ventricular septal defect (VSD) showing sinus rhythm, leftward QRS axis (–45) and high-voltage mid-precardial leads.

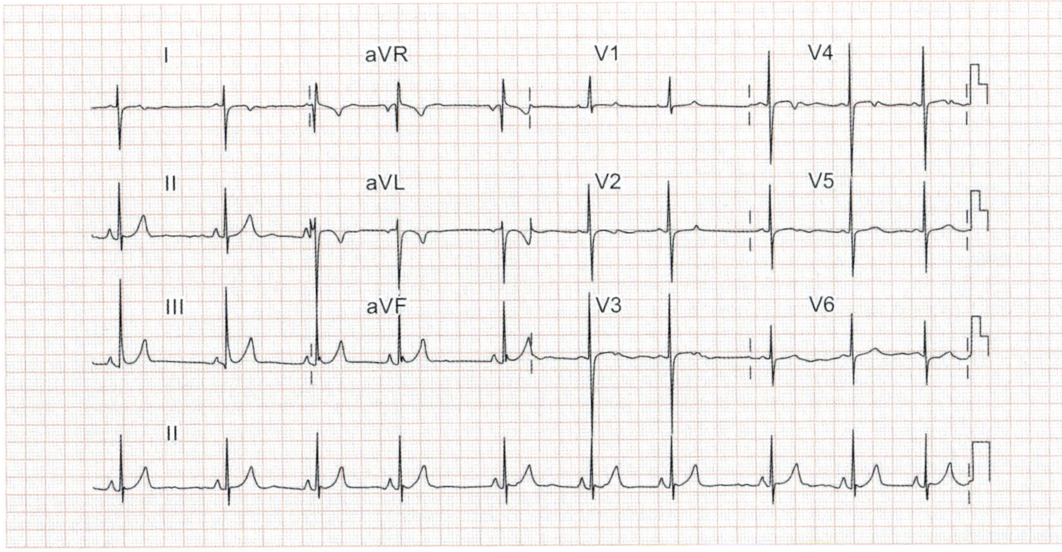

Fig. 6: A 12-lead electrocardiogram of an adult with Eisenmenger syndrome [large ventricular septal defect (VSD) with right-to-left shunt] showing sinus rhythm, right axis deviation (QRS axis +120), "R" wave in V1, and presence of "S" wave in V6 suggests right ventricular hypertrophy due to pulmonary hypertension.

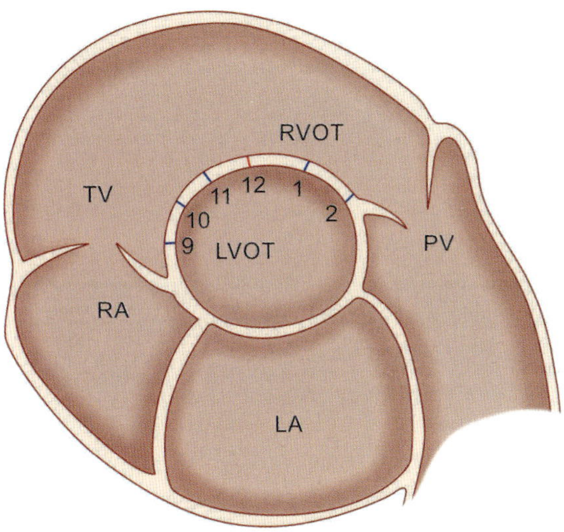

Fig. 7: Schematic diagram of short axis view of transthoracic echocardiogram at the level of aortic valve representing the clock. Please see the text for the description
(LA: left atrium; LVOT: left ventricular outflow tract; PV: pulmonary valve; RA: right atrium; RVOT: right ventricular outflow tract; TV: tricuspid valve)

regarding the size, location, pressure gradient across the VSD, suitability for the transcatheter closure, and other associations such as development of aortic regurgitation, right ventricular outflow tract abnormalities, and tricuspid regurgitation. Parasternal short axis and long axis views provide valuable information. The cross section at the level of aortic valve provides information regarding the location of VSD.[36] The defects at 8 o'clock are posterior in location such as inlet VSDs. Perimembranous VSDs are located between 9 and 11 o'clock and subpulmonary between 12 and 2 o'clock (**Fig. 7**). Muscular VSDs should be assessed in multiple views including subxiphoid sagittal and coronal planes (**Figs. 8A to D**). Assessment of location, size, and number of muscular defects are crucial and utmost important in planning for either surgical or transcatheter closure. Perimembranous VSD with partial closure due to septal tricuspid leaflet aneurysm can be seen in apical views and parasternal long axis view with posterior tilt (**Figs. 9A to D**). Subpulmonic VSDs can be assessed in long axis and short axis views (**Figs. 10A and B**). Development of aortic regurgitation due to aortic cusp prolapse needs assessment in multiple views including long axis and apical views (**Figs. 11A and B**).[37] Acquired RVOTO either due to infundibular or mid cavity of right ventricle can be better assessed by subxiphoid views or long axis view with anterior sweep (**Figs. 12A and B**). Color flow mapping with appropriate Nyquist limits demonstrate the shunt pattern, presence of tricuspid regurgitation, or aortic regurgitation in case of aortic leaflet prolapse. Turbulent jet across the defect suggests restrictive VSD. Often, it is difficult to differentiate between a restrictive VSD jet and RVOTO jet in a single view. Color flow mapping with interrogation by pulse Doppler helps in differentiating the two jets. Continuous Doppler assessment of the flow across the VSD gives idea about the pressure difference between left ventricle and right ventricle. Gradient above 60 mm Hg is seen in restrictive small VSDs, gradient <40 mm Hg in moderate-to-large defects (**Figs. 13A and B**).

Cardiac Catheterization and Angiography

Cardiac catheterization in VSD is indicated (1) to decide operability when there is suspicion of elevation in PVR and (2) trans-catheter intervention. In large defects, the increase in pulmonary flow causes remodeling of pulmonary vasculature leading to the development of pulmonary arterial hypertension (PAH). In the long-term, this process leads to the development of pulmonary vascular occlusive disease with right-to-left shunt and cyanosis.[38]

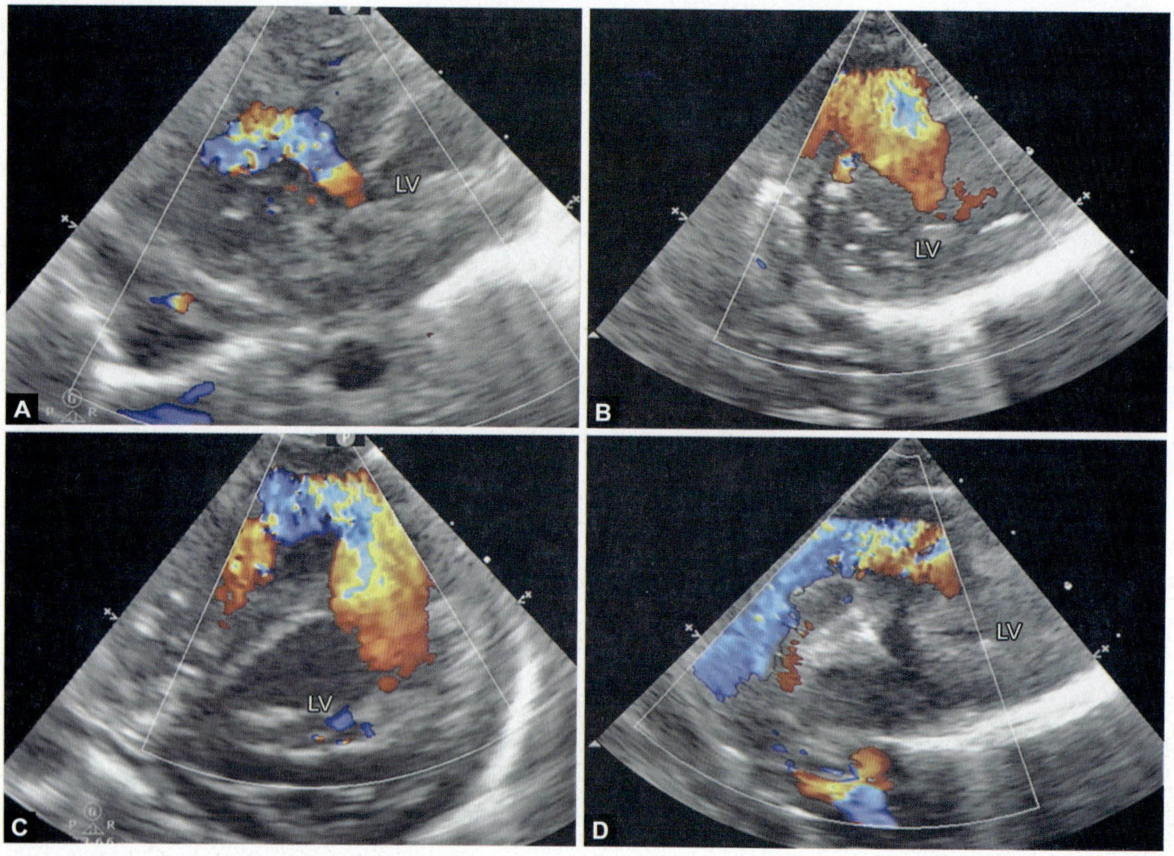

Figs. 8A to D: Subxiphoid views of transthoracic echocardiogram with color flow mapping showing multiple muscular ventricular septal defects (VSDs) at various levels.
(LV: left ventricle)

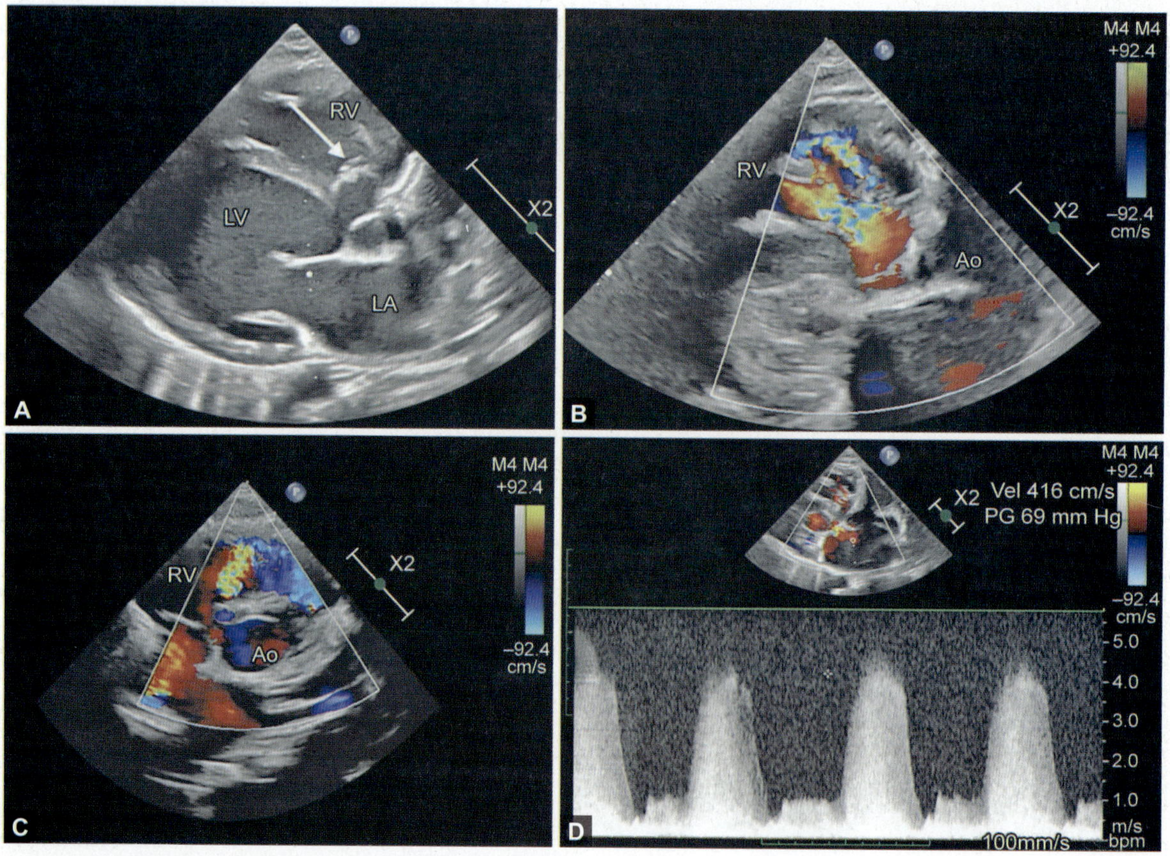

Figs. 9A to D: Transthoracic echocardiogram. (A and B) Parasternal long axis views showing perimembranous ventricular septal defect (VSD) with septal aneurysm (white arrow); (C) Short axis view showing shunt cross the defect; (D) Demonstrating the high gradient across the defect.
(Ao: aorta; LA: left atrium; LV: left ventricle; RV: right ventricle;)

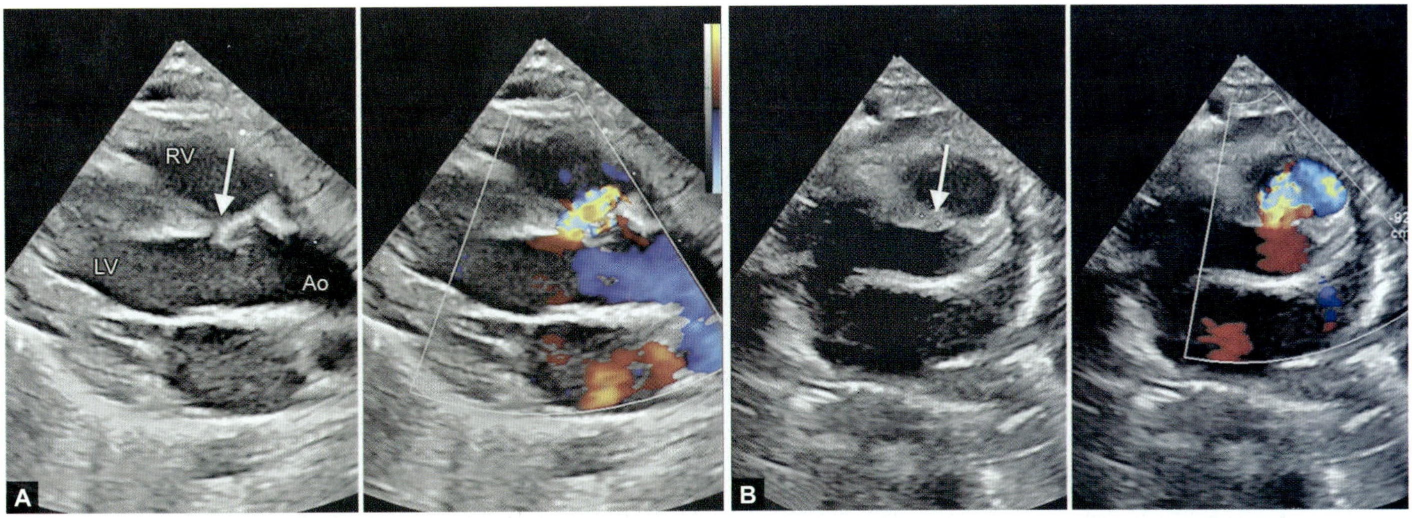

Figs. 10A and B: Parasternal long axis (A) and short axis (B) showing subpulmonic ventricular septal defect (VSD) with left-to-right shunt (white arrows).
(Ao: aorta; LV: left ventricle; RV: right ventricle)

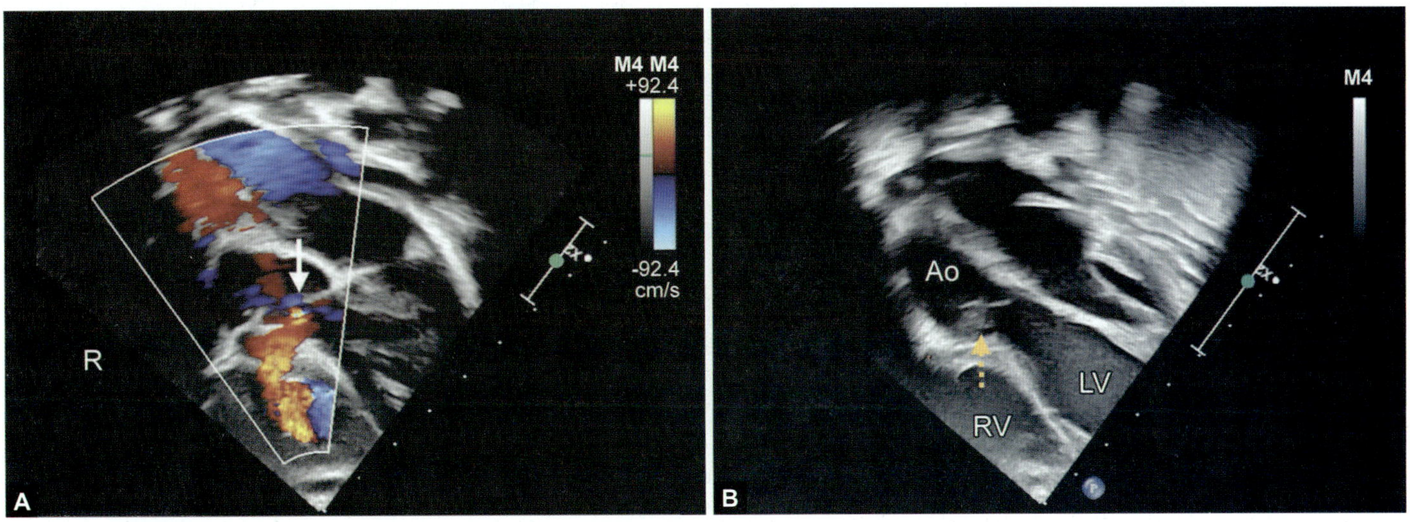

Figs. 11A and B: Transthoracic apical view showing perimembranous ventricular septal defect (VSD) with left-to-right shunt. There is aortic valve prolapse (B: yellow broken arrow) with trivial aortic regurgitation (A: white arrow).
(Ao: aorta; LV: left ventricle; RV: right ventricle)

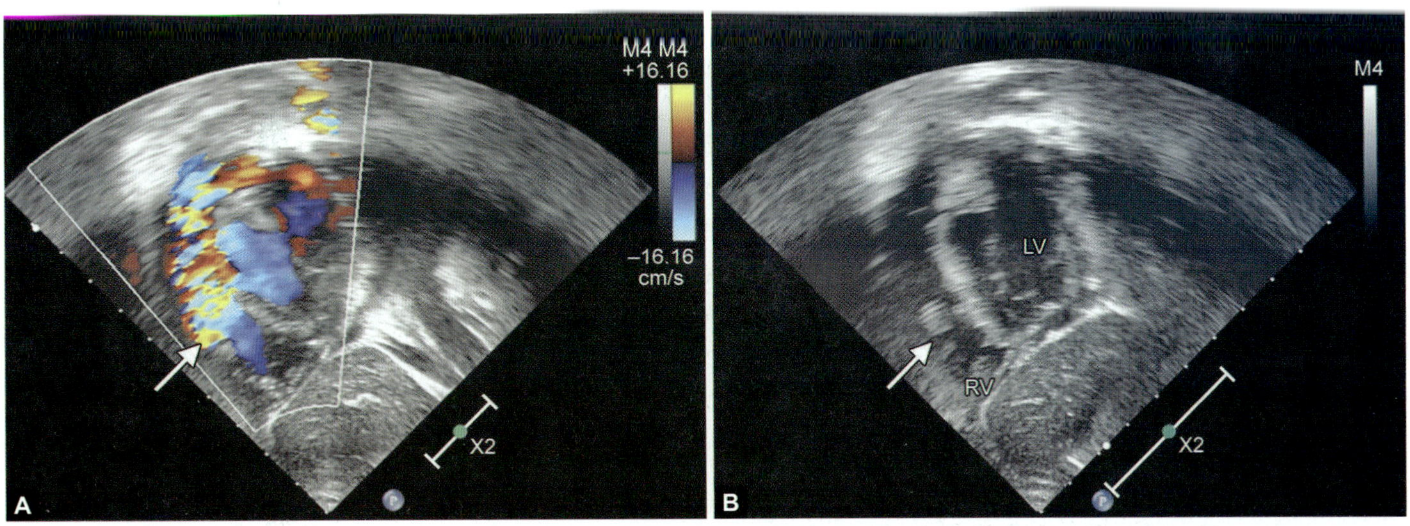

Figs. 12A and B: Subxiphoid coronal view showing right ventricular outflow tract obstruction in a child with perimembranous ventricular septal defect (VSD). White arrow in (A) showing turbulent jet due to obstruction (B) hypertrophied infundibular muscles (white arrow).
(LV: left ventricle; RV: right ventricle)

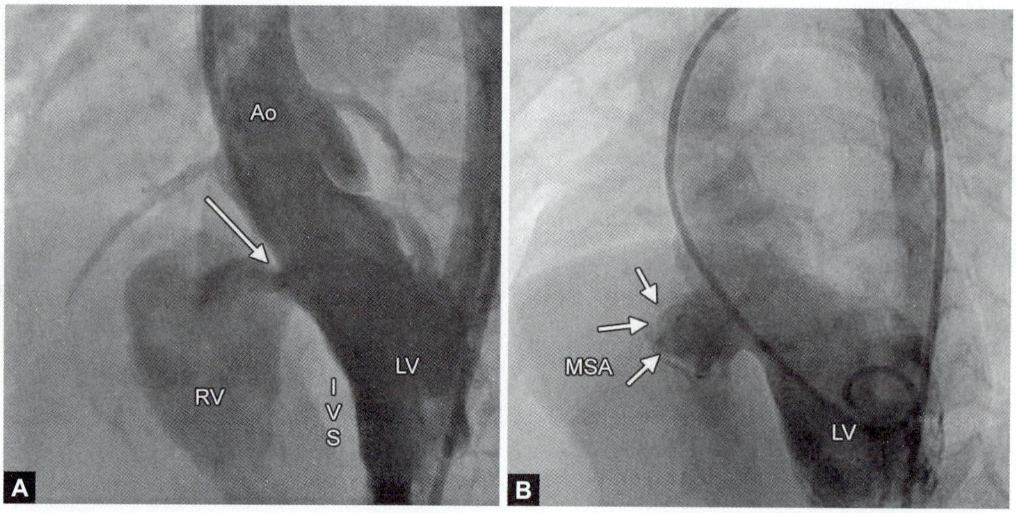

Figs. 13A and B: Left ventricular angiogram in long axis view (left anterior oblique view with cranial tilt) showing (A) Perimembranous ventricular septal defect (VSD) away from the aortic valve (single white arrow); (B) Membranous aneurysm with multiple openings in a grown-up child (multiple short arrows).
(Ao: aorta; LV: left ventricle; RV: right ventricle; IVS: interventricular septum)

TABLE 1: Hemodynamic criteria for assessment of operability.

Condition	*Hemodynamics*
Baseline	PVRI <6 Wood Units.m^2 (WU.m^2), PVR:SVR ratio <0.3
Acute vasodilator challenge (O_2, nitric oxide inhalation)	• Baseline PVRI 6–9 WU.m^2, PVR:SVR 0.3–0.5 • Decrease in PVR index of 20% • PVR:SVR decrease of 20% • Final PVR index <6 WU/m^2 • Final PVR/SVR <0.3

(PVR: pulmonary vascular resistance (indexed); PVRI: pulmonary vascular resistance index; SVR: systemic vascular resistance)

The response of the pulmonary vasculature to high pulmonary blood flow is not uniform and does not occur in a predictable fashion.[39,40] This results in difficulties in decision-making regarding operability of these defects, particularly in patients who present beyond infancy and early childhood. It is important to determine the operability before surgery as after development of PVOD, the patient would persist having PAH even after correction of defect. There can be a stormy postoperative course due to the development of PAH crisis. The persistent PAH causes long-term morbidity and early mortality as compared to patients living with Eisenmenger syndrome in which the defect is not corrected.

Cardiac catheterization is needed for quantitative assessment of pulmonary blood flow and PVR in borderline cases. The hemodynamic criteria for operability are given in **Table 1**.[41]

During diagnostic catheterization, the shunt should be quantified precisely and comprehensive pressure data including the PA pressures, capillary wedge pressures, and LV end-diastolic pressures should be obtained. Pulmonary vascular and systemic vascular resistance and their ratio should be calculated to assess operability. The responsiveness to vasodilator in the form of nitric oxide or intravenous sildenafil may allow for an in-depth assessment. However, the basal data offers the best prediction of operability. LV angiogram is routinely done in long axis view to profile the perimembranous VSD (**Figs. 14A and B**). Inlet VSDs can be profiled better in hepatoclavicular view. Subpulmonary VSD and outflow VSDs can be visualized well in either left lateral or right anterior oblique views. In estimating the suitability for operability clinical examination, basic investigations such as ECG, chest X-ray, and echocardiography play an important role (**Table 2**). Decisions should be ideally made after considering all these variables together with the cardiac catheterization data.

MANAGEMENT

Medical Management of Heart Failure

Medical treatment includes control of heart failure, prevention, and prompt treatment of respiratory infections, providing adequate nutrition and nutritional supplementation.

- *Control of heart failure*: Diuretics play a major role in controlling heart failure due to left-to-right shunts. Furosemide therapy is indicated between 1 and 3 mg/kg twice daily. Addition of spironolactone (1–4 mg/kg) may be recommended in case of prolonged use of furosemide therapy or in severe heart failure while waiting for surgery. Commencement of diuretic therapy is recommended when infant develops typical features of heart failure usually between 4 and 6 weeks of age. Diuretic therapy should be continued till the time of surgical closure.[42] Vasodilator therapy such as angiotensin converting enzyme inhibitors (ACEI) have a potential role in reducing the systemic vascular resistance so that the net left-to-right shunt will come down.[43] These second-line medications are usually initiated when surgery is delayed due to various reasons. ACEI (captopril: 0.3–0.5 mg/kg/dose; enalapril: 0.1–0.5 mg/kg/day)

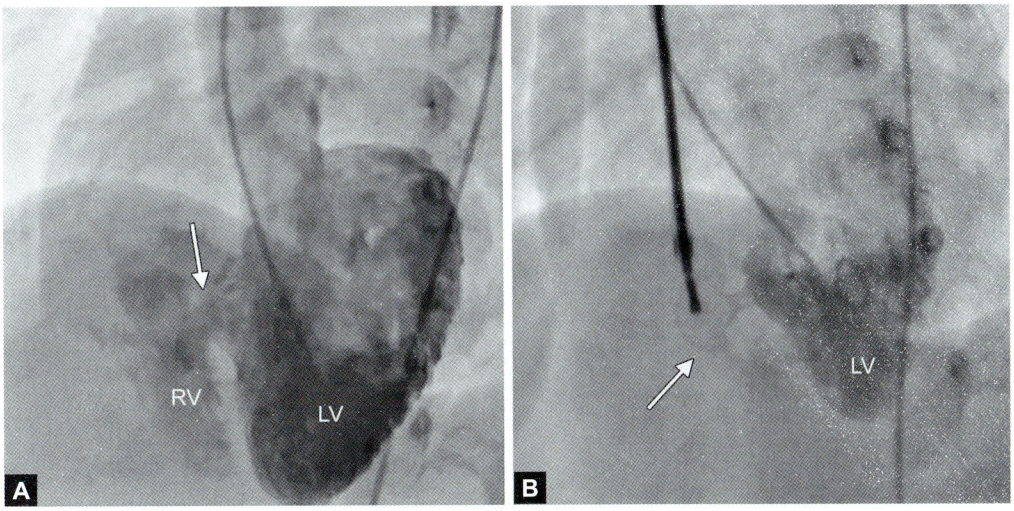

Figs. 14A and B: Left ventricular angiogram in left anterior oblique (LAO) view cranial tilt showing (A) Midmuscular ventricular septal defect (VSD); (B) Angiogram showing complete closure of muscular device (arrow).
(LV: left ventricle; RV: right ventricle)

TABLE 2: Clinical and echocardiographic correlates of operability.

Operable	• *Clinical*: Failure to thrive ↑ precordial activity, mid-diastolic murmur (MDM) at apex • *Chest X-ray*: Cardiac enlargement, ↑pulmonary blood flow • *ECG*: Q in lateral leads, good LV forces • *Echocardiography*: Left atrial and left ventricular enlargement, exclusively left–right flows across the defect
Inoperable	• *Clinical*: Cyanosis, quiet precordium, no MDM • *Chest X-ray*: Normal heart size, peripheral pruning • *ECG*: No Q in lateral leads, predominant RV forces • *Echocardiography*: No left atrial and left ventricular enlargement, significant right–left flows across the defect

can cause renal failure in infants, especially when add along with stiff diuretic therapy and therefore it is recommended purely based on the physician experience. Role of digoxin is very limited to cases with dilated left heart and presence of ventricular dysfunction. The dose is 10 µg/kg in two divided doses. Electrolytes should be monitored periodically in all patients with full doses of diuretic therapy.

- *Lower respiratory infections*: Infants with VSDs are high risk for developing respiratory infections due to various mechanisms described in this chapter in the section on pathophysiology. Respiratory infections contribute substantially to morbidity and mortality due to VSDs. All children with VSDs should be immunized completely including pneumococcal, *Haemophilus*, and *Influenza*. Prompt treatment of all respiratory infections are essential while waiting for the surgery.
- *Nutrition*: Feeding can aggravate heart failure in infants with significant left-to-right shunt due to post-tricuspid shunt. Nonresponders with diuretics need change from breastfeeding to nasogastric feeds. Expressed breast milk can be given with pallada spoon. High calorie formulas or preterm formulas may be used as per the individual case scenario. Patients with additional problems such as gastroesophageal reflex disorder should be managed carefully. Gastrostomy feeds can be considered in selected refractory cases where surgery is delayed in preterm low birth weight babies. However, with improvements in surgery, younger and smaller babies can be operated with good results and therefore the need for gastrostomy or prolonged nasogastric feeds is seldom required.
- *Supplementation*: Fortification of milk with medium chain triglyceride oils may be done within permissible limits. Physiological anemia of infancy and poor nutrition due to hypercatabolic state can exaggerate CHF in infants. Iron supplementation is needed to maintain hemoglobin above 10 g.

It is important to recognize that medical management has a limited role and early surgery is warranted when infants with large VSD develop heart failure.

Surgical Treatment

Indications for surgical closure is recommended for all large VSDs with left-to-right shunt. The Indian guidelines (modified) for the surgical closure are:[44]

- Small VSD (no symptoms, normal PA pressures, normal left heart chambers):
  - VSD closure is indicated if one episode of endocarditis
  - Development of aortic regurgitation
  - Development of RVOTO
- Moderate VSD:
  - *Left heart dilation (LV end-diastolic dimension by TTE "z" > +2.5)*: After 1st year
  - *Symptomatic on medication*: Elective closure

- Large VSD:
  - *Poor weight gain, CHF on medication*: After 2–3 months of age
  - *Small/moderate subpulmonic VSD with cusp prolapse*: Elective closure after 2 years of age.

Several methods had been described based on the location of the defect. Surgical patch closure is done under cardiopulmonary bypass.[45] Perimembranous VSDs can be effectively closure from the right atrial approach visualizing through tricuspid valve. In small babies with large defects or posterior extension, usually closure by detaching the tricuspid leaflet for better visualization. Subpulmonic VSDs are usually closed by both transatrial and transpulmonary approach. Some surgeons prefer to close the VSD with aortic prolapse and aortic regurgitation from the transaortic route while repairing the aortic valve.

Muscular VSDs closure is quite challenging even in experienced hands. The location and number of VSDs in a small infant is difficult. Several methods described include RV exclusion, double patch technique, and sandwich method; however, each procedure has got both advantages and disadvantages. Swiss-chees VSDs are not amenable for the closure and hence a palliative pulmonary artery banding (PAB) is recommended in cases with heart failure and not responding to conventional diuretic therapy. PAB is also indicated in large VSDs amounting to single ventricle to prevent the pulmonary hypertension.[46] In preterm infants with large VSD, the trend is now toward closing the defects surgically rather than performing a PA band.

Interventional Closure

Transcatheter closure is limited to only selected cases with perimembranous VSD and adequate subaortic rim.[47] The chances of complete heart block after transcatheter closure is higher than surgical closure and therefore should be done in carefully selected cases. Amenable muscular VSDs such as midmuscular and some anterior muscular can be closured using muscular VSD devices.[48]

Hybrid Closure

Selected cases with large muscular defects can be closed in the operating room or hybrid laboratories using limited sternotomy approach. Direct needle puncture of right ventricle using a needle and crossing with guidewire under transesophageal echocardiography are the important steps.[49] The short delivery sheath is exchanged with the guide wire for deployment of muscular device. The procedure carries less morbidity and complications if it is performed by the experienced people.

SPECIAL CHALLENGES IN VSD

VSD with Pneumonia

- For infants with large VSDs who develop a pneumonia, it is generally advisable to operate at the first "window" of opportunity rather than wait for complete resolution of infection. This is especially true for ventilated infants who may never improve enough to be extubated. Using the following criteria developed at the Amrita Institute of Medical Sciences, it is possible to identify a suitable window for surgical closure in ventilated babies with pneumonia.[50]
  - Absence of fever for 48 hours or longer
  - Decreasing leukocyte counts, if initially increased, and increasing platelet counts, if initially reduced
  - At least partial radiologic clearance of lung infiltrates
  - Improved arterial blood gases using pressure-controlled ventilation with maximum peak inspiratory pressures of 30–35 mm Hg and tidal volumes of 10 mL/kg
  - Unequivocal documentation of predominant left-to-right systolic shunting on color Doppler echocardiography.

VSD with Undernutrition

A series of studies from India have consistently shown that in a well-developed pediatric cardiac surgical program, undernutrition is no longer a risk factor for surgery. These babies should be operated at the earliest instance without the need for prolonged nutritional supplementation preoperatively. In general, it is no longer acceptable to target weight thresholds for VSD closure surgery.[51,52] After surgery, these babies show impressive early catch up growth[53]; however, late growth may be suboptimal especially in those who were severely undernourished initially.[54,55]

CONCLUSION

The VSD is one of the most common congenital heart malformations that present variably depending on the size of the defect. It is essential to appreciate the anatomy of the defect as it has an important bearing on natural history and treatment approaches. While this lesion is a source for considerable mortality and morbidity especially in the Indian setting, it is possible now to address almost all clinical challenges with VSD and enable an excellent long-term outlook. The approach for a large VSD in a young infant is now clearly shifted toward early closure to minimize the complications relating to undernutrition from feeding difficulty, recurrent respiratory infections, and development of PVOD.

REFERENCES

1. Moller JH, Moodie DS, Blees M, Norton JB, Nouri S. Symptomatic heart disease in infants: comparison of three studies performed during 1969–1987. Pediatr Cardiol. 1995;16(5):216-22.
2. Hoffman JIE, Kaplan S. The incidence of congenital heart disease. J Am Coll Cardiol. 2002;39(12):1890-900.
3. Garg V, Kathiriya IS, Barnes R, Schluterman MK, King IN, Butler CA, et al. GATA4 mutations cause human congenital heart defects and reveal an interaction with TBX5. Nature. 2003; 424(6947): 443-7.

4. Nora JJ, Nora AH. The genetic contribution to congenital heart disease. In: Nora JJ, Takao A, (Eds). Congenital Heart Disease Mount Kisco. New York: Futura Publishing Company; 1984.
5. Lamers W, Moorman A. Cardiac septation. Circ Res. 2002;91(2): 93-103.
6. Wenink A. Embryology of the ventricular septum. Separate origin of its components. Virchows Archiv A Pathological Anatomy and Histology. 1981;390(1):71-9.
7. Franco D, Meilhac S, Christoffels V, Kispert A, Buckingham M, Kelly R. Left and right ventricular contributions to the formation of the interventricular septum in the mouse heart. Dev Biol. 2006;294(2):366-75.
8. Ya J, van den Hoff M, de Boer P, Tesink-Taekema S, Franco D, Moorman A, et al. Normal development of the outflow tract in the rat. Circ Res. 1998;82(4):464-72.
9. Webb S, Qayyum S, Anderson R, Lamers W, Richardson M. Septation and separation within the outflow tract of the developing heart. J Anat. 2003;202(4):327-42.
10. Soto B, Becker AE, Moulaert AJ, Lie JT, Anderson RH. Classification of ventricular septal defects. Br Heart J. 1980;43(3):332-43.
11. Kirklin JK, Castaneda AR, Keane JF, Fellows KE, Norwood WI. Surgical management of multiple ventricular septal defects. J Thorac Cardiovasc Surg. 1980;80(4):485-93.
12. Jacobs JP, Burke RP, Quintessenza JA, Mavroudis C. Congenital Heart Surgery Nomenclature and Database Project: ventricular septal defect. Ann Thorac Surg. 2000;69(4 Suppl):S25-35.
13. Rabinovitch M, Haworth SG, Castaneda AR, Nadas AS, Reid LM. Lung biopsy in congenital heart disease: a morphometric approach to pulmonary vascular disease. Circulation. 1978; 58(6):1107-22.
14. Keith JD, Rose V, Collins G, Kidd BS. Ventricular septal defect. Incidence, morbidity, and mortality in various age groups. Br Heart J. 1971; 33(Suppl):81-7
15. Kirklin J, Kouchoukos N. Kirklin/Barratt-Boyes Cardiac Surgery. Philadelphia: Elsevier/Saunders; 2013.p. 16.
16. Freedom R. The natural and modified history of congenital heart disease. Elmsford: Blackwell Pub./Futura; 2004.
17. Nir A, Weintraub Z, Oliven A, Kelener J, Lurie M. Anatomic evidence of spontaneous intrauterine closure of a ventricular septal defect. Pediatr Cardiol. 1990;11(4):208-10.
18. Mesko Z, Jones J, Nadas A. Diminution and closure of large ventricular septal defects after pulmonary artery banding. Circulation. 1973, 48(4):[illegible].
19. Anderson R, Lenox C, Zuberbuhler J. Mechanisms of closure of perimembranous ventricular septal defect. Am J Cardiol. 1983; 52(3):341-5.
20. Krovetz L. Spontaneous closure of ventricular septal defect. Am J Cardiol. 1998;81(1):100-1.
21. Pongiglione G, Freedom R, Cook D, Rowe R. Mechanism of acquired right ventricular outflow tract obstruction in patients with ventricular septal defect: an angiocardiographic study. Am J Cardiol. 1982;50(4):776-80.
22. Corone P, Doyon F, Gaudeau S, Guérin F, Vernant P, Ducam H, et al. Natural history of ventricular septal defect. A study involving 790 cases. Circulation. 1977;55(6):908-15.
23. Nadas AS. Report from the Joint Study on the Natural History of Congenital Heart Defects. I. General introduction. Circulation. 1977;56(1 Suppl):I3-I4.24.
24. Gasul BM, Dillon RF, Vrla V, Hait G. Ventricular septal defects; their natural transformation into the cyanotic or noncyanotic type of tetralogy of Fallot. J Am Med Assoc. 1957;164(8):847-53.
25. Momma K, Toyama K, Takao A, Ando M, Nakazawa M, Hirosawa K, et al. Natural history of subarterial infundibular ventricular septal defect. Am Heart J. 1984;108(5):1312-7.
26. Cox K, Algaze-Yojay C, Punn R, Silverman N. The natural and unnatural history of ventricular septal defects presenting in infancy: an echocardiography-based review. J Am Soc Echocardiography. 2020;33(6):763-70.
27. Shah P, Singh WS, Rose V, Keith JD. Incidence of bacterial endocarditis in ventricular septal defects. Circulation. 1966; 34(1):127-31.
28. Zakrzewski T, Keith J. Bacterial endocarditis in infants and children. J Pediatr. 1965;67:1179.
29. Van Hare GF, Soffer LJ, Sivakoff MC, Liebman J. Twenty-five-year experience with ventricular septal defect in infants and children. Am Heart J. 1987;114(3):606-14.
30. Lucas RV Jr, Adams P Jr, Anderson RC, Meyne NG, Lillehei CW, Varco RL. The natural history of isolated ventricular septal defect. A serial physiologic study. Circulation. 1961;24:1372-87.
31. Neumayer U, Stone S, Somerville J. Small ventricular septal defects in adults. Eur Heart J. 1998;19(10):1573-82.
32. Campbell M. Natural history of ventricular septal defect. Heart. 1971;33(2):246-57.
33. Spicer DE, Hsu HH, Co-Vu J, Anderson RH, Fricker FJ. Ventricular septal defects. Orphanet J Rare Dis. 2014;9:144.
34. Weidman WH, Blount Jr. SG, Dushane JW, Gersony WM, Hayes CJ, Nadas AS. Clinical course in ventricular septal defect. Circulation. 1977;56(1 Suppl):I56-69.
35. Minette MS, Sahn DJ. Ventricular septal defect. Circulation. 2006;114:2190-7.
36. Cheatham JP, Latson LA, Gutgesell HP. Ventricular septal defect in infancy: detection with two dimensional echocardiography. Am J Cardiol. 1981;47(1):85-9.
37. Sutherland GR, Godman MJ, Smallhorn JF, Guiterras P, Anderson RH, Hunter S. Ventricular septal defects: two dimensional echocardiographic and morphological correlations. Br Heart J. 1982;47(4):316—28.
38. Kumar RK, Sandoval J. Advanced pulmonary vascular disease: the Eisenmenger syndrome. Cardiol Young. 2009;19 Suppl 1: 622-6.
39. Viswanathan S, Kumar RK. Assessment of operability of congenital cardiac shunts with increased pulmonary vascular resistance. Catheter Cardiovasc Interv. 2008;71(5):665-70.
40. Walker WJ, Garcia-Gonzalez E, Hall R, Czarnecki SW, Franklin RB, Das SK, et al. Interventricular septal defect: analysis of 41 catheterized cases, ninety with serial hemodynamic studies. Circulation. 1965;31:54-[illegible]
41. Myers PO, Tissot C, Beghetti M. Assessment of operability of patients with pulmonary arterial hypertension associated with congenital heart disease. Circ J. 2014;78(1):4-11.
42. Artman M, Graham TP Jr. Congestive heart failure in infancy: recognition and management. Am Heart J. 1982;103(6):1040-55.
43. Montigny M, Davignon A, Fouron JC, Biron P, Fournier A, Elie R. Captopril in infants for congestive heart failure secondary to a large ventricular left-to-right shunt. Am J Cardiol. 1989;63(9): 631-3.
44. Saxena A, Relan J, Agarwal R, Awasthy N, Azad S, Chakrabarty M, et al. Indian guidelines for indications and timing of intervention for common congenital heart diseases: revised and updated consensus statement of the Working Group on Management of Congenital Heart Diseases. Ann Ped Card. 2019;12(3):254-86.
45. Lun K, Li H, Leung MP, Chau AK, Yung T, Chiu CS, et al. Analysis of indications for surgical closure of subarterial ventricular septal defect without associated aortic cusp prolapse and aortic regurgitation. Am J Cardiol. 2001;87(11):1266-70.
46. Brown S, Boshoff D, Rega F, Eyskens B, Meyns B, Gewillig M. Dilatable pulmonary artery banding in infants with low birth

weight or complex congenital heart disease allows avoidance or postponement of subsequent surgery. Eur J Cardiothorac Surg 2010;37(2):296-301.

47. Butera G, Carminati M, Chessa M, Piazza L, Micheletti A, Negura DG, et al. Transcatheter closure of perimembranous ventricular septal defects: early and long-term results. JACC. 2007;50(12):1189-95.
48. Holzer R, Balzer D, Cao QL, Lock K, Hijazi ZM. Device closure of muscular ventricular septal defects using the Amplatzer muscular ventricular septal defect occluder: immediate and mid-term results of a U.S. registry. JACC. 2004;43(7):1257-63.
49. Crossland DS, Wilkinson JL, Cochrane AD, D'udekem Y, Brizard CP, Lane GK. Initial results of primary device closure of large muscular ventricular septal defects in early infancy using perventricular access. Cathet Cardiovasc Interv. 2008;72(3): 386-91.
50. Bhatt M, Roth S, Kumar RK, Gauvreau K, Chengode S, Nair SG, et al. Management of infants with large, unrepaired left-to-right shunts and respiratory infection requiring mechanical ventilation. J Thorac Cardiovasc Surg. 2004;127(5):1466-73.
51. Vaidyanathan B, Roth SJ, Rao SG, Gauvreau K, Shivaprakasha K, Kumar RK. Outcome of ventricular septal defect repair in a developing country. J Pediatr. 2002;140(6):736-41.
52. Reddy SN, Kappanayil M, Balachandran R, Sudhakar A, Sunil GS, Raj BR, et al. Preoperative determinants of outcomes of infant heart surgery in a limited-resource setting. Semin Thorac Cardiovasc Surg. 2015;27(3):331-8.
53. Banerji N, Sudhakar A, Balachandran R, Sunil G, Kotayil B, Krishna Kumar R. Early weight trends after congenital heart surgery and their determinants. Cardiology in the Young. Cardiol Young, 2020;30(1):89-94.
54. Vaidyanathan B, Radhakrishnan R, Aravindakshan DS, Sundaram KR, Kumar RK. What determines nutritional recovery in malnourished children undergoing correction of congenital heart defects? A prospective study. Pediatrics. 2009;124(2): e294-9.
55. Vaidyanathan B, Roth S, Gauvreau K, Shivaprakasha K, Rao SG, Kumar RK. Somatic growth after ventricular septal defect repair in malnourished infants. J Pediatr. 2006;149(2): 205-9.

23 CHAPTER

Patent Ductus Arteriosus

Anand Subramanian, M Jayranganath

HISTORY AND BACKGROUND

The ductus arteriosus, derived from the upper portion of the sixth arterial arch, connects the pulmonary artery to the descending aorta. Although known to Galen as early as 131 AD, and beautifully illustrated by Rokitansky in 1844, it has been erroneously named after the 16th century Italian physician, L Bottalo.[1] The vessel is an essential part of fetal circulation in terrestrial vertebrates and diverts the right (or single) ventricular output to the placenta via the descending aorta for oxygenation. Absence of the ductus in the human fetus has been shown to play a role in the pathogenesis of certain cardiac conditions such as tetralogy of Fallot with absent pulmonary valve and persistent truncus arteriosus.[2,3] While its postnatal patency is essential for survival of a newborn in the setting of congenital heart disease with a duct-dependent pulmonary or systemic circulation, continued patency in others is undesirable. The present chapter focuses on the patent ductus arteriosus (PDA) in term infants.

EMBRYOLOGY AND ANATOMY

The proximal portions of the sixth pair of embryonic arches persist as the right and left pulmonary arteries. The distal portion of the left sixth arch persists as the ductus arteriosus while the distal portion of the right sixth arch involutes. The ductus arteriosus in most is thus a left-sided structure, which connects the main pulmonary trunk near the origin of the left pulmonary artery to the descending aorta, 5–10 mm distal to the origin of the left subclavian artery.[4] Variations do exist in infants with arch anomalies. The ductus still remains left-sided in the majority of those with a right aortic arch; its aortic attachment in these cases is usually from the base of the innominate artery.[5] In 10% of those with a right aortic arch, the ductus may be right-sided and connect the main pulmonary artery to the descending aorta.[6] A left aortic arch with a right ductus is extremely rare. Bilateral ducts have been described.[7] The ductal diameter in intrauterine life is nearly the same as the descending aorta. Postnatal constriction begins at the pulmonic end and progresses to the aortic end; hence, most patent ducts have a funnel-shaped appearance. Histologically, the ductus arteriosus has a greater proportion of spirally arranged smooth muscle in its media as against elastic fibers in the two adjacent great arteries that it connects. The ductus arteriosus is more sensitive to higher pO_2 at increasing gestational ages, which constricts the ductus at birth in term neonates by mechanisms involving inhibition of Kv channels, membrane depolarization and activation of the L-type, and voltage-gated calcium channel.[8] Functional closure is achieved within 12 hours of birth and anatomic closure by the next 2–3 weeks.[9] A ductus that does not close by 3 months in a term infant does not do so later. Initial closure is by formation of intimal cushions which protrude into the lumen and migration of smooth muscle cells into the wall of the ductus. This is followed by endothelial infolding, disruption of the internal elastic lamina, subintimal cytolytic necrosis with hemorrhage, and formation of mucoid lakes in the medial wall.[10] Eventually, fibrosis sets in to form the ligamentum arteriosum. Prostaglandins have the opposite effect and maintain patency of the duct. PGE2, produced by the placenta is more potent than PGI2 in maintaining ductal patency and this is again more pronounced in preterm neonates.[11] The commercially available PGE1 is equally effective in keeping the ductus open. Loss of the placental source of prostaglandins at birth and their removal by the lung vascular bed promote normal ductal closure. The closure of the ductus is thus dependent on the interplay of several factors such as oxygen and vasoconstrictors on one hand and prostaglandins on the other. The incidence of patent ductus has been found to be 10 times greater at an altitude of 4,700 meters above sea level.[12] Pulmonary diseases, including meconium aspiration syndrome, may delay ductal closure in term neonates.

INCIDENCE AND GENETICS

The incidence of PDA in term infants is 1:2,000 and constitutes up to 10% of all congenital heart diseases.[13] PDA is two times more common in females. 5% of the siblings of an index case will also have PDA, suggesting a genetic component.[14] An epidemiological study from India showed a 78% prevalence of congenital heart disease among 137 laboratory confirmed congenital rubella syndrome infants; of these 63% were PDA.[15] Heritable PDAs have been described in animal models and 8–11% of humans with PDA have a chromosomal abnormality.[16] Trisomy 21, Noonan syndrome, Cri-du-chat, and CHARGE syndrome have been associated with PDA. Char syndrome consists of PDA, facial anomalies, and minor skeletal anomalies with mutations in the transcription factor TFAP2B, expressed in neural crest cells.[8] The higher prevalence of PDA in Iran (15%) has been attributed to consanguinity and a single locus on chromosome 12q24p.[17] Congenital ductal aneurysms may be seen in the third trimester and are characterized by abnormal dilatation of the aortic end and a stenosed pulmonary end. They may also be seen following surgical ligation or catheter interventions. Marfan syndrome, Loeys-Dietz, and Ehlers–Danlos syndromes have been associated with ductal aneurysms. Mutations in genes encoding vascular smooth muscle cell (VSMC) contractile proteins have been associated with familial thoracic aortic aneurysm, aortic dissection, and PDA.[18]

NATURAL HISTORY

Spontaneous closure of ducts in term infants is very rare beyond 3 months of age.[13] However, in 1968, Campbell published a follow-up of children and adults (11 examples in 1,842 patient-years) with a clinical diagnosis of PDA and estimated the rate of spontaneous closure as 0.6% per annum during the first four decades.[19] The rate of spontaneous closure in preterm ducts is also much higher than previously thought and is inversely proportional to gestational age and birth weight. Clyman et al. reported spontaneous closure in 98% of preterms born at a gestational age >30 weeks, a week after birth while only 13% with a gestational age of 24 weeks had closed by day 7.[20] Symptoms of heart failure in infancy are dependent on the rapidity with which the pulmonary vascular resistance (PVR) declines. Those with a more gradual decline in PVR have fewer manifestations of heart failure, even with moderate-to-large shunts, as the left ventricle adapts to the volume overload. The ductus, being a dynamic structure, may have a varied presentation with respect to the age of onset of symptoms and development of fixed pulmonary hypertension. Hence, one may occasionally see a large PDA in an adolescent or young adult shunting left-to-right with features of left ventricular volume overload. Such patients may be symptomatic with exercise-induced fatigue or dyspnea and be largely asymptomatic at rest. If a moderate-to-large PDA has not been treated in childhood, they may present with symptoms of heart failure by the 3rd to 6th decades of life.[21] Chronic atrial dilatation may predispose to atrial fibrillation in 25% of adults over the age of 50 years.[22] Congestive cardiac failure has been the most common cause of death in moderate-to-large ducts in various natural history studies in the postantibiotic era.[19-22]

The Eisenmenger syndrome in PDA is usually established within the first 2 years of life and this did not occur if the diameter of the ductus was <5 mm.[23] The length of the ductus is inversely related to the age of occurrence of irreversible pulmonary hypertension as ductal length confers inherent resistance to flow (Poiseuille's law) and also contributes to periods of relatively reduced flow from intermittent contraction. The average age of presentation in PDA with Eisenmenger syndrome was 19 years and average age of death was 33 years.[24] Survival in this subset is around 87% at 5 years and 77% at 20 years since diagnosis.[25] Clinical features may include exertional fatigue (due to fixed cardiac output), hemoptysis, and right heart failure. Breathlessness is less often described, as oxygenated blood still reaches the cerebral circulation, unlike those with atrial or ventricular septal defects with Eisenmenger syndrome.[24]

The cumulative incidence of infective endocarditis (IE) in children (0–18 years) with PDA was found to be 0.32% with an incidence rate of 3.5/10,000 person-years.[26] IE risk is usually limited to children <4 years of age and is probably due to most children having undergone closure of the defect by that time. According to Lloyd and Beekman, the risk of IE in a silent PDA was 1,000-fold lesser than in those with a continuous murmur.[27] A Swedish study of 3 million deaths from 1960 to 1993 in their country, reported only 2 deaths attributable to IE in PDA.[28]

Ductus arteriosus aneurysm is a localized saccular or tubular dilatation of the ductus arteriosus. Congenital aneurysms of the ductus may be seen in the third trimester of pregnancy and most occur within the first 2 months after birth. They may be seen in association with connective tissue disorders such as Ehlers–Danlos and Marfan syndromes. Most have a narrow pulmonary artery end with minimal flow. Complications include rupture, thrombosis with thrombus extension into the pulmonary artery or aorta, stridor or erosion into the airways.[29]

PATHOPHYSIOLOGY

The effects of a PDA are determined by the diameter of the ductus at its pulmonary end, ductal length, and pulmonary and systemic vascular resistance. At birth, the PVR is high. It falls precipitously with the onset of respiration and continues to decline over the next 4–6 weeks. The mean pulmonary artery pressure declines to half systemic pressure by the end of the first day and drops to the adult level by the end of 2 weeks.[30] Thus, PDA flows may be noted soon after birth. The direction of flow may be transiently bidirectional in the first few days of life and eventually becomes fully left to right with the fall in PVR.[31] A small PDA has a Qp:Qs of <1.5 and does not cause volume overload of the left heart. The pulmonary artery pressure is normal in those with a small PDA. A moderate-sized ductus with Qp:Qs of 1.5–2.2 causes significant increase in pulmonary venous return and leads to left atrial and ventricular volume overload. The pulmonary artery pressure is elevated but is less than two-thirds of the systemic arterial pressure. A large PDA has a shunt fraction exceeding 2.2:1, leads to left atrial and ventricular volume overload with pulmonary artery pressures more than two-thirds the systemic arterial pressure, at times being equisystemic.[32]

Symptoms of heart failure may become less pronounced even with moderate and large ducts as the child grows older, as the left ventricle adapts and remodels to the chronic volume overload. If a large ductus has not been diagnosed and treated in infancy, obliterative changes begin to develop in the pulmonary vascular bed, eventually leading to fixed pulmonary vascular obstructive disease. The shunt becomes bidirectional once again before getting abolished, and the ductus may start shunting predominantly right to left. Disappearance of heart failure signs beyond infancy should thus not be erroneously construed to indicate spontaneous closure. A large ductus would rarely, if ever, close spontaneously.

Although the incidence has declined, small and moderate-sized ducts have a risk of developing infective endarteritis. The high velocity jet needed to cause endothelial damage is not seen with large ducts and silent ducts (small ducts with minimal flow detected only on echocardiogram) and these two opposite extremes of ductal flow would not usually predispose to development of infective endarteritis. Besides involvement of the ductal tissue and adjacent pulmonary artery wall, endocarditis involving the pulmonary valve is well documented.[33]

CLINICAL FEATURES AND SIGNS[34]

Small Patent Ductus Arteriosus

Infants with a small PDA are asymptomatic and usually come to medical attention due to a murmur. They may be prone to development of infective endarteritis. The heart sounds are normal, there is no cardiomegaly and the murmur may be continuous; more often predominantly systolic (the diastolic component not being well appreciated due to the small amount of shunt flow) in the first and second intercostal space.

Moderate-sized Patent Ductus Arteriosus

They may become symptomatic after the first 2 months of life and present with mild tachypnea, interrupted feeding, head sweating, failure to thrive, and recurrent chest infections.

The wide pulse pressure leads to bounding peripheral pulses and is one of the hallmark physical signs in an infant or child with a moderate-to-large PDA. The pulse has a brisk rise and collapses rapidly. Diastolic pressure in the aorta falls due to run off from the descending aorta to pulmonary artery and increased force of ventricular contraction due to left ventricular volume overload (which counters the effect of systolic run off) maintains a higher systolic pressure head in the aorta to cause a wide pulse pressure. There is a hyperdynamic left ventricular apex. The apex may be shifted downward and outward due to cardiomegaly. A restrictive ductus may have a palpable thrill, often continuous. The first heart sound is normal and the second heart sound may be normally split, often less discernible due to the continuous murmur. Gibson precisely characterized the murmur of the patent ductus and the continuous machinery murmur with eddy sounds rightfully bears an eponym. The timing and configuration of the murmur reflect the pressures and resistances across the pulmonary and systemic circuits. When the neonatal PVR is still high, the flow is predominantly systolic and only a faint systolic murmur may be appreciated. With the fall in neonatal PVR, the murmur becomes truly continuous. Although a pressure gradient exists between the aorta and pulmonary artery throughout the cardiac cycle, the murmur gets reinforced during mid systole and this delay following left ventricular contraction is due to the time taken for blood to reach the descending aorta. The murmur peaks around the second heart sound for this reason and gradually fades away toward the end of diastole. A small and moderate-sized ductus would have a continuous murmur. It is important to note that a continuous murmur only envelops the second heart sound and need not be present in the initial period of systole or toward the end of diastole. Eddy sounds are generated due to a collision of wave fronts from forward flow into the ductus from the right ventricular outflow tract and retrograde flow into the pulmonary artery from the descending aorta.

Large Patent Ductus Arteriosus

Symptoms of heart failure, as mentioned above for a moderate-sized ductus, are more pronounced with a large ductus. A long-standing moderate-to-large ductus may have a precordial bulge due to a volume overloaded left ventricle and pressure overloaded right ventricle. Prominent pulmonary artery pulsations may be palpable in the left second intercostal space. A left parasternal heave suggests a hypertensive ductus with equisystemic right ventricular pressures. The first heart sound is normal. The second heart sound may be paradoxically split in children with a large PDA (P2 occurs earlier than A2). The increased pulmonary venous return must traverse the aortic valve and ascending aorta before the shunt occurs at the descending aortic level through the ductus. This leads to prolonged left ventricular ejection and a delayed A2. P2 occurs earlier as there is a rapid increase in pulmonary artery pressure after right ventricular systole due to additional retrograde pressure transmitted from ductal flow.

A large ductus with equisystemic pulmonary artery pressures may again have only a faint systolic murmur as diastolic pressures in the two great arteries are equal and flow in diastole diminishes. Although flow in systole also reduces in these situations, augmented left ventricular contraction aids in some forward flow, giving rise to the systolic component of the murmur. A mid-diastolic flow murmur may be heard at the mitral area due to increased pulmonary venous return and transmitral flow.

Patent Ductus Arteriosus with Eisenmenger Physiology

This is recognized by differential cyanosis andclubbing with pink hands and fingers and blue toes. If the right subclavian artery arises anomalously from the descending aorta, the right arm may also be blue in addition to the lower extremities. Differential saturation in borderline situations may be better appreciated by asking the child to walk briskly or climb a flight of stairs. The normal increase in pulmonary blood flow during exercise would not occur once the pulmonary microvascular bed has developed obliterative changes, leading to increased right-to-left shunt and differential saturation.

The pulse pressure may normalize when the shunt decreases due to pulmonary vascular obstructive disease. The pulse pressure may again become wide in a child with a large PDA with irreversible pulmonary vascular changes with the onset of pulmonary regurgitation. The diastolic run off in this case happens across the incompetent pulmonary valve into the right ventricle. The disappearance of heart failure symptoms with reappearance of a wide pulse pressure is an ominous symptom–sign combination.

With fixed pulmonary vascular hypertension, there is no cardiomegaly, the apex may be formed by the right ventricle and the left parasternal heave becomes more prominent.

The jugular venous pulse is unremarkable. Right heart failure in PDA with Eisenmenger is a late occurrence as the ductus acts as a pop-off and prevents the right ventricular pressure from becoming suprasystemic. Such young adults may have an elevated jugular venous pressure; although wave forms usually remain normal. With the onset of irreversible pulmonary hypertension, the second heart sound may be narrowly split or single, with a loud pulmonary component. With established pulmonary vascular occlusive disease, the hypertensive right ventricle pumps as vigorously as the left ventricle and the contributory effect of the left ventricle to systolic flows is lost and no murmur is heard. An early diastolic, high-pitched sound from pulmonary regurgitation may then be audible in the second intercostal space. As a corollary, the presence of a continuous murmur in the setting of a patent ductus rules out severe pulmonary arterial hypertension.

DIAGNOSTIC EVALUATION

Chest X-ray

Moderate-to-large shunts would manifest with cardiomegaly, the left ventricle forming the apex, with features of increased pulmonary vascularity (**Fig. 1**). The increased pulmonary venous return has to traverse the ascending aorta before shunting at the level of the duct. The degree of ascending aortic dilation would be proportional to the shunt. Even in cases where the ascending aortic shadow may not conspicuously form the right heart border, its junction with the transverse arch (aortic knob) is conspicuous on the left. The ductus per se, may form a shadow between the arch and the pulmonary trunk (**Figs. 2A and B**). The ductal hump might be more conspicuous with an aneurysm of the ductus. Older adults may have a calcified ductus.[35]

When the shunt reverses due to fixed pulmonary hypertension, the cardiac size may be normal and the apex may be formed by the right ventricle. The central pulmonary artery would appear dilated with peripheral pruning. The ascending aorta stays dilated and may help in differentiating from Eisenmenger complex with ventricular septal defect, where the aorta does not dilate.

Electrocardiogram

The QRS axis may be superior in children with rubella; else the axis is usually normal. Features of left atrial abnormality and left ventricular volume overload, suggested by deep Q waves in left precordial leads, are seen with moderate and large shunts. These Q waves may be lost once the shunt becomes bidirectional and their absence is an important sign, suggesting inoperability. Similarly, features of combined ventricular hypertrophy may be replaced by prominent right ventricular forces, right axis deviation, and right atrial

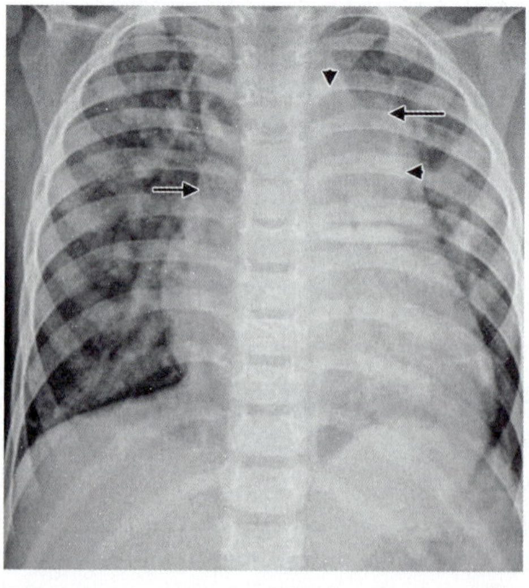

Fig. 1: Chest X-ray posteroanterior (PA) view from a child with a large patent ductus arteriosus (PDA). The arrow on the right heart border is the dilated ascending aorta. The aortic knob and enlarged pulmonary artery are depicted by arrowheads along the left heart border with the ductal shadow (arrow) in between.

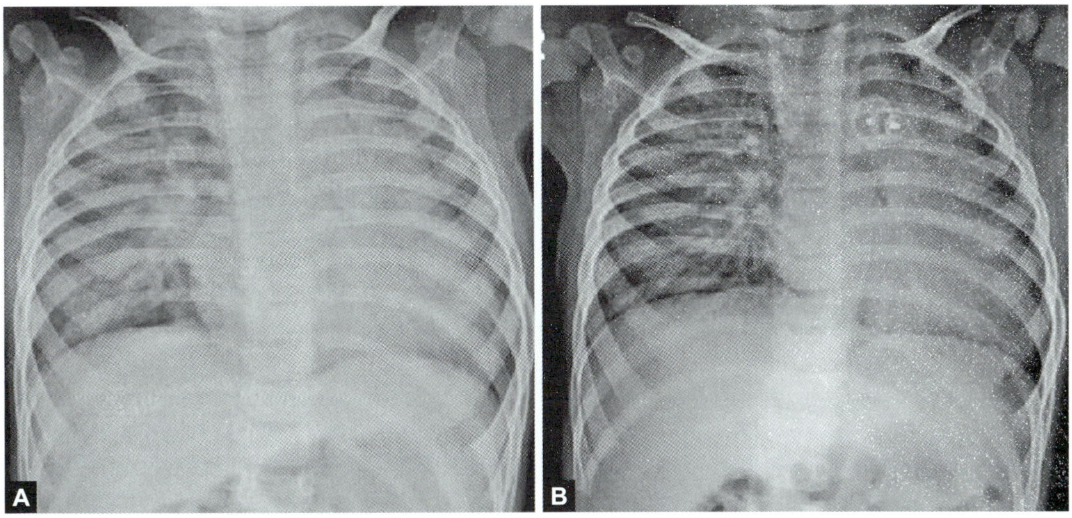

Figs. 2A and B: Chest X-ray PA view in a child pre (A) and postdevice closure (B) of a large PDA. Note the immediate decrease in vascularity in the chest X-ray (B), taken a day after the procedure.

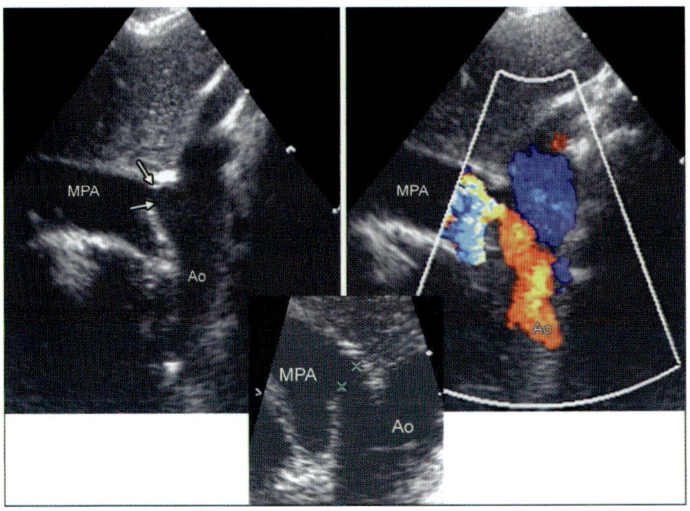

Fig. 3: Two-dimensional echocardiogram depicting the ductal view. The panel on the left shows the various structures visualized in this view. The two small arrows point to the pulmonary arterial end of the ductus. Color Doppler on the right shows the red flow indicating left-to-right shunt. The enlarged figure (middle) shows the measured size of the PDA (green cross marks).
(Ao: aorta; MPA: main pulmonary artery)

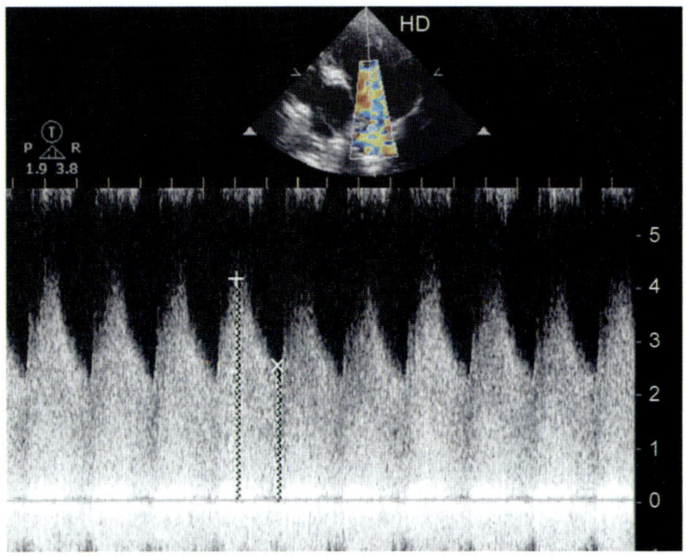

Fig. 4: Spectral Doppler pattern showing continuous flow and gradient in a moderate-sized, restrictive ductus. Systolic peak gradient approaches 64 mm Hg (4 m/s), while the diastolic gradient approaches 25 mm Hg (2.5 m/s).

abnormality in children with large ducts and irreversible pulmonary hypertension.

Echocardiogram

The ductus can be visualized in the short axis view at the level of the great arteries, especially with the use of color Doppler. The high parasternal "ductal view" precisely defines the ductal anatomy as it visualizes the descending aorta, the entire length of the ductus, its insertion into the pulmonary artery, and relation to the left pulmonary artery (**Fig. 3**). Suprasternal arch views help determine the sidedness of the arch and variations in ductal anatomy in those situations. The ductal flow is seen as a red flow from the descending aorta to the pulmonary artery, when it shunts left to right. The main and branch pulmonary arteries appear dilated. The left ventricle and atrium will be dilated in moderate and large shunts and long-standing volume overload may lead to mitral regurgitation. Doppler interrogation shows a continuous Doppler spectral pattern throughout the cardiac cycle in restrictive ducts and the peak systolic velocity helps determine the gradient and indirectly gives an estimation of the pulmonary artery systolic pressure (**Fig. 4**). With large ducts, diastolic gradients progressively diminish and only a low velocity systolic flow may be appreciated. Reversal of shunt with severe pulmonary hypertension may show the Doppler spectrum to appear below the baseline. Post ligation or device closure, it is important to look at device position, assess residual flow, and ensure unobstructed flow in the left pulmonary artery and descending aorta.

Computed tomography (CT) and cardiac magnetic resonance (CMR) studies are not required in the vast majority of cases. Cardiac CT is more often useful in adults presenting with pulmonary hypertension to rule out a large ductus as the cause of the condition as echocardiographic windows may be suboptimal and color flow may not be helpful as flows are minimal in these patients. Ductus arteriosus aneurysms and unusual ductal morphologies, especially in patients with arch anomalies, may also be better visualized using cardiac CT or CMR. A ligamentum arteriosum or diverticulum of the ductus may also contribute to the formation of a vascular ring and precise characterization prior to surgery is usually done with these imaging modalities. CMR gives more precise measurements of pulmonary and systemic blood flow (Qp/Qs) compared to those obtained in the cardiac catheterization laboratory using the Fick principle. For the same reason, diagnostic cardiac catheterization for PDA has become obsolete and a child with PDA undergoes cardiac catheterization only with an intention to treat.

MANAGEMENT

Small ducts usually require no management in infancy and may be observed. They may be considered for closure toward the end of the first year to mitigate the risk of infective endarteritis. Silent ducts should not be closed. Indomethacin and similar agents have no role in closure of a PDA in term babies. Moderate and large ducts may need diuretics as part of decongestive therapy to minimize symptoms. Angiotensin-converting enzyme inhibitors (ACEI) have no proven role in the management of heart failure symptoms as the systemic vascular resistance is already reduced due to diastolic run off. The use of digoxin for heart failure due to shunt lesions is again controversial.[36] Moderate and large ducts can both be safely closed surgically, but most ducts are currently amenable to transcatheter closure using various occluder devices (**Figs. 2B and 5**). Although the ADO-II AS and Piccolo devices are recently available for closure of PDA in preterms and low birth weight babies, surgical ligation may be preferred in this subset, especially if the PDA is larger than 4 mm. Mortality rates following these procedures are almost close to nil in the current era and procedural complication rates are usually <2%.[37-39] Hence, a symptomatic baby with a large ductus should have ductal closure as soon as possible. Moderate-sized ducts are usually closed in the cardiac catheterization laboratory between 6 months and 1 year of age. Coils are made of stainless steel with embedded Dacron fibers to increase thrombogenicity. They are delivered using detachable delivery systems and can be safely used for ducts measuring <3 mm at the pulmonary arterial end. For larger ducts, most operators now use duct occluder devices made of nitinol with polyester fibers sewn into the device to increase thrombogenicity. Complications following device closure of PDA are rare and include device migration, infection, impingement on surrounding structures leading to aortic coarctation or stenosis of the left pulmonary artery, residual shunts with hemolysis, and rarely dissection of the ductus. IE prophylaxis is recommended for a period of 6 months after device closure or surgical ligation to allow for endothelialization and complete cessation of flow. Transient hypertension (secondary to the Branham effect) and transient left ventricular dysfunction (secondary to sudden increase in afterload) may complicate closure of moderate and large ducts. They usually respond to a short course of ACEI or systemic vasodilators. Post-PDA ligation

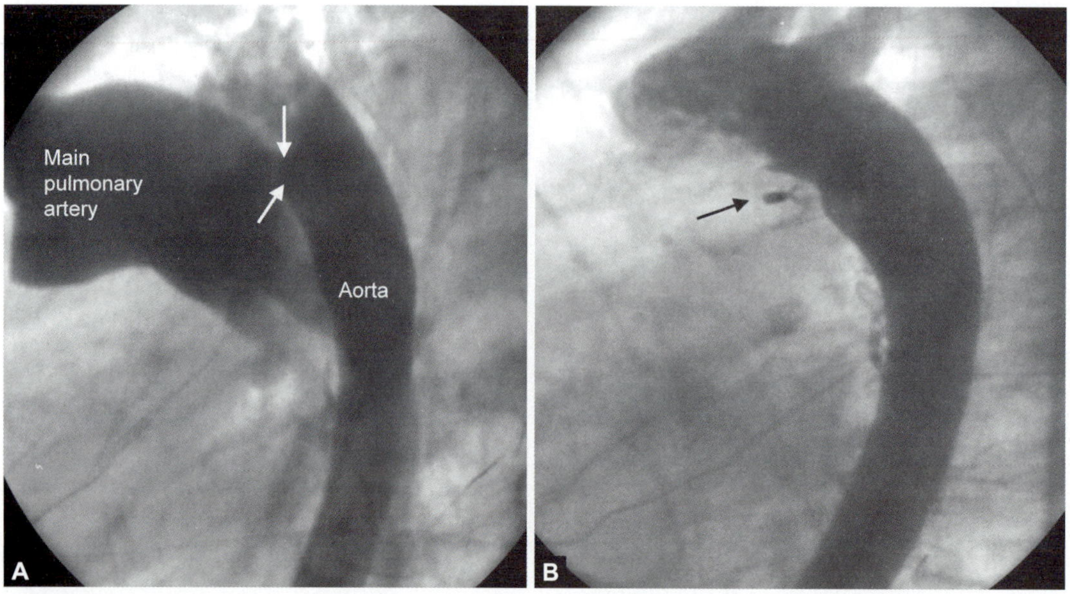

Figs. 5A and B: Lateral descending aortic angiogram depicting a large, short patent ductus arteriosus (PDA) (A) closed successfully with an Amplatzer duct occluder device (B). White arrows in (A) indicate the duct and a black arrow in (B) points to the duct occluder device that has completely occluded the PDA.

syndrome seen in neonates after surgical ligation results in ventricular dysfunction and hypotension, needing transient inotropic support.[40] Surgical ligation is usually carried out by a lateral thoracotomy and triple ligation is the standard procedure across most centers worldwide. Symptomatic ductal aneurysms and those with impending complications need surgical excision. Video-assisted thoracoscopic procedures are carried out in some centers to minimize scar and morbidity.

Large PDAs with borderline operability are best managed in tertiary referral centers and the decision to close such ducts needs to be individualized and calls for a comprehensive approach. Due to the inherent fallacies in oximetry with a PDA, trial occlusion using a balloon or device to document a fall in mean pulmonary artery pressures without a corresponding drop in systemic pressures may be a better guide to operability. However, the long-term outcome following closure in such cases is still unknown. In those who are deemed inoperable, standard pulmonary hypertension treatment medications such as phosphodiesterase inhibitors (sildenafil and tadalafil), endothelin receptor antagonists (bosentan, ambrisentan and macitentan), inhaled prostanoids, and other supportive therapy provides symptomatic benefit and helps improve functional capacity.

REFERENCES

1. Boyer NH. Patent ductus arteriosus: some historical highlights. Ann Thorac Surg. 1967; 4(6):570-3.
2. Van Praagh R, Van Praagh S. The anatomy of common aorticopulmonary trunk (truncus arteriosus communis) and its embryologic implications. A study of 57 necropsy cases. Am J Cardiol. 1965;16(3):406-25.
3. Emmanoulides GC, Thanopoulos B, Siassi B, Fishbein M. "Agenesis" of ductus arteriosus associated with the syndrome of tetralogy of Fallot and absent pulmonary valve. Am J Cardiol. 1976;37(3):403-9.
4. Véronique G. The ductus arteriosus: physiology, regulation, and functional and congenital anomalies. Arch Cardiovasc Dis. 2011;104(11):578-85.
5. Hanneman K, Newman B, Chan F. Congenital variants and anomalies of the aortic arch. Radio Graphics. 2017;37(1):32-51.
6. Bronshtein M, Zimmer EZ, Blazer S, Blumenfeld Z. Right ductus arteriosus: facts and theory. Eur J Obstet Gynecol Reprod Biol. 2011;159(2):282-8.
7. Barger JD, Creasman RW, Edwards JE, Bilateral ductus arteriosus associated with interruption of the aortic arch. Am J Clin Pathol. 1954;24(4):441-4.
8. Bökenkamp R, DeRuiter MC, van Munsteren C, Gittenberger-de Groot AC. Insights into the pathogenesis and genetic background of patency of the ductus arteriosus. Neonatology. 2010;98(1):6-17.
9. Gillam-Krakauer M, Mahajan K. Patent ductus arteriosus. In: StatPearls Treasure Island (FL): StatPearls Publishing; 2020.
10. Gittenberger-de Groot AC, van Ertbruggen I, Moulaert AJ, Harinck E. The ductus arteriosus in the preterm infant: histologic and clinical observations. J Pediatr. 1980;96(1):88-93.
11. Clyman RI, Campbell D, Heymann MA. Persistent responsiveness of the neonatal ductus arteriosus in immature lambs: a possible cause for reopening of patent ductus arteriosus after indomethacin-induced closure. Circulation. 1985;71(1):141-5.
12. Zheng J, Qiu Y, Li D, He J, Chen Y, Cao Y, et al. Prevalence and composition of CHD at different altitudes in Tibet: a cross-sectional study. Cardiol Young. 2017;27(8):1497-503.
13. Schneider DJ, Moore JW. Patent ductus arteriosus. Circulation. 2006;114(17):1873-82.
14. Patel PM, Momany AM, Schaa KL, Romitti PA, Druschel CD, Cooper ME, et al. Genetic modifiers of patent ductus arteriosus in term infants. J Pediatr. 2016;176:57-61.e1.
15. Murhekar M, Verma S, Singh K, Bavdekar A, Benakappa N, Santhanam S, et al. Epidemiology of congenital rubella syndrome (CRS) in India, 2016-18, based on data from sentinel surveillance. PLoS Negl Trop Dis. 2020;14(2):e0007982.
16. Stoll C, Alembik Y, Roth MP, Dott B, De Geeter B. Risk factors in congenital heart disease. Eur J Epidemiol. 1989;5(3):382-91.
17. Mani A, Meraji S, Houshyar R, Radhakrishnan J, Mani A, Ahanger M, et al. Finding genetic contributions to sporadic disease: a recessive locus at 12q24 commonly contributes to patent ductus arteriosus. Proc Nat AcadSci U S A. 2002;99(23):15054-9.
18. Zhu L, Vranckx R, Khau Van Kien P, Lalande A, Boisset N, Mathieu F, et al. Mutations in myosin heavy chain 11 cause a syndrome associating thoracic aortic aneurysm/aortic dissection and patent ductus arteriosus. Nat Genet. 2006; 38(3):343-9.
19. Campbell M. Natural history of persistent ductus arteriosus. Br Heart J. 1968;30(1):4-13.
20. Clyman RI, Couto J, Murphy GM. Patent ductus arteriosus: are current neonatal treatment options better or worse than no treatment at all? Semin Perinatol. 2012;36(2):123-9.
21. Gross RE. The patent ductus arteriosus: observations on diagnosis and therapy in 525 surgically treated cases. Am J Med. 1952;12(4): 472-82.
22. Ng AS, Vlietstra RE, Danielson GK, Smith HC, Puga FJ. Patent ductus arteriosus in patients more than 50 years old. Int J Cardiol. 1986;11(3):277-85.
23. Wood P. The Eisenmenger syndrome or pulmonary hypertension with reversed central shunt. Br Med J. 1958;2(5099):755-62.
24. Wood P. The Eisenmenger syndrome or pulmonary hypertension with reversed central shunt. I. Br Med J. 1958;2(5098):701-9.
25. Saha A, Balakrishnan KG, Jaiswal PK, Venkitachalam CG, Tharakan J, Titus T, et al. Prognosis for patients with Eisenmenger syndrome of various etiology. Int J Cardiol. 1994;45(3):199-207.
26. Rushani D, Kaufman JS, Ionsescu-Ittu R, Mackie AS, Pilote L, Therrien J, et al. Infective endocarditis in children with congenital heart disease cumulative incidence and predictors. Circulation. 2013;128(13):1412-9.
27. Lloyd T, Beekman RH. Clinically silent patent ductus arteriosus. Am Heart J. 1994;127(6):1664-5.
28. Thilén U, Åström-Olsson K. Does the risk of infective endarteritis justify routine patent ductus arteriosus closure? Eur Heart J. 1997; 18(3):503-6.
29. Dyamenahalli U, Smallhorn JF, Geva T, Fouron JC, Cairns P, Jutras L, et al. Isolated ductus arteriosus aneurysm in thefetus and infant: a multi-institutional experience. J Am Coll Cardiol. 2000;36(1):262-9.
30. Rudolph AM. The changes in the circulation after birth: their importance in congenital heart disease. Circulation. 1970;41(2);343-59.
31. Kang C, Zhao E, Zhou Y, Zhao H, Liu Y, Gao N, et al. Dynamic changes of pulmonary arterial pressure and ductus arteriosus in human newborns from birth to 72 hours of age. Medicine (Baltimore). 2016;95(3):e2599.
32. Webb GD, Smallhorn JF, Therrien J, Reddington A. Congenital heart disease in the adult and pediatric patient. In: Zipes DP, Libby P, Bonow RO, Mann DL, Tomaselli GF, (Eds); founding

editor and online editor Eugene Braunwald. Braunwald's Heart Disease: A Textbook of Cardiovascular Medicine, 11th edition. Philadelphia, PA: Elsevier/2019. pp. 1519-73.

33. Tekin R, Acet H, Ertas F, Ceylan Tekin R, Albudak B. An unusual case of endocarditis: isolated pulmonary valve endocarditis in patient with patent ductus arteriosus. J Med Cases. 2012;3(6): 340-3.
34. Perloff J. The Clinical Recognition of Congenital Heart Disease, 5th edition. Philadelphia, PA: Elsevier Saunders; 2009. pp. 403-29.
35. Gu, X, Zhang, Q, Sun, H, Fei, J, Zhang, X, Kutryk, MJ. Transcatheter closure of calcified patent ductus arteriosus in older adult patients: Immediate and 12-month follow-up results. Congenit Heart Dis. 2017;12(3):289-93.
36. Jain S, Vaidyanathan B. Digoxin in management of heart failure in children: should it be continued or relegated to the history books? Ann Pediatr Cardiol. 2009;2(2):149-52.
37. El-Said HG, Bratincsak A, Foerster SR, Murphy JJ, Vincent J, Holzer R, et al. Safety of percutaneous patent ductus arteriosus closure: An unselected multicenter population experience. J Am Heart Assoc. 2013;2(6):e000424.
38. Behjati-Ardakani M, Rafiei M, Behjati-Ardakani MA, Vafaeenasab M, Sarebanhassanabadi M. Long-term results of transcatheter closure of patent ductus arteriosus in adolescents and adults with amplatzer duct occluder. North Am J Med Sci. 2015;7(5):208-11.
39. Morville P, Akhavi A. Transcatheter closure of hemodynamic significant patent ductus arteriosus in 32 premature infants by amplatzer ductal occluder additional size-ADOIIAS. Catheter Cardiovasc Interv. 2017;90(4):612-7.
40. Rios DR, Bhattacharya S, Levy PT, McNamara PJ. Circulatory insufficiency and hypotension related to the ductus arteriosus in neonates. Front Pediatr. 2018;6:62.

24 CHAPTER

Aortopulmonary Window and Other Aortic Shunts

MK Usha, M Jayranganath

INTRODUCTION

This chapter deals with four relatively uncommon congenital heart diseases (CHDs) that involve the aorta. They are all in many ways quite unrelated but have been brought together in this chapter for the sake of convenience. Aortopulmonary (AP) window presents in early infancy as a large left-to-right shunt. The origin of one of the branch pulmonary arteries from the aorta also typically presents early with heart failure and pulmonary hypertension. Aneurysms sinus of Valsalva typically presents in adulthood and aorta to left ventricle (LV) tunnel is an extremely rare congenital communication between aorta and LV that presents early with features resembling severe aortic regurgitation (AR).

AORTOPULMONARY WINDOW

Introduction

An abnormal communication between the ascending aorta and the main pulmonary artery in the presence of two distinct aortic and pulmonary valves is described as AP window. It is a rare congenital anomaly accounting for 0.2–0.6% of all congenital heart defects. It was first described by in 1830 by Elliotson during an autopsy. In 1948, Robert Gross first ligated it surgically and Cooley and colleagues performed the first surgical closure of AP window under cardiopulmonary bypass in 1957.[1]

Embryology

The presumed basis for AP window is defective septation of the truncus arteriosus is responsible for formation of AP window.

Anatomy

Aortopulmonary window is often an isolated anomaly. It can also be associated with other defects like coarctation of aorta, interrupted aortic arch, tetralogy of Fallot, abnormal origin of right coronary artery, abnormal origin of right pulmonary artery or atrial septal defect (ASD). Rare associations are transposition of great arteries, pulmonary, aortic or tricuspid atresia.

Mori's classification (**Figs. 1A to D**) is used to classify the anatomic subtypes of AP window.[2] It is as follows:

- *Type I (**Fig. 1A**)*: Proximal defect above sinus of Valsalva. Most common type

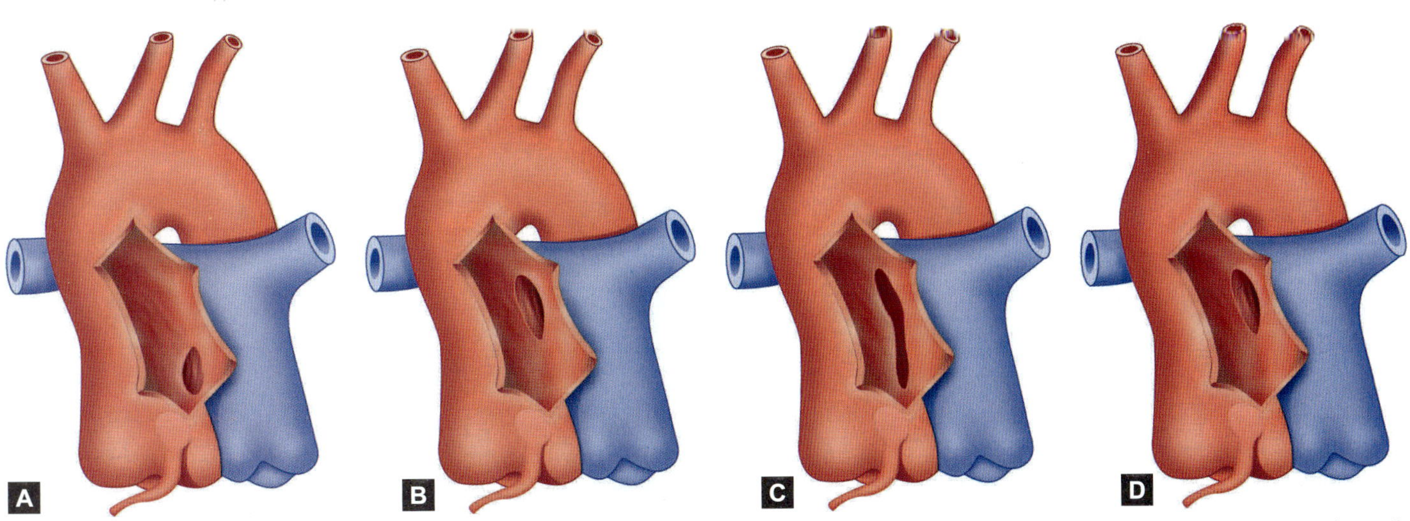

Figs. 1A to D: Mori's classification of aortopulmonary (AP) window. (A) Proximal defect above sinus of Valsalva. Most common type (type I); (B) Type II, distal defect just before the branches of aortic arches; (C) Type III, combined large defect which is combination of type I and type II. Least common type; (D) Society of Thoracic Surgeons Congenital Heart Surgery Database Committee recommend a fourth subtype of AP window called the intermediate type which consists of smaller central defects.

- *Type II* (***Fig. 1B***): Distal defect just before the branches of aortic arches
- *Type III* (***Fig. 1C***): Combined large defect which is combination of type I and Type II. Least common type
- Society of Thoracic Surgeons Congenital Heart Surgery Database Committee recommend a fourth subtype of AP window called the intermediate type (**Fig. 1D**) which consists of smaller central defects.

Pathophysiology

The hemodynamic effect depends upon two factors, the size of the lesion and the pulmonary vascular resistance. In initial 2 weeks of life when the pulmonary vascular resistance is elevated the magnitude of shunt is limited. As the resistance falls, the left-to-right shunt progressively increases. The larger the defect, higher is the shunt and pulmonary blood flow. Increased pulmonary venous return leads to dilatation of left atrium and LV and features of congestive heart failure. Increased flow leads to hyperkinetic pulmonary hypertension in large defects. Progressive increase in pulmonary vascular resistance occurs with time due to proliferative changes in pulmonary vasculature. This leads to reversal of shunt like any other form of Eisenmenger physiology. An additional consideration in AP window is the fact that there is aortic run off and "steal" from the descending aorta just as in a large patent arterial duct. It is important to be mindful of this physiology in neonates. Overzealous oxygen administration can result in excessive steal and reduced gut perfusion and predisposition to necrotizing enterocolitis.

Clinical Presentation

Clinical features are similar to any large left-to-right shunt such as ventricular septal defect (VSD) or patent ductus arteriosus (PDA). Symptoms of pulmonary overcirculation and congestive heart failure in large defects are seen. Infants with AP window tend to present at an early age because of a large shunt. They present with feeding difficulties, suck-rest-suck cycles, diaphoresis, fast breathing, and poor weight gain. Recurrent episodes of lower respiratory infections can be life-threatening. Small defects remain asymptomatic and come to light due to incidental murmurs, but these are rare. Large defects have clinical findings like that of a large unrestrictive patent arterial duct. The pulses are bounding with wide pulse pressure and there is tachycardia when large and moderate defects are present. The precordium is hyperdynamic with prominent pulsations. Systolic thrill may be present when the defect is restrictive. The second heart sound tends to have a narrow split from delay in A2. The pulmonary component of second sound is prominent. Large defects produce early systolic murmur, whereas restrictive defects cause continuous murmurs. Associated defects such as coarctation of aorta or interruption will accelerate the clinical worsening and worsen the heart failure.

Chest X-ray and Electrocardiogram

Chest X-ray shows cardiomegaly with dilated main pulmonary artery and plethoric lung fields when shunt is large (**Fig. 2**). Electrocardiogram (ECG) may show features of left atrium and LV volume overload in the form of broad p waves and tall R waves with q waves in V5 and V6.

Echocardiography and Other Investigations

Echocardiography is the most important tool for evaluation of AP window. It delineates the size, location of the defect, and associated features. Dilatation of left atrium and LV is observed. Computed tomography (CT) scan may be useful to delineate large AP windows and to confirm arch and coronary anomalies when suspected (**Fig. 3**).

Management

Diuretics are necessary to initially manage heart failure symptoms. Furosemide in the dose 1–2 mg/kg/day in

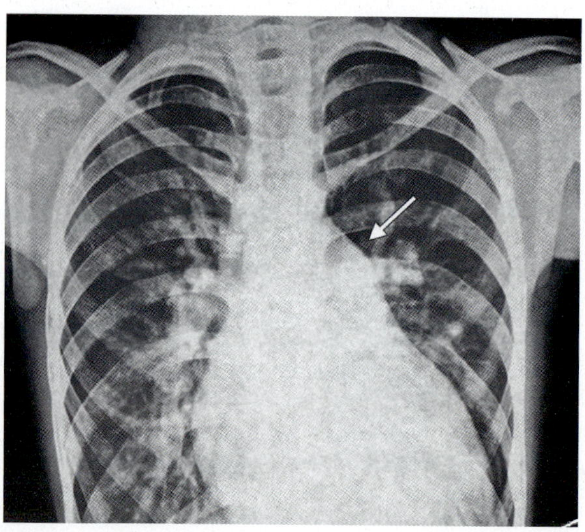

Fig. 2: Chest X-ray showing cardiomegaly with dilated pulmonary artery (arrow) and plethoric lung fields.

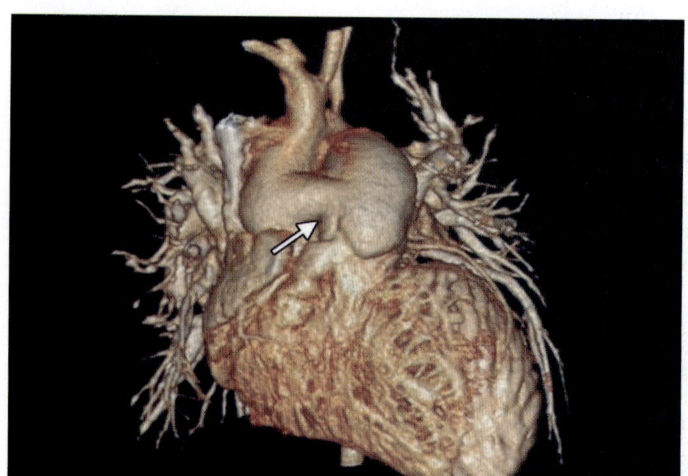

Fig. 3: Computed tomography (CT) scan showing large aortopulmonary (AP) window clearly seen between the aorta and the pulmonary artery (arrow).

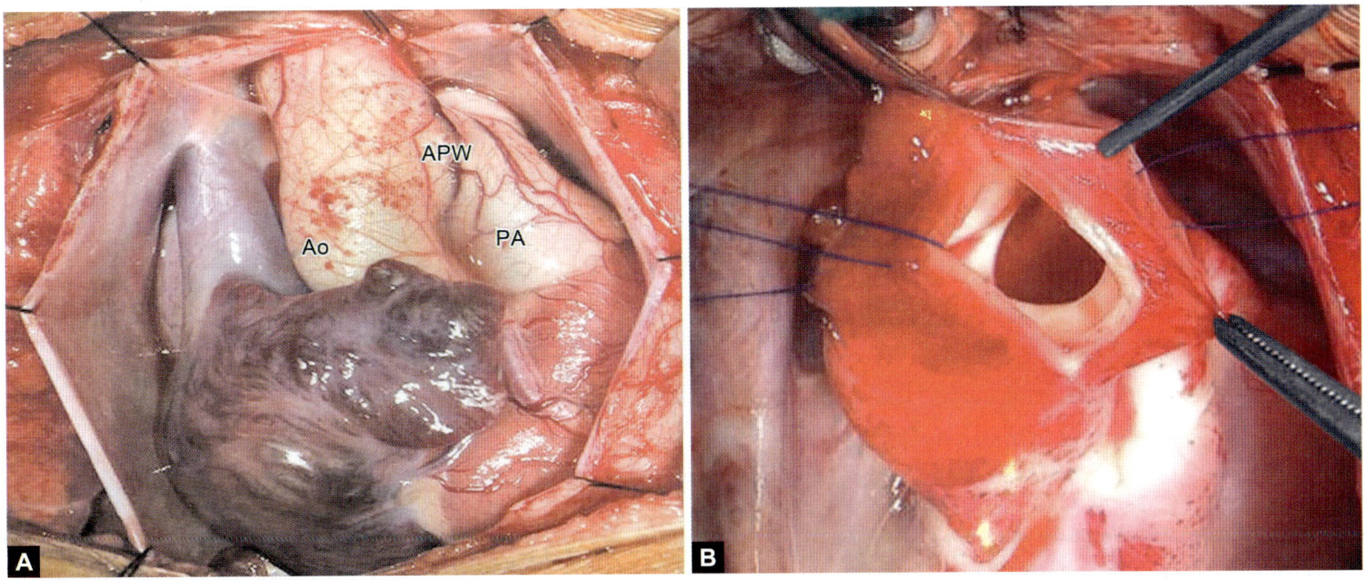

Figs. 4A and B: Surgery for aortopulmonary (AP) window. (A) The external findings; (B) The window seen through the aortic approach. (Ao: aorta; APW: aortopulmonary window; PA: pulmonary artery)

divided doses should be given in large defects till surgery is performed. Early surgical closure is essential to prevent the progression to pulmonary vascular obstructive disease and the detrimental effects of increased pulmonary flow. In most modern centers, operation is planned soon after diagnosis. It may be necessary to operate in the neonatal period itself to prevent the inevitable development of heart failure and mitigate rapid worsening of status. Midline sternotomy followed by closure is performed on cardiopulmonary bypass usually by transaortic approach (**Fig. 4**). Restrictive defects are rare and they may be amenable to device closure in cathetrization laboratory. Patients presenting late are often inoperable. However, surgery can be contemplated in selected rare instances where there is still evidence of markedly increased pulmonary blood flow after detailed evaluation for operability. The immediate and long-term mortality is increased and may need long-term pulmonary vasodilators.[4]

Prognosis

Without treatment 40–50% of children die in first year of life due to congestive heart failure. Isolated AP windows when operated early in life have an excellent outcome. Complex anatomy with associated arch abnormalities carry increased surgical risk.

ORIGIN OF ONE PULMONARY ARTERY FROM AORTA

Introduction

The pulmonary arteries are a part of right heart circulation and are not usually connected with the aorta other than by a PDA. However, in rare cases, one of the pulmonary artery can arise anomalously from the ascending aorta. The other pulmonary artery arises from the right ventricle and is the continuation of main pulmonary artery with the presence of aortic and pulmonary valves. Anomalous right pulmonary artery is 5–6 times more frequent than left. The anomalous pulmonary artery originates from the wall of the ascending aorta, 5–30 mm above the aortic valve. Rarely the origin can be high from the distal part of ascending aorta close to innominate artery. This lesion was previously referred to as "hemitruncus" and accounts for 0.1% of all congenital heart diseases.[4]

Embryology

Kutsche and Van Mierop proposed that abnormal migration of pluripotent cells is important in the development of the anomalous origin of pulmonary arteries. On the left side, this occurs due to failure of development of the left sixth arch leading to the failure of fusion of left pulmonary artery to the main pulmonary artery. On the right side, it may be due to the incomplete migration of the right sixth aortic arch to the left side.

Hemodynamics

The right ventricle pumps the entire systemic venous return to one lung. This normally connected lung has volume overload which poses a risk for development of pulmonary vascular obstructive disease. The lung supplied by the anomalous pulmonary artery is exposed to both pressure and volume overload. Hence, both lung fields are exposed to increased flow. The normally connected lung also has elevated pulmonary pressures.[5] The underlying mechanism may be circulating vasoconstrictor substances and neurogenic crossover from the unprotected lung. These children have severe pulmonary hypertension at presentation.

Elevated vascular resistance happens early in life if not surgically corrected. The 1-year unoperated survival may be as low as 30%.

Associated Lesions

Anomalous pulmonary artery is usually an isolated condition. But it can be associated with various lesions, most common being tetralogy of Fallot. Others are PDA, ASD, VSD, coarctation, interrupted aortic arch, or subvalvar aortic stenosis.

Clinical Presentation

The disease is more common in males. The condition usually presents in the newborn period or in early infancy with complaints of difficulty in feeding, fast breathing, and poor weight gain. On examination, the child will have failure to thrive with tachypnea and respiratory distress. Pulses are bounding with tachycardia. The pulmonary component of the second sound is loud and a short systolic murmur may be heard.

Diagnosis

The chest radiograph shows cardiomegaly with differential vascularity. There is plethora bilaterally, but is more pronounced on the side of the anomalous connection. The differential vascularity is exaggerated in the presence of pulmonary stenosis such as tetralogy of Fallot. Electrocardiogram might show right axis deviation with biventricular hypertrophy.

Echocardiography enables accurate diagnosis of the condition along with associated lesions. But this needs to be done meticulously. This condition should be specifically excluded in patients being evaluated for unexplained pulmonary hypertension. A CT angiogram will clearly depict the anatomy if doubts persist after echocardiography (**Figs. 5A and B**).

Management

The acutely sick child should be managed in an acute care setting with judicious use of diuretics and inotropes if needed. There is no role of pulmonary vasodilators prior to surgery. Corrective repair should be arranged as early as possible. Neonatal repair has shown good outcomes with near complete resolution of pulmonary hypertension.[6] Surgical reimplantation of the anomalous pulmonary artery to the main pulmonary artery is performed along with correction of associated lesions. In the immediate postoperative period, the children can have pulmonary hypertensive crises that may need pulmonary vasodilators.[6] Those who present late beyond 1 year of life with desaturation may need careful evaluation including catheterization before contemplating surgery.

Prognosis

The prognosis is very good with normalization of pulmonary pressures if operated early during infancy.[4-6] Long-term follow-up shows survival of 93% at 20 years.[7] Anomalous origin of one pulmonary artery must be considered in all cases of severe neonatal pulmonary hypertension. If not diagnosed in early infancy, death may ensue due to heart failure. Development of pulmonary vascular obstructive disease is a strong possibility in those operated late.[4]

ANEURYSM OF SINUS OF VALSALVA

Introduction

Sinus of Valsalva is the normal bulge in the aortic root which is located immediately above the hinge point of the valve leaflets. There are three sinuses right, left, and posterior sinus as three leaflets are present. The coronary arteries arise from the right and the left sinus. The posterior sinus is the noncoronary sinus (**Fig. 6**). The sinuses prevent complete opposition of the leaflets to the aortic wall during systole thus

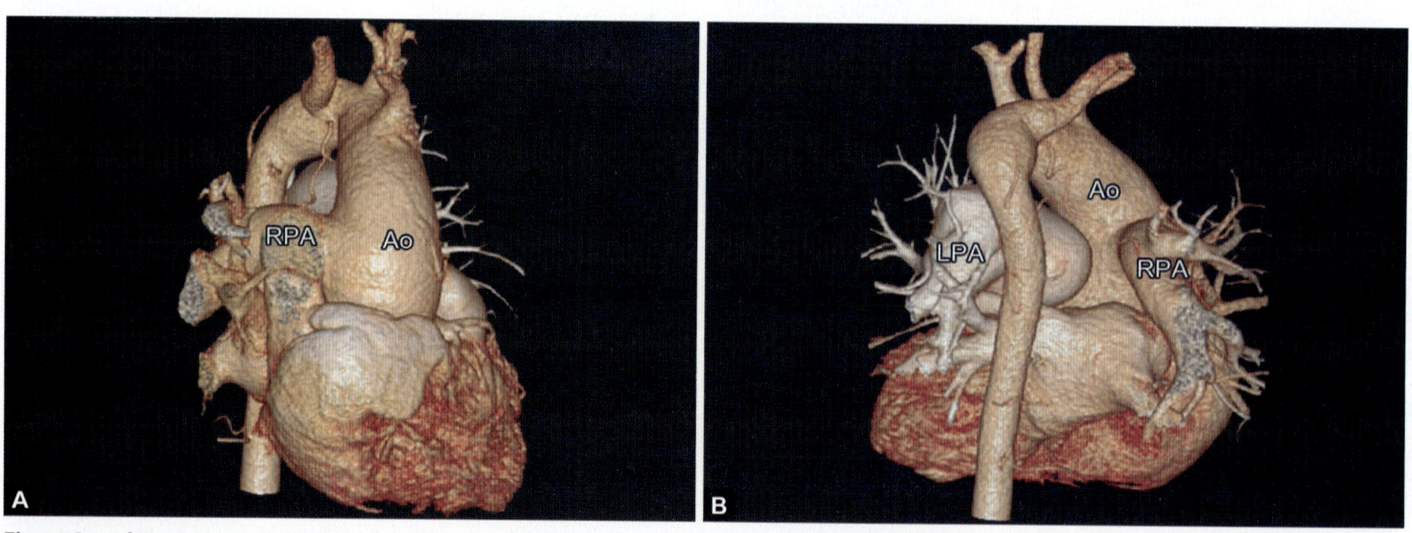

Figs. 5A and B: Computed tomography (CT) reconstruction in a patient with aortic (Ao) origin of the right pulmonary artery (RPA). The main pulmonary artery continues as left pulmonary artery (LPA).

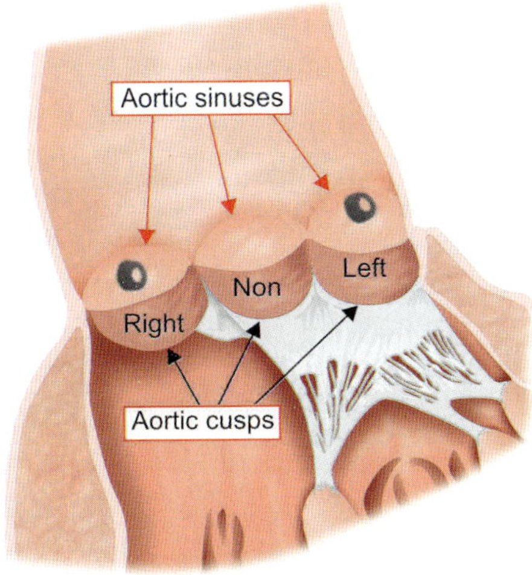

Fig. 6: Normal aortic root and anatomy of the sinuses.

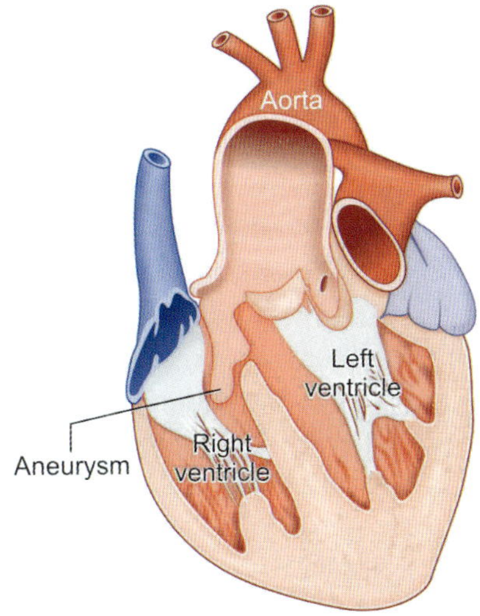

Fig. 7: Aneurysmally dilated sinus of Valsalva.

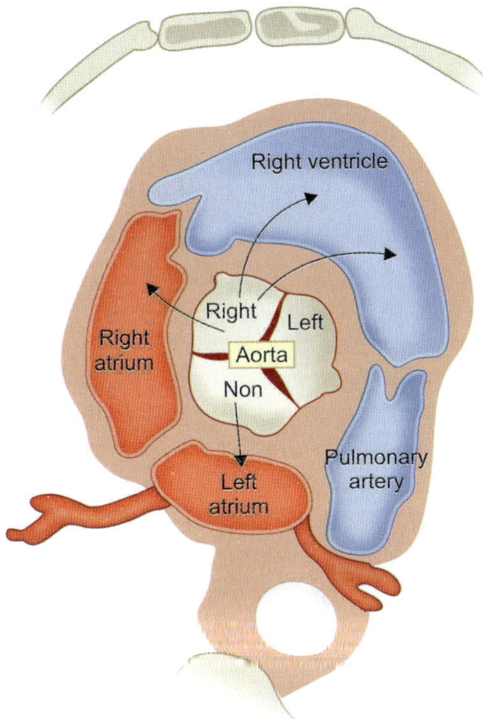

Fig. 8: Schematic representation of rupture of different sinuses of Valsalva into various chambers of the heart—Axial section—as seen from below.

preventing closure of the coronary ostia. Weakness of the elastic lamina of the sinus leads to separation of the aortic media from annulus fibrosus causing dilatation or aneurysm of the sinus of Valsalva. Progressive dilatation can lead to rupture of the aneurysm into various cardiac chambers leading to potentially catastrophic heart failure and even death (**Figs. 7 and 8**).

Etiology

Etiology can be congenital or may be acquired. It is rare in infancy and early childhood. Bicuspid aortic valve, connective tissue disease, infective endocarditis, and trauma are usual causes. Takayasu arteritis, syphilis, Behçet's syndrome, iatrogenic and Marfan syndrome are some rare causes.

Pathoanatomy and Pathophysiology

About 70–80% of aneurysms originate in right sinus and 10–25% arise from noncoronary sinus. Less than 5% arise from left sinus. They appear as windsock deformities. Nearly 30–50% are associated with VSD. There can be associated aortic regurgitation (AR) in nearly 30–40%. Coarctation of aorta, atrial septal defect, tetralogy of Fallot, and PDA are other associations. Rupture is most commonly into right ventricle from right coronary sinus. Noncoronary sinus usually ruptures into the right atrium. This leads to volume overload of chambers resulting in congestive heart failure. Rarely, rupture can be into pericardium causing tamponade and sudden death. The unruptured aneurysm can obstruct the right ventricle outflow tract, compress on a coronary causing ischemia or can cause heart block due to compression on conduction system.[8-11]

Clinical Features

The usual age of presentation in second or third decade of life. There is a distinct male predominance (M:F ratio: 4:1). Though rare, it can occur in young children as young as 10 months.[12] Symptom onset depends on the rate of rupture. Around 30% of patients develop sudden large rupture causing chest pain and catastrophic heart failure. Slow rupture and small shunts can remain asymptomatic for few months before cardiac failure sets in. Dyspnea, palpitation, and chest pain are the most common symptoms. There will be wide pulse pressure with collapsing pulse and hyperdynamic precordium. The jugular venous pressure may be elevated in presence of heart failure. S1 will be normal and P2 component of S2 may be accentuated. A loud continuous murmur is heard in parasternal border.

With rupture into right atrium, there is often a prominent murmur in right sternal border. Rupture to RV or right ventricular outflow tract (RVOT) will cause murmur to be best heard in left second or third space, respectively. Rupture into LV can cause a to-and-fro murmur. PDA, coronary artery fistula, systemic arteriovenous fistula, and restrictive AP window are differential diagnosis of continuous murmurs.

Investigations

Chest X-ray will show cardiomegaly with pulmonary plethora. The ECG will show corresponding chamber enlargement. Echocardiogram shows dilated chambers downstream to the chamber into which the fistula ruptures. The dilated aortic sinus with wind sock deformity protruding into corresponding chamber is seen. Color Doppler shows the flow across the windsock into cardiac chamber, presence of AR, VSD, and associated lesions. Transesophageal echocardiogram can give a better anatomical definition and sizing of the defect. Cardiac CT may define the size of deformity and accurate location of opening aiding in planning of management.

Management

Survival is often <1 year without treatment. Death occurs due to heart failure. Heart failure should be alleviated with the use of diuretics and afterload reducing agents that include angiotensin-converting enzyme (ACE) inhibitors (enalapril). All rupture of sinus of Valsalva (RSOV) require closure which is the definitive treatment. Acute heart failure warrants immediate intervention. Transcatheter device closure in catheterization laboratory is possible if the anatomy is suitable and there is no associated significant AR.[13] Presence of VSD or significant AR necessitates surgical correction. Long-term follow-up shows good outcomes once there is complete closure and recurrences are relatively rare.

AORTO-LEFT VENTRICULAR TUNNEL

Introduction

A rare anomaly which consists of an extracardiac channel which connects ascending aorta above the sinotubular junction to the cavity of left ventricular (90%) or right ventricle (10%) (**Fig. 9**). They form 0.03–0.4% of all CHDs. The aortic opening usually lies above right coronary sinus of Valsalva. The tunnel courses down along the base of the aortic valve toward the LV entering the LV immediately below the right coronary cusp (**Fig. 9**). Loss of support for right coronary cusp can lead to AR. Coronary anomalies in the form of stenosis or atresia may be present. Bicuspid aortic valve with stenosis or regurgitation can occur in 20% of patients. Rarely, it can open to the right ventricle or the right atrium. Histologically, the aortic end resembles aorta with elastic fibers and smooth muscle cells. Ventricular end has collagen tissue with hyaline and myocardial muscle.[14]

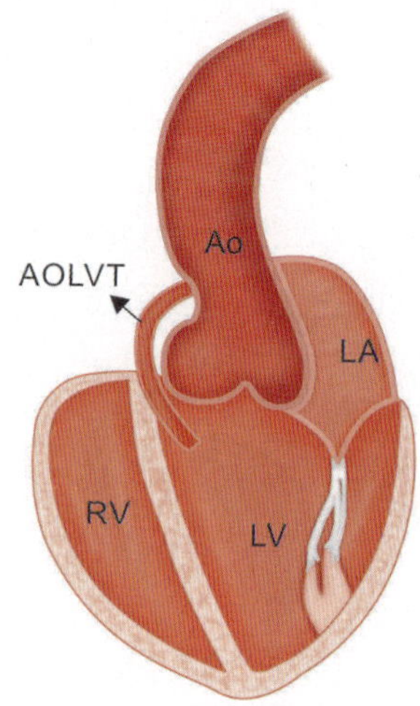

Fig. 9: Line diagram demonstrating aorto-left ventricular tunnel. (Ao: aorta, AOLVT: aorto-left ventricular tunnel; LA: left atrium; LV: left ventricle; RV: right ventricle)

Embryologically aortic and pulmonary sinuses are formed from cushions with encasing muscular tissue. As they develop, the muscular tissue involutes leaving behind the fibrous structure of sinuses. Persistence of this muscular cuff may lead to formation of tunnel.[15]

Clinical Picture

The clinical picture is due to nonvalvular severe AR causing left ventricular volume overload. Valvular AR may also accompany when associated aortic valve anomalies are present. Clinical presentation is in the form of heart failure in half the patients in early infancy. Bounding pulses with wide pulse pressure is found on examination. There may be palpable systolic and diastolic thrills and auscultation reveals to-and-fro murmur.

Chest X-ray shows cardiomegaly with left ventricular apex. ECG shows LV volume overload in the form of prominent R waves in V5 and V6 with deep q waves. Echocardiogram is diagnostic. The anatomy of the tunnel, flow across, LV dimensions, and function can be accurately assessed. Associated lesions such as AR and dilatation of ascending aorta can be identified. Large dilated tunnels can narrow the RVOT. CT scan can give improved definition of the extent of tunnel, coronary involvement, and ascending aortic dimensions. This will aid in the comprehensive surgical management (**Fig. 10**).

Differential Diagnosis

Presence of bounding pulses and wide pulse pressure with hyperdynamic apex and to-and-fro murmur can also be seen in few other conditions.

- *VSD with AR*: Moderate AR with moderate VSD. But the murmur is pan systolic and early diastolic.
- *Truncus arteriosus*: Desaturation will be present on oximetry readings. Babies present early in life with failure.
- Bicuspid aortic valve with aortic stenosis and AR.

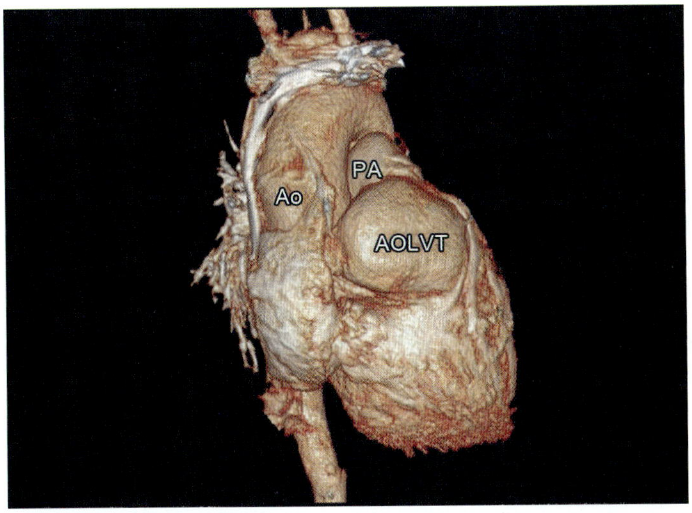

Fig. 10: Computed tomography (CT) angiogram with 3D reconstruction showing aorta to left ventricular tunnel—patient was 5-year-old boy who presented in cardiac failure.
(Ao: aorta; AOLVT: aorto-left ventricular tunnel; PA: pulmonary artery)

Treatment

Surgery is the mainstay of therapy. Medical stabilization with diuretics and afterload reducing agents such as ACE inhibitors will be required. Surgery should be performed in infancy to prevent cardiac failure and progressive distortion of aortic valve. Closure of both aortic end and of LV opening with patch is required as the redundant pouch may enlarge, distort the LV, and lead to LV dysfunction. Coronaries may require reimplantation if arising from the tunnel. Aortic valve repair should be performed if significant AR is present. Older children can present with progressive ascending aortic dilatation in later life requiring aortic root replacement. Surgery has good outcome with <5% mortality.[16]

CONCLUSION

Congenital anomalies of the aortic root are a rare group of disorders. The common presentation is that of hyperdynamic circulation with bounding pulses and wide pulse pressure. Aortopulmonary window is the prototype anomaly which also has features of increased pulmonary circulation. Early recognition is crucial for early repair. All lesions are amenable to surgery. Surgery is curative with excellent outcomes in immediate and long-term follow-up.

REFERENCES

1. Taggart MW, Qureshi MY. Patent ductus arteriosus and aortopulmonary window. In: Allen HD, Shaddy RE, Penny DJ, Feltes TF, Cetta F, (Eds). Moss and Adam's Heart Disease in Infants, Children and Adolescents, 9th edition. Philadelphia: Wolters Kluwer; 2016. pp. 1479-509.
2. Mori K, Ando M, Takao A, Ishikawa S, Imai Y. Distal type of aortopulmonary window. Report of 4 cases. Br Heart J. 1978;40(6):681-9.
3. Talwar S, Siddharth B, Gupta SK, Choudhary SK, Kothari SS, Juneja R, et al. Aortopulmonary window: results of repair beyond infancy. Interact Cardiovasc Thorac Surg. 2017;25(5):740-4.
4. Garg P, Talwar S, Kothari SS, Saxena A, Juneja R, Choudhary SK, et al. The anomalous origin of the branch pulmonary artery from the ascending aorta. Interact Cardiovasc Thorac Surg. 2012;15(1):86-92.
5. Amir G, Frenkel G, Bruckheimer E, Dagan T, Katz J, Berant M, Vidne B, et al. Anomalous origin of the pulmonary artery from the aorta: early diagnosis and repair leading to immediate physiological correction. Cardiol Young. 2010;20(6):654-9.
6. Agati S, Sousa CG, Calvaruso FD, Zanai R, Campanella I, Poli D, et al. Anomalous aortic origin of the pulmonary arteries: case series and literature review. Ann Pediatr Cardiol. 2019;12(3):248-53.
7. Nathan M, Rimmer D, Piercey G, del Nido PJ, Mayer JE, Bacha EA, et al. Early repair of hemitruncus: excellent early and late outcomes. J Thorac Cardiovasc Surg. 2007;133:1329-35.
8. Moustafa S, Mookadam F, Cooper L, Adam G, Zehr K, Stulak J, et al. Sinus of Valsalva aneurysms—47 years of a single center experience and systematic overview of published reports. Am J Cardiol. 2007;99(8):1159-64.
9. Gupta M, Shoeb M, Mishra PK, Bathala A, Prasad J. Management of the ruptured sinus of Valsalva aneurysmsa. Int Surg J. 2017;4(6):1873-7.
10. Choudhary SK, Bhan A, Sharma R, Airan B, Kumar AS, Venugopal P. Sinus of Valsalva aneurysms: 20 years' experience. J Card Surg. 1997;12(5):300-8.
11. Diwakar A, Patnaik SS, Hiremath CS, Chalam KS, Dash P. Rupture of sinus of Valsalva - A 15 years single institutional retrospective review: Preoperative heart failure has an impact on post operative outcome? Ann Card Anaesth. 2019;22(1):24-9.
12. Steflik D, Churchill T, Chowdhury S. Sinus of Valsalva aneurysm rupture in an infant. Cardiol Young. 2018;28(2):338-40.
13. Mahimarangaiah J, Chandra S, Subramanian A, Srinivasa KH, Usha MK, Manjunath CN. Transcatheter closure of ruptured sinus of Valsalva: different techniques and mid-term follow-up. Cathet Cardiovasc Intervent. 2016; 87(3):516-22.
14. Hovaguimian H, Cobanoglu A, Starr A. Aortico-left ventricular tunnel: a clinical review and new surgical classification. Ann Thorac Surg. 1988;45(1):106-12.
15. Anderson RH, Cook A, Brown NA, Henderson DJ, Chaudhry B, Mohun T. Development of the outflow tracts with reference to aortopulmonary windows and aorto-ventricular tunnels. Cardiol Young. 2010;20 Suppl 3:92-9.
16. Spicer DE, Hraska V, Anderson RH, Ginde S, Block JR. Congenital anomalies of the aortic valve and left ventricular outflow tract. In: Wenovsky G, Anderson RH, Krishna K, Mussato KA, Andrew R, Tweddell JS, Tretter J, (Eds). Anderson's Pediatric Cardiology, 4th edition. Philadelphia: Elsevier; 2019. pp. 3557-9.

25 CHAPTER

Atrioventricular Septal Defect

Navaneetha Sasikumar

INTRODUCTION

Atrioventricular septal defects are also known as endocardial cushion defects or atrioventricular canal defects.

In the normal heart, the septal leaflet of the tricuspid valve is attached more toward the apex than the mitral valve. This divides the membranous part of the interventricular septum into an "atrioventricular part" between the right atrium and left ventricle and the "interventricular part" (**Fig. 1**). Atrioventricular septal defects are characterized by complete or partial deficiency of the atrioventricular part of the membranous septum.

Atrioventricular septal defects have a prevalence of 0.19 per 1,000 live births and account for 2.9–5% of congenital heart disease. Down syndrome has a major association with atrioventricular septal defects. About 40–45% of children with Down syndrome have congenital heart disease. Among these, approximately 45% have an atrioventricular septal defect. Conversely, approximately 50% of patients with atrioventricular septal defect have Down syndrome. In more than 75% of patients with Down syndrome, atrioventricular septal defect presents in the complete form.[1,2] Ellis-Van Creveld syndrome has been associated with common atrium. The heterotaxy syndromes also are associated with atrioventricular septal defect. Unbalanced atrioventricular septal defect is one of the commoner complex lesions associated with right isomerism.

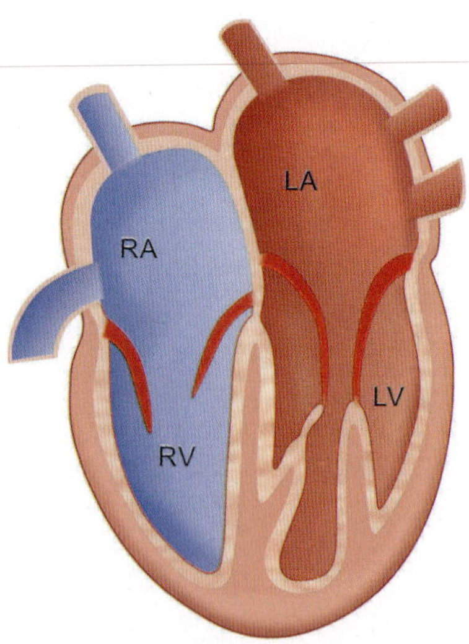

Fig. 1: Normal heart. The mitral and the tricuspid valve leaflets are attached to the septum at different levels. The tricuspid valve is attached more towards the apex, thus dividing the membranous part of the interventricular septum into an "atrioventricular part" between the right atrium and left ventricle and the "interventricular part".
(LA: left atrium, LV: left ventricle, RA: right atrium, RV: right ventricle)

PATHOLOGY

These defects are classically considered as a result of failure of the primitive endocardial cushions to fuse and form the normal crux of the heart. Complete failure of fusion results in a complete atrioventricular septal defect, while partial failure results in a partial defect. The accompanying array of complex abnormalities as described here suggests that failure of fusion could be a starting point for the development of the malformation. This is likely followed by abnormal delamination and development of the atrioventricular valvar leaflets from the abnormal ventricular mass with a common atrioventricular junction.

When the atrioventricular septum is absent or deficient, there are accompanying inevitable pathological changes. These changes, in addition to the first and basic abnormality—deficiency of atrioventricular septum—characterize all hearts with atrioventricular septal defects. An oval-shaped common atrioventricular junction is the hallmark of these hearts.

The presence of a common atrioventricular junction and the absence of septal atrioventricular contiguity ensure that the leaflets that guard the common atrioventricular junction are arranged abnormally. The common atrioventricular valve has five leaflets (**Fig. 2**). The left lateral or the mural leaflet belongs exclusively to the left ventricle. The right antero-superior and the right mural leaflets belong exclusively to the right ventricle. Two lateral leaflets correspond to the posterior tricuspid and posterior mitral leaflets in a normal heart. The right antero-superior leaflet represents the normal anterior tricuspid leaflet. The other two leaflets extend across the ventricular septum into both ventricles and are called the superior and the inferior bridging leaflets. The size of the inferior bridging leaflet remains constant. The superior bridging leaflet on the other hand can vary significantly in size and its attachments to the structures below. Based on this the complete atrioventricular septal defects have been historically classified into Rastelli types A, B, and C. In type A, the superior bridging leaflet is divided and attached to the crest of the interventricular septum. In Type B, it is partially divided and attached to papillary muscles in the right ventricular side of the interventricular septum. In Type C, it is nondivided and attached to papillary muscles in the right ventricular free wall.

The left ventricular component of this valve closes in a trifoliate fashion quite unlike the normal mitral valve that has a bifoliate arrangement. The commissure between the left anterior and the left posterior bridging leaflets is referred to as the "cleft". The invariable presence of a cleft in these hearts make them vulnerable to regurgitation. Over time, the regurgitant leaflets can become thickened and myxomatous. The left ventricular components of the bridging leaflets have unusual chordal attachments to the ventricular septum, which also can contribute to narrowing of the left ventricular outflow tract and obstruction. The papillary muscles in the left ventricle are abnormally rotated counterclockwise and spaced supero-inferiorly rather than in the normal anterolateral and posteromedial positions. Abnormal arrangement of papillary muscles can lead to a parachute like deformity or a double orifice of the left atrioventricular valve component, both of which predispose to obstruction to left ventricular inflow.

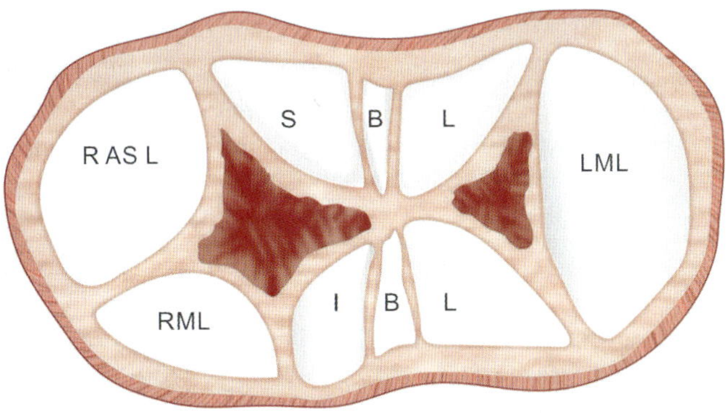

Fig. 2: Leaflets guarding the common atrioventricular junction, as seen in the subcostal en face view on echocardiography. (LML: left mural leaflet; SBL: superior bridging leaflet; IBL: inferior bridging leaflet; RML: right mural leaflet; RASL: right antero-superior leaflet)

The fibrous skeleton of the heart is also abnormal. The left ventricular outflow tract, instead of being wedged normally between the right and left atrioventricular valves, is now unwedged and "sprung anteriorly." The aortic valve is more antero-superior in position (**Fig. 3**). The crest of the inlet ventricular septum is deficient, apically displaced, and has a scooped out appearance. The septal attachment of the left- and right-sided atrioventricular valve components are at the same level in contrast to normal hearts, where the septal tricuspid leaflet is attached more apically than the mitral. The distance from the crux to the apex is shortened. The left ventricular outlet is longer than the inlet, while in normal hearts, it is the same. These features together give rise to the elongated and narrow "goose neck" shape of the left ventricular outflow tract, which is prone to outflow tract obstruction. Absence of the central fibrous body alters the normal conduction axis. The atrioventricular node is positioned postero-inferior to the coronary sinus and the penetrating bundle of His lies on the postero-inferior rim of the ventricular component of the atrioventricular septal defect.

In addition to abnormalities of left-sided component of the atrioventricular valve and left ventricular outflow tract obstruction, other commonly associated abnormalities include common atrium, additional muscular ventricular septal defect, tetralogy of Fallot, and coarctation or interruption of the arch when the left ventricle is hypoplastic.

TYPES OF ATRIOVENTRICULAR SEPTAL DEFECTS

Atrioventricular septal defects can be categorized into different types based on two distinct features. These are

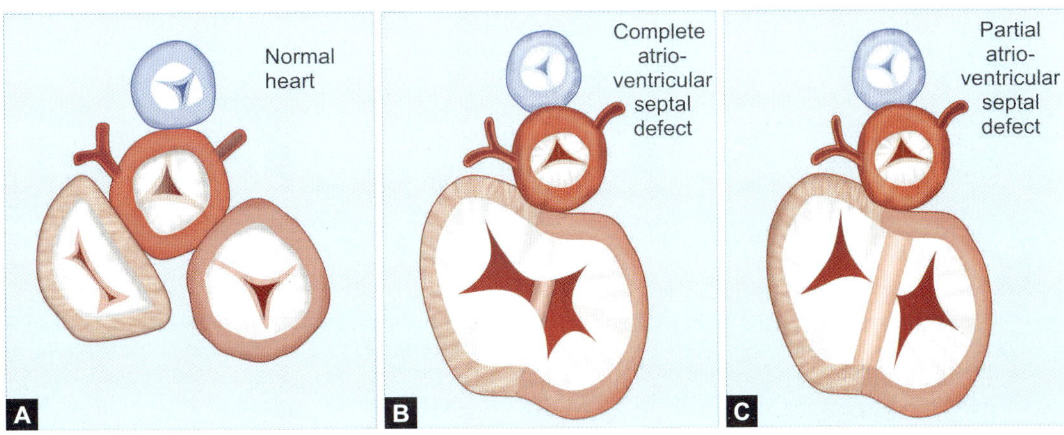

Figs. 3A to C: In the normal heart (A) the aorta/left ventricular outflow tract is wedged between the mitral and the tricuspid valves. In complete (B) as well as partial (C) atrioventricular septal defects, the aorta/left ventricular outflow tract is unwedged and pushed or "sprung" anteriorly.

based on the arrangement of the individual leaflets of the common atrioventricular valve relative to the right and left orifices and the relationship of the bridging leaflets to the atrial and ventricular septal defects. When there is a space between the superior and inferior bridging leaflets, separating them, there is a single, common atrioventricular orifice. When the superior and inferior bridging leaflets are connected by a tongue of valvular tissue, there are two atrioventricular orifices. Partial atrioventricular septal defects differ from the complete variety in that the former has two distinct atrioventricular valve orifices although contiguous.

When the bridging leaflets are attached to the interventricular septum, the shunting is at the atrial level. This is a type of partial atrioventricular septal defect and is called ostium primum atrial septal defect (ASD) (**Fig. 4**). When the bridging leaflets are attached to the distal end of the atrial septum, shunting is at the ventricular level. This is another type of partial atrioventricular septal defect called inlet ventricular septal defect (**Fig. 4**). When the bridging leaflets are free floating, shunting occurs at both the atrial and ventricular level. When this happens with a common atrioventricular orifice, this is called complete atrioventricular septal defect (**Fig. 5**).

Apart from the partial and complete atrioventricular septal defects as described above, classically two other types have also been described. These are called transitional and intermediate type defects. Transitional atrioventricular septal defect is a subtype of partial atrioventricular septal defect. Here, a partial atrioventricular septal defect (primum ASD) is associated with an inlet ventricular septal defect, which is small, partially occluded by dense chordal attachments to the ventricular septum (**Fig. 4**). Intermediate atrioventricular septal defect is a form of complete atrioventricular septal defect that has distinct right and left atrioventricular valve orifices (tongue of valvular tissue joining the bridging leaflets) despite having only one common annulus (**Fig. 5**).

Generally, irrespective of the number of orifices, the left and right components of the common atrioventricular junction are similar in circumference and the ventricles are similar in size. This type of arrangement is called a balanced atrioventricular septal defect. Less commonly, either component of the common atrioventricular junction can be dominant along with the corresponding ventricle. The other ventricle and its corresponding outflow tracts would then be hypoplastic, the arrangement being called unbalanced atrioventricular septal defect. Careful assessment needs to be done as to whether such a heart is amenable to biventricular corrective surgery or univentricular palliation.

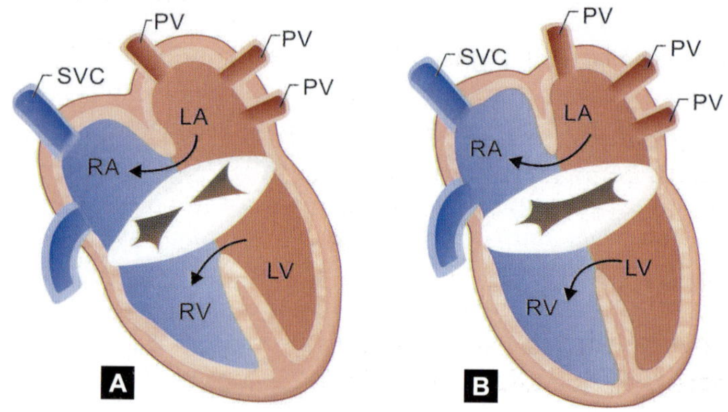

Figs. 5A and B: Intermediate (A) and complete (B) types of atrioventricular septal defects. The common atrioventricular junction is guarded by a single atrioventricular valve with five leaflets as described previously. There is non-restrictive left to right shunt at the ventricular level, in addition to atrial level shunt. In the Intermediate type of atrioventricular septal defect (A), a tongue of tissue connects the superior and inferior bridging leaflets. In the complete variety (B), the superior and inferior bridging leaflets are separate.

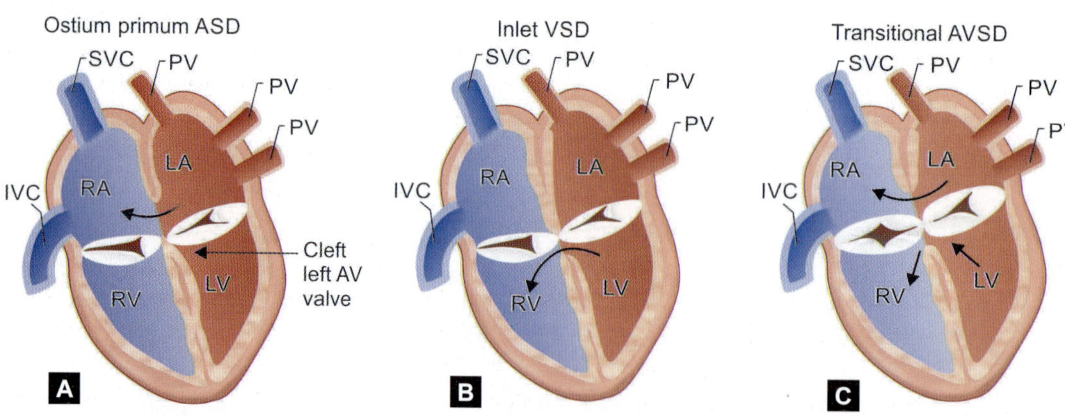

Figs. 4A to C: Partial atrioventricular septal defects. There are two separate atrioventricular valves. (A) Ostium primum type of atrial septal defect. Shunt occurs at the atrial level; (B) Inlet type of ventricular septal defect. Large shunt occurs through the non-restrictive ventricular septal defect; (C) Transitional type of atrioventricular septal defect. Atrial level shunt occurs through the primum type of atrial septal defect. The ventricular level shunt is typically small, as it is restricted by dense chordal attachments to the crest of the interventricular septum. The cleft of the left atrioventricular valve can lead to regurgitation.

(AVSD: atrioventricular septal defect; IVC: inferior vena cava; PV: pulmonary vein; LA: left atrium; LV: left ventricle; RA: right atrium; RV: right ventricle; SVC: superior vena cava; VSD: ventricular septal defect)

PATHOPHYSIOLOGY

The physiological consequences of atrioventricular septal defect depends essentially on the individual components of the lesion.

Ostium Primum Atrial Septal Defect

Degree of left-to-right shunting across an ostium primum ASD depends on its size. The shunt leads to volume loading of the right ventricle.

Inlet Ventricular Septal Defect

When the ventricular level shunt is nonrestrictive, the physiology is like that of any large ventricular septal defect. The shunt depends on the relative resistances of the pulmonary and systemic circulations, is generally large and left to right, resulting in volume overload of the left ventricle.

Complete Atrioventricular Septal Defects

The atrial component as well as the ventricular component are generally nonrestrictive, leading to large left-to-right shunts. Both ventricles are volume loaded. The atrial level shunt leads to right ventricular volume overload while the ventricular level shunt leads to left ventricular volume overload.

Intermediate and Transitional Atrioventricular Septal Defects

Although there are separate left and right orifices to a common atrioventricular valve in intermediate atrioventricular septal defect, shunts at both atrial and ventricular level are often nonrestrictive and resemble the complete form. In a transitional atrioventricular septal defect, the ventricular level shunt is small, restricted by the chordal attachments of the bridging leaflets to the crest of the ventricular septum. Major shunt is at atrial level, through the ostium primum defect.

In essence, partial and transitional atrioventricular septal defects behave such as ASD with or without a restrictive ventricular septal defect. Complete and intermediate varieties behave like combination of large atrial and ventricular septal defects.

Influence of Atrioventricular Valve Regurgitation

Irrespective of the presence or absence of separate left and right orifices, the leaflets guarding the common atrioventricular junction are frequently regurgitant. It can happen on both sides. Left-sided regurgitation is far more significant clinically than right-sided. It can add to volume load of the left ventricle, augment shunting at the atrial level and also raise pulmonary artery pressure. Regurgitant jets from left ventricle to the right atrium can occur through regurgitant leaflets and are not uncommon in atrioventricular septal defects.

Pulmonary Artery Pressure and Pulmonary Vascular Obstructive Disease

Isolated primum ASDs behave like other pretricuspid shunts, which takes quite large shunts persistent for significant duration for pulmonary pressures to rise. Also they generally do not develop pulmonary vascular obstructive disease in childhood. Presence of left-sided regurgitation or obstruction at the atrioventricular valve level or at left ventricular outflow tract can contribute to pulmonary hypertension.

As in any large ventricular septal defect, hyperkinetic pulmonary hypertension resulting from increased flow is invariably present when there is a nonrestrictive shunt at the ventricular level. Long-standing high flow to the lungs leads to pulmonary vascular obstructive disease. Large shunt at both atrial and ventricular levels are believed to bring in early onset of pulmonary vascular obstructive disease, compared to isolated ventricular septal defects. Patients with Down syndrome and atrioventricular septal defect are particularly prone to early onset of pulmonary vascular obstructive disease. This results from a multitude of factors ranging from upper airway obstruction resulting in alveolar hypoventilation and sleep apnea to faulty lung development resulting in decreased number of alveoli.

CLINICAL PRESENTATION

Prenatal detection of rates of complete atrioventricular septal defect is high as it is easily identified in the basic four-chamber view. Babies with Down syndrome are generally screened for heart disease. That is another setting where atrioventricular septal defects are commonly brought to medical attention.

Isolated ostium primum defects may present for the first time in older children or adults, like ostium secundum defects. Common presentation is with an incidentally detected murmur. Recurrent chest infections can sometimes be present. The presentation is markedly altered by the presence of moderate-to-severe left atrioventricular valve regurgitation or associated lesions like left ventricular inflow or outflow obstruction. These patients present with earlier and more severe symptoms including heart failure and failure to thrive. Infantile presentation is not uncommon in such a situation.

Isolated large shunts at the inlet ventricular level present with heart failure like any other large ventricular septal defect, around 4–6 weeks of age when the pulmonary vascular resistance falls. Babies with complete atrioventricular septal defects and shunting at both atrial and ventricular levels tend to present earlier. Severe left atrioventricular valvar regurgitation and significant left ventricular hypoplasia with aortic coarctation are other situations where heart failure can set in during early infancy. Nevertheless, in some babies, the pulmonary vascular resistance does not fall and they remain asymptomatic, presenting much late. This is more so in children with Down syndrome. Presentation with Eisenmenger syndrome later in life is not uncommon in low-middle-income counties where treatment is not accessible or affordable to many.

PHYSICAL EXAMINATION

The distinctive phenotype that is associated with atrioventricular septal defects is that of Down syndrome. Mild desaturation can be seen in those with a common atrium. Visible cyanosis is uncommon except in Eisenmenger syndrome and tetralogy of Fallot associated with atrioventricular septal defect. A low volume pulse and tachycardia are expected in heart failure. Prominent v waves in jugular venous pulse is typically identified in older children when there is large regurgitant jet from the left ventricle into the right atrium.

Clinical examination findings in an isolated ostium primum ASD is similar to ostium secundum ASD. The second heart sound has a wide and fixed split. A grade 2 or 3 ejection systolic murmur is best heard at the left upper sternal border, resulting from increased flow across the pulmonary valve. When the interatrial shunt is large, a mid-diastolic flow murmur across the tricuspid valve can be auscultated at the left sternal border.

Those with a nonrestrictive shunt at the ventricular level as an isolated lesion or with a common atrioventricular septal defect with large shunts at the atrial and ventricular level present with feeding difficulty and failure to gain weight which are characteristic of heart failure in infancy. History of recurrent chest infections is also common. On examination, these babies are generally underweight. Tachycardia, tachypnea, and hepatomegaly are present. Subcostal and intercostal retractions can be noted. The precordium is hyperactive. The apical impulse is hyperkinetic secondary to left ventricular volume load from shunt and or regurgitation from left atrioventricular component. Systolic thrill can be palpated at the lower sternal border.

The first heart sound and the aortic component of the second heart sound could be obscured in a pansystolic murmur from a ventricular septal defect or from left atrioventricular valve regurgitation, when the latter is present. The pulmonary component of the second heart sound is loud. Murmurs can vary markedly. When the shunts are nonrestrictive and or the pulmonary vascular resistance is high, soft, short systolic murmurs might be heard. When there is left-to-right shunt across a restrictive ventricular septal defect component, a harsh grade 4 or louder pansystolic murmur can be heard at the left sternal border. The presence of severe regurgitation from the left atrioventricular valve component results in a pansystolic murmur, best heard at the apex. This frequently radiates to the left sternal border, following the direction of the jet from the left ventricle to the right atrium. A mid-diastolic flow murmur at the apex can result from a large shunt at ventricular level or from severe left atrioventricular valve regurgitation. An ejection systolic murmur can be heard at the left upper sternal border, from increased flow across the pulmonary valve.

INVESTIGATIONS

Electrocardiogram

A quarter to half of patients with complete and partial defects have prolonged PR interval. The QRS axis is affected by the displacement of atrioventricular conduction tissues along with the loss of ventricular myocardium. Resultantly, a north-west or superior axis is seen (–30 to –120 degrees, mostly –30 to –90 in partial defects and –90 to –120 in complete atrioventricular septal defect). Extreme left axis deviation is seen in Down syndrome. Left-, right-, or biatrial enlargement can be noted. Right ventricular volume load from atrial level shunt leads to right ventricular hypertrophy seen mostly as a variation of RSR pattern or as qR pattern in precordial leads. Left ventricular volume load (Q waves and well-developed R waves in left precordial leads) can be seen in complete defects, partial defects with a nonrestrictive shunt at ventricular level and partial defects with significant left atrioventricular valve regurgitation.

Chest X-ray

Isolated primum ASDs lead to right atrial and right ventricular enlargement. The right ventricle forms the apex. The right ventricular outflow tract and the pulmonary trunk is enlarged. The increased pulmonary blood flow can be noted as increased vascularity extending into the peripheral one third of the lung fields. Left atrial enlargement does not occur unless there is significant left atrioventricular valve regurgitation, when the left ventricle will also be enlarged. Pulmonary venous congestion can also be noted in that situation. In complete atrioventricular septal defects, cardiomegaly is typical. All four chambers are enlarged. Left ventricle is apex forming. Increased convexity of right heart border due to right atrial enlargement and straightening of left heart border due to left atrium enlargement can be seen. Pulmonary blood flow is also increased and pulmonary trunk is enlarged.

Echocardiography

In addition to being the primary diagnostic modality, echocardiography can provide a gamut of information when planning management of atrioventricular septal defects.

Partial Atrioventricular Septal Defect

Characteristic diagnostic feature is the visualization of the cardiac crux from the apical four chamber view. Both atrioventricular valves are attached at the same level in contrast to the normal distal attachment of the septal leaflet of the tricuspid valve. The primum ASD is seen as a deficiency of

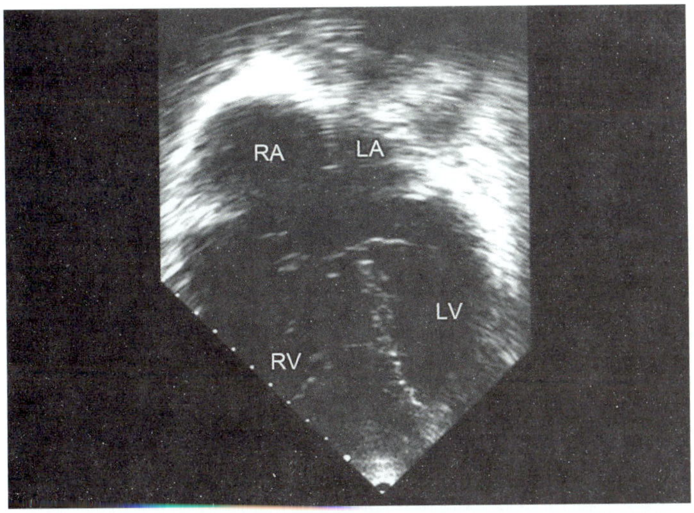

Fig. 6: Transthoracic echocardiographic image from apical 4-chamber view in a patient with transitional type of atrioventricular septal defect. There is a large ostium primum atrial septal defect and a small ventricular septal defect. Note that both atrioventricular valves are attached at the same level.
(LA: left atrium; LV: left ventricle; RA: right atrium; RV: right ventricle)

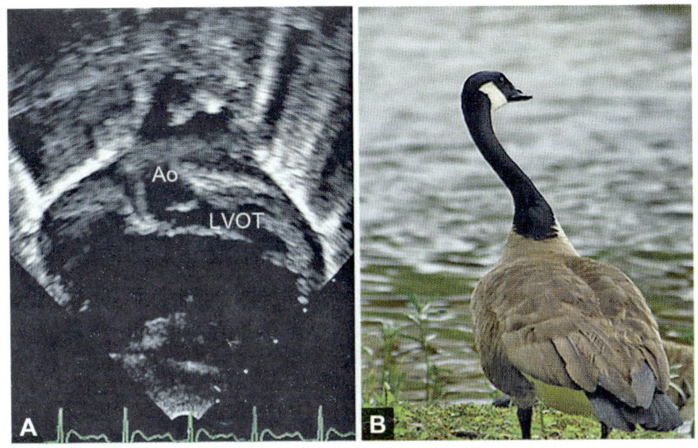

Figs. 7A and B: Elongated and narrow left ventricular outflow tract in atrioventricular septal defect, which resembles a "goose neck".
(Ao: aorta; LVOT: left ventricular outflow tract)

the lower atrial septum (**Fig. 6**). Color flow Doppler imaging visualizes the left-to-right shunt at the atrial level. Right atrial and ventricular enlargement accompanies the atrial level left-to-right shunt. In addition, in the transitional form, the bridging leaflets attach to the crest of the interventricular septum, forming a "tricuspid pouch", small ventricular level shunts can be seen through the interchordal spaces. The sizes of the ventricles are assessed in comparison to each other as well as based on Z scores.

Left atrioventricular valve abnormalities can be assessed in detail. The cleft of the left atrioventricular valve, the functional commissure between the superior and inferior bridging leaflets is best visualized in the parasternal and subcostal short axis views, directed to the ventricular septum. This is the most common, but not the only pathology leading to regurgitation. Others like papillary muscle and chordal abnormalities, myxomatous changes with or without prolapse and details of same are invaluable information which needs to be communicated to the surgeon who would be repairing the valve. Left atrioventricular valve regurgitation directed to the right atrium is generally taken care of by closing the primum defect and repairing the cleft which is a relatively straightforward proposition. On the other hand, regurgitation to the left atrium implies other abnormalities mentioned above and is a demanding task for the surgeon to repair. Presence of left ventricular inflow obstruction from valvar (double orifice) or subvalvar (abnormal chordal attachments, single papillary muscle, abnormally oriented papillary muscles) pathology needs interrogation. Other pathologies include discrete subaortic fibromuscular ridge and septal hypertrophy. The long and narrow left ventricular outflow tract, which has a "goose neck" appearance can be easily identified (**Fig. 7**). Left ventricular outflow obstruction is more common when two separate atrioventricular orifices are present.

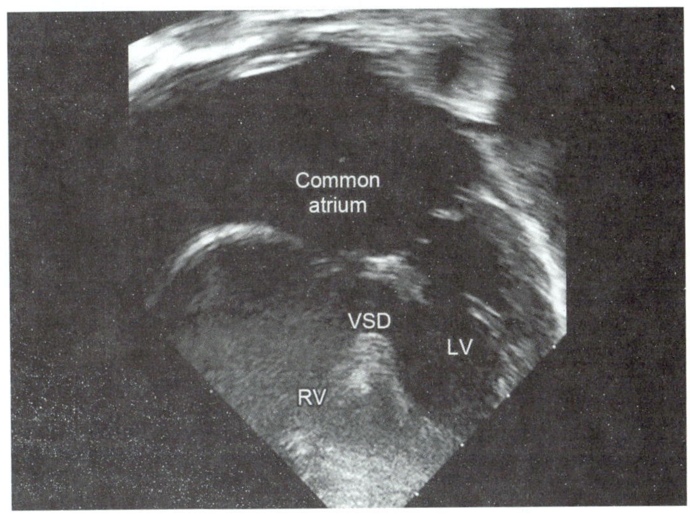

Fig. 8: Transthoracic echocardiographic image from apical four chamber view in a patient with complete atrioventricular septal defect. Note the large defect at atrial level in the ostium primum position as well as a large defect in the inter ventricular septum.
(LV: left ventricle, RV: right ventricle, VSD: ventricular septal defect)

Complete Atrioventricular Septal Defect

Diagnosis of the complete variety is a straightforward proposition as the atrial and ventricular components as well as the common atrioventricular junction can be readily noted from the apical four-chamber view (**Fig. 8**). A thorough anatomical and hemodynamic assessment takes expertise and skill and is an absolute necessity to plan appropriate management. The size and degree of shunting at both levels vary considerably and need to be assessed, from the apical four chamber and subcostal views using two-dimensional (2D) echo as well as color Doppler imaging. The ventricular septal defect is characteristically located posteriorly, where there is deficiency of inlet ventricular septum.

Additional secundum ASDs and ventricular septal defects scan also be assessed.

Commitment of the common atrioventricular valve to either ventricles and associated hypoplasia of the other ventricle as well as malalignment of the atrial and ventricular septae can also be assessed in the apical four-chamber view. This information as to whether the atrioventricular septal defect is a balanced one or an unbalanced one which precludes biventricular repair is also an essential point in preoperative assessment. 10% of all atrioventricular septal defects can be unbalanced. Presence and severity of atrioventricular valve regurgitation can be assessed using color flow mapping at ideal scales. Underlying pathology can be assessed using a combination of 2D imaging and color flow mapping, and should be communicated to the surgeon to aid in preparing with repair techniques. In addition, obstruction at the left ventricular outflow as well as inflow needs to be interrogated in multiple views. Severity and pathology as described earlier has surgical implications.

The subcostal sagittal (en face) view is ideal for interrogating the common atrioventricular orifice, leaflets guarding same as well as the subvalvar apparatus. The size of the leaflets and their attachments; the size, number, and orientation of papillary muscles, commitment of the common valve to either ventricular chambers are all essential for surgical planning. The relative sizes of both ventricles can also be assessed in this view (**Fig. 9**).

Associated Lesions

Tetralogy of Fallot, double-outlet right ventricle, and pulmonary atresia are more commonly associated with the complete form of atrioventricular septal defect. Coarctation of aorta can occur with the partial or complete forms. Patent ductus arteriosus is a common association of the complete form.

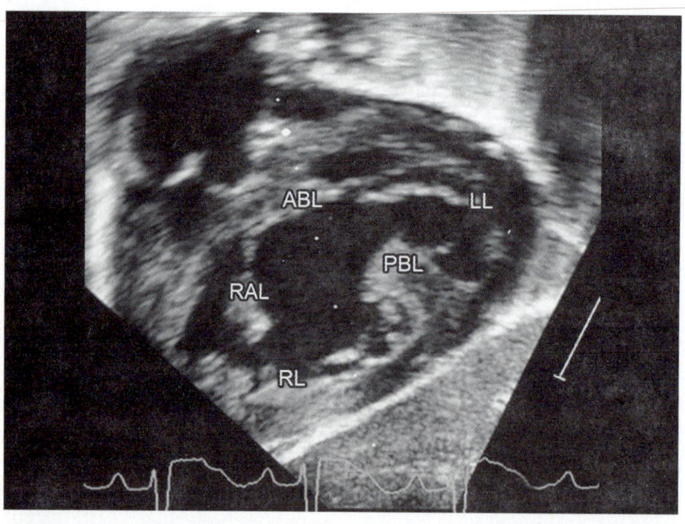

Fig. 9: Subcostal en face view of the common atrioventricular valve and leaflets.
(ABL: anterior/superior bridging leaflet; LL: left mural leaflet; PBL: posterior/inferior bridging leaflet; RL: right mural leaflet; RAL: right antero-superior leaflet)

Additional Imaging and Diagnostic Work Up

Computed tomography or magnetic resonance imaging can be particularly helpful in complex types of atrioventricular septal defects, e.g., ventricular hypoplasia, pulmonary atresia to delineate pulmonary artery anatomy, heterotaxy syndromes to confirm diagnosis and to delineate pulmonary and systemic venous drainage. Cardiac catheterization is required when pulmonary vascular obstructive disease has set in and patient presenting with borderline features of operability, to assess pulmonary vascular resistance and response to pulmonary vasodilators.

MANAGEMENT

Medical management is not an alternative to surgical correction, but is an integral part of preoperative stabilization. This involves heart failure management with diuretics and digoxin and, in some instances, angiotensin-converting enzyme (ACE) inhibitors. Attention should be paid to weight gain, calorie intensification being an integral part of preoperative management. With current standards of care, weight is not a limitation to infantile cardiac surgery when the clinical situation of the baby demands it.

All atrioventricular septal defects need open heart surgery under cardiopulmonary bypass for correction. Isolated primum defects with no significant atrioventricular valve regurgitation can be electively corrected at preschool age. Partial atrioventricular septal defects with significant left atrioventricular valve regurgitation are particularly challenging to manage. They do need corrective surgery which includes restoration of competency of the left atrioventricular valve and closure of the primum defect. Timing of surgery is variable and depends on the clinical presentation, best achievable physiology with medial management, underlying pathology, availability of expert hands for surgical correction, chances of technical success at surgery and an estimated reoperation risk. In the widely quoted Pediatric Heart Network study, 31% of patients had moderate or greater left atrioventricular valve regurgitation 6 months after surgery. Unless the patient is symptomatic from uncontrolled heart failure in spite of optimal medical management or there is severe regurgitation, elective surgery at a later age is preferred. The risk of hospital death after surgery for partial atrioventricular canal defects is <1%.[3]

Complete, intermediate, and the nonrestrictive inlet ventricular septal type defects invariably have large left-to-right shunts and need to undergo corrective surgery between 3 and 6 months, no later than 6 months of age. When heart failure and failure to thrive is uncontrollable, earlier surgery should be considered. At surgery, the interatrial and interventricular communications need be closed, two separate atrioventricular valves needs to be constructed from available leaflet tissue and competency of the valves restored. There are various techniques described for same.

In the double-patch technique, separate patches are used to close the communications at the ventricular and atrial level

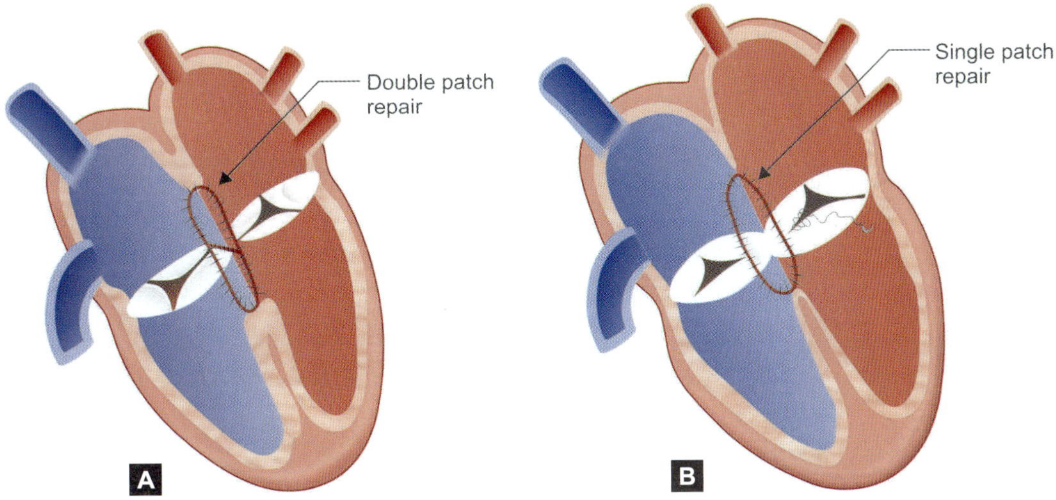

Figs. 10A and B: (A) Double patch technique for surgical repair of complete atrioventricular septal defect. The atrial and ventricular level communications are closed by two different patches; (B) Single patch repair for complete atrioventricular septal defect. The same patch is used to close the atrial and ventricular level communications, necessitating division and re attachment of the bridging leaflets.

(**Fig. 10A**). In the single-patch technique, the same patch is used for both, this necessitates that the bridging leaflet be divided and reattached (**Fig. 10B**). The "Australian" single-patch technique is suited for those with shallow ventricular components. Here, the bridging leaflets are sutured to the crest of the septum, closing the ventricular component without a patch. The atrial septal component is closed using a patch. The cleft is closed by majority of the surgeons, whichever technique they prefer. Additional techniques such as annuloplasty, leaflet extension/augmentation, chordal shortening, transfer, creation of neochordae, papillary muscle splitting can be utilized to restore left atrioventricular valve competency. When valve repair techniques fail, replacement is considered, although not preferred in infants and small children owing to attendant risks and long-term implications.

Hospital mortality for surgical correction of complete atrioventricular septal defects is 2.5–3%.[3,4] Complete heart block necessitating permanent pacemaker implantation occurs in another 3%. Younger age (<2.5 months) and lesser weight (<3.5 kg) have been identified to be associated with higher mortality, longer postoperative hospital stay, and increased frequency of major complications.[3] Most common reason for reoperation was left atrioventricular valve regurgitation, 4% in 6 months. At 6 months after surgery, 25% patients will have at least moderate left atrioventricular valve regurgitation.[3]

LONG-TERM OUTCOMES AND FOLLOW-UP

Regular follow-up with a pediatric cardiologist, followed by transition to an adult congenital heart disease specialist is recommended for repaired patients. The frequency should be dictated by patient status and severity of residual lesions. Common indications for reoperation include left atrioventricular valve regurgitation or stenosis, left ventricular outflow tract obstruction, right atrioventricular valve regurgitation, and residual shunt.

Pregnancy is well-tolerated in operated patients without significant residual lesions. Patients with unoperated partial atrioventricular canal defects will also generally tolerate pregnancy. Obstruction at left ventricular inflow or outflow levels will not be well-tolerated in pregnancy. Pulmonary vascular obstructive disease is a contraindication for pregnancy, considering the high maternal and fetal mortality rates.

The recurrence rate in children of parents with atrioventricular septal defects is 3–5%. Fetal echocardiography is advisable for early detection of congenital heart disease in offspring when repaired patients conceive.

ACKNOWLEDGMENT

Illustrations, as in Figures 1 to 5 and Figure 10 were kindly done particularly for this chapter by Dr Sowmya Ramanan, Assistant Professor, Pediatric Cardiac Surgeon, Department of Cardiothoracic and Vascular Surgery, SCTIMST, Trivandrum, Kerala, India.

REFERENCES

1. Cetta F, Truong D, Minich LL. Atrioventricular septal defects. In: Allen HD, Shaddy RE, (Eds). Moss and Adams' Heart Disease in Infants, Children and Adolescents Including the Fetus and Young Adult, 9th edition. Philadelphia: Lippinkot Williams and Wilkins; 2013. pp 757–82.
2. Narayanan DL, Yesodharan D, Kappanayil M, Kuthiroly S, Thampi MV, Hamza Z, et al. Cardiac spectrum, cytogenetic analysis and thyroid profile of 418 children with Down syndrome from South India: a cross-sectional study. Indian J Pediatr. 2014;81(6):547-51.
3. Atz AM, Hawkins J A, Lu M, Cohen MS, Colan SD, Jaggers J, et al. Surgical management of complete atrioventricular septal defect: associations with surgical technique, age, and trisomy 21 Subjects and Clinical Outcomes at Surgery. J Thorac Cardiovasc Surg. 2014;141(6):1371-9.
4. St Louis JD, Jodhka U, Jacobs JP, He X, Hill KD, Pasquali SK, et al. Contemporary outcomes of complete atrioventricular septal defect repair: analysis of the Society of Thoracic Surgeons Congenital Heart Surgery Database. J Thorac Cardiovasc Surg. 2014;148(6):2526-31.

26
CHAPTER

Pulmonary and Systemic Venous Anomalies

Arun Gopalakrishnan, Harikrishnan KN

ANOMALIES OF PULMONARY VENOUS DRAINAGE

INTRODUCTION

Anomalies of pulmonary venous drainage affect 9 per 100,000 live births and constitutes 1.5–2.5% of all congenital heart defects (CHDs).[1] There needs to be a clarity in the terms used for description of these entities. Total or partial anomalous pulmonary venous *connection* refers to the *anatomic* abnormality where pulmonary veins do not connect to the morphological left atrium (LA). Total or partial anomalous *return* (or *drainage*) is a *physiological* state in which pulmonary venous blood enters the systemic venous atrium. Usually, these are concordant. However, there are noteworthy exceptions. Anomalous return with normal connection of pulmonary veins to LA occurs in displacement of septum primum such that pulmonary veins are connected to left-sided atrium with drainage into right heart. In left heart inflow obstructions, there may be a large levoatrial cardinal vein that decompresses the pulmonary venous return to the right side (although anatomic connections are to LA). In the rare instance where all pulmonary veins join to form a common chamber draining into the LA, the connection is anomalous although drainage is normal. The pulmonary venous anomalies which will be subsequently described in this chapter are as given further:

- Total anomalous pulmonary venous connection (TAPVC)
- Partial anomalous pulmonary venous connection (PAPVC)
- Cor triatriatum
- Pulmonary vein stenosis and atresia.

EMBRYOLOGY OF PULMONARY VEINS

The lung buds develop from the trachea (foregut mesenchyme). The intrapulmonary veins are formed within the lung parenchyma from the splanchnic plexus and they establish connections with the primary pulmonary vein. The primary pulmonary vein is formed by canalization of the dorsal mesenchymal tissue in the mediastinum. This vein is engulfed by the posterior wall of the LA and the membrane separating them disappears, thus establishing connections between the pulmonary veins and the LA. TAPVC is a result of failure of canalization of the dorsal mesenchyme. Since the pulmonary veins do not establish connections to the LA, the connections with the systemic veins (also formed from foregut mesenchyme) persist and this leads to the anomalous connections to the systemic veins and to the right heart. This event occurs later in development. The site of this anomalous return depends on the level of persistence of systemic vein connections. Thus, in supracardiac TAPVC, the connections are established with anterior cardinal vein system. Similarly, the persistence of connections of pulmonary veins with left horn of sinus venosus constitutes cardiac TAPVC, and that with omphalomesenteric system leads to infracardiac TAPVC.

TOTAL ANOMALOUS PULMONARY VENOUS CONNECTION

The incidence of TAPVC ranges from 0.6 to 1.3 per 10,000 live births.[2] A recent Indian study reported that TAPVC accounts for 1.2% of all CHDs, 6% of cyanotic CHDs with a birth prevalence of 0.09/1,000 live births.[3] This group of anomalies presents at birth or within the first 6 months of life in the majority of patients.

Total anomalous pulmonary venous connection has been known to be associated with syndromes such as Holt-Oram and Klippel-Feil syndromes. There is a male preponderance in infracardiac TAPVC with males affected almost four times as frequently as females.

Sites of Drainage and Classification

The classification of TAPVC (**Table 1**) is based on:

- The pathway taken by the pulmonary venous return to drain to the LA
- Whether there is an obstruction to the pathway or not.

TABLE 1: Classification of total anomalous pulmonary venous connection (TAPVC).

	Anomalous drainage sites	
Darling's classification based on the level of anomalous venous return	Supracardiac	Left brachiocephalic vein (commonest) Right SVC, azygos system, left SVC
	Cardiac	Coronary sinus Right atrium
	Infracardiac	Portal veins Hepatic veins Rarely IVC, left gastric vein
	Mixed	Separate drainage of pulmonary veins or drainage of confluence to different sites
Smith's classification	Supradiaphragmatic • With or without pulmonary venous obstruction Infradiaphragmatic • With or without pulmonary venous obstruction	

(IVC: inferior vena cava; SVC: superior vena cava)

Neil's classification based on embryology and Burroughs and Edwards classification based on length (long, intermediate, short) of anomalous channel is of historical importance.

Supracardiac type accounts for 45–55% of cases of TAPVC. Cardiac type is seen in 20–30%, and infracardiac in 13–25% of TAPVC. The four pulmonary veins usually join to form a common chamber (confluence) just behind the LA. This chamber is horizontally oriented in most cases except for infracardiac TAPVCs where it may be oriented vertically and assume an "inverted fir tree" configuration. Supracardiac and infracardiac TAPVCs commonly have a vertical vein which ascends or descends respectively for some distance, before joining their site of drainage. The ascending vertical vein in supracardiac TAPVC travels in the left paravertebral gutter either anterior or posterior to the left pulmonary artery. The descending vertical vein in infracardiac TAPVC courses through the esophageal orifice of the diaphragm and joins the portal vein or its tributaries.

Associations

Except for the invariably associated interatrial communication, most children with TAPVC have either no associated heart disease, or only a patent arterial duct. The patent foramen ovale or atrial septal defect (ASD) may occasionally be restrictive and contribute to pulmonary venous obstruction. TAPVC is seen in 30–50% of right isomerism (asplenia).[4] Right isomerism is also associated with a high incidence of atrioventricular septal defects and pulmonary atresia or stenosis. Unbalanced atrioventricular canal defects (AVCDs) and single ventricle physiology in association with TAPVC constitutes one of the conditions with worst prognosis in palliated univentricular hearts.[5,6] Other heart diseases less often associated with TAPVC include ventricular septal defect, coarctation, aortic arch interruption, and tetralogy of Fallot.

Hemodynamics

There is complete admixture of oxygenated and deoxygenated blood at the venous level. There is an obligatory left-to-right shunt because the entire pulmonary venous return comes to right atrium (RA) independent of the pulmonary vascular resistance. The right-to-left shunt across the interatrial communication constitutes the only source of blood to the left heart, thereby determining the cardiac output. Since the blood reaching the RA can take either routes (across the tricuspid valve or into the LA), the left-sided heart structures are often underfilled and smaller in size. There is volume overload of RA and right ventricle as it handles the entire pulmonary and systemic venous return. The quantum of left-to-right shunt is much higher in TAPVC, as opposed to an ASD, due to the obligatory nature of the shunt. This increased pulmonary blood flow causes early symptoms in infants and contributes to hyperkinetic pulmonary hypertension and progresses much faster to pulmonary vascular disease. The systemic saturation in babies with TAPVC is dependent on the amount of pulmonary blood flow. Many patients with unobstructed TAPVC do not have clinical cyanosis.

One of the most important determinants of TAPVC hemodynamics is the presence or absence of obstruction in the venous channel. Almost all infracardiac TAPVCs are obstructive because of the long channel, drainage commonly into the portal venous system which offers high resistance to blood flow, and due to closure of ductus venosus immediately after birth. Supracardiac and cardiac TAPVCs are commonly unobstructed. There may be obstruction at the level of hemodynamic vise in supracardiac TAPVC— at the site anteriorly bounded by the pulmonary artery and posteriorly by the left bronchus where the ascending vertical vein can get compressed, especially with dilated pulmonary arteries and elevated PA pressures.[7]

Other sites of obstruction include superior vena cava (SVC)–right atrial junction in supracardiac TAPVC, and ostium of the coronary sinus in cardiac TAPVC. A restrictive interatrial communication is, in effect, an obstruction at the cardiac level.

Obstructive TAPVC leads to pulmonary venous hypertension which causes further increase in pulmonary arterial pressures. This contributes to pressure overload of the right ventricle in addition to the volume overload imposed by the large left-to-right shunt. There is severe desaturation because of inadequate oxygenated blood available for mixing. Severe hypoxemia combined with reduction in cardiac output, results in tissue hypoxemia and metabolic acidosis.

Clinical Presentation

Routine pulse oximetry prior to discharge will identify most of the cases in the present era. However, TAPVC with a large left-to-right shunt may be missed if saturations are borderline and baby is otherwise well. The typical infant with unobstructed TAPVC presents with mild tachypnea and cyanosis. There is cardiomegaly, right ventricular apical impulse, with normal first sound, and a wide and fixed split second sound. Midsystolic murmur in the pulmonary area and a mid-diastolic murmur along the left lower sternal border are soft clinical indicators of large shunt fraction. Occasionally one may hear a soft venous hum in the left infraclavicular region due to the flow in the vertical vein. This is not louder during diastole and is not altered by change in position or pressure on the neck veins.

Patients with obstructive TAPVC usually present in the first week of life with tachypnea, feeding difficulty, and cyanosis. Marked breathlessness may be associated with features of low cardiac output—feeble pulses, delayed capillary refill, and often need respiratory support. Despite presentation in extremis, precordial examination findings are less remarkable. Cardiomegaly, split of second heart sound, and flow murmurs typical of unobstructed TAPVC may be conspicuously absent. Hepatomegaly and a loud pulmonary component of the second heart sound are virtually the only positive findings besides lung crackles.

Rare presentations reported include dysphonia due to recurrent laryngeal nerve compression by vertical vein or hematemesis in neglected TAPVC draining into left gastric vein. Feeding or crying may cause compression on the descending vertical vein that aggravates respiratory distress and increases the cyanosis.[8]

Electrocardiogram

Right ventricular hypertrophy and right axis deviation of the QRS are the common electrocardiogram (ECG) findings in the neonate with TAPVC. Right atrial abnormality, with peaked p waves, is notable in infants with obstructed TAPVC, but is unusual in unobstructed TAPVC in infancy. In older patients with pulmonary hypertension, ECG shows tall peaked p waves, right axis deviation, right ventricular enlargement manifested as tall right precordial R waves, and deep left precordial S waves (**Fig. 1**). Incomplete right

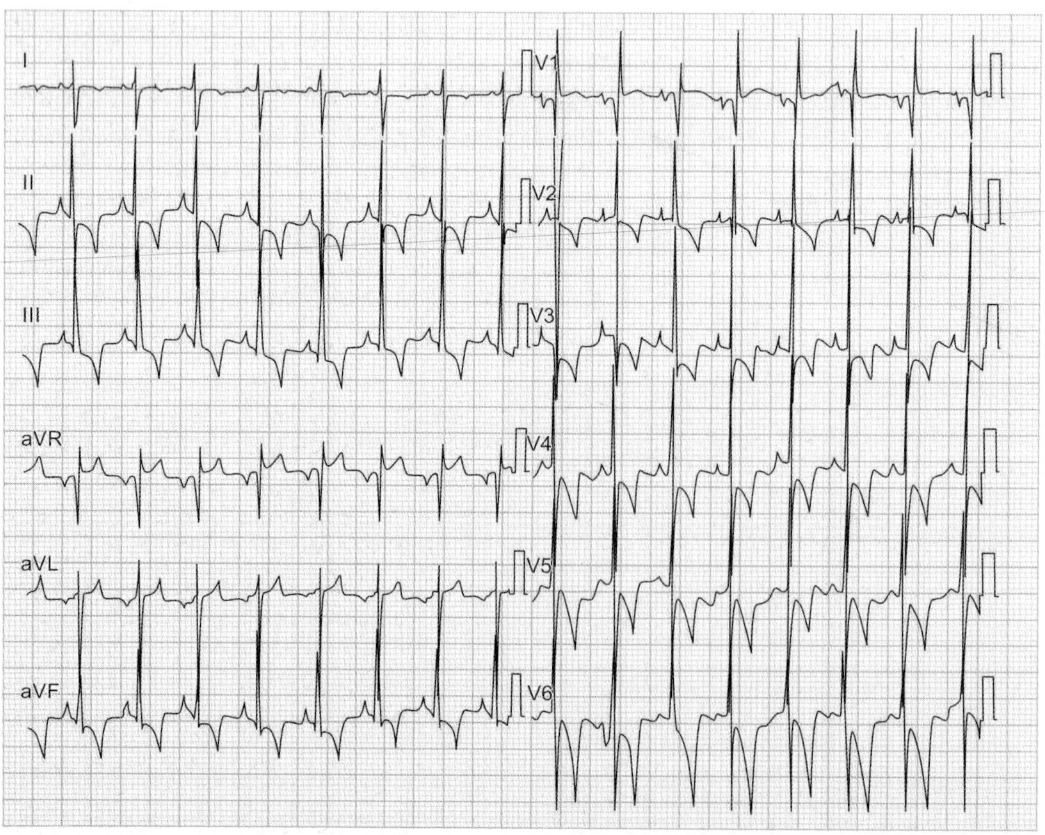

Fig. 1: A 12-lead electrocardiogram of a 24-year-old gentleman with unobstructed supracardiac total anomalous pulmonary venous connection (TAPVC) and severe pulmonary hypertension. Right axis deviation of the QRS, right atrial abnormality, and right ventricular hypertrophy with strain pattern are conspicuous.

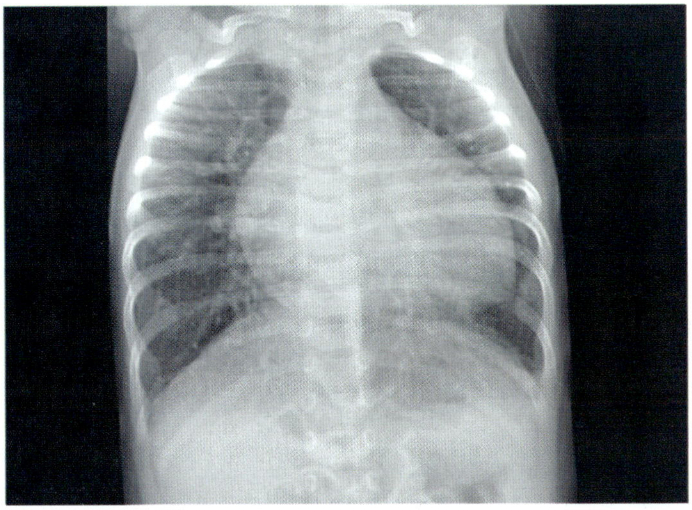

Fig. 2: Chest X-ray anteroposterior projection of a 10-week-old infant with unobstructed cardiac total anomalous pulmonary venous connection (TAPVC) to the coronary sinus. Cardiomegaly with right ventricular apical contour, right atrial enlargement, and increased pulmonary vascularity are notable.

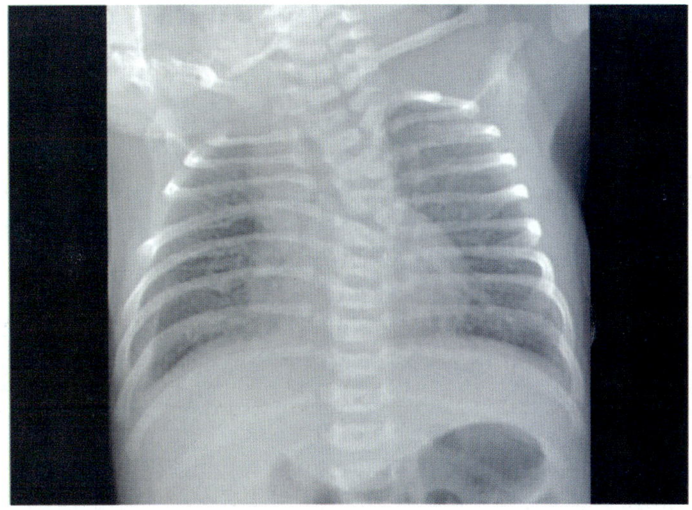

Fig. 3: Chest X-ray anteroposterior projection of a 24-hour-old neonate with obstructed infracardiac total anomalous pulmonary venous connection (TAPVC). Ground-glass appearance of the lungs is notable due to pulmonary venous congestion with pulmonary plethora rendering the right heart border quite inconspicuous. Multiple hemivertebrae are also seen.

bundle branch block pattern may also be noted. Patients with heterotaxy may exhibit low atrial rhythm and first-degree heart block.

Chest X-ray

Chest X-ray in the newborn with unobstructed TAPVC may be unremarkable or show only subtle signs of increased pulmonary blood flow. With increase in age, cardiomegaly due to right ventricular dilatation and prominent increased pulmonary vascularity herald the diagnosis (**Fig. 2**). In obstructed TAPVC, cardiac silhouette may become obscured because of the combination of severe pulmonary venous congestion and pulmonary plethora. This may lead to a characteristic ground-glass appearance or reticulonodular pattern (**Fig. 3**) and present a close radiological differential diagnosis to respiratory distress syndrome in the neonate. The older child with unobstructed TAPVC may demonstrate right atrial enlargement, cardiomegaly, and signs of increased pulmonary blood flow and resembles X-ray of children with large ASDs. Unoperated supracardiac TAPVC to the brachiocephalic vein in older children and beyond may reveal the classical "figure of 8" appearance or "snowman heart" (**Fig. 4**). The upper segment of the contour is formed by the left vertical vein and the right SVC. The lower portion is formed by the enlarged RA and right ventricle.

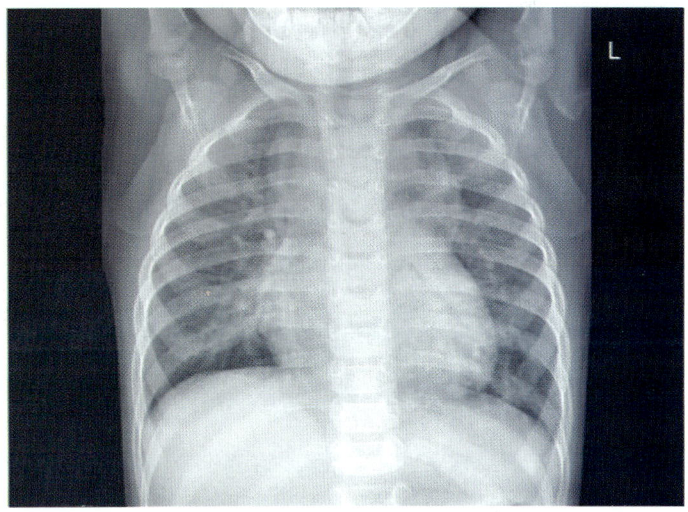

Fig. 4: Chest X-ray posteroanterior projection of a 12-month-old child with unobstructed supracardiac total anomalous pulmonary venous connection (TAPVC) to left brachiocephalic vein showing pulmonary plethora and the classical "figure of 8" appearance.

Echocardiography

Echocardiography helps delineate the drainage of the pulmonary veins, presence or absence of obstruction to the drainage, and presence of associated anomalies. The identification of an ASD shunting right-to-left should prompt screen for TAPVC (**Fig. 5**). The vertical vein in supracardiac TAPVC may be identified by imaging from the suprasternal window. The hemodynamic vise (**Fig. 6**), which is bounded anteriorly by the pulmonary artery and posteriorly by the left bronchus is also appreciated in this view. Analysis of the size of the individual pulmonary veins is important in preoperative evaluation as it predicts the long-term survival.

Additional imaging in the form of cardiac computed tomography (CT) or magnetic resonance imaging (MRI) is useful when echocardiography fails to delineate the anatomy fully. It is particularly useful in the setting of small-sized pulmonary veins, mixed TAPVC, and with associated aortopulmonary collaterals.[9] 3D reconstructed CT (**Fig. 7**) facilitates excellent understanding of the anatomy in TAPVC.[10]

Prenatal diagnosis is possible in almost 80% of cases. The diagnostic clues on fetal echocardiography include ventricular disproportion and increased distance posteriorly between the LA and the descending aorta. A vertical vein seen in up to 60% of cases.[11]

Natural History

Unoperated survival of TAPVC is bleak with only 20% surviving the first year of life.[12] Most deaths occur in the first 3 months of life in those with obstructed TAPVC due to pulmonary venous obstruction and/or low cardiac output. The median survival of supracardiac, cardiac, and infracardiac TAPVC is 2.5 months, 3 months, and 3 weeks, respectively.[13] Those who survive beyond the initial few months usually have unobstructed pulmonary venous return with increased pulmonary blood flow and minimal cyanosis. Most of them have some degree of pulmonary artery hypertension. The development of pulmonary vascular disease and Eisenmenger physiology is relatively earlier in TAPVC (second decade) as opposed to patients with ASDs (third and fourth decades).

Management

Corrective surgery should be offered as early as possible after a diagnosis of TAPVC. Stable children without obstruction

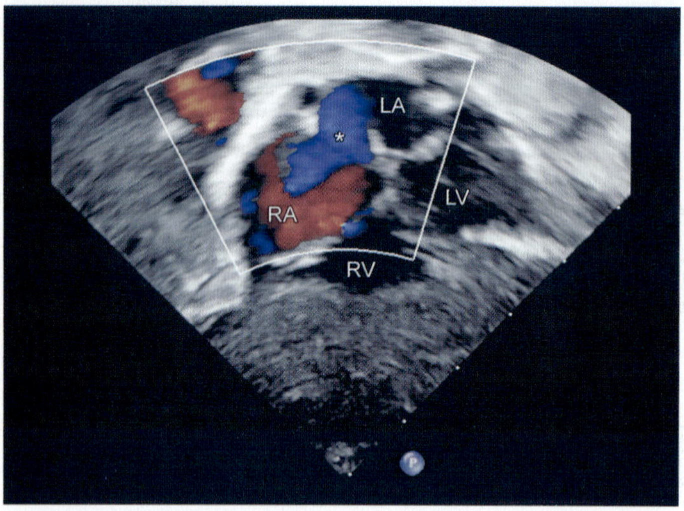

Fig. 5: Transthoracic echocardiographic still from the subxiphoid four chamber view in a 3-week-old infant showing the atrial septal defect (asterisk) shunting right-to-left as delineated by the blue flow away from the transducer. This should prompt a screen for total anomalous pulmonary venous connection (TAPVC).

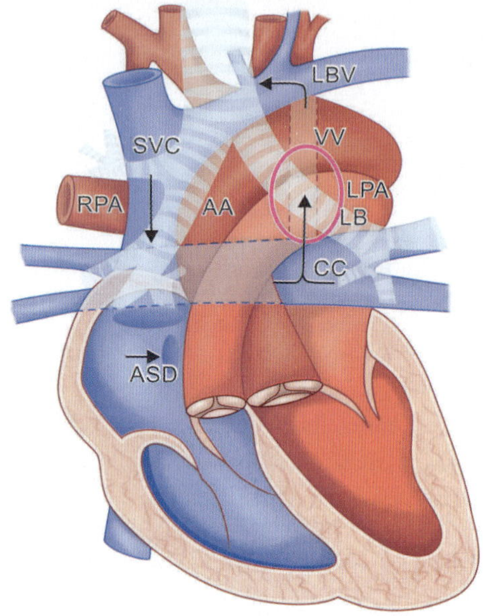

Fig. 6: Diagrammatic representation of supracardiac total anomalous pulmonary venous connection (TAPVC) to the left brachiocephalic vein (LBV) to superior vena cava (SVC). The "hemodynamic vise" (circled) is a potential site of compression of the vertical vein (VV) due to its compression by the proximal left pulmonary artery (LPA) against the left mainstem bronchus (LB).
(AA: ascending aorta; ASD: atrial septal defect).
Source: Reproduced by permission from Springer Nature: Gopalakrishnan A, Krishnamoorthy KM, Valaparambil A. Hemodynamic vise in obstructed total anomalous pulmonary venous connection. J Echocardiogr. 2019; 17(3):164-6.

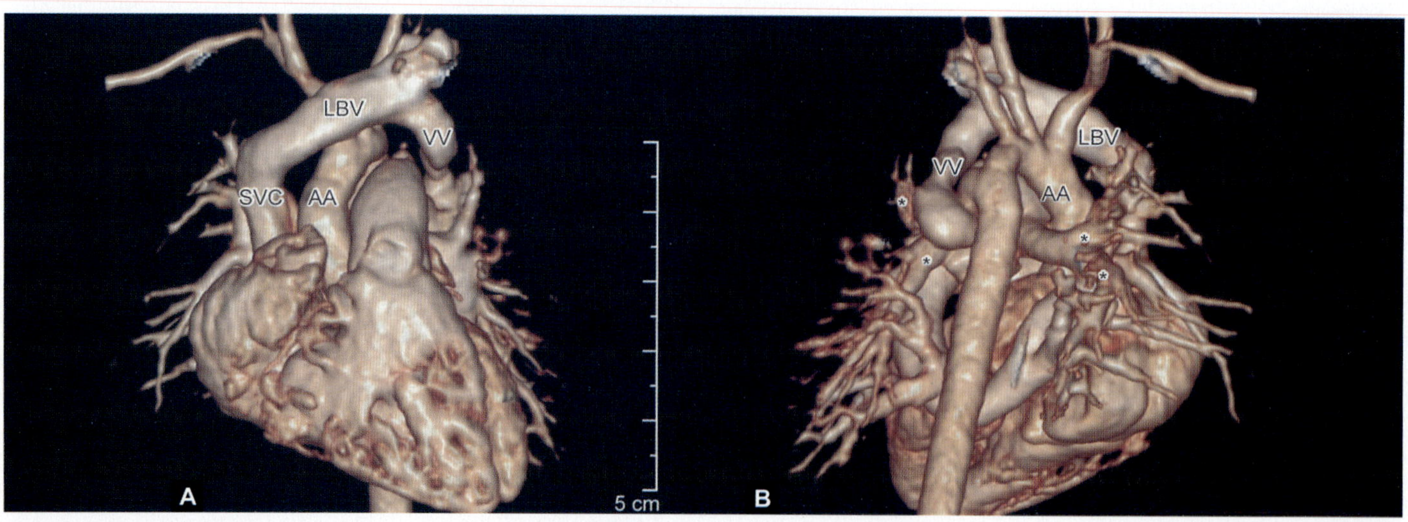

Figs. 7A and B: 3D reconstructed cardiac computed tomography showing supracardiac total anomalous pulmonary venous connection (TAPVC) to left brachiocephalic vein (LBV) to superior vena cava (SVC). Panel "A" is the view from anterior aspect, and "B" from the posterior aspect. The individual pulmonary veins (asterisks) join to give rise to the vertical vein (VV).
(AA: ascending aorta)

can be scheduled for elective surgical repair.[14] The surgical results have improved tremendously over the years to such a state that most operated patients have an event free survival resembling the normal population. The Pediatric Cardiac Care Consortium has reported excellent transplant-free survival after TAPVC repair with mortality or requirement for transplantation of 9.7% over 18 years.[15]

Obstructed TAPVC constitutes a pediatric cardiac surgical emergency. Preoperative medical stabilization is of paramount importance for the sickest child, with consideration for inotropes, mechanical ventilation and correction of acidosis, and other metabolic derangements. Diuretic use should be judicious, as overenthusiastic diuresis can reduce the cardiac output further. Ventilatory strategies include appropriate use of positive-end expiratory pressure to counteract pulmonary edema. A high inspired oxygen fraction can be detrimental as it can potentially worsen pulmonary edema. An arterial saturation of 85% in TAPVC offers a fair balance of pulmonary to systemic blood flow and limits pulmonary flooding.[16]

While prostaglandin infusion may be used in dire emergency to transport cyanotic babies to a cardiac surgical center, it may be considered a double-edged sword in obstructed TAPVC. The effect of prostaglandin E1 (PGE1) in an individual patient depends on its relative effects on the ductus arteriosus and the pulmonary vasculature.[17] If the action on the arterial duct predominates, opening up a closed ductus arteriosus can reduce suprasystemic pulmonary artery pressures but at the cost of desaturation due to the right-to-left shunt. If pulmonary vasodilation predominates, then the total pulmonary blood flow would increase, potentially increasing oxygen saturation but with a higher risk of pulmonary edema shortly thereafter. However, in infracardiac TAPVC, PGE1 can relieve obstruction to the ductus venosus and may offer temporary relief of pulmonary edema.

Balloon atrial septostomy was performed in the past for LA decompression in TAPVC with restrictive interatrial communication. This procedure is now obsolete for TAPVC.

The goals of surgery in TAPVC are as follows:

- To establish an unobstructed entry for pulmonary veins to the LA
- Interrupt the pulmonary venous connections with the systemic venous circulation
- Management of associated cardiac pathology.

Good outcomes are reported with surgery even in the neonatal period.[18] Multiple approaches have been used to reach the confluence which is subsequently anastomosed to the LA in supracardiac and cardiac TAPVC.[19] The overall results are good, and those with good pulmonary venous anatomy have excellent long-term results (**Figs. 8A and B**). In cardiac TAPVC to coronary sinus, the mouth of the sinus is cut back into the LA and the atrial septum is repaired in such a way as to leave the opening in the coronary sinus on its left side.[20] Alternatively, the muscular wall between the coronary sinus and LA is removed. Age at the time of surgery, the site of connection and presence of obstruction are the most important determinants of operative survival. The immediate postoperative period is complicated by existence of a low output state, persistence of pulmonary hypertension, and a highly reactive pulmonary vasculature which often responds well to inhaled nitrous oxide. Sutureless techniques adapted recently have a lower rate of postoperative pulmonary vein stenosis and need for reoperations although mortality is not significantly different.[21]

Postoperative Complications and Follow-up

Patients need to be on regular follow-up for evaluation of pulmonary artery pressures, pulmonary vein anatomy, and screening for atrial arrhythmias.

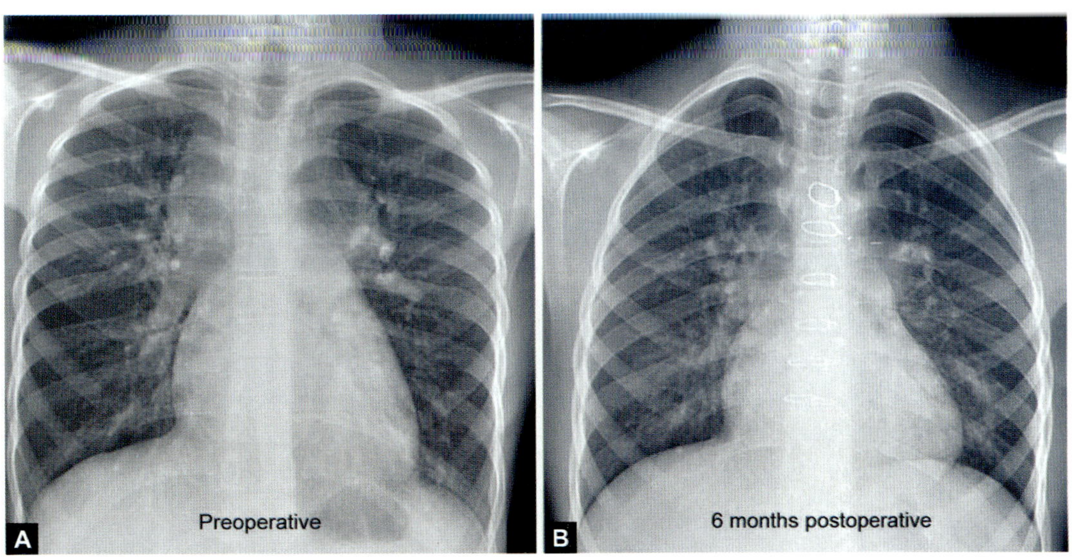

Figs. 8A and B: Serial chest X-rays of a child with unobstructed supracardiac total anomalous pulmonary venous connection (TAPVC) to left brachiocephalic vein. The "figure of 8" appearance in the preoperative X-ray (A) at 13 months of life is not seen at 6 months' follow-up (B).

The most common and difficult to treat complication after repair is pulmonary vein stenosis. The reported incidence is 5–18% across large series.[21] It is believed to be a reaction of tissues either to the operation or to prosthetic material used. Other theories include presence of unrelieved obstruction upstream to the pulmonary venous pathway, surgical errors, and flow disturbances leading to intimal proliferation. Freedom from reoperation was 82.6% at 11 years after repair, with increased risk associated with mixed connection type, hypoplastic pulmonary veins, and postoperative pulmonary venous obstruction.[22] In a series of 2,191 surgeries from Pediatric Cardiac Care Consortium, the overall in-hospital surgical mortality for simple TAPVC was 13%.[23] Mortality improved from 23% in the 1980s and 90s[24] to 8% in the first decade of the 21st century. The results of surgery performed later in life are also acceptable although there is a risk of persistent pulmonary hypertension and arrhythmias. Talwar et al. reported an event-free survival of 94.2% at 5 years and 90% at 20 and 30 years when surgery was performed after 10 years of age.[25] Age <2 months, obstructive TAPVC, pulmonary hypertensive crisis, and complex anatomy were the incremental risk factors for mortality in mixed TAPVC repair.[26]

PARTIAL ANOMALOUS PULMONARY VENOUS CONNECTION

When some of the pulmonary veins drain to systemic venous system and the rest are connected normally to the LA, the anomaly is termed PAPVC. Embryologically, this is a result of persistent connections between some of the intrapulmonary venous plexus and the systemic venous circulation. It is termed hemianomalous pulmonary venous connection if the entire venous drainage of one lung is anomalously connected to systemic veins. The left-sided pulmonary veins usually connect anomalously to derivatives of the left cardinal system (coronary sinus, left innominate vein). Anomalous drainage of the right pulmonary veins is usually to the right cardinal venous derivatives [SVC and inferior vena cava (IVC)]. The most common PAPVC is the anomalous drainage of RUPV to SVC as a part of sinus venosus defect, followed by PAPVC of left upper pulmonary vein to the left brachiocephalic vein. Patients with left atrial isomerism have a high incidence of PAPVC secondary to malposition of the septum primum. In this condition, pulmonary veins tend to drain to the ipsilateral atria.

Partial anomalous pulmonary venous connection results in obligatory left-to-right shunt as with TAPVC. In PAPVC with intact atrial septum, the various factors determining the quantum of shunt are the number of veins that are anomalously connected, the relative resistance of the normally and anomalously connected vascular beds, compliance of the atria, and the presence and degree of obstruction to pulmonary venous blood flow.

The clinical presentation depends on the quantum of shunt. If only one pulmonary vein drains anomalously, the shunt fraction would be small (~25%) and hence the patients are mostly asymptomatic. When the atrial septum is intact, the splitting of the second sound is usually normal and respirophasic. Cardiovascular examination is usually normal except for the occasional identification of a midsystolic murmur in the pulmonary area. In the presence of an ASD, clinical findings are similar to the latter.

Electrocardiographic findings are similar to that of an uncomplicated ASD. Pulmonary vascularity on chest X-ray gives a rough idea of the shunt fraction. It is a good practice to screen all cases of ASD for anomalous pulmonary venous drainage, more so in patients who are symptomatic disproportionate to the size of the ASD or present at an earlier age.

Partial anomalous pulmonary venous connection of a single pulmonary vein may be kept on medical follow-up in most instances as the shunt fraction is insignificant. When there is evidence of pulmonary overcirculation, shunt fraction >1.5, or right ventricular volume overload, surgical treatment is offered, as with HAPVC. The long-term survival results are excellent.

Two major entities in PAPVC merit further mention.

Sinus Venosus Defect

Sinus venosus defect is a consequence of a roofing defect of the right upper pulmonary vein (RUPV) such that the membranous wall between RUPV and SVC is absent. This leads to overriding of the SVC to both atria. There is a defect in the high atrial septum associated with left-to-right shunt and PAPVC of the RUPV to SVC. It constitutes around 5–10% of all ASDs. It may also be noted that PAPVC of the RUPV to SVC can occur even without a sinus venosus defect.

The clinical presentation of patients with sinus venosus defects is similar to any other ASD. The ECG may occasionally show a mild leftward frontal P-wave axis (less than +30 degrees) (inverted P wave in lead III).[27] Treatment is rerouting of the RUPV to the LA and closure of the ASD.[28] Warden procedure is one of the commonly employed strategy in the current era. It involves transection of the SVC above the level of drainage of RUPV and reconnection to the right atrial appendage. The distal segment along with RUPV is rerouted to the LA through closure of the ASD.

Scimitar Syndrome

Inferior vena cava type sinus venosus defects are located in the lower portion of the atrial septum with the IVC overriding the defect. This is a rare condition and is associated with abnormal drainage of the right lower pulmonary vein.

Scimitar syndrome refers to a complex of abnormalities of lung vasculature associated with PAPVC or hemianomalous drainage of right pulmonary veins to the IVC. It is often associated with right lung hypoplasia, dextroposition of heart, hypoplastic right pulmonary artery, and pulmonary sequestration, and is believed to be a developmental anomaly of right lung. The blood supply to the right middle and lower lobes also usually arise from the aorta or its branches. It constitutes 3–6% of patients with partial anomalous venous connection. The pulmonary venous drainage of the right lower lobe (and the middle lobe if present) is commonly abnormal (79%). In 20% of cases, the whole right lung drainage is anomalous into the IVC, either above or below the diaphragm. Around 20–30% of cases have associated cardiac anomalies including tetralogy of Fallot, ventricular septal defects, and hypoplasia of left heart. Left-sided Scimitar syndrome has also been described.

The patients may be asymptomatic or present predominantly with respiratory symptoms. A large surgical series reported 64% of patients to be symptomatic with recurrent upper respiratory tract infections (40%), congestive heart failure (35%), recurrent pneumonia (13%), and cyanosis in 6% of patients.[29] It has varied presentations with an infantile form with significant symptoms and pulmonary hypertension, an adult relatively benign condition, and a form with associated congenital cardiac anomalies.[30]

X-ray in Scimitar syndrome is notable for a vascular shadow in the right lung field that descends toward the diaphragm which resembles a "scimitar," a crescentic short Turkish sword (**Fig. 9**). Dextroposition of the heart due to right lung hypoplasia is characteristic. Relatively smaller right pulmonary artery, PAPVC of the right lower (+/- upper) pulmonary vein(s), and presence of aortopulmonary collaterals are other findings on echocardiography. Computed tomography is useful to delineate the right lung hypoplasia, pulmonary artery, and venous drainage of the right lung and aortopulmonary collaterals (**Fig. 10**).

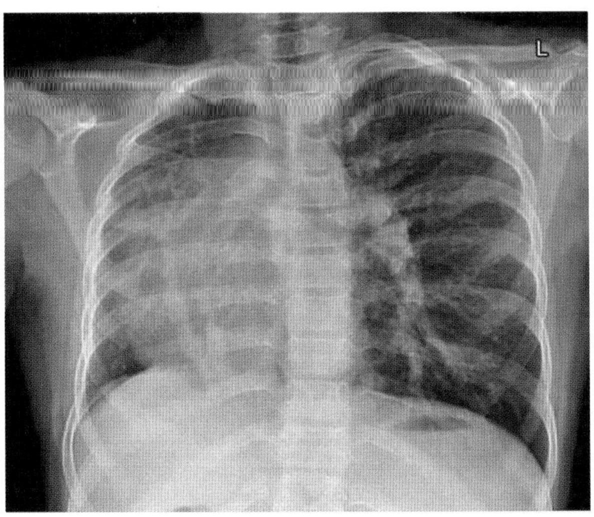

Fig. 9: Chest X-ray posteroanterior projection of a 4-year-old child with Scimitar syndrome. Cardiac dextroposition, right lung hypoplasia, and dilated pulmonary arteries consistent with pulmonary arterial hypertension are notable. The dilated right lower pulmonary vein assuming the "Turkish sword" contour is seen through the cardiac silhouette.

Surgical repair involves rerouting the anomalous pulmonary vein(s) with the use of an intra-atrial baffle or scimitar vein reimplantation. The early postoperative mortality of Scimitar syndrome is around 5.9% with either of the techniques.[29] Infantile presentation is associated with a poorer prognosis.[31]

Cor Triatriatum

Cor triatriatum, or cor triatriatum sinister, is an abnormality of development of the pulmonary veins where the absorption of the common pulmonary vein into the morphological LA is incomplete resulting in an appearance of "congenitally partitioned LA". If the membrane is obstructive, there is a left-to-right shunt by means of a superiorly placed ASD and a right-to-left shunt inferiorly through another interatrial communication. In classical cor triatriatum, the confluent pulmonary venous chamber communicates with the morphological LA through a narrow orifice **(Table 2)**. Subtotal cor triatriatum has part of the pulmonary veins connecting normally to LA and rest forming a proximal chamber which may or may not be connected to LA.[32] There are variants in which the pulmonary venous chamber does not communicate with the LA, but has connections with RA or is associated with TAPVC to systemic veins.

The clinical presentation depends on the adequacy of the communication between the proximal and distal chambers. In obstructive cor triatriatum, the clinical features are dominated by symptoms attributable to pulmonary venous congestion and pulmonary hypertension. These patients tend to present earlier in life with feeding difficulty, breathlessness, lower respiratory tract infections and, failure to thrive. Cyanosis may be seen in patients with associated TAPVC or with right-to-left shunt occurring at atrial level in certain subtypes of cor triatriatum.

Signs of pulmonary hypertension dominate the cardiac examination. Prominent right ventricular impulse, left parasternal leave, pulmonary ejection click, and accentuated pulmonary component of the second heart sound are typical.

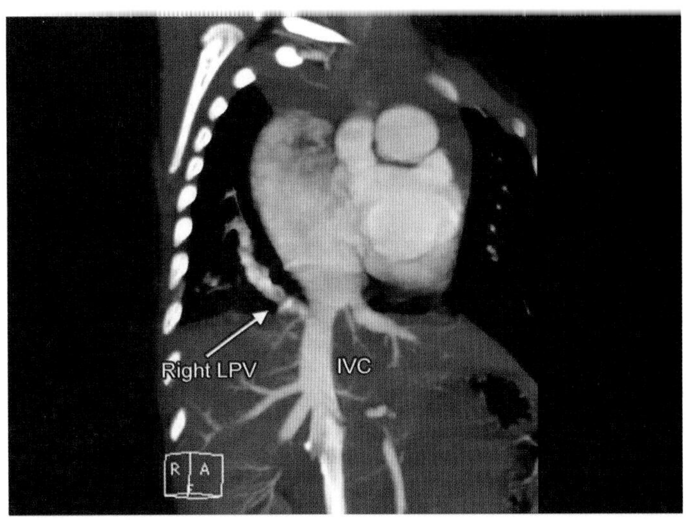

Fig. 10: Contrast computed tomography (CT) scan of an 11-month-old infant showing the Scimitar vein.

TABLE 2: Classification of cor triatriatum.[33]

Type	*Description*
I	Pulmonary venous chamber receives all pulmonary veins and communicates with LA
	• No other connection—classic cor triatriatum
	• With other anomalous connections – To RA directly – With TAPVC
II	Pulmonary venous chamber receives all pulmonary veins and does not communicate with LA
	• Anomalous connection to RA directly • With TAPVC
III	Subtotal cor triatriatum
	• Pulmonary venous chamber receives part of pulmonary veins and connects to LA – Remaining pulmonary veins connect normally – Remaining pulmonary veins connect anomalously • Pulmonary venous chamber receives part of pulmonary veins and connects to RA – Remaining pulmonary veins connect normally

(LA: left atrium; RA: right atrium; TAPVC: total anomalous pulmonary venous connection)

The usual cardiac murmur in obstructive cor triatriatum is a soft, blowing, systolic murmur along the left sternal border. Less often, a diastolic murmur is detected at the mitral area, or a continuous murmur is heard.

The identification of pulmonary venous congestion in chest roentgenogram in a child should prompt screen for pulmonary venous obstructive pathology such as obstructive cor triatriatum. Kerley B lines may be seen. Preferential venous engorgement of the upper lobe pulmonary veins can lead to the butterfly wing sign or the Staghorn sign. Concomitant dilatation of the pulmonary arteries (pulmonary plethora) is seen in patients with coexisting TAPVC.

The electrocardiographic findings are dominated by features of right ventricular hypertrophy, right axis deviation of the frontal QRS axis (+100 to +140 degrees), with or without right atrial abnormality.

Echocardiography is the diagnostic modality of choice. It permits direct visualization of a proximal and distal chamber along the pulmonary venous pathway before it traverses the mitral valve. Doppler is useful to quantify the degree of obstruction. Cor triatriatum may be associated with other congenital heart diseases including atrioventricular septal defect,[34] mitral regurgitation,[35] and tetralogy of Fallot.[36]

Cor triatriatum should be distinguished from supramitral ring, another cause of LV inflow obstruction. The membrane in cor triatriatum usually is more mobile, located proximal to the LA appendage and the region of oval fossa, and have the appearance of a windsock. A supramitral ring is located on the atrial surface of the mitral valve leaflets and is relatively immobile.

Surgical resection of the obstructive partition between the proximal and distal chambers is the treatment of choice for obstructive cor triatriatum. Any concomitant pathology such as anomalous pulmonary venous drainage or ASD is also corrected. Surgical outcomes are excellent with long-term survival comparable to the general population. Percutaneous management has been tried in selected patients.[37]

ATRESIA OF THE COMMON PULMONARY VEIN

This is an exceedingly rare anomaly where the confluence of the developing pulmonary vein fails to get access either to the LA or directly to the systemic veins. The physiological consequence would be marked elevation of pulmonary venous pressures. This markedly reduces the pulmonary blood flow over time. While deaths in early childhood are not unusual, there are reports of long-term survival. This is possible when these veins find an egress via bronchopulmonary venous anastomoses to the pleurohilar bronchial veins, which drain into the azygos, hemiazygos, and brachiocephalic veins.[38] Alternatively, blood could reflux from pulmonary capillaries into pulmonary arteries, and thence pass through bronchopulmonary arterial anastomoses and bronchial arteries into the systemic circuit.

The clinical presentation of this condition is similar to that of obstructive TAPVC. Deep cyanosis, breathlessness, and severe acidosis unresponsive to oxygen and medical therapy are typical. ECG would reveal right axis deviation of the QRS and right ventricular hypertrophy. Besides severe pulmonary hypertension and an atrial level right-to-left shunt, inability to visualize the confluence of the pulmonary veins or a definite channel draining under developed pulmonary veins on echocardiography suggests this condition. CT and invasive pulmonary angiography may fail to delineate the exit of the pulmonary veins. While pulmonary arterial wedge angiography may be necessary to fully define the anatomy, catheterization is often poorly tolerated.

Trisomy 21, asplenia, and ventricular septal defect are reported associations.[39] Survival beyond 4 weeks is exceptional. Untreated patients may develop secondary pulmonary lymphangiectasia. Surgical correction is similar to TAPVC repair, but long-term outcomes depend on the adequacy of individual pulmonary veins.

STENOSIS OF THE INDIVIDUAL PULMONARY VEINS

One or more of the pulmonary veins may have narrowing particularly at the entry to the LA. The more serious variant involves diffuse pulmonary venous narrowing or hypoplasia. The latter has particularly poor outcomes. They tend to present early with breathlessness, hemoptysis, pulmonary hypertension, and right heart failure. Surgical rehabilitative measures have not been consistently reassuring. Progressive reocclusion of the operated pulmonary veins is common and may necessitate lung transplantation.

SYSTEMIC VENOUS ANOMALIES

INTRODUCTION

Systemic veins are the blood vessels that carry blood toward the heart. The sole exception to definition of "vein" is the portal vein which directs blood to the liver, and is thereby part of a "portal system" and not entirely confined to the definition of systemic veins. Anomalies of the systemic veins are less frequently reported as opposed to pulmonary venous anomalies. Clinically relevant anomalies of the systemic veins are rare when the viscera and atria are normally lateralized, i.e., with usual arrangement of the viscera and atrial appendages and with mirror imaged arrangement of the same. However, the incidence of systemic venous anomalies is reported to be as frequent as 90% in heterotaxy.

It is imperative to have a thorough understanding of the normal anatomy of the systemic veins before trying to decipher its anomalies. The superior caval vein is right-sided in the vast majority of the population and drains the upper half of the body. The predominant venous return of the lower half of the body is through the inferior caval vein constituted by the confluence of the iliac veins. The posteriorly located azygos–hemiazygos system is usually diminutive and runs along the sides of the vertebrae and can serve as an alternative venous pathway in the case of obstruction to either caval veins.

EMBRYOGENESIS OF THE SUPERIOR CAVAL VEINS

The development of the SVC occurs later in embryological life as opposed to the IVC. There are two venous systems in the primitive venous network in the 4th-week embryo. The dorsal venous network consisting of the anterior and posterior cardinal veins carries the intraembryonic blood. The vitelline (omphalomesenteric) and umbilicoallantoic veins form the ventral nutritional extraembryonic venous system. The venous plexuses that drain the upper limb fuse to form the subclavian veins and ultimately open into the paired anterior cardinal veins. The anastomotic segment between the right and left anterior cardinal veins develop into the left brachiocephalic vein. The anterior cardinal veins cranial to the anastomosis become the internal jugular veins. The left anterior cardinal vein, below the anastomosis, loses its connection with the left common cardinal vein. The part that persists is a short segment which forms the left superior intercostal vein. The left common cardinal vein regresses, and the distal portion develops into the coronary sinus while the proximal vestigial portion may be left behind as a ligament of Marshall with the oblique vein of Marshall. The SVC is finally formed by the fusion of the right common cardinal vein and the proximal portion of the right anterior cardinal vein.

ANOMALIES OF UPPER BODY VENOUS RETURN

Persistent Left Superior Caval Vein with Normal Drainage

Failure of the left anterior and left common cardinal veins to involute leads to this anomaly, also known as SVC duplication. Autopsy studies reveal an incidence of 0.3% in the general population,[40] but it may be as common as 4% in the presence of other congenital heart diseases.[41] It is particularly common with some congenital heart diseases; tetralogy of Fallot (11%), atrioventricular septal defects (19%), mitral atresia (17%), and juxtaposition of the right atrial appendage (RAA) (34%).[42] The persistent left SVC courses to the left of the aortic arch, anterior to the left pulmonary hilum, and drains into the coronary sinus. A dilated coronary sinus is a usual echocardiographic clue to the diagnosis. The chest X-ray may occasionally show a shadow along the left superior mediastinum when the left SVC is prominent. The size of the left brachiocephalic (or innominate) vein tends to vary inversely with the size of persistent left SVC.

While most instances of persistent left SVC are clinically insignificant, it may occasionally be the choice of approach for insertion of a permanent pacemaker lead if the right SVC is small. Dilated coronary sinus associated with persistent left SVC may lead to mitral inflow obstruction and has association with Shone's complex. The diagnosis of a persistent left SVC is important to direct a bilateral bidirectional Glenn shunt in univentricular hearts.

Bilateral Superior Caval Veins with Unroofed Coronary Sinus

In this condition, the persistent left SVC opens to the roof of the LA as the coronary sinus is unroofed. The right SVC drains normally to the RA. This is seen in <10% of all instances of bilateral SVC. Heterotaxy is the usual association. Physiologically, it constitutes an isolated right-to-left shunt with desaturation at the left atrial level, presenting as cyanosis.

Absent Right Superior Vena Cava in Visceral Situs Solitus

This is a rare condition, and may occur even in the absence of associated cardiovascular malformations in 54%. It has been reported in 0.07–0.13% of congenital cardiac malformations.[43] Absent right SVC is almost invariably associated with persistent left SVC draining to the coronary sinus in the absence of heterotaxy. Although mostly benign, accurate diagnosis of this condition is required in permanent pacemaker implantation, venous cannulation for cardiopulmonary bypass or extracorporeal membrane oxygenator, and placement of a right ventricular or pulmonary arterial monitoring line through the subclavian or jugular veins, Glenn shunt, and orthotopic heart transplantation.

Total absence of both the superior caval veins is an extremely rare scenario where the primitive veins of the upper body gain access to the azygos system to drain sub-diaphragmatically to the IVC system.[44] The latter is invariably associated with congenital heart disease.

Anomalous Drainage of Right Superior Vena Cava to Left Atrium

Unlike most of the above-mentioned abnormalities, anomalous drainage of the right SVC to the LA can present with unexplained cyanosis or stroke due to paradoxical embolism in patients with no other congenital heart disease. The degree of cyanosis may be mild, and symptoms may not develop until late childhood or adolescence, or even adulthood. Van Praagh explains the origin of this condition to be analogous to that of SVC-type sinus venosus defect.[45] A deficiency of the common wall between the SVC and the RUPV causes the RUPV to drain to the SVC. The resultant defect in the roof of the LA serves as the site of drainage of the SVC to the LA **(Fig. 11)**. Concomitant atresia of the right SVC orifice completes the genesis of this anomaly. Transection of the right SVC above the entrance of the RUPV and anastomosis of the transected caval end to the RAA is the treatment of choice.

Retroaortic Innominate Vein

The normal course of left brachiocephalic (innominate) vein is from left to right, anterior to the aortic arch in the superior mediastinum, joins right innominate vein to form right SVC. It occasionally follows a deviant course, anterior to the left pulmonary artery turning rightward and crossing posterior to the ascending aorta, beneath the aortic arch, ending on the SVC caudal to the azygos vein **(Fig. 12)**. This anomaly called retroaortic innominate vein, or postaortic innominate vein, has been reported in 0.98% of patients with congenital heart disease. Associated cardiovascular malformations include tetralogy of Fallot with or without pulmonary atresia, truncus arteriosus, atrioventricular septal defect, heterotaxy syndrome, hypoplastic left heart syndrome, pulmonary atresia with intact ventricular septum, and coarctation of aorta. However, this is a benign condition and does not merit intervention.

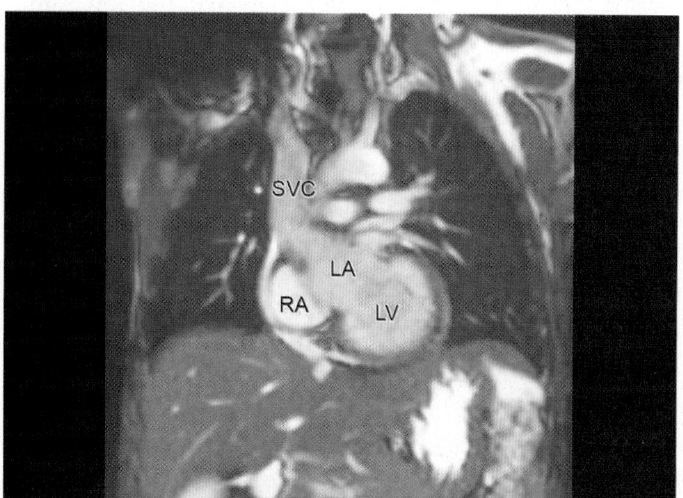

Fig. 11: Cardiac magnetic resonance imaging (MRI) showing right superior vena cava (SVC) draining to the left atrium (LA) in a 9-year-old boy.
(LV: left ventricle; RA: right atrium)

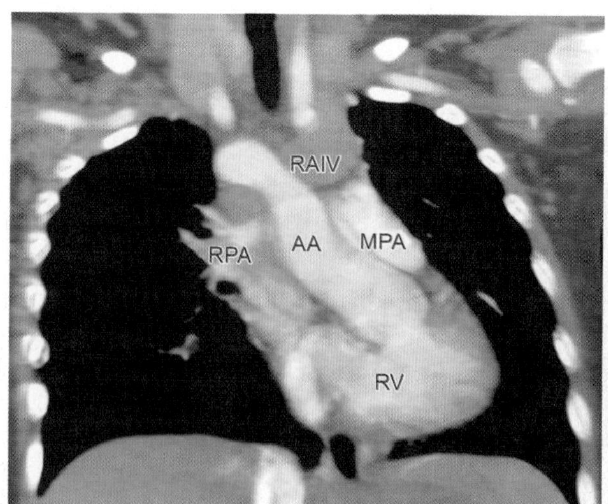

Fig. 12: Contrast computed tomography (CT) scan showing the course of retroaortic innominate vein (RAIV) in a 12-month-old infant with tetralogy of Fallot with right aortic arch.
(AA: ascending aorta; MPA: main pulmonary artery; RPA: right pulmonary artery; RV: right ventricle)

Levoatrial Cardinal Vein

The levoatrial cardinal vein (LACV) is the remnant of an early embryonic venous channel that connects the splanchnic plexus of the lungs with the cardinal system. This vestigial structure can open and provide an egress of left atrial blood to the systemic venous circuit in the absence of an alternate exit from the LA. It is most commonly reported in mitral atresia with highly restrictive interatrial communication.[46] Other reported associations include cor triatriatum and tetralogy of Fallot.[47] LACV typically takes a serpentine course ascending posterior to the left pulmonary artery to gain access to the SVC system.

ANOMALIES OF THE CORONARY SINUS

Coronary Sinus Septal Defect and Unroofed Coronary Sinus

Coronary sinus septal defect (CSSD) or unroofed coronary sinus syndrome, is reported in 0.1% of all congenital heart diseases.[48] Though often considered in the discussion of ASDs, it cannot be considered a true ASD. The morphology of this condition was lucidly elaborated by Raghib et al. in 1965.[49] CSSD may be classified into three types; type I, completely unroofed CS; type II, midportion partially unroofed type; type III, terminal portion partially unroofed type.[50] Subtype "a" is given to each type when associated with a persistent left SVC, and "b" in its absence. Completely unroofed coronary sinus with persistent left SVC and coronary sinus ASD (type Ia) is called Raghib syndrome.

In Raghib syndrome, the interatrial communication is located in the posteroinferior region of the interatrial septum at the usual location of the CS ostium. This defect may, on occasion, be confluent with a primum septal defect or common atrium. Besides the left-to-right shunt akin to an ASD, this condition presents an obligatory right-to-left shunt and desaturation at the left atrial level (**Fig. 13**). This constitutes another differential diagnosis in the evaluation of unexplained systemic desaturation in childhood or later in life. Demonstration of opacification of the left heart from saline contrast injection from the left upper limb venous access is useful in the diagnosis.

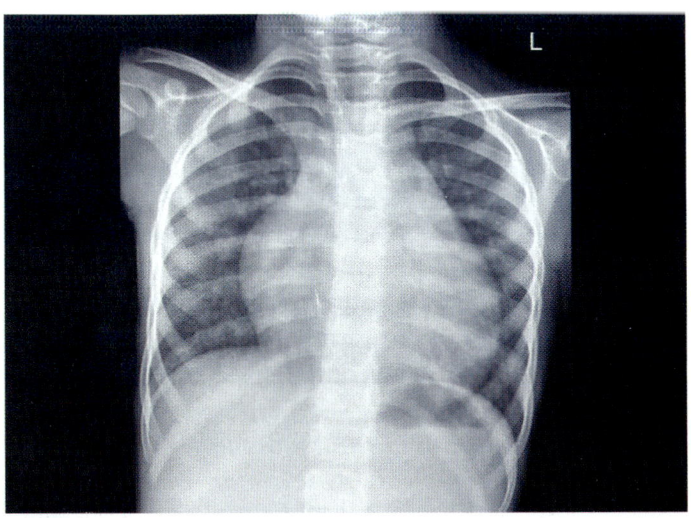

Fig. 13: Chest X-ray posteroanterior view of a 3-year-old boy with Raghib syndrome showing cardiomegaly and evidence of increased pulmonary blood flow. The oxygen saturation on room air was 93%.

Coronary Sinus Orifice Atresia

This is a rare anomaly where the coronary sinus does not have its expected opening into the RA. Myocardial ischemia is a sequel in the absence of an alternate egress for the coronary venous blood which limits long-term survival of these patients.[51] Some have alternative restrictive channels for exit of cesarean section (CS) blood. The identification of a persistent left SVC with retrograde flow toward the left brachiocephalic (innominate) vein warrants a careful screen for this condition.

Coronary Sinus Aneurysm or Diverticulum

The coronary sinus diverticulum is a pouch with its neck originating in the coronary sinus proximal to the entrance of the middle cardiac vein. It is an occasional site for accessory atrioventricular pathway and resultant supraventricular tachycardia. Most cases are benign and may be kept on medical follow-up.

ANATOMY AND EMBRYOGENESIS OF LOWER BODY VEINS

The IVC results from the confluence of the two common iliac veins at about the fifth lumbar vertebra. It develops between the 6th and 8th week of gestation. During the 5th week, paired subcardinal veins arise medial to inferior cardinal veins, and drain the developing urogenital sinuses. Cranially they drain into the caudal cardinal veins bilaterally. The right subcardinal vein becomes predominant, developing into *infrahepatic suprarenal segment* of IVC. The terminal *suprahepatic* portion of the IVC is formed by the right vitelline vein, which joins the right subcardinal vein. The infrarenal segment is formed by right supracardinal vein, while the posterior cardinal veins develop into terminal IVC and common iliac veins.

The azygos–hemiazygos system is a paravertebral venous pathway located in the posterior mediastinum. The azygos (meaning-unpaired) vein arises from the confluence of the right ascending lumbar vein and the right subcostal vein around T12-L2. It enters the thorax passing through the diaphragm via the aortic hiatus and ascends along the right paravertebral region, till the T4 level where it arches over the right main bronchus and terminates in the SVC. The hemiazygos vein develops similarly on the left side and turns at T8–T9 level to terminate in the azygos vein. The accessory hemiazygos vein drains the superior left hemithorax and left bronchial vein. It arises from the fourth to eighth left posterior intercostal veins and terminates in the azygos vein at T8 level.

ANOMALIES OF INFERIOR VENA CAVA

Interrupted Inferior Vena Cava with Azygos Continuation

Absence of the hepatic segment of the IVC with azygos continuation into the right or left SVC is referred to as an interrupted IVC. The hepatic veins drain directly to the RA carrying the portal venous return. While it can occur in the absence of any other intracardiac pathology, interrupted IVC has been reported in 86% of cases of left isomerism (polysplenia).[33] It may rarely occur in asplenia.

It is an asymptomatic anomaly as it does not cause any physiological disturbance. However, the diagnosis of the condition is relevant to plan cardiac catheterization or surgical management in isomeric hearts. Echocardiography is the imaging modality of choice. The absence of the infrahepatic portion of the IVC in the subxiphoid projection can be made out. A dilated azygos vein coursing with the abdominal and descending thoracic aorta is a usual accompaniment that can be identified by echocardiography. Care must be taken not to confuse a hepatic vein with the IVC. Other than its relevance with respect to management of the usually associated heart disease, no specific treatment is required.

Interruption of the infrarenal IVC with preservation of the suprarenal segment is a rarer condition which is also associated with hypertrophy of the azygos–hemiazygos system.[52]

Bilateral Inferior Vena Cava

Also called duplicated IVC, this anomaly may be explained by the development of the IVC which is related to the four bilateral venous systems that contribute to its formation. Bilateral suprahepatic IVC is more common in heterotaxy. It has been documented in 28% of asplenia and 6% of polysplenia in an autopsy series.[53] Bilateral infrarenal IVC may occur in patients with normal or abnormal visceral situs. This condition is usually benign, but becomes clinically relevant in the context of Fontan surgery.

Inferior Vena Cava to the Left Atrium

Whenever the IVC is noted to the left of spine, it is imperative to rule out anomalies of visceroatrial situs. In mirror imaged arrangement (situs inversus), the IVC on the left drains to the left-sided morphological RA and is physiologically normal. Anomalous drainage of the IVC to the pulmonary venous atrium can occur in several scenarios, most common being heterotaxy. With normal situs, the IVC blood can drain into the LA due to a prominent Eustachian valve at its atrial end which directs the blood across a patent foramen ovale or a low-lying ASD into the LA. Direct connection of the IVC to the LA in normal situs and intact atrial septum is exceedingly rare. Cyanosis and related complications are a concern and may necessitate IVC reimplantation.

ANOMALIES OF AZYGOS–HEMIAZYGOS SYSTEM

Azygos fissure and lobe is an anomaly found in 0.4–1% of the population due to an abnormal course of the azygos vein in the apex of the right lung subsequent to a failure of migration of the posterior cardinal vein.[54] The abnormally laterally located vein indents the lung and both parietal and visceral pulmonary pleura, resulting in the azygos meso fissure, a fissure with four pleural layers, similar to a mesentery structure.

Congenital absence of the azygos vein is rare and may be associated with enlargement of the paravertebral veins that drain to the SVC system.

ANOMALIES OF THE DUCTUS VENOSUS

Absent Ductus Venosus

The ductus venosus may rarely be absent and the umbilical veins may have anomalous extrahepatic termination.[55] Adverse perinatal outcomes including hydrops fetalis has been reported in one-third of cases.[56] It has been associated with varied genetic anomalies, intestinal obstruction, and CHDs. The diagnosis of the same is also relevant during umbilical venous cannulation in the newborn and upon cardiac catheterization.

Postnatal Persistence of Ductus Venosus

The ductus venosus is a fetal channel that permits oxygenated blood from the placenta to flow directly to the IVC—right atrial junction, bypassing the liver. It closes off in the first week of life in the vast majority of newborns. Persistent ductus venosus constitutes an intrahepatic portocaval shunt and can present with hyperammonemia and encephalopathy in affected neonates. The persistent ductus venosus has been postulated to decrease the perfusion of the neonatal liver, leading to neonatal cholestasis.[57] It can also impair ammonia detoxification, regulation of total bile acid concentration and production of vitamin K-dependent clotting factors with consequent hepatic dysfunction in neonates.[58]

CONGENITAL EXTRAHEPATIC PORTOSYSTEMIC VENOUS SHUNT (ABERNETHY MALFORMATION)

Congenital extrahepatic portosystemic venous shunt (CEPS) constitutes a venous anomaly of the portal vascular system where portal blood enters the caval return to the right heart bypassing the liver. It was first described by John Abernethy in the late 18th century.[59]

Morgan and Superina classified this anomaly into two types based on the absence or presence of an intrahepatic portal venous supply.[60] Type I CEPS refers to the condition when the liver is not perfused with portal blood, i.e., absent intrahepatic portal venous drainage. Partial shunts are classified as type II CEPS, where the intrahepatic portal veins are intact. Type 1 CEPS is further classified into those, in which splenic vein and superior mesenteric vein drain separately into systemic vein (Type 1a) and those in which superior mesenteric and splenic vein form a confluence and drain into systemic vein (Type 1b). Type 1 CEPS shows a female preponderance and tends to present early in life, unlike type 2 with no gender predilection.[61]

As the portal vein is formed by the selective involution of the peri-intestinal vitelline venous loop, abnormal patterns of involution may result in a preduodenal, prebiliary, or duplicated portal vein. Excessive involution may result in an absent portal vein. The absence of the portal vein thus results due to abnormal development in weeks 4–10 of gestation. Since the IVC develops from multiple venous channels, persistent connections between the right and left vitelline veins toward the liver can explain the development of CEPS.

Congenital extrahepatic portosystemic venous shunt may constitute an incidental diagnosis in some patients. However, it may also present with secondary complications of portosystemic shunt. Hepatopulmonary syndrome, with hepatic dysfunction, pulmonary abnormalities, and systemic desaturation, is a common presentation. It is probably related to altered hepatic synthesis or metabolism of vasoactive pulmonary substances, leading to pulmonary vasodilatation as well as diffusion perfusion defects.[62] The mean age of presentation of CEPS with heptopulmonary syndrome is between 6 and 8 years of life.[63] Pulmonary arteriovenous fistulae are often associated with CEPS causing intrapulmonary right-to-left shunt and resultant arterial desaturation. The presence of cyanosis and clubbing in patients without structural heart disease should prompt a screen for CEPS. With CEPS, the mesenteric blood bypasses hepatic detoxification, thereby entering the pulmonary and systemic circulation. Hyperammonemia is almost universal in CEPS, and rarely may lead to hepatic encephalopathy.[64]

Unexplained pulmonary artery hypertension can occasionally be a presentation of CEPS. This subset is usually not associated with pulmonary arteriovenous fistula. Regression of pulmonary arterial hypertension has been documented after closure of CEPS in patients with heterotaxy and congenital heart disease.[65]

Membranoproliferative glomerulonephritis with hematuria and proteinuria with no hepatic cirrhosis is another rare mode of presentation of CEPS.[66] This may present with nephrotic syndrome or chronic renal failure.

Diagnosis is made by ultrasound of the abdomen which can delineate the abnormal portosystemic connection with/without liver abnormality. The communication may be end-to-side or end-to-end. It is also important to rule out acquired causes of portal vein occlusion such as portal cavernoma and portal venous thrombosis before assigning a label of CEPS. As a rule, patients with congenital portosystemic shunts do not have features of portal hypertension, such as splenomegaly, varices, and collaterals.[67] CT can delineate the anomaly rapidly and with precision, but involves radiation. MRI avoids radiation, but offers lower spatial resolution and is time-consuming.

Agitated saline contrast injection from a large bore peripheral venous access can be used to screen for pulmonary arteriovenous fistula, in the absence of intracardiac shunt lesions. The appearance of saline contrast in the left heart between three to five cardiac cycles is suggestive of intrapulmonary right-to-left shunt.

Asymptomatic patients with incidentally detected CEPS with normal oxygen saturation and metabolic parameters may be managed medically. Liver transplantation is the only effective treatment for type 1 CEPS. Surgical interruption of the portosystemic connection and percutaneous occlusion of the shunt are the treatment modalities for type 2 CEPS.[64] Percutaneous strategies include the use of detachable coils, various device occluders, vascular plugs, and aortic endografts. Portal venous pressure must be assessed prior to occlusion. Those with portal venous pressures above 32 mm Hg upon test occlusion require staged interventions.[68] Long-term outcomes are good with both surgical occlusion[63] and device closure.[69] Intrahepatic portal ramification tends to improve over time following closure of the shunt.

TOTALLY ANOMALOUS SYSTEMIC VENOUS CONNECTION

The extremely rare situation where all the hepatic veins, coronary sinus, and both the caval veins connect to the LA constitutes totally anomalous systemic venous connection (TASVC). TASVC is a cyanotic heart disease and produces complete admixture of oxygenated and deoxygenated blood in LA. Left-to-right shunt across an atrial or ventricular septal defect is the most often source of pulmonary blood flow and decides the systemic saturation in TASVC.[70] It is associated with left atrial isomerism.

REFERENCES

1. Hoffman JIE, Kaplan S, Liberthson RR. Prevalence of congenital heart disease. Am Heart J. 2004;147(3):425-39.
2. Hoffman JIE, Kaplan S. The incidence of congenital heart disease. J Am Coll Cardiol. 2002; 39(12):1890-900.
3. Saxena A, Mehta A, Sharma M, Salhan S, Kalaivani M, Ramakrishnan S, et al. Birth prevalence of congenital heart disease: a cross-sectional observational study from North India. Ann Pediatr Cardiol. 2016;9(3):205-9.
4. Morales DLS, Braud BE, Booth JH, Graves DE, Heinle JS, McKenzie ED, et al. Heterotaxy patients with total anomalous pulmonary venous return: improving surgical results. Ann Thorac Surg. 2006;82(5):1621-7; discussion 1627-1628.
5. Khan MS, Bryant R, Kim SH, Hill KD, Jacobs JP, Jacobs ML, et al. Contemporary outcomes of surgical repair of total anomalous pulmonary venous connection in patients with heterotaxy syndrome. Ann Thorac Surg. 2015;99(6):2134-40.
6. White BR, Ho DY, Faerber JA, Katcoff H, Glatz AC, Mascio CE, et al. repair of total anomalous pulmonary venous connection: risk factors for postoperative obstruction. The Ann Thorac Surg. 2019;108(1):122-9.

7. Gopalakrishnan A, Krishnamoorthy KM, Valaparambil A. Hemodynamic vise in obstructed total anomalous pulmonary venous connection. J Echocardiogr. 2019;17(3):164-6.
8. Roy A, Agarwal S, Geelani MA, Tomar AS, Chauhan A, Raj N. Dysphagia lusoria with a supracardiac total anomalous pulmonary venous connection. J Card Surg. 2017;32(11): 724-6.
9. Dillman JR, Yarram SG, Hernandez RJ. Imaging of pulmonary venous developmental anomalies. Am J Roentgenol. 2009;192(5): 1272-85.
10. Oh KH, Choo KS, Lim SJ, Lee HD, Park JA, Jo MJ, et al. Multidetector CT evaluation of total anomalous pulmonary venous connections: comparison with echocardiography. Pediatr Radiol. 2009;39(9):950-4.
11. Paladini D, Pistorio A, Wu LH, Meccariello G, Lei T, Tuo G, et al. Prenatal diagnosis of total and partial anomalous pulmonary venous connection: multicenter cohort study and meta-analysis. Ultrasound Obstet Gynecol. 2018; 52(1):24-34.
12. Burroughs JT, Edwards JE. Total anomalous pulmonary venous connection. Am Heart J. 1960;59(6):913-31.
13. Hazelrig JB, Turner ME, Blackstone EH. Parametric survival analysis combining longitudinal and cross-sectional-censored and interval-censored data with concomitant information. Biometrics. 1982;38(1):1-15.
14. Kouchoukos NT, Blackstone EH, Hanley FL, Kirklin JK. Total anomalous pulmonary venous connection. In: Kirklin/Barratt-Boyes Cardiac Surgery, 4th edition. Philadelphia: Elsevier/ Saunders; 2013. pp. 1196-8.
15. Louis JDS, McCracken CE, Turk EM, Hancock HS, Menk JS, Harvey BA, et al. Long-term transplant-free survival after repair of total anomalous pulmonary venous connection. Ann Thorac Surg. 2018;105(1):186-92.
16. Tharakan JA. Admixture lesions in congenital cyanotic heart disease. Ann Pediatr Cardiol. 2011;4(1):53-9.
17. Rudolph A. Congenital Diseases of the Heart: Clinical-Physiological Considerations, 3rd edition. Chichester, UK; Hoboken, NJ: Wiley-Blackwell; 2009. p. 544.
18. Warrier G, Dharan BS, Koshy S, Kumar S, Krishnanaik S, Rao SG. Repair of total anomalous pulmonary venous connection in neonates. Indian J Thorac Cardiovasc Surg. 2004; 20(4):155-8.
19. Vanderlaan RD, Caldarone CA. Surgical approaches to total anomalous pulmonary venous connection. Semin Thorac Cardiovasc Surg Pediatr Card Surg Ann. 2018;21:83-91.
20. Koshy S, Kumar RK, Gururaja RS, Shivaprakasha K. Novel repair for obstructed total anomalous pulmonary venous connection to coronary sinus. Ann Thorac Surg. 2005;79(2):711-3.
21. Wu Y, Wu Z, Zheng J, Li Y, Zhou Y, Kuang H, et al. Sutureless technique versus conventional surgery in the primary treatment of total anomalous pulmonary venous connection: a systematic review and meta-analysis. J Cardiothorac Surg. 2018;13(1):69.
22. Karamlou T, Gurofsky R, Al Sukhni E, Coles JG, Williams WG, Caldarone CA, et al. Factors associated with mortality and reoperation in 377 children with total anomalous pulmonary venous connection. Circulation. 2007; 115(12):1591-8.
23. Louis JDS, Harvey BA, Menk JS, Raghuveer G, O'Brien JE, Bryant R, et al. Repair of "simple" total anomalous pulmonary venous connection: a review from the Pediatric Cardiac Care Consortium. Ann Thorac Surg. 2012;94(1):133-8.
24. Choudhary SK, Bhan A, Sharma R, Mathur A, Airan B, Saxena A, et al. Repair of total anomalous pulmonary venous connection in infancy: experience from a developing country. Ann Thorac Surg. 1999;68(1):155-9.
25. Talwar S, Arora Y, Gupta SK, Kothari SS, Ramakrishnan S, Saxena A, et al. Total anomalous pulmonary venous connection beyond the first decade of life. World J Pediatr Congenit Heart Surg. 2019;10(2):185-91.
26. Chowdhury UK, Airan B, Malhotra A, Bisoi AK, Saxena A, Kothari SS, et al. Mixed total anomalous pulmonary venous connection: anatomic variations, surgical approach, techniques, and results. J Thorac Cardiovasc Surg. 2008;135(1):106-16, 116.e1-5.
27. Davia JE, Cheitlin MD, Bedynek JL. Sinus venosus atrial septal defect: analysis of fifty cases. Am Heart J. 1973;85(2):177-85.
28. Jost CHA, Connolly HM, Danielson GK, Bailey KR, Schaff HV, Shen WK, et al. Sinus venosus atrial septal defect. Circulation. 2005; 112(13):1953-8.
29. Vida VL, Padalino MA, Boccuzzo G, Tarja E, Berggren H, Carrel T, et al. Scimitar syndrome. Circulation. 2010;122(12):1159-66.
30. Dupuis C, Charaf LA, Brevière GM, Abou P, Rémy-Jardin M, Helmius G. The "adult" form of the scimitar syndrome. Am J Cardiol. 1992; 70(4):502-7.
31. Brink J, Yong MS, d'Udekem Y, Weintraub RG, Brizard CP, Konstantinov IE. Surgery for Scimitar syndrome: the Melbourne experience. Interact Cardio Vasc Thorac Surg. 2015;20(1):31-4.
32. Nassar PN, Hamdan RH. Cor triatriatum sinistrum: classification and imaging modalities. Eur J Cardiovasc Med. 2011;1(3):84-7.
33. Moss & Adams' Heart Disease in Infants, Children, and Adolescents, Including the Fetus and Young Adult, 9th edition. Lippincott Williams & Wilkins; 2016. p. 1900.
34. Goel AK, Saxena A, Kothari SS. Atrioventricular septal defect with cor triatriatum: case report and review of the literature. Pediatr Cardiol. 1998;19(3):243-5.
35. Jayaprakash K, Madhavan S, Sudha Kumary V, George R, Cletus N, Baiju S. Wong's anomaly – a rare variant of cor triatriatum. Indian Heart J. 2015;67(5):469-71.
36. Gupta SK, Ramakrishnan S, Doshi S. Cor triatriatum. Catheter Cardiovasc Interv. 2013; 82(4):E507-10.
37. Sivakumar K, Satish R, Tailor K, Coelho R. Transcatheter management of subtotal cor triatriatum sinister: a rare anomaly. Pediatr Cardiol. 2008;29(4):812-5.
38. Anderson R, Krishna K, Mussato K, Redington A, Tweddell J, Tretter J, (Eds). Anderson's Pediatric Cardiology, 4th edition. S.L.: Elsevier; 2019. p. 1650.
39. Vaideeswar P, Tullu MS, Sathe PA, Nanavati R. Atresia of the common pulmonary vein—a rare congenital anomaly. Congenit Heart Dis. 2008;3(6):431-4.
40. Albert M, Geissler W. Persistent left superior vena cava and mitral stenosis. Z Gesamte Inn Med. 1956;11(19):865-74.
41. Cormier MG, Yedlicka JW, Gray RJ, Moncada R. Congenital anomalies of the superior vena cava: a CT study. Semin Roentgenol. 1989;24(2):77-83.
42. de Leval MR, Ritter DG, McGoon DC, Danielson GK. Anomalous systemic venous connection. Surgical considerations. Mayo Clin Proc. 1975; 50(10):599-610.
43. Bartram U, Van Praagh S, Levine JC, Hines M, Bensky AS, Praagh RV. Absent right superior vena cava in visceroatrial situs solitus. Am J Cardiol. 1997;80(2):175-83.
44. Demos TC, Posniak HV, Pierce KL, Olson MC, Muscato M. Venous anomalies of the thorax. Am J Roentgenol. 2004;182(5):1139-50.
45. Van Praagh S, Carrera ME, Sanders SP, Mayer JE, Van Praagh R. Sinus venosus defects: unroofing of the right pulmonary veins—anatomic and echocardiographic findings and surgical treatment. Am Heart J. 1994;128(2):365-79.
46. Beckman CB, Moller JH, Edwards JE. Alternate pathways to pulmonary venous flow in left-sided obstructive anomalies. Circulation. 1975; 52(3):509-16.
47. Fujiwara K, Naito Y, Komai H, Noguchi Y, Nishimura Y, Uemura S, et al. Tetralogy of Fallot with levoatrial cardinal vein. Pediatr Cardiol. 1999;20(2):136-8.
48. Xie M, Yang Y, Cheng TO, Wang X, Li K, Ren P, et al. Coronary sinus septal defect (unroofed coronary sinus): echocardiographic diagnosis and surgical treatment. Int J Cardiol. 2013;168(2): 1258-63.
49. Raghib G, Ruttenberg HD, Anderson RC, Amplatz K, Adams P, Edwards JE. Termination of left superior vena cava in left

atrium, atrial septal defect, and absence of coronary sinus; a developmental complex. Circulation. 1965; 31:906-18.

50. Ootaki Y, Yamaguchi M, Yoshimura N, Oka S, Yoshida M, Hasegawa T. Unroofed coronary sinus syndrome: diagnosis, classification, and surgical treatment. J Thorac Cardiovasc Surg. 2003;126(5):1655-6.
51. Yokota M, Kyoku I, Kitano M, Shimada I, Mizuhara H, Sakamoto K, et al. Atresia of the coronary sinus orifice. Fatal outcome after intraoperative division of the drainage left superior vena cava. J Thorac Cardiovasc Surg. 1989;98(1):30-2.
52. Bass JE, Redwine MD, Kramer LA, Huynh PT, Harris JH. Spectrum of congenital anomalies of the inferior vena cava: cross-sectional imaging findings. Radiographics. 2000;20(3):639-52.
53. Praagh van, Santini F, Sanders, S. P. Cardiac malpositions with special emphasis on visceral heterotaxy (asplenia and polysplenia syndromes). In: Nadas AS, Fyler DC, (Eds). Nadas' Pediatric Cardiology, 4th edition. Philadelphia: Hanley & Belfus; 1992. p. 589-608.
54. Oliveira JD, Martins I. Congenital systemic venous return anomalies to the right atrium review. Insights into Imaging. 2019;10(1):115.
55. Thomas A, Balakrishnan BK, Batra M, Kuriakose RR, Vikraman SK, Gopinathan KK. Varied presentations of absent ductus venosus, their associations, and outcomes. J Fetal Med. 2015;2(4):167-70.
56. Contratti G, Banzi C, Ghi T, Perolo A, Pilu G, Visentin A. Absence of the ductus venosus: report of 10 new cases and review of the literature. Ultrasound Obstet Gynecol. 2001; 18(6):605-9.
57. Gitzelmann R, Arbenz UV, Willi UV. Hypergalactosaemia and portosystemic encephalopathy due to persistence of ductus venosus Arantii. Eur J Pediatr. 1992;151(8):564-8.
58. Murayama K, Nagasaka H, Tate K, Ohsone Y, Kanazawa M, Kobayashi K, et al. Significant correlations between the flow volume of patent ductus venosus and early neonatal liver function: possible involvement of patent ductus venosus in postnatal liver function. Arch Dis Child Fetal Neonatal Ed. 2006;91(3):F175-9.
59. Abernethy J. Account of two instances of uncommon formation in the viscera of the human body. Med Facts Obs. 1797;7:100-8.
60. Morgan G, Superina R. Congenital absence of the portal vein: two cases and a proposed classification system for portasystemic vascular anomalies. J Pediatr Surg. 1994;29(9):1239-41.
61. Murray CP, Yoo S-J, Babyn PS. Congenital extrahepatic portosystemic shunts. Pediatr Radiol. 2003;33(9):614-20.
62. Alvarez AE, Ribeiro AF, Hessel G, Baracat J, Ribeiro JD. Abernethy malformation: one of the etiologies of hepatopulmonary syndrome. Pediatr Pulmonol. 2002;34(5):391-4.
63. Jain V, Sangdup T, Agarwala S, Bishoi AK, Chauhan S, Dhua A, et al. Abernethy malformation type 2: varied presentation, management and outcome. J Pediatr Surg. 2019;54(4):760-5.
64. Venkateshwaran S, Krishnamoorthy KM, Sivasankaran S. Percutaneous device closure of Abernethy malformation—a treatable cause of hepatopulmonary syndrome. Catheter Cardiovasc Interv. 2014;83(6):968-70.
65. Raghuram KA, Bijulal S, Krishnamoorthy KM, Tharakan JA. Regression of pulmonary vascular disease after therapy of abernethy malformation in visceral heterotaxy. Pediatr Cardiol. 2013;34(8):1882-5.
66. Karashima S, Hattori S, Nakazato H, Awata H, Seguchi S, Ikeda S, et al. Membranoproliferative glomerulonephritis in congenital portosystemic shunt without liver cirrhosis. Clin Nephrol. 2000;53(3):206-11.
67. Park JH, Cha SH, Han JK, Han MC. Intrahepatic portosystemic venous shunt. AJR Am J Roentgenol. 1990;155(3):527-8.
68. Franchi-Abella S, Branchereau S, Lambert V, Fabre M, Steimberg C, Losay J, et al. Complications of congenital portosystemic shunts in children: therapeutic options and outcomes. J Pediatr Gastroenterol Nutr. 2010;51(3):322-30.
69. Azad S, Arya A, Sitaraman R, Garg A. Abernethy malformation: our experience from a tertiary cardiac care center and review of literature. Ann Pediatr Cardiol. 2019;12(3):240-7.
70. Gupta SK, Juneja R, Anderson RH, Gulati GS, Devagorou V. Clarifying the anatomy and physiology of totally anomalous systemic venous connection. Ann Pediatr Cardiol. 2017; 10(3):269-77.

27
CHAPTER

Coronary Artery Abnormalities

Jayashree Mishra

INTRODUCTION

Multiple variations in coronary artery anomalies exist that may occur in isolation or in association with other congenital anomalies. Overall, anomalies of the coronary arteries are rather rare. The incidence of primary congenital coronary anomalies varies from 0.3% in a necropsy series reported by Alexander and Griffith to 1.6% of patients undergoing cardiac catheterization in a series of >38,000 patients. A higher incidence (~6%) is found in coronary computed tomography (CT) angiographic series due to higher sensitivity of coronary CT.

Knowledge of normal and variant anatomy and physiology of coronary circulation is an increasingly vital component in managing congenital and acquired pediatric heart diseases. Much of acquired coronary artery diseases in children are in the context of Kawasaki disease (*see* Chapter 44). Additionally, lifestyle-related conditions in children set the stage for atherosclerotic coronary artery disease which is dealt with in Chapter 8.

Coronary anomalies are important because they have the potential to cause myocardial ischemia. A rare but potentially lethal coronary artery anomaly is anomalous origin of left coronary artery from pulmonary artery (ALCAPA). The origin of left coronary artery (LCA) from the right coronary artery (RCA) or proximal right aortic sinus with subsequent passage between aorta and right ventricular outflow tract has been associated with sudden death during or shortly after exercise in the young, particularly in athletes. The most common hemodynamically significant coronary artery abnormalities are coronary artery fistulae. Small fistulae may be asymptomatic and present with incidentally detected murmur, while large fistulae result in significant left-to-right shunts and can present with heart failure.

Variations in coronary artery anomalies are associated with many congenital heart diseases. Certain cardiac surgical repairs demand precise understanding of these variations to ensure good operative outcomes. Inability to do so can result in potentially serious consequences. Examples of these operations include those involving coronary translocations such as the arterial switch operation (ASO), Ross operation, and root translocations along with certain relatively common surgeries such as the tetralogy of Fallot (TOF) repair when a major coronary artery crosses the right ventricular outflow tract.

ANATOMY OF CORONARY ARTERIES AND COMMON ANATOMIC VARIANTS

The entire blood flow to the myocardium is derived from two main coronary arteries arising from the right and left aortic sinuses of Valsalva (**Fig. 1**). The left main coronary artery (LMCA) gives rise to the circumflex branch which courses posteriorly in the left atrioventricular (AV) groove before continuing as left anterior descending branch. The RCA gives rise to a small conal branch and then courses in the right AV groove. The septum is supplied by perforating branches from anterior and posterior descending arteries. In 69% of cases, the RCA is dominant, giving rise to the posterior descending coronary artery. In 11% cases, the LCA is dominant, usually associated with bicuspid aortic valve and aortic stenosis.[1] In rest, coronary supply is codominant.

Normally, there are connections between coronary artery branches that are known as collaterals. These collaterals are

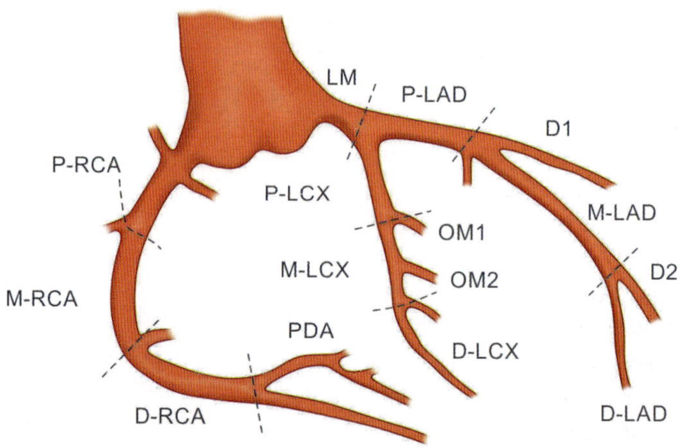

Fig. 1: Normal coronary artery anatomy.
(RCA: right coronary artery; LCX: left circumflex; LAD: left anterior descending artery; PDA: patent ductus arteriosus)

capable of enlarging in primary arterial occlusion, in which case they allow reperfusion of affected myocardium.

Usually, the coronary arteries arise from the middle of the aortic sinuses, but they may arise from the sinotubular junction or above it. The position of the ostium does not affect the flow through it. Separate origin of the conus branch of the RCA occurs commonly.[2] The corresponding anomaly on the left side occurs in about 1% of people and is more frequent with bicuspid aortic valve.[1]

CORONARY ARTERY ANOMALIES

Anomalous Origin of Left Coronary Artery from Pulmonary Artery

Anomalous origin of left coronary artery from pulmonary artery is the most common major congenital malformation of the coronary circulation with an incidence of 1/300,000 live births.[3] In this anomaly, the LCA arises from the pulmonary artery, usually from the left posterior sinus. The first report relating clinical and autopsy findings in a 3-month-old boy were by Bland et al.[4] The anomaly has thus been called Bland-White-Garland syndrome.

Pathophysiology and Hemodynamics

In fetal life, the pressures and oxygen saturations are similar in aorta and pulmonary artery. Consequently, myocardial perfusion in unaffected without ischemia or collateral formation.

In the early neonatal period, the relatively high pulmonary artery pressures allow perfusion of the LCA territory that arises from the pulmonary artery. In spite of the reduced oxygen saturation of the pulmonary arterial blood, there is usually no ischemia.

Beyond neonatal period: There is a progressive decline in pulmonary artery pressure as a result of fall in pulmonary vascular resistance. This results in a progressive decline in perfusion via the LMCA. There is variable compensation by collateral flow from the RCA. There also some compensation by dilation of myocardial vessels that dilate to reduce resistance and increase perfusion. However, these compensatory mechanisms are often inadequate and progressive myocardial ischemia sets in. The collaterals are also relatively ineffective because they flow into the low-pressure pulmonary artery and this "steals" blood away from the myocardium. Initially, the ischemia is transient but this soon gives way to frank infarction and scarring that often involves the anterior-lateral free wall and the anterolateral papillary muscle with ventricular dysfunction and a variable degree of mitral valve regurgitation (**Flowchart 1**).

There are variations in the manner in which ALCAPA presents depending on the rate at which the pulmonary vascular resistance falls vis-à-vis development of collaterals. In select infants, the damage to papillary muscle occurs early and this results in severe mitral regurgitation (MR) with pulmonary venous and pulmonary artery hypertension that may allow left ventricular (LV) systolic function to be preserved.[5] Survival to adulthood with minimal ventricular dysfunction is described in a small and highly select group of patients who have the fortuitous situation where extensive collaterals develop and take over the left coronary circulation.[4] In the majority, however, severe myocardial dysfunction with variable degrees of MR sets in early in infancy as a result of infarction of LV wall and papillary muscle with accompanying heart failure.

Flowchart 1: Pathophysiology of anomalous origin of left coronary artery from pulmonary artery (ALCAPA) beyond neonatal period.

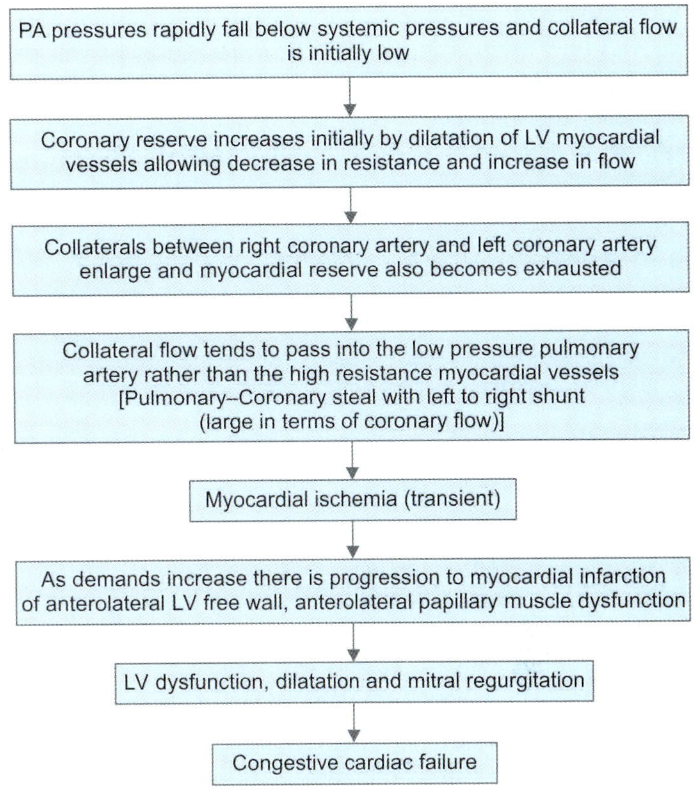

Anatomic Description

The LCA arises from the main pulmonary artery usually in the left posterior pulmonary sinus but rarely arises from a branch pulmonary artery. The anomalous LCA is small and thin-walled and in adults resembles a venous channel. The RCA originates normally from its aortic sinus, is dilated and tortuous, and rarely aneurysmal because it supports additional collateral circulation. Multiple large collaterals may be visible on the surface of the heart. In infancy, the heart is enlarged and the left ventricle in particular is dilated and hypertrophied. The anterolateral papillary muscle is scarred and atrophied with shortened chordae. There may be diffuse endocardial fibroelastosis (EFE) of the left ventricle and the anterior mitral leaflet is often thickened. Thinning and scarring of the anterolateral LV wall and apex owing to infarction are seen. In adults, the heart is usually enlarged but not as much as in infants and usually there is no EFE.

This anomaly is usually isolated but it has been associated with patent ductus arteriosus, ventricular septal defect, TOF, or coarctation of aorta.[6] The presence of pulmonary hypertension as in a large VSD may prevent ischemia by maintaining LV perfusion; however, closure of defect without correcting the anomalous coronary origin results in fall in pulmonary artery pressure which can be catastrophic.

Clinical Presentations

The common clinical presentations are listed in **Box 1**. The most common presentation is of heart failure in a young infant. Many of these babies may carry a label of myocarditis or cardiomyopathy. Additional presentations include isolated MR that is otherwise unexplained in infancy or later in childhood. As stated above, exceptional survival to adulthood is well described.

Physical Examination

In infants, the heart is usually enlarged, the left ventricle being the predominant ventricle affected. Often there are signs and symptoms of congestive heart failure. If there is significant pulmonary hypertension due to LV failure or severe MR, the pulmonary component of second heart sound will be loud. The first heart sound is soft or absent (in the presence of MR) and apical gallop rhythm is common. There may be no murmurs, or the murmur of MR at apex. A soft continuous murmur at the upper left sternal border which is due to the continuous flow from the anomalous coronary artery into the pulmonary artery can be heard under exceptional circumstances in selected older patients who have well-developed collaterals.

BOX 1: Common clinical presentations of anomalous origin of left coronary artery from pulmonary artery.

- Congestive cardiac failure in infancy and childhood: Patients might have been previously labeled as myocarditis or idiopathic dilated cardiomyopathy
- Episodes of excessive crying, pallor, and sweating precipitated by feeding during early infancy
- Murmur of mitral regurgitation
- Dyspnea and angina of effort in older children
- Syncope and sudden death in older children and adults
- Asymptomatic with an abnormal ECG or exercise stress test

(ECG: electrocardiogram)

Diagnosis

The diagnosis of ALCAPA should always be considered and specifically excluded in any infant with heart failure and ventricular dysfunction or isolated MR. There are valuable clues from the ECG (electrocardiogram) and echocardiography that enable accurate diagnosis in almost all patients. Exceptionally, coronary angiography is needed to confirm the diagnosis.

Electrocardiography: There are three electrocardiographic patterns described in ALCAPA (**Fig. 2**). Of these, the first is considered most specific and often enables accurate diagnosis. *Deep but narrow q waves* in limb leads I and aVL and precordial leads V4 to V6 (lateral and apical) are often accompanied by ST segment (elevation or depression) and T wave changes (inversion). The q waves are typically >1/4 the height of the R wave in the same lead. This ECG finding in an infant raises a very strong suspicion. This is the most common pattern.

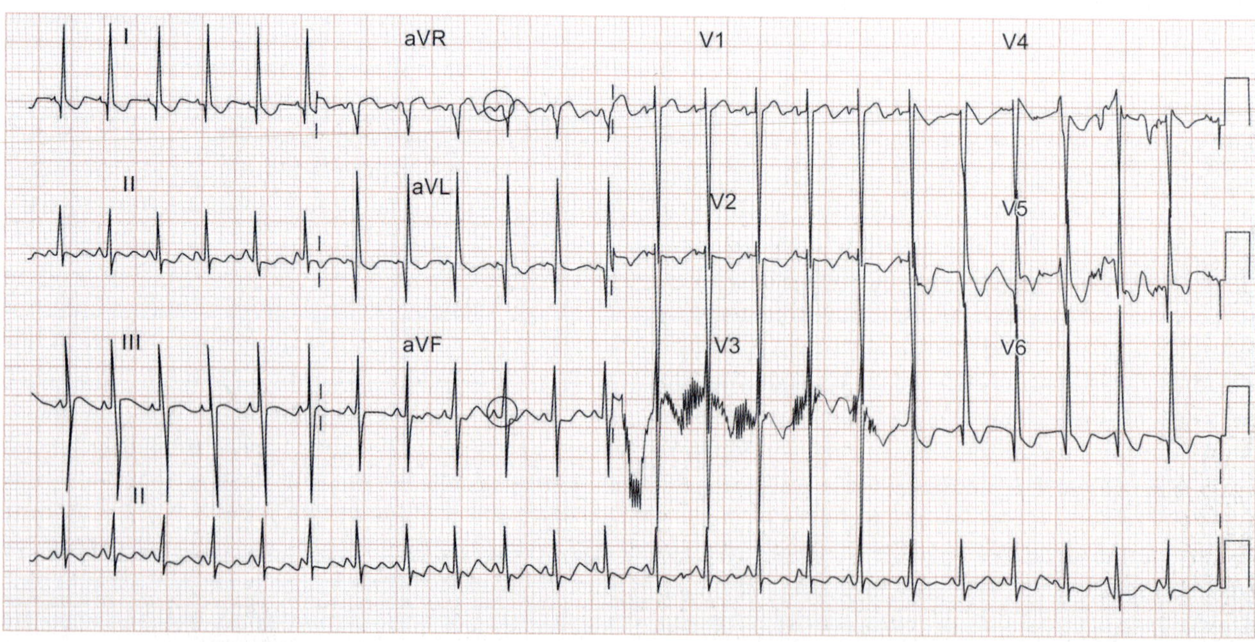

Fig. 2: Electrocardiogram (ECG) in a 2-month-old patient with anomalous origin of left coronary artery from pulmonary artery (ALCAPA). Note the deep, narrow q waves in leads I, aVL, V5, and V6. There is left QRS axis, left ventricular hypertrophy, and ST-T wave changes in lateral precordial leads.

Left ventricular hypertrophy (LVH) is represented in the ECG by typical voltage and repolarization criteria. This is seen in older patients. Often the ventricular function is preserved in these patients. Even in the presence of LVH, it is necessary to look for q waves in the apicolateral leads as described above. *Left axis deviation* as a result of disproportionate increase in posterobasal LV muscle mass that attracts the depolarization vector in the left superior direction. In addition, prominent left atrial P waves may result from left atrial enlargement secondary to MR. This sign, however, is not very sensitive. ECG recorded during exercise stress test may show ischemic ST segment depression and T wave inversions.[7]

Chest radiography: The cardiac shadow shows marked cardiomegaly in symptomatic infants predominantly of the left ventricle and the left atrium. The size may be normal or mildly enlarged in occasional older child or adult. Pulmonary venous hypertension (*see* Chapter 8) is secondary to congestion from LV failure and/or MR. The severe and long-standing LV enlargement often results in collapse of the adjacent left lung segments that take some time to resolve even after surgery.

Echocardiography: With the advent of improved resolution current echocardiographic equipment, two-dimensional (2D) echocardiography with color Doppler is the standard method of diagnosis for ALCAPA.[8] 2D echocardiography identifies the origin of the anomalous LCA from the pulmonary trunk as well as an enlarged but normally originating RCA. It also shows the size and function of the cardiac chambers, particularly the left ventricle, as well as reduced contractility of the apical and lateral portions of the left ventricle (regional wall motion abnormalities). Increased echogenicity of the papillary muscles and adjacent endocardium due to fibrosis and fibroelastosis (**Fig. 3**) is a characteristic sign that strongly suggests ALCAPA. Color flow imaging demonstrates reverse direction of blood flow in the left anterior descending and left circumflex (LCX) coronary arteries and establishes the presence of continuous or diastolic flow entering the pulmonary trunk (**Fig. 4**) just distal to the pulmonary valve and adhering to the medial wall of the pulmonary trunk. It also detects the presence and severity of the MR.

Angiography: When there are persistent doubts after meticulous echocardiography, it may be necessary to do a coronary angiography or an aortic root angiography to demonstrate the anomalous origin of LCA. This situation may arise when the coronary artery arises from one of the branch pulmonary arteries. The aortic root angiogram shows filling of the RCA alone and the LCA fills late via collaterals. The drainage into the pulmonary artery is consistently demonstrated.

Cardiac CT: Cardiac CT can be used to define coronary artery anatomy and origin in selected older patients. However, this is not as accurate as aortic or right coronary angiography.

Natural History

Approximately 87% of children born with ALCAPA present in infancy[6] and of these, 65–85% die before 1 year of age from intractable congestive cardiac failure,[9] usually after 2 months of age, if they are untreated. At the other end of the spectrum are occasional patients who never have symptoms, perhaps due to extensive collaterals. They are at risk, however, of exercise-induced angina and sudden death.[10]

Management

The diagnosis of ALCAPA alone is a definitive indication for surgical repair. Currently recommended practice is to translocate the LCA from pulmonary artery to adjacent aorta.[11,12] This restores normal left coronary blood flow and enables recovery of LV function in the following weeks or months. The speed of recovery is often related to the age of

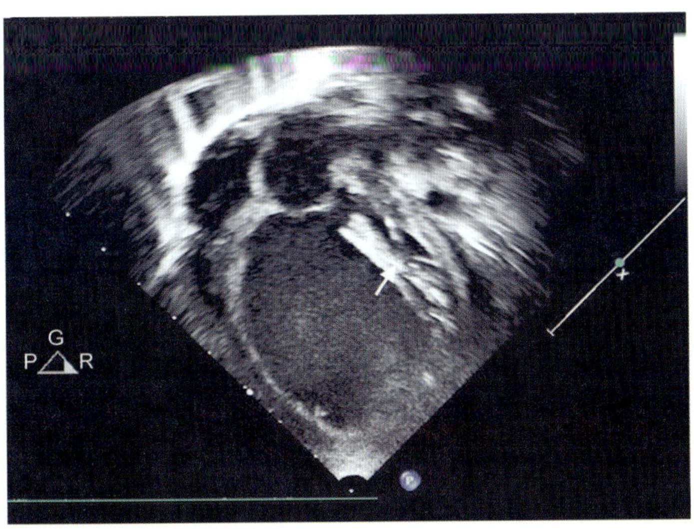

Fig. 3: Dilated left ventricle (LV) with hyperechoic anterolateral papillary muscle (arrow). The LV is dilated and dysfunctional.

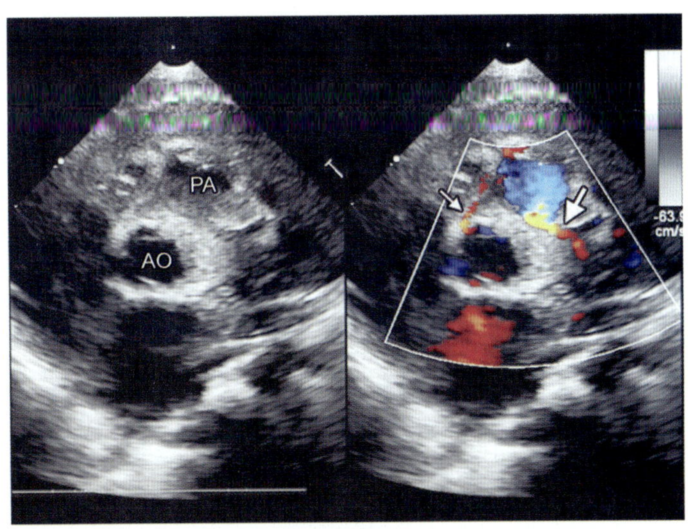

Fig. 4: Anomalous left coronary artery (LCA) entering the left posterior sinus of pulmonary artery (bold arrow). Note the flow reversal in coronary artery marked by red flow indicating flow toward the transducer. Right coronary artery arising normally from the right aortic sinus (thin arrow).

operation, extent of ventricular dysfunction, and severity of MR. Postoperative recovery is prolonged in many patients and selected patients require extracorporeal membranous oxygenation (ECMO) support.[13] Operations that are seldom performed and mostly of historical importance include ligation of the LCA at its origin to prevent the steal,[10] ligation of the origin of LCA, and revascularization with an internal mammary arterial or saphenous venous graft.[14] The Takeuchi procedure in which an aortopulmonary window is created and then a tunnel is fashioned that directs blood from the aorta to the left coronary ostium[15] is seldom performed today. The current era success rate following ALCAPA repair exceeds 90%. However, requirement of mitral valve repair or replacement predicts a less favorable outcome.

Rare Coronary Artery Anomalies that can Present like ALCAPA

Stenosis and Atresia of a Coronary Ostium

Stenosis or atresia of coronary ostium or first few millimeters of the LMCA is very rare. The more distal branches are normal and receive multiple collaterals from the RCA which may be inadequate to maintain perfusion. This condition often coexists with supravalvular aortic stenosis and other congenital cardiac defects. Patients present between 3 months and 60 years of age with angina, sudden death, myocardial infarction, or congestive heart failure. Treatment included coronary artery bypass graft or surgical reconstruction of left main origin.

Left anterior descending coronary artery from pulmonary artery is very rare with only few reported cases. It presents with angina and ECG evidence of myocardial ischemia. Treatment by ligation of the anomalous artery and connecting it to the aorta has been recommended.

Abnormal Origin of Right or Left Coronary Artery from Contralateral Sinus

A coronary artery that originates from the contralateral sinus of Valsalva can follow five potential paths toward its perfusion territory: (1) prepulmonic, anterior to the right ventricular outflow tract (usually benign, though rarely associated with angina); (2) retroaortic, posterior to the aortic root (no hemodynamic consequences); (3) trans-septal, with a subpulmonic and intramyocardial course; (4) retrocardiac, behind the mitral and tricuspid valves, in the posterior AV groove; and (5) interarterial, between the aorta and the pulmonary artery.[16,17]

Abnormal origin of either coronary artery is of interest because of its potential association with sudden cardiac death (SCD) in young athletes,[17] especially when the anomalous coronary artery crosses inter-arterially between the aorta and the pulmonary artery. Death is almost certainly due to myocardial ischemia but the causes are not clear and several explanations have been proposed:

- An acute angle in the take-off of the anomalous coronary artery with a slit-like ostium
- Exercise-induced expansion of the aortic and the pulmonary trunk compresses and exacerbates the slit-like ostium, resulting in further ischemia during exercise[18]
- An intramural course of the anomalous coronary within the aortic wall with resultant stretching as aortic root distends in systole
- The intramural segment has thin inner and outer aortic wall layers. Therefore, the section of the aorta that is penetrated by the ectopic artery is a localized weak spot, prone to extensive distensibility during strenuous exercise, which further exacerbates stenosis and ischemia[19]
- The intramural coronary artery may show intussusception of variable lengths and has a cross section which is ovoid instead of circular. These parameters lead to lateral luminal compression which is present throughout the cardiac cycle but more pronounced in systole.[19,20]

Presumably, the severe myocardial ischemia that occurs from any of these mechanisms produces either ventricular fibrillation or electromechanical dissociation.

Incidence

Anomalous origin of RCA from the left sinus of Valsalva is relatively common with frequency of 0.03–0.92% making up about 30% of all major coronary arterial anomalies and has a significantly higher incidence in Asians and Hispanics.[16] Ectopic origin of the LCX from the right sinus of Valsalva is the most common coronary artery anomaly,[21] with a frequency of 0.37%, but it is considered benign as the course of the ectopic LCX is usually retroaortic or retrocardiac. Much less frequent (0.03%) but of greater clinical significance is origin of the LMCA from the right sinus of Valsalva.[16]

Clinical Presentation

Anomalous origin of a coronary artery from an opposite sinus of Valsalva is related with sudden death mostly in young athletes <35 years old but less frequently in older patients. Symptoms such as angina, syncope, heart failure, and myocardial infarction may appear in both age groups but are seen more frequently in older patients. It has been proposed that stiffening of the aortic wall in older adults is the reason why sudden death is less frequent in this age group.[22]

Diagnosis

The diagnosis of this entity is difficult since most of the patients are asymptomatic prior to SCD. However, there have been reports of premonitory symptoms such as syncope and chest pain prior to SCD. Diagnostic work-up in patients with the above symptoms (especially young athletes) must include electrocardiography, Holter monitoring, and focused expert

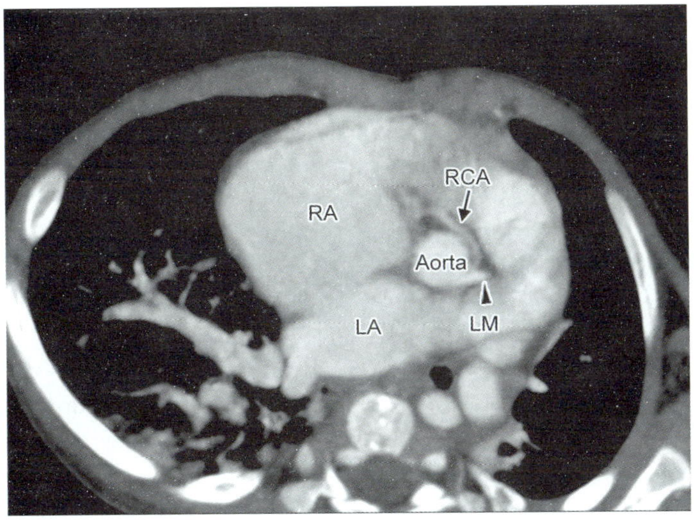

Fig. 5: Abnormal origin of right coronary artery from contralateral sinus and coursing between the aorta and right ventricular outflow tract.

echocardiography. If at least two normally located coronary ostia can be identified with echocardiography, no further investigations are needed.[22] Because most patients are older children and adults, the resolution of the transthoracic echocardiogram may not be adequate to show the anomalies. If transthoracic echocardiography is inconclusive, further investigations with TEE, CT, or magnetic resonance imaging are recommended.[22,23] Treadmill evaluation is unfortunately hampered by a high incidence of false positive and false negative results. Coronary angiography may reveal additional obstructive coronary disease, and intracoronary imaging [intravascular ultrasound (IVUS)] establishes the severity of the condition.[22] However, CT remains the most accurate method to characterize the course of ectopic coronary arteries (**Fig. 5**).

If the anomaly is confirmed, the patients need to undergo nuclear stress testing to evaluate exercise-induced ischemia and to establish baseline for follow-up.

Treatment

Patients with anomalous left coronary arising from the right sinus of Valsalva should undergo surgical repair regardless of symptoms, if younger than 35 years old. Older patients should undergo surgery if they develop symptoms or if they have positive nuclear stress test. Asymptomatic patients with RCA arising from the left sinus of Valsalva with negative nuclear stress test need regular follow-up only. Symptomatic patients and asymptomatic ones with positive nuclear stress test should be further evaluated with IVUS and if significant stenosis is found should be offered surgical repair.

Surgical options include osteoplasty (creation of a new ostium at the end of the ectopic artery's intramural segment) and unroofing of the intramural segment (excising of the common wall located between the aorta and the anomalous coronary).[24,25] Currently, unroofing is the most favored procedure.

Single Coronary Artery

In 5–20% of all major coronary arterial anomalies, a single coronary artery may originate from the left or right sinus of Valsalva and may sometimes coexist with other congenital anomalies.[16] About 40% of these anomalies are associated with other cardiac malformations, including transposition of the great vessels, TOF, truncus arteriosus, coronary-cameral fistulas, and bicuspid aortic valves. Most are benign in the absence of a severe atheroma affecting the proximal artery.

When the single coronary has an origin from the left sinus, the RCA may originate from the proximal or midportion of the anterior descending artery (LAD) and follows a course anterior to the pulmonary artery or between the aorta and pulmonary artery to reach the right AV groove. It is usually benign, however, if the RCA has an interarterial course, myocardial ischemia and SCD may occur. When the single coronary artery arises from the right sinus, the LCA has an anterior or interarterial course to reach its perfusion territory. Prevalence is around 0.02–0.05%, and this condition is associated with SCD more frequently than a single coronary arising from the left sinus, interarterial one being the potentially most life-threatening.

Left and Right Coronary Arterial Branches Arising from the Posterior Sinus of Valsalva

These are very rare and have not been associated with premature or sudden death.

Coronary Artery Fistulae

Coronary fistulae are persistent and abnormal connection between one or more than one coronary artery and one of the cardiac chambers or pulmonary artery, coronary sinus, vena cava, or a pulmonary vein. The right and left coronary arteries arise from their respective aortic sinuses. In the modern era of high resolution ultrasound imaging, they are frequently discovered incidentally and if small pose no significant burden to the patient. However, less commonly, they may be large and impose a significant hemodynamic burden or future risk of cardiovascular events. Reported prevalence is 0.3–0.87% in the general population.

Anatomic Variants

Types according to drainage site are as follows:

- *Arteriovenous (>90%)*: When the fistula drains into a right cardiac chamber *(referred to as coronary-cameral fistula)* or pulmonary trunk. The majority in approximate order of frequency enters the right ventricle (RV) (40%), or right atrium (25%), less commonly the pulmonary trunk (15%) or coronary sinus (7%) and most rarely the superior vena cava.
- *Coronary fistula (3%)*: When it drains into the left atrium or the left ventricle.[26] The drainage site of fistula consists of either single or multiple vascular channels or a maze

of fine channels that form a diffuse network or plexus. Approximately half of these fistulas arise from the RCA, somewhat less than half from the LCA, and a minority 5% from both coronary arteries. The coronary artery that gives rise to the fistula is characteristically dilated, elongated, and tortuous but the coronary arteries distal to it are of normal caliber. The fistulous coronary artery often contains saccular aneurysms that may rupture. They occasionally harbor calcification of the wall and thrombi with distal embolization. Coronary fistulae may develop significance over time. Some small- to moderate-sized fistulae have demonstrated the capacity to grow over time, while other small ones remain trivial.

Physiology

The physiologic response to coronary arterial fistulas are related to the volume of blood flowing through the fistula, the chamber or vascular bed into which the fistula drains, and the myocardial ischemia that results from the coronary steal caused by low resistance vascular channels. A left-to-right shunt is established when the fistula drains into right atrium, RV, or coronary sinus.[27] If drainage is into the right ventricular outflow tract, pulmonary trunk, left atrium, or left ventricle, the hemodynamic burden is borne by the left ventricle alone. If the fistula drains into inflow of RV directly or indirectly via right atrium or coronary sinus, volume overload of the RV coexists along with LV volume overload. When the fistula drains into the left ventricle, the aortic-to-left ventricular flow occurs during diastole and hence the hemodynamic result is analogous to aortic regurgitation. Myocardial ischemia occurs when the coronary arterial fistula functions as a low-resistance pathway that constitutes a coronary steal.[28,29]

In summary, following are three pathophysiologic consequences of a significant coronary fistula:

1. Pulmonary over circulation
2. Diastolic aortic run off, presents similar to aortic insufficiency
3. Distal coronary insufficiency.

Presentation

The male-to-female ratio is about 1:1. A small acoustically silent coronary arterial fistula comes to light during coronary angiography or echocardiography done for other reasons. The majority of patients, especially those younger than 20 years of age are asymptomatic when coronary arterial fistulas are first diagnosed.[30] The initial suspicion is likely to be a continuous murmur in the asymptomatic child or young adult. Infants and young children may present with heart failure due to the presence of a hemodynamically significant fistula with a large left-to-right shunt. Symptoms are complications in approximate order of frequency include dyspnea, fatigue, myocardial ischemia, congestive heart failure, sudden death, infective endocarditis, and rupture.[31]

Clinical Features

Physical appearance, the arterial pulse, and the jugular venous pressure (JVP) are usually normal. Precordial palpation detects the impulses of either or both ventricles depending on the drainage site of the coronary arterial fistula. A precordial continuous murmur which is not at the site of patent ductus arteriosus murmur is the most common presenting feature. Newborns and young infants with large coronary fistula present with clinical findings of congestive cardiac failure such as increased precordial LV impulse, cardiomegaly, and gallop rhythm.

Investigations

The chest X-ray reflects the response of individual chambers to the size and duration of left-to-right shunt. ECG changes such as atrial enlargement and ventricular hypertrophy are related to the chamber/s receiving the shunt and the volume of blood flowing through the fistula. Fistulas draining into the right atrium cause biatrial enlargement and biventricular hypertrophy. Those draining into right ventricular outflow tract, pulmonary trunk, left atrium or left ventricle cause left atrial enlargement and LV hypertrophy. A coronary steal may induce ischemic ST and T wave changes at rest or with exercise.[31] Echocardiography identifies the origin and drainage site of the fistula and the physiologic effects on the heart-like chamber enlargements and ischemic effects of coronary steal. Cardiac CT and magnetic resonance imaging provide excellent delineation of the location and anatomy of coronary fistula as well as the degree of associated chamber enlargement.

Management

Therapeutic interventions on coronary fistulae are indicated for those with pathophysiologic burden to the fistula. Given the potential risks associated with coronary fistula intervention, it is not recommended to close fistulas in the absence of documented physiologic burden.[32] Interventions on coronary fistulae include transcatheter occlusion and open surgical ligation. The majority are amenable to transcatheter occlusion. This usually involves delineation of the fistula anatomy from retrograde transarterial approach, to delineate the neck of the fistula proximal to its entry into the right-sided chamber or pulmonary trunk. Care is taken not to compromise circulation to viable myocardial territory. The occluding plug or coil can then be delivered from either the aortic side, or a through and through wire rail can be achieved to allow the plug to be delivered from the right side of the heart (**Figs. 6A and B**).

Natural History and Outcomes after Occlusion

Without treatment survival to adulthood is expected, although lifespan is not normal. Longevity has been observed from the sixth to ninth decade[30] and death may be

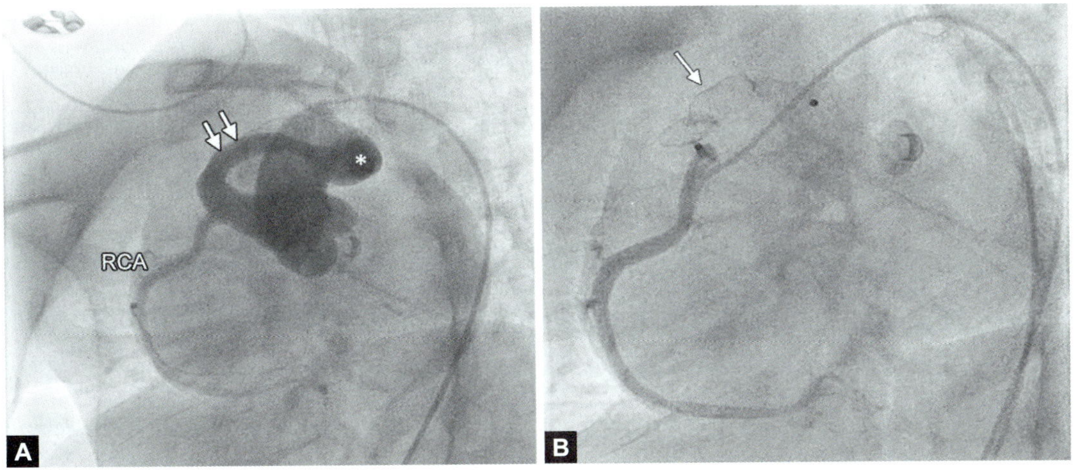

Figs. 6A and B: (A) Right coronary artery fistula (arrows) draining into the right ventricular outflow tract (RVOT) (asterix); (B) A 12-mm Amplatzer vascular plug II positioned inside the fistula with complete occlusion of the fistula and unobstructed right coronary artery flow.

due to acquired coronary artery disease or from noncardiac causes.

Following transcatheter occlusion of the fistula or ligation, usually there is significant decrease in the proximal coronary artery size. However, there is known persistence of coronary microvascular dysfunction after fistulae therapy by either approach, and long-term follow-up as well as lifelong healthy habits to prevent atherosclerosis are recommended.

Myocardial Bridges

It is common for part of the epicardial coronary artery to dip beneath the epicardial muscle for several millimeters so that there is a muscle bridge over the large artery.[33] During coronary angiography, a portion of the coronary artery appears to be narrowed in systole but widely patent in diastole, distinguishing it from a partially occlusive lesion of the artery. Most myocardial bridges are not functionally important, particularly if they are superficial. Ischemia may be due to long, thick bridges that compress the epicardial artery in systole and relax slowly to impair filling of artery in diastole. Myocardial bridges are rare in children with normal heart but can be the cause of significant morbidity and mortality in children with hypertrophic cardiomyopathy (HCM).[34] In HCM, they have been associated with chest pain, exercise intolerance, ventricular arrhythmias, and cardiac arrest in some but debated in others. Patients with above symptoms should be evaluated and consideration should be given for unroofing the bridges if detected and felt to be causative.

Coronary Artery Abnormalities in the Context of Common Congenital Heart Defects

Transposition of the Great Arteries

Arterial switch operation done in the neonatal period has transformed the outcome of patients with transposition of the great arteries (TGA). This operation requires translocation of coronary arteries to the neo-aorta, as the most important and intricate step. The two sinuses facing the pulmonary artery are called facing sinuses. In almost all the patients coronary arteries arise from the facing sinuses.[35] In 60%, the coronary arteries arise from the appropriate sinuses. However, there are many variations of origin and course including the intramural course of coronary artery or its branches. Anomalies of coronary artery are important to identify because some patterns are more difficult to transfer with the ASO. Patients also require continued long-term follow-up with ECG and echocardiogram which can reveal ischemic changes due to ostial stenosis like abnormal q waves or hyperechoic papillary muscles. Coronary arterial abnormalities can present late after ASO and are not infrequent (11.3%). These patients usually present without preceding symptoms and often after negative noninvasive screening. Hence, routine coronary imaging in all patients after ASO before they participate in competitive sports is advocated.[36]

Tetralogy of Fallot

In some patients, a conal branch or left anterior descending coronary artery arising from the RCA passes across the right ventricular outflow tract. In this situation, surgery with traditional transannular incision becomes more difficult and interferes with the effectiveness of the surgery. In a small infant, it may lead to a decision to palliate rather than perform a complete repair. A detailed delineation of the anatomy preoperatively by echocardiogram or cardiac CT or coronary angiography can help plan the procedure more effectively.

Truncus Arteriosus

Large diagonal branches of the RCA may cross over the anterior aspect of the RV and supply anterobasal parts of both ventricles and upper part of interventricular septum.

These arteries are at special risk in surgical procedures utilizing a conduit anastomosis to a right ventriculotomy.[37]

CONCLUSION

This chapter has presented an overview of congenital coronary artery anomalies. There is considerable diversity in the abnormalities and variations in clinical manifestations. Those abnormalities that are considered to be of greater clinical significance and those that occur with a higher relative frequency have received greater attention. The less common variants have been discussed in brief. Additional details are available in the references provided.

REFERENCES

1. Hutchins GM, Nazarian IH, Bulkley BH. Association of left dominant coronary arterial system with congenital bicuspid aortic valve. Am J Cardiol. 1978;42(1):57-9.
2. Baroldi G, Scomazzoni G. Coronary Circulation in Normal and Pathologic Heart. Washington DC: Office of Surgeon General; 1967.
3. Keith JD. Anomalous origin of left coronary artery from pulmonary artery. Br Heart J. 1959; 21:149.
4. Bland EF, White PD, Garland J. Congenital anomalies of the coronary arteries: report of an unusual case associated with cardiac hypertrophy. Am Heart J. 1933;8(6):787-801.
5. Kurup RP, Daniel R, Kumar RK. Anomalous origin of the left coronary artery from the pulmonary artery in infancy with preserved left ventricular function: potential pitfalls and clues to diagnosis. Ann Pediatr Cardiol. 2008;1(1):65-7.
6. Neufeld HN, Schneweiss A. Coronary Artery Disease in Infants and Children. Philadelphia, PA: Lea and Febiger;1983.
7. Vesterlund T, Thomsen PEB. Anomalous origin of the left coronary artery from the pulmonary artery in an adult. Br Heart J. 1985;54(1):110-2.
8. King DH, Danford DA, Huhta JC, Gutgesell HP. Noninvasive detection of anomalous origin of left coronary artery from pulmonary trunk by pulsed Doppler echocardiography. Am J Cardiol. 1985;55(5):608-9.
9. Wesselhoeft H, Fawsett JS, Johnson AL. Anomalous origin of left coronary artery from pulmonary trunk. Its clinical spectrum, pathology, and pathophysiology, based on review of 140 cases with seven further cases. Circulation. 1968;38(2):403-25.
10. Moodie DS, Faye D, Gill CC, Cook SA, Lytle BW, Taylor PC, et al. Anomalous origin of the left coronary artery from the pulmonary artery (Bland-White-Garland syndrome) in adult patients: long term follow-up after surgery. Am Heart J. 1983;106(2):381-8.
11. Schwartz MI, Jonas RA, Colan SD. Anomalous origin of left coronary artery from pulmonary artery: recovery of left ventricular function after dual coronary repair. J Am Coll Cardiol. 1997;30(2):547-53.
12. Ando M, Mee RB, Duncan BW, Drummond-Webb JJ, Seshadri SG, Mesia CII. Creation of a dual coronary system for anomalous origin of left coronary artery from pulmonary artery utilizing the trapdoor flap method. Eur J Cardiothorac Surg. 2002;22(4): 576-81.
13. Del Nido PJ, Duncan BW, Mayer JE, Wessel DL, LaPierre RA, Jonas RA. Left ventricular assist device improves survival after repair of anomalous origin of the left coronary artery from the pulmonary artery. Ann Thorac Surg. 1999;67(1):169-72.
14. Cooley DA, Hallman GI, Bloodwell RD. Definitive surgical treatment anomalous origin of left coronary artery from pulmonary artery: indications and results. J Thoracic Cardiovasc Surg. 1966;52(6):798-808.
15. Takeuchi S, Imamura H, Kasumoto K, Hayashi I, Katohgi T, Yozu R, et al. New surgical method for repair of anomalous left coronary artery from pulmonary artery. J Thorac Cardiovasc Surg. 1979;78(1):7-11.
16. Villa AD, Sammut E, Nair A, Rajani R, Bonamini R, Chiribiri A. Coronary artery anomalies overview: the normal and the abnormal. World J Radiol. 2016;8(6):537-55.
17. Basso C, Maron BJ, Corrado D, Thiene G. Clinical profile of congenital coronary artery anomalies with origin from the wrong aortic sinus leading to sudden death in young competitive athletes. J Am Coll Cardiol. 2000;35(6):1493-501.
18. Taylor AJ, Rogan KM, Virmani R. Sudden cardiac death associated with isolated congenital coronary artery anomalies. J Am Coll Cardiol. 1992;20(3):640-7.
19. Angelini P. Coronary artery anomalies—current clinical issues: definitions, classification, incidence, clinical relevance, and treatment guidelines. Tex Heart Inst J. 2002;29(4):271-8.
20. Angelini P, Velasco JA, Ott D, Khoshnevis GR. Anomalous coronary artery arising from the opposite sinus: descriptive features and pathophysiologic mechanisms, as documented by intravascular ultrasonography. J Invasive Cardiol. 2003;15(9):507-14.
21. Ogden JA. Congenital anomalies of the coronary arteries. Am J Cardiol. 1970;25(4):474-9.
22. Angelini P. Coronary artery anomalies: an entity in search of an identity. Circulation. 2007; 115(10):1296-305.
23. Hejmadi A, Sahn DJ. What is the most effective method of detecting anomalous coronary origin in symptomatic patients? J Am Coll Cardiol. 2003;42(1):155-7.
24. Van Son JA, Haas GS. Anomalous origin of left main coronary artery from right sinus of Valsalva: modified surgical treatment to avoid neocoronary ostial stenosis. Eur J Cardiothorac Surg. 1996;10(6):467-9.
25. Angelini P, Walmsley RP, Libreros A, Ott DA. Symptomatic anomalous origination of the left coronary artery from the opposite sinus of Valsalva. Clinical presentations, diagnosis, and surgical repair. Tex Heart Inst J. 2006;33(2):171-9.
26. Papaioannou A, Agorogiannis S, Nihoyanopoulos J, et al. Congenital coronary artery fistula. Am J Cardiol. 1962;10:588.
27. Neufeld HN, Lesser RG, Adam PJr, Anderson RC, Lilehei CW, Edwards JE. Congenital communication of a coronary artery with a cardiac chamber or the pulmonary trunk. Circulation. 1961;24(2):171.
28. Rowe GG. Inequalities of myocardial perfusion in coronary artery disease. Circulation. 1970; 42:193.
29. Edis AJ, Schattenberg TT, Feldt RH, Danielson GK. Congenital coronary artery fistula. Mayo Clin Proc. 1972;47(8):567-71.
30. Liberthson RR, Sagar K, Berkoben JP, Weintraub RM, Lrvine FH. Congenital coronary arteriovenous fistula. Circulation. 1979;59:849.
31. Perloff JK. Clinical Recognition of Congenital Heart Disease, 5th edition. Philadelphia: W.B. Saunders; 2003. pp. 442-53.
32. Lim DS, Matherne GP. Congenital anomalies of the coronary vessels and the aortic root. In: Moss and Adams Heart Disease in Infants, Children, and Adolescents, 9th edition. Philadelphia: Wolters Kluwer; 2016. pp. 827.
33. Angelini P, Trivellato M, Donis J, Leachman RD. Myocardial bridges: a review. Prog Cardiovasc Dis. 1983;26(1):75-88.
34. Yetman AT, McCrindle BW, MacDonald C, Freedom RM, Gow R. Myocardial bridging in children with hypertrophic cardiomyopathy—a risk factor for sudden death. N Engl J Med. 1998;339:1201-9.
35. Wernosky G, Sander SP. Coronary artery anatomy and transposition of great arteries. Coron Artery Dis. 1993;4:148-58.
36. Tsuda T, Bhat AM, Robinson B, Baffa JM. Coronary artery problems late after arterial switch operation for transposition of great arteries. Circ J. 2015; 79(11):2372-9.
37. Anderson KR, McGoon DC, Lie JT. Surgical significance of the coronary arterial anatomy in truncus arteriosus communis. Am J Cardiol. 1978;41(1):76-81.

28 CHAPTER

Left Heart Outflow Obstruction

Nikhil Thatte

INTRODUCTION

Obstruction to left ventricular (LV) outflow can occur at three levels (**Fig. 1**), i.e., below the level of the aortic valve (subaortic stenosis), at the level of the aortic valve [valvar aortic stenosis (AS)], or distal to the aortic valve [supravalvar aortic stenosis (SVAS)]. Left ventricular outflow tract obstruction (LVOTO) exists on a spectrum of severity, the most extreme form of which is aortic atresia and variants of hypoplastic left heart syndrome (HLHS). The present chapter will discuss forms of left heart outflow obstruction in which there remains a two-ventricle circulation while HLHS is discussed separately in this chapter.

EPIDEMIOLOGY

The incidence of valvar AS is estimated at around 400 cases per million live births.[1] Nonstenotic bicuspid aortic valves (BAVs) are not included within this number. The incidence of such cases is much larger, around 13,500 cases per million live births[1]—larger than all other congenital heart diseases combined. These patients can go on to develop AS or aortic regurgitation (AR) as well as ascending aortopathy independent of AS in adulthood but since they are asymptomatic in childhood, they are typically excluded from discussions of congenital AS. Valvar AS is much more common in males than females (4:1).

Subaortic stenosis and SVAS are less common than valvar AS; good incidence data are difficult to obtain due to the rarity and asymptomatic nature of these diseases. The most extensive report from 1991[2] reports incidence of ~83 cases per million live births for SVAS and ~47 cases per million live births for subvalvar AS.

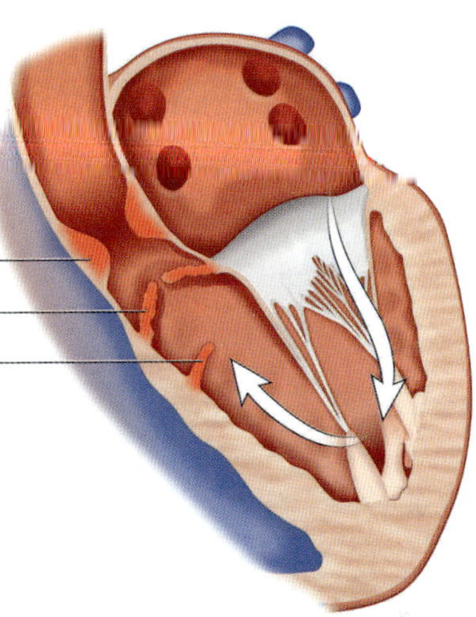

Fig. 1: Multiple levels of left ventricular outflow tract (LVOT) obstruction. The arrows indicate direction of blood flow from the left atrium into the left ventricle and then into the ascending aorta via the LVOT. Obstruction can be at the subvalvar (1), valvar (2), or supravalvar (3) levels.
(AS: aortic stenosis)

PATHOPHYSIOLOGY

The LV outflow tract is bounded medially by the interventricular septum, laterally by the anterior leaflet of the mitral valve and superiorly by the aortic valve. This smooth cylindrical pathway provides an efficient outlet for blood ejected by ventricular contraction. Under normal physiology, there exists no resistance to ventricular outflow between the apex of the left ventricle (LV) and the ascending aorta. This is characterized in pressure waveforms as absence of any pressure gradient between the LV apex and the ascending aorta during systole (**Fig. 2A**). Obstruction to outflow leads to generation of a pressure gradient between the LV apex and the ascending aorta (**Fig. 2B**). The gradient generated across the area of obstruction is proportional to the severity of obstruction as well as the amount of flow passing through the area. Therefore, pressure gradients can underestimate the severity of obstruction in situations where cardiac output is diminished such as in neonates with AS who have LV systolic dysfunction.

Despite anatomic variations between the different types of LVOTO, similar compensatory changes occur in the LV when faced with LVOTO. The principle response is concentric hypertrophy of the LV. LV afterload is directly proportional to end-systolic pressure and inversely proportional to ventricular wall thickness. Initially, LV afterload is tremendously increased in the face of high LV end-systolic pressure. However, compensatory left ventricular

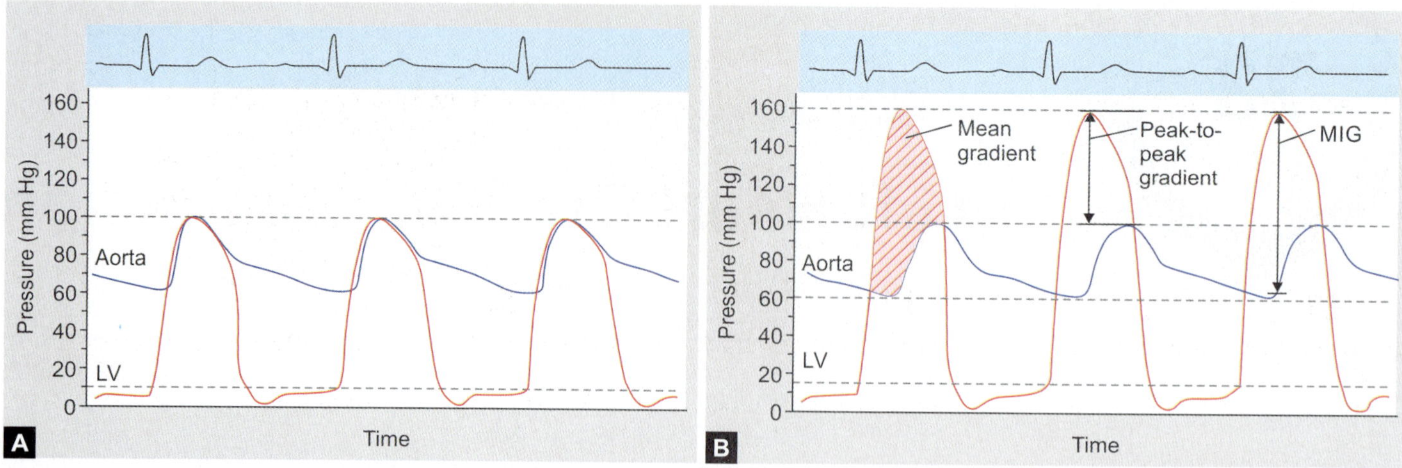

Figs. 2A and B: Simultaneous pressure tracings from the left ventricle (LV) in red and aorta in blue. (A) A normal tracing with no pressure gradient between the LV and the aorta during systole. The left ventricular end-diastolic pressure (LVEDP) is normal (~10 mm Hg); (B) A scenario with aortic stenosis. The aortic systolic pressure pulse is delayed compared to the LV systolic pressure pulse due to obstruction to LV ejection. There is a pressure gradient between the LV and the aorta during systole. Different ways of measuring and reporting the LV to aorta pressure gradient are shown in the three heart beats depicted (see text for explanation). The LVEDP is elevated (~18 mm Hg) due to long-standing outflow obstruction leading to left ventricular hypertrophy.
(MIG: maximum instantaneous gradient)

hypertrophy (LVH) begins to occur and continues until there is normalization of LV afterload such that the increase in wall thickness offsets the increase in ventricular end-systolic pressure. Therefore, contrary to intuitive thinking, LVs faced with LVOTO operate under normal afterload once adequate compensatory hypertrophy has occurred. As a result, such ventricles typically maintain normal systolic function for several years even in the presence of obstruction. However, these compensatory mechanisms cannot compensate indefinitely if obstruction persists for long periods or becomes more severe.

The increasing thickness of the LV leads to increasing myocardial stiffness and insidious diastolic dysfunction manifested as elevation of the left ventricular end-diastolic pressure (LVEDP). Though systolic function is normal, the myocardial oxygen (O_2) consumption required to maintain contractile function at the higher systolic pressures is significantly increased. Myocardial perfusion occurs predominantly in diastole and is driven by myocardial perfusion pressure, defined as the difference between coronary artery blood pressure and LV pressure. In the setting of LVH and elevated LVEDP, there is a relative decrease in the perfusion pressure of LV myocardium during diastole. Additionally, LV systolic pressure in these patients is much higher than aortic systolic pressure, so coronary perfusion cannot occur at all during systole. As a result, there is limited coronary reserve to augment myocardial perfusion at times of stress. Thus, in patients with LVOTO, there is increased myocardial O_2 demand and decreased supply reserve at baseline. This leaves such patients susceptible to ischemia at times of even modest stress such as exercise or tachycardia and eventually forms the common final pathway to adverse outcomes such as ventricular arrhythmia and sudden cardiac death.

Patients with Williams syndrome and other elastin gene mutations additionally often demonstrate narrowing of coronary ostia due to generalized thickening of the walls of the sinuses of Valsalva, along with a tendency of adherence between the tips of aortic valve leaflets and the sinotubular junction, leading to further diminished coronary supply. This puts patients with Williams syndrome and SVAS at high-risk of sudden cardiovascular collapse during any procedure involving induction of anesthesia, and specifically during cardiac catheterizations if the coronary ostia are directly engaged for angiograms.[3]

PATHOLOGY

Valvar Aortic Stenosis

A normal aortic valve is comprised of three thin and mobile leaflets or cusps which are named on the basis of the coronary artery arising from the corresponding sinus of Valsalva, as the right, left, and noncoronary cusps (**Fig. 3A**). These three cusps form three commissures at sites of coaptation which are referred to as the right-left or intercoronary commissure, right noncommissure, and left noncommissure. Congenital valvar AS most commonly occurs due to partial or total fusion of one or more of these commissures leading to a bicommissural or unicommissural valve. The most common commissure that is fused in bicommissural aortic valves (BAVs) is the intercoronary commissure.[4] However, fusion of this commissure is most likely to be asymptomatic during childhood (leading to the nonstenotic BAV described above). Aortic coarctation is most commonly associated with this type of BAV even in the absence of AS. On the other hand, fusion of the right noncommissure is most likely to be involved in cases of congenital AS (**Fig. 3B**).[4] The worst form is the unicommissural valve in which there is either only a

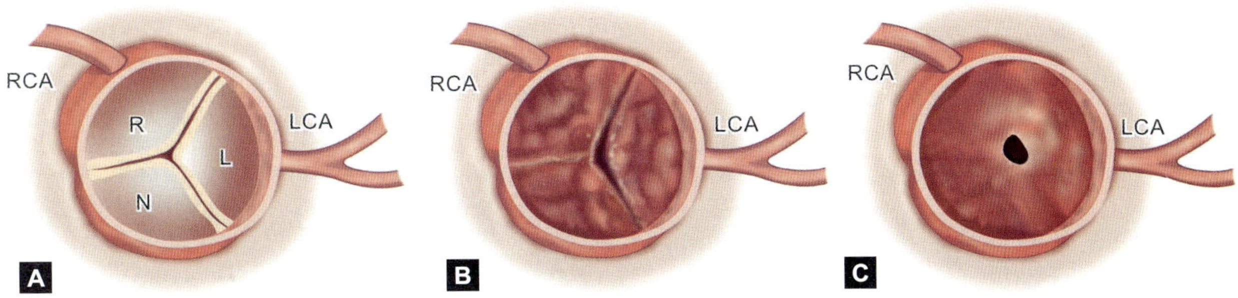

Figs. 3A to C: A normal aortic valve (A), a bicommissural aortic valve with right noncommissure fusion (B) and a unicommissural "volcano"-type valve (C).
(L: left coronary cusp; LCA: left coronary artery; N: non-coronary cusp; R: right coronary cusp; RCA: right coronary artery)

pinhole opening with doming myxomatous leaflet tissue ("volcano" type valve, *see* **Fig. 3C**) or a single commissure between the left and noncoronary leaflet with fusion of the other two commissures. The "volcano" type valve is most often seen in cases of critical AS in neonates.

Subvalvar Aortic Stenosis

There are two major types of subaortic stenosis. The majority of cases involves a discrete subaortic membrane. This is a layer of fibrous tissue that forms proximal to the aortic valve. The membrane can appear to be attached solely to the ventricular septum but is often circumferential in nature with attachments to the anterior leaflet of the mitral valve; the membrane can also grow toward and encroach upon the aortic valve leaflets. The remaining cases are related to more complex obstruction due to some combination of septal muscular hypertrophy, tunnel-like narrowing of the left ventricular outflow tract (LVOT), and abnormal septal attachments of the mitral valve or accessory mitral valve tissue that billows into the LVOT during systole. The latter variety is important to recognize and distinguish from discrete subaortic membranes due to the more complex nature of surgery needed for its relief. All cases of subaortic stenosis can be associated with AR. The acceleration of the blood flow jet in subaortic stenosis occurs below the aortic valve so the blood flow reaching the aortic valve is already traveling at high velocity. This jet of blood is thought to damage the valve leaflets over time leading to AR.

Supravalvar Aortic Stenosis

Supravalvar aortic stenosis refers to the obstruction to blood flow at the level of the aortic root, sinotubular junction, or proximal ascending aorta. This type of obstruction is strongly related to Williams syndrome and other diseases involving mutations of the elastin (ELN) gene together referred to as elastinopathies. This gene is involved in the formation of the walls of blood vessels throughout the body and therefore patients with SVAS who are suspected to have Williams syndrome should undergo screening of blood vessels in other parts of the body as well, including the descending aorta, renal vessels, and cerebral vessels.

GENETIC PREDISPOSITION AND SCREENING

A number of syndromes are associated with high prevalence of left-sided obstructive lesions (including isolated coarctation of the aorta which is discussed separately in Chapter 29); the most common syndrome known to cause left-sided cardiac anomalies is Turner syndrome or monosomy X in which >50% of patients have some type of cardiovascular involvement, and >50% of this is comprised of coarctation and BAV.[5] There is a high degree of heritability amongst nonsyndromic patients with left-heart obstructive lesions, much more so than most other congenital heart diseases. First-degree relatives of patients with left-heart obstruction are likely to have congenital heart disease at a rate that is significantly higher than that expected in the general population. The most common condition diagnosed on screening echocardiograms of first-degree relatives is asymptomatic BAV.[6] Due to the significant cost of echocardiograms, and the most common screening echocardiographic diagnosis being asymptomatic BAV, it is unclear whether routine screening of first-degree relatives should be undertaken for all patients with left-heart obstruction in a resource-limited setting. A potential resource-efficient strategy is to screen relatives for only those index patients who have severe disease (i.e., HLHS or critical AS).

CLINICAL FEATURES AND DIAGNOSIS

Symptoms

The presentation of LVOTO varies depending on the severity of obstruction. Neonates with severe obstruction present with cardiogenic shock once the ductus arteriosus closes as they are dependent on ductal flow to maintain systemic perfusion due to inadequate forward flow from the left heart. This is known as "critical aortic stenosis". Older children and adults with mild-to-moderate LVOTO are usually asymptomatic for the reasons mentioned under Pathophysiology above. Symptoms of worsening LVOTO include fatigue, dyspnea on exertion, anginal chest pain, and syncope. Sudden cardiac death, typically during exercise, can be the first manifestation of LVOTO.

Physical Examination

Vital signs are usually normal in patients with subaortic and valvar AS. Patients with Williams syndrome and other elastinopathies can have systemic hypertension due to stiffening of their large elastic arteries as well as concomitant renal artery stenoses. Stiffening of the large elastic arteries leads to a diminished ability to "cushion" the force of systolic ventricular contraction—a major function of the large elastic arteries—which then manifests as elevated systolic blood pressure with normal or decreased diastolic pressure thereby producing a wide pulse pressure even in the absence of AR. Occasionally, patients with SVAS can also have right arm blood pressure measure higher than left arm and leg blood pressure. This is thought to be due to preferential streaming of the jet of accelerated flow from the area of stenosis toward the right innominate artery. Patients with Williams syndrome also have developmental delay, characteristic elfin facies, and typical friendly or "cocktail party" personalities.

Cardiac examination reveals a prominent and laterally displaced apical impulse due to LVH. Palpation of the precordium shows a systolic thrill at the left sternal border in cases of moderate-to-severe and severe AS. Palpation in the suprasternal notch reveals a thrill in even milder cases due to direct radiation of the accelerated flow jet toward the palpating finger. In severe outflow obstruction, peripheral pulses show a low peak and delayed upstroke compared to the first heart sound, a finding which is described as "*pulsus parvus et tardus*". On auscultation, an ejection click can be heard in valvar AS but not in subaortic or supra-aortic stenosis. A harsh crescendo-decrescendo ejection systolic murmur is easily audible. It is best appreciated at the right upper sternal border and radiates toward the carotid arteries. The intensity of the murmur and presence of a palpable thrill correlate well with severity of obstruction, assuming normal cardiac output. Patients with subaortic stenosis can have associated AR which results in an early to mid-diastolic decrescendo murmur. Due to a delay in the closure of the aortic valve compared to the pulmonary valve, the second heart sound is narrowly split and may become single with expiration. With more severe AS, there can be "paradoxical splitting" of S2 in which P2 occurs before A2 during expiration, i.e., in contrast to physiologic splitting which is seen most prominently during inspiration, these patients have splitting of S2 that is appreciable during expiration with S2 becoming single during inspiration.

Electrocardiography

The electrocardiogram (ECG) is usually normal with mild obstruction. The typical ECG changes observed are markedly elevated voltages of S waves in V1/V2 and R waves in V5/V6. A typical LV strain pattern consisting of T wave inversion and ST segment depression in left-sided leads (I, aVL, V6) can be seen (**Fig. 4**). While ECG changes of LVH and LV strain are known to correspond to increased risk of adverse outcomes in adults,[7] the same has not been demonstrated in pediatrics and the ECG is not highly sensitive or specific either for detecting severity of disease or for predicting adverse outcomes in pediatric patients.

Cardiac Imaging

Echocardiography is the mainstay of diagnosis. Two-dimensional and Doppler transthoracic echocardiography can diagnose the level of outflow obstruction, define the anatomic cause, and also estimate severity of disease. Although estimation of outflow gradients is important, it is equally important to carefully delineate the anatomic

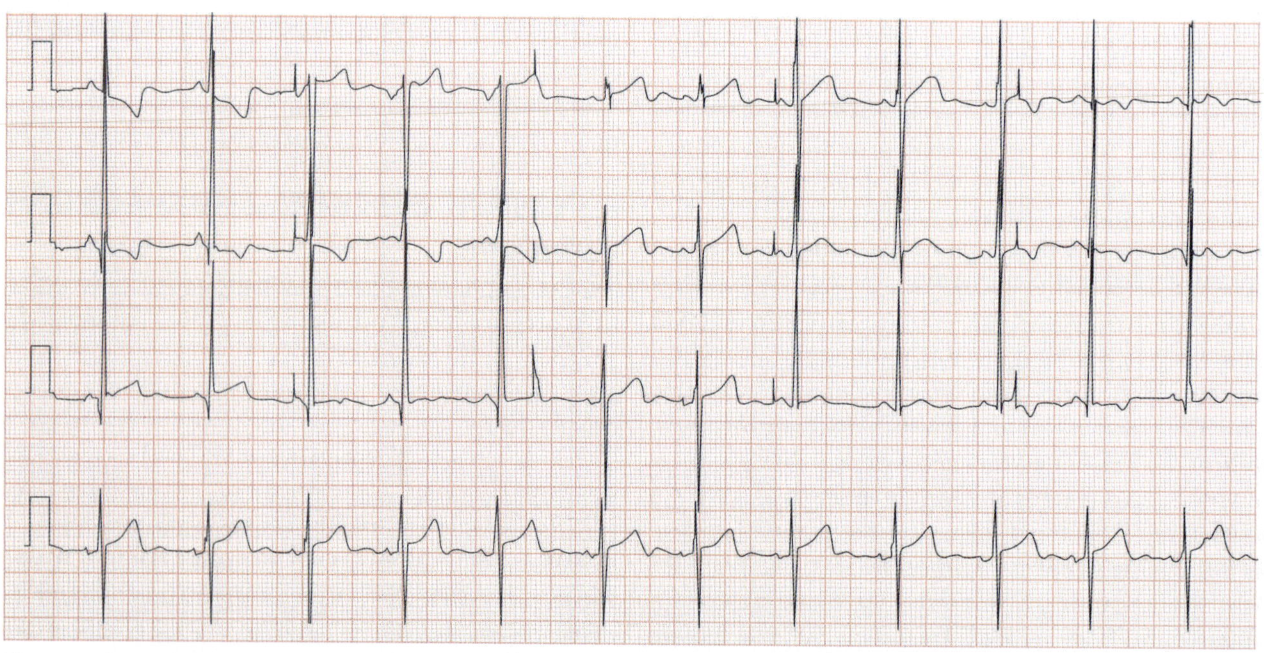

Fig. 4: Electrocardiogram showing typical features of left ventricular hypertrophy and left ventricular strain pattern.

substrate causing the obstruction as this determines the best mode of therapy (surgical versus transcatheter) as well as type of surgery required. Use of pulsed wave Doppler at the different levels of the outflow tract allows distinction of subvalvar, valvar, and supravalvar stenosis. Next, the echocardiogram should evaluate for the effect of the obstruction on the ventricle, i.e., to determine if there has been LVH and whether the systolic or diastolic function of the ventricle is affected. In most cases, systolic function as determined by ejection fraction is normal or sometimes hyperdynamic. Diastolic dysfunction can be detected using tissue Doppler imaging and combining it with mitral valve inflow Doppler measurements.[8] Using mitral valve inflow Doppler ratio of E wave to A wave velocity can lead to erroneous results due to the phenomenon of "pseudonormalization" of mitral inflow patterns in patients with left atrial hypertension. Instead, the E/E' ratio (i.e., the ratio of the early diastolic filling velocity of the mitral inflow Doppler to the velocity of the E' wave at the mitral valve annular septal or lateral wall tissue Doppler) provides a more reliable estimate of diastolic function. An E/E' ratio of >10 is abnormal and a ratio >14 indicates significant diastolic dysfunction.[8] Cardiac magnetic resonance imaging (MRI) and cardiac computed tomography (CT) scans can provide additional data regarding anatomy, flow dynamics as well as details of coronary artery ostia and supply which can supplement echocardiographic data. These studies are becoming more relevant in the current era of transcatheter aortic valve replacement, although this procedure has been mostly limited to adult patients with AS at this time.

GRADING SEVERITY OF AORTIC STENOSIS

Severity of disease is assessed by estimating the pressure gradient across the obstruction using the modified Bernoulli equation and blood flow velocity as measured by Doppler echocardiography as well as by assessing the chronic effects of the obstruction on the ventricle in terms of presence or absence of ventricular hypertrophy and ventricular systolic or diastolic dysfunction. The apical three-chamber or five-chamber view is the best echocardiographic window to determine the gradient, as the suprasternal or high-parasternal windows often produce significant overestimates. Maximum instantaneous gradient (MIG) as measured by Doppler echocardiography frequently overestimates the degree of obstruction when compared to peak-to-peak gradient measured in the catheterization laboratory. Therefore, the mean Doppler gradient is also calculated by outlining the area under the curve of the outflow tract spectral Doppler tracing. The catheter-derived peak-to-peak gradient usually falls somewhere between the MIG and the mean gradients measured by Doppler. Multiple factors contribute to the Doppler MIG overestimation compared to catheter gradients. The two principal factors are the phenomenon of pressure recovery and the fact that the MIG is measuring a value that is fundamentally different than a peak-to-peak gradient. The MIG occurs when LV pressure is at its peak but at this point in the cardiac cycle the aortic pressure has not yet reached its peak (*see* **Fig. 2B**). The instantaneous difference between LV and aortic pressure (and consequently flow velocity) at this time point is therefore higher than the calculated difference between a measured peak LV pressure and separately measured peak aortic pressure, as is done in the catheterization laboratory. The grading of severity of AS using Doppler estimates is listed in **Table 1**.[9]

TABLE 1: Grading severity of aortic stenosis (AS) using Doppler echocardiography.

Severity	*Maximum instantaneous gradient, mm Hg*	*Mean gradient, mm Hg*
Mild	15–34	<20
Moderate	35–64	20–39
Severe	≥65	≥40

Cardiac Catheterization

Cardiac catheterization is primarily utilized as a treatment modality and has been largely replaced by noninvasive imaging modalities for diagnostic purposes. However, in cases of multilevel obstruction, careful measurement of pressures at different levels of the outflow tract remains the gold standard for defining the degree of obstruction at different levels of the outflow tract. In cases of Williams syndrome, evaluation of the coronary ostia with an aortic root injection is important because these patients often have narrowing of the coronary ostia due to thickening of the walls of the sinuses of Valsalva. They are also at risk for adherence of the tips of aortic valve leaflets to the thickened sinotubular junction which predisposes them to diminished coronary blood flow even in the absence of ostial narrowing. Direct coronary angiograms should be avoided due to risk of precipitating ischemia and cardiovascular collapse.

Exercise Stress Testing

Exercise testing is restricted to those patients who are asymptomatic at rest. The presence of ischemic ST-T wave depression with exercise in otherwise asymptomatic patients is important to determine need for intervention.

Natural History

Left ventricular outflow tract lesions tend to be progressive in nature regardless of the level of obstruction. Unlike valvar pulmonary stenosis which tends to stabilize after 1 year of age, valvar AS tends to worsen over time and most patients with greater than mild stenosis will require intervention. The risk of sudden cardiac death in patients with untreated AS is estimated to be ~1% per year.

Subvalvar AS is more likely to be associated with development of AR. Subvalvar membranes also tend to recur after surgical resection with a rate of ~1% per year despite good acute results of surgery.

Management

The management strategies vary depending on the severity of the disease, level of obstruction, and presence of associated lesions such as AR. The impact of the lesions on the LV—specifically presence of LVH or LV dilation in cases with AR—is also carefully tracked and can be an indication for intervention in cases where it is difficult to determine the need for intervention.

SUBVALVAR STENOSIS

There is no significant role of medical management in subvalvar AS. It is difficult to clearly define indications for surgical intervention in subaortic stenosis. This is in part due to the fact that there is a risk of recurrence of the subaortic membrane after surgical resection even though acute results of surgery are excellent with low mortality. Factors associated with increased risk of recurrence include high gradient at time of initial operation (≥60 mm Hg by Doppler) and low valve-to-membrane distance (<6 mm),[10] while earlier reports have also suggested young age (<10 years) at the time of initial operation to be a risk factor for recurrence. Indication for intervention in subvalvar AS is usually considered to be at least moderate stenosis (Doppler MIG ≥35 mm Hg, i.e., maximum velocity ≥ 3 m/s) and/or any new-onset AR, though there is no clear consensus on this topic.[11] More significant stenosis or regurgitation by themselves can also be considered indications for surgery. Surgery involves complete resection of the subaortic membrane or fibromuscular ridge. Patients with more complex subvalvar lesions such as tunnel-like stenosis with associated hypoplasia of the outflow tract, or those with significant associated aortic valve disease, require more complex operations such as the Ross–Konno procedure which involves using the patient's pulmonary valve as a neoaortic valve, placement of a right ventricle (RV) to pulmonary artery (PA) conduit in place of the native pulmonary valve (i.e., the Ross procedure), and incising the interventricular septum in the outflow region to enlarge this area (i.e., the modified Konno procedure). Results of surgery for discrete subaortic membranes are good with significant improvement in both outflow obstruction as well as AR, but there is a tendency toward recurrence of gradients due to regrowth of the membrane. A large series from All India Institute of Medical Sciences, New Delhi showed freedom from a significant postoperative gradient, defined as a Doppler MIG of ≥30 mm Hg, at 93.2 ± 0.23% at 5 years follow-up,[12] which is in keeping with other studies that report a ~10% recurrence rate after surgery.

VALVAR STENOSIS

The treatment of choice for isolated valvar AS has become transcatheter balloon valvuloplasty with almost no indications for surgical valvotomy for valvar AS alone. Surgery is still indicated in cases with associated lesions such as AR, subvalvar or supravalvar obstruction, or other congenital heart disease such as coarctation and ventricular septal defect.

In cases of typical valvar AS with bicuspid valve, balloon valvuloplasty causes tearing of the valve leaflets preferentially along the fused commissural line thereby recreating a commissure where there was previously a fused raphe. This procedure can be performed with minimal morbidity and mortality outside the neonatal period. Indications for balloon aortic valvuloplasty in the non-neonatal age group are based on catheter peak-to-peak gradients and presence or absence of "symptoms" which are defined as angina, syncope, or presence of ST-T wave changes suggestive of ischemia at rest or with exercise stress testing.[13] Accordingly, indication for balloon aortic valvuloplasty include catheter-derived gradient of ≥50 mm Hg, or gradient ≥40 mm Hg in the presence of symptoms. If the patient has circumstances in which there is an anticipated increase in physiological demands, such as desire for pregnancy or participation in competitive sports, the threshold for intervention can be decreased to ≥40 mm Hg, even in the absence of symptoms. It is important to note that the measured gradient can be lower if the patient is heavily sedated or under general anesthesia; therefore, it is reasonable to proceed with valvuloplasty if the measured gradient is <50 mm Hg in the catheterization laboratory, but there has been documentation of Doppler-derived *mean* gradients of >50 mm Hg in the nonsedated state. Presence of pre-existing AR is a contraindication to transcatheter intervention, and such patients should instead be referred for surgical aortic valve repair or replacement.[13]

The above guidelines for Doppler gradient thresholds for intervention do not apply in the neonate with "critical" AS as these patients have a state of low output from the LV with low measured gradients but still require immediate intervention to relieve AS. A subset of these patients with hypoplasia of left heart structures may require univentricular palliation with a Stage 1 Norwood-type operation. Among those felt to be candidates for biventricular circulation—a complex decision usually based on a combination of Z-scores of left heart structures such as mitral and aortic valve annuli, LV volume, and whether the LV is apex-forming—a balloon valvuloplasty is considered reasonable.[13] The initial procedure in these patients is performed less aggressively with one or at most two dilations, with a plan for repeat intervention once the child is older.

RESULTS OF BALLOON AORTIC VALVULOPLASTY

Balloon aortic valvuloplasty has excellent short-term results with reduction in the peak systolic gradient by at least 20–35 mm Hg and usually 40–50 mm Hg.[14] Complications include injury to the femoral arterial access site, inadequate relief of AS (which tends to occur if a small diameter balloon was used with balloon-to-annulus ratio <0.9) or tearing of the aortic valve causing AR (which is seen more commonly if a large diameter balloon was used with balloon-to-annulus ratio >1.0). Other complications such as mitral valve injury and myocardial perforation are rare and mostly confined to the neonatal age group. It is important to note that this procedure should be considered a palliative rather than curative technique. A series of 165 patients from New Delhi, India with a median age of 9 years showed a transcatheter reintervention rate of 13% for the entire cohort,[14] whereas a review of 92 patients from Puducherry, India[15] showed that the rate of surgical reintervention was 10% among patients with successful initial dilation, 50% amongst those with partially successful initial dilation and 100% amongst those with failed initial dilation. These and multiple other reports indicate that families should be counseled that there is a significant chance that another intervention—surgical or transcatheter—is likely to be required in the future even with acute success. Reinterventions include repeat dilations for residual AS or surgical valve repair or replacement in cases with progressive regurgitation after balloon dilation.

FETAL INTERVENTIONS FOR AORTIC STENOSIS

Aortic stenosis that occurs in utero can progress toward HLHS by the time of birth. The idea that this could be intervened upon during the fetal period was first introduced by Maxwell et al. in 1991 in London[16] and then reintroduced and popularized by Tworetzky et al. at Boston Children's Hospital.[17] The procedure involves maternal transuterine needle puncture followed by fetal transthoracic perventricular insertion of this same needle to gain access to the fetal LV under ultrasound guidance, followed by introduction of a guidewire that is passed across the aortic valve. This is used to guide placement of a standard coronary balloon (typically ~3 mm in diameter) via the bore of the needle to achieve balloon dilation of the fetal aortic valve. Results from Boston Children's Hospital are encouraging[18] with the technical success rate at 82% over the entire experience since 2000, rising to 94% in the recent era (2008 onward). There was a 10% risk of fetal loss. Of the live-born patients, 40% of fetuses had a biventricular circulation at neonatal hospital discharge after fetal aortic valvuloplasty, with the remainder undergoing univentricular palliation. Further research is ongoing to better define ideal candidates and timing of intervention for this procedure as well as to refine the procedural technique.

SURGICAL AORTIC VALVE INTERVENTION

Surgery is indicated in those patients in whom balloon dilation has failed to relieve stenosis, or there is coexisting regurgitation. Surgery for AS consists of aortic valve repair or replacement. Aortic valve repair for stenotic valves involves a combination of commissurotomy, debridement of thickened leaflets, and/or enlargement of the aortic annulus and outflow tract in cases of annular hypoplasia (modified Konno procedure). If there is significant coexisting regurgitation, the techniques of valve repair depend on the mechanism of regurgitation which has to be carefully studied by echocardiography. The Ross operation is the next option in which the patient's own pulmonary valve serves as the neoaortic valve. The Ross procedure has excellent outcomes in terms of the longevity of the neoaortic valve with minimal need for reintervention on it. However, the Ross procedure requires placement of a conduit from the RV to the PA which is typically made of cadaveric pulmonary homograft material. This conduit cannot accommodate for somatic growth and tends to degenerate over time; it is this conduit that often requires multiple reinterventions over the lifespan of a pediatric patient treated with a Ross procedure.

The final option for aortic valve disease not amenable to the above repairs is replacement with a bioprosthesis, aortic allograft, or mechanical valve. They each have their own advantages and disadvantages which make them better or worse suited to specific patients (**Table 2**). In general, valve replacement is avoided in pediatric patients due to the inability of such valves to accommodate somatic growth and, in case of mechanical valves, the need for lifelong anticoagulation which can significantly hamper quality of life in growing children and in females who desire pregnancy. Outside of these situations, mechanical valve replacement has excellent longevity and minimal need for reintervention.

TABLE 2: Advantages and disadvantages of aortic valve replacement with a bioprosthesis or aortic allograft versus a mechanical (tilting disk) valve in pediatric patients.

Bioprosthesis or allograft	*Mechanical (tilting disk) valve*
Risk of accelerated calcification in pediatric patients leading to early valve failure	No risk of calcification
Minimal risk of thromboembolism	Higher risk of thromboembolism
Does not require anticoagulation	Lifelong anticoagulation recommended
Limited longevity, usually require multiple replacements over lifespan	Excellent longevity, can last several decades once placed
Cannot accommodate for somatic growth	Cannot accommodate for somatic growth

SUPRAVALVAR AORTIC STENOSIS

The management of SVAS is primarily surgical with only a diagnostic role for cardiac catheterization. However, among patients with Williams syndrome and other elastinopathies, cardiac catheterization continues to play a major role in the rehabilitation of coexisting branch PA stenoses and narrowing of the descending aorta.

The surgical management of SVAS involves patch augmentation of the aortic root and sinotubular junction to relieve the obstruction. The surgery is extended to augment the ascending aorta and aortic arch if concomitant hypoplasia of these structures is present. Coronary ostial unroofing or patch plasty is also required in cases involving significant narrowing of the ostia. In a large series from Mayo Clinic, Rochester, Minnesota,[19] acute surgical outcomes were good, whereas long-term survival was reported to be 90, 84, and 82% at 5, 10, and 20 years, respectively. Freedom from reoperation was 86% at 20 years follow-up. Factors associated with worse outcome include diffuse vasculopathy and coexisting aortic valve pathology. Williams syndrome by itself is not a risk factor for worse outcome in patients with SVAS.

SHONE'S COMPLEX AND HYPOPLASTIC LEFT HEART SYNDROME

Shone's complex consists of a constellation of left-heart anomalies including annulo-leaflet mitral ring (often referred to as a "supra-mitral ring" though the ring is not truly supra-annular), parachute mitral valve, discrete subaortic stenosis, and coarctation of the aorta. HLHS consists of various anomalies of the left heart such as mitral and aortic stenosis or atresia that together lead to underdevelopment of the LV, such that it can no longer supply the systemic circulation. While both Shone's complex and HLHS can present with LV outflow obstruction as part of the overall clinical picture, their management differs substantially from those patients that have isolated obstruction of the LV outflow. In some cases of Shone's complex and all cases of HLHS, a univentricular palliation with an eventual Fontan circulation is required. These patients are discussed separately in Chapter 39.

CONCLUSION

Obstruction to outflow from the left heart can occur at multiple levels. It is well tolerated when mild but can lead to symptoms such as dyspnea, fatigue, exertional chest pain or sudden cardiac death when moderate or severe. Treatment involves transcatheter or surgical relief of obstruction after careful delineation of the mechanism of obstruction using echocardiography.

ACKNOWLEDGMENT

The author would like to thank Kai-ou Tang for preparing the figures in this chapter.

REFERENCES

1. Hoffman JIE, Kaplan S. The incidence of congenital heart disease. J Am Coll Cardiol. 2002; 39(12):1890-900.
2. Kitchiner D, Jackson M, Malaiya N, Walsh K, Peart I, Arnold R. Incidence and prognosis of obstruction of the left ventricular outflow tract in Liverpool (1960-91): a study of 313 patients. Br Heart J. 1994;71(6):588-95.
3. Matisoff AJ, Olivieri L, Schwartz JM, Deutsch N. Risk assessment and anesthetic management of patients with Williams syndrome: a comprehensive review. Paediatr Anaesth. 2015;25(12):1207-15.
4. Fernandes SM, Sanders SP, Khairy P, Jenkins KJ, Gauvreau K, Lang P, et al. Morphology of bicuspid aortic valve in children and adolescents. J Am Coll Cardiol. 2004;44(8):1648-51.
5. Sybert VP. Cardiovascular malformations and complications in Turner syndrome. Pediatrics. 1998;101(1):E11.
6. Loffredo CA, Chokkalingam A, Sill AM, Boughman JA, Clark EB, Scheel J, et al. Prevalence of congenital cardiovascular malformations among relatives of infants with hypoplastic left heart, coarctation of the aorta, and d-transposition of the great arteries. Am J Med Genet. 2004;124A(3):225-30.
7. Greve AM, Boman K, Gohlke-Baerwolf C, Kesäniemi YA, Nienaber C, Ray S, et al. Clinical implications of electrocardiographic left ventricular strain and hypertrophy in asymptomatic patients with aortic stenosis: the simvastatin and ezetimibe in aortic stenosis study. Circulation. 2012;125(2):346-53.
8. Nagueh SF, Smiseth OA, Appleton CP, Byrd BF, Dokainish H, Edvardsen T, et al. Recommendations for the evaluation of left ventricular diastolic function by echocardiography: an update from the American Society of Echocardiography and the European Association of Cardiovascular Imaging. J Am Soc Echocardiogr. 2016;29(4):277-314.
9. Nishimura RA, Otto CM, Bonow RO, Carabello BA, Erwin JP, Guyton RA, et al. 2014 AHA/ACC guideline for the management of patients with valvular heart disease: Executive summary: a report of the American College of Cardiology/American Heart Association Task Force on Practice Guidelines. Circulation. 2014;129(23):2440-92.
10. Geva A, McMahon CJ, Gauvreau K, Mohammed L, del Nido PJ, Geva T. Risk factors for reoperation after repair of discrete subaortic stenosis in children. J Am Coll Cardiol. 2007;50(15):1498-504.
11. Lupinetti FM, Pridjian AK, Callow LB, Crowley DC, Beekman RH, Bove EL. Optimum treatment of discrete subaortic stenosis. Ann Thorac Surg. 1992;54(3):467-71.
12. Talwar S, Anand A, Gupta SK, Ramakrishnan S,Kothari SS, Saxena A, et al. Resection of subaortic membrane for discrete subaortic stenosis. J Card Surg. 2017;32(7):430-5.
13. Feltes TF, Bacha E, Beekman RH, Cheatham JP, Feinstein JA, Gomes AS, et al. Indications for cardiac catheterization and intervention in pediatric cardiac disease: a scientific statement from the American Heart Association. Circulation. 2011;123(22):2607-52.
14. Awasthy N, Garg R, Radhakrishnan S, Shrivastava S. Long-term results of percutaneous balloon valvuloplasty of congenital aortic stenosis in adolescents and young adults. Indian Heart J. 2016;68(5):604-11.
15. Pillai AA, Balasubramanian VR, Sharma DK. Immediate and long-term follow-up results of balloon aortic valvuloplasty in congenital bicuspid aortic valve stenosis among young patients. J Heart Valve Dis. 2018;27(1):17-23.
16. Maxwell D, Allan L, Tynan MJ. Balloon dilatation of the aortic valve in the fetus: a report of two cases. Br Heart J. 1991;65(5): 256-8.
17. Tworetzky W, Wilkins-Haug L, Jennings RW, Van Der Velde ME, Marshall AC, Marx GR, et al. Balloon dilation of severe aortic stenosis in the fetus: potential for prevention of hypoplastic left heart syndrome. Candidate selection, technique, and results of successful intervention. Circulation. 2004;110(15):2125-31.
18. Friedman KG, Sleeper LA, Freud LR, Marshall AC, Godfrey ME, Drogosz M, et al. Improved technical success, postnatal outcome and refined predictors of outcome for fetal aortic valvuloplasty. Ultrasound Obstet Gynecol. 2018;52(2):212-20.
19. Deo SV, Burkhart HM, Schaff HV, Li Z, Stensrud PE, Olson TM, et al. Late outcomes for surgical repair of supravalvar aortic stenosis. Ann Thorac Surg. 2012;94(3):854-9.

29
CHAPTER

Aortic Arch Obstruction: Coarctation and Aortic Arch Interruption

Sangeetha Viswanathan

INTRODUCTION

This chapter will provide a broad overview of aortic arch obstruction, which includes coarctation of aorta (CoA) and aortic arch interruption (AAI).

BACKGROUND AND EPIDEMIOLOGY

In order to understand the abnormalities of the arch, let us first familiarize ourselves with the normal left aortic arch and its branches as shown in **Figure 1**.

Note that the part of the arch between the left common carotid artery and the left subclavian artery is called the transverse arch and the part of the aorta just distal to the left subclavian artery is known as the isthmus.

Coarctation of aorta is a narrowing of the aorta, which usually occurs at the junction between the aortic arch and the descending thoracic aorta (isthmic region) in close proximity to the patent ductus arteriosus (PDA) (if present). The isthmic region is the part of the aorta that receives the least blood flow during fetal life and therefore it is logical that this region is the most prone to narrowing to produce coarctation of the aorta. Although traditionally coarctation has been classified into pre and postductal coarctation in real life, we often find the narrowing to be peri or juxtaductal. The portion of the arch between the left subclavian artery and the coarctation is known as the isthmus and is often hypoplastic or small in patients with CoA. Sometimes the origin of the left subclavian artery may also be involved in the coarctation and found to be narrowed.

Coarctation may be discrete and localized or associated with hypoplasia of the transverse arch illustrated in **Figures 2A and B**. The transverse arch is the segment of the aortic arch between the left common carotid artery and the left subclavian artery and is usually hypoplastic in patients with coarctation of aorta. The degree of hypoplasia of the transverse arch has important implications on the management strategy in these patients. In addition, there is usually dilatation of the aorta seen distal to the coarctation, which is sometimes referred to as poststenotic dilatation. Abdominal aortic coarctation can also occur but is rare and will not be addressed in this chapter.

Coarctation of aorta occurs in approximately 4 in 10,000 live-born babies with a slight male preponderance.[1] Although it is mostly sporadic, there is reported familial occurrence with a possibly autosomal dominant

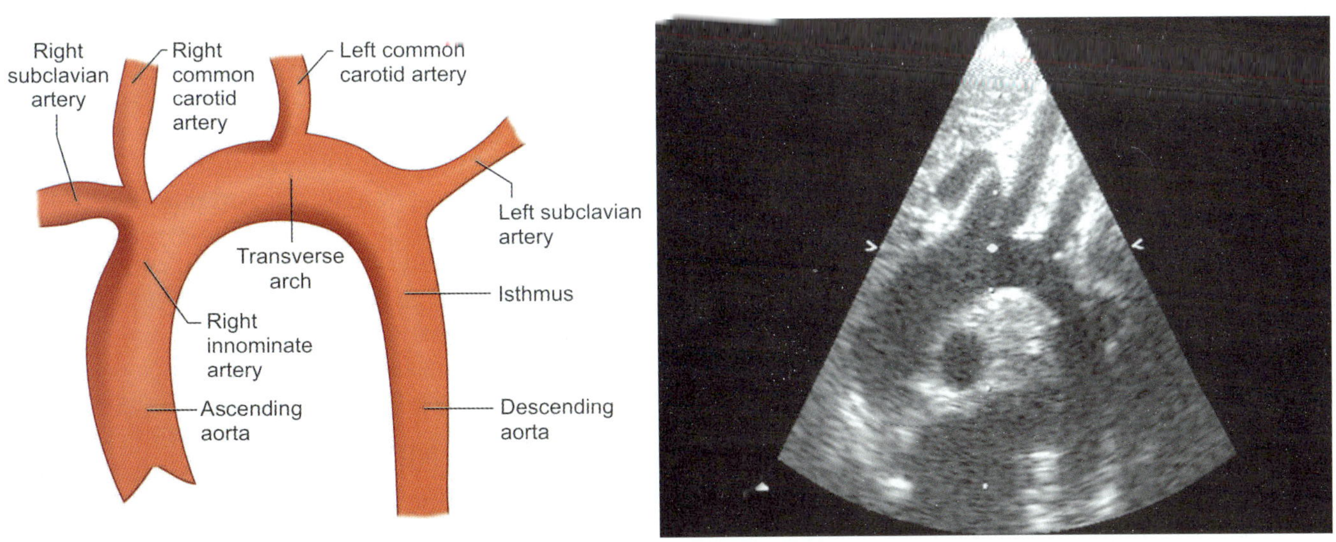

Fig. 1: Labeled sketch of normal branching pattern of the left aortic arch with corresponding echocardiographic image.

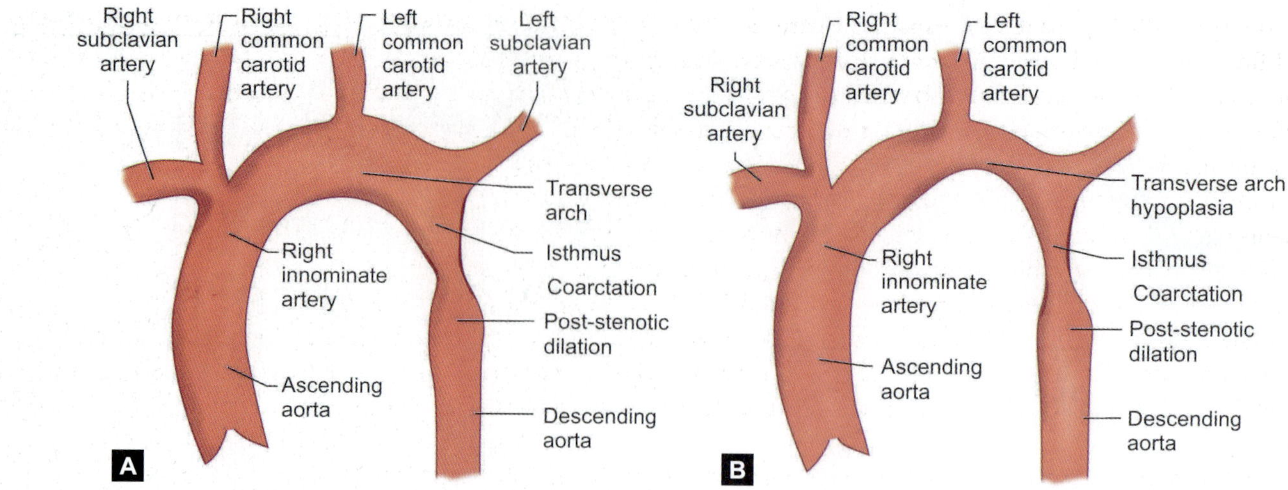

Figs. 2A and B: Labeled sketch of left aortic arch with a discrete coarctation (A) and with associated transverse arch hypoplasia (B).

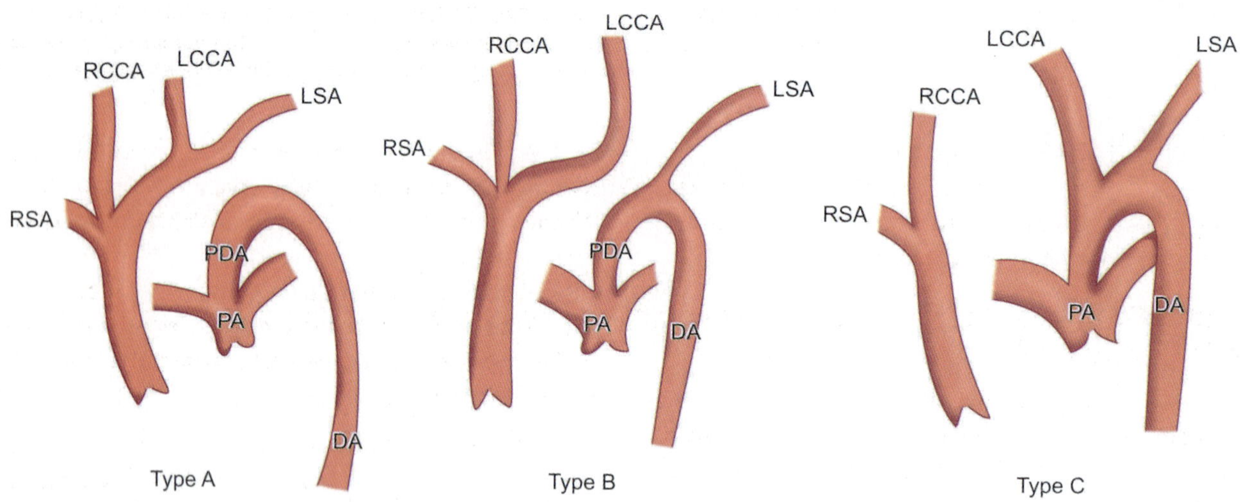

Fig. 3: Labeled sketch of types of aortic arch interruption.
(DA: descending aorta; LCCA: left common carotid artery; LSA: left subclavian artery; PA: pulmonary artery; PDA: patent ductus arteriosus; RCCA: right common carotid artery; RSA: right subclavian artery)

inheritance pattern.[2] There is also a fairly strong association with Turner syndrome with a reported 7–18% of patients with Turner syndrome having coarctation of the aorta.[3]

Left heart lesions often coexist and a combination of left ventricular inflow, outflow and arch obstruction is commonly referred to as Shone's complex. The obstruction at the mitral and aortic level can be supravalvar, valvar, or subvalvar in nature. The original description of the complex in fact involved a patient with supramitral membrane, subaortic membrane, and coarctation. Coarctation often coexists with a bicuspid aortic valve and vice versa and this is particularly common in patients with Turner syndrome.

Aortic arch interruption refers to a complete discontinuity in the aortic arch. This can occur at multiple sites and AAI is classified accordingly into types A, B, and C with type B being the most common (**Fig. 3**).

Type A interruption refers to interruption at the isthmus distal to the left subclavian artery, type B interruption occurs between the left common carotid artery and the left subclavian artery, and type C interruption refers to interruption between the carotid arteries.

Arch interruption is relatively rare and is often associated with DiGeorge syndrome with two-thirds of patients with interruption between the left carotid artery and the subclavian artery (type B) having the 22q11 deletion.[4] Interruption of aorta between the left common carotid and subclavian arteries (type B) accounts for 50–75% of cases, followed by interruption of the isthmus (type A), while interruption between the carotids (type C) is rare.[5]

Interruption rarely occurs in isolation and is commonly associated with a ventricular septal defect (VSD).[5] Also, patients with truncus arteriosus (TA), not infrequently, have associated arch interruption and this can be easily missed. Usually, these patients have associated DiGeorge syndrome.

EMBRYOGENESIS

There are several theories regarding the embryogenesis of arch obstruction, which include a low-flow theory, a ductal theory, and abnormal embryogenesis theory.

- The low-flow theory proposes that a decrease in blood flow through the left heart in the fetus results in hypoplasia and narrowing at the arch in the region of the isthmus, which receives the lowest fraction of the cardiac output during fetal life. It is thought that a restriction of the foramen ovale results in reduced flow of blood in the left heart resulting in poor growth of left-sided structures with the already vulnerable isthmic area being most prone for narrowing and development of coarctation.
- The ductal theory proposes that ductal tissue that often encircles the aorta in the region of the PDA constricts postnatally when the PDA closes resulting in arch narrowing.
- Abnormal embryogenesis implies that the problem arises much earlier in fetal life during aortic arch development.

The substrate for coarctation can often be identified in utero through fetal echocardiography. Subtle clues include ventricular disproportion with a small left ventricle and relative smallness of the aortic arch.

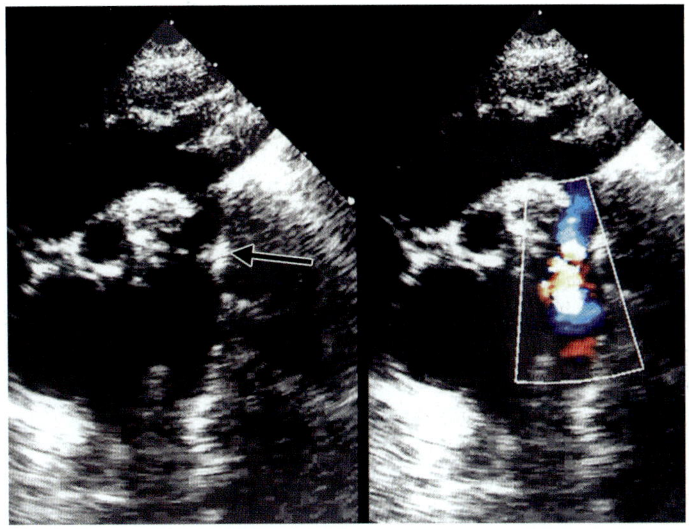

Fig. 4: A still image from an echocardiographic view of the aortic arch with a discrete coarctation (note clear posterior shelf indicated with a black arrow giving an appearance of the number "3"). The color frame shows aliasing due to flow acceleration at the level of the coarctation.

CLINICAL PRESENTATION

Clinical presentation of arch obstruction can be highly variable as illustrated by the cases discussed here. The common clinical presentations are described here.

Circulatory Collapse due to Duct-dependent Systemic Outflow Obstruction

This presentation may be seen in arch interruption and severe coarctation. In this scenario, the problem manifests in the early neonatal period when the PDA, which mainly supplies the descending thoracic aorta, constricts resulting in poor lower extremity pulses, poor peripheral perfusion (prolonged capillary refill, cool peripheries, and pallor), metabolic acidosis, and respiratory distress. The common differential diagnosis is neonatal sepsis. Upper extremity pulses are preserved and this points toward arch obstruction. The right upper extremity pulse is more consistently preserved as compared to the left because the left subclavian may be downstream to the obstruction (type B interruption) or involved in the coarctation.

Case Example

A 2-day-old neonate presents to the emergency department unwell with pallor, respiratory distress, poor pulses, and cool peripheries. Parents give history of early discharge at 6 hours after a normal delivery. A routine neonatal examination was unremarkable but neonatal pulse oximetry screening was not carried out. There is no history of fever and there are no risk factors for neonatal sepsis. On examination, the baby is in shock with no palpable femoral pulses and well felt brachial pulses. There is a soft systolic murmur heard over the left axilla. Lower limb saturation (SpO_2) and blood pressure (BP) are unrecordable.

What is the likely diagnosis in this baby?

Duct-dependent arch obstruction; although sepsis is a differential diagnosis in this scenario and needs to be ruled out.

The baby receives oxygen by mask and an intravenous cannula is inserted. A partial septic screen is done and is negative. There is no pediatric cardiologist available at the hospital.

What would the next management step be?

Start prostaglandin infusion at 50–100 ng/kg/min and arrange to shift the patient to a center with pediatric cardiac facilities.

The baby is started on prostin with improvement in overall condition and reappearance of femoral pulses and is transferred to the nearest pediatric cardiac facility. Echocardiography confirms the diagnosis of severe CoA (**Fig. 4**) and surgical repair is carried out successfully with the patient being discharged from hospital within 10 days.

Incidental Detection on Neonatal Screening

Routine neonatal examination should include palpation of femoral pulses and can detect absent or weak femoral pulses. It is useful to simultaneously feel the right brachial pulse for comparison. It is recommended not to use the left brachial pulse as sometimes the left subclavian artery can be involved in the coarctation and give false results.

Neonatal pulse oximetry is a useful adjunct to physical examination as it can pick up duct-dependent systemic circulation in the first few days of life when the PDA may be wide open. When the PDA is open in the first few days of life, it supplies the lower body in the presence of a significant coarctation or arch interruption. Therefore, the femoral pulses which are supplied by the duct might actually be

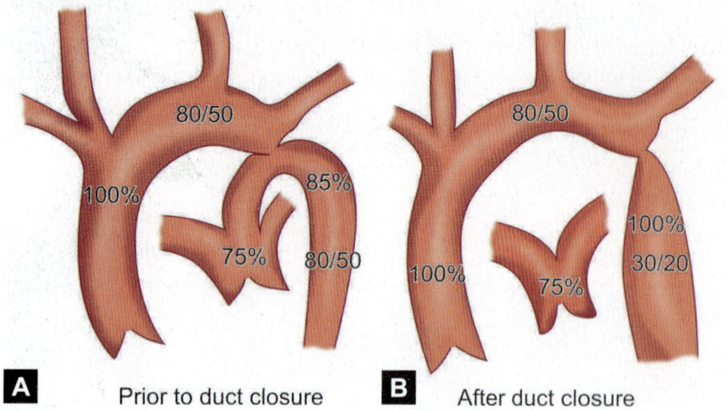

Figs. 5A and B: (A) The difference in saturation (SpO_2) between upper and lower limb although there is no difference in the blood pressure (BP) and femoral pulse when the patent ductus arteriosus (PDA) is open; (B) The difference in BP with a weak femoral pulse which becomes evident after the PDA closes. Note that there is no longer a difference in the SpO_2 between the upper and lower limb once the PDA closes.

well felt leading to a "missed diagnosis" of arch obstruction. In this situation, pulse oximetry screening will detect differential saturations with the lower limb saturation being lower than the upper limb saturation. Once the PDA closes, the saturations will become equal but the femoral pulses will become weak or absent (**Figs. 5A and B**). It is therefore critical to use a combination of physical examination and pulse oximetry to maximize clinical pick up.

Four-limb BP measurement can be a useful adjunct but in neonates this may be a technical challenge due to nonavailability of appropriate cuff sizes and poor patient cooperation with the procedure. A difference in lower limb BP of 20 mm Hg or more is considered significant with the lower limb pressure being less than the upper limb. Practically, palpation often provides a more convenient guide than BP measurement in the neonatal age group.

Case Example

A 24-hour-old neonate undergoes routine saturation screening and the right upper limb saturation is measured at 98% while the lower limb saturation is 80%. The baby is asymptomatic but in view of the saturation findings, kept under close observation. Two more readings are repeated at hourly intervals and reveal similar results. The child is referred for echocardiography and is noted to have AAI with a large PDA supplying the descending aorta. There is in addition a large VSD. Prostaglandin infusion is commenced at 20 ng/kg/min and the child is transferred to a pediatric cardiac center. It is essential to not be overzealous about oxygen administration in these situations because of the risk of pulmonary vasodilation resulting in steal of blood from systemic circulation with resultant necrotizing enterocolitis and renal injury. Often room air is adequate in ventilated children and children breathing spontaneously need not receive supplemental oxygen, where aortic arch reconstruction and VSD closure is carried out. The child is discharged after 2 weeks in hospital with good flow in the aortic arch and no residual VSD.

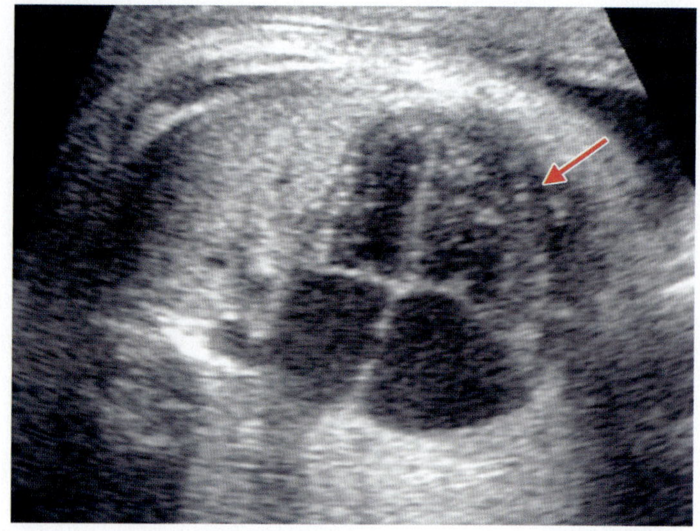

Fig. 6: A still frame of a fetal echocardiogram at 18 weeks' gestation showing a four-chamber view of the heart with a dilated right heart indicated by the red arrow.

Antenatal Detection on Fetal Echocardiography

Antenatal ultrasound can detect possible arch obstruction during fetal life. This is usually suspected due to dilatation of the right ventricle in early pregnancy. If this is detected during routine anomaly screening carried out at 18–20 weeks' gestation, the patient is usually referred for detailed fetal echocardiography. This finding of right heart dilatation may not be as useful in advanced pregnancy as it can be a normal finding at late gestation. In addition, experienced fetal echocardiographers can also directly delineate the arch and demonstrate the coarctation/arch interruption in fetal life. If a potential aortic arch obstruction is picked up in fetal life, delivery should be planned at a center where postnatal echocardiography is readily available and where neonatal care can be provided promptly including initiation of prostaglandin infusion.

Case Example

A 32-year-old primigravid woman undergoes routine anomaly screening at 20 weeks and the fetus is found to have right heart dilation on the scan (**Fig. 6**). An urgent referral is made to a fetal cardiologist who diagnoses coarctation of aorta. The family is counseled and opts to continue the pregnancy and the baby is delivered at term by normal vaginal delivery at a facility with pediatric cardiology services. A postnatal echocardiogram is carried out to confirm the diagnosis and as the PDA is wide open low dose, prostin is started (10–20 ng/kg/min) to maintain ductal patency. The child then undergoes coarctation repair on day 3 of life with a good operative outcome and is discharged home on no medications.

Incidental Detection in Older Children

In milder forms of arch obstruction, detection might be incidental due to a murmur, weak femoral pulses, or unexplained hypertension. The murmur of coarctation is usually best heard in the left axillary region as a soft ejection systolic murmur. In older patients with established collaterals, a continuous murmur may be appreciated in the back. It is important to make it a routine practice to palpate the femoral pulses in children as significant coarctation may be otherwise missed. Coarctation must be suspected if femorals are absent or weak compared to the radial pulse. Also, simultaneous palpation of the radial and femoral pulses in older children may help detect radiofemoral delay where there is delayed peaking of the femoral pulse when compared with the radial. Note that this finding may not be appreciated in infants and very young children.

Four-limb BP may be more useful in the older age group as the patients are able to cooperate better with the procedure. A difference of 20 mm Hg or more between upper and lower limb BP (upper > lower) is considered abnormal.

Unexplained hypertension in children and young adults should prompt thorough evaluation of the aortic arch for undetected coarctation. Although the incidence of primary hypertension is increasing in younger individuals due to early-onset obesity and metabolic syndrome, it is critical to rule out secondary hypertension due to renal and cardiovascular abnormalities.

Case Example

A 15-year-old girl presents with hypertension, which was incidentally detected during a visit to pediatric outpatient clinic for poor growth. She is yet to attain menarche and has short stature, poor sexual development. On further examination, she has cubitus valgus, a broad chest, and a webbed neck. Her BP is above the 99th centile for her age and sex. Cardiovascular examination reveals poor femoral pulses with well felt radial pulses. She has radiofemoral delay and a continuous murmur is heard on auscultation of her back. In addition, there is an ejection click that is well heard over the aortic area and apex.

What is the likely cardiac diagnosis of this patient?
Coarctation of the aorta with bicuspid aortic valve.

What is the likely underlying genetic diagnosis?
Turner syndrome.

How can the cardiac diagnosis be confirmed?
Transthoracic echocardiogram and if required cardiac computed tomography (CT) or cardiac magnetic resonance imaging (MRI).

She undergoes echocardiography and is diagnosed with a bicuspid aortic valve, dilated ascending aorta, and CoA with significant left ventricular hypertrophy (LVH) (**Figs. 7A to C**).

What is the treatment of choice for coarctation in this patient?
Transcatheter stenting of the coarctation with a covered stent due to concerns regarding aortic fragility associated with Turner syndrome.

She underwent transcatheter coarctation stenting with a covered stent, which resulted in significant reduction in her BP. She was also confirmed to have Turner syndrome by karyotyping and counseled accordingly.

Adult Presentation of Arch Obstruction

Usually adults with undetected coarctation present with unexplained hypertension.

This may be an incidental finding during a medical examination or may be associated with symptoms and/or

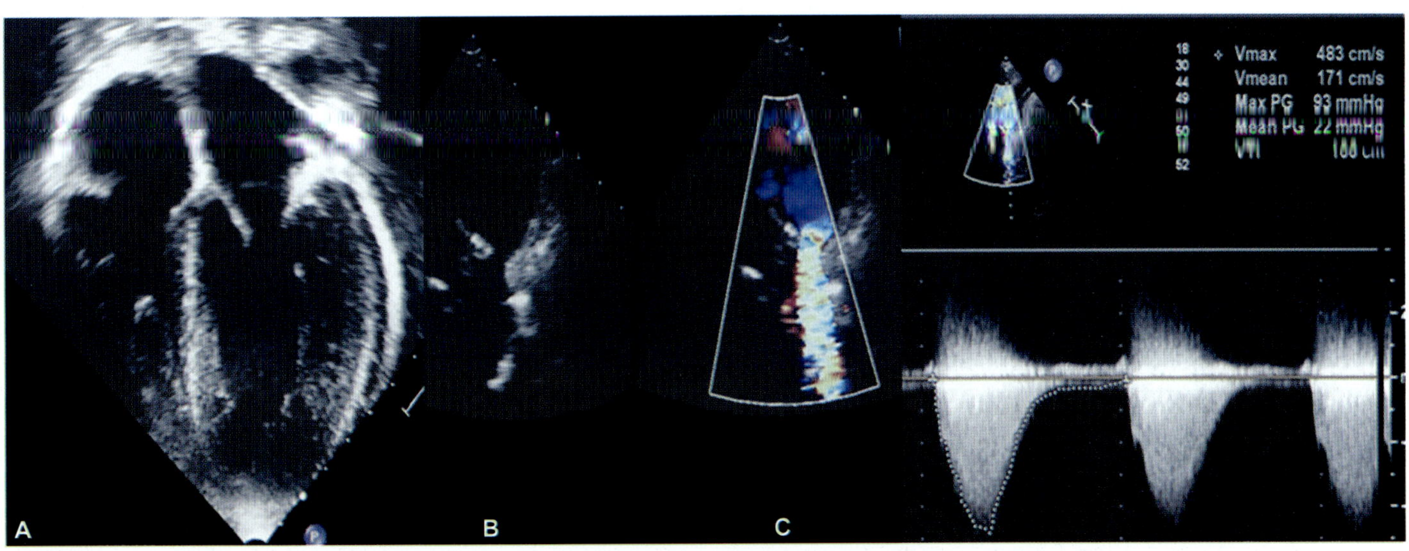

Figs. 7A to C: (A) Four-chamber view of the heart with significant left ventricular hypertrophy (LVH); (B) Suprasternal view of the aortic arch showing a severe, discrete narrowing with flow acceleration on color Doppler; (C) Continuous wave Doppler image showing a high pressure gradient across the narrowed segment with diastolic tailing.

complications, which include intracranial hemorrhage and early atherosclerotic disease. A specific association seen in patients with coarctation is berry aneurysms in the circle of Willis, which can rupture giving rise to subarachnoid hemorrhage. It is important to examine the femoral pulses in all young patients with hypertension and to pay attention to the aortic arch during echocardiography.

DIAGNOSTIC MODALITIES

A wide range of imaging options have greatly enhanced the ease with which coarctation can be diagnosed and characterized.

Transthoracic Echocardiography, Chest X-ray, and ECG

In neonates, infants, and young children, transthoracic echocardiography is the gold standard for diagnosis of arch obstruction and delineates both the anatomy and severity of the lesion. As with any other congenital heart defect, it is important that the pediatric echocardiographer follows a sequential segmental approach so that other associated lesions are not missed. As left-sided lesions frequently occur together, careful examination of the mitral and aortic valves is essential.

Coarctation of the aorta is usually seen on the echocardiogram as an area of narrowing of the aortic arch in the vicinity of the PDA (periductal). This is usually appreciated as a posterior shelf giving rise to the 3-sign or inverted E sign on echocardiography (*see* **Fig. 4**). Note that an anterior shelf is commonly seen in neonates with large PDAs and should not be mistaken for coarctation. Coarctation may be difficult to diagnose in the presence of a large PDA and repeated assessments may be required in order to make the diagnosis. Some neonates and infants with severe coarctation may have left ventricular dysfunction of varying severity. In older children, there is usually poststenotic dilatation distal to the coarctation, which is thought to be due to the jet effect. Measurements are taken at multiple sites to aid in planning management and include the narrowest segment of the aorta, transverse arch, isthmus, and descending aorta at the level of the diaphragm. Older children may have significant LVH due to significant long-standing aortic obstruction (*see* **Fig. 7**).

Color Doppler imaging shows flow turbulence across the coarctation site with aliasing (*see* **Fig. 7**) and the width of the color jet gives a rough estimation of the severity of the narrowing. Continuous wave (CW) Doppler examination of the jet gives an estimation of the gradient across the coarctation. A peak gradient of 35 mm Hg or more on echocardiography is considered to be significant with a characteristic Doppler tracing showing the phenomenon of diastolic tailing as seen in **Figure 7**. Note that the gradient may be underestimated if there is poor left ventricular function, significant stenosis of the mitral or aortic valves, or significant collateralization.

Arch interruption can be easily missed on echocardiography and should be looked for carefully. An inability to visualize the arch in its entirety and the presence of a large PDA with right-to-left flow supplying the descending thoracic aorta should raise suspicion of arch interruption (**Fig. 8**). There is a typical appearance of the ascending aorta heading sharply upward as the head and neck vessels with an inability to visualize the aortic arch in its entirety. Depending on the site of interruption, the lesion is classified into one of three types as discussed previously with type B interruption between the left common carotid artery and the left subclavian artery being the most common type. Each head and neck vessel should be clearly identified and the gap between the proximal and distal segments of the aorta measured to assist the surgeon in planning surgical strategy.

Aortic arch interruption is usually associated with a muscular VSD and this should be looked for on

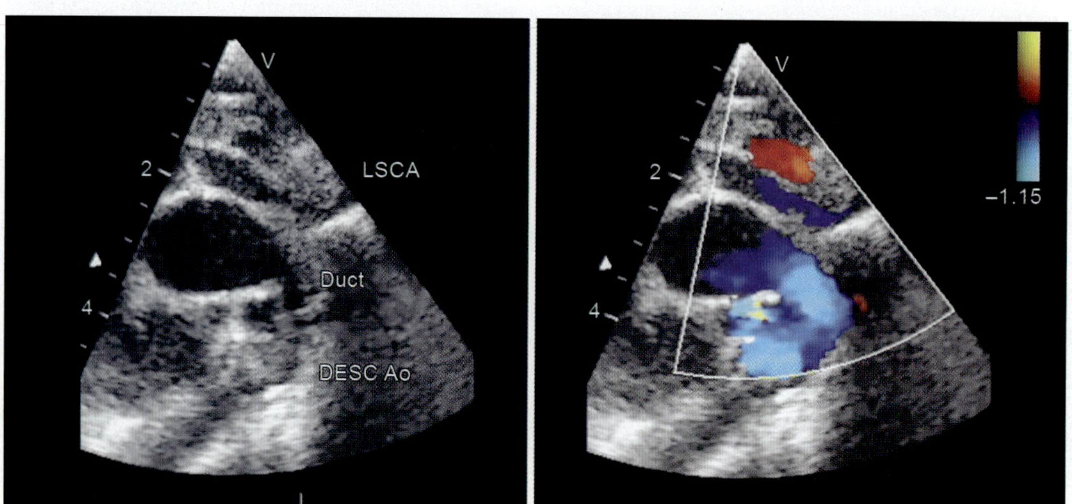

Fig. 8: Type A interruption distal to the left subclavian artery (LSCA) with a large patent ductus arteriosus (PDA) with right-to-left flow supplying the descending aorta (DESC Ao).

echocardiography. AAI is commonly seen in patients with TA and can be easily missed. One of the clues to picking up these patients is the presence of a PDA as patients with TA usually do not have a PDA and the only situation when they do have a PDA shunting right-to-left is when the TA is associated with AAI.

Other routine investigations include ECG and chest X-ray which are usually carried out preprocedurally. The ECG in a neonate with coarctation shows right axis deviation with right ventricular hypertrophy (RVH) pattern whereas in an older child or adult with coarctation, we see LVH.

Chest X-ray is not particularly diagnostic but may be of benefit if there are additional lesions like a VSD, TA, etc. In adults with untreated coarctation who have significant collateralization, the hallmark chest X-ray finding of rib notching may be seen (**Fig. 9**).

Advanced Imaging

Advanced imaging including CT and cardiac magnetic resonance imaging (CMRI) is particularly useful in older patients with poor echocardiographic windows and in patients with complex anatomy such as TA with interruption (**Fig. 10**).

Computed tomography is a very good tool to image the aortic arch but carries the risk of radiation exposure, especially when serial imaging is required. Cardiac MRI (CMRI) may therefore be a better modality in the long-term follow-up of these patients, although it is more resource intensive (**Fig. 11**).

Cardiac Catheterization

Cardiac catheterization is not routinely required to make a diagnosis of arch obstruction and is often a prelude to transcatheter therapy. A pressure gradient of 20 mm Hg or more is considered significant. Angiography demonstrates the site of coarctation and allows measurement of the transverse arch and descending aorta at the level of the diaphragm to aid in stent/balloon selection **(Fig. 12)**.

Ambulatory BP Monitoring and Exercise Testing

Older children and adults with coarctation may benefit from 24-hour ambulatory BP monitoring to uncover "masked" hypertension. Patients with coarctation fail to exhibit the nocturnal dip in BP that is usually seen in normal individuals and tend to have an exaggerated BP response to exercise. These abnormalities may be detected by ambulatory BP monitoring and exercise testing and are particularly useful in decision-making regarding the management of hypertension that often accompanies CoA in older patients, which may not fully resolve even after the arch obstruction is treated satisfactorily.

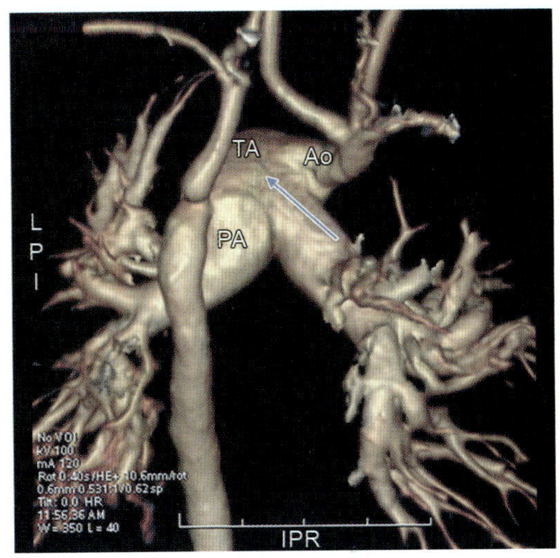

Fig. 10: 3D reconstruction of a computed tomography (CT) angiogram showing truncus arteriosus with aortic arch interruption (AAI) (the blue arrow points to the gap in the aortic arch).
(Ao: aorta, PA: pulmonary artery; TA: truncus arteriosus)

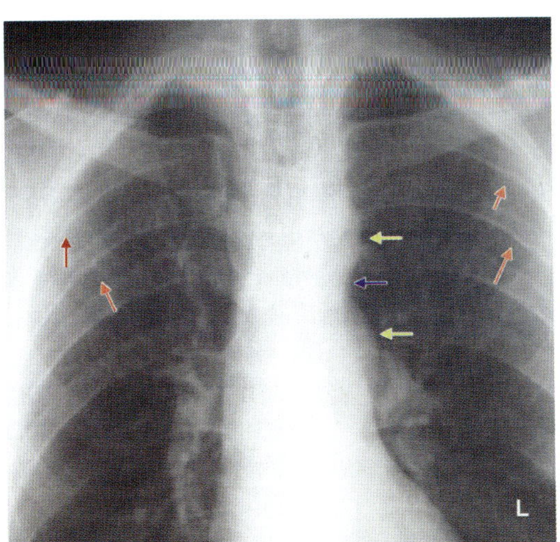

Fig. 9: Chest X-ray (CXR) with rib notching as indicated by the red arrows and the "3" sign or "inverted E" sign typical of aortic coarctation.

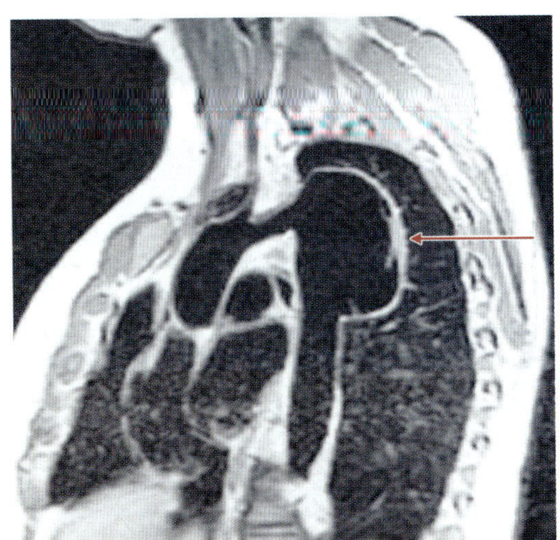

Fig. 11: Cardiac magnetic resonance (MR) of a patient following surgical patch repair of coarctation showing aneurysmal dilatation of repair site (red arrow) with transverse arch hypoplasia.

TREATMENT

Treatment of aortic arch obstruction varies based on the severity of obstruction and the age at presentation. Neonatal presentation usually represents the severe end of the spectrum and requires immediate/early treatment, which is usually surgical. In older children (usually with coarctation), transcatheter options including balloon dilation and stent implantation may be equally efficacious or superior.

Treatment of Neonatal Arch Obstruction

Medical Stabilization

Neonatal arch obstruction is usually duct-dependent and initial management includes prostaglandin infusion to maintain ductal patency. The dose required depends on the clinical scenario with higher doses (50–100 ng/kg/min) required in sick neonates where the PDA has closed and needs to be reopened who present with circulatory shock and lower doses (10–20 ng/kg/min) required in well neonates with antenatal or incidental detection of arch obstruction who have a patent duct which needs to be maintained. It is believed that in addition to actually opening the duct, prostaglandin may open the coarctation segment by relaxing the ductal tissue encircling the aorta. There is therefore value to administering the medication even if there is no evidence of opening of a closed duct.

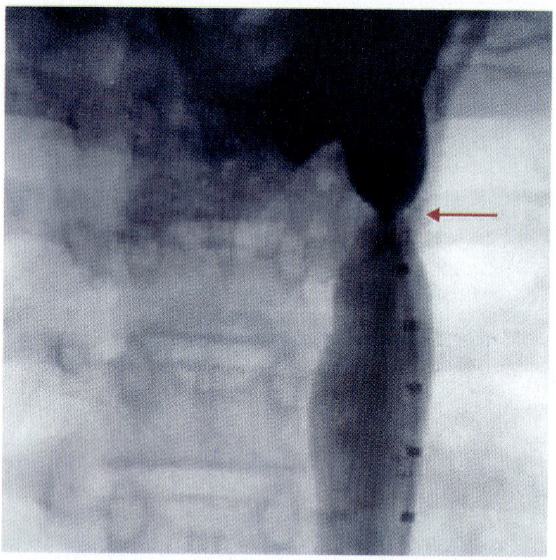

Fig. 12: An aortogram with a pigtail catheter that demonstrates a discrete coarctation (red arrow) with poststenotic dilatation.

Surgical Repair

Surgery is the mainstay of treatment in neonatal arch obstruction and may require

- End-to-end or end-to-underside anastomosis (most common technique)
- Patch aortoplasty
- Subclavian flap aortoplasty (not commonly used).

Surgery is based on the anatomy and extent of coarctation and arch hypoplasia/interruption **(Fig. 13)**.

Treatment of discrete coarctation without significant transverse arch hypoplasia can be carried out through a left lateral thoracotomy without cardiopulmonary bypass or circulatory arrest. In the presence of significant transverse arch hypoplasia or in AAI, more extensive arch repair may be required with circulatory arrest involving cooling the patient down to 20°C and temporarily arresting brain circulation for 20–30 minutes in order to carry out arch repair. Aortic interposition graft may be rarely required in patients with a long segment interruption where the arch cannot be adequately mobilized to complete an effective repair.

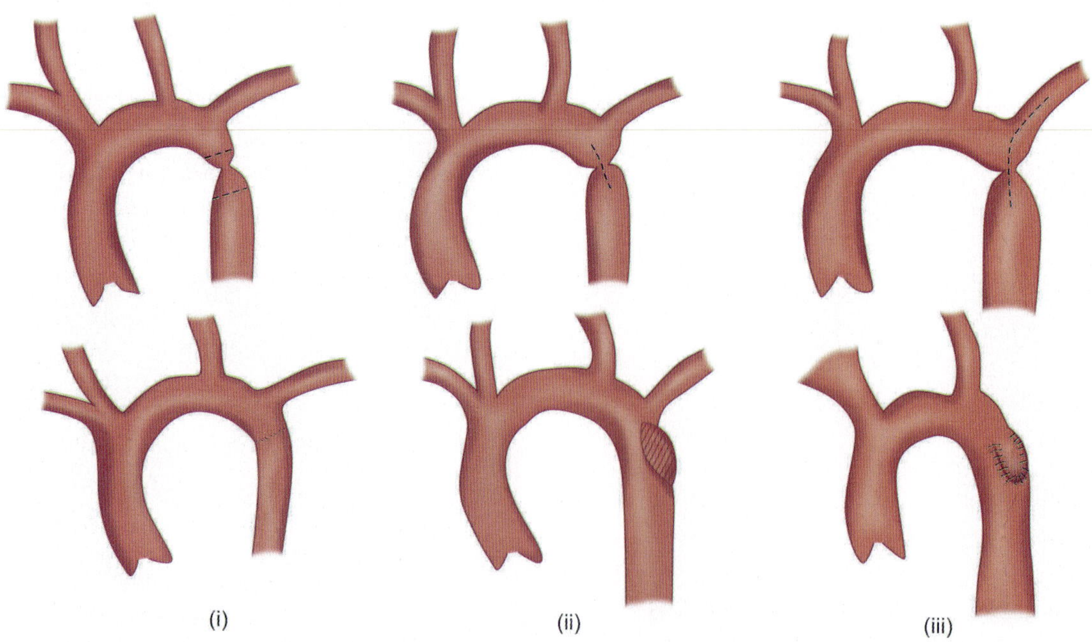

Fig. 13: Surgical techniques used to treat neonatal coarctation of aorta (i) end-to-end anastamosis; (ii) patch aortoplasty; (iii) subclavian flap repair.

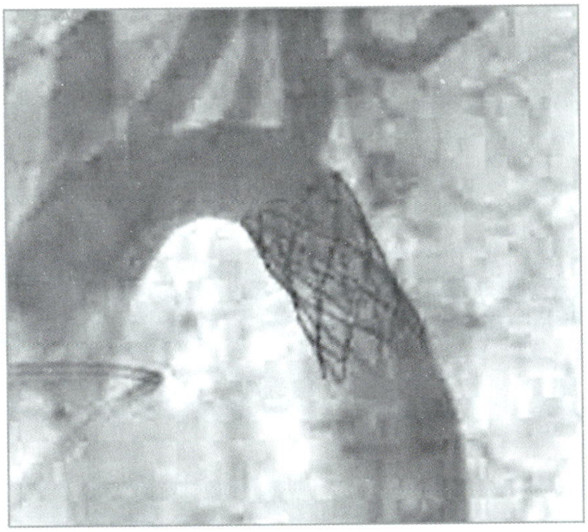

Fig. 14: A still frame of an angiogram poststent implantation to treat coarctation.

Balloon Angioplasty

Balloon angioplasty is not routinely used to treat neonatal coarctation due to a very high likelihood of recoarctation and is used only as a salvage procedure in sick neonates with severe myocardial dysfunction and acidosis where surgery is high risk. Balloon dilation can be used as a temporizing measure and is usually followed by definitive surgical repair after the overall condition of the patient has improved.

Treatment of Coarctation in Older Children and Adults

Although surgery is still an option in older infants and young children, transcatheter techniques are often preferred in older children and adults. Transcatheter techniques include balloon dilation and transcatheter stent implantation **(Fig. 14)**.

COMPLICATIONS AND LONG-TERM OUTCOME

Early surgical results of coarctation repair during infancy are excellent in most large volume pediatric cardiac centers with surgical mortality being well under 5%. A recent study published by the Pediatric Cardiac Consortium[6] reported the long-term results of coarctation repair with excellent overall survival at 20 years postoperatively. 94.5% of all patients and 95.8% of those discharged after initial operation remained alive with significant multivariable predictors of mortality including surgical weight <2.5 kg, presence of a genetic syndrome, and repair before 1990. None of the other factors examined including age at repair, gender, coarctation type, or surgical approach were found to be statistically significant. However, patients do experience small continued survival attrition throughout early adulthood and ongoing monitoring of this cohort is necessary to assess late mortality risk.[7] Long-term complications include recoarctation and aneurysm formation requiring reintervention with redo surgery or stent implantation. In a study looking at early to mid-term outcomes, freedom from aortic arch reintervention was 90% at 1 year and 88.5% at 5 years; however, longer term follow-up studies have revealed a need for arch reintervention of up to 30%.[7,8] Surgery for interruption of the aortic arch carries a slightly worse outcome due to associated intracardiac defects and genetic abnormalities.

Coarctation stenting in older children and adults carries good immediate results with a mortality of <2% and a complication rate of around 10% with complications including aortic rupture, dissection, thromboembolism, and access site complications.[9] Freedom from reintervention at 5 years was around 85%. Patients with additional risk factors such as Turner syndrome have a higher mortality and complication rate and should be electively treated with covered stents.[10]

Hypertension in Patients with Treated Arch Obstruction

Patients who have undergone effective treatment for aortic arch obstruction continue to have a higher propensity for hypertension on long-term follow-up. This is particularly true when the treatment is carried out beyond infancy and early childhood. In one study looking at patients who had undergone treatment for coarctation during adulthood nearly 60% of patients eventually developed hypertension by 50 years of age.[7]

CONCLUSION

Aortic arch obstruction has variable clinical presentations some of which can be life-threatening. The pediatrician must therefore have a high degree of suspicion and a low threshold for referral of patients with suspected arch obstruction. Advanced imaging along with modern day interventional and surgical therapies provides good immediate and long-term outcomes in these patients. Hypertension remains a long-term complication despite adequate anatomical correction in a significant proportion of patients and requires careful surveillance and aggressive treatment to prevent long-term cardiovascular morbidity and mortality.

REFERENCES

1. Reller MD, Strickland MJ, Riehle-Colarusso T, Mahle WT, Correa ASO. Prevalence of congenital heart defects in metropolitan Atlanta, 1998-2005. J Pediatr. 2008;153(6):807-13.
2. Wessels MW, Berger RM, Frohn-Mulder IM, Roos-Hesselink JW, Hoogeboom JJM, Mancini GS, et al. Autosomal dominant inheritance of left ventricular outflow tract obstruction. Am J Med Genet A. 2005;134A(2):171-9.
3. Silberbach M, Roos-Hesselink JW, Andersen NH, Braverman AC, Brown N, Collins RT, et al. Cardiovascular Health in Turner Syndrome: A Scientific Statement From the American Heart Association. American Heart Association Council on

Cardiovascular Disease in the Young; Council on Genomic and Precision Medicine; and Council on Peripheral Vascular Disease. Circ Genom Precis Med. 2018;11(10):e000048.
4. Momma K. Cardiovascular anomalies associated with chromosome 22q11.2 deletion syndrome. Am J Cardiol. 2010; 105(11):1617-24.
5. Freedom RM, Bain HH, Esplugas E, Dische R, Rowe RD. Ventricular septal defect in interruption of aortic arch. Am J Cardiol. 1977; 39(4):572-82.
6. Oster ME, McCracken C, Kiener A, Aylward B, Cory M, Hunting J, et al. Long-term survival of patients with coarctation repaired during infancy (from the Pediatric Cardiac Care Consortium). Am J Cardiol. 2019;124(5):795-802.
7. Lee MGY, Babu-Narayan SV, Kempny A, Uebing A, Montanaro C, Shore DF, et al. Long-term mortality and cardiovascular burden for adult survivors of coarctation of the aorta. Heart. 2019;105(15):1190-6.
8. Lehnert A, Villermain O, Gaudin R, Meot M, Raisky O, Bonnet D. Risk factors of mortality and recoarctation after coarctation repair in infancy. Interact Cardiovasc Thorac Surg. 2019; 29(3):469-75.
9. Erben Y, Oderich GS, Verhagen HJM, Witsenburg M, Lawrence PF, van den Hoven AT, et al. Multicenter experience with endovascular treatment of aortic coarctation in adults. J Vasc Surg. 2019;69(3):671-9.
10. Van den Hoven AT, Duijnhouwer AL, Eicken A, de Bruin C, Roos-Hesselink JW, Aboulhosn J, et al. Adverse outcome of coarctation stenting in patients with Turner syndrome. Catheter Cardiovasc Interv. 2017;89(2):280-7.

30 CHAPTER

Vascular Rings and Slings

Shweta Bakhru

INTRODUCTION

The *vascular ring* (VR), a term coined by Gross in 1945, is a congenital anomaly where the trachea and esophagus are entirely surrounded by an aortic arch or its remnants, giving rise to compressive symptoms.[1,2] High degree of clinical suspicion and timely identification of this anomaly is essential in a symptomatic patient. Untreated patients can suffer significant mortality and morbidity.[1-4] *Vascular sling* (VS) is a congenital malformation where the left pulmonary artery (LPA) arises from the right pulmonary artery (RPA) and travels in between the trachea and esophagus. Since vascular structures do not completely encircle the trachea, it is labeled as a sling.[5] Computed tomography (CT) angiogram or magnetic resonance imaging (MRI) is a gold standard imaging modality for diagnosis.[6-8]

APPLIED ANATOMY OF AORTIC ARCH

The thoracic part of the aorta is composed of ascending aorta, proximal transverse arch, distal transverse arch, and thoracic part of descending aorta. Ascending aorta arises from the left ventricle, and then transverse arch turns posteriorly and leftward to the trachea. The arch of aorta passes on the left bronchus. The transverse arch has three neck vessels; they are right brachiocephalic artery, left carotid artery, and left subclavian artery (LSA). Occasionally left vertebral artery can arise from the arch of aorta as an independent vessel instead of the LSA, which is a standard variant. 10% of the population can have the right brachiocephalic artery and left carotid artery arising together, giving the two-vessel appearance from the arch of the aorta. Again, these findings are normal variants.[9]

The relation of the pulmonary artery (PA) and aorta is vital to understand. The PA is left and anterior to the aorta and bifurcates into the right and left pulmonary arteries. The RPA is underneath the arch of the aorta and anterior to the trachea and right bronchus. The LPA is leftward and posterior and enters the left hilum.

Ductus Arteriosus

The left-sided ductus arteriosus (DA) arises after the distal arch closes to the LSA and joins the main pulmonary artery (MPA) close to LPA. During fetal circulation, DA plays a significant role, and it regresses soon after birth. A remnant of DA called as ligament arteriosum persists even after spontaneous closure. Ligament arteriosum, although non-patent fibrous stand, contributes to several VRs, as discussed in subsequent literature.

IDENTIFICATION OF LEFT OR RIGHT ARCH

Left or right aortic arch is defined by which side of bronchus does the arch passes. If it passes on left bronchus, then left aortic arch and vice versa. The definition of the aortic arch has no relation with the sidedness of descending aorta.

INCIDENCE AND EPIDEMIOLOGY

Vascular rings are rare congenital malformations with an incidence of around 1%.[10] However, VR may remain asymptomatic, and therefore the exact incidence is unpredictable. Double aortic arch (DAA) and right aortic arch (RAA) with the aberrant left subclavian artery (ALSA) and diverticulum of Kommerell (DOK) account for 60–80% of VR. Patients who were antenatally diagnosed as VRs have a bias in the incidence for obvious reasons. Several studies demonstrated that VRs might remain asymptomatic for the initial few years.[11,12]

EMBRYOLOGY

Truncus arteriosus forms the proximal part of great arteries. Truncus arteriosus connects the ventricle (heart) to aortic sac. The development of pharyngeal arches occurs around the fourth-fifth gestational week. The aortic arches are within pharyngeal arches and ultimately terminate as right and left dorsal aorta. In the proximal region, the dorsal aortas are in a pair, whereas distally they fuse to form a single vessel. The aortic sac provides arteries to each pharyngeal arch from cranial to caudal. Therefore, all arches do not form simultaneously.

The first aortic arch that disappears by Day 27 of life forms a small portion of the maxillary artery. The second aortic arch forms hyoid and stapedial arteries. Third, fourth, and sixth

TABLE 1: Derivative of primitive aortic arches.

Arches	*Left*	*Right*
Third	Common carotid artery (CCA)	CCA
Fourth	Arch of aorta [between left CCA and left subclavian artery (SA)]	Most proximal segment of right SA
Fifth	Regresses	Regresses
Sixth (proximal)	Proximal left pulmonary artery	Proximal right pulmonary artery
Sixth (distal)	Ductus arteriosus	Regresses
Dorsal aortae	Persist to form descending aorta	Regresses from seventh intersegmental artery till junction of left dorsal aortae
Aortic sac	(Left horn) proximal arch	(Right horn)—right brachiocephalic artery

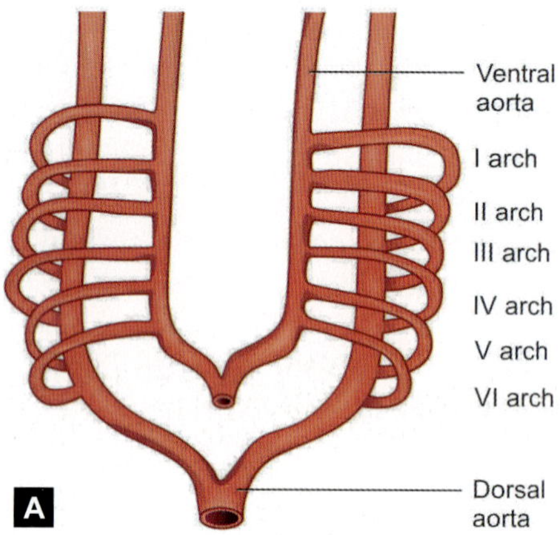

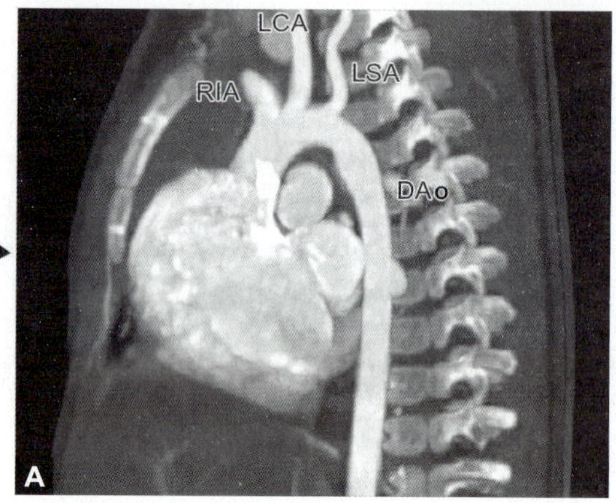

Figs. 1A and B: Normal embryology of aortic arch.
(DAo: descending aorta; LCA: left carotid artery; LSA: left subclavian artery; RIA: right innominate artery)

aortic arches persist and soon lose their symmetric form. Fifth aortic arch is often not formed or regresses soon after its formation without its remnants.[13,14] The outcome of various arches is discussed in **Table 1** (**Fig. 1**).

HYPOTHETICAL DOUBLE ARCH MODEL OF EDWARD

Vascular rings are an outcome of the abnormal derivative of embryological aortic arches. Jesse Edwards, in 1948, proposed a hypothetical DAA model that encircles the trachea and esophagus.[15] The DAA model described will eventually transform into its derivatives or regresses. Almost all kinds of VRs can be described based on this model. The VR is the eventuality of abnormal regression or persistence of arch that should have usually disappeared. However, this model does not discuss slings. In this chapter, the embryological basis of various VRs is described in Edward's model (**Fig. 2**).

GENETIC ASSOCIATION

22q11.2 is the most common deletion known with an incidence of 1 in 4,000–5,000 live births. It has 70–80% association with congenital heart defects (CHDs). Chromosome 22q11 microdeletion is commonly associated with VRs as shown by several series. A study by McElhenny showed 24% of patients with this chromosomal anomaly had a defect of the aortic arch with the maximum occurrence of DAA or RAA with ALSA. Genetic testing should be performed during the antenatal period when a VR is suspected. The incidence of antenatal positive genetic testing varies between 8 and 25% in various studies. Multiple studies have demonstrated that the association of intracardiac anomaly with abnormal aortic arch has a higher incidence of microdeletion. CHDs commonly associated with 22q11 deletion are truncus arteriosus, interrupted aortic arch, tetralogy of Fallot (TOF), and conotruncal ventricular septal defect (VSD). The genes responsible for CHD manifestations are TBX1, CRKL, and ERK2 gene. 6–10% are familial and inherited from parents.[16-18]

The PHACE (posterior fossa brain malformations, hemangioma, arterial lesions, cardiac abnormalities, and eye abnormalities) syndrome, which has 90% association with CHD, can also have an aortic arch anomaly. Notably associated anomalies are RAA, DAA, or cervical aortic arch. Extracardiac anomalies include posterior fossa malformation, hemangiomas, and eye anomalies.[19]

CLINICAL PRESENTATION

Symptomatology in the isolated VR is quite heterogeneous. Variable degree of breathlessness, stridor, wheezing

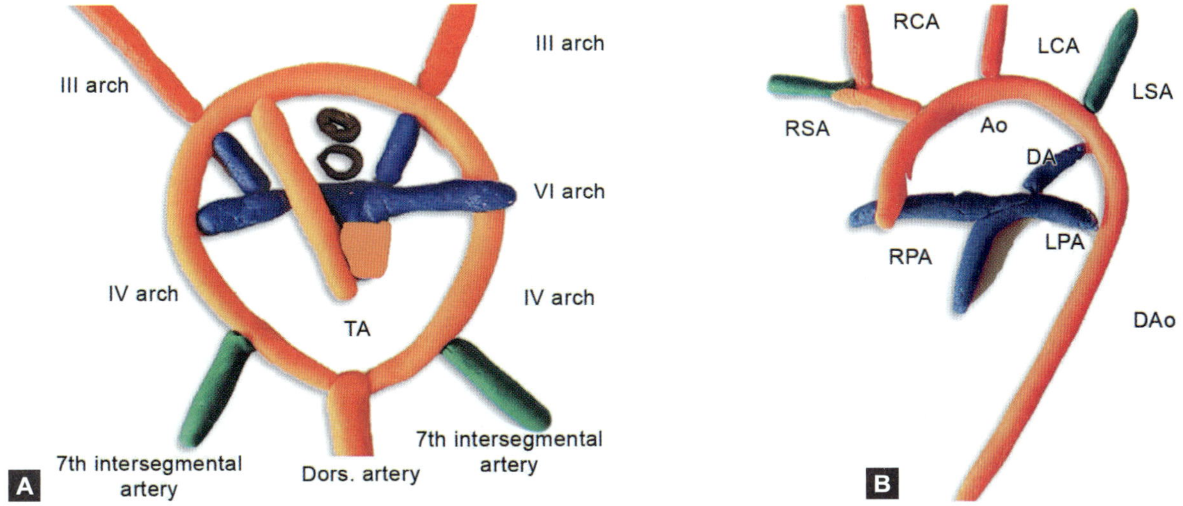

Figs. 2A and B: Edward model. Color coding for various arches and its outcome: Orange: IV aortic arch and dorsal aorta; Red: III aortic arch; Blue: VIth aortic arch; Green: seventh intersegmental artery; Brown: trachea and esophagus.

(Ao: aorta; DA: ductus arteriosus; DAo: descending aorta; Dors: dorsal; LCA: left carotid artery; LPA: left pulmonary artery; LSA: left subclavian artery; RCA: right carotid artery; RPA: right pulmonary artery; RSA: right subclavian artery; TA: truncus arteriosus)

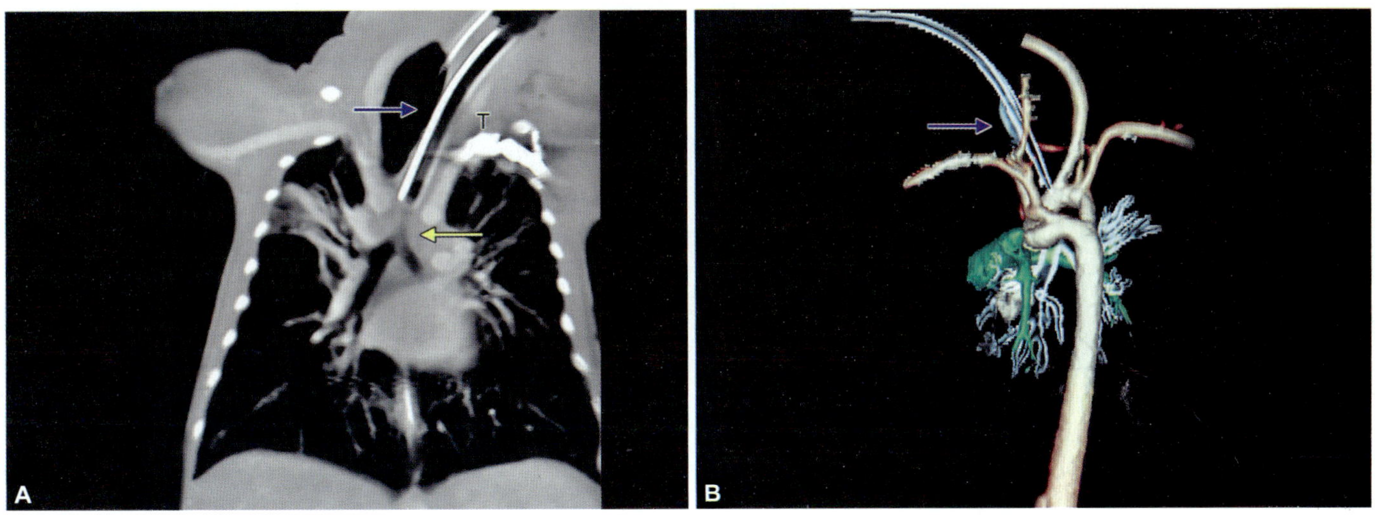

Figs. 3A and B: Double aortic arch in a newborn; 3 days old baby came with severe respiratory distress, difficult intubation. Preintubation arterial blood gas (ABG) showed PCO_2 180 mm Hg, PO_2 58 mm Hg, and pH of 7.009. After intubation PCO_2 109 mm Hg, PO_2 107 mm Hg, and pH of 7.29. (A) Computed tomography (CT) scan suggests severe tracheal stenosis distal to endotracheal (ET) tube; (B) Strenuous to cross ET tube beyond tracheal obstruction showed by 3D volume rendered CT image.

(Blue arrow: ET tube; yellow arrow: site of obstruction in trachea; T: trachea)

episodes, and feeding difficulty is encountered in the young. Among respiratory symptoms, stridor is predominant. The tighter the ring, the earlier are the symptoms. A DAA can lead to severe respiratory compromise and may require intubation in the neonatal period. Intubation is often challenging as the required endotracheal tube size may not cross the stenotic segment of the trachea and often an undersized endotracheal tube is needed. Blood gas during respiratory failure is marked by severe hypercarbia and borderline hypoxia. Unidentified, this situation can lead to significant mortality. It can cause life-threatening events that parents often describe as a choking episode (**Figs. 3A and B**).

In children, VR can also present as recurrent respiratory tract infection with wheezing episodes due to aspiration. Infant, therefore, suffer from failure to thrive and repeated admissions due to persistent and/or repeated pneumonia. Stridor may or may not be seen during this phase. A high degree of suspicion is needed for VR when patients present with recurrent wheezing episodes. Baker et al. found out that 74% cases of VR are symptomatic, but often diagnosis is delayed until 1–84 months.[20-24]

Another type of presentation is dysphagia and gastric regurgitations. Tighter rings, like a DAA, can have coexisting symptoms of stridor and dysphagia. Right circumflex aorta can lead to isolated dysphagia due to predominant esophageal compression. The RAA with ALSA may remain asymptomatic but may develop dysphagia typically to solid food. Shah et al. showed in their study that 47% of patients with symptomatic VR have esophageal symptoms in the form of dysphagia, whereas 94% have predominantly respiratory symptoms.[3,25-28]

Vascular ring may remain undiagnosed till adulthood, and patients are often treated such as asthma, bronchitis, and unspecified respiratory ailments or rarely dysphagia.[11] Age-related changes in compliance of thoracic aorta and progressive increase in vascular resistance may lead to adult onset of symptoms in VR. RAA and ALSA are the most common VRs (56%) that may remain asymptomatic due to lighter ring formation.[11,12] Although the DAA presents with acute respiratory symptoms soon after birth, literature review showed that DAA can rarely survive till adult life.[28] This bias might be due to the overall more incidence of these two types of VRs than the other types. Diverticulum of Kommerell remains at risk of developing dissection in adulthood owing to systemic hypertension.

CERTAIN RULES OF VASCULAR RING

- Ductus or ligament arteriosum should be on the contralateral side of the aortic arch.
- The aberrant vessel is contralateral to the aortic arch.
- Descending aorta contralateral to the aortic arch.
- 3 Ds (dimple, diverticulum, and descending aorta) contralateral to arch.

ANATOMICAL SUBTYPES OF VASCULAR RINGS (TABLE 2)

Double Aortic Arch

Embrylogically, persistence of both right and left fourth aortic arches with patency of distal dorsal aorta leads to the formation of a double arch (**Fig. 4**). Hence, it is one of the most malignant from of VR. DAA is the most common symptomatic VR, accounting for 40–55%. A DAA is defined as the persistence of both right and left arches, which might be either patent or atretic.

It is subdivided into the following:
- Both arches widely patent
- Hypoplasia of one arch (usually left, rarely right)
- Atresia of one arch.

TABLE 2: List of complete and incomplete vascular rings.

Complete vascular ring	Double aortic ach RAA with ALSA RAA ALSA DOK Right circumflex aorta Left circumflex aorta with right ductus Left arch ALSA DOK right ductus
Incomplete vascular ring	Vascular slings Left arch ARSA left duct Innominate artery compression syndrome

(ALSA: aberrant left subclavian artery; ARSA: aberrant right subclavian artery; DOK: diverticulum of Kommerell; RAA: right-sided aortic arch)

In DAA, the branching pattern is characteristically different from a normal branching pattern. There is no brachiocephalic artery; instead, each aortic arch gives symmetrical two neck vessels. The left aortic arch gives the left carotid and subclavian artery. The RAA gives the right carotid and subclavian artery. Usually, the RAA is dominant in 75–80% of cases and crosses behind the trachea to join the left side of descending aorta.[29,30] The second variation is the unequal sizes of aortic arches. Commonly left aortic arch is hypoplastic, and the RAA is dominant (70–80%) (**Figs. 5A to D**). Unobstructed flow is maintained through the dominant right arch. Neck vessel pattern is similar to the first variant. Rarely distal or proximal segment of each aortic arch can be atretic (**Figs. 6A to C**). Mirror image branching pattern is seen when left aortic arch distal to LSA is atretic. When proximal left arch is atretic, it gives impression of RAA with ALSA.[31] Sometimes, DAA may be associated with conotruncal anomalies such as TOF, VSD, and rarely truncus arteriosus (**Figs. 7A to E**).

Double aortic arch is always symptomatic sooner or later. According to a single large series of 81 patients, the median age of presentation was 5 months. They become symptomatic early due to formation of the tight ring with patent large vascular structures. Predominant respiratory symptoms of stridor, breathing difficulty are noticed in neonatal age. They may rarely present with wheezing episodes at a later stage. Choking episodes are noticed in 46% of cases.[24]

Investigations

Chest X-ray: Chest X-ray provides a subtle clue of the indentation of the trachea from both the right and left sides. Usually, the right indentation is superior to left as the right arch is superior (**Figs. 7A to E**).

Barium swallow: Barium swallow is an obsolete test but, if done, would show classic reverse S-shaped indentation in frontal view and posterior indentation in lateral view.

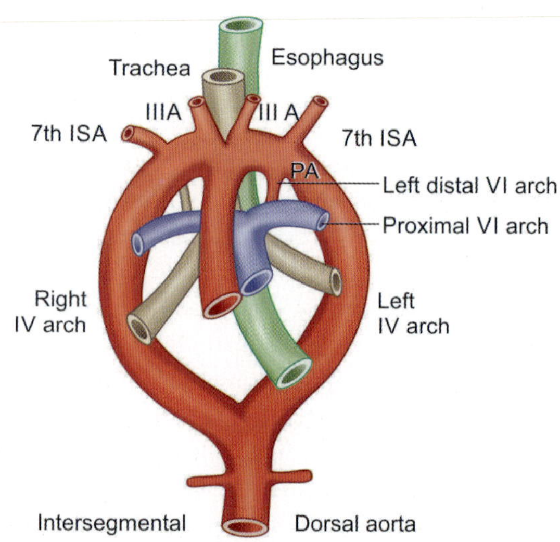

Fig. 4: Embryology of double arch.
(ISA: intersegmenta artery; PA: pulmonary artery)

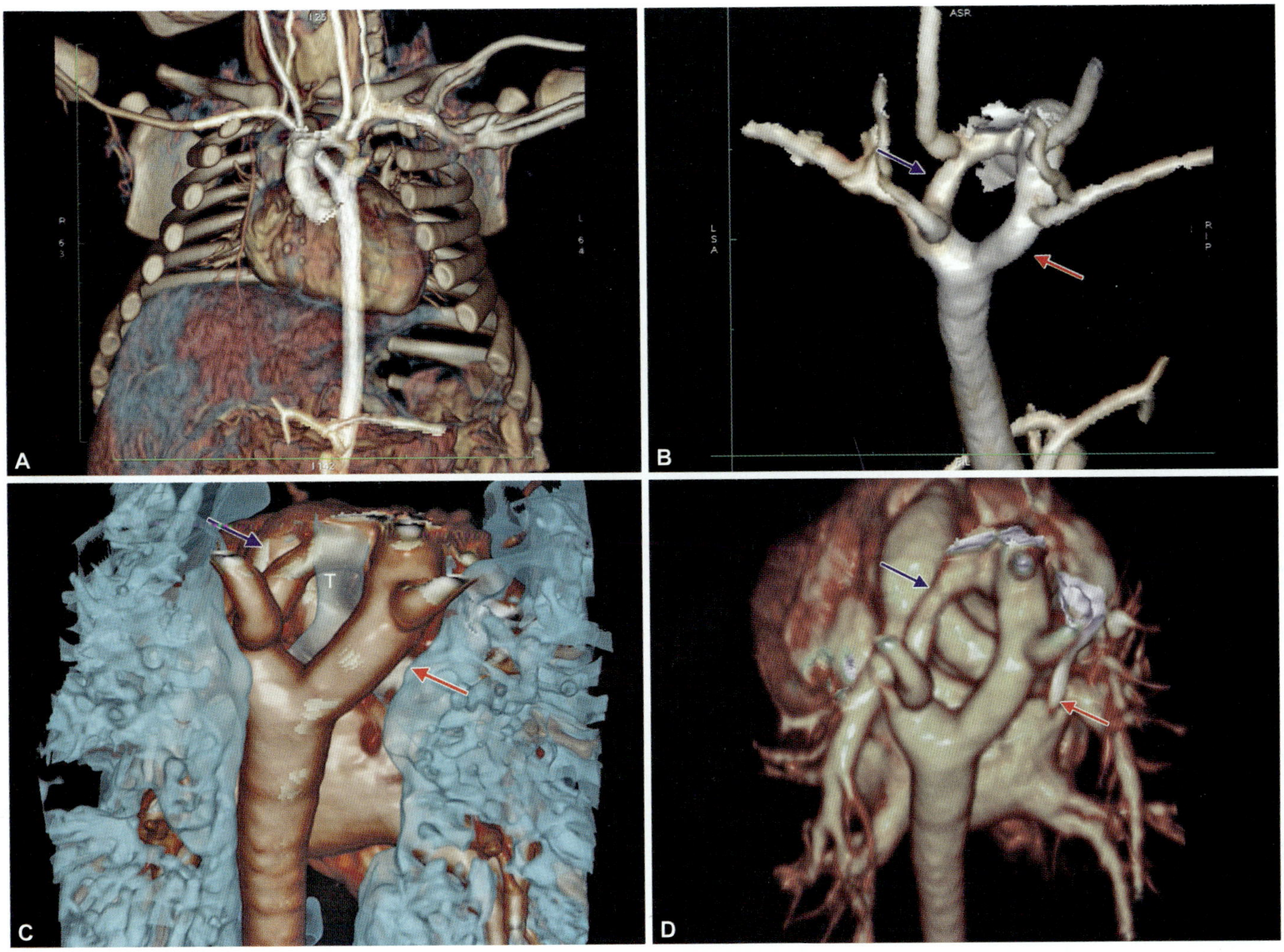

Figs. 5A to D: Double aortic arch computed tomography (CT) images. (A) CT angiogram of double aortic arch child who was diagnosed during fetal life shows two arches within thorax and descending aorta (DAo) on the left side; (B) Three-dimensional (3D) reconstruction of same baby showing double arch with each arch giving two neck vessels; (C) A ring formation (between left and right arch around trachea due two double arch; (D) Left aortic arch smaller than right.

(Blue arrow: left arch; red arrow: right arch; T: trachea)

Transthoracic echocardiogram is a useful bedside equipment to suspect DAA. In an experienced hand, it can diagnose both aortic arches in different planes, encircling trachea. Cardiologists must always evaluate for VR in clinically suspected cases. It can also show associated CHD to plan the type of surgery.

Computed tomography angiogram with contrast study or MRI angiogram is the gold standard for diagnosing DAA. They can easily demonstrate both the arches with 3D reconstruction to confirm the diagnosis. An additional advantage of CT and MRI is to demonstrate the dominant arch and sidedness of descending aorta. Virtual bronchoscopy on CT scan is useful to identify the level and degree of tracheal compression. The level of esophageal compression can also be seen. However, both these modalities cannot image the atretic segment fibrous cord part of DAA in type C variety. Subtle clues such as the symmetric appearance of the carotid and subclavian artery around the trachea or presence of DOK can help in differentiating between double arch (with atretic segment) and RAA with mirror image branching pattern.[31-33]

Often a patient undergoing an angiogram for the intracardiac defect can also reveal DAA. Nevertheless, noninvasive techniques such as CT scan and MRI have almost avoided the need for angiograms.

Treatment

Surgical division of nondominant aortic arch to relive the ring is the treatment of choice. It should be performed as soon as the diagnosis is established (*see* **Figs. 7A to E**). CT scan or MRI is mandatory prior to surgery to decide the segment of the division. The surgical approach is usually through thoracotomy in isolated cases and sternotomy if intracardiac defect needs to be repaired simultaneously. Various studies have showed excellent outcomes with a mortality of <2%. Postsurgery symptoms are relieved and patients tend to have normal life expectancy.[34,35]

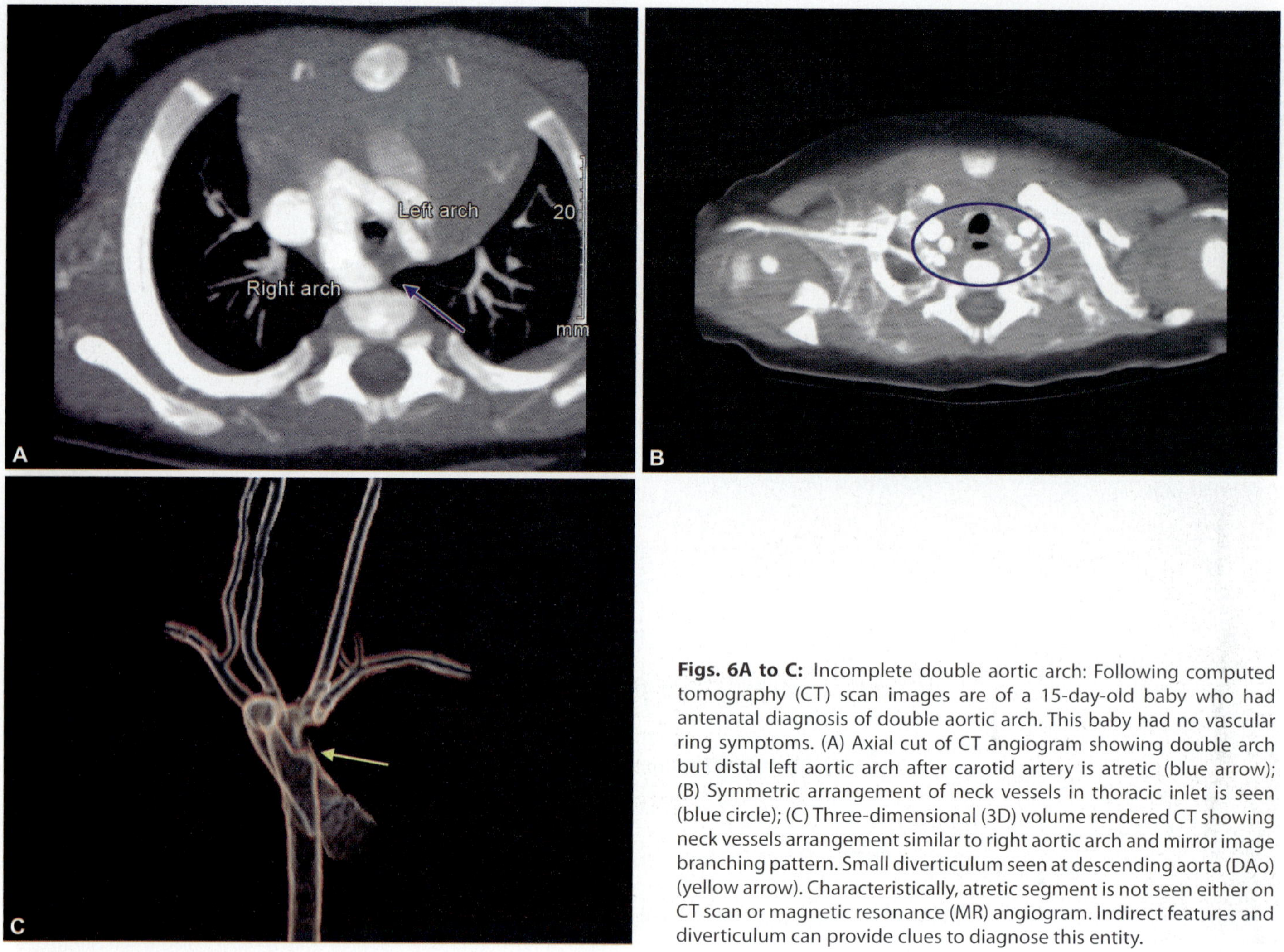

Figs. 6A to C: Incomplete double aortic arch: Following computed tomography (CT) scan images are of a 15-day-old baby who had antenatal diagnosis of double aortic arch. This baby had no vascular ring symptoms. (A) Axial cut of CT angiogram showing double arch but distal left aortic arch after carotid artery is atretic (blue arrow); (B) Symmetric arrangement of neck vessels in thoracic inlet is seen (blue circle); (C) Three-dimensional (3D) volume rendered CT showing neck vessels arrangement similar to right aortic arch and mirror image branching pattern. Small diverticulum seen at descending aorta (DAo) (yellow arrow). Characteristically, atretic segment is not seen either on CT scan or magnetic resonance (MR) angiogram. Indirect features and diverticulum can provide clues to diagnose this entity.

Right Aortic Arch

There are four subvarieties of RAA are as follows:

1. RAA with mirror image branching pattern
2. RAA with ALSA
3. RAA with ALSA and DOK
4. RAA with aberrant left brachiocephalic artery.

Except RAA and mirror-image branching, all other subtypes can form VR. These lesions can be associated with a tracheoesophageal fistula.

Right Aortic Arch with Mirror Image Type

This is an anomaly where aortic arch passes on the right main bronchus, and the branching pattern is mirror image of a left aortic arch. This means the first neck vessel, from left to right, is left brachiocephalic artery, right carotid artery, and right subclavian artery. This is usually associated with conotruncal anomalies such as TOF, truncus arteriosus, and VSD pulmonary atresia or as a part of situs inversus dextrocardia. This does not form a complete VR, as no vascular structure is retrotracheal. This type of vascular anomaly does not need treatment.

Right Aortic Arch with Aberrant Left Subclavian Artery with or without Diverticulum of Kommerell[36]

Right aortic arch with retroesophageal ALSA and left DA and RAA and retroesophageal ALSA with DOK are most prevalent forms of VR. In this setting, the aortic arch passes on the right main bronchus, but the branching pattern is different. The order of the origin of vessels is left carotid artery, right carotid artery, right subclavian artery, and LSA as the last vessel. The aberrant LSA travels retroesophageal and produces compression. Aortic arch on the right, ALSA retroesophageal, and ligament arteriosus on the left complete the VR. In our experience, isolated RAA always form VR most possibly due to ALSA.

Embryologically, RAA is seen due to the persistence of the right fourth aortic arch and regression of the left fourth arch (**Figs. 8A and B**). Part of the left dorsal aorta that comes in proximity to the subclavian artery forms the LSA. By this etiology, the subclavian artery does not connect to the brachiocephalic artery and becomes the last vessel of the aortic arch. Right dorsal aorta forms the thoracic aorta.

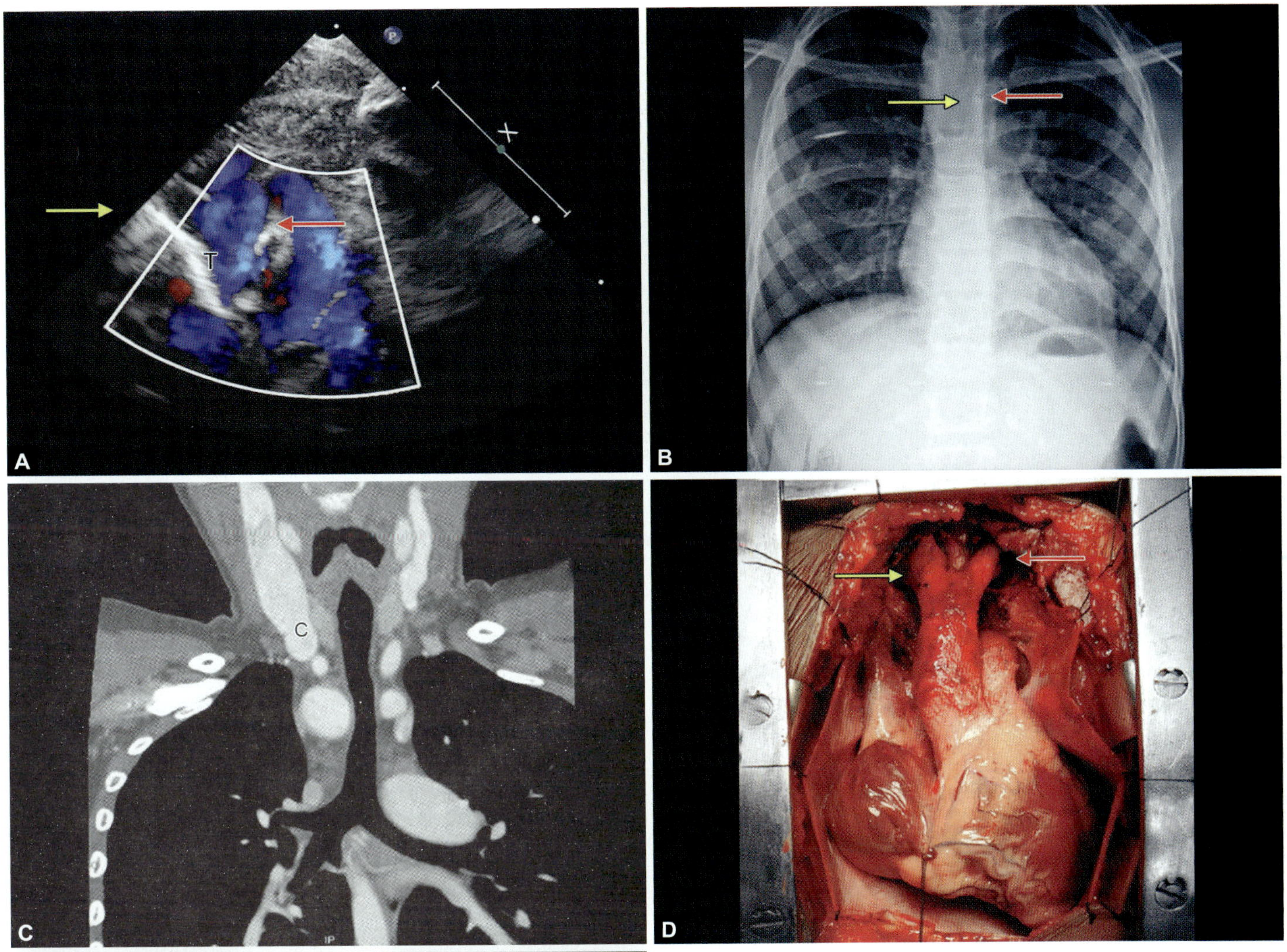

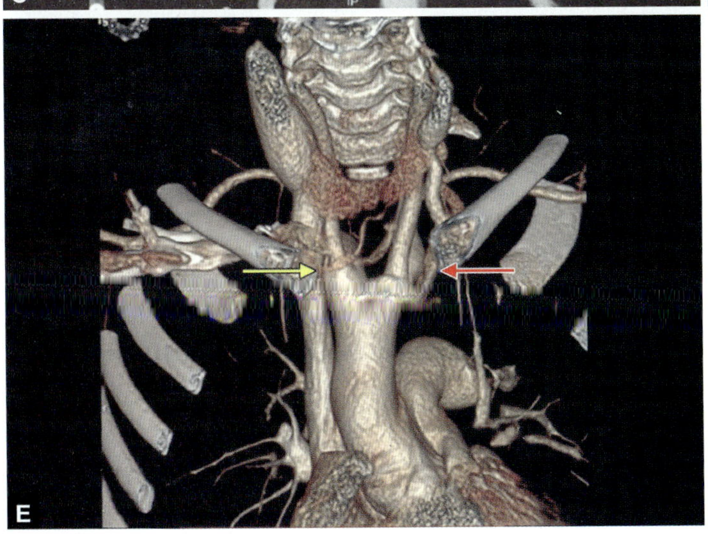

Figs. 7A to E: This is an 8 year-patient of tetralogy of Fallot with double aortic arch. This patient had no vascular ring symptoms and double arch was detected during echocardiographic scanning. (A) Echocardiography image showing left and right aortic arch around trachea; (B) Chest X-ray showing indentation around trachea due to bilateral arches; (C) Computed tomography (CT) scan comparison of chest X-ray showing tracheal indentation; (D) Intraoperative image of double aortic arch; (E) CT scan depiction mimicking intraoperative image.

(Yellow arrow: right arch; red arrow: left arch; T: trachea).

If this is associated with patency of left sixth arch (future DA), this anomaly would turn into the vascular anomaly. Also, left dorsal aorta, therefore, connects with the left sixth arch. Normal DA during fetal life carries significant RV cardiac output that would cause dilation of the left dorsal aorta. Hence, the proximal part of the subclavian artery (left dorsal aorta) becomes aneurysmal and referred to as the DOK (**Fig. 8**).

Clinical features and investigations: Our experience and review of the literature show that this form of the VR may remain asymptomatic as it forms a loose ring. Most of these patients, when symptomatic, have a variable degree of

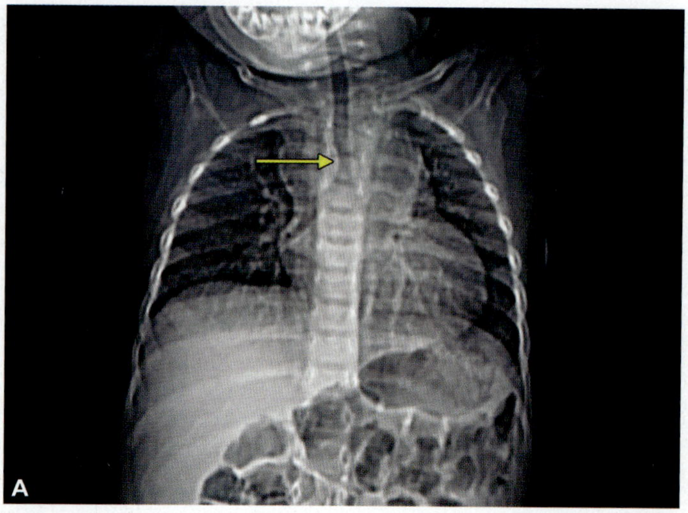

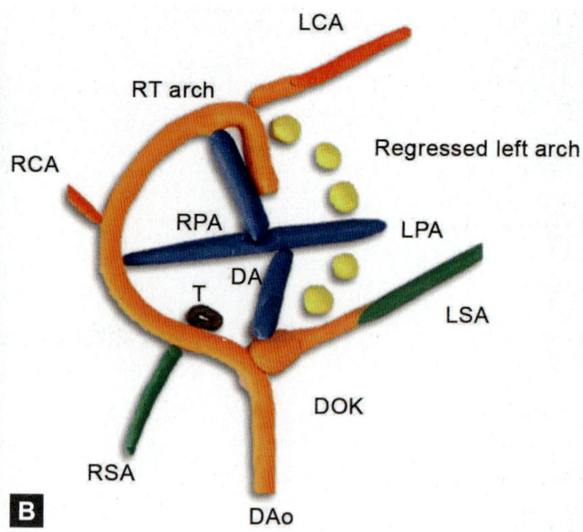

Figs. 8A and B: (A) Chest X-ray of right aortic arch infant. Indentation on right side of trachea is seen (yellow arrow); (B) Embryology of right aortic arch and diverticulum of Kommerell. (Color coding as shown in Figure 2).

(DA: ductus arteriosus; DAo: descending aorta; DOK: diverticulum of Kommerell LCA: left carotid artery; LPA: left pulmonary artery; LSA: left subclavian artery; RCA: right carotid artery; RPA: right pulmonary artery; RSA: right subclavian artery; T: trachea)

respiratory symptoms.[24] At our center, 35 consecutive cases of fetal VRs were evaluated. 80% of the fetus had RAA with ALSA with or without DOK. They remained asymptomatic in infancy and early childhood. Dysphagia is predominantly seen when solid food is introduced in the young.

Chest X-ray is the first test that provides a subtle clue about the indentation of the trachea on the right side (**Figs. 8A and B**). Echocardiogram is an easily accessible tool that can accurately pick up RAA. ALSA is suspected either by direct visualization or indirectly when the first neck vessel on the left fails to bifurcate. CT angiogram or MRI angiogram is the gold standard test and also provides information about tracheal and esophageal compression (**Figs. 9 and 10**). Barium swallow, if performed, shows posterior indentation on the lateral view and right indentation on the frontal view.

Treatment: Symptomatic patients must undergo a VR division. It is done by ligation and division of ligament arteriosus. This surgery can be performed through a lateral thoracotomy and has an excellent prognosis **(Figs. 11A and B)**. Some authors advise surgical resection of DOK and reimplantation of the subclavian artery to prevent the occurrence of symptoms. Surgical results are excellent, with a mortality of <1%.[20]

Right Aortic Arch with Aberrant Left Brachiocephalic Artery and Left Ductus Arteriosus

This anomaly is more or less similar to RAA with ALSA. Instead of ALSA, the left brachiocephalic artery is retroesophageal and is the last vessel to arise from the aortic arch. So, the order of neck vessels is the right carotid artery, right subclavian artery, and left brachiocephalic artery. A complete ring is formed by the aortic arch on the right side, the brachiocephalic artery posterior to the esophagus, and DA on the left side.

This condition can be suspected or diagnosed by echocardiogram and confirmed on CT angiogram/MRI (**Fig. 12**). Treatment is surgical where the brachiocephalic artery is relocated anterior to trachea, and ligament (or ductus) is divided.

RAA with Left Descending Aorta and Left Ductus Arteriosus (Right Circumflex Aorta)

This anomaly is rare than other forms of the RAA. Usually, the right arch has the right descent of thoracic aorta, and then it crosses to the left side after T4-T5 vertebrae. However, in the circumflex aorta, the distal aortic arch itself crosses to left before T4, T5 vertebra, and hence arch of the aorta itself becomes retrotracheal. The ring is completed with left-sided DA, aortic arch retroesophageal, and on the right side. Often LSA arises aberrantly as the last vessel.

This anomaly happens when the right dorsal aorta migrates leftward and posteriorly and left dorsal aorta regresses like in RAA. Another hypothesis is that the left dorsal aorta persists and right regresses leading to the left seventh intersegmental artery to originate from the proximal descending aorta. This forms an ALSA. Persistence of left sixth aortic arch forms left DA.

Clinical Features and Investigations

Symptoms are related to the VR. In contrast to RAA with ALSA, this vascular anomaly becomes symptomatic soon after birth as a large vessel of arch compresses the esophagus and trachea. We have observed that dysphagia is more common than respiratory symptoms. This might be due to the muscular esophagus being easily compressible than trachea, which is rigid due to the presence of cartilaginous tracheal rings.

Chest X-ray shows indentation on the trachea on the right side. Echocardiography is a crucial first tool to diagnose

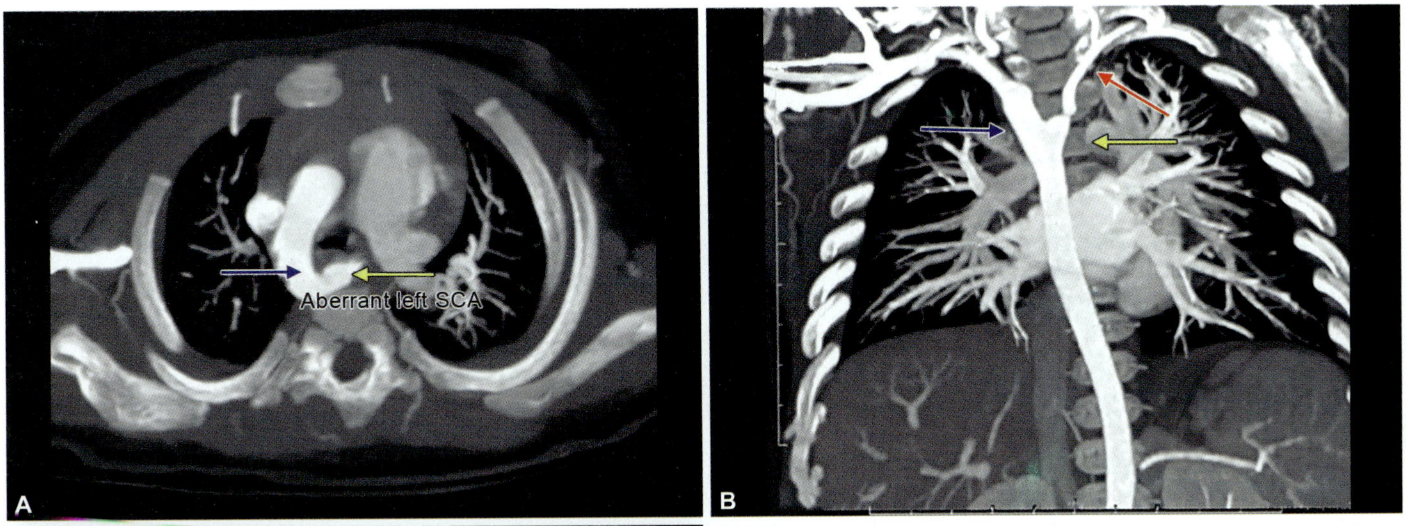

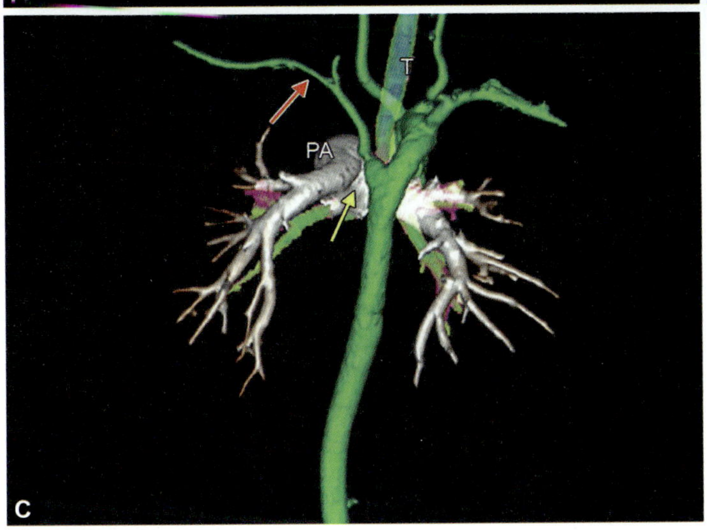

Figs. 9A to C: Right aortic arch with aberrant left subclavian artery: Images of 1-year-old boy who had antenatal diagnosis. He had dysphagia to solid foods. (A) Computed tomography (CT) angiogram showing right aortic arch (blue arrow) and diverticulum of Kommerell (DOK) (yellow arrow); (B) Coronal plain of CT angiogram showing right aortic arch, right descent, DOK, and aberrant left subclavian artery (ALSA) (red arrow); (C) Three-dimensional (3D) volume rendered CT angiogram, showing right aortic arch (RAA) DOK with ALSA. Vascular ring around trachea is seen.
(PA: pulmonary artery; T: trachea)

the RAA and locate its branching pattern. All suspected cases must undergo a CT angiogram, which is diagnostic and clarifies anatomy. It shows that aortic arch crosses the midline above the T4 level to become retrotracheal (**Figs. 13A to D**).

Treatment

All cases of the right circumflex aorta must undergo surgery. Aortic arch translocation and ligament division is the surgery of choice to relieve symptoms completely. The aortic arch is relocated anterior to the trachea to relieve the compression. The surgical and long-term outcome is good.[37,38]

Rare Vascular Anomalies of the Left Aortic Arch

This can be divided into following subtypes:

- *Left aortic arch with DOK and right aberrant subclavian artery and right ductus arteriosus*: This is a rare anomaly where the ring is formed by the arch on the left side, DOK with aberrant right subclavian artery (ARSA) posterior to esophagus and DA on the right side. Symptoms and clinical presentations are like RAA counterparts. The diagnosis is confirmed by CT angiogram or MRI (**Figs. 14A and B**). Treatment is surgical division of right ligament and resection of DOK with relocation of the ARSA.
- *Left aortic arch and right retroesophageal descending aorta with right ductus arteriosus (left circumflex aorta)*: This is a mirror image of what we discussed in the right circumflex aorta. The ring is formed by a right-sided proximal arch, retroesophageal distal arch with left thoracic aorta and right-sided DA. Often right subclavian artery is aberrant. Diagnosis is suspected on echocardiography when a complete arch cannot be profiled in suprasternal view. CT angiogram or MRI confirms the diagnosis (**Fig. 15**). Surgical repositioning or keeping interposed graft between ascending and descending aorta is the treatment of choice.

*Anatomical parts that contribute to various VRs are displayed in **Table 3**.*

RARE AORTIC ARCH ANOMALY WITHOUT A VASCULAR RING

Cervical Arch

This is an aortic anomaly where the aortic arch is within the thoracic inlet or neck. Characteristically aortic pulsations are

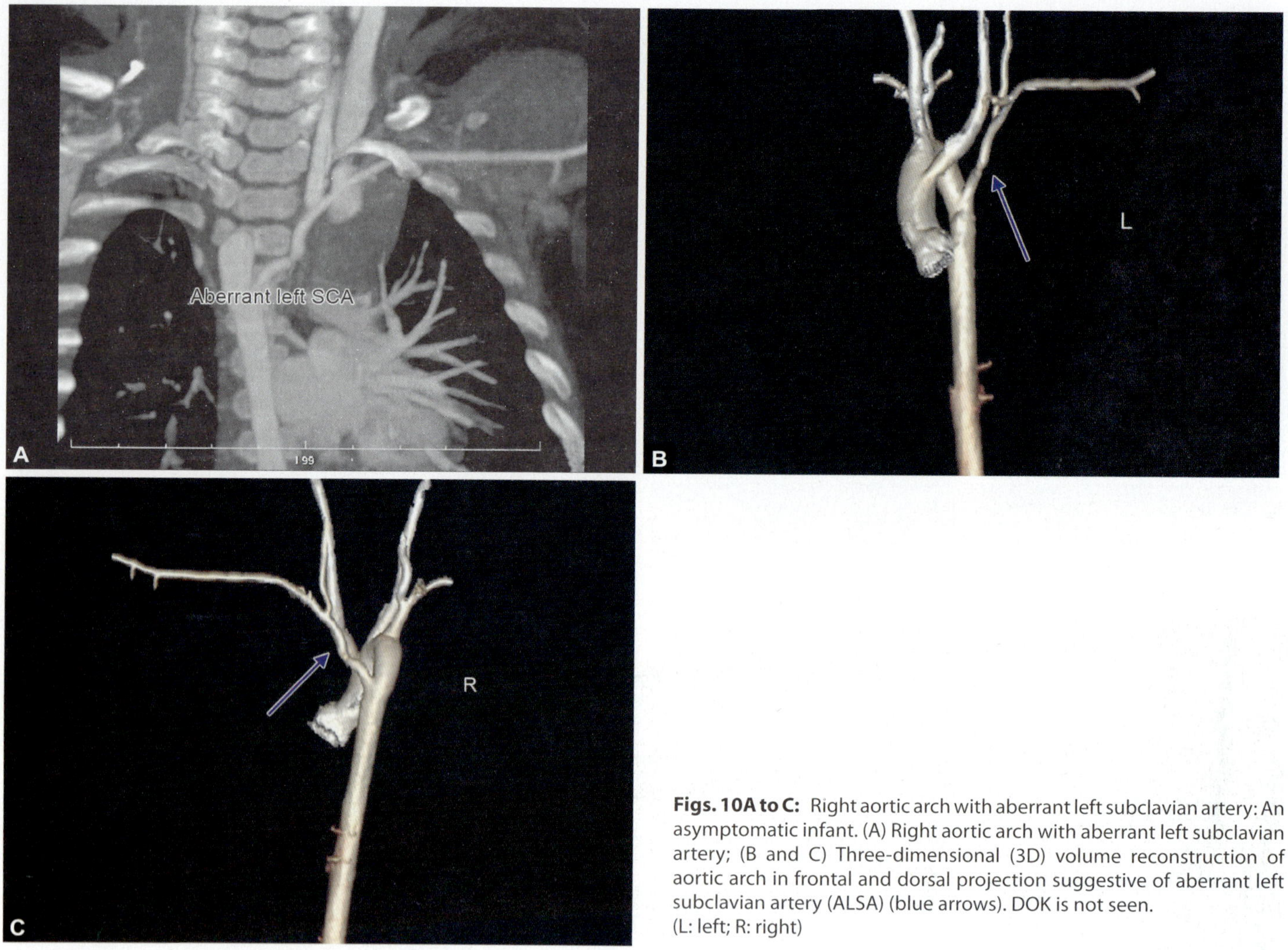

Figs. 10A to C: Right aortic arch with aberrant left subclavian artery: An asymptomatic infant. (A) Right aortic arch with aberrant left subclavian artery; (B and C) Three-dimensional (3D) volume reconstruction of aortic arch in frontal and dorsal projection suggestive of aberrant left subclavian artery (ALSA) (blue arrows). DOK is not seen.
(L: left; R: right)

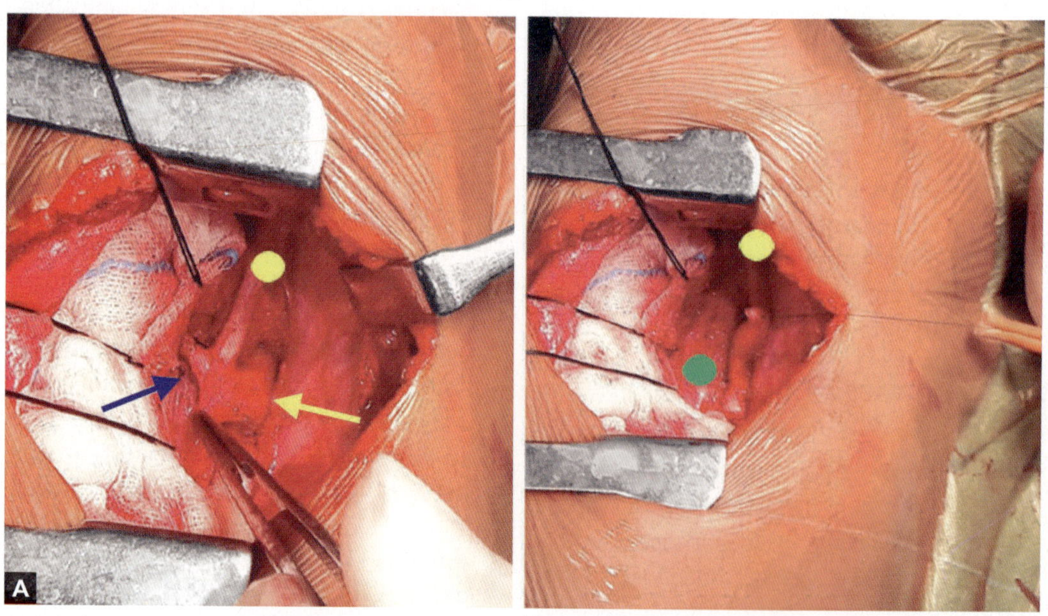

Figs. 11A and B: Intraoperative images of right aortic arch (RAA) with aberrant left subclavian artery. (A) Preoperative image through left lateral thoracotomy showing ring formation around esophagus; (B) After ligament arteriosus division and diverticulum resection, esophagus can be well visualized now as vascular ring is resected.

(Yellow circle: left subclavian artery; blue arrow: left ligament arteriosus; yellow arrow: aortic arch; green circle: esophagus)

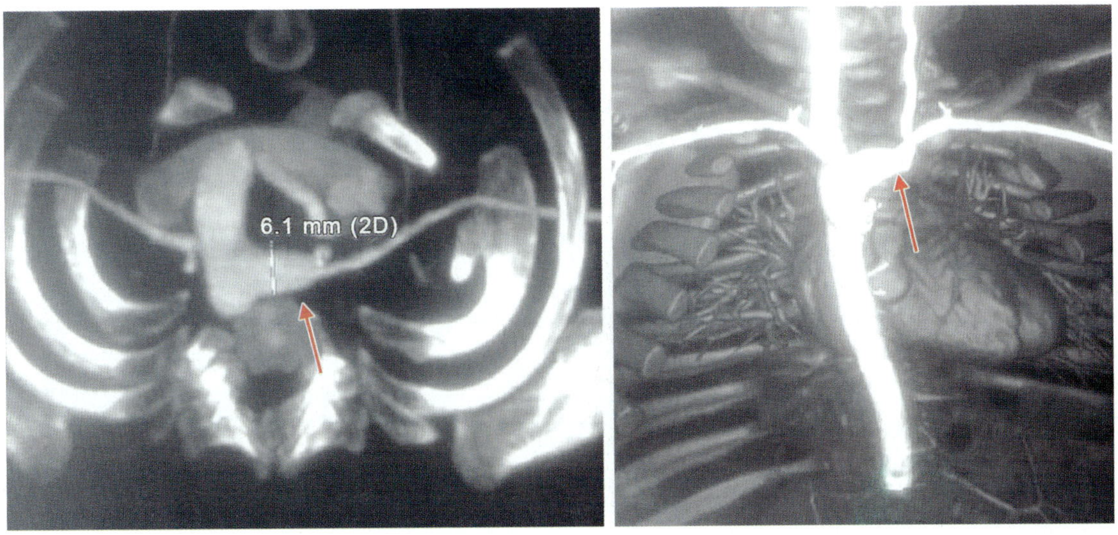

Fig. 12: Right aortic arch aberrant brachiocephalic artery (red arrows).

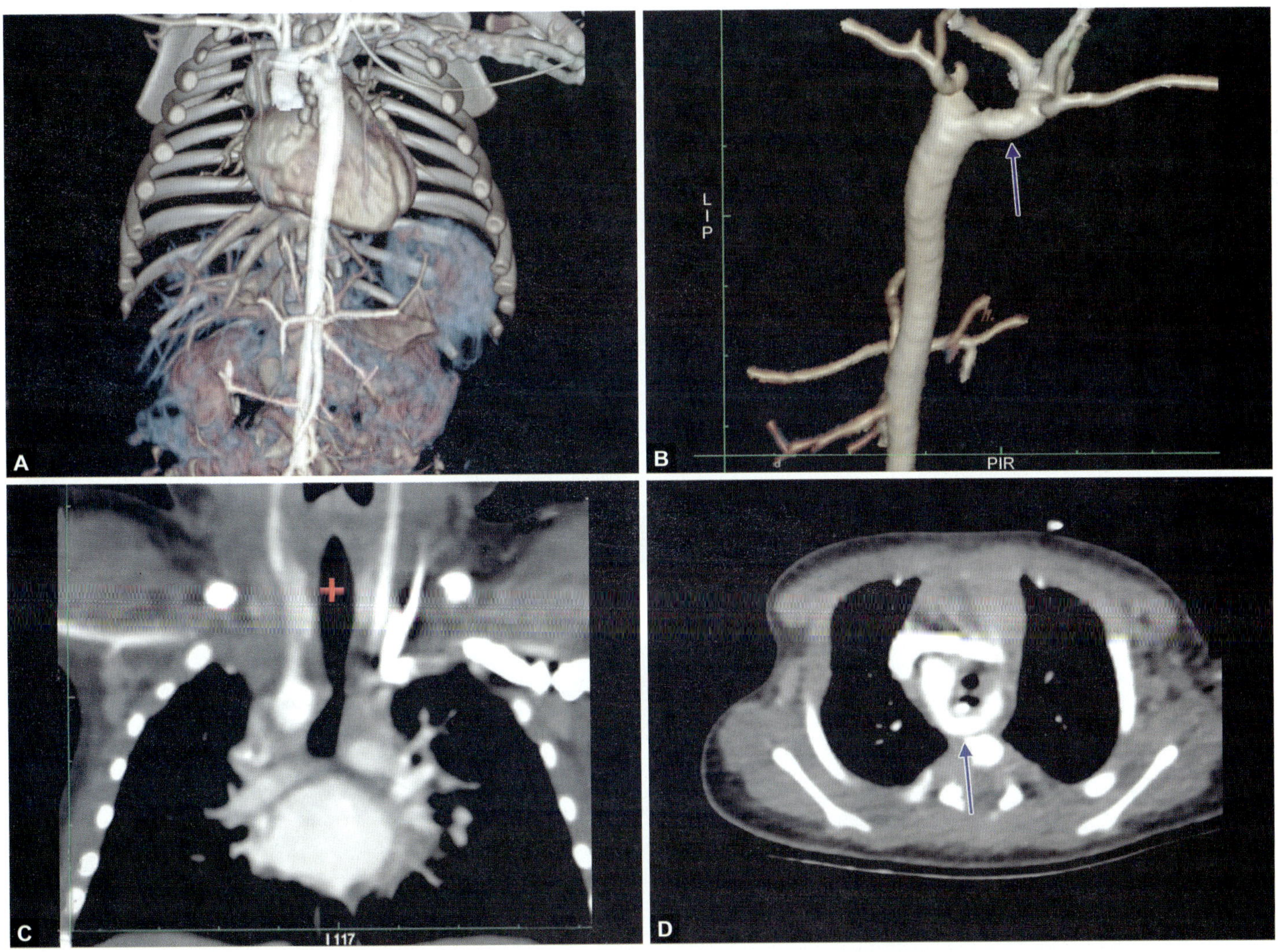

Figs. 13A to D: A newborn who had dysphagia to milk, persistent vomiting. Echocardiographic evaluation showed right aortic arch with vascular ring. Computed tomography (CT) scan showed right circumflex aorta with aberrant left subclavian artery causing severe esophageal compression. (A, B, and D) Three-dimensional (3D) volume rendered image of aortic arch showing right arch with distal transverse arch coursing retrotracheal with aberrant left subclavian artery. Aortic arch contributes to compression of esophagus; (C) Esophageal compression noticed on CT scan.

(Blue arrows: aortic arch; red plus: esophagus)

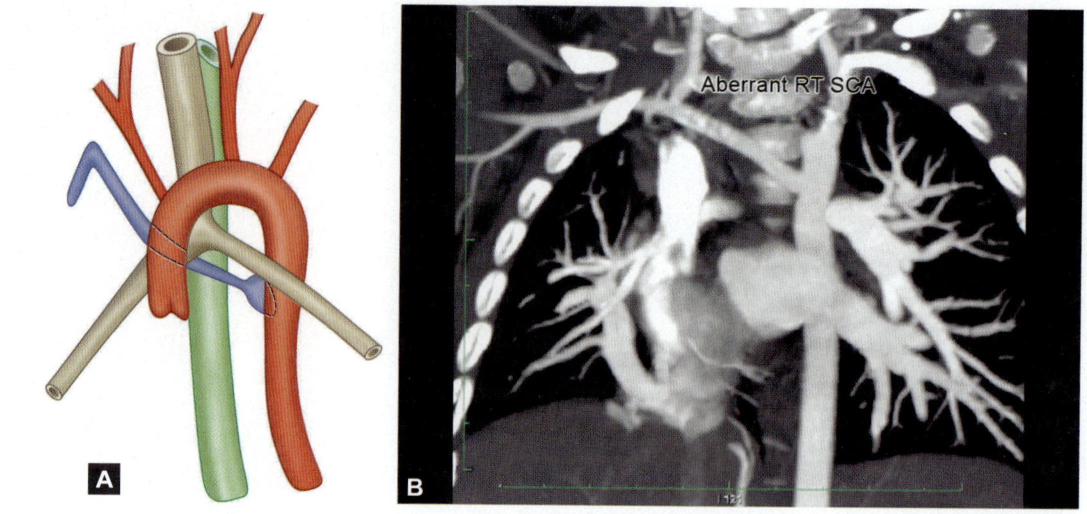

Figs. 14A and B: (A) Pictorial representation of left aortic arch with aberrant right subclavian artery (ARSA). This anomaly does not form complete vascular ring if it is associated with left ductus. (Color codes—brown: trachea; green: esophagus, pink: aorta; blue: ARSA); (B) Computed tomography (CT) scan image of left aortic arch with aberrant right subclavian artery.

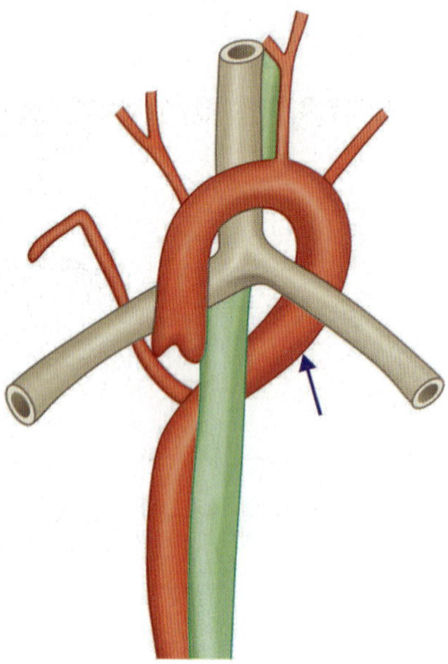

Fig. 15: Left circumflex aorta.
(Brown configuration: trachea; green: esophagus)

seen in the right or left of the neck. This lesion is due to the persistence of the third aortic arch and abnormal regression of fourth aortic arches. Without an aberrant vessel, this lesion does not form a VR. This kind of aortic arch is prone to kink and coarctation. Surgery is indicated in cases with anatomical and physiological obstruction[39] (**Figs. 16A and B**).

Isolation of the Subclavian Artery

In this anomaly, subclavian artery contralateral to aortic arch arises from the PA. Embryologically persistence of bilateral ductus leads to the continuation of the sixth distal aortic arch to the proximal sixth aortic arch. Isolated subclavian artery develops when there is regression of the ipsilateral 4th arch. The seventh intersegmental artery (which develops into the subclavian artery) is attached to the ipsilateral sixth aortic arch via the intervening portion of dorsal aorta. So the subclavian artery is discontinuous with the aorta and proximally connects to PA through DA.

TABLE 3: Anatomical parts of various vascular ring.

Types of VR	*Right*	*Left*	*Posterior*
DAA	RAA	LAA	Desc Ao and part of RAA
RAA ALSA	RAA	Ductus Art	ALSA
RAA ALSA DOK	RAA	Ductus Art	DOK and ALSA
Right circumflex Ao	RAA	Ductus Art	Distal right arch
LAA ARSA DOK	Right duct	LAA	ARSA and DOK
Left circumflex Ao	Right duct	LAA	Distal left arch
Cervical arch	RAA	Ductus Art	ALSA

(Ao: aorta; ALSA: aberrant left subclavian artery; Art: arteriosus; ARSA: aberrant right subclavian artery; DAA: double aortic arch; Desc: descending; DOK: diverticulum of Kommerell; LAA: left aortic arch; RAA: right aortic arch)

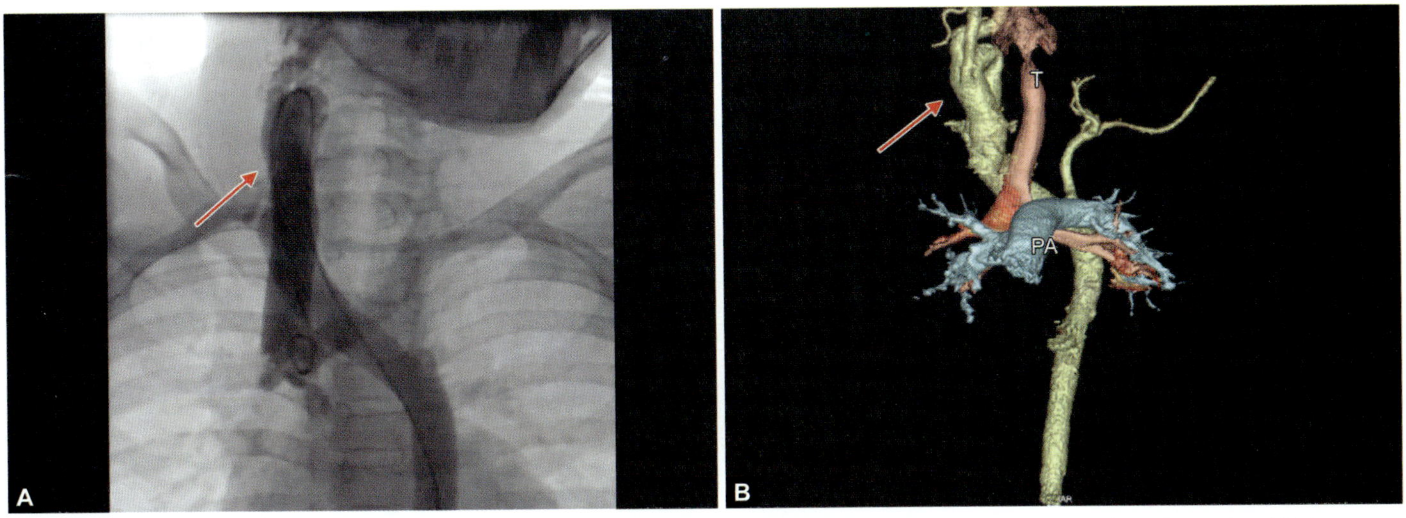

Figs. 16A and B: Cervical arch: A 9-year-old boy with dysmorphic facies complained of pulsation on right supraclavicular region. (A) Aortogram shows cervical arch (arch is seen in supraclavicular region); (B) Three-dimensional (3D) volume rendered image shows right cervical arch (red arrow) with obstruction and aberrant left subclavian artery.

(PA: pulmonary artery; T: trachea)

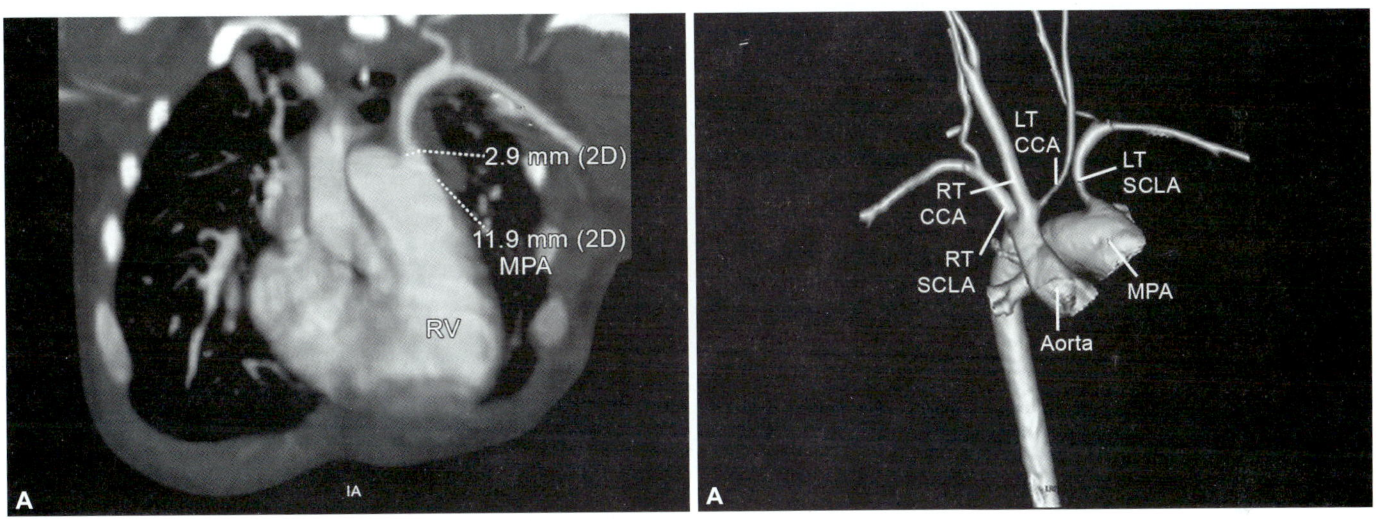

Figs. 17A and B: A 1-month-old baby who had large patent ductus arteriosus (PDA) and differential saturations in right and left arm; CT angiogram revealed isolated left subclavian artery mean its origin from pulmonary artery.

(LTCCA: left common carotid artery; LTSCLA: Left subclavian artery; MPA: main pulmonary artery; RTSCLA: right subclavian artery; RTCCA: right subclavian artery; RV: right ventricle)

In this anomaly, blood flow in the subclavian is retrograde through the vertebral artery. There is stealing of blood from the cerebral and subclavian circulation into the PA as latter is a low-pressure circuit (**Figs. 17A and B**).

Persistence of Fifth Aortic Arch

Usually, fifth aortic arch regresses soon, or it is not developed at all (**Fig. 18**). However, when it persists, it gives additional channel between ascending and descending aorta. It remains asymptomatic if not associated with a CHD. Diagnosis is confirmed by CT angiogram and MRI, which shows an additional channel inferior to the true arch. Characteristically, no neck vessel arises from this channel. Since this lesion is asymptomatic, treatment is not warranted.[40]

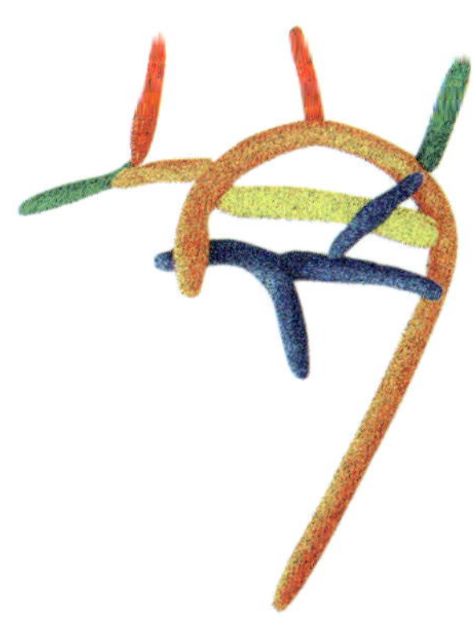

Fig. 18: Pictorial representation of persistent 5th arch. This image suggests embryologic explanation—orange: left aortic arch formed by left IV aortic arch; red: Bilateral carotid arteries formed by III aortic arch; green: Seventh intersegmental artery; yellow: V aortic arch that usually regresses; blue: VI aortic arch forming right and left pulmonary artery and left ductus arteriosus.

VASCULAR SLINGS (TABLE 4)

In this anomaly, the LPA arises from the RPA instead of the MPA and travels between the trachea and the esophagus. Therefore, the trachea is trapped anteriorly by the MPA and right and posteriorly by the LPA.[41]

Since the trachea is not entirely encircled by vascular structure, this lesion is called a sling and not a ring. This is the only compressive vascular lesion where esophageal indentation is anterior. Partial PA sling is a lesion where the LPA arises from MPA, but a branch of left PA arises from RPA and travels between trachea and esophagus. This anomaly can be associated with an intracardiac defect like TOF, VSD, and patent ductus arteriosus (PDA).

Embryology

Proximal PAs are derivatives of proximal right and left sixth aortic arch. Distal PAs develop from capillary plexus in respective lung bed. LPA sling occurs due to the failure of the connection between the left capillary plexus to the left proximal sixth arch. Instead, it gets connected to the sixth right arch through postbronchial vessels.

TABLE 4: Embryology of various vascular anomalies.

Vascular anomaly	*Embryology*
Double aortic arch	Persistent right and left fourth aortic arch
Right aortic arch with ALSA and DOK	Persistence of right fourth aortic arch and regression of left fourth arch. Part of left dorsal aorta forms ALSA. Patency of left sixth distal arch to form ductus arteriosus
Right circumflex aorta	Persistence of 4th aortic arch with migration of right dorsal aorta behind esophagus
Left circumflex aorta	Migration of left dorsal aorta rightward and behind esophagus
Cervical arch	Persistence of 3rd aortic arch and abnormal regression of 4th aortic arches
Persistent fifth aortic arch	Persistence of fifth aortic arch along with left 4th aortic arch
LPA sling	Failure of connection between capillary plexus in lung bed and left sixth proximal arch leading to abnormal coarse of LPA

(ALSA: aberrant left subclavian artery; DOK: diverticulum of Kommerell; LPA: left pulmonary artery)

Clinical Features

This anomaly leads to various respiratory ailments due to tracheal compression, such as stridor, wheezing episodes, and repeated respiratory infections. Rarely this anomaly is associated with right lung hypoplasia.

Investigations

An echocardiogram shows that LPA is not arising from the MPA. Instead, LPA can be seen originating from distal RPA. Since LPA is often elongated, it can lead to a variable degree of stenosis. CT angiogram is diagnostic and provides detailed anatomy including LPA size and stenosis if present (**Figs. 19 and 20**). Since this anomaly can have abnormal right bronchus and lungs, CT angiogram acts vital in assessing lungs and bronchi. Tracheal stenosis can also be analyzed by virtual bronchoscopy.

Treatment

The LPA is divided from RPA and anastomosed with the MPA anterior to the trachea. It is often associated with tracheal stenosis and should be repaired at the same time. This surgery is accomplished by sternotomy, unlike some of the other VRs. Morbidity is higher with a sling if tracheal stenosis is present as it tends to persist even after surgery. In our experience of 8 patients of LPA sling, tracheal stenosis was not seen, and the surgical outcome was excellent. LPA stenosis may need future stenting if it recurs after surgery.[42]

OUTCOME OF THE VASCULAR RING AFTER SURGERY

The three-dimensional (3D) reconstruction of the VR provides virtual orientation and helps in planning

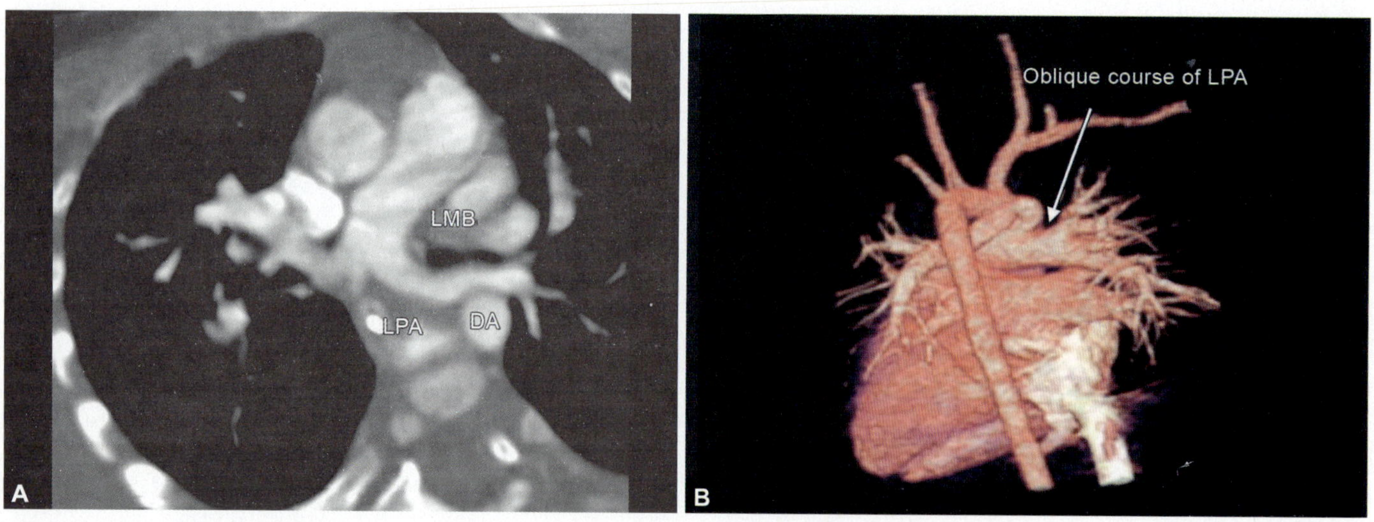

Figs. 19A and B: Pulmonary artery (PA) sling. (A) Left main pulmonary artery (LPA) coursing posterior to trachea and left main bronchus (LMB); (B) 3D construction of left pulmonary artery from right pulmonary artery [known as left pulmonary artery (LPA) sling].

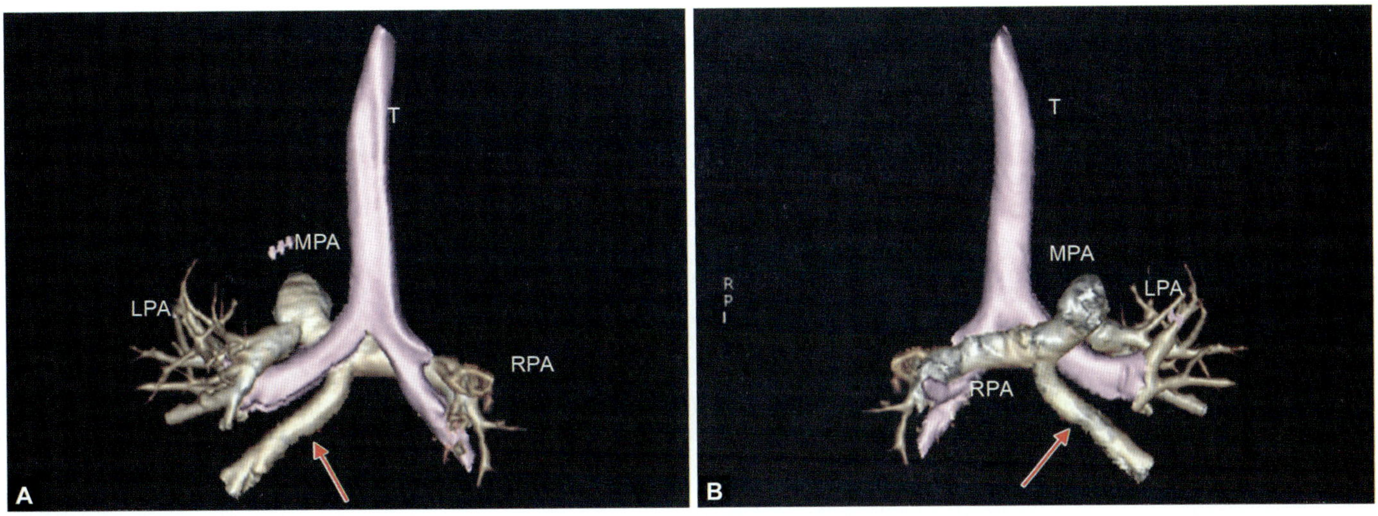

Figs. 20A and B: Partial pulmonary artery (PA) sling. (A and B) Frontal and dorsal projection of PA reveals left pulmonary artery (LPA) from main pulmonary artery (MPA) but left lower branch of LPA (red arrow) arising from RPA (right pulmonary artery). It shows left lower branch encircles left bronchus.
(T: trachea)

surgical repair. Surgical outcomes are excellent. In our experience, once surgery relieves VR, 90–95% of patients become free of aerodigestive symptoms. In instances where the concomitant trachea bronchomalacia is present, patients may have residual or recurrent symptoms. However, the degree of symptoms improves even in these cases. Woods et al. showed freedom of symptoms in 90% of cases; 10% had respiratory ailments due to tracheomalacia which persisted for 4–6 months.[2,3] This concludes that timely identification and treatment of VR is crucial and lifesaving.

REFERENCES

1. Gross RE. Surgical relief for tracheal obstruction from a vascular ring. N Engl J Med. 1945;233:586-90.
2. Woods RK, Sharp RJ, Holcomb GW 3rd, Snyder CL, Lofland GK, Ashcraft KW, et al. Vascular anomalies and tracheoesophageal compression: a single institution's 25-year experience. Ann Thorac Surg. 2001;72(2):434-8.
3. Shah RK, Mora BN, Bacha E, Sena LM, Buonomo C, Del Nido P, et al. The presentation and management of vascular rings: an otolaryngology perspective. Int J Pediatr Otorhinolaryngol. 2007;71(1):57-62.
4. Humphrey C, Duncan K, Fletcher S. Decade of experience with vascular rings at a single institution. Pediatrics. 2006;117(5): e903-8.
5. Bertolini A, Pelizza A, Panizzon G, Moretti R, Bava CL, Calza G, et al. Vascular rings and slings. Diagnosis and surgical treatment of 49 patients. J Cardiovasc Surg (Torino). 1987;28(3):301-12.
6. Hernanz-Schulman M. Vascular rings: a practical approach to imaging diagnosis. Pediatr Radiol. 2005;35(10):961-79.
7. Hellinger JC, Daubert M, Lee EY, Epelman M. Congenital thoracic vascular anomalies: evaluation with state-of-the-art MR imaging and MDCT. Radiol Clin N Am. 2011;49(5):969-96.
8. Dillman JR, Attili AK, Agarwal PP, Dorfman AL, Hernandez RJ, Strouse PJ. Common and uncommon vascular rings and slings: a multi-modality review. Pediatr Radiol. 2011;41(11): 1440-54; quiz 1489-90.
9. Edward JE. An Atlas of Acquired Diseases of the Heart and Great Vessels. Philadelphia: WB Saunders; 1961.
10. Licari A, Manca E, Rispoli GA, Mannarino S, Pelizzo G, Marseglia GL. Congenital vascular rings: a clinical challenge for the paediatrician. Pediatr Pulmonol. 2015;50(5):511-24.
11. Grathwohl WK, Affi AY, Dillard TA, Olson JP, Heric BR. Vascular rings of the thoracic aorta in adults. Am Surg. 1999;65(11): 1077-83.
12. Rohit S. Natural history of asymptomatic and unrepaired vascular ring: is watchful waiting a viable option? A new case and review of previously reported cases. Children (Basel). 2016; 3(4):44.
13. Sadler TW (Ed). Langham Medical Embryology, 12th edition. Philadelphia: Lippincott Williams and Wilkins; 2011.
14. Anderson RH, Moorman AFM, Brown NA, Bamforth SD. Normal and abnormal development of heart. London: Springer; 2013. pp. 151-77.
15. Edwards JE. Anomalies of the derivatives of the aortic arch system. Med Clin North Am. 1948;32:925-49.
16. McElhinney DB, Clark BJ 3rd, Weinberg PM, Kenton ML, McDonald-McGinn D, Driscoll DA, et al. Association of chromosome 22q11 deletion with isolated anomalies of aortic arch laterality and branching. J Am Coll Cardiol. 2001;37(8): 2114-9.
17. Momma K. Cardiovascular anomalies associated with chromosome 22q11.2 deletion syndrome. Am J Cardiol. 2010; 105(11):1617-24.
18. Weinberg PM. Aortic arch anomalies. J Cardiovasc Magn Reson. 2006;8(4):633-43.
19. Bayer ML, Frommelt PC, Blei F, Breur JM, Cordisco MR, Frieden IJ, et al. Congenital cardiac aortic arch and vascular bed anomalies in PHACE syndrome. (From International PHACE syndrome Registry). Am J Cardiol. 2013 15;112(12):1948-52.
20. Backer CL, Mavroudis C, Rigsby CKM, Holinger LD. Trends in vascular ring surgery. J Thorac Cardiovasc Surg. 2005;129(6): 1339-47.
21. Turner A, Gavel G, Coutts J. Vascular rings—presentation, investigation and outcome. Eur J Pediatr. 2005;164(5):266-70.
22. Valletta EA, Pregarz M, Bergamo-Andreis IA, Boner AL. Tracheoesophageal compression due to congenital vascular anomalies (vascular rings). Pediatr Pulmonol. 1997;24(2):93-105.
23. McLaren CA, Elliott MJ, Roebuck DJ. Vascular compression of the airway in children. Pediatr Respir Rev. 2009;9(2):85-94.
24. Alsenaidi K, Gurofsky R, Karamlou T, Williams WG, McCrindle BW, et al. Management and outcome of double aortic arch in 81 patients. Pediatrics. 2006;118(5):e1336-41.

25. Ruzmetov M, Vijay P, Rodefeld MD, Turrentine MW, Brown JW, et al. Follow up of surgical correction of aortic arch anomalies causing trachea esophageal compression: a 38-year single institution experience. J Pediatri Surg. 2009;44(7):1328-32.
26. Fernandez-Valls M, Arnaiz J, Lui D, Arnaiz-Garcia ME, Canga A, Martin-Duran R. Double aortic arch presents with dysphagia as initial symptom. J Am Coll Cardiol 2012;60(12):1114.
27. Ochi N, Yasugi M, Takigawa N. Asymptomatic double aortic arch with compressed oesophagus in an adult. BMJ Case Rep. 2012;2012:bcr 1220115315.
28. Ikenouchi H, Tabei F, Itoh N, Nozaki A. Images in cardiovascular medicine. Silent double aortic arch found in an elderly man. Circulation. 2006; 114(8):e360-1.
29. Kocis KC, Midgley FM, Ruckman RN. Aortic arch anomalies: 20 year experience with symptoms, diagnosis, associated cardiac defect, and surgical repair. Pediatr Cardiol. 1997;18(2):127-32.
30. Lowe GM, Donaldson JS, Backer CL. Vascular rings: 10-year review of imaging. Radiographics.1991;11(4):637-46.
31. Schlesinger AE, Krishnamoorthy R, Sena LM, Guillerman RP, Chung T, DiBardino DJ, et al. Incomplete double aortic arch with atresia of distal left arch: distinctive imaging appearance. AJR Am J Roentgenol. 2005;184(5):1634-9.
32. Etesami M, Ashwath R, Kanne J, Gilkeson RC, Rajiah P. Computed tomography in the evaluation of vascular rings and slings. Insights Imaging. 2014;5(4):507-21.
33. Türkvatan A, Büyükbayraktar FG, Ölçer T, Cumhur T. Congenital anomalies of the aortic arch: evaluation with the use of multidetector computed tomography. Korean J Radiol. 2009; 10(2):176-84.
34. Yilmaz M, Ozkan M, Dogan R, Demircin M, Ersoy U, Boke E, et al. Vascular anomalies causing tracheoesophageal compression: a 20-year experience in diagnosis and management. Heart Surg Forum. 2003;6(3):149-52.
35. Sebening C, Jakob H, Tochtermann U, Lange R, Vahl CF, Bodegom P, et al. Vascular tracheobronchial compression syndromes-experience in surgical treatment and literature review. Thorac Cardiovasc Surg. 2000;48(3):164-74.
36. Van Son JAM, Konstantinov IE. Burkhard F. Kommerell and Kommerell's diverticulum. Tex Heart Inst J. 2002;29:109-12.
37. Whiteman G, Stephenson LW, Weinberg P. Vascular ring left cervical arch, right descending aorta,and right ligament arteriosum. J Thorac Cardiovasc Surg. 1982;83(2):311-5.
38. Bleakney CA, Zafar F, Fraser Jr CD. Circumflex right aortic arch with hypoplasia and coarctation: repair by aortic arch advancement and end to side anastomosis. Ann Thorac Surg. 2011;91(2):624-6.
39. Predey TA, McDonald V, Demos TC, Moncada R. CT of congenital anomalies of the aortic arch. Semin Roentgeneol. 1989;24(2): 96-113.
40. Kirsch J, Julsrud PR. Magnetic resonance angiography of an ipsilateral double aortic arch due to persistent fourth and fifth aortic arch. Pediatri Radiol. 2007;37(5):501-2.
41. Quail MA, Ho SY, et al. Vascular rings, pulmonary slings, and other vascular abnormalities. In: Gatzoulis M, Webb G, Daubeney P (Eds). Diagnosis and Management of Adult Congenital Heart Disease, 3rd edition. Elsevier, USA. 2018. pp 429-39.
42. Backer CL, Idriss FS, Holinger LD, Mavroudis C. Pulmonary artery sling. Results of surgical repair in infancy. J Thorac Cardiovasc Surg. 1992;103(4):683-91.

31
CHAPTER

Right Ventricular Outflow Obstruction

Edwin Francis, Annu Jose

INTRODUCTION

Right ventricular (RV) outflow obstruction is one of the common cardiac problems presenting in the pediatric age group and has an incidence of 0.7/1,000 livebirths.[1] In isolation or in association with other cardiac anomalies, it accounts for about 20–30% of congenital heart diseases (CHDs). Though majority of cases are congenital, a small percentage is acquired. Over the last few decades, with advances in the treatment of various CHDs, there is however an increase in the cases of acquired RV obstruction.

Right ventricular outflow obstruction may occur at different anatomical levels. Accordingly, it could be infundibular, valvular, supravalvular, or at the level of peripheral pulmonary artery (PA) (**Fig. 1**). Obstruction may be associated with other cardiac anomalies of which an unrestrictive ventricular septal defect (VSD) is the most common. Tetralogy of Fallot (TOF) is the most common example in this category (*see* Chapter 34).

INCIDENCE AND EMBRYOLOGY

Morgagni was the first to describe pulmonary stenosis (PS) in 1761.[2] It is not uncommon and comprises about one-tenth of all congenital cardiac malformations. Development of RV outflow tract is complex and beyond the scope of this chapter. Initial development involves migration of subset of endothelial cells lining the inner layer of developing heart tube. Final development involves migration of neural crest cells to the outflow tract.[3] There are separate vascular components contributing to the development of PA. The proximal main pulmonary artery (MPA) arises from bulbus cordis, distal MPA from the truncus arteriosus, proximal branch pulmonary arteries from the 6th branchial arch, and the peripheral portion from the postbranchial pulmonary vascular plexus.

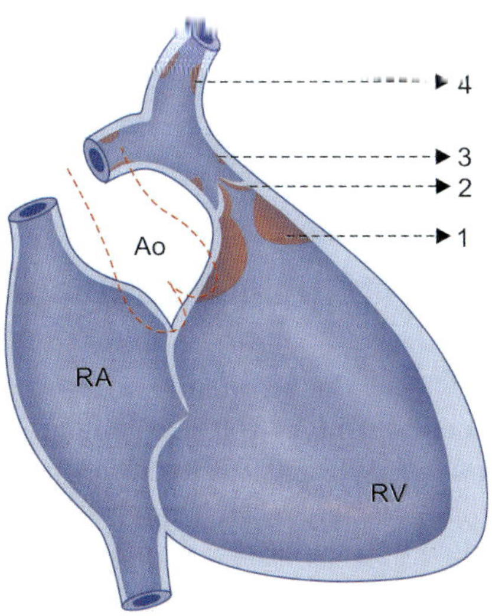

Fig. 1: Different levels of obstruction. (1) Infundibular, (2) valvular, (3) supravalvular, and (4) peripheral pulmonary artery.
(Ao: aorta: RA: right atrium; RV: right ventricle)

ANATOMICAL LEVELS OF RIGHT VENTRICULAR OUTFLOW TRACT OBSTRUCTION

The various levels of right ventricular outflow tract obstruction (RVOTO) are listed here:

- Valvular PS
- Subvalvular PS
- Supravalvular PS
- Peripheral pulmonary stenosis (PPS)
- Absence of PA.

Valvular Pulmonary Stenosis

This is the most common type of isolated RV obstruction.

Morphology

Pulmonary valve is normally comprised of three equally sized, semilunar cusps of leaflets that are joined by three commissures (**Fig. 2**). The cusps namely right, left, and anterior are made of a thin layer of endocardium that is surrounded by a tough fibrous annular ring. Each leaflet is attached at its two extremities along the sinotubular junction, while the basal attachment is supported by the infundibular musculature. There are three rings, which are described in relation with the pulmonary valve. Two anatomical rings are one at the level of sinotubular junction and the other at the anatomic ventriculoarterial junction. The third is a virtual ring constructed by joining together the basal attachments of leaflets. Normally, the free edge of each leaflet is significantly longer than the circumference of the sinus it supports, allowing the leaflets to close competently with some overlap during closure. Valvular PS is caused by fusion of leaflets along the commissures.

*Clinical Features (**Table 1**)*

The clinical symptoms vary according to the age of presentation, severity of stenosis, and associated lesions. In the neonate, critical PS may present like any other cyanotic heart lesions with severe cyanosis caused by right-to-left shunting across atrial septal defect (ASD). Beyond neonatal period, patients with mild-to-moderate PS are mostly asymptomatic. In severe PS, symptoms appear with increasing age. Exertional dyspnea and fatigue are the most common complaints due to the inability of the RV to increase cardiac output in response to exertion. Few may present with chest pain, syncope, or sudden death on exercise. Cyanosis may be present in those with right-to-left shunt through the ASD or a widely open patent foramen ovale.

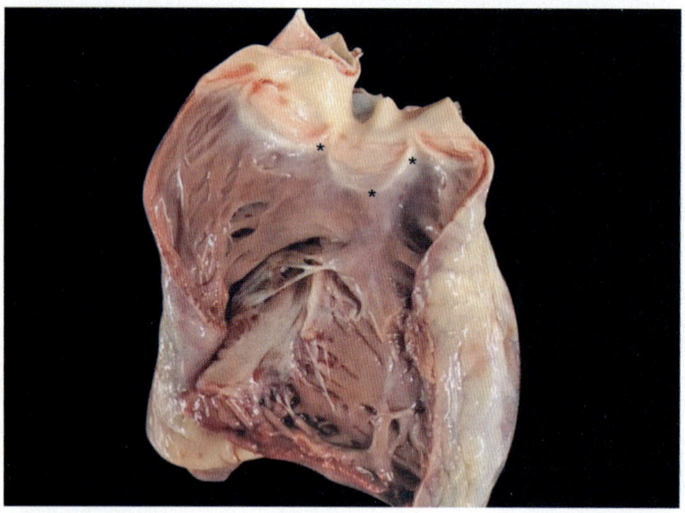

Fig. 2: Pulmonary valve. Normal pulmonary valve shown with the semilunar attachment of the cusps up to the level of sinotubular junction (*).

Physical examination reveals normal jugular venous pressure (JVP) in children with mild-to-moderate PS. Prominent "a" wave is a feature of severe PS. This reflects the prominent atrial systolic wave caused by restrictive filling of the hypertrophied right ventricle due to downstream outflow obstruction. With increase in severity, there are presystolic pulsations palpable in the liver. The JVP is elevated when there is associated RV dysfunction and tricuspid regurgitation.

Prominent left parasternal impulse with a systolic thrill can be felt in patients with severe PS due to hypertrophied right ventricle ejecting against stenotic pulmonary valve. Classically, a thrill is felt in the second to third intercostal space and may be felt in the suprasternal notch also. The thrill may be absent in infants with severe stenosis.

First heart sound is normal, second heart sound is usually widely split with the degree of splitting proportional to the degree of stenosis. Wide splitting is caused by the delay in pulmonary component of second sound (typically quite soft), which is in turn caused by the delayed closure of valve leaflets. The factors contributing to delayed closure include prolonged mechanical systole and continued forward flow of blood in the branch pulmonary arteries even after RV pressures have fallen below PA pressures (prolonged hang out interval). The split may become fixed in severe stenosis as a result of fixed stroke volume. With increasing obstruction, the intensity of pulmonary component of the second heart sound decreases further and may be inaudible altogether.

TABLE 1: Summary of clinical findings and investigations in mild, moderate, and severe stenosis.

	Mild pulmonary stenosis	*Moderate pulmonary stenosis*	*Severe pulmonary stenosis*
Symptoms	Asymptomatic	Asymptomatic	Majority asymptomatic Right heart failure in advanced stages
Cyanosis	Absent	Absent	Mostly absent except in cases having ASD with R→L shunt
JVP	Normal	Normal	Prominent "a" wave
RV heave	Absent	Absent	Present
Ejection click	Present	Present	Merges with first heart sound
Second sound	Normal	Normal to wide split	Wide split, soft or absent P2; S2 split may be fixed when heart failure sets in
Murmur	2/6 MSM	3/6 MSM, mid peaking	>grade 3/6 MSM, late peaking
ECG	Normal	Right ward axis R/S V1 >1	Right axis deviation R/S V1 >4 Right atrial enlargement
CXR	Normal	Dilated pulmonary trunk	Dilated pulmonary trunk Right atrial enlargement
Hemodynamics	Gradient <40 mm Hg	Gradient 41–60 mm Hg	Gradient >60 mm Hg

(ASD: atrial septal defect; CXR: chest X-ray; ECG: electrocardiogram; JVP: jugular venous pressure; MSM: midsystolic murmur; RV: right ventricle)

An ejection click precedes the onset of murmur. The click is caused when the doming pulmonary valve leaflets reaches the open position. The more severe the stenosis, the earlier the click occurs and in severe cases, it merges with first heart sound. It is best heard separate from the area of maximal intensity of murmur and more toward the apex or the left lower sternal border. Contrary to a constant click noted in aortic valve stenosis, pulmonary valve stenosis classically causes a variable click with the intensity of click varying with respiration. It decreases during inspiration and increases during expiration, unlike other events of the right heart. During inspiration, there is increased venous return to the right heart resulting in more forceful right atrial contraction, which in turn produces a rise in RV end-diastolic pressure. RV late diastolic pressure exceeds the PA diastolic pressure and thus pulmonary valve cusps get pushed open in the late diastole. Consequently, the actual excursion of pulmonary valve leaflets is reduced during inspiration resulting in softer or absent ejection click.[4] When PS is severe, the first heart sound appears to show varying intensity with respiration and becomes louder in expiration.

The murmur of PS is ejection in character and maximally heard at the left upper sternal border and is also well heard all over precordium. The intensity and duration of murmur are related to the severity of obstruction. Grade 2 or 3 systolic murmur is heard in mild stenosis, while more than grade 3 murmur is associated with severe stenosis. Higher degrees of stenosis are associated with longer period of ejection by the right ventricle. In severe obstruction, the murmur may extend beyond the aortic closure sound and murmur peaks late in systole. Those with severe stenosis and RV dysfunction, the murmur may be soft because of reduced RV output.

Electrocardiographic Features

In mild stenosis, electrocardiogram will be essentially normal. Moderate-to-severe PS is associated with right axis deviation and evidence of RV hypertrophy. In severe PS, pure R, RS, or QR patterns are seen in right precordial leads. The R:S ratio in V6 may be <1 in most cases. It is possible to roughly estimate the RV pressure in patients between 2 and 20 years of age if a pure R wave is present in lead V4R or V1 (**Fig. 3**). The height of R wave in millimeters multiplied by 5, approximates the RV systolic pressure in millimeters of mercury.[5] In infants with hypoplastic RV, QRS axis may have a more leftward axis than expected. In patients of Noonan syndrome, a superior axis is sometimes seen.

Radiological Features

Prominent MPA segment due to poststenotic dilatation of the MPA and left PA is the most common chest X-ray finding in patients with valvar PS (**Fig. 4**). This feature is absent in infants and patients with Noonan syndrome. In patients with significant tricuspid regurgitation, there may be evidence of right atrial enlargement.

Echocardiography

Echocardiography is the gold standard for the assessment of a patient with PS. Detailed echocardiographic evaluation provides accurate information regarding the morphology and site of obstruction, anatomy of pulmonary valve and its

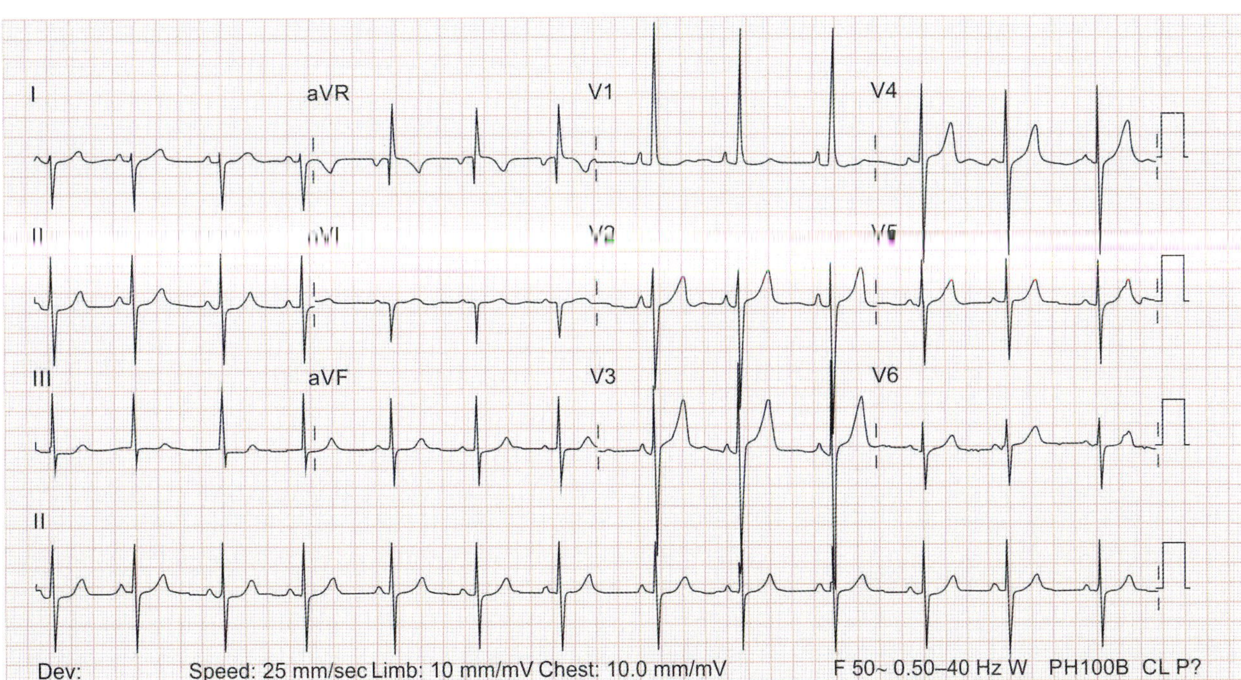

Fig. 3: Electrocardiogram (ECG) of a 10-year-old showing severe pulmonary stenosis. Findings include right axis deviation (QRS axis + 150), right atrial enlargement, and right ventricular hypertrophy.

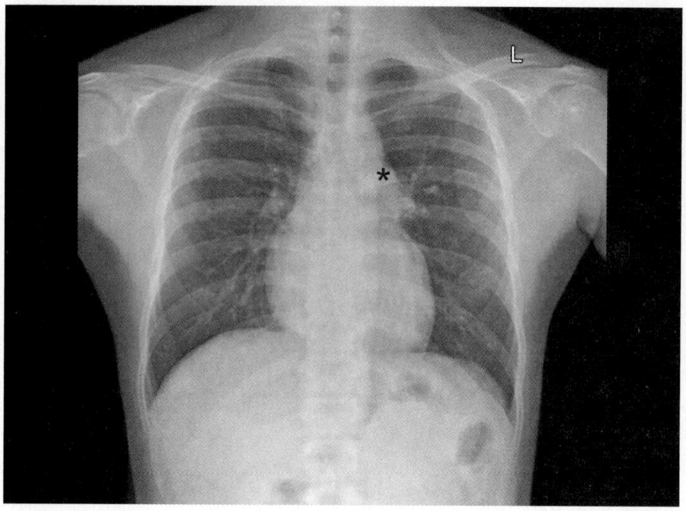

Fig. 4: Chest X-ray. Chest X-ray posteroanterior (PA) view showing dilated pulmonary artery segment (*) due to poststenotic dilatation of main pulmonary artery (MPA) and left pulmonary artery (LPA).

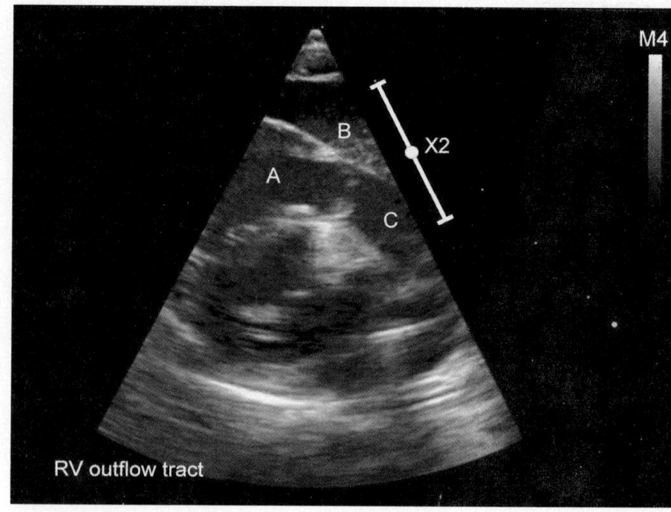

Fig. 5: Echocardiographic image. Parasternal long axis view showing doming pulmonary valve. A—right ventricular outflow, B—pulmonary annulus, and C—main pulmonary artery.

leaflets, severity of obstruction, and any associated cardiac abnormalities (**Fig. 5**).

Detailed assessment of the morphology of the pulmonary valve and measurement of annulus can be done in parasternal long axis and short axis views. Characteristics of the pulmonary valve leaflets should be noted like the thickness and supravalvular tethering as they also help in predicting the results of balloon dilatation. Thin, doming leaflets with no evidence supravalvular tethering indicates likelihood of good result with ballooning. Associated anomalies such as poststenotic dilatation, branch PA stenosis, RV size and hypertrophy, and presence of ASD should also be assessed.

Dysplastic pulmonary valve appears thickened and immobile, without the characteristic doming. It may be associated with hypoplastic pulmonary annulus and supravalvular main pulmonary artery narrowing. The classical poststenotic dilatation is absent.

Pressure gradients across pulmonary valve can be accurately estimated with Doppler measurements. It is done using simplified Bernoulli equation, which estimates the pressure drop across the pulmonary valve, $P = 4\ V^2$. P is the peak instantaneous pressure gradient (mm Hg) across the pulmonary valve and V is the peak flow velocity (m/s) distal to the obstructive orifice. If there is associated significant subpulmonary obstruction, V1 (peak flow velocity proximal to the obstruction) should be considered while calculating pressure gradients. Another important consideration is that the Doppler beam should be aligned parallel to the direction of flow to get accurate results.

There is good correlation between the Doppler-derived gradient and that obtained by direct pressure measurement at cardiac catheterization.[6,7] Doppler-derived gradient measures peak instantaneous gradient, while during cardiac catheterization what is measured is the peak-to-peak gradients. In pulmonary valve stenosis, the differences are not important in clinical decision-making and they correlate reasonably well.

Echocardiography may underestimate the severity of stenosis in two situations. One, when there is RV dysfunction that fails to generate high RV pressures in relation to the severity of stenosis. Second situation is when there is elevated PA pressure, as in a neonate with critical PA stenosis.

Cardiac Computed Tomography and Magnetic Resonance Imaging

Advanced imaging techniques of cardiac computed tomography (CT) and magnetic resonance imaging (MRI) allow comprehensive examination of the heart in a single examination. But its use in the assessment of the pulmonary valve is still limited as compared to a good echocardiography. A CT pulmonary angiogram however is superior in the assessment of supravalvular and peripheral PA anatomy and also helps in planning mode of treatment and intervention (**Fig. 6**).

Cardiac Catheterization and Hemodynamics

Cardiac catheterization was previously the gold standard. Today, it is almost never done for diagnostic purpose alone. All the information required on PS can be obtained noninvasively through a detailed echocardiogram. Pull-back gradients can be measured from the PA to right ventricle when the patient is taken for balloon pulmonary valvotomy. A rare indication for diagnostic cardiac catheterization is when there are inadequate echocardiographic images or there is a need for further delineation of associated anomalies such as branch PA stenosis that cannot be clearly defined on echocardiography.

Hemodynamic measurements made during cardiac catheterization are RV and PA pressure measurements. The normal RV and PA systolic pressure are <30 mm Hg.

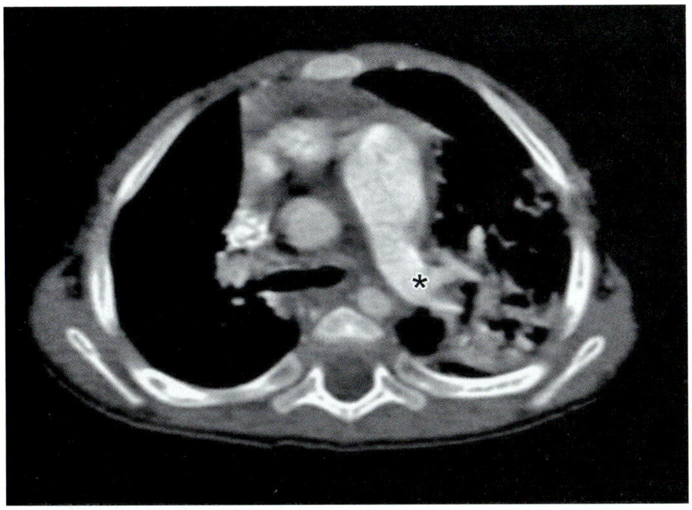

Fig. 6: Computed tomography (CT) showing absent right pulmonary artery (RPA). Axial CT scan cut showing main pulmonary continuing as left pulmonary artery (*) and absent right pulmonary artery.

TABLE 2: Management of pulmonary stenosis.

Indications	*Procedure*
Mild pulmonary stenosis	Medical follow-up
• Moderate–severe valvular pulmonary stenosis • Critical pulmonary stenosis in newborns • Dysplastic pulmonary valve with moderate or severe stenosis	Balloon valvuloplasty
• Infundibular stenosis • Dysplastic pulmonary valve with failed balloon • Postoperative supravalvular or peripheral pulmonic stenosis	Surgery
• Peripheral pulmonary stenosis • Postoperative supravalvular or peripheral pulmonic stenosis	Balloon dilation with stenting

Normal mean arterial pressure (MAP) is <20 mm Hg. Systolic pressure gradients between right ventricle and PA ≤10 mm Hg may be seen with structurally normal pulmonary valves. Thus, RV systolic pressure of >30 mm Hg and a pressure gradient across pulmonary valve >10 mm Hg are considered abnormal.

*Treatment (**Table 2**)*

Balloon pulmonary valvotomy is the treatment of choice in valvular PS. Jean Kan and coworkers first described the percutaneous technique of pulmonary valvuloplasty.[8] This is one of the first few pediatric catheter interventions to have been performed after the iconic Rashkind balloon atrial septostomy.

Transcatheter intervention is indicated in all patients with moderate or severe valvular PS. Balloon dilatation may be considered even with lower gradients in symptomatic patients or with evidence of RV dysfunction. Similarly, valvuloplasty is also indicated in neonates with critical PS.

It is reasonable to perform pulmonary valvuloplasty on a patient with valvar PS who meets the above criteria in the setting of a dysplastic pulmonary valve (AHA, 2011).

Pulmonary valvuloplasty involves measurement of hemodynamic data followed by angiography. RV angiogram done in lateral view and/or anteroposterior view with cranial tilt will demonstrate the RV outflow and pulmonary valve anatomy (**Fig. 7**). Classical findings include thickened and doming pulmonary valve leaflets, narrow jet of contrast crossing the pulmonary valve, and post-stenotic dilatation.

Technique of balloon valvuloplasty involves crossing the stenotic valve with the help of an end-hole catheter and exchange length guidewire. The wire is positioned deep in the branch PA. A balloon with a diameter about 20% more than the echocardiographic or angiographic pulmonary annular measurement is positioned across the stenotic valve and inflated till the disappearance of the waist.

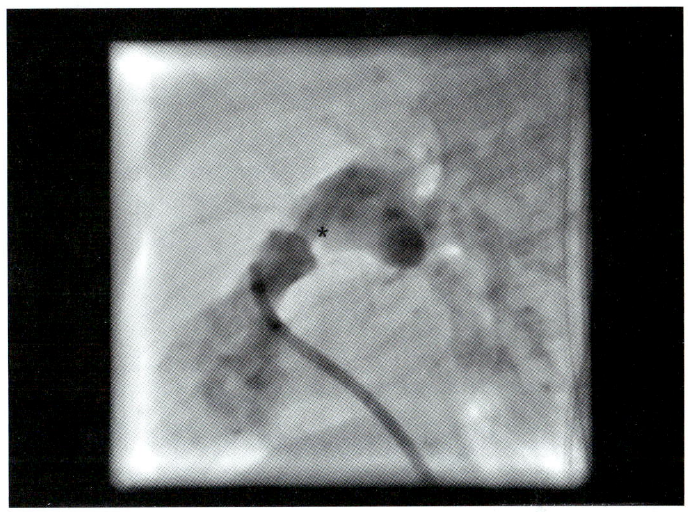

Fig. 7: Right ventricular (RV) angiogram. Right ventricular outflow angiography done in lateral view showing doming pulmonary valve, narrow contrast jet (*) and dilated main pulmonary artery.

Surgical pulmonary valvotomy is done in cases that are not amenable to balloon valvotomy and in those cases with dysplastic pulmonary valve and multiple sites of obstruction. PPS can be tackled by either surgery or balloon dilatation with or without stenting in the catheterization laboratory.

Subvalvular Pulmonary Stenosis

Subvalvular PS accounts for 5% of all cases with RVOTO and usually occurs due to hypertrophy of muscle bands within the right ventricle, dividing the RV cavity into two chambers. It may result due to an arrested incorporation of the primitive bulbus cordis into the RV body.[9] This condition, which is commonly known as double-chambered right ventricle, is characterized by a high-pressure proximal chamber and a lower pressure distal chamber. Rarely, subvalvular PS may also be due to a narrowing of the infundibulum as a result of fibromuscular thickening of the infundibular wall. Clinical features are similar to isolated valvular PS with the exception of an ejection click. Though the condition can be easily diagnosed by echocardiography, a cardiac MRI has proven to be superior in patients with poor echocardiographic windows. The treatment usually is surgical resection of the abnormal muscle bundles.

Peripheral Pulmonary Stenosis

The entity of PPS was first reported by Maugars et al.[10] It is commonly associated with other cardiac lesions such as valvar PS and TOF but can also occur as an isolated lesion in 2–3% of cases with CHD. Isolated PPS was further classified by Gay et al.[11] into four types based on the level of stenosis, which may be at the main trunk or proximal branches, at the bifurcation, at multiple peripheral branches or a combination type. Williams syndrome, Noonan syndrome, Alagille syndrome, cutis laxa, and Ehlers–Danlos syndrome are known to have associated PPS. Clinically other than the features of any associated syndrome, there will be an ejection systolic murmur in the pulmonary area. The presence of a continuous murmur is suggestive of very significant stenosis. The treatment modality is transcatheter rehabilitation of the affected vessels by balloon dilation and stenting.

Isolated Unilateral Absence of Pulmonary Artery

Unilateral absence of either right or left PA could be associated with other complex cardiac anomalies. Absence of right PA is more frequently seen in otherwise normal heart unlike absence of left pulmonary, which is often accompanied with other lesions.[12] Two types of presentation are described. One example is seen in infants where they usually present with pulmonary hypertension and congestive heart failure. The other presentation is in older patients, who do not develop pulmonary hypertension and may be asymptomatic or have symptoms of exercise intolerance, hemoptysis, etc.[13] Chest X-ray shows differential vascularity in majority of cases. A cardiac MDCT can confirm the diagnosis and delineate any hilar PA along with the presence of any collaterals.

If there are well-developed intrapulmonary arteries, a primary anastomosis with central pulmonary arteries can be considered. Infants presenting with severe pulmonary hypertension tend to have very diminutive PA are not surgical candidates and tend to have very poor prognosis.[14]

GENETIC AND NONGENETIC ASSOCIATIONS OF PULMONARY STENOSIS

There are a lot of environmental, genetic, and stochastic factors contributing to the cause of CHD in the population. Few factors associated with RVOTO lesions are as follows:

Chromosome Abnormalities Associated with RVOTO

- *Williams-Beuren syndrome* or commonly known as Williams syndrome has an occurrence of 1/20,000 live births and is due to microdeletion of 7q11.23. The cardiac manifestation of the disease is due to haploinsufficiency of the elastin gene (ELN) and typically includes supravalvar aortic stenosis and PPS.[15,16] The PPS in Williams syndrome may improve with time. They can also have hypercalcemia, skeletal and renal anomalies, cognitive deficits, social personality, and elfin facies. The genetic abnormality is not usually seen on routine karyotyping but can be easily diagnosed with fluorescence in situ hybridization (FISH), multiplex ligation-dependent probe amplification (MLPA), and microarray tests.
- *8p23.1 Deletion syndrome* occurs due to interstitial or terminal deletions in *GATA4* gene and is associated with PS, ASD, atrioventricular septal defect (AVSD), VSD, and left ventricular (LV) noncompaction as well as genitourinary (GU) anomalies, abnormal ears and minor hand anomalies and diaphragmatic hernia.[17,18]
- *Deletion 4qter* is also associated with RVOTO and PS along with abnormal pinnae, cleft palate, and Pierre-Robin sequence.

Single Gene Mutations and Genetic Syndromes Associated with RVOTO

- *The RASopathies or Noonan syndrome spectrum* [*Noonan syndrome, LEOPARD, cardiofaciocutaneous (CFC) syndrome, and Costello syndrome*] results due to mutations in the RAS/MAPK pathway.[19] Noonan syndrome has an occurrence of 1/1,000 to 1/2,500 live births and is characterized by the typical facial appearance associated with ptosis, hypertelorism, low-set posteriorly rotated ears, arch eyebrows, low posterior hairline, excessive nuchal thickness, neck webbing, and short stature (**Fig. 8**). It is

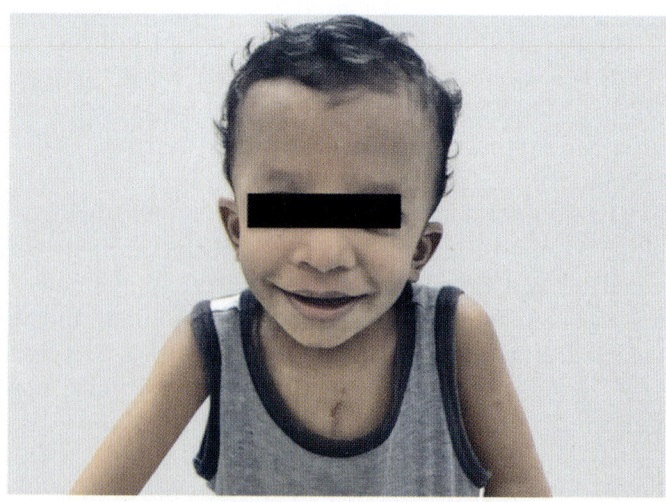

Fig. 8: Noonan syndrome. Noonan syndrome is associated with dysplastic pulmonary valve, with valvular and supravalvular pulmonary stenosis. Typical facial appearance includes ptosis, hypertelorism, low-set posteriorly rotated ears, and arch eyebrows.

associated with abnormality in the genes associated with RAS-MAPK signaling pathway such as PTPN11 (the most common), SOS1, RAF1, KRAS, NRAS, BRAF, and SHOC2. PS is the most common cardiac lesion followed by ASD and hypertrophic cardiomyopathy. CFC syndrome can be caused by BRAF, MEK1, MEK2 mutations, and Costello by *HRAS* gene mutation.

- *Alagille syndrome* is an autosomal dominant disorder occurring due to lesions in notch signaling pathway genes *JAG1* and *NOTCH2* and has an occurrence of 1/70,000 live births. It commonly presents with cholestasis due to bile duct paucity, CHDs, skeletal or ocular abnormalities, and typical facial features. It is most commonly associated with right-sided heart lesions including PPS, pulmonary valve stenosis, and TOF.[20,21]
- *Neurofibromatosis* with NF1 mutation can be associated with valvar PS, aortic stenosis, coarctation, and hypertrophic cardiomyopathy.[22]
- *Keutel syndrome,* which occurs due to MGP mutation, is associated with PPS.[23]

Nongenetic Causes for Pulmonary Stenosis

- *Congenital rubella syndrome* is known to be associated with PPS and patent ductus arteriosus (PDA) along with sensory neural deafness and ocular abnormalities.
- *The teratogenicity of fever and flu-like illness* is uncertain but studies show that it may be associated with a relative high risk for right-sided obstructive lesions.
- Rarely, Takayasu arteritis may involve branch pulmonary arteries.

REFERENCES

1. Bruneau BG. The developmental genetics of congenital heart disease. Nature. 2008; 451(7181):943-8.
2. Morgagni JB. The seats and causes of diseases investigated by anatomy. Padua 1761. Alexander B, translator (from latin). London: Milar, Cadell, Johnson and Payne.
3. Hutson MR, Kirby ML. Model systems for the study of heart development and disease. Cardiac neural crest and conotruncal malformations. Semin Cell DivBiol. 2007;18(1):101-10.
4. Wernovsky G, Anderson R, Krishna K, Mussatto K, Redington A, Tweddell J (Eds). Anderson's Pediatric Cardiology, 4th edition. Philadelphia: Elsevier; 2019. pp. 3319-97.
5. Rudolph A. Congenital Diseases of the Heart. Chicago: Yearbook Medical; 1974.
6. Lima CO, Sahn DJ, Valdes-Cruz LM, Goldberg SJ, Barron JV, Allen HD, et al. Non-invasive prediction of transvalvular pressure gradient in patients with pulmonary stenosis by quantitative two-dimensional echocardiographic Doppler studies. Circulation. 1983;67(4):866-71.
7. Currie PJ, Hagler DJ, Seward JB, Reeder GS, Fyfe DA, Bove AA, et al. Instantaneous pressure gradient: a simultaneous Doppler and dual catheter correlative study. J Am Coll Cardiol. 1986;7(4):800-6.
8. Kan JS, White RI, Mitchell SE, Gardner TJ. Percutaneous balloon valvuloplasty: a new method for treating congenital pulmonary-vale stenosis. N Engl J Med. 1982;307(9):540-2.
9. Keith A. The Hunterian lectures on malformations of the heart. Lancet. 1909;2:359.
10. Maugars A. Description d'unearterepulmonaire considerable naissantdel'aorteabdominale. Rec Period Soc Med Paris. 1802; 13:74.
11. Gay BB Jr, French RH, Shuford WH, Rogers Jr JV. The roentgenologic features of single and multiple coarctations of the pulmonary artery and branches. Am J Roentgenol Radium Ther Nucl Med. 1963;90:599-613.
12. Cucci CE, Doyle EF, Lewis EW. Absence of a primary division of the pulmonary trunk: an ontogenetic theory. Circulation. 1964;29:124-31.
13. Shakibi JG, Rastan H, Nazarian I, Paydar M, Aryanpour I, Siassi B. Isolated unilateral absence of the pulmonary artery. Review of the world literature and guideline for surgical repair. Jpn Heart J. 1978;19(3):439-51.
14. Singhi AK, Francis E, Kumar RK. Isolated absence of right pulmonary artery. Ann Pediatr Cardiol 2010;3(2):119-22.
15. Eronen M, Peippo M, Hiippala A, Raatikka M, Arvio M, Johansson R, et al. Cardiovascular manifestations in 75 patients with Williams syndrome. J Med Genet. 2002;39(8):554-8.
16. Kececioglu D, Kotthoff S, Vogt J. Williams-Beuren syndrome: a 30-year follow-up of natural and postoperative course. Eur Heart J. 1993;14(11):1458-64.
17. Ballarati L, Cereda A, Caselli R, Selicorni A, Recalcati MP, Maitz S, et al. Genotype-phenotype correlations in a new case of 8p23.1 deletion and review of the literature. Eur J Med Genet. 2011;54(1):55-9.
18. Pehlivan T, Pober BR, Brueckner M, Garrett S, Slaugh R, Van Rheeden R, et al. GATA4 haploinsufficiency in patients with interstitial deletion ofchromosome region 8p23.1 and congenital heart disease. Am J Med Genet. 1999;83(3):201-6.
19. Tidyman WE, Rauen KA. Noonan, Costello and cardio-facio-cutaneous syndromes: dysregulation of the Ras-MAPK pathway. Expert Rev Mol Med. 2008;10:e37.
20. McDaniell R, Warthen DM, Sanchez-Lara PA, Pai A, Krantz ID, Piccoli DA, et al. NOTCH2 mutations cause Alagille syndrome, a heterogeneous disorder of the notch signaling pathway. Am J Hum Genet. 2006;79(1):169-73.
21. Goldmuntz E, Moore E, Spinner NB. The cardiovascular manifestations of Alagille syndrome and JAG1 mutations. Methods Mol Med. 2006;126:217-31.
22. Lin AE, Birch PH. Korf BR, Tenconi R, Niimura M, Poyhonen M, et al. Cardiovascular malformations and other cardiovascular abnormalities inneurofibromatosis 1. Am J Med Genet. 2000; 95(2):108-17.
23. Hur DJ, Raymond GV, Kahler SG, Riegert-Johnson DL, Cohen BA, Boyadjiev SA. A novel MGP mutation in a consanguineous family: review of the clinical and molecular characteristics of Keutel syndrome. Am J Med Genet A. 2005;135(1):36-40.

32
CHAPTER

Pulmonary Atresia with Intact Ventricular Septum

Preeti Ramachandran, Vasu Gooty

INTRODUCTION

Pulmonary valve atresia with intact ventricular septum (PA/IVS) is a unique form of cyanotic congenital heart disease (CHD), in which the pulmonary valve (PV) is atretic with no interventricular communication. This type of CHD is rare and accounts for 1–3% of all cardiac defects with a prevalence at 4–8 births per 100,000 live birth.[1]

ANATOMY

The combination of defects in PA/IVS can present with a wide spectrum with varying degrees of tricuspid valve (TV), PV, and right ventricular (RV) hypoplasia (**Figs. 1A and B**). Degree of PV atresia can range from membranous to plate-like atresia. In the membranous type, valve leaflets are well-formed but fused at their commissures. In the more severe form of "plate-like" atresia, the PV may not be formed at all and severe infundibular hypoplasia is present.[2,3] Along with the valve abnormality, different degrees of RV hypoplasia may exist. A normal RV cavity comprises of the inlet component, trabecular component, and the conus or infundibulum. In PA/IVS, the RV may be normal-sized and tripartite with well-developed inflow, trabecular and infundibular portion; however, in more severe cases, it may be bipartite (hypoplastic infundibulum with normal-sized inlet and trabecular portion) or unipartite (only inlet developed, remaining parts are hypoplastic). The RV cavity may be hypoplastic, especially when the TV is hypoplastic. A unique feature of PA/IVS is the presence of abnormal coronary artery fistulas which communicate with the RV cavity. These ventricular-coronary sinusoids can be present in 31–61% of patients.[4-9] Due to heterogeneity of available data, a small proportion of patients (9–34%) may exhibit "RV-dependent coronary circulation" when stenosis of the coronary artery system is present (typically proximal stenosis or ostial atresia).[4,9-12] As a result, instead of antegrade perfusion through the aorta, the most of the myocardium is perfused retrograde by deoxygenated blood from the high-pressure RV via the RV ventricular sinusoidal connections (**Fig. 2**).

PATHOPHYSIOLOGY

In PA/IVS, there is complete mixing of systemic and pulmonary venous return. Blood returns from superior vena

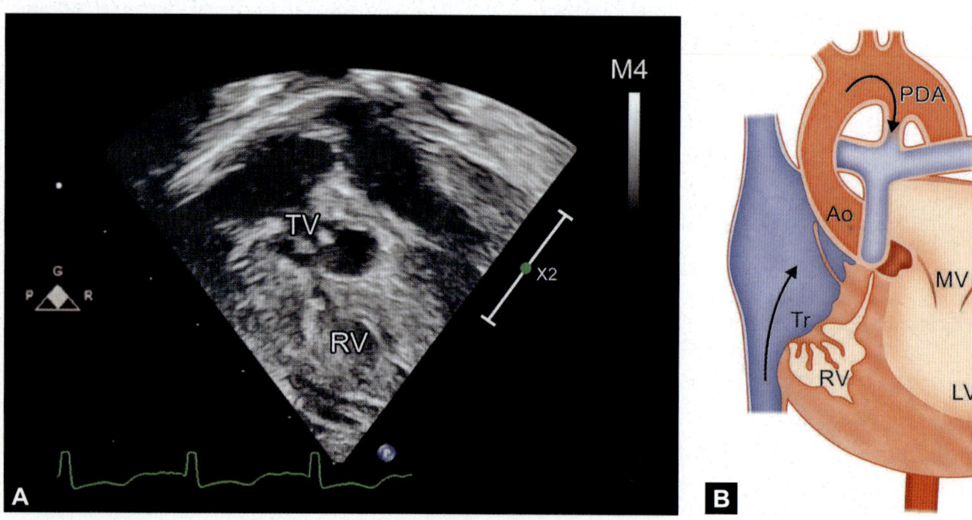

Figs. 1A and B: (A) Apical four-chamber view of heart with severe hypoplasia of the right ventricle (RV) with severe tricuspid valve (TV) hypoplasia in a patient with pulmonary atresia intact ventricular septum; (B) Pulmonary atresia with intact ventricular septum physiology.
(PDA: patent ductus arteriosus; LV: left ventricle; Ao: aorta; ; MV: mitral valve)

cava (SVC) and inferior vena cava (IVC) into the right atrium. Due to a lack of egress into the pulmonary circulation, there is right-to-left shunting across an obligatory atrial septal defect. There is mixing of systemic and pulmonary venous return in the left atrium and this mixed blood travels into the left ventricle and is pumped to the body via aorta. The mixed deoxygenated blood flowing through the aorta is the sole source of pulmonary blood supply via a left-to-right shunting patent ductus arteriosus (PDA) (**Figs. 3A and B**). Severe TV regurgitation may be present at which time care must be taken if a PV perforation via catheterization is attempted, since patients may develop a "circular" ineffective shunt resulting in worsening heart failure due to poor systemic perfusion (**Fig. 4**).

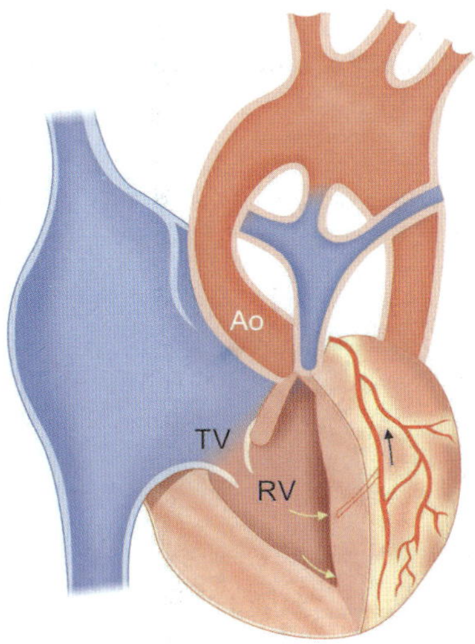

Fig. 2: Right ventricle (RV)-dependent coronary circulation where there is systolic flow of blood from RV into abnormal ventriculocoronary sinusoids.
(Ao: aorta; TV: tricuspid valve)

CLINICAL PRESENTATION

Due to ductal-dependent pulmonary circulation, majority of PA/IVS patients present with cyanosis within first few hours to days of life. Physical examination reveals the presence of central cyanosis, single second heart sound (due to single outflow). Typically, no cardiac murmur can be auscultated, especially if the duct is constricted; however, if severe tricuspid regurgitation is present, a holosystolic murmur may be heard over the left lower sternal border. Acidosis may result from persistent hypoxia if the presenting diagnosis is late or if there is a delay in the initiation of prostaglandin infusion.

DIAGNOSIS

- *Chest radiograph (CXR) findings*: CXR may demonstrate normal to mildly enlarged heart, along with reduced pulmonary vascular markings secondary to reduced

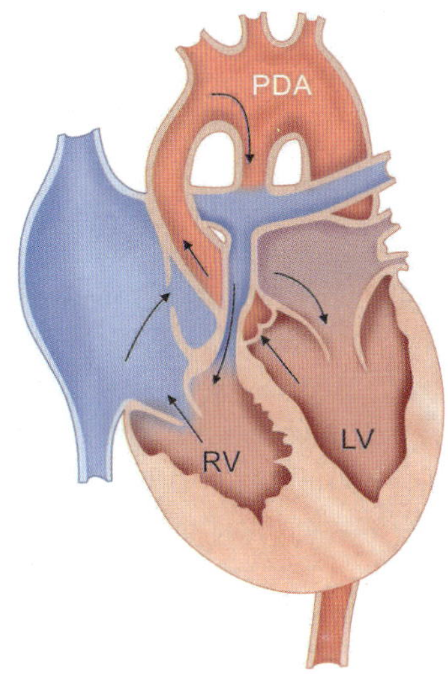

Fig. 4: Circular shunt physiology.
(PDA: patent ductus arteriosus; RV: right ventricle; LV: left ventricle)

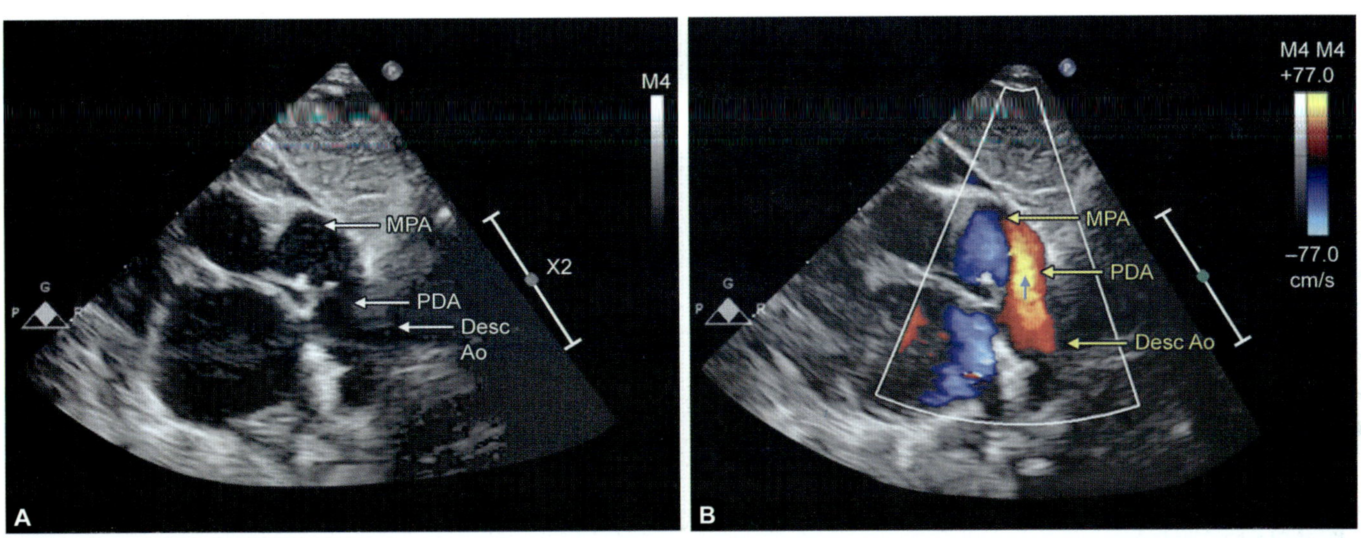

Figs. 3A and B: (A) Two-dimensional (2D) view of the large patent ductus arteriosus (PDA) connecting the descending thoracic aorta to pulmonary artery; (B) Color Doppler flow showing PDA flow direction from descending thoracic aorta to pulmonary artery.
(Desc Ao: descending aorta; MPA: mean pulmonary artery)

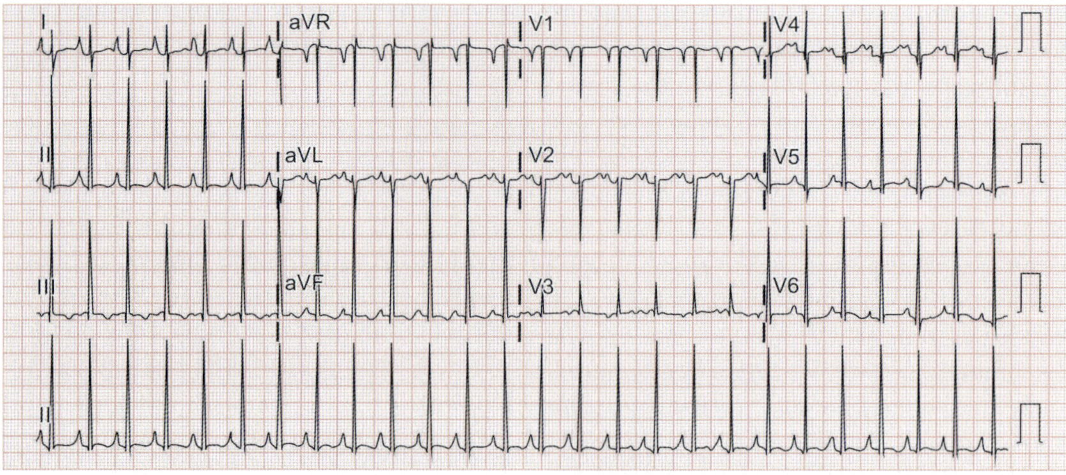

Fig. 5: A 12-lead electrocardiogram (ECG) shows increased left ventricular voltage with reduced right ventricular forces.

pulmonary blood flow. When there is severe TV regurgitation or atrial septal restriction, massive cardiomegaly may be seen.

- *Electrocardiogram (ECG)*: This typically shows increased left-sided forces and reduced right-sided forces secondary to poor development of the RV (**Fig. 5**). There may be ST-T wave changes associated with ischemia secondary to abnormal coronary development.
- *Echocardiography*: Echocardiographic evaluation is the crucial first step toward confirming the diagnosis of PA-IVS. Evaluation comprises assessing for the presence of adequate atrial level shunt, size, and function of TV and RV size, the anatomy of the RV outflow tract and confluence of branch pulmonary arteries and patency of ductus arteriosus. The echocardiogram is vital in planning catheter intervention for the initial management. Another vital element of echocardiographic evaluation comprises assessment of coronary origins and the presence of abnormal ventriculoarterial sinusoids.
- *Computed tomography (CT)*: Cardiac CT is seldom necessary but may be performed to obtain high resolution images of intracardiac anatomy, main pulmonary artery, and branch pulmonary artery size when anatomical evaluation is limited or unclear by echocardiography. It may also help with excellent three-dimensional anatomic visualization prior to undergoing surgical or catheterization intervention.[13]
- *Cardiac catheterization*: Cardiac catheterization is the gold standard in determining coronary anatomy and RV-dependency of the coronary circulation (**Fig. 6**). Depending on coronary anatomy, PV perforation and dilation may or may not be performed. Other palliative interventions may include PDA stent placement and an atrial septal balloon septostomy.

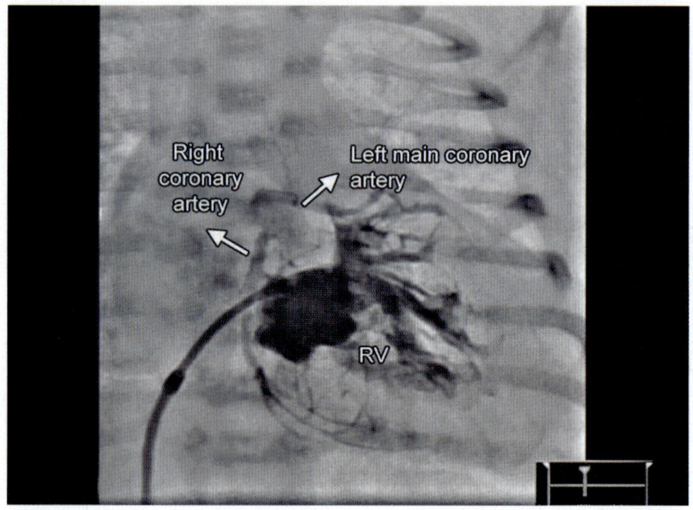

Fig. 6: Cardiac catheterization with right ventriculogram shows suprasystemic right ventricle (RV) with abnormal coronary connections and areas of severe stenosis of the proximal left main coronary artery and associated RV-dependent coronary circulation.

MANAGEMENT

Patients require prostaglandin infusion immediately after birth due to duct-dependent pulmonary circulation. Based on imaging and catheterization studies, the patient is determined to be a candidate for complete biventricular repair versus single ventricle palliation. Risk factors precluding biventricular repair or catheter-based intervention include presence of RV-dependent coronary circulation, severe hypoplasia of RV or TV, and low birth weight or prematurity.[4,6,9,14-16] If RV decompression is not contraindicated in the patient, then either catheter-based intervention consisting of perforation of the atretic PV using a radiofrequency energy or using certain specific coronary guidewires followed by pulmonary balloon valvuloplasty. Often the PDA will need to be stented in the same setting because even after opening up of the outflow tract, the thick noncompliant RV may not fill well enough to ensure adequate pulmonary blood flow. Surgical pulmonary valvotomy is a potential alternative. The RV outflow tract may need to be enlarged with a patch.

For patients who are determined to be poor biventricular repair candidates, single ventricle pathway is pursued. Within the first few weeks of life, a Blalock–Taussig shunt

(BT shunt) or central shunt is surgically placed for maintaining pulmonary blood flow. Alternatively, the PDA may be stented to provide a reliable source of pulmonary blood flow. This procedure is increasingly preferred because it is less invasive and is perhaps associated with better immediate survival. Following this, a bidirectional Glenn anastomosis (SVC to branch pulmonary artery anastomosis) is performed around 4–6 months of life. This is followed by the Fontan procedure (IVC to branch pulmonary artery connection via conduit) which is usually performed >4 years of age. For patients with RV-dependent coronary circulation, the options are much more limited. Due to risk of myocardial ischemia from RV decompression with biventricular repair, typically single ventricle palliation with placement of BT shunt and stenting of PDA is considered as the first palliative option. Surgical treatment of those with TV regurgitation is challenging with these patients eventually requiring single ventricle palliation. Cardiac transplantation may be required in those with more severe forms of PA/IVS such as RV-dependent coronary circulation with coronary stenosis or atresia or severe TV regurgitation.

LATE MANAGEMENT

In general, these patients should be followed by a cardiologist who specializes in congenital cardiac disease every 1–2 years; however, those with significant residual lesions should be followed very closely. As patients who underwent single ventricle palliation get older, typical long-term complications associated with the Fontan circulation such as, chronic low cardiac output state, elevated systemic venous pressure leading to thrombotic events, protein losing enteropathy, plastic bronchitis, arrhythmias, and liver dysfunction could occur. Exercise limitations may be required based on the type of surgical procedure performed and underlying hemodynamics. Although endocarditis prophylaxis is not routinely recommended, high level of dental hygiene is necessary.

PROGNOSIS

Although it is difficult to accurately assess the prognosis of patients, due to heterogeneity of available data across different institutions, overall survival into adolescents based on the gathered data is ~60–86%.[4,16-18] Most of the studies report excellent survival and quality after the first year of life. Lifelong surveillance is needed for these patients to assess chronic issues as mentioned above. Patients with RV-dependent coronary circulation need lifelong surveillance of the coronary arteries. Patients needing interventions to reduce morbidity must be attended in a proactive fashion when clinically applicable.

REFERENCES

1. Talner CN. Report of the New England Regional Infant Cardiac Program. Pediatrics. 1980;65(2 Pt 2):375-461.
2. Quail MA, Anderson RH, Spicer DE, Daubeney PEF. Hypoplasia of the right ventricle. In: Anderson's Pediatric Cardiology, Anderson RH, (Ed). Philadelphia, PA: Churchill Livingstone Elsevier; 2010. pp. 803-18.
3. O'Leary PW, Edwards WD, Julsrud PR, and Burkhart HMD (2013). Pulmonary atresia and ventricular septal defect. In: Moss and Adams' Heart Disease in Infants, Children, and Adolescents: Including the Fetus and Young Adult, 8th edition (Vol. 2-2). Wolters Kluwer Health Adis (ESP).
4. Ashburn DA, Blackstone EH, Wells WJ, Jonas RA, Pigula FA, Manning PB, et al. Determinants of mortality and type of repair in neonates with pulmonary atresia and intact ventricular septum. J Thorac Cardiovasc Surg. 2004;127(4):1000-7; discussion 1007-8.
5. Calder AL, Co EE, Sage MD. Coronary arterial abnormalities in pulmonary atresia with intact ventricular septum. Am J Cardiol. 1987; 59(5):436-42.
6. Coles JG, Freedom RM, Lightfoot NE, Dasmahapatra HK, Williams WG, Trusler GA, et al. Long-term results in neonates with pulmonary atresia and intact ventricular septum. Ann Thorac Surg. 1989;47(2):213-7.
7. Fenton KN, Pigula FA, Gandhi SK, Russo L, Duncan KF. Interim mortality in pulmonary atresia with intact ventricular septum. Ann Thorac Surg. 2004;78(6):1994-8; discussion 1998.
8. Giglia TM, Mandell VS, Connor AR, Mayer Jr JE, Lock JE. Diagnosis and management of right ventricle-dependent coronary circulation in pulmonary atresia with intact ventricular septum. Circulation. 1992;86(5):1516-28.
9. Hanley FL, Sade RM, Blackstone EH, Kirklin JW, Freedom RM, Nanda NC. Outcomes in neonatal pulmonary atresia with intact ventricular septum. A multiinstitutional study. J Thorac Cardiovasc Surg. 1993;105(3):406-23, 424-7; discussion 423-4.
10. Jahangiri M, Zurakowski D, Bichell D, Mayer JE, del Nido PJ, Jonas RA. Improved results with selective management in pulmonary atresia with intact ventricular septum. J Thorac Cardiovasc Surg. 1999;118(6):1046-55.
11. Powell AJ, Mayer JE, Lang P, Lock JE. Outcome in infants with pulmonary atresia, intact ventricular septum, and right ventricle-dependent coronary circulation. Am J Cardiol. 2000;86(11): 1272-4, A9.
12. Rychik J, Levy H, Gaynor JW, DeCampli WM, Spray TL. Outcome after operations for pulmonary atresia with intact ventricular septum. J Thorac Cardiovasc Surg. 1998;116(6): 924-31.
13. Gatzoulis M, Webb G, Daubeney P. Pulmonary atresia with intact ventricular septum. In: Diagnosis and Management of Adult Congenital Heart Disease, 3rd edition. Philadelphia: Elsevier; 2018. p. 503-12.
14. Bull C, Kostelka M, Sorensen K, de Leval M. Outcome measures for the neonatal management of pulmonary atresia with intact ventricular septum. J Thorac Cardiovasc Surg. 1994; 107(2): 359-66.
15. Daubeney PE, Wang D, Delany DJ, Keeton BR, Anderson RH, Slavik Z, et al. Pulmonary atresia with intact ventricular septum: predictors of early and medium-term outcome in a population-based study. J Thorac Cardiovasc Surg. 2005;130(4):1071.
16. Dyamenahalli U, McCrindle BW, McDonald C, Trivedi KR, Smallhorn JF, Benson LN, et al. Pulmonary atresia with intact ventricular septum: management of, and outcomes for, a cohort of 210 consecutive patients. Cardiol Young. 2004;14(3):299-308.
17. Ekman Joelsson BM, Sunnegårdh J, Hanseus K, Berggren H, Jonzon A, Jögi P, et al. The outcome of children born with pulmonary atresia and intact ventricular septum in Sweden from 1980 to 1999. Scand Cardiovasc J. 2001;35(3):192-8.
18. Odim J, Laks H, Plunkett MD, Tung TC. Successful management of patients with pulmonary atresia with intact ventricular septum using a three tier grading system for right ventricular hypoplasia. Ann Thorac Surg. 2006; 81(2):678-84.

33 CHAPTER

Ebstein Anomaly of Tricuspid Valve

Renu P Kurup

INTRODUCTION

Ebstein anomaly of the tricuspid valve (TV) refers to an embryological derangement of TV formation associated with right ventricular myopathy.[1] The tricuspid leaflets are tethered to varying degrees to the right ventricular free wall and the ventricular septum, often resulting in significant tricuspid regurgitation and a small functioning right ventricular chamber.

Though Wilhelm Ebstein gave the first description of the disease in 1866, it was much later in 1951 that Soloff and colleagues reported a confirmed case in a living patient.[2,3] Ebstein anomaly had a uniformly poor prognosis in earlier days. Improvements in medical and surgical management of this condition have led to progressively better outcomes over the years.

EPIDEMIOLOGY

Ebstein anomaly is a rare congenital heart disorder with a wide spectrum of anatomical and clinical presentations that perhaps account for the variable estimates in the population. Although the prevalence of Ebstein anomaly was earlier reported as 1–5 per 200,000 live births,[4,5] more recent population studies have reported a prevalence of 1 in 13,800–25,600 live births.[4,6] The etiology of Ebstein anomaly is uncertain. Most cases are sporadic; familial recurrence and heterogeneous genetic factors account for a small number of cases.[6]

Various studies have shown an association between Ebstein anomaly and left ventricular noncompaction cardiomyopathy (LVNC) with mutations in the sarcomeric protein gene *MYH7*, encoding β-myosin heavy chain.[7,8]

The association between use of lithium by the mother during pregnancy and Ebstein anomaly has remained conflicting. While a meta-analysis by McKnight et al. published in The Lancet did not record any association, a cohort study by Paterno et al. concluded that there is an increased risk of cardiac malformations including Ebstein anomaly with lithium use in the first trimester of pregnancy.[9-11]

EMBRYOLOGY

The leaflets of the TV develop equally from the endocardial cushion tissues and the myocardium. The leaflets and tensor apparatus of the atrioventricular (AV) valves seem to be formed by a process of delamination—splitting of the tissue by detachment of the inner layers of the inlet zone of the ventricles. In Ebstein anomaly, the delamination (primarily of the septal and posterior leaflets of TV) is incomplete. The exact reasons for the incomplete lamination are poorly understood. As there are no chords to suspend the leaflets, they arise from the cavity of the ventricle and are attached directly to the wall.[12-14]

PATHOLOGICAL ANATOMY

In a normal heart, the TV has three unequal leaflets. The anterior leaflet (ATL) is the largest with greatest mobility. The septal tricuspid leaflet (STL) is the shortest and is attached to the annulus directly above the interventricular septum. The posterior tricuspid leaflet (PTL) may have multiple scallops and may not be completely separated from the ATL in 10% cases.[15]

These leaflets are suspended from the muscular AV junction and from a small area of membranous septum with attachments to the papillary muscles through the chordae.

Ebstein anomaly is characterized by a spectrum of several features which include:

- *Adherence of the TV leaflets to the underlying myocardium* (failure of delamination).
- *Downward (apical) displacement of the functional annulus (septal > posterior > anterior)*: In normal human hearts, septal and posterior tricuspid leaflets are displaced apically by <8 mm/m² body surface area in relation to the anterior mitral leaflet.[16]
- *Dilation of the "atrialized" portion of the right ventricle (RV)* (***Figs. 1A and B***): Normal RV is constituted by an inlet portion (in relation to AV valve), apical trabecular portion, and outflow area. In Ebstein anomaly, the RV has only two components due to apical displacement of the functional annulus. The inlet portion is functionally

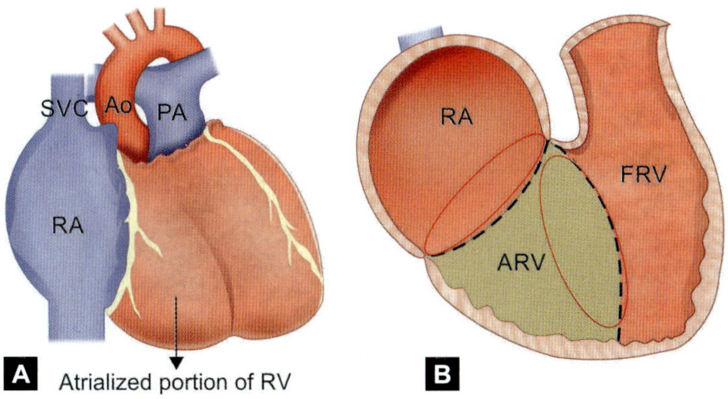

Figs. 1A and B: (A) External appearance of a heart with Ebstein malformation; (B) A cartoon showing the plane of displacement of the tricuspid annulus (red circle).
(Ao: aorta; ARV: atrialized right ventricle; FRV: functional right ventricle; PA: pulmonary artery; RA: right atrium; SVC: superior vena cava)

integrated with the right atrium (RA) forming the atrialized RV, and the trabecular and outlet portions together constitute the functional RV. The wall of atrialized RV shows variable degrees of hypertrophy and thinning. The atrialized RV can get disproportionately dilated resulting in a small functional RV. The ATL is usually not displaced but is often redundant and has multiple fenestrations. The tendinous cords are often short and poorly formed as a part of the "tethering" of the leaflet. The ATL is usually long and forms a sail like intracavitary curtain. This significantly deformed ATL tissue can cause RV outflow obstruction.

- *Dilation of the right AV junction (true tricuspid annulus)*: The true tricuspid annulus is not displaced and is demarcated by right coronary artery, which courses in the right AV groove.[14] The true annulus gets markedly dilated. The atrialized RV separates the true annulus from functional RV. Often the functional RV can also get significantly dilated causing bowing of interventricular septum that compresses the left ventricle (LV) cavity.[12]
- *Accessory bypass tracts*: Accessory AV conduction pathways tend to cluster along the septal and posterior aspects of the true AV ring, accounting for the extraordinarily high incidence of re-entrant tachycardias in Ebstein anomaly.[17]

ASSOCIATED ANOMALIES

A patent foramen ovale or true atrial septal defect (ASD) is present in 80–94% of patients with Ebstein anomaly.[13] In utero, the reduced flow passing through the right ventricular outflow tract affects the development of the pulmonary annulus, the main pulmonary arteries or its branches, sometimes resulting in pulmonary atresia or hypoplastic pulmonary artery (PA).[14] Additional associated anomalies include left-sided lesions such as bicuspid or atretic aortic valves, subaortic stenosis, coarctation, mitral valve prolapse, accessory mitral valve tissue, or muscle bands of the LV and ventricular septal defects (VSDs).[13] Lesions affecting left ventricular myocardium (noncompaction) or valves can affect the prognosis. RV volume overload and low arterial oxygen levels leading to left ventricular interstitial fibrosis and diastolic dysfunction, have been described in adults with Ebstein anomaly.[14]

EBSTEIN ANOMALY AND CONGENITALLY CORRECTED TRANSPOSITION OF GREAT ARTERIES

Most patients with congenitally corrected transposition of the great arteries have an abnormal systemic TV, fulfilling the Ebstein anomaly criteria in 15–50% of patients.[13] Left-sided Ebstein anomaly differs from the classical right-sided Ebstein anomaly in the following criteria: the AV sulcus circumference is not increased; the anterior leaflet of the valve is smaller and not sail like, with a cleft in 30% of cases. Additionally, the atrialization of the inlet portion of the morphological RV is minimal. Here, the extent of regurgitation across the valve decides the symptom status.[18]

PHYSIOLOGY

The forward flow across the pulmonary valve is determined by many factors, among which are the adequacy of functional RV, severity of tricuspid regurgitation, PA pressure, and the presence of RV outflow obstruction. During atrial systole, the atrialized RV acts as a passive reservoir resulting in reduced amount of blood reaching functional RV. The tricuspid regurgitation also adds on to the dilatation of the RA and atrialized RV. Presence of an interatrial communication results in right-to-left shunt at the atrial level.[4] Functional pulmonary atresia occurs when the pulmonary arterial pressure exceeds the pressure that the RV is able to generate and the pulmonary valve leaflets fail to open.

CLASSIFICATION

In 1988, Carpentier proposed a classification for Ebstein anomaly based on the degree of severity of various components of the anomaly and with a surgical perspective (**Figs. 2A to D**).

- *Type A*: The volume of the true RV is adequate.
- *Type B*: There is a large atrialized component of the RV but the ATL moves freely.
- *Type C*: The ATL is severely restricted in its movement and may cause significant obstruction of the right ventricular outflow tract.
- *Type D*: Almost complete atrialization of the RV with the exception of a small infundibular component.[19]

This classification lost its initial significance with the introduction of newer surgical techniques.

A simpler and subjective way of expressing the severity as anatomically mild, moderate, or severe, is based on the echocardiographic image. It is derived from an impression

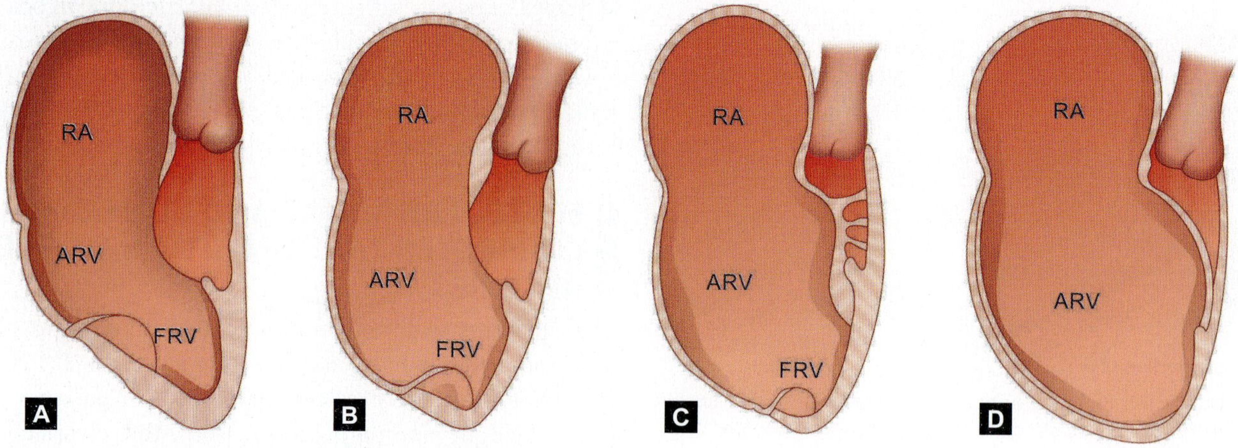

Figs. 2A to D: Carpentier classification of Ebstein anomaly.
(ARV: atrialized right ventricle; FRV: functional right ventricle; RA: right atrium)

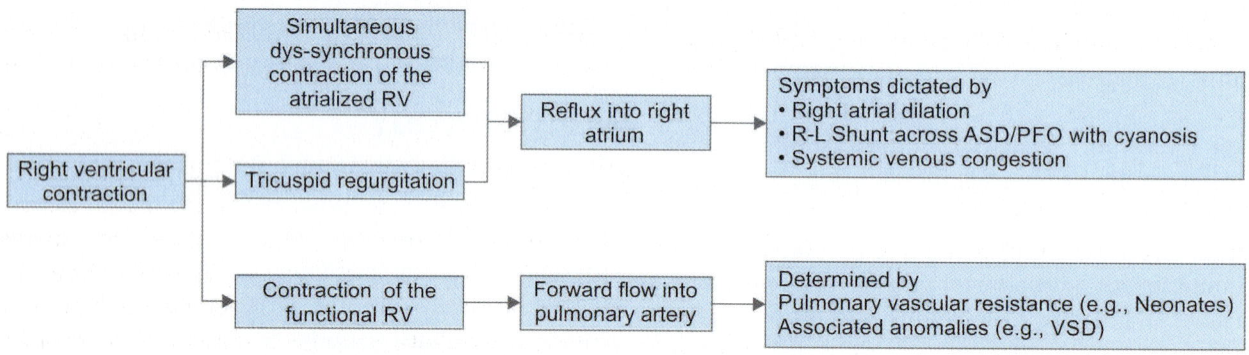

Fig. 3: Physiology of Ebstein's anomaly. The most significant physiological alterations are shown here. Additional features that impact clinical manifestations include tachyarrhythmias from re-entrant circuits.
(ASD: atrial septal defect; PFO: patent foramen ovale; RV: right ventricle; VSD: ventricular septal defect)

formed by summation of the degree of displacement of the leaflets, tethering of the ATL, size of atrialized RV, and the functional RV.[4]

CLINICAL PRESENTATION

Ebstein anomaly has a wide spectrum of clinical presentation depending on the age at presentation and anatomical severity. The hemodynamics is determined by the amount of tricuspid regurgitation, right-to-left shunt across the atrial septum and degree of RV dysfunction (**Fig. 3**).

Ebstein Anomaly in the Fetus

Ebstein anomaly can lead to severe TV regurgitation and cardiac dysfunction in utero, resulting in fetal cardiomegaly, heart failure, pulmonary hypoplasia, hydrops, and even intrauterine demise.[20] Fetal tachyarrhythmias can be the presenting symptom as accessory pathways are common. Severe cardiac enlargement can result in the heart occupying most of the intrathoracic space needed for lung growth. This, along with reduced pulmonary blood flow, can contribute to severe pulmonary hypoplasia, which may complicate neonatal resuscitation.[21]

Neonate

Clinical presentation in neonates can vary from an asymptomatic newborn to a critically ill cyanotic neonate. They can present as congestive heart failure due to tricuspid regurgitation and ventricular dysfunction. This may also be associated with cyanosis due to right-to-left shunt across the atrial septum.

The condition can be duct-dependent due to functional/anatomical pulmonary atresia. Functional pulmonary atresia results from a dysfunctional RV failing to pump against a pulmonary vascular bed with high resistance (RV contractility—afterload mismatch).[22] Such patients are likely to improve once the pulmonary vascular resistance decreases and forward flow across the pulmonary valve improves.

The neonates with most severe forms are the ones with a spiral hemodynamic failure. A "circular shunt" is maintained by a patent ductus arteriosus (PDA) that results in an ineffective circulation of aortic blood back to the aorta without crossing the capillary bed (**Fig. 4**).[14] Pulmonary regurgitation results in retrograde flow down the RV into the LV via the ASD. It creates a hemodynamically unstable

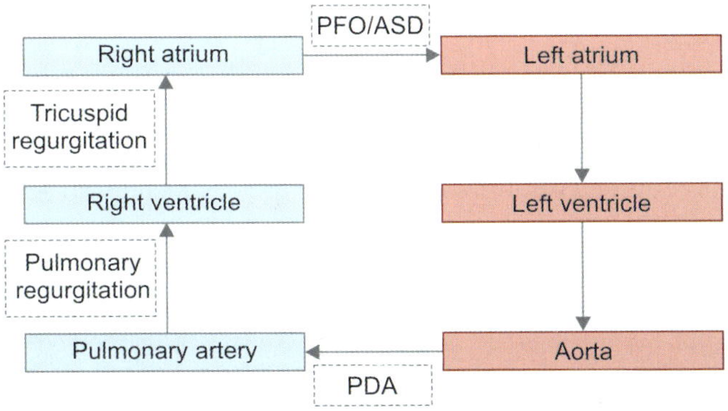

Fig. 4: Circular shunt in Ebstein anomaly. The blood leaving the aorta takes the route through a patent ductus, to the pulmonary arteries, to the right ventricle due to pulmonary insufficiency, to the right atrium through the dysplastic tricuspid valve, to the left atrium through the foramen ovale, then to the left ventricle whereupon it returns to the aorta.
(ASD: atrial septal defect; PDA: patent ductus arteriosus, PFO: patent foramen ovale)

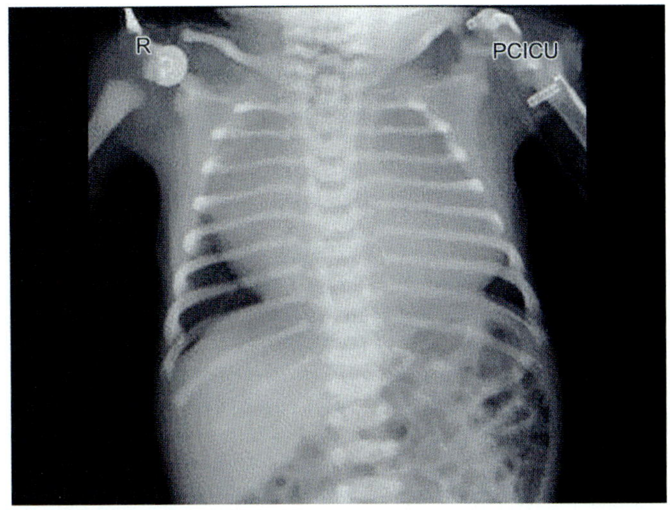

Fig. 5: Massive cardiomegaly on chest X-ray in a newborn with Ebstein anomaly.

condition with severe hypoxia and diminished systemic cardiac output. Prostaglandin E1 to maintain duct patency in such patients can worsen the hemodynamics and lead to clinical deterioration.[23]

Childhood to Adolescence

The common symptoms in childhood and adolescence are exercise intolerance, fatigue, palpitation, and cyanosis. The exercise capacity is reduced due to the effect of tricuspid regurgitation, ventricular dysfunction, right-to-left shunt, and reduced cardiac output.

The predominant symptom in adolescents and adults is related to arrhythmias. Supraventricular re-entrant tachyarrhythmias (accessory pathway-mediated reciprocating tachycardia, AV nodal re-entrant tachycardia) or atrial flutter or fibrillation due to progressive atrial dilatation or the association of both can occur. More than 75% of the accessory pathways identified in Ebstein anomaly are capable of bidirectional conduction and can present as narrow QRS (orthodromic conduction) or wide QRS (antidromic conduction) short RP tachycardia. These arrhythmias tend to be recurrent and are often resistant to drug treatment.[illegible]

Tachyarrhythmia, if associated with right to left across the atrial septum, can lead onto paradoxical embolization, brain abscess, and death. Sudden death due to ventricular arrhythmias can occur even in asymptomatic patients, especially if atrial fibrillation is associated with pre-excitation.[24]

In milder forms of the disease, pregnancy is well tolerated. Maternal cyanosis increases the chance of fetal loss and low birth weight.[14]

PHYSICAL EXAMINATION

Physical findings depend on the anatomical severity and right-to-left shunting. Children with milder forms are usually missed; a murmur or systolic click may be the only finding. Cyanosis and clubbing can be present in older patients with right-to-left shunting. The large V-wave of jugular venous pressure (JVP) (due to tricuspid regurgitation) is not manifested because the wave gets dampened in the significantly dilated RA.

Auscultation often reveals multiple heart sounds. First heart sound is widely split due to increased excursion of abnormally large anterior tricuspid leaflet and delayed closure.[25] Right bundle branch block can result in a widely-split second heart sound. Early systolic click or sail sound may be heard, which most likely occurs when the large, sail-like TV reaches the limit of systolic excursion.[26] Prominent S3/S4 may be present during ventricular filling. Together they result in triple/quadruple gallop. Pansystolic murmurs of tricuspid regurgitation are not always audible because of the low velocity to and fro flow in the presence of a dilated RA. It may be audible in less severe forms and adults. Soft systolic murmur is more often heard which increases with inspiration.

INVESTIGATIONS

Chest X-ray

Ebstein anomaly is one of the few cardiac lesions, which can present with massive cardiomegaly. A critically ill neonate can present with a wall-to-wall heart with the cardiac silhouette filling the thorax (box-shaped heart)[27] (**Fig. 5**). In severe forms, the heart becomes globe-shaped with a narrow pedicle (similar to large pericardial effusion). A cardiothoracic ratio >0.65 is prognostic for poor outcomes in a symptomatic neonate.[20]

The most consistent feature is right atrial enlargement; the RA and atrialized RV may be huge and fill the entire right hemithorax. Pulmonary vascularity can be normal or decreased depending on the forward flow across RV outflow tract and lung hypoplasia. Chest X-ray can be near normal in milder forms of the disease (**Fig. 6**).

Electrocardiogram

The common electrocardiogram (ECG) findings in Ebstein anomaly include tall and broad P-waves (right atrial enlargement), prolonged PR-interval, right bundle branch block pattern, fragmented QRS complex, evidence of accessory pathways, and tachyarrhythmias (**Fig. 7**).[13]

The fragmented QRS complex ("splintered," "fractionated", or "second QRS") is described as a normal-shaped R-wave directly followed by a broad positive deflection (R′) of lower amplitude.[28] The progressive myocardial fibrosis and scarring within the atrialized RV wall may represent the morphologic substrate for QRS prolongation and fractionation.[29]

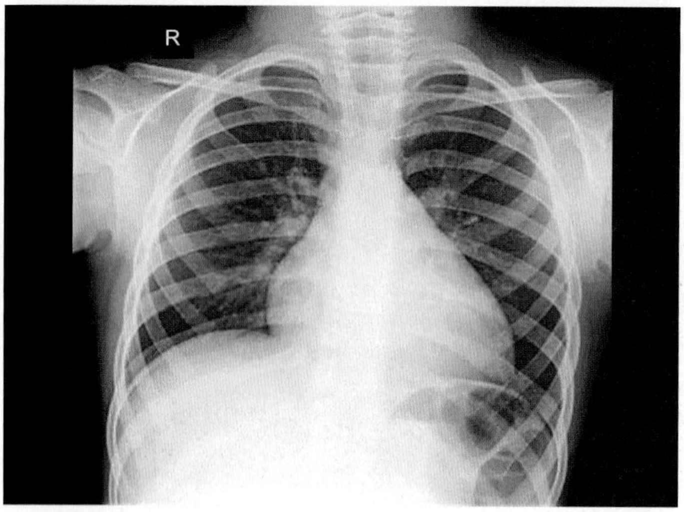

Fig. 6: Ebstein anomaly chest X-ray with mild cardiomegaly in a relatively older child. The characteristic appearance of the cardiac contour results from right atrial enlargement.

Arrhythmia Evaluation

Incidence of accessory pathways in Ebstein anomaly far exceeds the general population and is estimated to be between 10 and 38%. Majority of them are capable of bidirectional conduction and generate pre-excitation (delta wave) (**Fig. 8**) on the electrocardiogram.[17] In the current era, a comprehensive electrophysiology study can be considered as a part of preoperative evaluation in older children and adults with Ebstein anomaly. Arrhythmia evaluation is recommended in view of occurrence of postoperative arrhythmias even in patients with concealed pathways and the fact that electrophysiologic study and ablation can be problematic in the postoperative setting.

Echocardiography

Echocardiography forms the primary modality in diagnosing Ebstein anomaly. It helps to identify the abnormal tricuspid valvar complex and to guide management. Two-dimensional (2D) echocardiography can show displacement of the proximal attachments of the TV leaflets, distal attachments of the TV leaflets, tricuspid regurgitation, right heart size, and ventricular function.

The single most important feature in the diagnosis of Ebstein anomaly is the rotational and downward displacement of the attachment of STL in apical four-chamber view (**Fig. 9A**). The degree of apical displacement of STL by ≥8 mm/m^2 body surface area (displacement index) differentiates Ebstein anomaly from other congenital causes of tricuspid regurgitation.[30] This displacement into the right ventricular apex mainly involves the STL and PTL; the ATL is not usually displaced.

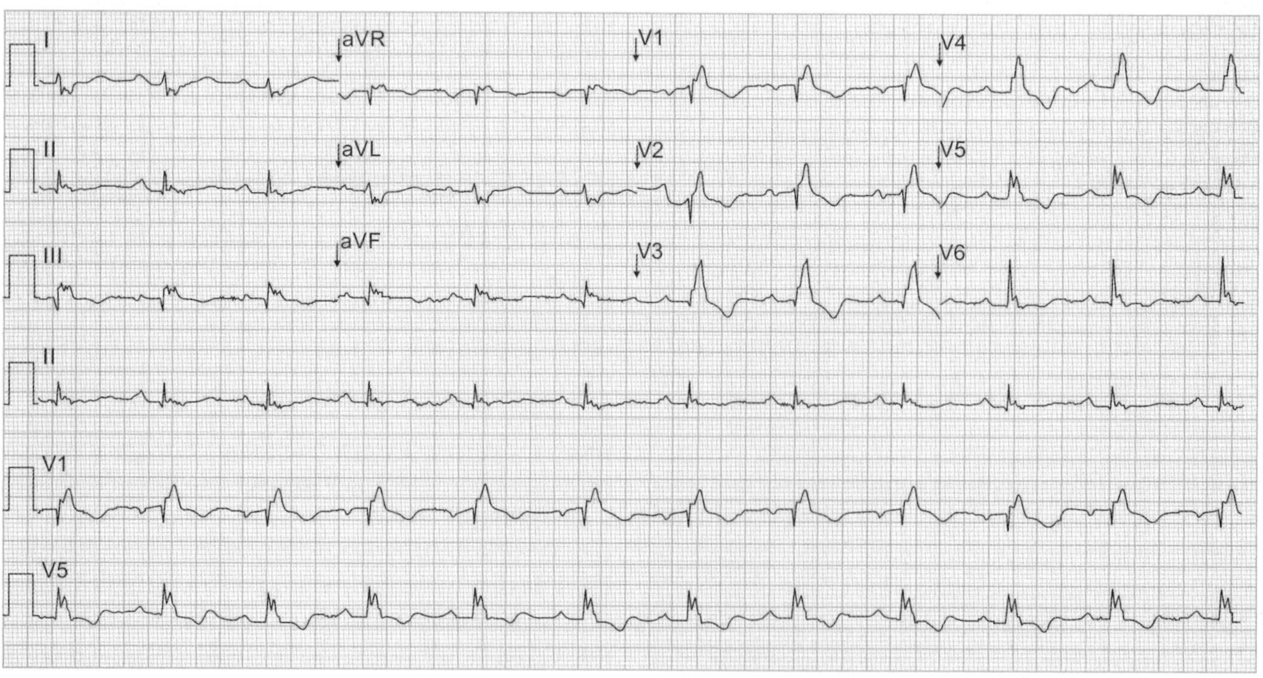

Fig. 7: Electrocardiogram (ECG) from an adult with Ebstein anomaly. The features evident here are the tall P waves in lead II, P waves are fragmented in lead III, QRS complexes show a right bundle branch block pattern with low voltages and fragmented terminal vectors.

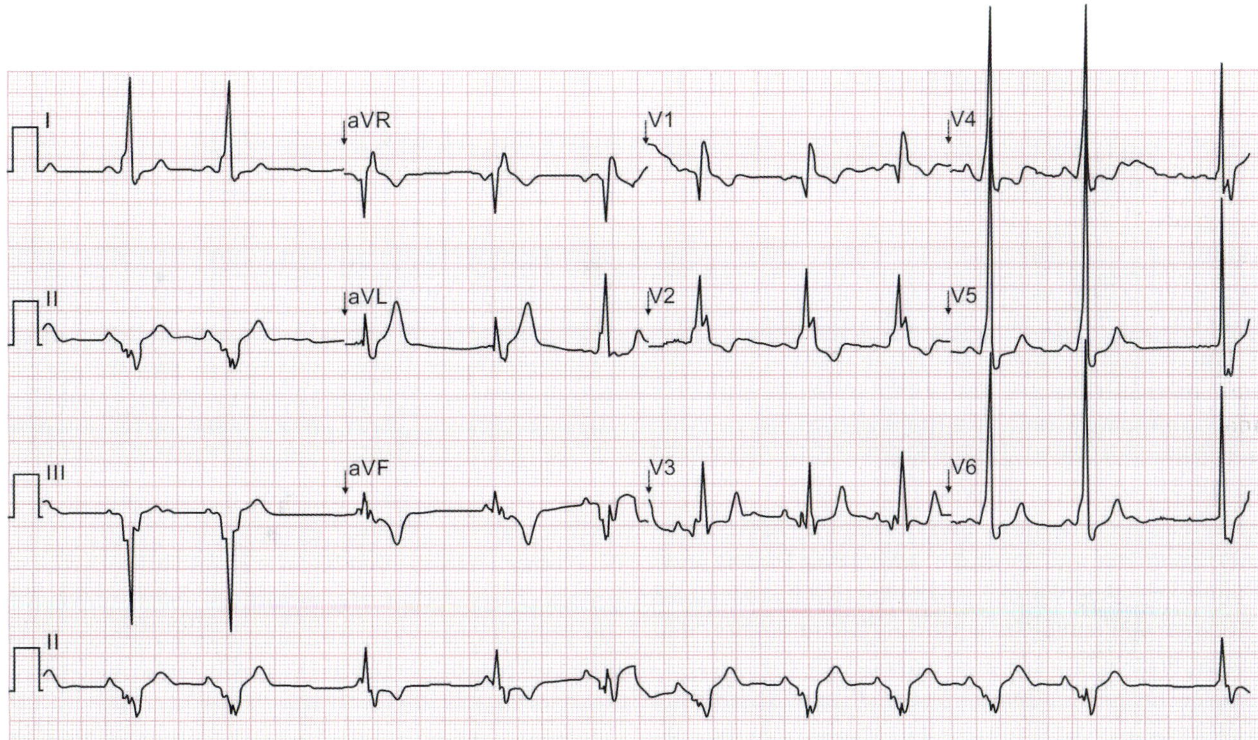

Fig. 8: Electrocardiogram (ECG) from a patient with Ebstein anomaly with pre-excitation resulting from a right-sided accessory pathway. Note the delta waves in leads I, V2-V6 together with short PR interval.

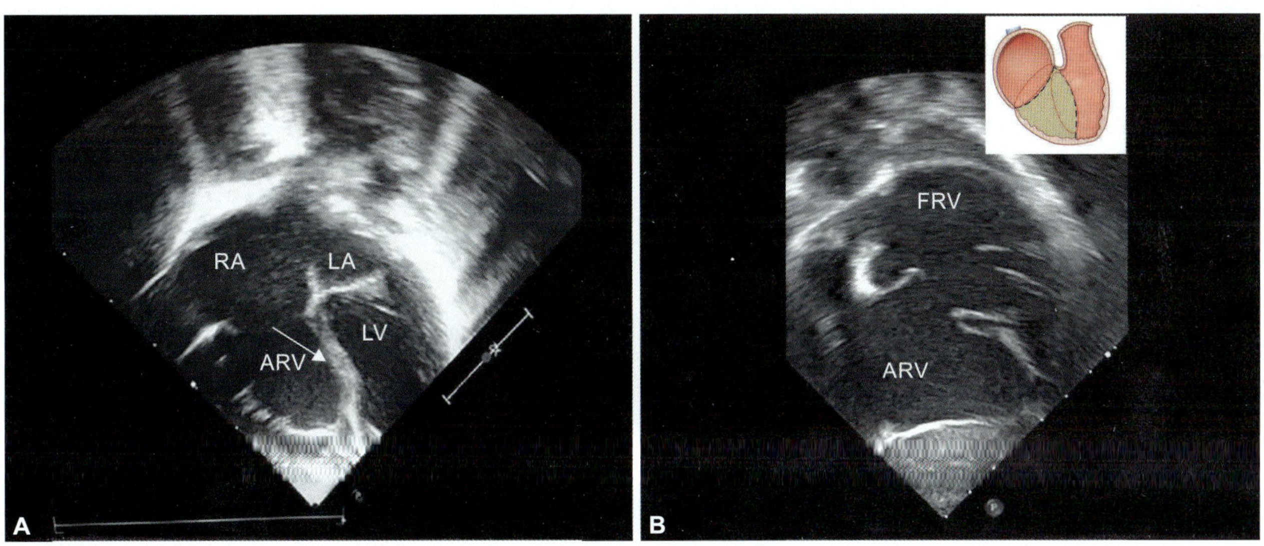

Figs. 9A and B: Apical four-chamber view (A) and subcostal view (B) of a child with severe Ebstein anomaly showing a grossly displaced and tethered septal leaflet (arrow). The anterior leaflet is long and sail-like. Functional RV (FRV) is small.
(ARV: atrialized right ventricle; RA: right atrium; LA: left atrium; LV: left ventricle)

Failure of delamination results in points of tethering (chordal attachments from the body or free edge of the TV) to the underlying myocardium, which results in restricted leaflet excursion. In severe forms of the disease, the leaflets can be dysplastic and plastered to the myocardium further restricting the mobility. The displaced leaflets and sail-like ATL displaces coaptation point into the RV cavity. The restricted mobility of leaflets results in defective coaptation and tricuspid regurgitation. The distal attachment of the leaflets and motion of the ATL affects prognostic outcome and surgical management.[13]

The subcostal view also reveals a significantly dilated RA and atrialized RV, defined by the wall separating the true from the functional annulus of the RV (**Fig. 9B**).

The GOSE (Glasgow Outcome Score Extended) Score or (Great Ormond Street Score) or Celermajer Index described by Celermajer et al. is commonly used as a measure to express the severity of the lesion.[31] This includes the combined area of the RA and atrialized RV relative to the combined area of the functional RV, left atrium (LA), and LV, as measured in the apical four-chamber view at end-diastole (ratio <0.5: grade 1; ratio 0.5–0.99: grade 2; ratio 1.0–1.49: grade 3; and if ratio ≥1.5: grade 4). Risk of mortality increases with the value of this ratio.

The pulmonary valve can be atretic along with hypoplasia of the pulmonary arteries. Often the valve apparatus is well-formed and atresia is functional in neonates. Presence of pulmonary regurgitation and circular shunt supports functional pulmonary atresia. Right ventricle can be dysplastic with wall thickening, dilatation, and dyskinesia of the atrialized or functional RV. Paradoxical motion of the interventricular septum causes alteration in the right and left ventricular geometry and function. Associated lesions such as ASD, mitral valve prolapse, ventricular septal defect, and left ventricular abnormalities such as noncompaction can also be identified.

Assessing Ebstein anomaly using three-dimensional (3D)-transthoracic echocardiography provides additional information about the leaflet surface, tethering of the leaflets, and the right ventricular volume and function.

Exercise Testing

In patients with Ebstein anomaly, exercise testing is done to assess exercise capacity, exercise-induced desaturation, and tachyarrhythmias.

One of the major contributing factors to preoperative exercise intolerance is hypoxemia. The presence of an ASD significantly influences the oxygen saturation at rest and at peak exercise. However, in patients with an insignificant shunt, right ventricular dysfunction may be a contributing factor to the lower cardiac output response relative to oxygen uptake. Oxygen saturation at rest and exercise help in risk stratification and assessing functional limitation. Definitive surgery for Ebstein anomaly results in improved exercise tolerance.[32]

Cardiac Catheterization

Cardiac catheterization is rarely necessary and is used mostly for hemodynamic analysis in selected situations. The main parameters that are assessed are left ventricular end-diastolic pressure (measure of LV dysfunction) and PA sizes and pressures when a bidirectional cavopulmonary shunt is being considered.

Cardiac Magnetic Resonance

Cardiac magnetic resonance imaging (MRI) helps in better visualization of the PTL of the TV and quantitative assessment of the right atrial and ventricular size and function as compared to echocardiography. Cardiac magnetic resonance (CMR) data compliments the information obtained by echocardiography and allows more accurate assessment of disease severity, risk stratification, surgical planning, and postoperative evaluation and follow-up.[33]

MEDICAL MANAGEMENT

Ebstein anomaly can be diagnosed prenatally by fetal echocardiography. The physiology is tolerated in utero by most of the fetuses. However, they need close monitoring as the disease can progress with advancing gestation. High-risk fetuses can be identified by features such as extreme cardiomegaly, severe tricuspid regurgitation, pulmonary atresia, evidence of circular shunt (pulmonary regurgitation), tachyarrhythmia, and hydrops. Fetal tachyarrhythmia can be managed by transplacental or fetal therapy. Refractory tachyarrhythmias with evolution of heart failure carry a poor prognosis.

Prenatal counseling has to be individualized depending on the severity of the spectrum of Ebstein anomaly. Termination of pregnancy may be considered in selected cases with poor prognosis (risk of intrauterine fetal demise). It is preferable to deliver the high-risk fetuses at a tertiary neonatal care unit as they are likely to be critically ill, needing ventilatory support and prostaglandin infusion to maintain duct patency soon after birth.

Neonatal management depends on the pathophysiology (**Flowchart 1**). In the less severe forms with reasonable functional RV and stable hemodynamics, the neonates are managed with oxygen and pulmonary vasodilators (sildenafil) and prostaglandin infusion if antegrade pulmonary blood flow is not adequate. The goal of medical management is to support functional RV and improve antegrade pulmonary blood flow by reducing pulmonary vascular resistance.[34] Such neonates are closely followed up into infancy with plan for elective surgery.

Unstable critically ill neonates require tertiary neonatal support with ventilation, inhaled nitric oxide, prostaglandin infusion, and inotropic support. Neonate with functional pulmonary atresia might need a trial of prostaglandin withdrawal to enable duct constriction and establish antegrade pulmonary blood flow. The prognosis is generally quite poor in such neonates.

Neonate with circular shunt is a rare, but serious scenario with hemodynamic instability. The neonate is usually very sick, with metabolic acidosis and elevated filling pressures. Frequently, these babies are born prematurely as a result of intrauterine stress and hydrops, which makes their management even more difficult. There is volume overload on the heart with low cardiac output and severe hypoxia which is worsened by prostaglandin infusion as it keeps the duct open. If anatomic pulmonary atresia is ruled out, this group might benefit from withdrawal of prostaglandin infusion.[35]

In patients who are hypoxic despite ventilation and using pulmonary vasodilators, it is reasonable to try extracorporeal

Flowchart 1: Management algorithm of a newborn with Ebstein anomaly (EA), PA (pulmonary atresia), PBF (pulmonary blood flow), PVR (pulmonary vascular resistance), and PGE1 (prostaglandin E1).

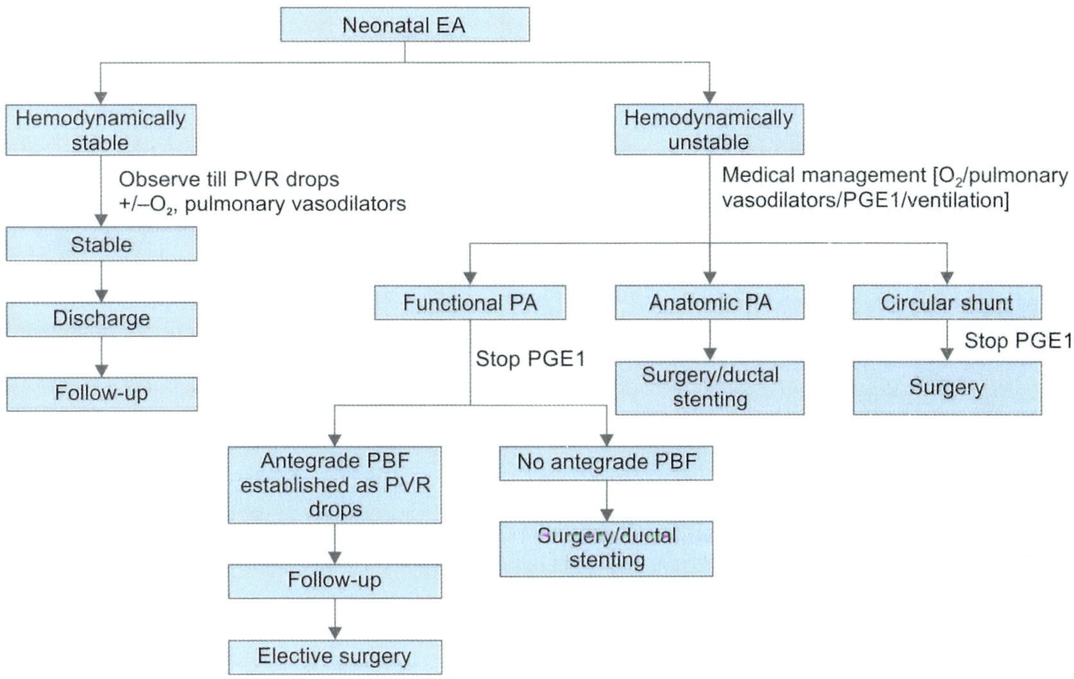

membrane oxygenation (ECMO) for few days to allow remodeling of the RV as the pulmonary vascular resistance decreases.

Infants and children are kept on regular follow-up for evolution of symptoms, cardiomegaly, and arrhythmias. Apart from surgery, prevention and management of tachyarrhythmias form the mainstay of treatment. Infective endocarditis prophylaxis is recommended despite its low risk. Athletes with severe form of the anomaly are restricted from sports unless the lesion has been optimally repaired and is arrhythmia free. Patients with severe forms of the disease who are in cardiac failure and are not candidates for surgery should be treated with standard heart failure medications.[12]

CATHETER ABLATION

Electrophysiological evaluation and radiofrequency ablation should be performed preoperatively or intraoperatively when feasible, in patients with Ebstein anomaly associated with tachyarrhythmias.

SURGICAL MANAGEMENT

The goals of surgical treatment of Ebstein anomaly include correction of TV regurgitation, restoration of right ventricular function, and treatment of other comorbid cardiac conditions such as arrhythmias.[36]

The decision for a biventricular repair/single ventricle pathway is taken depending on the anatomical and functional assessment and the clinical status.

The key steps in a biventricular repair are TV repair with reduction in the size of RA and atrialized RV along with establishment of RV-PA continuity in case of pulmonary valve atresia.

The two tricuspid valvuloplasty techniques described are Knott-Craig monocusp technique (ATL is adequately mobilized to help coaptation with the ventricular septum to achieve valvular competency) and Da Silva's cone repair.

Cone Repair

Though numerous techniques of valve repair have been described for Ebstein anomaly, the cone reconstruction as described by Dr da Silva and coworkers is different in that it is the closest to an "anatomic repair"[37] with leaflet-to-leaflet tissue coaptation and the hinge point at the true AV junction. Since the introduction of this technique, there has been a paradigm shift in the surgical approach to Ebstein anomaly.[38]

It provides the most anatomic repair with a 360-degree circumferential presence of coapting tricuspid valvular tissue with a central flow of blood as compared to the eccentric flow with the monocusp technique. There is leaflet-to-leaflet coaptation rather than a leaflet-to-ventricular septum coaptation, with a more symmetric distribution of the closing pressure to the leaflets. Since it utilizes all the three leaflets of the TV, it can be used in surgical correction of wide morphological variations that are seen in Ebstein anomaly.[34,37]

The key steps **(Figs. 10A and B)** include:

- *Mobilization of the leaflets from the functional annulus*: All three leaflets, except certain portions of the ATL are disconnected from the functional annulus leaving a 1–2 mm rim of valvular tissue retained on the annulus in

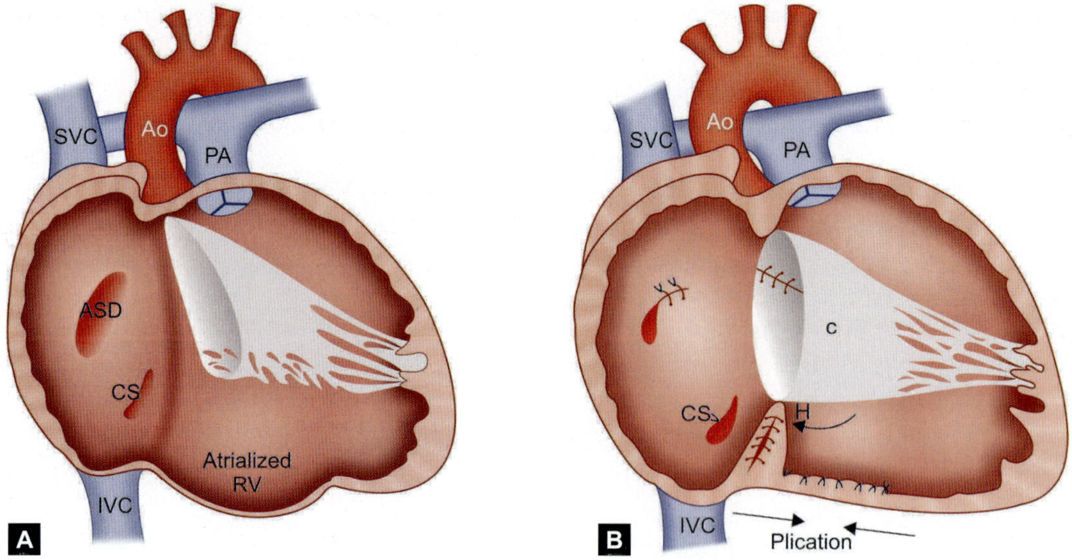

Figs. 10A and B: The cone repair for Ebstein anomaly. (A) The mobilized tricuspid valve tensor apparatus; (B) The recreated cone (c) with resuspension of the tensor apparatus at the level of the normal tricuspid valve annulus.
(Ao: aorta; ASD: atrial septal defect; CS: coronary sinus; IVC: inferior vena cava; PA: pulmonary artery; RV: right ventricle; SVC: superior vena cava)

order to facilitate reattachment. This edge is called the "cut edge."

- *Delamination of the leaflets*: The body of the leaflets is mobilized off the ventricular wall and the septum by dividing fibromuscular adhesions.
- Creation of a freely mobile and supported leading edge or the coapting edge subtended by existing primary chordae or newly created autologous chordae.
- *Creation of the cone*: Once all the three leaflets have been mobilized, the cut edge of the PTL is brought to the cut edge of the STL by a clockwise rotation to create a 360-degree "cone" of tricuspid tissue. This represents a "cone", the base of which is formed by the mobilized cut edges of the leaflet and the apex by the coapting edge with the subtending chordal structures.
- Plication of the atrialized RV longitudinally from an apex-to-base fashion and reduction of the anatomic annulus.
- Attachment of the "cut edge" to the plicated true annulus.
- *Closure of ASD*: The ASD is closed in a valved or fenestrated fashion when concerns exist about adequacy of RV and right heart dysfunction, thus acting as a "pop-off" with a right-to-left shunt.
- *Reduction atrioplasty*: Redundant portion of the enlarged RA is resected before atrial closure.[34]

One and a Half Ventricle Repair

A 1.5 ventricle repair (valvuloplasty + bidirectional Glenn) may be needed in case there is significant RV dilation or dysfunction or the TV orifice area (after repair) is inadequate to accommodate a full systemic venous return. Glenn shunt reduces the volume load on the RV by 35–45%.

Univentricular Repair

Single ventricle repair is considered in patients with severe RV dysfunction and in more progressive disease such as Carpentier's types C and D.

The key steps in univentricular repair include the following:

- Ligation of the main PA if the valve is incompetent and ligation of the PDA with creation of a systemic-to-pulmonary artery shunt.
- Fenestrated patch closure of the TV (modified Starnes procedure)[39] to allow for RV decompression. Alternatively, a Sano-RV exclusion procedure[40] can be performed. The principle here is to create functional tricuspid atresia, which is tolerated better.
- Creation of an unrestrictive interatrial communication for exit of blood from RA.
- Reducing right atrial size to allow for growth of the lungs.

This initial stage is followed by completion of single ventricle palliation by bidirectional Glenn procedure and Fontan procedure. However, the RV should be reassessed at each step for conversion to 1.5 ventricle or biventricular repair.

Indications for surgery in the neonate with Ebstein anomaly include anatomic pulmonary atresia, a circular shunt, dependency on prostaglandins or mechanical ventilation, worsening cyanosis or heart failure with inability to tolerate feeds due to mesenteric congestion, and severe forms such as Carpentier type C/D or GOSE Score >3.[34]

Neonates with Circular Shunt

The aim of managing these patients with a high mortality risk should be to allow survival, rather than trying to achieve a biventricular repair. The management approach should be individualized to each patient and decided after a detailed echocardiographic assessment soon after birth. Surgical option should essentially be considered in patients with circular shunts with evidence of low cardiac output and metabolic acidosis who do not respond to medical management.

A trial of ductal ligation should be done if the RV has an adequate muscle mass and can generate a pressure gradient of >30 mm Hg across the TV. If the patient becomes hypoxic despite using pulmonary vasodilators, then it is reasonable to try ECMO for few days to allow remodeling of the RV as the pulmonary vascular resistance drops. If the RV fails to generate forward flow after a week, then Starnes procedure is preferred.[35]

Indications for surgery in older children and adults include increasing cardiomegaly, deepening cyanosis, exercise intolerance and fatigue, heart failure, paradoxical embolism, progressive RV dilatation on echocardiography, and new onset of atrial and ventricular arrhythmias. TV repair should be the goal in younger patients, whereas selective TV replacement is considered for older and adult patients. Severe RV dilatation, severe TV annular dilatation, complete absence of STL tissue, and high degree of leaflet muscularization make the valve repair more difficult. Heart transplant should be considered in patients with severe LV dysfunction, especially if associated with structural left heart lesions.[34]

NATURAL HISTORY AND OUTCOME

Fetus

It is likely that more severe forms of the disease are detected in early pregnancy as a result of cardiomegaly (right atrial dilatation) or evidence of hydrops. The longer a fetus is exposed to the progressive pathophysiological aberrations of Ebstein anomaly in utero, the more likely is the patient to experience its adverse sequelae.[41] Thus, an earlier diagnosis indicates a severe form of the disease and a poor outcome.

Reduced LV filling occurs as a result of direct compression of LV by the dilated right-sided chambers as well as by distortion of the atrial septal anatomy that diminishes right-to-left flow at the atrial level. This can lead to reduced systemic cardiac output, diminished end-organ perfusion, acidosis, and ultimately, fetal demise.

Presence of pulmonary regurgitation (circular shunt) at the time of diagnosis is a powerful hemodynamic indicator of systemic steal and is associated with adverse outcomes. Severe tricuspid regurgitation in the fetus may lead to cardiomegaly, hydrops, and arrhythmia, with demise rates as high as 48%.[21] Pulmonary hypoplasia as a result of significant cardiomegaly can lead to deleterious cardiorespiratory compromise in the postnatal period. As per a multicenter study by Freud et al., independent predictors of mortality at the time of diagnosis were gestational age <32 weeks, higher TV annulus diameter Z score, pulmonary regurgitation, and a pericardial effusion.[41]

Ebstein anomaly in the fetus is a progressive lesion where hemodynamic compromise can occur as the gestation advances. A multicenter, retrospective study by Tierney et al. highlights that great caution must be taken in counseling before 24 weeks, as the absence of factors associated with poor outcome early in pregnancy may be falsely reassuring.[42]

Neonates and Children

The true "natural history" of Ebstein anomaly cannot be determined in the current era as it is modified by surgical treatment.

In one of the largest studies of over 500 patients with Ebstein anomaly, published >30 years ago (in the pre-echocardiographic era); a high mortality rate was noted during first few months of life followed by plateauing of mortality to an average of 12%, scattered uniformly throughout childhood and adolescence.[43]

The natural history of Ebstein anomaly is summarized by Celermajer et al.[44] Death hazard in neonates is due to heart failure and intrauterine cardiomegaly leading to pulmonary hypoplasia. Those surviving the first month of life are at high risk of late hemodynamic deterioration, perioperative mortality, or even sudden cardiac death. In contrast, childhood Ebstein anomaly usually presents with an incidental murmur and the outlook is good. Adolescents and adults with Ebstein anomaly usually present with arrhythmia due to pre-excitation, progressive atrial dilation, or the association of both. Actuarial survival for all live-born patients was 67% at 1 year and 59% at 10 years.

The GOSE Score provides information about prognosis: when the ratio is 1.5, 100% mortality is likely; a ratio of 1–1.4 indicates a decreased risk of death, with an early mortality of 10% but a mortality rate in early childhood of 45%; and a ratio of <1 indicates 92% survival.[44,45] Cardiothoracic ratio of >85% and presence of cyanosis associated with GOSE score >1 were predictors of mortality in 100% neonates.[45]

Surgical Outcome

Most patients with Ebstein anomaly undergo surgical repair at some point in their life. The earlier approach was to delay intervention, which resulted in operating on advanced stages of the anomaly with high mortality and poor valve durability.

There have been significant advances in the operative management of Ebstein anomaly and the most contemporary repair—the cone repair provides a near anatomic result compared to the earlier repairs that were based on ATL monocusp coaptation with the ventricular septum.[38] Although monocusp repairs were effective in the short term, many patients eventually required reoperation and TV replacement.

A retrospective analysis of 235 patients who underwent cone repair between June 2007 and October 2015 by

Holst et al.[38] inferred that there was a sustained reduction in tricuspid regurgitation and a clear reduction in RV size that also showed progressive improvement over time and had an advantageous impact on RV remodeling. Overall survival at 6 years in this study was 98%. Freedom from TV replacement and late reoperation were 97.1% and 97.3%, respectively at 6 years.

Analysis of multi-institutional data concerning operations and outcomes in neonates and infants with Ebstein anomaly by Holst et al.[46] revealed an overall mortality of 18.6% with notably higher rates for neonates (27.4%) than for infants (9.2%). They conclude that patients with Ebstein anomaly who present symptomatically in infancy, particularly in the neonatal period are at high operative risk, and operative outcomes were relatively similar to historical cohorts.[47,48]

CONCLUSION

Ebstein anomaly is a complex congenital heart disease (CHD) with a wide spectrum of anatomical and clinical presentations. Echocardiography supplemented by novel imaging techniques enables precise anatomical and functional assessment. Improvement in knowledge about the anatomy and hemodynamics has brought significant changes in the medical and surgical management strategies. The management has to be highly individualized as the presetation varies from a symptomatic fetus to an asymptomatic adult. The cone repair (anatomical repair) has revolutionized the surgical management and outcome with the follow-up results that appear promising. However, the prognosis continues to be poor in a sick fetus and critically ill neonate.

ACKNOWLEDGMENT (SURGICAL FIGURE)

Dr Balaji Srimurugan, Amrita Institute of Medical Sciences, Kochi, Kerala, India.

REFERENCES

1. Morray B. Preoperative physiology, imaging, and management of Ebstein's anomaly of the tricuspid valve. In: Seminars in Cardiothoracic and Vascular Anesthesia. Los Angeles: SAGE Publications; 2016. pp. 74-81.
2. Mazurak M, Kusa J. The two anomalies of Wilhelm Ebstein. Tex Heart Inst J. 2017;44(3): 198-201.
3. Soloff LA, Stauffer HM, Zatuchni J. Ebstein's disease: report of the first case diagnosed during life. Am J Med Sci. 1951;222(5):554.
4. Attenhofer Jost CH, Connolly HM, Dearani JA, Edwards WD, Danielson GK. Ebstein's anomaly. Circulation. 2007;115(2): 277-85.
5. Correa-Villaseñor A, Ferencz C, Neill CA, David Wilson P, Boughman JA. Ebstein's malformation of the tricuspid valve: genetic and environmental factors. Teratology. 1994;50(2): 137-47.
6. Sicko RJ, Browne ML, Rigler SL, Druschel CM, Liu G, Fan R, et al. Genetic variants in isolated Ebstein anomaly implicated in myocardial development pathways. PLoS One. 2016;11(10): e0165174.
7. Budde BS, Binner P, Waldmüller S, Höhne W, Blankenfeldt W, Hassfeld S, et al. Noncompaction of the ventricular myocardium is associated with a de novo mutation in the β-myosin heavy chain gene. PloS One. 2007; 2(12):e1362.
8. van Engelen K, Postma AV, Van De Meerakker JB, Roos-Hesselink JW, Helderman-Van Den Enden AT, Vliegen HW, et al. Ebstein's anomaly may be caused by mutations in the sarcomere protein gene MYH7. Neth Heart J. 2013;21(3):113-7.
9. Patorno E, Huybrechts KF, Bateman BT, Cohen JM, Desai RJ, Mogun H, et al. Lithium use in pregnancy and the risk of cardiac malformations. N Engl J Med. 2017;376(23):2245-54.
10. McKnight RF, Adida M, Budge K, Stockton S, Goodwin GM, Geddes JR. Lithium toxicity profile: a systematic review and meta-analysis. Lancet. 2012;379(9817):721-8.
11. Poels EM, Bijma HH, Galbally M, Bergink V. Lithium during pregnancy and after delivery: a review. Int J Bipolar Disord. 2018;6(1):26.
12. Attenhofer CJ, Connolly HM, Edwards WD, Hayes D, Warnes CA, Danielson GK. Ebstein anomaly-review of a multifaceted congenital cardiac condition. Swiss Med Weekly. 2005; 135(19-20):269-81.
13. Paranon S, Acar P. Ebstein's anomaly of the tricuspid valve: from fetus to adult. Heart. 2008;94(2):237-43.
14. Lamers WH, Virágh S, Wessels A, Moorman AF, Anderson RH. Formation of the tricuspid valve in the human heart. Circulation. 1995;91(1):111-21.
15. Dahou A, Levin D, Reisman M, Hahn RT. Anatomy and physiology of the tricuspid valve. JACC Cardiovasc Imaging. 2019;12(3): 458-68.
16. Holst KA, Connolly HM, Dearani JA. Ebstein's anomaly. Methodist DeBakey Cardiovasc J. 2019;15(2):138.
17. Walsh EP. Ebstein's anomaly of the tricuspid valve: a natural laboratory for re-entrant tachycardias. JACC Clin Electrophysiol. 2018; 4(10):1271-88.
18. Wallis GA, Debich-Spicer D, Anderson RH. Congenitally corrected transposition. Orphanet J Rare Dis. 2011;6(1):22.
19. Carpentier A, Chauvaud S, Macé L, Relland J, Mihaileanu S, Marino JP, et al. A new reconstructive operation for Ebstein's anomaly of the tricuspid valve. J Thorac Cardiovasc Surg. 1988;96(1):92-101.
20. Roberson DA, Silverman NH. Ebstein's anomaly: echocardiographic and clinical features in the fetus and neonate. J Am Coll Cardiol. 1989;14(5):1300-7.
21. Hornberger LK, Sahn DJ, Kleinman CS, Copel JA, Reed KL. Tricuspid valve disease with significant tricuspid insufficiency in the fetus: diagnosis and outcome. J Am Coll Cardiol. 1991;17(1):167-73.
22. Baek JS, Yu JJ, Im YM, Yun TJ. Outcomes of neonatal Ebstein's anomaly without right ventricular forward flow. J Thorac Cardiovasc Surg. 2016;152(2):516-21.
23. Wald RM, Adatia I, Van Arsdell GS, Hornberger LK. Relation of limiting ductal patency to survival in neonatal Ebstein's anomaly. Am J Cardiol. 2005;96(6):851-6.
24. Frescura C, Angelini A, Daliento L, Thiene G. Morphological aspects of Ebstein's anomaly in adults. Thorac Cardiovasc Surg. 2000; 48(04):203-8.
25. Willis PW, Craige E. First heart sound in ebstein's anomaly: observations on the cause of wide splitting by echo-phonocardiographic studies before and after operative repair. J Am Coll Cardiol. 1983;2(6):1165-8.
26. Fontana ME, Wooley CF, Goodwin RS, Rieser GF. Sail sound in Ebstein's anomaly of the tricuspid valve. Circulation. 1972;46(1):155-64.
27. Ferguson EC, Krishnamurthy R, Oldham SA. Classic imaging signs of congenital cardiovascular abnormalities. Radiographics. 2007; 27(5):1323-34.
28. Acharya P, Ang JR, Gitler B. Ebstein anomaly with QRS fragmentation on electrocardiogram. J Investig Med High Impact Case Rep. 2017; 5(1):2324709616688710.

29. Egidy Assenza G, Valente AM, Geva T. QRS duration and QRS fractionation on surface electrocardiogram are markers of right ventricular dysfunction and atrialization in patients with Ebstein anomaly. Eur Heart J. 2013;34(3):191-200.
30. Shiina A, Seward JB, Edwards WD, Hagler DJ, Tajik AJ. Two-dimensional echocardiographic spectrum of Ebstein's anomaly: detailed anatomic assessment. J Am Coll Cardiol. 1984;3(2 Part 1):356-70.
31. Celermajer DS, Cullen S, Sullivan ID, Spiegelhalter DJ, Wyse RK, Deanfield JE. Outcome in neonates with Ebstein's anomaly. J Am Coll Cardiol. 1992;19(5):1041-6.
32. MacLellan-Tobert SG, Driscoll DJ, Mottram CD, Mahoney DW, Wollan PC, Danielson GK. Exercise tolerance in patients with Ebstein's anomaly. J Am Coll Cardiol. 1997;29(7):1615-22.
33. Attenhofer Jost CH, Edmister WD, Julsrud PR, Dearani JA, Tepe MS, Warnes CA, et al. Prospective comparison of echocardiography versus cardiac magnetic resonance imaging in patients with Ebstein's anomaly. Int J Cardiovasc Imaging. 2012;28(5):1147-59.
34. Sainathan S, da Silva LD, da Silva JP. Ebstein's anomaly: contemporary management strategies. J Thorac Dis. 2020; 12(3):1161-73.
35. Elzein C, Subramanian S, Ilbawi M. Surgical management of neonatal Ebstein's anomaly associated with circular shunt. World J Pediatr Congenit Heart Surg. 2019;10(1):116-20.
36. Kim MS, Lim HG, Kim WH, Lee JR, Kim YJ. Long-term results after surgical treatment of Ebstein's anomaly: a 30-year experience. Korean Circ J. 2016;46(5):706-13.
37. Dearani JA, Bacha E, da Silva JP. Cone reconstruction of the tricuspid valve for Ebstein's anomaly: anatomic repair. Oper Tech Thorac Cardiovasc Surg. 2008;13(2):109-25.
38. Holst KA, Dearani JA, Said S, Pike RB, Connolly HM, Cannon BC, et al. Improving results of surgery for Ebstein anomaly: where are we after 235 cone repairs? Ann Thorac Surg. 2018; 105(1):160-8.
39. Reemtsen BL, Fagan BT, Wells WJ, Starnes VA. Current surgical therapy for Ebstein anomaly in neonates. J Thorac Cardiovasc Surg. 2006; 132(6):1285-1290.
40. Sano S, Fujii Y, Kasahara S, Kuroko Y, Tateishi A, Yoshizumi K, et al. Repair of Ebstein's anomaly in neonates and small infants: impact of right ventricular exclusion and its indications. Eur J Cardiothorac Surg. 2014;45(3):549-555.
41. Freud LR, Escobar-Diaz MC, Kalish BT, Komarlu R, Puchalski MD, Jaeggi ET, et al. Outcomes and predictors of perinatal mortality in fetuses with Ebstein anomaly or tricuspid valve dysplasia in the current era: a multicenter study. Circulation. 2015; 132(6):481-9.
42. Tierney ES, McElhinney DB, Freud LR, Tworetzky W, Cuneo BF, Escobar-Diaz MC, et al. Assessment of progressive pathophysiology after early prenatal diagnosis of the Ebstein anomaly or tricuspid valve dysplasia. Am J Cardiol. 2017;119(1):106-11.
43. Watson H. Natural history of Ebstein's anomaly of tricuspid valve in childhood and adolescence. An international co-operative study of 505 cases. Br Heart J. 1974;36(5):417.
44. Celermajer DS, Bull C, Till JA, Cullen S, Vassillikos VP, Sullivan ID, et al. Ebstein's anomaly: presentation and outcome from fetus to adult. J Am Coll Cardiol. 1994;23(1):170-6.
45. Knott-Craig CJ, Overholt ED, Ward KE, Razook JD. Neonatal repair of Ebstein's anomaly: indications, surgical technique, and medium-term follow-up. Ann Thorac Surg. 2000;69(5):1505-10.
46. Holst KA, Dearani JA, Said SM, Davies RR, Pizarro C, Knott-Craig C, et al. Surgical management and outcomes of Ebstein anomaly in neonates and infants: a society of thoracic surgeons congenital heart surgery database analysis. Ann Thorac Surg. 2018;106(3):785-91.
47. McElhinney DB, Salvin JW, Colan SD, Thiagarajan R, Crawford EC, Marcus EN, et al. Improving outcomes in fetuses and neonates with congenital displacement (Ebstein's malformation) or dysplasia of the tricuspid valve. Am J Cardiol. 2005;96(4):582-6.
48. Dearani JA, Mora BN, Nelson TJ, Haile DT, O'Leary PW. Ebstein anomaly review: what's now, what's next? Expert Review of Cardiovasc Ther. 2015;13(10):1101-9.

34 CHAPTER

Tetralogy of Fallot

Sushil Azad

INTRODUCTION

Tetralogy of Fallot (TOF) is the most common form of cyanotic congenital heart disease (CHD). It consists of a wide range of anatomic malformations leading to varied clinical expressions and management strategies.

EPIDEMIOLOGY

Tetralogy of Fallot makes up to 16.8% of all CHDs. Of all infants born with CHD, approximately 3.5% will have TOF, giving a figure of 0.28 per 1,000, or 1 in 3,600 live births.[1] A 2002 meta-analysis of the incidence of CHD, which included 41 studies pertaining to TOF, suggested the best estimate of incidence would be 577 cases per million live births.[2] TOF has a nearly equal sex distribution with a slight male preponderance. A patient with TOF has approximately 2–3% chance of having a sibling with any form of CHD but not necessarily TOF. And a patient with TOF has a 3–4% chance of having a child with CHD.[3]

ETIOLOGY

The etiology can be broadly divided into genetic and environmental factors. Familial causes make up only a very small fraction of the total TOF cases, but its frequency is increased in consanguineous populations. A chromosomal duplication or a microdeletion at the 22q11.2 locus occurs in approximately 20% of patients with TOF and single gene mutations have been identified in others.[4] Trisomy syndromes such as Down syndrome, Edwards syndrome, and Patau syndrome make up to 5–7% of syndromic TOF. But in at least 50–60% of patients with TOF, the causal genetic influences remain unidentified.[5] Among the environmental exposures that contribute a modest increase in the risk for TOF include maternal pregestational diabetes, febrile or viral illnesses, vitamin A exposure, and exposure to organic solvents.[6]

ANATOMY AND EMBRYOLOGY

The first anatomical description of TOF was done by a Danish anatomist named Niels Stensen in 1671. However, it was in 1888 that, Etienne-Louis Arthur Fallot gave the classical description of four cardiac malformations, i.e., stenosis of the pulmonary artery (PA), a ventricular septal defect (VSD), hypertrophy of the right ventricle, and rightward deviation of the origin of the aorta. The eponym "tetralogy of Fallot" was coined by Maude Abbott, the early 20th century pediatric cardiology pioneer in a 1924 article that classified congenital heart defects.[7] More recently it is believed that TOF should be basically considered as a single malformation ("monology") from which all the four characteristic features occur. The defining morphology is the failure of the development of the subpulmonary infundibulum that results in anterior-cephalad deviation of the outlet septum (infundibulum) relative to the rest of the ventricular septum which is easily seen on echocardiography. The identification of this anatomy is the key to diagnosis.[8]

CLINICAL FEATURES

Patients with TOF most often present in infancy with cyanosis due to right-to-left shunting of blood at the level of the VSD. The degree of right ventricular (RV) outflow tract obstruction often correlates with the degree of cyanosis and the timing of presentation. Thus, patients with mild pulmonary obstruction present late, the so-called "pink TOF," with some infants presenting with features of congestive heart failure at 4–6 weeks of life due to increasing pulmonary flow as their pulmonary vascular resistance drops and they shunt left-to-right across the VSD. On the other hand, patients with severe obstruction may present soon after birth on closure of the ductus arteriosus.

Almost two-thirds of newborns with TOF appear healthy at birth, and by 6 months of age over half will have become desaturated at rest. This occurs due to worsening of infundibular stenosis and right ventricular hypertrophy (RVH), which leads to further reduction in pulmonary blood flow and increase in right-to-left shunting across the VSD. Intermittent cyanotic episodes are one of the defining features of TOF.[9] A typical spell is characterized by a progressive increase in the rate and depth of breathing and leads to paroxysmal hyperpnea, deepening of cyanosis, limpness, syncope, and occasionally convulsions, cerebrovascular accidents, and if left untreated may lead to death. Peak incidence is between the second and sixth month of life, with comparatively few spells after the age of 2 years, and only rarely in adults. Spells in infants are typically initiated by the stress of feeding, crying, or a bowel movement and also seen after awakening from a long deep sleep.[10] The mechanism for cyanotic spells remains unknown but the previous assumption that they were related to "infundibular spasm" fails to explain the frequent recognition of identical clinical features in those lacking a subpulmonary infundibulum (e.g., tetralogy with a doubly committed VSD) and those with pulmonary atresia.

The physiologic cause of spells can be explained by the following:

- Acute increase in inotropy due to release of endogenous catecholamine in response to pain
- Pain and anxiety lead to an increase in the systemic oxygen consumption thereby reducing the mixed venous oxygen content
- An acute reduction in systemic vascular resistance (they are more frequent during febrile illness)
- Decreased circulating blood volume (RV preload) resulting from dehydration (precipitated by a diarrhea episode) and tachycardia (atrial tachycardia leads to further reduction in pulmonary blood flow).

It is hypothesized that cyanotic spells may result from mechanoreceptor stimulation from the right ventricle quite like as in neurocardiogenic syncope. Increased contractility (due to catecholamines) and decreased RV size (due to various factors) can trigger a reflex resulting in hyperventilation, some peripheral vasodilation without bradycardia, and this may initiate a spell. This mechanism explains most of the precipitating events and many other issues about cyanotic spells more satisfactorily.[11]

Older children present with exertional dyspnea which usually worsens with age. A characteristic posture of squatting is seen in this age group. Squatting increases peripheral vascular resistance and thus decreases the magnitude of the right-to-left shunt across the VSD. With longstanding reduction in oxygen saturation, erythrocytosis develops with a number of clinical consequences. Brain abscess is more common in older patients and is associated with the extent of polycythemia. On the other hand, stroke for cerebrovascular accidents occurs in infants with associated iron deficiency. Rarely, hemoptysis may occur in the older child due to rupture of bronchial collaterals.

Physical Examination

An infant with TOF on auscultation will have a normal first heart sound, a single second heart sound, and a systolic ejection murmur audible at the left upper and middle sternal border. This murmur originates from turbulent blood flow across the narrowed right ventricular outflow tract (RVOT). The loudness of the murmur is proportional to, and the length of the murmur inversely proportional to, the degree of right ventricular outflow tract obstruction (RVOTO). The murmur may become virtually inaudible in those who are experiencing a spell. The patient who has aortopulmonary collaterals may have continuous murmur heard loudest over the back.

INVESTIGATIONS

It is necessary to obtain a complete blood count and correct iron deficiency early. Additionally, it is important to identify the presence of 22q11 deletion (CATCH 22) in patients with TOF at the earliest convenient opportunity. The high prevalence of 20% perhaps merits routine testing in all patients. This has significant implications that include requirement of irradiated blood during heart surgery, delayed postoperative recovery because of airway-related issues, hypocalcemia, delayed development, late learning difficulties, and a high prevalence of psychiatric illnesses in adulthood. Also, it has important bearing on the recurrence risks in future pregnancies. A higher likelihood of 22q11 microdeletion is indicated by specific dysmorphic features and by a high mean platelet volume in the complete blood counts.[12]

Electrocardiogram Findings

Preoperatively, the ECG (electrocardiogram) in TOF shows sinus rhythm with normal or rightward axis deviation and RVH. RVH is characterized by a tall monophasic R wave often confined to lead V1, with an abrupt change to an rS pattern in V2 signifying early transition **(Fig. 1)**. The presence and depth of Q waves and the amplitude of R waves in leads V5-V6 are indicative of the magnitude of pulmonary blood flow and of left ventricular (LV) filling. Reduced pulmonary flow with an underfilled left ventricle is accompanied by rS patterns in leads V2-V6. A balanced shunt is accompanied by small q waves and well-developed R waves in lead V5-V6. A left to right shunt is accompanied by deeper left precordial Q waves and relatively tall R waves.[13] There may be left axis deviation in TOF associated with atrioventricular septal defect (AVSD).

Chest X-ray

The chest radiograph findings in TOF consist of a normal cardiac size but with an upturned apex, also known as a boot-shaped heart **(Fig. 2)**. This is due to RVH, deficiency of the main PA segment (seen as a notch in the upper left cardiac border), and reduced pulmonary vascularity. There is a right aortic arch in 20–30% of patients with TOF.

Echocardiography

Echocardiography plays a pivotal role in the diagnosis and follow-up of patients with TOF. All of the characteristic

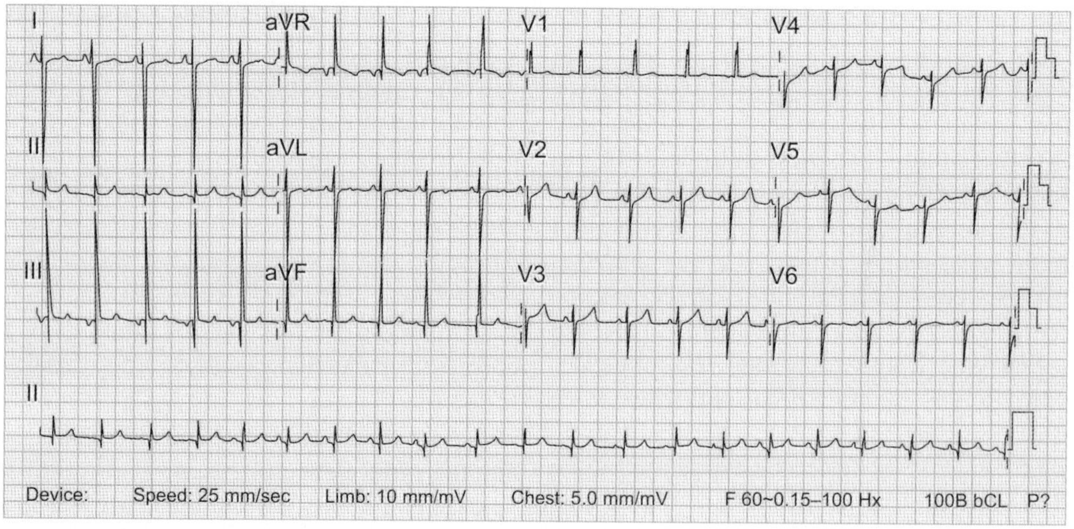

Fig. 1: Electrocardiogram from a 3-year-old girl with Fallot's tetralogy. There is moderate right axis deviation. Right ventricular hypertrophy is represented by a tall monophasic R wave in lead V1 with a typical abrupt change to an rS complex in lead V2 representing early transition.

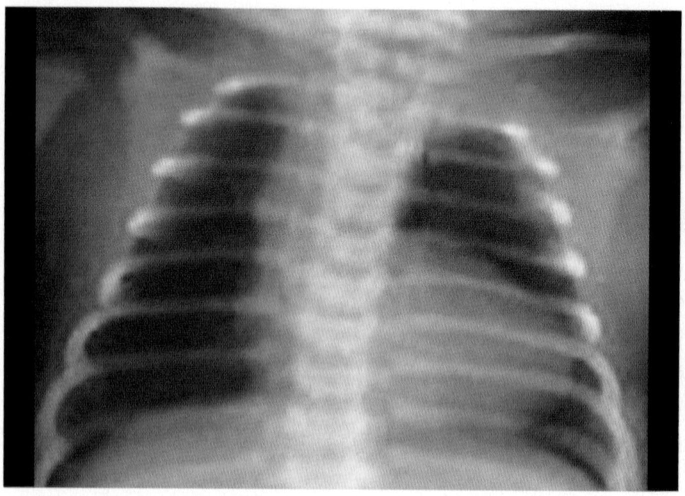

Fig. 2: A chest X-ray anteroposterior (AP) view of a 1-year-old girl with tetralogy of Fallot (TOF). The heart is typically boot-shaped. The ascending aorta is prominent, the main pulmonary artery segment is concave, and the lungs are oligemic.

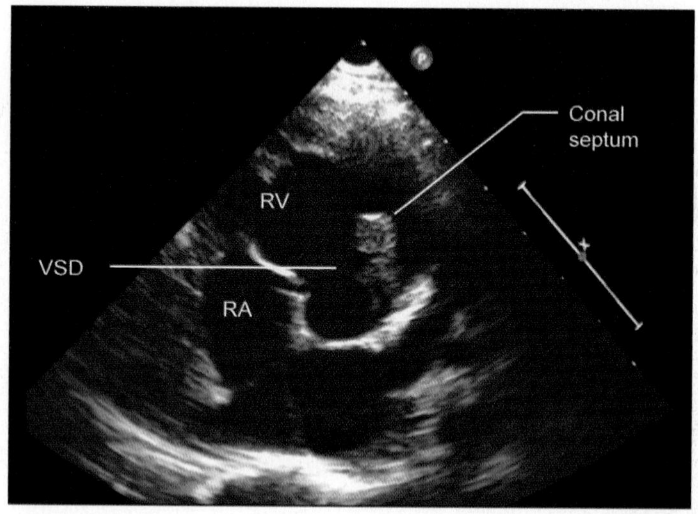

Fig. 3: Two-dimensional (2D) echocardiography (parasternal short axis view) of a case of tetralogy of Fallot (TOF) showing perimembranous ventricular septal defect (VSD) with anterior deviation of conal septum which is the hallmark of TOF.
(RA: right atrium; RV: right ventricle)

features of the anatomy and physiology can be obtained from a transthoracic echocardiography **(Figs. 3 to 6)**.

A preoperative assessment must include the following:

- The location and number of VSDs.
- The anatomy and severity of obstruction of the RVOT. The obstruction can be at the level of infundibulum, pulmonary valve and the pulmonary annulus, and the adjacent main PA.
- The size and anatomy of the main PA, the pulmonary arterial confluence, and the branch pulmonary arteries.
- The coronary arteries must be imaged, specifically looking for any major branch crossing the RVOT.
- The presence of any associated anomalies such as atrial septal defect, patent ductus arteriosus (PDA), and AVSD must also be looked for. Additionally, selected patients may have aortopulmonary collaterals that can potentially impact the postoperative course.

Echocardiography also plays a major role at the time of corrective surgery, particularly in checking the completeness of VSD closure and relief of RVOTO. During the immediate postoperative phase, it is routinely used to assess LV and RV functions and the status of the RVOT. Its role in postoperative follow-up is primarily in the surveillance for late complications, particularly in patients with pulmonary regurgitation (PR).

Other Imaging Modalities

High-resolution computed tomography (CT) **(Fig. 7)** scan is used in those cases where the coronary anatomy or the peripheral branch pulmonary arteries are not well visualized

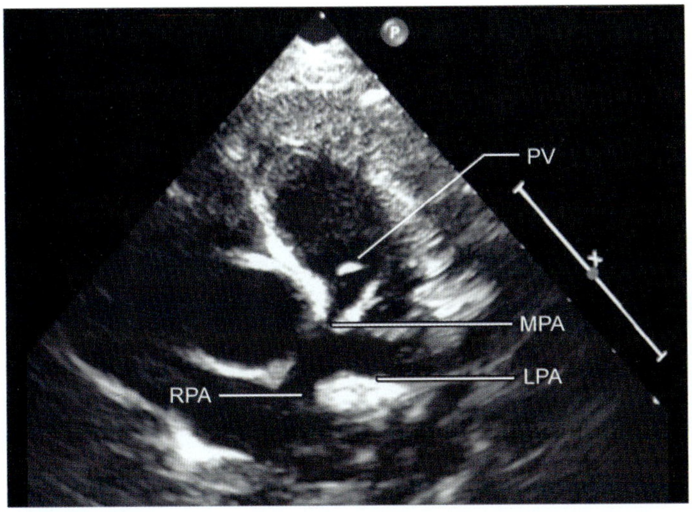

Fig. 4: Color Doppler two-dimensional (2D) echocardiography (parasternal short axis view) of a case of tetralogy of Fallot (TOF) showing valvular and supravalvular obstruction with confluent branch pulmonary arteries.
(LPA: left pulmonary artery; MPA: main pulmonary artery; PV: pulmonary valve; RPA: right pulmonary artery)

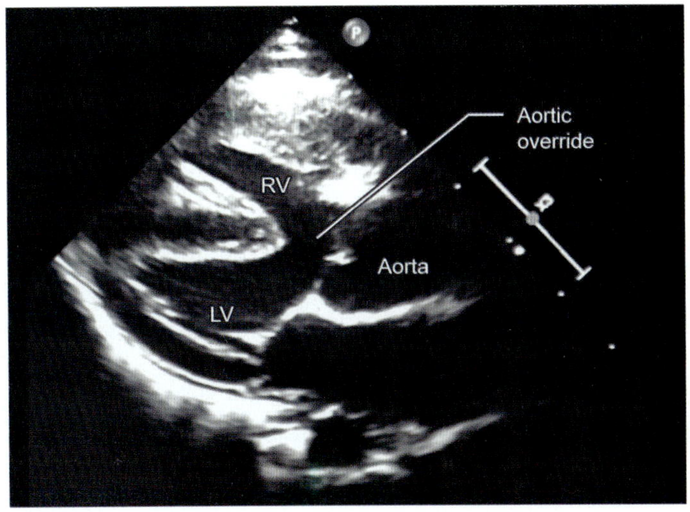

Fig. 5: Two-dimensional (2D) echocardiography (parasternal long axis view) of a case of tetralogy of Fallot (TOF) showing overriding of aorta with a large perimembranous ventricular septal defect (VSD).
(LV: left ventricle; RV: right ventricle)

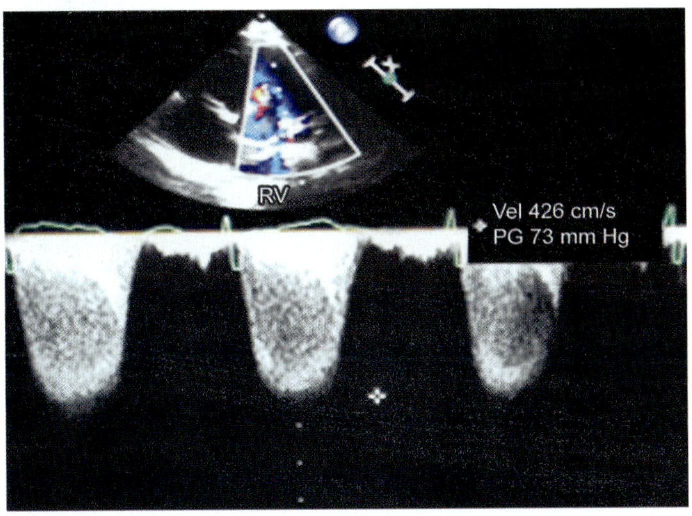

Fig. 6: Continuous wave Doppler echocardiography of right ventricular outflow tract (RVOT) showing severe pulmonary stenosis in a case of tetralogy of Fallot (TOF).

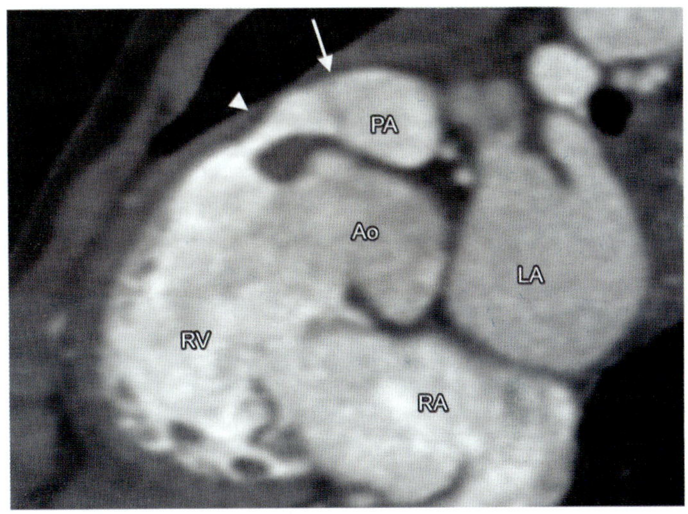

Fig. 7: Sagittal oblique computed tomography (CT) image showing infundibular (arrowhead) and valvular (arrow) stenosis.
(Ao: aorta; LA: left atrium; PA: pulmonary artery; RA: right atrium; RV: right ventricle)

by echocardiography. Magnetic resonance imaging (MRI) has become an important component of postoperative follow-up, particularly in the older adolescent and adult with repaired TOF. The poor acoustic windows generally found in adults do not limit MRI and, furthermore, the ability to accurately quantify RV volumes and PR is an important advantage. MRI can also be used to quantify RV and LV systolic functions, assess differential pulmonary blood flow, and quantify PR. It is used to monitor the potentially deleterious effects of chronic PR on RV volume and function. It is used in clinical decision-making regarding interventions such as pulmonary valve replacement (PVR) in postoperative TOF patients.[14]

Cardiac Catheterization and Angiography

Preoperative cardiac catheterization and invasive angiography have almost entirely been replaced by imaging modalities such as echocardiography and cardiac CT. However, cardiac catheterization and angiography may be indicated in the following situations:

- Suspicion of multifocal PA supply, aortopulmonary collaterals, anomalous origin of one PA, and anomalous pulmonary venous drainage. Cardiac catheterization also allows preoperative occlusion of aortopulmonary collaterals to enable a smooth postoperative course in selected patients.

- Patients where complete preoperative information is not possible by echocardiography or cardiac CT.
- Postsurgical repair patients who have a residual VSD or PA branch stenosis.

NATURAL HISTORY

Although two-thirds of the newborns with TOF have normal saturation at birth, by 6 months of age more than half develop resting cyanosis. This is due to the progressive pulmonary stenosis that decreases the pulmonary blood flow. The natural history of TOF is better than that of many other cyanotic congenital heart defects. A cyanotic toddler is four times as likely to have a TOF than all the other forms of cyanotic heart disease combined. Nevertheless, the natural survival is substantially reduced. There are two retrospective studies that considered autopsy data from fixed geographical populations during time periods prior to the availability of any cardiac surgery that serve to illustrate the natural history of TOF. One of them, conducted in Denmark, found that without surgical intervention only 66% of babies born with TOF survived to 1 year of age, 49% until 3 years of age, and only 24% lived to the age of 10 years. Deaths are seldom from congestive heart failure in children but occur more often in adults. In the most severely affected infants and young children, death is usually due to hypoxemia (with or without acute spells), infective endocarditis, brain abscess, intercurrent infections, and cerebrovascular accidents.

MEDICAL MANAGEMENT

Surgical correction is the definitive treatment for TOF, but in certain cases, a brief period of medical therapy is needed. The main aims of medical management are as follows:

- Prevention of cyanotic spells
- Correction of anemia to maintain Hb >14 g/dL
- Preventing complications from infection such as brain abscess or infective endocarditis.

General supportive measures include iron-folic acid supplementation along with nutritional management and a close watch on growth. Infants who develop gradual worsening of cyanosis usually do so as a result of increasing RVOTO and will benefit little from medical therapy. Cyanotic spells warrant institution of a specific treatment plan that is usually effective in controlling the episode. Additionally, beta-blockers such as oral propranolol in a dose of 0.25–1 mg/kg 2–3 times per day is used for prevention of cyanotic spells. Although most consider that even a single cyanotic spell is an indication for early surgery.

Management of Cyanotic Spells

The basic pathophysiology of cyanotic spells should be thought of as an acute imbalance between systemic and pulmonary blood flows resulting from a vicious spiral of changes in inotropy secondary to endogenous catecholamine release, increased systemic oxygen consumption, reduced systemic vascular resistance, and reduced RV preload due to increased heart rate. Thus, the aim of therapy must be directed to reverse this imbalance and disrupt the pathophysiologic spiral by relieving pain and anxiety (to reduce heart rate and systemic oxygen consumption), increase systemic vascular resistance, and increase pulmonary blood flow.

The following treatment is used to manage a typical cyanotic spell[15]:

- Since most cyanotic spells are provoked by crying, the infant should be picked up and comforted as soon as an episode begins, ideally while being held in a knee-chest position that kinks or compresses the femoral arteries and increases peripheral systemic vascular resistance.
- If no improvement is seen within a few minutes, oxygen should be administered, and intravenous access obtained. Administration of oxygen may provide some increase of oxygen uptake, but this is of limited value when pulmonary blood flow is very low.
- An intravenous bolus (5–10 mL/kg) of crystalloid fluid is often sufficient to increase intravascular volume, maximize preload, and improve cardiac output. Colloids are seldom indicated. Blood transfusion is indicated in anemic infants with cyanotic spells.
- Morphine (0.1–0.2 mg/kg) should be given to relieve pain and anxiety. It reverses the endogenous catecholamine release, reducing heart rate and lowering respiratory rate. Intravenous route is preferable but intramuscular route can also be used.
- Intravenous beta-blockers in the form of propranolol (0.015–0.02 mg/kg), metoprolol (1–4 μg/kg/min), or the shorter-acting esmolol (0.5 mg/kg given over 1 minute, thereafter, continued as an infusion). These agents lower the heart rate and improve diastolic ventricular filling thus increasing preload. It is seen that propranolol shifts the blood oxygen dissociation curve to the right and thus could increase the release of oxygen from hemoglobin at the tissue site.[16] Also, blockade of β-adrenoceptors could result in vasoconstriction and increase peripheral vascular resistance, thus elevating systemic arterial pressure, or preventing reductions of pressure. This would help to maintain pulmonary blood flow.
- Intravenous sodium bicarbonate (1 mEq/kg) may be required if there is evidence of worsening acidosis despite the measures above. It is best administered after sufficient dilution as a part of volume resuscitation.
- In cases not responding to the above measures, intravenous systemic vasoconstrictors in the form of phenylephrine (boluses of 0.005–0.001 mg/kg), or norepinephrine (0.05–1.0 mg/kg/min), may be required. They have predominantly α-adrenoceptor stimulant effects and produces marked systemic vasoconstriction thereby improving the pulmonary blood flow.

- Ultimately anesthesia, intubation, and ventilation remain the last resort to reduce the work of breathing and reduce oxygen consumption and improve mixed venous oxygen content. This needs to be followed by surgical correction or palliation (if not suited). In selected situations, it may be possible to improve pulmonary blood flow by means of a catheter procedure such as balloon pulmonary valvotomy, stenting of the PDA, or RVOT.

SURGICAL MANAGEMENT

Surgical options for TOF can be divided into palliative procedures and definitive surgery. The definitive surgical procedure for TOF consists of closing the VSD and relieving the right ventricular outflow obstruction. Closure of the VSD is accomplished with a patch of flexible synthetic material such as Dacron or using pericardium. Relief of RVOTO may require removal of hypertrophied muscle in the infundibulum together with a surgical valvotomy of the pulmonary valve, if required. In most modern cardiac surgical programs, every effort is made to retain the competence of the pulmonary valve (valve sparing repair). However, in about a third of cases, particularly in older patients, it may be necessary to insert a patch over the incision (the transannular patch). If the pulmonary valve annulus is very narrow, it may be necessary to open the annular region and to extend the patch to the main PA. It may also be necessary to enlarge the main PA and the junction of the branch pulmonary arteries with the patch. The resultant PR has an important bearing on the long-term outcomes.

Timing of the Surgery

The timing of the corrective surgery varies among the centers depending on their experience and also the condition of the patient. But most centers perform elective repair of TOF in asymptomatic infants between 3 and 12 months of age, with a trend toward a younger age of surgery in many large centers across the globe. Recently, Indian guidelines have been published in 2010 to guide the timing of the surgery.[17] They are as follows:

- *Patients who are stable and minimally cyanosed*: Total repair at 6–12 months of age or earlier according to the institutional policy
- Symptomatic children of <6 months of age with significant cyanosis or history of spells despite therapy can undergo one of the following depending on the anatomy and the centers experience:
  - Systemic-to-pulmonary artery shunt in the form of modified BT shunt
  - Stenting of the ductus arteriosus or RVOT
  - Pulmonary valve balloon valvuloplasty
  - Total repair depending on anatomy and center's experience.

Outcome of Surgery and Long-term Prognosis

With the advent of better surgical techniques and postoperative ICU care, there is a >96% chance of survival to hospital discharge. Of the surviving infants, >90% are expected to be alive 30 years after repair. Around 5% of patients require reoperation and 6% will need a catheter intervention during the childhood. It is important to note that although TOF repair is associated with little short- or medium-term mortality, long-term survival is not equal to that of the general population. It is seen that in a 30-year-old patient with repaired TOF, there is a 0.5% annual risk of death and that the annual mortality increases by 0.1% per decade.[18] Chronic PR is by and far the most important complication, which affects the long-term survival in a patient with TOF. A common sequel of TOF repair, PR is especially likely, and most severe in patients with a transannular patch. PR tends to increase with time and places a volume load on the RV that is exacerbated by any distal PA stenosis. In the face of chronic PR, compensatory RV dilation and hypertrophy maintain forward flow and wall stress. Initially, the RV dilates but the RV systolic function remains normal. Ultimately, RV compensatory adaptations become inadequate and TOF patients with severe PR begin to develop RV contractile dysfunction. For a period of time, RV dysfunction remains reversible with intervention to abolish PR but, eventually, the damage progresses, and permanent myocardial injury ensues. Thus, timely intervention in the form of PVR is very important. Late follow-up studies have shown a 0.8% risk per year of requiring PVR.[19] Another problem is the presence of electrical disturbance such as right bundle branch block which could be a result of RV dilatation or ventricular fibrosis. QRS duration on ECG >180 ms has been identified as an important predictor of adverse outcome. The European, American, and Canadian guidelines for the care of adults with CHD all recommend lifelong follow-up of patients with TOF in a specialist center by physicians with expertise in adult CHD.[20] The purpose of routine follow-up is to anticipate and monitor potential complications and, when necessary, to intervene before these become clinically important.

VARIANTS OF TETRALOGY OF FALLOT

The following variants of TOF exist which differ significantly on the basis of physiology, clinical presentation, and surgical management.

Tetralogy of Fallot with Absence of the Pulmonary Valve

This variant is characterized by the absence of pulmonary valve leaflet tissues or only a rudimentary ridge of tissue is present. It is seen in 3–6% of patients with TOF.[21] The cause for RVOTO is predominantly due to a ring of tissue present

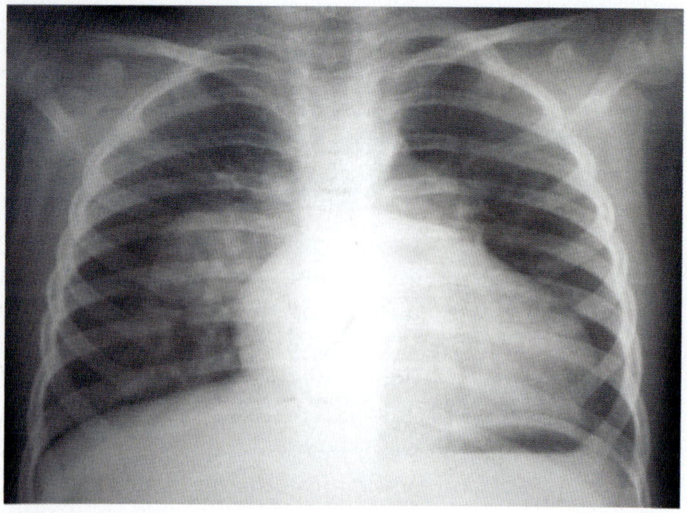

Fig. 8: Chest X-ray of a 1-year-old boy shows cardiomegaly with dilated proximal branch pulmonary arteries (PAs) and normal pulmonary vascular markings.

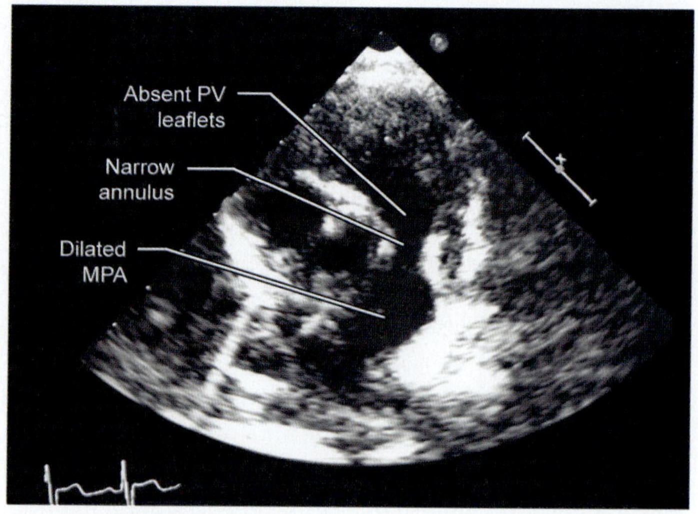

Fig. 9: Two-dimensional (2D) echocardiography (parasternal short axis view) in a case of tetralogy of Fallot (TOF) with absent pulmonary valve showing absent pulmonary valve (PV) leaflets with hypoplastic annulus and the typical dilated main pulmonary artery (MPA).

at the level where the pulmonary valve leaflets would be expected. In about 50% of patients with TOF and absent pulmonary valve, there is also a right-sided aortic arch, and the condition may also be associated with absent or aortic origin of a branch PA. An important feature in this variant is the aneurysmal dilation of the main and branch pulmonary arteries that may compromise the airways and respiratory function and can lead to varying degrees of tracheobronchial malacia and air trapping. This can be attributed either abnormality of the tissues of the pulmonary vessel, the orientation of the subpulmonary infundibulum, or to severe in utero PR.[22] There also exists abnormal branching of the pulmonary arteries with "tufts" of arteries that entwin and compress the intrapulmonary bronchi.

On examination, patients with TOF and absent pulmonary valve exhibit a characteristic "to-and-fro" systolic and diastolic murmurs and a single second heart sound. As the pulmonary vascular resistance falls, infants usually develop signs of increased pulmonary blood flow. The chest X-ray **(Fig. 8)** shows a moderately enlarged cardiac silhouette that has a prominent bulge at the upper left cardiac border, caused by the massively dilated proximal pulmonary arteries, and usually normal peripheral vascular markings. Some infants also demonstrate lobar emphysema. Echocardiography typically shows absent pulmonary valve leaflets with hypoplastic annulus causing severe obstruction and free pulmonary regurgitation with dilated main pulmonary artery and branch pulmonary arteries **(Fig. 9)**.

The clinical course can be divided into two groups. The first is those patients who present early in life (first few days to weeks of age) with severe respiratory symptoms and need early surgical intervention and have poor prognosis. The second group presents later with only mild respiratory symptoms. These patients are symptomatically managed till 1 year of age and then taken for surgery.[17] Surgical strategies usually focus on intracardiac TOF repair along with plication and reduction of the pulmonary arteries where necessary.

Tetralogy of Fallot with an Atrioventricular Septal Defect

It is seen in around 2% of patients with TOF. This variant has a higher incidence in Down syndrome patients. The clinical picture is like the patients with isolated TOF than isolated AVSD, since the RVOTO limits pulmonary overcirculation and prevents symptoms of heart failure. ECG will show a left axis deviation. Primary surgical repair of both the AVSD and TOF may be performed, often at an older age (>1 year), and interim catheter or surgical palliation is needed for cyanotic babies. Surgical repair is a challenge as it involves division of the inlet valve as well as closure of the interatrial and interventricular septal defects and reconstruction of the RVOT.[23]

Tetralogy of Fallot with Origin of One Pulmonary Artery from the Right Ventricle and One from the Ascending Aorta

This is a very rare variant of TOF where there is a discontinuity of the branch pulmonary arteries with one PA (more often the left) originating from the ascending aorta. There is a high change of early development of PA hypertension in the lung which is connected to the ascending aorta. Thus, it is important to identify patients with this abnormality and undertake surgical repair early, to prevent the development of pulmonary arterial hypertension.[23,24] Occasionally, there may be apparent complete absence of the left PA in the setting of TOF.

REFERENCES

1. Bhardwaj R, Rai SK, Yadav AK, Lakhotia S, Agrawal D, Kumar A, et al. Epidemiology of congenital heart disease in India. Congenit Heart Dis. 2015;10(5):437-46.

2. Hoffman JI, Kaplan S. The incidence of congenital heart disease. J Am Coll Cardiol. 2002; 39(12):1890-900.
3. Burn J, Brennan P, Little J, Holloway S, Coffey R, Somerville J, et al. Recurrence risks in offspring of adults with major heart defects: results from first cohort of British collaborative study. The Lancet. 1998;351(9099):311-6.
4. Goldmuntz E, Clark BJ, Mitchell LE, Jawad AF, Cuneo BF, Reed L, et al. Frequency of 22q11 deletions in patients with conotruncal defects. J Am Coll Cardiol. 1998;32(2):492-8.
5. Pierpont ME, Basson CT, Benson Jr DW, Gelb BD, Giglia TM, Goldmuntz E, et al. Genetic basis for congenital heart defects: current knowledge: a scientific statement from the American Heart Association Congenital Cardiac Defects Committee, Council on Cardiovascular Disease in the Young: endorsed by the American Academy of Pediatrics. Circulation. 2007; 115(23): 3015-38.
6. Jenkins KJ, Correa A, Feinstein JA, Botto L, Britt AE, Daniels SR, et al. Non-inherited risk factors and congenital cardiovascular defects: current knowledge: a scientific statement from the American Heart Association Council on Cardiovascular Disease in the Young: endorsed by the American Academy of Pediatrics. Circulation. 2007;115(23):2995-3014.
7. Neill CA, Clark EB. Tetralogy of Fallot. The first 300 years. Tex Heart Inst J. 1994;21(4):272.
8. Anderson RH, Weinberg PM. The clinical anatomy of tetralogy of Fallot. Cardiol Young. 2005 Feb;15(S1):38-47.
9. Bonchek LI, Starr A, Sunderland CO, Menashe VD. Natural history of tetralogy of Fallot in infancy: clinical classification and therapeutic implications. Circulation. 1973;48(2):392-7.
10. Wood P. Attacks of deeper cyanosis and loss of consciousness (syncope) in Fallot's tetralogy. Br Heart J. 1958;20(2):282-6.
11. Kothari SS. Mechanism of cyanotic spells in tetralogy of Fallot—the missing link? Int J Cardiol. 1992;37(1):1-5.
12. Anilkumar A, Kappanayil M, Nampoothiri S, Thampi MV, Vasudevan DM, Kumar RK. Screening for TBX1 gene in children with or without microdeletion of chromosome 22q11 and conotruncal defect. Lab Med. 2012; 43(2):11-3.
13. Pileggi F, Bocanegra J, Tranchesi J, Macruz R, Borges S, Portugal O, et al. The electrocardiogram in tetralogy of Fallot: a study of 142 cases. Am Heart J. 1960;59(5):667-80.
14. Geva T. Indications and timing of pulmonary valve replacement after tetralogy of Fallot repair. In: Seminars in Thoracic and Cardiovascular Surgery: Pediatric Cardiac Surgery Annual. 2006;9(1):11-22.
15. Van Roekens CN, Zuckerberg AL. Emergency management of hypercyanotic crises in tetralogy of Fallot. Ann Emerg Med. 1995;25(2):256-8.
16. Abraham M. Pulmonary stenosis and atresia with ventricular septal defect (tetralogy of Fallot). In: Abraham M, (Ed). Congenital Diseases of the Heart Clinical-Physiological Considerations. West Sussex: Blackwell Publishing; 2009. p. 379.
17. Saxena A, Relan J, Agarwal R, Awasthy N, Azad S, Chakrabarty M, et al. Indian guidelines for indications and timing of intervention for common congenital heart diseases: revised and updated consensus statement of the Working group on management of congenital heart diseases. Ann Pediatr Cardiol. 2019;12(3):254.
18. Ooi A, Moorjani N, Baliulis G, Keeton BR, Salmon AP, Monro JL, et al. Medium term outcome for infant repair in tetralogy of Fallot: indicators for timing of surgery. European journal of cardio-thoracic surgery. 2006;30(6):917-22.
19. Hickey E, Veldtman G, Bradley TJ, Gengsakul A, Manlhiot C, Williams WG, et al. Late risk of outcomes for adults with repaired tetralogy of Fallot from an inception cohort spanning four decades. Eur J Cardiothorac Surg. 2009; 35(1):156-64.
20. Stout KK, Daniels CJ, Aboulhosn JA, Bozkurt B, Broberg CS, Colman JM, et al. 2018 AHA/ACC guideline for the management of adults with congenital heart disease: a report of the American College of Cardiology/American Heart Association Task Force on Clinical Practice Guidelines. J Am Coll Cardiol. 2019; 73(12): e81-192.
21. Lev M, Eckner FA. The pathologic anatomy of tetralogy of Fallot and its variations. Chest. 1964;45(3):251-61.
22. Fouron JC. Tetralogy of Fallot with absent pulmonary valve. Clarification of a complex malformation and of its therapeutic challenge. Circulation. 1990;82(4):1531-2.
23. Najm HK, Van Arsdell GS, Watzka S, Hornberger L, Coles JG, Williams WG. Primary repair is superior to initial palliation in children with atrioventricular septal defect and tetralogy of Fallot. J Thorac Cardiovasc Surg. 1998;116(6): 905-13.
24. Robin E, Silberberg B, Ganguly SN, Magnisalis K. Aortic origin of the left pulmonary artery: variant of tetralogy of Fallot. Am J Cardiol. 1975;35(2):324-9.

35

CHAPTER

Persistent Truncus Arteriosus

Saileela Rajan

INTRODUCTION

Persistent truncus arteriosus, also referred to simply as truncus arteriosus, is a congenital cardiovascular malformation in which a single arterial trunk arises from the heart, giving origin sequentially to the coronary arteries, one or more pulmonary arteries, and the systemic arterial circulation. This cyanotic heart defect, which accounts for approximately 1.2% of all congenital heart defects,[1-3] was first described by Wilson in 1798 and subsequently by Buchanan in 1864, based on the autopsy findings of a neonate and 6-month-old infant, respectively.[4,5] It is equally prevalent in both genders.

EMBRYOLOGY

Normally, the embryonic truncus arteriosus lies between the conus cordis proximally and the aortic sac and arch distally. During the 5th week of fetal development, two ridges namely truncal swellings or cushions appear on opposite walls of truncus arteriosus. Migration of cells from the neural crest contributes to the normal development of these cushions.[6] Fusion of these cushions results in the formation of a spiral septum called truncal septum or aortopulmonary septum. The conal swellings, which appear on opposite walls of conus cordis, fuse to form the conal septum. The conal septum divides the conus into an anterolateral portion called conus arteriosus (infundibulum)of the right ventricle and a posteromedial portion namely aortic vestibule of the left ventricle. When the proximal portion of the truncal septum joins the conal septum, the ventricular origins of pulmonary trunk and aorta are established. The spiral nature of the aortopulmonary septum produces the normal intertwinement of the great arteries. The semilunar valves develop at the line of fusion of truncal and conal swellings. The complete failure of aortopulmonary septum to contribute to the separation process results in common arterial trunk, common arterial orifice, and juxta-arterial ventricular septal defect (VSD).[6,7] The deficient or absent conal septum is responsible for VSD. Vestigial development of the distal truncal septum is responsible for the short main pulmonary artery (PA) segment in truncus type I.

PATHOLOGY

There is a single trunk from the heart supplying the systemic, pulmonary, and coronary circulation. The VSD is most often large and located in the subtruncal region (conotruncal). The trunk is committed to both ventricles equally in 42%, predominantly to the right ventricle (RV) in 42%, and to the left ventricle (LV) in 16% of cases.[8] Usually, there is fibrous continuity between the truncal valve and mitral valve; but sometimes there may be a discontinuity, especially when trunk is more committed to RV. The number of cusps in the truncal valve may vary from 2 to 6, most common being tricommissural valve (in 60% of cases).[8] Truncal valves are dysplastic, deformed, and thickened in 50%. In one quarter to one half of the patients, truncal valve regurgitation occurs due to the dysplastic nature of the valve and prolapse of the unsupported valve leaflets in a dilated arterial trunk. Truncal valve stenosis may be seen in up to 33% of patients. Pulmonary arterial origin stenosis and crossed pulmonary arterial origins are rarely seen.[9] Ductus arteriosus is absent in 50–75% of cases. It is present in Van Praagh type A3 and A4. Various coronary artery anomalies have been reported including single coronary artery origin, high origin of coronary artery, and ostial stenosis of coronaries. Right-sided aortic arch is present in 30% and interruption of arch in 11–20% of truncus arteriosus.[8] Type B interruption is the most common, where the aorta is interrupted between the left common carotid artery and the left subclavian artery. Atrial septal defect and aberrant subclavian artery may be present. Other rare anomalies that have been associated are common atrioventricular valve, tricuspid atresia, single ventricle, and partial anomalous pulmonary venous return. Extracardiac anomalies, which are present in 20–30% of cases, include bowel malrotation, absence of gallbladder, hydroureter, renal agenesis, duodenal atresia, tracheoesophageal fistula, and cleft palate.[7,10]

GENETIC ASSOCIATIONS

Deletion 22q11.2 (DiGeorge/velocardiofacial syndrome) is detected in 30–50% of the patients with truncus arteriosus.

TABLE 1: Associated anomalies and their prevalence in truncus arteriosus.

Anomaly	Prevalence
Dysplastic truncal valve	50%
Truncal valve regurgitation	25–50%
Truncal valve stenosis	33%
Coronary artery anomalies	50%
Right aortic arch	30%
Interruption of aorta	11–20%
Atrial septal defect	9–20%
Aberrant subclavian artery	4–10%
Persistent left superior vena cava	4–9%
DiGeorge syndrome	30–50%
Extracardiac anomalies	20–30%

Those with right-sided aortic arch and abnormal branching pattern of arch are more likely to be associated with 22q11 deletion.[11,12] CHARGE association, trisomy 18, and trisomy 21 are also known to be associated with truncus arteriosus. **Table 1** lists the associated anomalies in truncus arteriosus.

CLASSIFICATION

The most commonly used classifications are described here **(Fig. 1)**:

Collett and Edward Classification (Fig. 1A)[10]

- *Type 1*: Main PA segment arises from the common arterial trunk, and divides into right and left pulmonary arteries.
- *Type 2*: Right and left pulmonary arteries arise as separate but adjacent orifices from posterior aspect of common arterial trunk.
- *Type 3*: Right and left pulmonary arteries arise as separate distant orifices from opposite lateral sides of common arterial trunk.
- *Type 4*: Is no more considered as truncus arteriosus; classified as pulmonary atresia with multiple aorto-pulmonary collaterals. Some authors call this pseudotruncus
- Type 1 truncus is present in 48–68% of patients, type 2 in 29–48%, and type 3 in 6–10%.[10,13]

Van Praagh Classification (Fig. 1B)[7]

There are two basic types in this classification: *type A*, those with VSD, which is more common; and *type B*, those without VSD, which is extremely rare.

They are subdivided into four types:

1. *Type A1*: Main PA arises from the common arterial trunk and divides into two branches (corresponds to Collett and Edwards type I).
2. *Type A2*: No main PA segment; both branch pulmonary arteries arise directly from the arterial trunk (includes both type II and type III of Collett and Edwards).

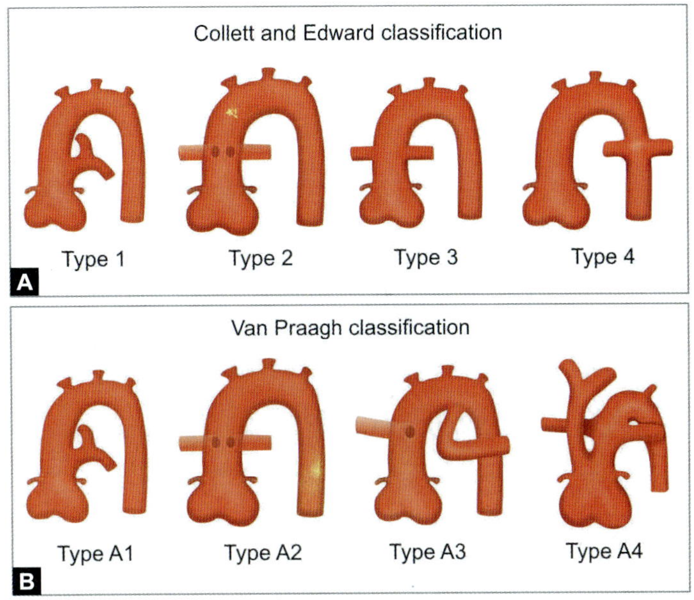

Figs. 1A and B: Classifications of persistent truncus arteriosus. (A) Collett and Edward classification; (B) Van Praagh classification.

3. *Type A3*: One PA arises from the ascending portion of the trunk, while the other lung is supplied by the ductus arteriosus or aortopulmonary collateral from descending aorta.
4. *Type A4*: Truncus arteriosus associated with hypoplastic aortic arch, coarctation or interruption of aorta; and large ductus arteriosus supplying the descending aorta.

Calder et al. reported an incidence of 50, 21, 12, and 8% for A1, A2, A4, and A3 respectively.[14]

PATHOPHYSIOLOGY

In truncus arteriosus, the pressure in both ventricles is equal due to the presence of unrestrictive VSD. There is admixture of oxygenated and deoxygenated blood in the single arterial trunk, resulting in similar oxygen saturation in both great arteries. Sometimes, the systemic arterial saturation may be more than the pulmonary arterial saturation due to preferential streaming of pulmonary venous blood into aorta. The pulmonary blood flow increases when the pulmonary vascular resistance drops in the late neonatal period. This results in a relatively better oxygen saturation of above 85%, at the expense of heart failure symptoms. There is left ventricular volume overload due to the increased pulmonary blood flow. The diastolic run-off into pulmonary arteries results in low diastolic arterial pressure and hence low coronary perfusion pressure. The increased pulmonary blood flow, coronary arterial insufficiency, and volume overload makes the left ventricle highly vulnerable to the hemodynamic burden of truncal valve stenosis/regurgitation and/or aortic arch interruption (**Flowchart 1**).

There is early development of pulmonary vascular obstructive disease (PVOD) (irreversible pulmonary hypertension) in truncus arteriosus, as the pulmonary

Flowchart 1: The basic pathophysiology in truncus arteriosus.

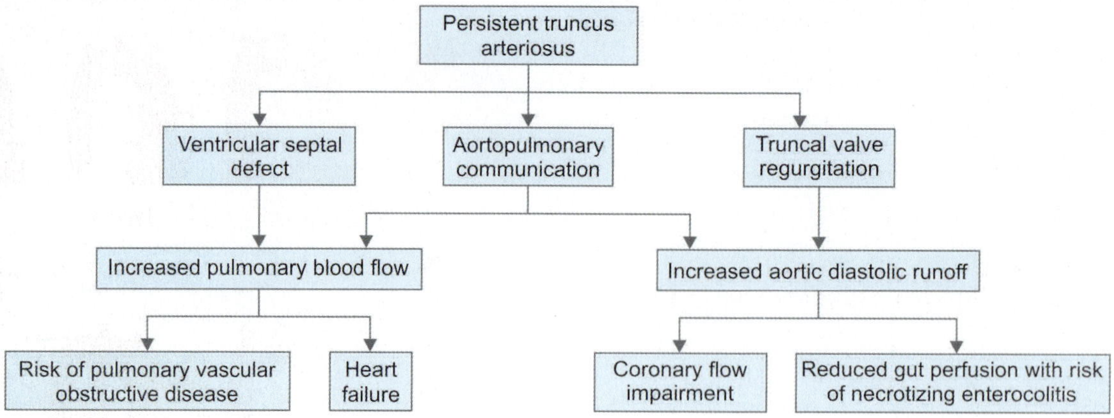

vasculature is constantly exposed to the hemodynamic insult of increased flow in the setting of hypoxia. There is more rapid progression of PVOD when one PA is absent.

In rare instances of pulmonary arterial origin stenosis or hypoplasia, the pulmonary blood flow is balanced or reduced. This prevents volume overload of the heart, but systemic desaturation is more pronounced in them.

CLINICAL PRESENTATION

The most common presentation of truncus arteriosus is congestive cardiac failure. Symptoms usually start after 2 weeks of life, when neonatal pulmonary vascular resistance decreases. They present with feeding difficulty, suck-rest-suck cycle, diaphoresis, subcostal and intercostal chest retractions, poor weight gain, and recurrent respiratory infections. Heart failure symptoms are exaggerated in infants with truncal valve regurgitation. Symptoms may manifest earlier in the neonatal period if the regurgitation is severe.

They have cyanosis, but most often it is mild in infancy. This is because of the increased pulmonary blood flow in this condition. Hence, the oxygen saturation is above 85% in early infancy. In many instances, the saturations are in excess of 90% which may result in the diagnosis being missed in neonatal units. Those associated with significant stenosis of PA branches may present with early cyanosis.

Heart failure symptoms are directly proportional to the pulmonary flow, while cyanosis is inversely proportional to it. If the child survives beyond infancy, pulmonary hypertension progresses and PVOD is established. Then the quantum of pulmonary blood flow decreases, resulting in worsening of cyanosis and alleviation of heart failure symptoms. Thus, an oxygen saturation level below 85% is often suggestive of PVOD in older children with truncus arteriosus.

Truncus arteriosus with interrupted aortic arch has duct-dependent systemic circulation and hence may present in neonatal period with shock and acidosis when ductus arteriosus decreases in size.

PHYSICAL EXAMINATION

General Examination

Child is often undernourished due to the catabolic state of heart failure. Subcostal and intercostal retractions are present. Cyanosis and clubbing are more obvious if there is associated PA stenosis or PVOD. One should look for features of DiGeorge syndrome that includes the characteristic square nose tip, micrognathia, short philtrum, narrow palpebral fissures, palate abnormalities, and long fingers.

Vital Signs

There is tachycardia and tachypnea. Pulse is bounding and high volume. Pulse pressure is wide, due to the diastolic run-off into the pulmonary arteries and/or associated truncal valve regurgitation. Bounding pulses may be absent in bilateral PA stenosis. Manifestations of congestive cardiac failure in the form of hepatomegaly are present.

Cardiovascular Examination

There are signs of hyperdynamic circulation. Apical impulse is shifted downward and outward due to the cardiomegaly. Parasternal impulse is present due to systemic right ventricular pressure. First heart sound is normal. Second heart sound is single and loud as there is only one semilunar valve, which closes at systemic pressure. Sometimes, the second heart sound may be split, attributed to the asynchronous closure of multiple leaflets of truncal valve. Second heart sound may be palpable in some. Often, a systolic ejection click is heard following the first heart sound that coincides with the truncal valve opening. An ejection systolic murmur is heard along the left sternal border, due to the increased flow across the single semilunar valve. A longer and louder systolic murmur is heard in the presence of truncal valve stenosis. An early diastolic murmur is heard along the left sternal border, when truncal valve regurgitation is present. A short mid-diastolic murmur and third heart sound heard at apex represent increased transmitral flow, secondary to increased pulmonary blood flow and pulmonary

TABLE 2: Salient clinical features in truncus arteriosus.

Symptoms	Failure to thrive, feeding difficulty, diaphoresis, and recurrent respiratory infections
General examination	Subcostal/intercostal retractions, mild cyanosis, bounding pulses, wide pulse pressure, hepatomegaly, and dysmorphic features (if associated DiGeorge syndrome)
Cardiovascular examination	Hyperdynamic apex Parasternal and epigastric impulse S1 normal S2 single and loud (may be split sometimes) S3 ± Systolic ejection click Ejection systolic murmur at left sternal border Early diastolic murmur at upper left sternal border (if truncal regurgitation present) MDM at apex ±
Chest X-ray	Cardiomegaly, pulmonary plethora hilar comma sign Right arch ±
Electrocardiogram	Biventricular hypertrophy Left atrial enlargement
Truncus arteriosus with pulmonary arterial stenosis	Heart failure symptoms less Cyanosis more obvious Continuous bruite (murmur) present Heart size normal or mild cardiomegaly Pulmonary vascularity normal
Truncus arteriosus with PVOD	Heart failure symptoms absent Cyanosis more obvious (SpO_2 <85%) Quiet precordium, hyperdynamic features absent RV type apex S3 and MDM absent No cardiomegaly Dilated proximal pulmonary arteries with peripheral pruning on X-ray RV hypertrophy on ECG

(S1: first heart sound; S2: second heart sound; S3: third heart sound; MDM: mid-diastolic murmur; RV: right ventricle; PVOD: pulmonary vascular obstructive disease)

venous return. Presence of this flow murmur in an older child with truncus arteriosus is a favorable sign and an indication that pulmonary flow is still large and PVOD is not established. Mid-diastolic murmur may also occur in the presence of severe truncal valve regurgitation (Austin Flint murmur). A continuous murmur in truncus arteriosus is most often due to bilateral branch PA stenosis. **Table 2** summarizes the salient clinical features of truncus arteriosus.

DIAGNOSIS

X-ray

Cardiomegaly and increased pulmonary vascularity are the common features noted on chest X-ray of a child with truncus arteriosus (**Fig. 2**). Cardiomegaly is due to biventricular and left atrial enlargement. The left PA arises more medially and has a high arching course over the left bronchus. This is called the "hilar comma sign". In type A3, there may be differential vascularity to the lungs, as the pulmonary flow to each lung

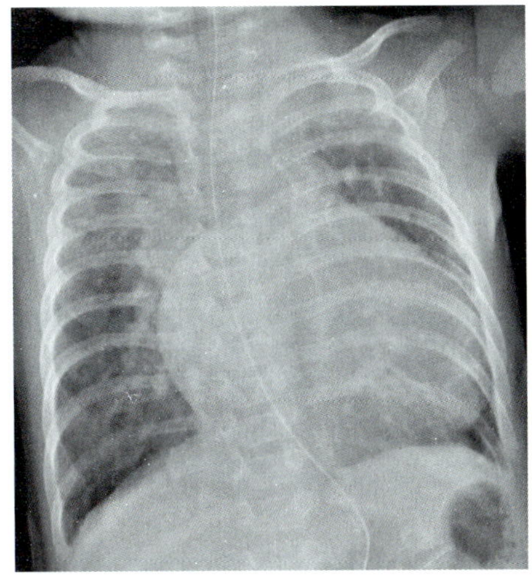

Fig. 2: Chest X-ray of an infant showing significant cardiomegaly and pulmonary plethora.

differs. Right aortic arch may be noted in some cases. In older children, when PVOD is established, there are dilated central pulmonary arteries while peripheral pulmonary vasculature is pruned. Superior mediastinum may be narrow in children with associated thymic hypoplasia. One should strongly suspect truncus arteriosus when there is a combination of pulmonary plethora and right-sided aortic arch on the X-ray of a cyanotic child.

Electrocardiogram

Most often, the rhythm is sinus. The QRS axis is normal or may have a mild right axis deviation. There is evidence of biventricular hypertrophy, evidenced by tall equiphasic QRS complexes in midprecordial leads (**Fig. 3**). Deep q waves and tall R waves in V5, V6 are suggestive of left ventricular volume overload. Bifid wide P waves suggestive of left atrial enlargement may be seen but it is not a sensitive sign. When PVOD establishes, there is right ventricular hypertrophy and decrease in left ventricular forces.

Echocardiography

Echocardiography is diagnostic and provides complete information in most cases. Type of truncus arteriosus, morphology of truncal valve, presence of stenosis or regurgitation, origin and course of pulmonary arteries, location and extent of VSD, presence of additional defects, size of ventricles, aortic arch sidedness, presence of arch abnormality such as interruption, and presence of ductus arteriosus, aortopulmonary collaterals, and coronary artery abnormalities can be assessed on echocardiography (**Figs. 4 and 5**). Antenatal diagnosis of truncus arteriosus is possible on fetal echocardiography.

Cardiac Catheterization and Angiography

Cardiac catheterization is performed in children with late presentation for estimating pulmonary vascular resistance. Children with elevated pulmonary vascular

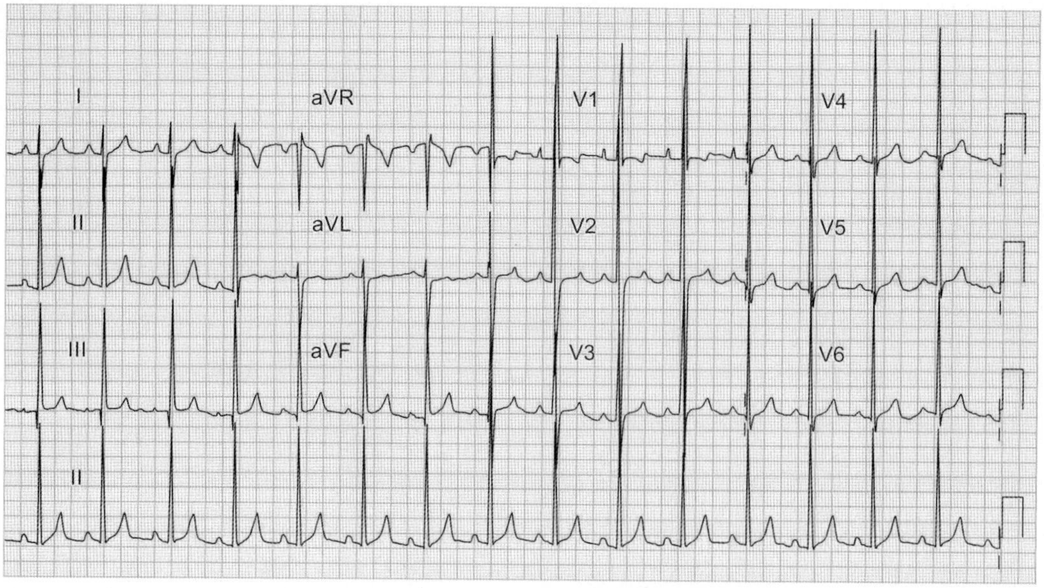

Fig. 3: Electrocardiogram of a child with truncus arteriosus showing biventricular hypertrophy. Note the tall equiphasic QRS complexes in midprecordial leads.

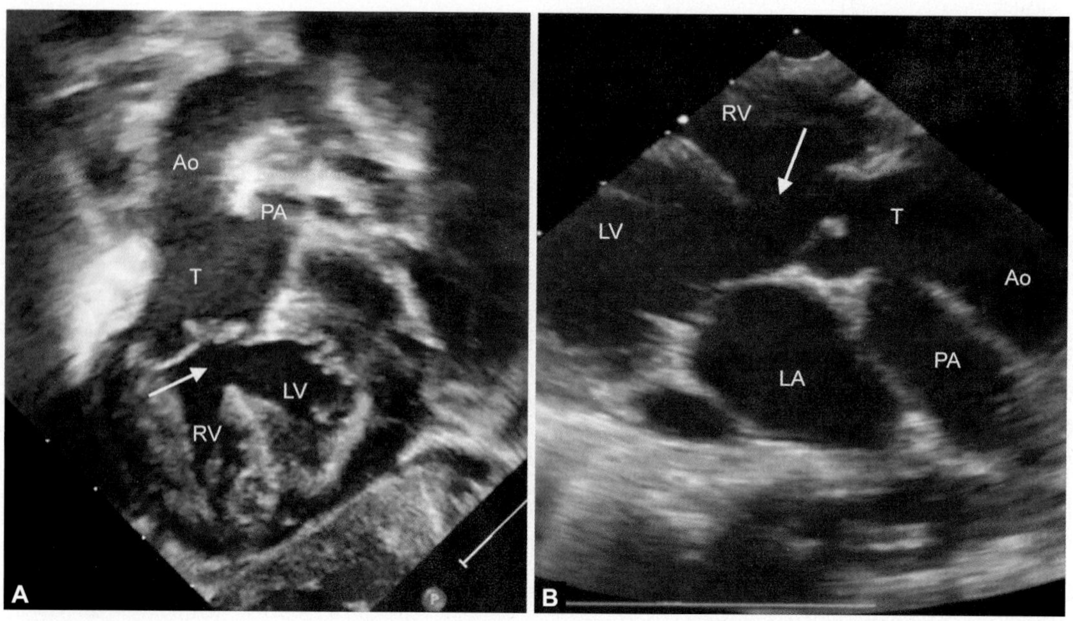

Figs. 4A and B: (A) Echocardiographic subcostal view showing an unrestrictive conoventricular septal defect (arrow), single arterial trunk (T) committed to both ventricles, main pulmonary artery (PA) arising from the leftward aspect of the trunk, after which the trunk continues as aorta (Ao); (B) Echocardiographic parasternal long axis view showing an unrestrictive conoventricular septal defect (arrow), single arterial trunk (T) committed to both ventricles, main pulmonary artery (PA) arising from the trunk, after which the trunk continues as aorta (Ao).
(LA: left atrium; LV: left ventricle; RV: right ventricle)

resistance (>6–8 Wood units) are inoperable and advised conservative management. As cardiac catheterization has limitations in accurately measuring flows and resistances in admixture lesions such as truncus arteriosus, relying on catheterization data alone for determining operability is not advisable. Clinical signs of increased pulmonary flow such as hyperdynamic circulation, signs of left ventricular volume overload, relatively high oxygen saturation (>90%), and radiological signs of cardiomegaly and pulmonary plethora favor operability. Some authors have reported lower pulmonary-to-systemic arterial diastolic pressure ratio and high pulmonary-to-systemic flow ratio to be significant predictors of a good postoperative outcome.[15] Angiography may delineate the PA origins/course, coronary artery origin/course, and presence of collaterals (**Fig. 6**).

Computed Tomography or Magnetic Resonance Imaging

Computed tomography (CT) angiogram or magnetic resonance imaging (MRI) may be required in few cases, to delineate associated interrupted arch, pulmonary origin abnormalities, and coronary abnormalities.

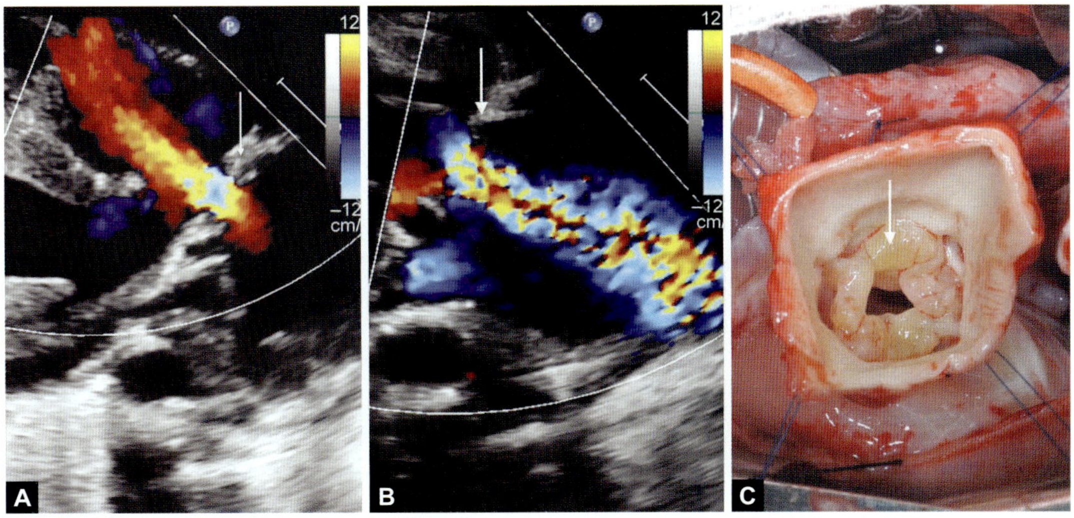

Figs. 5A to C: (A) Echocardiographic parasternal view showing a dysplastic truncal valve (arrow) resulting in valve regurgitation (red jet); (B) Truncal valve stenosis seen as blue mosaic jet; (C) Intraoperative image of a dysplastic quadricuspid truncal valve. Note the thickened valve leaflets.

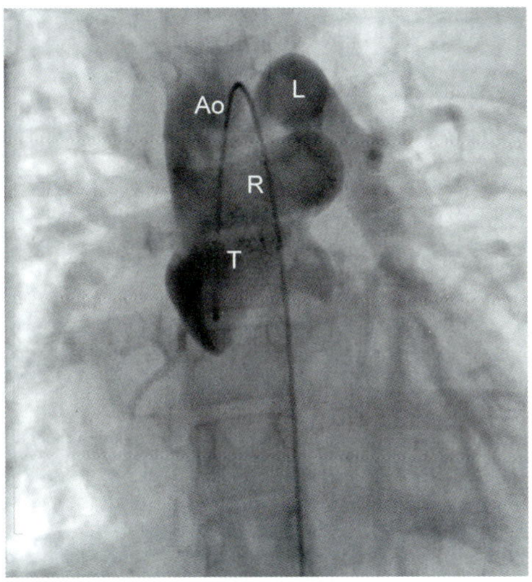

Fig. 6: Angiographic view of truncus arteriosus showing the common arterial trunk (T), right (R) and left (L) pulmonary arteries arising from the trunk, beyond which the trunk continues as aorta (Ao). Note that the left pulmonary artery has a high arching course, the reason for hilar comma sign on X-ray.

Genetic Analysis

Fluorescence in situ hybridization (FISH) study is needed to confirm presence of 22q11 deletion and should be strongly considered in all cases. This has several important implications in the immediate postoperative management, follow-up, and parental counseling. If the patient is found to be FISH positive, it is necessary to do a close follow-up of developmental status with early intervention and targeted speech therapy. Parental screening for carrier status is necessary to predict risk of 22q11 deletion in future pregnancies.

Antenatal Diagnosis

Truncus arteriosus can be reliably diagnosed by fetal echocardiography. A detailed fetal anomaly scan is advised in them to rule out associated extracardiac anomalies. The parents need to be counseled about fetal karyotyping and FISH analysis for 22q11 deletion.

NATURAL HISTORY

Infants with truncus arteriosus develop early heart failure between 2 and 6 weeks of age. Those with severe truncal valve stenosis may present with shock and acidosis in neonatal period. Similarly, those with associated arch anomalies may present earlier in neonatal period. Without treatment, 80% of children with truncus arteriosus die in infancy.[16] Median age of death ranges from few weeks to 6 months. The cause of death in infancy is congestive cardiac failure. If they survive beyond infancy, they develop progressive PVOD, and succumb to it by late childhood or adolescence. There are rare reports of natural survival till fifth decade of life.[17]

DIFFERENTIAL DIAGNOSIS

Truncus arteriosus has to be differentiated from other cyanotic heart diseases with increased pulmonary blood flow that present with similar clinical features of heart failure and mild cyanosis. They include unobstructed total anomalous pulmonary venous connection, double-outlet right ventricle without pulmonary stenosis, single ventricle without pulmonary stenosis, transposition of the great arteries with VSD, tricuspid atresia without pulmonary stenosis, and pulmonary atresia with large aortopulmonary collaterals. Echocardiography is the gold standard to differentiate these conditions.

Morphologically, the following are the differential diagnosis:

- *Hemitruncus* is a condition where there are two semilunar valves, but the main PA gives rise to only one branch. The other PA branch arises from the ascending aorta. The nomenclature of "hemitruncus" is now replaced by "anomalous origin of pulmonary artery (right or left) from ascending aorta", to differentiate this condition from truncus arteriosus.

- *Tetralogy of Fallot with pulmonary atresia* is also characterized by a single semilunar valve and arterial trunk from the heart, but pulmonary arteries do not arise from the ascending portion of the great artery. Pulmonary arteries are either supplied by the ductus arteriosus or by aortopulmonary collaterals from descending aorta.
- *Aortopulmonary window* is differentiated from truncus arteriosus by the presence of two semilunar valves. The great arteries arise from the respective ventricles, but there is a large window like communication between the ascending portion of the great arteries.
- Aortic atresia with a large VSD is often confused for truncus because the large PA is seen overriding the VSD and the diminutive aorta may not be seen during echocardiography. It is important to specifically exclude this possibility by looking at the coronary origins and ensuring that all the branches from the aorta are imaged.

MANAGEMENT

Medical Management

Heart failure management is initiated when the infants present with symptoms, most often beyond 2 weeks of age. Furosemide and spironolactone are started in all infants presenting with heart failure. Digoxin may be added if significant tachycardia is present. Angiotensin-converting enzyme (ACE) inhibitors may be added beyond neonatal age. Truncus arteriosus with arch interruption may become symptomatic in neonatal period if patent ductus arteriosus decreases in size. They may require prostaglandin E1 infusion, followed by early surgery. Neonates or infants associated with DiGeorge syndrome may have hypocalcemia and require calcium supplementation and sometimes, calcitriol.

Surgical Management

The first successful complete repair for truncus arteriosus was reported by McGoon et al. in 1968.[18] Since PVOD can develop as early as 6 months of age in truncus arteriosus, early surgery is the norm. Palliative procedures, such as banding of main PA or bilateral branch pulmonary arteries, are seldom performed in the present surgical era. Single-stage complete biventricular repair, at 2–6 weeks of age, is the treatment of choice at most cardiac centers. This comprises of patch closure of VSD, reconstruction of right ventricular outflow tract, separation of branch pulmonary arteries from the common trunk, and committing them to right ventricle using a valved conduit. Nonconduit options (Barbero-Marcial technique) may be possible in select cases.[19] When truncal valve stenosis or regurgitation is present, valve repair is performed. Valve replacement is done whenever repair is not feasible but this is very challenging in small infants. Truncal root replacement with homograft is adopted in extreme situations when neither valve repair nor replacement is possible. Arch reconstruction is performed when there is associated interrupted arch. Surgical outcome depends on the degree of pulmonary vascular disease, truncal valve regurgitation, presence of aortic arch abnormalities, and associated 22q11 deletion. Perioperative mortality ranges from 4 to 12.5% with 1-year survival of 84–92%.[20-22]

Transcatheter Interventions

Role of transcatheter interventions in truncus arteriosus is most often postoperative. The following are the instances where interventional procedures have a role in truncus arteriosus:[23]

- Balloon angioplasty or stent implantation in pulmonary arterial stenosis (postsurgical pulmonary arterial stenosis or native stenosis of distal pulmonary arteries)
- Balloon angioplasty or stent placement for RV to PA conduit stenosis
- Balloon angioplasty of truncal valve re-stenosis after surgical repair
- Device closure of residual defects after surgery
- Transcatheter pulmonary valve placement for conduit stenosis/regurgitation late in the follow-up period.

LONG-TERM PROGNOSIS AND FOLLOW-UP

Late survival rates are reported to be 90, 85, and 83% at 5, 10, and 15 years, respectively.[21] Determinants of long-term prognosis include residual or progressive pulmonary hypertension, need for conduit replacement, progressive truncal or neoaortic valve regurgitation, aortic root dilatation/aneurysm, and recurrent arch obstruction in truncus type A4. Almost all patients require reoperation for conduit replacement. Growth of patient relative to conduit size, valvular calcification, and formation of fibrin peel are the causes for conduit stenosis. Median age for conduit replacement ranges between 5 and 6 years.[20,21] In the present era, transcatheter pulmonary valve placement is an option in adolescents and adults, and reduces the burden of reoperations. Another common indication for reoperation is truncal valve regurgitation. Following truncal valve repair, freedom from reoperation was 89% at 5 years and 85% at 10 years. Overall, only about 30% of patients remain without reoperation 10 years after truncus arteriosus surgery. Nonetheless, the quality of life in treated patients is reported to be near normal. The presence of 22q11 deletion has an important bearing on long-term follow-up. Speech and development delays initially and psychiatric challenges later are particularly common.

Lifelong follow-up is required in view of need for reoperations. Exercise restriction is not required for those who have undergone corrective surgery with no residual defects. However, if they develop RV to PA conduit stenosis or RV dysfunction, they may be advised exercise restriction based on hemodynamics. Pregnancy is well tolerated in those without any residual defects.

CONCLUSION

Truncus arteriosus is a cyanotic heart disease that manifests with bounding pulses, congestive cardiac failure, and mild cyanosis in early infancy. Deletion of 22q11.2 is a common genetic association that has important postoperative and long-term implications. They require surgery early in infancy due to early development of PVOD. If left untreated, most children die by 1 year of age. With advancement in the field of cardiology and cardiothoracic surgery, most of these patients have good survival rate and long-term prognosis if surgery is done in early infancy. However, they have to remain on lifelong follow-up, as they may require reoperations for RV to PA conduit stenosis/regurgitation and truncal valve regurgitation.

REFERENCES

1. Saxena A, Mehta A, Sharma M, Salhan S, Kalaivani M, Ramakrishnan S, et al. Birth prevalence of congenital heart disease: a cross-sectional observational study from North India. Ann Pediatr Cardiol. 2016;9(3):205-9.
2. Samanek M, Slavik Z, Zborilova B, Hrobonová V, Voríšková M, Skovránek J. Prevalence, treatment and outcome of heart disease in liveborn children: a prospective analysis of 91823 liveborn children. Pediatr Cardiol. 1989; 110(4):205-11.
3. Samanek M, Voriskova M. Infants with critical heart disease in a territory with centralized care. Int J Cardiol. 1987;16(1):75-92.
4. Wilson J. A description of a very unusual malformation of the human heart. Philos Trans R Soc London. 1798;18:346.
5. Buchanan G. Malformation of the heart, undivided truncus arteriosus. Heart otherwise double. Trans Path Soc Lend. 1864:15:89-91.
6. Bartelings MM, Gittenberger-de Groot AC. Morphogenetic considerations on congenital malformations of the outflow tract. Part I: Common arterial trunk and tetralogy of Fallot. Int J Cardiol. 1991;32:213-230.
7. Van Praagh R, Van Praagh S. The anatomy of common aorticopulmonary trunk (truncus arteriosus communis) and its embryologic implications. Am J Cardiol. 1965;16:406-25.
8. Butto F, Lucas RV Jr, Edwards JE. Persistent truncus arteriosus: pathologic anatomy in 54 cases. Pediatr Cardiol. 1986;7(2): 95-101.
9. Talwar S, Rajashekar P, Gupta SK, Gulati GS, Airan B. Crossed pulmonary arteries in a patient with persistent truncus arteriosus. Ann Thorac Surg. 2016;101(6):2377-9.
10. Collett RW, Edwards JE. Persistent truncus arteriosus: a classification according to anatomic types. Surg Clin North Am. 1949;29(4):1245-70.
11. Goldmuntz E, Clark BJ, Mitchell LE, Jawad AF, Cuneo BF, Reed L, et al. Frequency of 22q11 deletions in patients with conotruncal defects. J Am Coll Cardiol. 1998;32(2):492-8.
12. McElhinney DB, Driscoll DA, Emanuel BS, Goldmuntz E. Chromosome 22q11 deletion in patients with truncus arteriosus. Pediatr Cardiol. 2003;24(6):569-73.
13. Bharati S, McAllister HA Jr, Rosenquist GC, Miller RA, Tatooles CJ, Lev M. The surgical anatomy of truncus arteriosus communis. J Thorac Cardiovasc Surg. 1974;67(4):501-10.
14. Calder L, Van Praagh R, Van Praagh S, Sears WP, Corwin R, Levy A, et al. Truncus arteriosus communis. Clinical, angiocardiographic and pathologic findings in 100 patients. Am Heart J. 1976;92(1): 23-38.
15. Arslan AH, Ugurlucan M, Yildiz Y, Ay S, Bahceci F, Besikci R, et al. Surgical treatment of common arterial trunk in patients beyond the first year of life. World J Pediatr Congenit Heart Surg. 2014;5(2):211-15.
16. Stark J, Gandhi D, de Leval M, Macartney F, Taylor JF. Surgical treatment of persistent truncus arteriosus in the first year of life. Br Heart J. 1978;40(11):1280-7.
17. Ginelliova A, Farkas D, Farkasova lannaccone S. Truncus arteriosus communis with survival to the age of 46 years: case report. Soud Lek. 2015;60(3):37-9.
18. McGoon DC, Rastelli GC, Ongley PA. An operation for the correction of truncus arteriosus. JAMA. 1968;205(2):69-73.
19. Barbero-Marcial M, Riso A, Atik E, Jatene A. A technique for correction of truncus arteriosus types I and II without extracardiac conduits. J Thorac Cardiovasc Surg. 1990;99(2):364-9.
20. Tlaskal T, Chaloupecky V, Hucin B, Gebauer R, Krupickova S, Reich O, et al. Long-term results after correction of persistent truncus arteriosus in 83 patients. Eur J Cardiothorac Surg. 2010; 37(6):1278-84.
21. Reddy VM, Hanley F. Late results of repair of truncus arteriosus. Semin Thorac Cardiovasc Surg Pediatr Card Surg Annu. 1998; 1:139-46.
22. Rajasinghe HA, McElhinney DB, Reddy VM, Mora BN, Hanley FL. Long-term follow-up of truncus arteriosus repaired in infancy: a twenty year experience. J Thorac Cardiovasc Surg. 1997;113(5):869-78.
23. Benson L, Freedom R. Catheterization interventions in the management of common arterial trunk. Prog Pediatr Cardiol. 2002;15(1): 73-80.

36

CHAPTER

Transposition of Great Arteries

R Suresh Kumar, John Valliattu

INTRODUCTION

Transposition of the great arteries (TGA) is a condition in which the great arteries arise from the wrong ventricles—aorta from the right ventricle (RV) and pulmonary artery (PA) from the left ventricle (LV). In terms of segmental anatomy, there is ventriculoarterial (VA) discordance with preserved atrioventricular (AV) concordance. Transposition could occur with either situs solitus or situs inversus.

EPIDEMIOLOGY

Transposition of the great arteries accounts for 5% of all congenital cardiac malformations.[1] TGA was found in 4.3% of all newborns with significant congenital heart disease when 20,307 consecutive newborns were screened in Northern India.[2] This is the most common cardiac cause for cyanosis on the first day of life.

ETIOLOGY

Like most congenital heart diseases, etiology of TGA is uncertain. Males are affected more often than females in ratios ranging from 1.5:1 to 3.2:1.[1] Unlike other conotruncal anomalies, TGA can be considered as a stand-alone lesion, association with chromosomal anomalies or other organ anomalies being extremely uncommon.[1] Association with genetic mutations has been reported only in isolated cases. The disease carries a recurrence risk of 1.7% in siblings. The reported risk factors in pregnant women include diabetes, high intake of vitamin A and, exposure to drugs such as ibuprofen and viral infections.[1]

MOLECULAR GENETICS

Last two decades have seen exciting developments unraveling the molecular genetic pathways involved in the morphogenesis of TGA.[3] In humans, the genes *CFC1*, *GDF1*, *PROSIT240*, and *ZIC3* have been linked to TGA. Experimental global deletion of CFC1 and GDF1 in mice has been reported to result in TGA. Mutations in mouse genes, such as *PITX2* and type IIB activin receptor, result in TGA and defects of left-right asymmetry, suggesting a common genetic lineage for these disorders. An animal model close to human TGA has been developed by global inactivation of HSPG2 in mice. In HSPG2-null mice, the endocardial cushions of the distal outflow tract become hyperplastic possibly due to increased cardiac neural crest cell migration, altering the orientation of the developing great arteries over the chambers resulting in TGA.[3]

EMBRYOLOGY

Van Praagh has observed that both the great arteries are above the developing RV in the embryo—with the aortic valve to the right of the pulmonary valve—when the straight heart tube has taken the rightward loop.[4] Then the right-sided (subaortic) infundibular free wall undergoes involution, while the left-sided (subpulmonary) infundibular free wall grows and expands. As a result, the pulmonary valve is pushed upward and is connected to the RV. With the pulmonary valve out of the way, the aortic valve moves leftward, backward, and inferiorly to open into the LV and establishes fibrous continuity with the mitral valve. This differential conal growth is the key factor that determines VA concordance.[4] In TGA, the subaortic infundibulum grows and expands, while the subpulmonary infundibulum undergoes involution. As a result, the pulmonary valve moves inferiorly and posteriorly, opening into the LV establishing fibrous continuity with the mitral valve.[4] Anderson has proposed that it is the formation of the intrapericardial arterial trunks in parallel, rather than spiral, fashion that leads to the morphogenesis of TGA. According to him, the fusion of the outflow cushions in a straight (rather than spiral) fashion is the key determinant of discordant VA connection.[5]

PATHOLOGIC ANATOMY

Transposition of the great arteries is characterized by VA discordance in the presence of AV concordance.[6] The term complete transposition has been traditionally employed to distinguish this entity from congenitally corrected transposition.[1] As the aorta is to the right of the PA, this form of TGA is designated D-TGA. Most often, this is in the setting of situs solitus with levocardia, but this can also happen with situs inversus and dextrocardia. The segmental anatomy would be S,D,D-Transposition or I,L,L-Transposition. The aortic valve is commonly located right and anterior to the pulmonary valve, but it may also be directly anterior. Extremely uncommonly, the aortic valve may be left and anterior to the pulmonary valve (S,D,L-Transposition).[7]

It is important to recognize that the defining feature of transposition is VA discordance—not the spatial arrangement of the semilunar valves.[6] There is mitral pulmonary continuity and aortic-tricuspid discontinuity due to the presence of subaortic conus with no subpulmonary conus. The most common associated lesions are ventricular septal defect (VSD) (40%) and LV outflow obstruction (5–10%).[1] The presence of a patent foramen ovale (PFO), small atrial septal defect (ASD) or a patent ductus arteriosus (PDA) in the newborn does not merit description as an additional lesion. Transposition of the great arteries with intact ventricular septum (TGA-IVS) denotes intact ventricular septum with D-TGA. VSD, when present, is usually conoventricular (perimembranous). Additional muscular VSDs may occur. LV outflow obstruction is more likely in presence of a VSD and results from posterior deviation of the infundibular septum. It may also result from pulmonary valve stenosis, subvalvar muscular stenosis or from abnormal insertion of mitral chordae. In presence of a large VSD, there is possibility for straddling of either AV valve. Coarctation of the aorta or interruption of the aortic arch occurs in 5%; it is much more common with anterior malalignment type of VSD, especially in Taussig–Bing anomaly.[1] Left juxtaposition of right atrial (RA) appendages has been reported. Abnormalities of the AV valves, particularly mitral regurgitation, may occur in 4%.[1]

Coronary artery anomalies have been reported in about a third of patients undergoing arterial switch operation (ASO).[8] The common abnormalities of coronary anatomy are described in the section on echocardiography.

Taussig–Bing anomaly is a form of double-outlet right ventricle (DORV), where the VSD is subpulmonary and the PA is overriding it. The semilunar valves are side by side and at the same level. There is a conus below both the semilunar valves. The LV pumps preferentially into the PA, while the RV pumps into the aorta giving a physiology of TGA. Coarctation or interruption of the arch occurs in >50% in surgical series.[8] Subvalvar pulmonary stenosis (PS) is also common. Coronary anomalies are also more common with this variant.[8]

PATHOPHYSIOLOGY

The normal circulation is in series. This means that the systemic venous blood returning to the RV is pumped into the PA and that the pulmonary venous blood coming into the LV is pumped into the aorta. As against this, in transposition, the circulation becomes parallel. The systemic venous blood is pumped back into the aorta from the RV without oxygenation.[6] Similarly, the pulmonary venous blood is recirculated into the lungs as LV pumps into the PA. Survival is possible, if only the parallel circulations have connections at one or more levels for intercirculatory mixing. The usual levels of connection are ASD/PFO and PDA. The PDA allows desaturated aortic blood to reach the PA to improve oxygenation. The increased pulmonary venous return encourages left-to-right shunt across the atrial septum delivering the much-needed pulmonary venous blood into RV and aorta. As a result, neonates with TGA-IVS have much better systemic arterial oxygen saturation, if they have a PDA and ASD.[6] In the absence of such a communication, arterial PO_2 will fall markedly, often to levels below 20 mm Hg. This results in tissue hypoxia, increased anaerobic metabolism and lactate production leading to severe metabolic acidosis.[6] The baby can be helped by administering prostaglandin E1 (PGE1) infusion to keep the ductus open. Creating an ASD by balloon atrial septostomy (BAS) further helps the baby.

When there is a large VSD, intercirculatory mixing is even better, especially when there is additional atrial communication. Cyanosis in such cases tends to be minimal. Such babies progress into heart failure by 2–6 weeks of life. TGA with a large VSD is prone to accelerated development of pulmonary vascular obstructive disease.[6]

As discussed before, left ventricular outflow tract (LVOT) obstruction (PS) is common in infants with a VSD. The anatomic substrate is usually complex and tends to occur at multiple levels. The hemodynamics depend on the size of the VSD and the severity of the PS. With a large VSD and severe PS, the presentation would resemble that of tetralogy of Fallot (TOF), but with more desaturation.[1,6]

CLINICAL FEATURES

Transposition of the Great Arteries with Intact Ventricular Septum

Babies with TGA-IVS typically present on day 1 with profound cyanosis.[1,6] The baby is tachypneic and cyanosed without any overt distress ("peaceful cyanosis"). The birth weight is normal. There are no dysmorphic features and other organ systems are usually normal. On cardiovascular examination, S1 is normal and S2 is single. Murmurs are uncommon; a faint systolic murmur due to PDA may be audible at the upper left sternal border. If the diagnosis is missed, the baby would present with severe metabolic acidosis in a few days. When TGA-IVS is associated with coarctation and PDA, the upper limbs will have lower saturation than the lower limbs-reverse differential cyanosis.[1]

Transposition of the Great Arteries with Large Ventricular Septal Defect

Careful examination and pulse oximetry screening will demonstrate mild desaturation (SpO_2 <94%) in these babies. It is not uncommon for these babies to be missed in the initial evaluation. As heart failure sets in by the second month, the diagnosis becomes more evident. Rapid breathing, excessive sweating, and feeding difficulty are common features. On examination, cyanosis is mild. There is tachycardia and tachypnea with prominent precordial pulsations. S1 is normal; S2 is single. There is a short early systolic murmur at the left sternal border, the murmur is louder if the VSD is restrictive. S3 and mid-diastolic murmur may be audible over the apex beat. Crepitations in the lungs fields and tender hepatomegaly may be noticed in infants in frank heart failure.

Transposition of the Great Arteries, Ventricular Septal Defect with Pulmonary Stenosis

These babies tend to have features similar to TOF. Cyanosis appears earlier than TOF and tends to be more severe.[1,6] If PS is severe, cyanosis appears early. Hypoxic spells may occur and older children may squat to relieve dyspnea. There are no features of cardiac failure. Precordium is quiet. S1 is normal, S2 is single. There is an ejection systolic murmur of variable intensity and duration depending on the severity of LVOT obstruction.

DIFFERENTIAL DIAGNOSIS

Transposition of the great arteries needs to be differentiated from other causes of cyanosis in the newborn.[1,6] To begin with, absence of respiratory distress in the cyanotic baby helps to rule out primary respiratory pathology. TOF and pulmonary atresia with intact ventricular septum top the list of cardiac differential diagnosis. The presence of a murmur and reduced lung vascularity on chest X-ray favor TOF. Critical PS will also have a murmur in the pulmonary area. If the baby presents with heart failure (TGA with VSD), other cyanotic heart diseases with increased pulmonary blood flow [truncus arteriosus, single ventricle, total anomalous pulmonary venous connection (TAPVC), and tricuspid atresia] will need to be excluded.

Electrocardiogram (ECG)

In TGA-IVS, there is right ventricular hypertrophy (RVH) with right axis deviation (**Fig. 1**). T wave in V1 is likely to be upright. When there is a large VSD, ECG may show biventricular thypertrophy in a few months. TGA/VSD/PS will show RVH and right axis deviation.

Chest X-ray

Mild cardiomegaly, narrow superior mediastinum, and increased lung vascularity are the characteristic radiologic features of TGA (**Fig. 2**). The posterior main pulmonary artery (MPA) segment is not seen in the X-ray. The cardiac silhouette is described as "egg-on side." More importantly, an X-ray showing increased lung vascularity, when the SpO_2 is very low, is highly suggestive of TGA in the neonate. TGA/VSD will show cardiomegaly with markedly increased vascularity by 2–3 months of age. TGA/VSD/PS will have normal sized heart with reduced lung vascularity as in TOF.

Echocardiography

The principal imaging tool to establish the diagnosis of TGA is echocardiography.[1] The key echocardiographic feature is VA discordance. Parasternal long axis view will

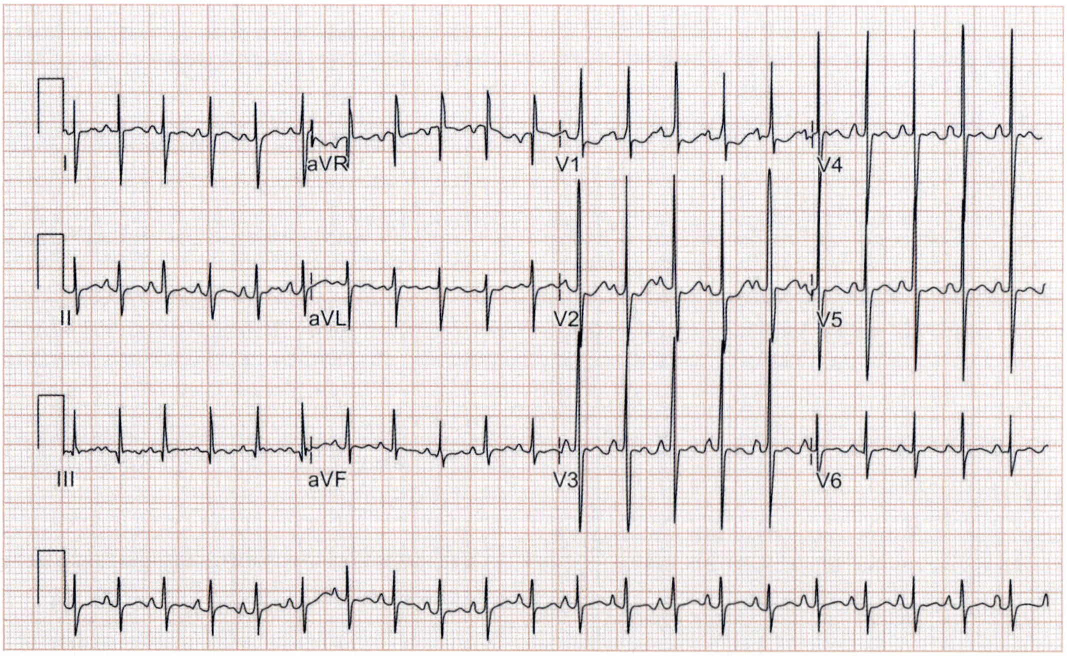

Fig. 1: Electrocardiogram (ECG) in a newborn with transposition of the great arteries with intact ventricular septum (TGA-IVS). Note right ventricular hypertrophy (RVH) with right axis deviation.

show parallel great vessels; the vessel originating from the posterior ventricle courses posteriorly and bifurcates showing that it is the PA (**Fig. 3A**). In the same view aorta, bearing the coronary arteries, courses anterior to the PA. Color Doppler evaluation may show ductal flow into the left PA. Parasternal short axis view shows cross sections of two vessels, aorta being right and anterior or directly anterior in relation to the PA (**Fig. 3B**). Uncommonly, aorta may be left and anterior. Parasternal short axis view also helps to delineate coronary artery anatomy. Apical and subcostal long axial views demonstrate VA discordance and the subvalvar outflow tracts. Additional lesions such as VSD and AV valve regurgitation can also be made out in these views.

Detailed evaluation of cardiac segmental anatomy is required. Situs is usually solitus with levocardia. Atrial septum should be looked at in subcostal and apical views to assess the presence and adequacy of interatrial shunt. An ASD measuring at least 5 mm is a reassuring sight in the neonate with TGA. Uncommonly, the saturations may be low even with an adequate ASD in TGA in the newborn. This is a sign of severe pulmonary arterial hypertension. The AV valves must be assessed for adequacy of the annulus (with Z scores), tricuspid regurgitation, mitral regurgitation, and straddling (if there is a VSD). Ventricular septum is evaluated for the presence, location, and number of VSDs. Commonly VSD is conoventricular (perimembranous). The echocardiographer measures the annulus of the semilunar valves and the diameter of the arteries, comparing the values against Z scores. Branch pulmonary arteries are also measured. Presence and size of PDA and the direction of blood flow must be evaluated. PDA is likely to be present as the baby might well be on PGE1 infusion.

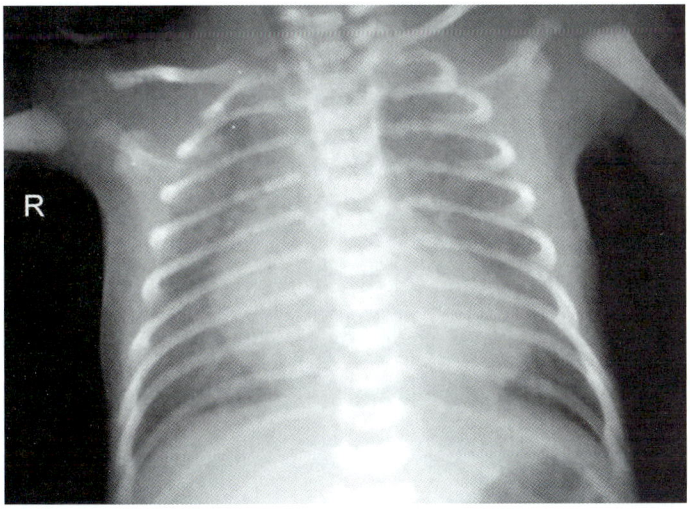

Fig. 2: Chest X-ray in a newborn with TGA-IVS. Note cardiomegaly, narrow superior mediastinum and increased lung vascularity.

Left ventricular outflow tract must be assessed for any narrowing. This may happen from posterior malalignment of the outlet septum, or simply from the bowing IVS in the older infant. It may be related to diffuse/discrete narrowing (fibrous or muscular) of the LVOT. Anomalous insertion of mitral chordae is another cause for LVOT obstruction.[1] In presence of a VSD, posterior displacement of the IVS is the most common cause for LVOT obstruction, but any of the forgoing mechanisms could also be present. When there is TGA/VSD/LVOT obstruction, it is common to find hypoplasia of the pulmonary annulus/MPA and branches.

The aortic arch is usually left-sided in situs solitus. Arch obstruction must be carefully looked for. This may be in the form of isthmial coarctation with transverse arch hypoplasia or complete interruption (type B being most common). Interruption or coarctation is a common association of Taussig–Bing anomaly.[8]

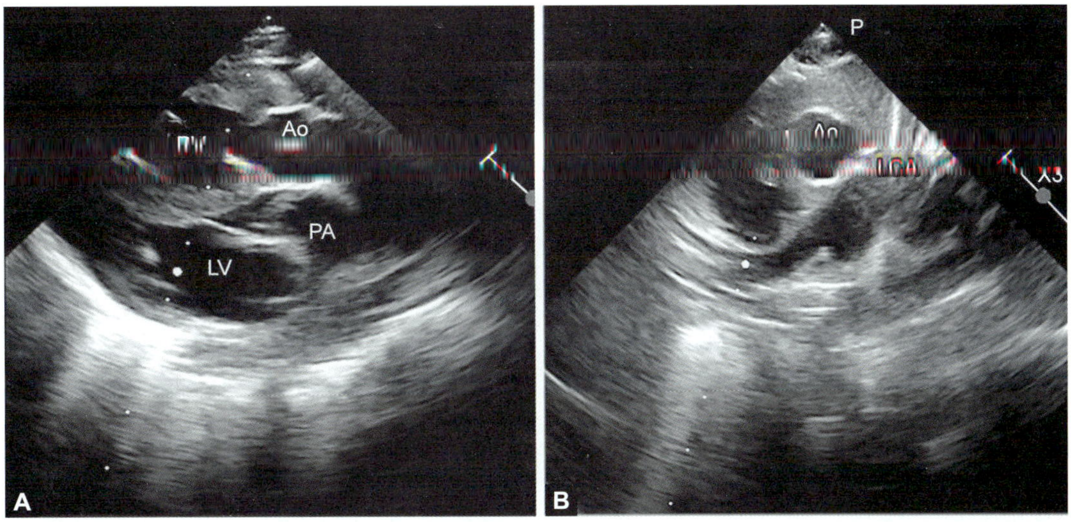

Figs. 3A and B: Echocardiogram in transposition of the great arteries with intact ventricular septum (TGA-IVS). (A) Parasternal long axis view of a 42-day old baby with TGA-IVS. Note that aorta (Ao) and pulmonary artery (PA) are parallel. The posterior vessel is bifurcating; (B) Parasternal short axis view in the same baby. Note that the "circle and sausage " appearance is replaced by aortic cross section (Ao) that is right and anterior, with PA bifurcation posteriorly and to the left. Note the beginning of left coronary artery (LCA).
(LV: left ventricle; RV: right ventricle)

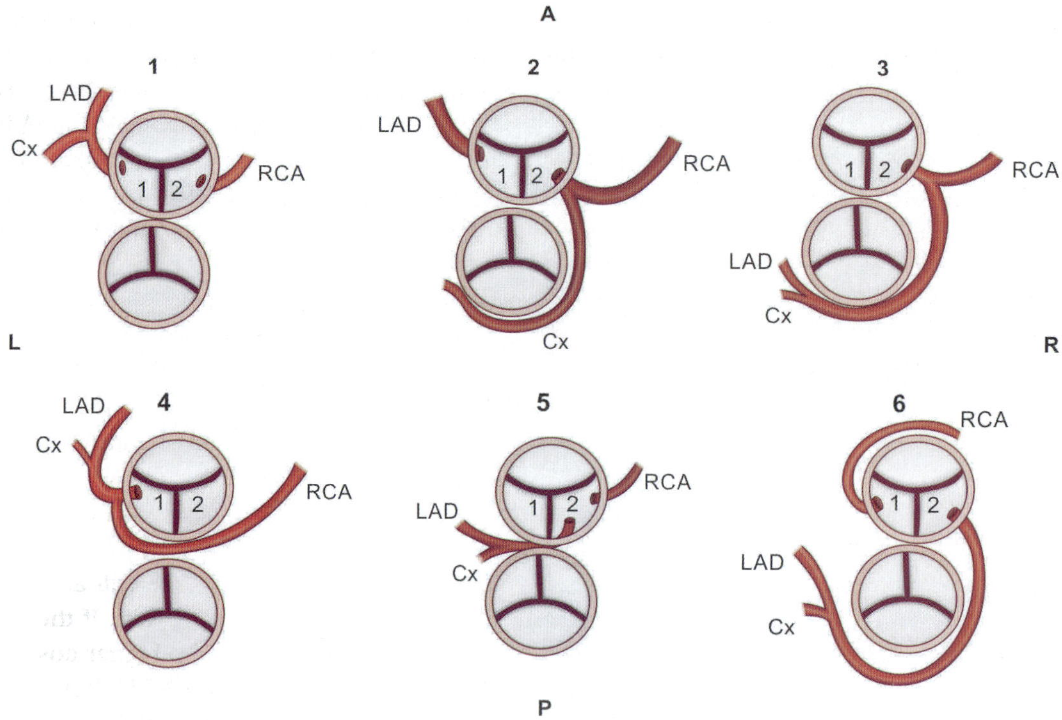

Fig. 4: Some surgically important patterns of coronary anatomy in dextro-transposition of the great arteries (D-TGA).
1. Usual. LCA from Sinus 1; RCA from Sinus 2.
2. LAD from Sinus 1; RCA from Sinus 2. Cx is from RCA with a posterior, circum-arterial loop.
3. Single coronary from Sinus 2; LCA has posterior circum-arterial loop.
4. Single coronary from Sinus 1; RCA is inter-arterial.
5. Both coronaries from Sinus 2 from separate ostia. LCA has first an intramural course and then an inter-arterial course.
6. Inverted coronaries: RCA from Sinus 1 with anterior loop, LCA from Sinus 2 with posterior circum-arterial loop.
(A: anterior; P: posterior; R: right; L: left. 1: Sinus 1; 2: Sinus 2; RCA: right coronary artery. LCA: left coronary artery; LAD: left anterior descending; Cx: circumflex)

Assessment of the coronary arteries is an important part of the echocardiographic evaluation of TGA. This is best done from parasternal short axis view, identifying the aortic sinuses and the coronary arteries that arise from them. Angulated views from parasternal short axis and subcostal long axis views will further help in delineating the origin and course of coronary arteries. There are different classifications for coronary anatomy in TGA (e.g., that of Yacoub and Radley Smith and Leiden Group).[9,10] The coronaries usually arise from the facing sinuses—left coronary from the left and posterior facing sinus (Sinus 1 in the Leiden classification) and the right coronary from the right and posterior facing sinus (Sinus 2 in the Leiden classification). Please note that the echocardiographer would find Sinus 1 to his right on the screen and Sinus 2 to his left. Most units prefer to describe the sinus of origin and the course (interarterial/intramural, anterior/posterior loop) of the coronaries, rather than follow any of the classifications. Some of the important coronary patterns are illustrated in **Figure 4**.

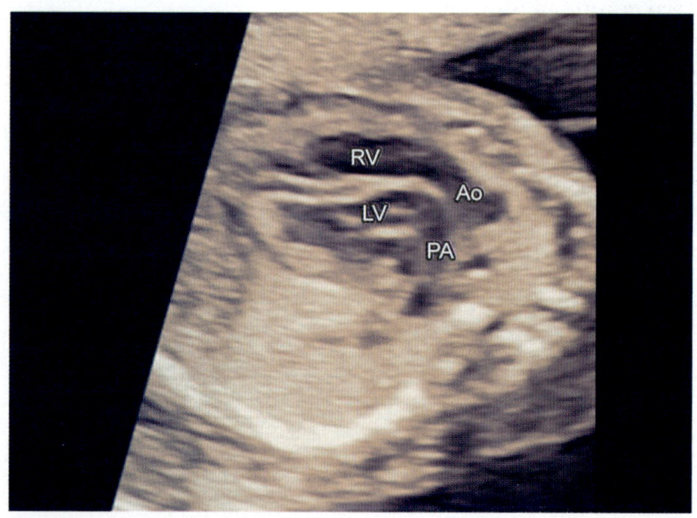

Fig. 5: Fetal echocardiogram. Echocardiographic image of an 18-week-old fetus showing parallel great vessels.
(Ao: aorta; PA: pulmonary artery; LV: left ventricle; RV: right ventricle)
Courtesy: Dr Rekha R Kuriakose, Department of Fetal Medicine, Believers Church Medical College Hospital, Thiruvalla, Kerala.

PRENATAL DIAGNOSIS

The diagnosis of TGA can be made in a fetal echocardiography by 16 weeks of gestation. It is important to add outflow views to four-chamber views during routine antenatal ultrasound scans to avoid missing TGA.[11] Demonstrating parallel outflows (not crossing) is the cornerstone of TGA diagnosis in the fetus (**Fig. 5**). VA discordance is easily demonstrated by showing that the anatomic RV (with moderator band) is connected to the aorta. Presence or absence of VSD and LVOT obstruction must be made out.

Once TGA is suspected, it should be confirmed by a pediatric cardiologist and family counseled regarding the diagnosis, prognosis, management of delivery, and perinatal management. Fetal karyotyping is usually not indicated, unless the fetal medicine specialist has a specific reason to do so on an individual basis. There must be at least one repeat scan in the few weeks prior to delivery to look for high-risk features.[11]

CARDIAC CATHETERIZATION

In the neonate with TGA, cardiac catheterization is undertaken, if only there is an indication for BAS.[1] Most centers do not perform hemodynamic evaluation at the time of BAS. LV pressures are subsystemic in TGA with intact IVS, RV being the systemic ventricle. Oximetry characteristically shows oxygen saturations to be higher in PA than in aorta. Angiography is seldom performed during BAS. However, if coronary arteries need to be demonstrated, a steep caudal anteroposterior (AP) view—"laid back" view—aortic root angiogram is done, entering the aorta from the RV with a balloon catheter.[1] In the older child with TGA/VSD/PS, ventricular angiograms may be required to demonstrate routability of VSD, ventricular adequacy, anatomy of LVOT obstruction, and branches of PA.

Cardiac catheterization is more often required during the long-term follow-up after ASO.[8] This may be for demonstration of coronary artery obstruction, right ventricular outflow tract (RVOT) obstruction, or other long-tern complications discussed later.

NATURAL HISTORY

The outcome of untreated TGA has been documented in the era before the advent of BAS. If untreated, about 30% of babies with TGA (all groups) die in the first week, 50% by first month, 70% by 6 months, and 90% by first year.[1,12] TGA-IVS fares still worse, with about 70% dying in the first month and almost none surviving the first year. [12]

PERINATAL MANAGEMENT

Antenatal diagnosis facilitates streamlined perinatal management of TGA. Delivery is planned in an obstetric unit close to a tertiary pediatric cardiac service. In utero transport of the fetus ensures optimal management of the baby right from birth. Indeed, current data suggest that preoperative and postoperative mortality and morbidity are lower in babies with antenatal diagnosis.[11] Normal vaginal delivery is recommended, with cesarean section being reserved for obstetric reasons. Postnatal oxygen saturation (SpO_2) measurement and monitoring are essential. In the absence of antenatal diagnosis, it is the investigation of hypoxia, which will lead to echocardiography and diagnosis of TGA. Other parameters to be monitored include ECG, noninvasive blood pressure (NIBP), respiration, tissue perfusion, urine output, and lactate levels. It is ideal to have umbilical venous and arterial lines inserted soon after delivery for medication and monitoring.

It is best to start prostaglandin infusion at the earliest, pending detailed evaluation. Prostaglandin in TGA (PGE1 or E2, the former more commonly used) maintains ductal patency, causes circulatory mixing at ductal level, improves pulmonary venous return, distends left atrium (LA), and causes more vigorous left-to-right shunt across the PFO, all leading to significant improvement in arterial oxygen saturation.[6] LA pressure increases, if PFO is restrictive. PGE1 is used in a dose ranging from 0.01 to 0.1 µg/kg/min as an infusion. Combining balloon septostomy with PGE1 infusion gives better systemic oxygen saturation. Side effects of PGE1 include apnea, tachycardia, hypotension, fever, and tissue edema. Employing lower doses helps to minimize side effects. Early initiation of PGE1 will allow employing very low doses such as 0.01 µg/kg/min. If the duct has already closed, you would need much higher doses, like 0.1 µg/kg/min.[1,6] Babies who were on PGE1 have been reported to require longer intensive care unit (ICU) stay after ASO.

Babies without prenatal diagnosis reaching a tertiary care center by suboptimal transportation systems present with deep hypoxemia, acidosis, and shock. Such babies would require intensive resuscitation including volume infusion, ventilation, inotropes, and sedation in addition to PGE1 infusion.

BALLOON ATRIAL SEPTOSTOMY

Rashkind and Miller, in 1966, introduced balloon atrial septostomy (BAS) as a palliative measure for the neonate with TGA. This heralded the era of interventional pediatric cardiology. Today BAS is indicated in all infants with TGA and severe hypoxemia due to inadequate intercirculatory mixing. Increasingly, it is being done at the bedside in the neonatal intensive care unit (NICU). The procedure can be done from femoral or umbilical venous access, the latter being the preferred route in the NICU. The older Rashkind septostomy catheters needed at least 7 F introducer sheath and had a latex balloon at the tip. The NuMed Z-5 atrioseptostomy catheter.

NuMed, Cornwall, ON, Canada, more readily available in India now, is a low-profile, dual lumen catheter that comes in 4F or 5F sizes, each requiring one size higher introducer sheaths. Z-5 catheter is introduced over a 0.014" coronary guidewire, parked in the left upper pulmonary vein. The balloon is made of polytetrafluoroethylene (PTFE) and is sturdy. The balloon is inflated in the LA and a sharp downward pull is given to the catheter. The septum tears and an ASD of at least 4–5 mm is created. Free fluttering of the torn margin of the defect and smooth flow from LA to RA across the ASD on color Doppler interrogation indicate successful septostomy. Arterial oxygen saturation improves significantly. Beattie and Mcleod noted an average rise of arterial oxygen saturation from 61.4±11.5% to 81.5±9.4% in a series of 26 newborns following BAS. However, 54% needed restarting of prostaglandin later to maintain good saturations till ASO.[13] Reported complications include balloon rupture, access site problems, arrhythmias, systemic embolism, and stroke.

The last decade has seen some concern and confusion regarding the role of BAS in neonates with TGA. In a series of 29 neonates who underwent brain magnetic resonance imaging (MRI) before ASO, McQuillen et al. found features of brain injury in 41%.[14] All the patients with brain injury had preceding BAS, and the incidence of stroke was 61% in babies who had BAS. However, Petit et al. strongly refuted these findings and showed that postoperative brain injury in TGA was associated with oxygenation and time to surgery, not BAS.[15] In their study of 64 newborns (44 with TGA), MRI revealed brain injury prior to surgery in 30%—occurring at similar rates in TGA, hypoplastic left heart syndrome (HLHS), and pulmonary atresia. BAS was not a risk factor for brain injury; the three cases of stroke in the study were distributed between TGA with BAS, TGA without BAS, and HLHS. The authors found no reason to change the established clinical practice of performing BAS in all hypoxic neonates with TGA.

It has been the authors' practice to do a BAS in cases of TGA with intact IVS presenting within the first week, unless there is a generous ASD. If ASO is being planned within 24 hours, as is increasingly the case now, the baby is maintained on prostaglandin infusion and BAS is not required. In late presenters, BAS may be needed for emergency palliation, while the management strategy is being finalized.

MANAGEMENT OF TRANSPOSITION OF THE GREAT ARTERIES WITH INTACT VENTRICULAR SEPTUM

History

Early attempts at surgical repair of TGA were uniformly unsuccessful, not in the least because cardiac surgery and related technology were in the early stages of evolution. Ake Senning in Europe (1957) and William Mustard in Canada (1963) introduced the first definitive operations for this condition—atrial switch—that bear their respective names. In the 1970s, Brom and Senning popularized the Senning operation in Europe, while Mustard remained popular in North America, both techniques carrying very low surgical mortalilty.[9]

The turning point in surgical history was when Jatene performed anatomical correction in a young infant with TGA and VSD in Brazil in 1975. Pioneers such as Aldo Castaneda, Roger Mee, Magdi Yacoub, AG Brom, and William Brawn took the concept rapidly forward and by 1990s, ASO became the standard of care in the surgical management of TGA.[9]

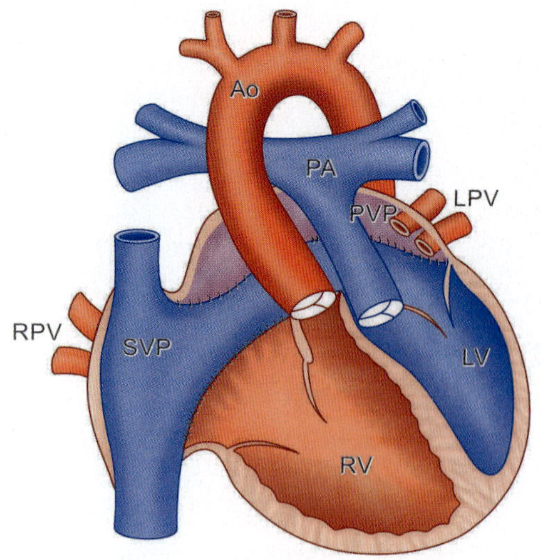

Fig. 6: Diagrammatic representation of atrial switch procedure. Systemic venous pathway (SVP), connecting vena caval orifices to the mitral valve; pulmonary venous pathway (PVP), connecting the entry of right pulmonary veins (RPV); left pulmonary veins (LPV) to the tricuspid valve). (Ao: aorta; LV: left ventricle; PA: pulmonary artery; RV: right ventricle)

Atrial Switch Procedures

The atrial switch procedures create two venous pathways within the atrium—the pulmonary venous pathway connecting the pulmonary veins to the tricuspid valve and the systemic venous pathway connecting the orifices of the venae cavae to the mitral valve.[1] This is illustrated in **Figure 6**. Whereas the Mustard procedure uses glutaraldehyde treated pericardium to create the systemic venous baffle, the baffles are constructed with flaps of the atrial septum and atrial wall in the Senning operation.

Results of Atrial Switch Procedures

The atrial switch operation, Senning or Mustard, was the preferred surgery for TGA until the early 1990s. These procedures gave excellent functional outcome in the intermediate term with low operative mortality for a condition that carried such dismal prognosis hitherto. Congenital Heart Surgeons Society (CHSS) data from 20 centers that performed atrial switch procedures in 281 patients (108 Mustard and 173 Senning) during 1985-89 showed survival at 1 month, 5 years, and 10 years to be 90, 85, and 84%, respectively, with Mustard patients doing better than Senning at all intervals.[16] Risk factors for poor outcome included VSD, lower weight, younger age, cardiac malposition, and LVOT surgery. Reoperations (n = 19; 2 for RV failure, 12 for Baffle obstruction, and 5 for baffle leak) carried a 36% overall mortality. At 10 years, freedom from baffle obstruction was 95% and freedom from pacemaker insertion 91%. For both surgeries, 60% of patients were in New York Heart Association (NYHA) functional Class I with the remainder in Class II.[16] However, two European studies did not find any difference in mortality or arrhythmias between Mustard and Senning operations and observed better functional class in Senning patients.[17,18]

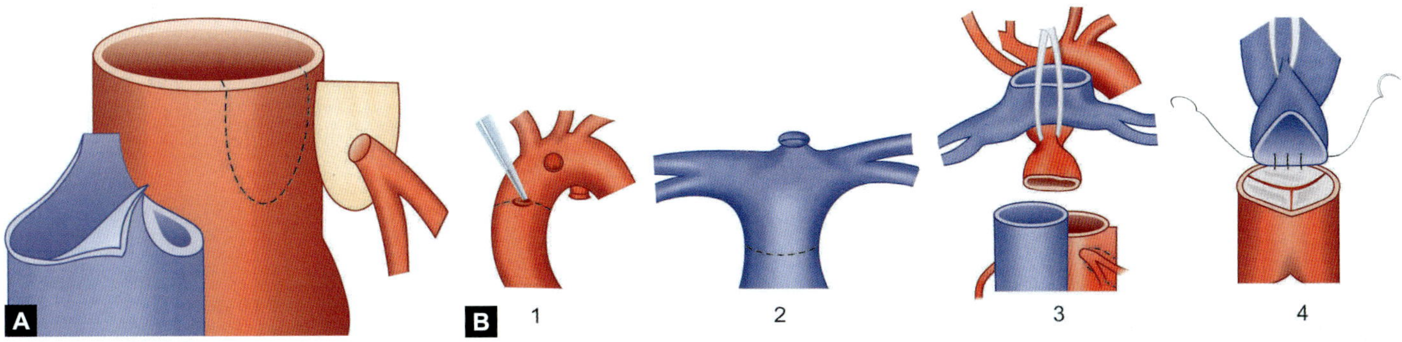

Figs. 7A and B: Arterial switch operation—Main steps. (A) Aorta and pulmonary arteries have been divided. Coronary buttons removed from the aorta. A U-shape segment of the left facing neo-aortic sinus has been removed to accommodate the left coronary button. Right coronary button is similarly harvested and anastomosed to a U-shaped incision in the right facing sinus (not shown in the image); (B) 1 and 2 Note the transection lines in aorta and PA; PA is transected lower. 3. The LeCompte maneuver has been done. The coronary buttons have been transferred to the neo-aorta. 4. The aortic anastomosis has started at the middle of the posterior sinus of Valsalva.
Courtsey: This diagrammatic representation follows techniques as practiced by the surgical author (modified from Lacour Gayet[10]). Computer graphics by Nandini Suresh Kumar (San Francisco, USA).

Arterial Switch Operation

The arterial switch operation (ASO) aims to achieve anatomic and physiologic correction of TGA by switching the great vessels to their appropriate ventricles.

*The surgery is done under cardiopulmonary bypass with moderate hypothermia. The aorta is transected at a higher level than the PA, in order to shorten the neoaorta and to prevent stretching of the anteriorly placed PA bifurcation. The coronaries are transferred to the neoaorta. PA bifurcation is placed in front of the aorta (LeCompte maneuver) to ensure smooth unobstructed pulmonary blood flow. Any intracardiac lesion is repaired. The defects in the neo-PA, caused by the removal of coronary arteries, are repaired with a quadrangular patch of fresh native pericardium. The neo-PA is reconstituted by connecting the neopulmonary root with the distal PA (**Figs. 7A and B**).*[9,10]

Results of Arterial Switch Operation

Arterial switch operation is hailed as one of the greatest achievements of pediatric cardiac surgery.[8] Different long-term studies attest to the success of this operation. Following ASO done in 1982-99, Losay et al. reported early mortality of 9.2% and survival of 88% at 15 years. Significant supravalvar PS and/or neoaortic regurgitation was present in 9%, the former being the most common cause for redo surgery. LV function was well preserved and arrhythmias were uncommon.[19]

Today the operative mortality for this procedure has dropped to 1–3%, with higher mortality only for complex forms of TGA such as Taussig–Bing anomaly and TGA with aortic arch interruption. Melbourne data from 1983 to 2009 showed operative mortality of 2.8% in 618 children with TGA, those with a VSD faring worse than those with IVS (3.8% vs. 1.8%). Challenging subgroups included patients with anomalous coronary anatomy, concomitant aortic arch obstruction, Taussig–Bing anomaly, VSD, low operative weight, and patients with an intact IVS who presented late. 20-year survival was 96% in this study.[20]

Reoperations are not uncommon after ASO. Most reoperations occur after the first postoperative year. Freedom from reoperation has been reported in a range of 79–97% at 10 year, 76–87% at 15 years, and 86% at 25 years.[20] The most common indication for reoperation is supravalvar PS, at the suture line along the neo-PA or at the post-LeCompte branch pulmonary arteries. 2.6% each had reoperation and catheter intervention for supravalvar PS in the Melbourne cohort of 618 patients over a 10-year period.[20] Mayo Clinic Group reported 10.9% reoperations in their series.[21] Of the 32 reoperations over a 27-year period, the most common was PA patch plasty (n = 18) followed by different aortic operations in eight (valve replacement in four, root replacement in three, repair in one), pulmonary valve replacement in four, coronary artery bypass grafting in three, and mitral valve repair in three. 15 patients required multiple reoperations.[21]

Early experience of ASO in India showed overall mortality of 8.8% for TGA-IVS and 33% for TGA-VSD including Taussig–Bing anomaly.[22] Coexisting arch anomalies, longer cross-clamp time, late presentation, and prolonged [illegible] were incremental risk factors. On follow-up for 1–10 years, 91% of the patients were asymptomatic. There were three late deaths and five patients required reoperation.[22] The results of TGA surgery in the developing world were analyzed by Schidlow et al. in 778 cases (50% above 30 days) done during 2010–2013 in 26 centers. 80% was primary arterial switch; 20% Senning, or two-stage arterial switch. Early survival was 85%. Poor nutrition and small surgical volume were most strongly associated with mortality.[23]

MANAGEMENT OF LATE PRESENTERS

With every passing week, LV in TGA loses its muscle mass and has less chance of supporting systemic circulation, following the ASO. Norwood considered ASO improbable after 3 weeks.[24]

TABLE 1: Which LV is unsuitable for ASO?[25-29]

Parameter	*Cut-off value*
Banana-shaped LV	Subjective
IVS moving with RV	Subjective
Posterior wall thickness of LV	<3.0 mm
LV mass	<35 g/m^2
LV end-diastolic volume	<90%
LV mass/volume ratio	<1.5
LV minor axis ratio **(Fig. 8)**	>3.0
LV/RV pressure ratio	<0.7

(ASO: arterial switch operation; IVS: intact ventricular septum; LV: left ventricle; RV: right ventricle)

If the older infant with regressed LV undergoes ASO, coming off bypass is stormy with high LA pressure and low cardiac output, unless mechanically supported. Presence of a small VSD, PDA, or aortopulmonary collaterals and the absence of too generous an ASD may help in preserving the LV beyond 3 weeks. In India and the developing world, it is quite common to encounter TGA-IVS for the first time beyond 3 weeks of age. Great Ormond Street Group was the first to show that it might be possible to do ASO in selected cases of TGA-IVS up to 2 months, and even up to 6 months.[25] Careful assessment of the LV is the key to success in such cases.

Diligent assessment of multiple parameters is required to assess left ventricular adequacy. **Table 1** lists different parameters which have been used for this purpose.

Response to PA band on the operating table maintaining hemodynamics with adequate PA band (shifting the ventricular septum to midline, achieving an LV pressure 50–70% systemic) has also been used to support the decision for primary ASO.[29] The infant unsuitable for primary ASO may undergo pulmonary arterial banding with a Blalock–Taussig (BT) shunt to prepare the LV to cope with the increased workload, followed by ASO after a few weeks to few months (two-stage arterial switch).[27-30] However, the strategy of two-stage arterial switch, with the attendant stormy ICU course between the stages, is not very popular in low- and middle-income countries. Most units in such settings would do an atrial switch beyond 3 months of age.[29] Some centers have performed primary ASO in older infants with good results, especially when supported by extracorporeal membrane oxygenation (ECMO). Bisoi et al. reported encouraging mid-term outcomes of 109 children with median age of 60 days (range 42–3,000 days), with regressed LV who underwent primary ASO. ECMO was used in 20%. There were 10 early deaths and 2 late deaths over a mean follow-up period of 28 months.[31]

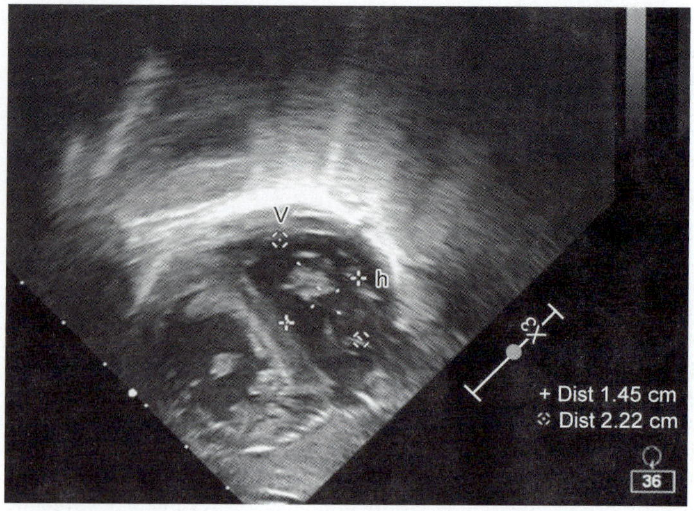

Fig. 8: Minor axis (v/h) ratio. End-systolic subcostal short axis view showing the minor axis (v/h) ratio in a 42-day old baby who had successful primary ASO. (h-anteroposterior "height" of LV, v-lateral dimension. v/h ratio 1.53 is in the favorable range).

FOLLOW-UP AFTER SURGERY FOR TRANSPOSITION OF THE GREAT ARTERIES

Follow-up after Atrial Switch Procedures

Patients who have undergone atrial switch procedures need regular follow-up, keeping in mind long-term issues such as failure of the systemic RV, systemic AV valve regurgitation, baffle leaks, baffle obstruction, and pulmonary hypertension.[1] Atrial tachyarrhythmias are common—usually due to intra-atrial reentry. If not controlled with medication, such patients would need radio frequency (RF) ablation. Bradycardia is usually due to sinus node dysfunction and often requires pacemaker implantation.[1]

Management of the atrial switch patient, who has developed severe RV dysfunction and/or severe tricuspid regurgitation, is a challenging proposition. PA band to retrain the LV over several months, Mustard/Senning takedown and eventual ASO have been done successfully in some cases.[32] The age at which LV ceases to be retrainable is uncertain, some people suggesting 12 years as the cut-off age.[33] Tricuspid valve repair/replacement may be the option for some such patients while some require heart transplantation.[1]

Follow-up after Arterial Switch Operation

Patients who have undergone ASO need regular follow-up all through their life. Neurodevelopmental evaluation is an important component of long-term follow-up after ASO.[34] Reports on neurodevelopmental outcome are conflicting. Whereas Frick et al. found quality of life in ASO survivors similar to normal population,[35] Kalfa et al. found young adult ASO survivors to suffer from cognitive impairment twice as frequently compared to normal population.[36]

All patients need clinical assessment, ECG, and echocardiography evaluation yearly. Exercise testing may be done in older children and adults. Many will need supplemental imaging with CT angiogram or cardiac MRI for problems such as coronary obstructive lesions and PA stenosis. Catheter interventions may be required for such problems. Surgical indications have already been referred to.[21]

SURGERY FOR TRANSPOSITION OF THE GREAT ARTERIES WITH VENTRICULAR SEPTAL DEFECT AND PULMONARY STENOSIS

Rastelli Operation

The most common surgery for TGA/VSD/LVOT obstruction has been the Rastelli operation. Through a right ventriculotomy, the VSD is closed with a patch in such a way as to connect the LV to the aorta. Using the same ventriculotomy, the RV is connected to the pulmonary arteries with a valved conduit. This conduit is extracardiac and is usually placed leftward of the ascending aorta.[37,38]

The Rastelli repair carries only a very low early mortality. Boston Children's Hospital Group has reported a drop in early mortality from 7 to 0% in their 25-year experience. However, there is considerable late morbidity and mortality due to conduit obstruction, left ventricular outflow tract obstruction, and arrhythmias. Estimated freedom from death or transplantation in the Boston data was 82, 80, 68, and 52% at 5, 10, 15, and 20 years, respectively. Freedom from death or reintervention (catheterization or surgical treatment) was 53, 24, and 21 at 5, 10, and 15 years of follow-up, respectively.[37] Mayo Clinic data of 231 patients over a 30-year period, beginning from the early era, showed 10% early mortality and 20-year survival of 48%.[38]

Two other surgical techniques dealing with TGA/VSD/PS need mention, even though only a fewer number of cases have been treated this way and the long-term results are not available.[39] **Table 2** compares the pros and cons of the different techniques vis-à-vis Rastelli operation.

Reparation À L'etage Ventriculaire

In this procedure, the infundibular septum is resected liberally and the pulmonary trunk is connected directly to the RV. A LeCompte maneuver is part of the reparation à l'etage ventriculaire (REV) procedure. REV results in a straighter LV to aorta connection than Rastelli operation.[39]

Nikaidoh–Bex Operation

In this procedure, aorta is detached from the RV and translocated posteriorly onto the LVOT. The advantage is the straight connection between LV and aorta with much less reduction of RV volume. A conduit is used to connect the RV to PA.[39]

In patients undergoing a REV procedure, a European Congenital Heart Surgeons Association study found freedom from death, reoperation, or catheter reintervention at 1, 5, and 10 years to be 90, 78, and 64%, respectively.[40] With the Nikaidoh procedure in 18 patients, Yeh et al. reported 95% overall survival, 100% freedom from reoperations for left ventricular outflow tract obstruction (LVOTO), 64% freedom from reoperations for right ventricular outflow tract obstruction (RVOTO) at 15 years, and only nil/mild aortic regurgitation .[41]

CONCLUSION

- In a neonate, severe cyanosis, no murmur, and increased lung vascularity on chest X-ray are clinical clues to suspect TGA.
- Two-dimensional (2D) echocardiography is the gold standard for diagnosis.
- Prostaglandin infusion can help in stabilizing a severely hypoxic neonate, before transferring to a tertiary care center.
- BAS is indicated in all severely hypoxic neonates with TGA-IVS if ASO is not being done immediately. BAS significantly improves arterial oxygen saturation and usually allows the baby to stay with the mother.
- ASO, done in the first few weeks of life, is the standard of care in TGA. In established centers, this surgery carries <2% mortality. Higher mortality is observed for complex

TABLE 2: Surgical options for TGA/VSD/LVOTO.

Operation	*Procedure*	*Advantage*	*Problems*
Rastelli[37,38]	· VSD closed tunneling LV to aorta · RV to PA conduit	· Simplicity · Larger series	· Conduit replacement · Lower RV volume · 50% 20-year survival
REV[39]	Direct connection of PA to RV	Straight LV/aorta connection	· 64% 10-year freedom from death/reintervention · Smaller series
Nikaidoh–Bex[40,41]	Posterior translocation of aorta	· Straight LV/aorta connection · Ideal for smaller RV	· 64% 15-year freedom from RVOT reoperation · Smaller series

(LV: left ventricle; LVOTO: left ventricular outflow tract obstruction; PA: pulmonary artery; REV: reparation à l'etage ventriculaire; RV: right ventricle; RVOT: right ventricular outflow tract; TGA: transposition of the great arteries; VSD: ventricular septal defect)

ASO as in difficult coronary transfers, Taussig-Bing anomaly, and concomitant arch repair.

- Antenatal diagnosis by fetal echocardiography helps in planning in utero transport of the baby for better neonatal management.
- Long-term neurodevelopmental outcome needs close monitoring after neonatal arterial switch.
- Following ASO, life-long follow-up is required in all patients, with focus on RV outflow, branch PAs, coronary arteries, and the neoaortic valve. Need for redo surgeries and interventions must be kept in mind.
- Surgical outcomes from the developing world, including arterial switch results in late presenters, have been very encouraging.
- Long-term surgical outcomes for TGA/VSD/LVOT obstruction are adversely affected by the need for repeated redo surgeries. Surgical efforts to address these shortcomings are evolving.

REFERENCES

1. Wernovsky G. Transposition of great arteries. In: Allen HD, Driscoll DJ, Shaddy RE, Feltes TF, (Eds). Moss & Adams' Heart Disease in Infants, Children, and Adolescents Including the Fetus and Young Adult, 8th edition. Philadelphia: Wolters Kluwer; 2013. pp. 1097-146.
2. Saxena A, Mehta A, Sharma M, Salhan S, Kalaivani M, Ramakrishnan S, et al. Birth prevalence of congenital heart disease: a cross-sectional observational study from North India. Ann Ped Card. 2016;9(3):205-9.
3. Laforest B, Zaffran S. Genetics of conotruncal anomalies. In: Lacour-Gayet F, Bove E, Hraska V, Morell VO, Spray TL (Eds). Surgery of Conotruncal Anomalies. Switzerland: Springer; 2016. pp. 607-23.
4. Van Praagh R. Definition of conotruncal anomalies. In: Lacour-Gayet F, Bove E, Hraska V, Morell VO, Spray TL (Eds). Surgery of Conotruncal Anomalies. Switzerland: Springer; 2016. pp. 1-25.
5. Anderson RH, Bamforth SD, Spicer DE, Henderson DJ, Chaudhry B, Brown NA, et al. Development and maldevelopment of the ventricular outflow tracts. In: Lacour-Gayet F, Bove E, Hraska V, Morell VO, Spray TL (Eds). Surgery of Conotruncal Anomalies. Switzerland: Springer; 2016. pp. 27-59.
6. Rudolph AM. Aortopulmonary transposition. In: Congenital Diseases of the Heart: Clinical-Physiological Considerations, 3rd edition. UK: Wiley-Blackwell; 2009. pp. 465-505.
7. Houyel L, Van Praagh R, LacourGayet F, Serraf A, Petit J, Bruniaux J, et al. Transposition of great arteries [S,D,L]. J Thorac Cardiovasc Surg. 1995;110(3):613-24.
8. Fricke TA, Konstantinov IE. Arterial switch operation: operative approach and outcomes. Ann Thorac Surg. 2019;107(1):302-10.
9. Scheule AM, Jonas R. Management of transposition of great arteries with single coronary. Semin Thorac Cardiovasc Surg Pediatr Card Surg Annu. 2001;4:34-57.
10. LacourGayet F. Arterial switch in TGA-IVS: coronary transfer. In: Lacour-Gayet F, Bove EL, Hraska V, Morell, VO, Spray TL (Eds). Surgery of Conotruncal Anomalies. Switzerland: Springer; 2016. pp. 247-68.
11. Sarris GE, Balmer C, Bonou P, Comas JV, da Cruz E, Di Chiara L, et al. EACTS/AEPC Task Force. Clinical guidelines for the management of transposition of great arteries with intact IVS. Eur J Cardiothorac Surg. 2017;51(1):e1-32.
12. Liebman J , Cullum L, Belloc NB. Natural history of transposition of great arteries. Anatomy and birth and death characteristics. Circulation. 1969;40(2):237-62.
13. Beattie LM, McLeod KA. Prostaglandin E2 after septostomy for simple transposition. Pediatr Cardiol. 2009;30(4):447-51.
14. McQuillen PS, Hamrick SEG, Perez MJ, Barkovich AJ, Glidden DV, Karl TR, et al. Balloon atrial septostomy is associated with preoperative stroke in neonates with transposition of the great arteries. Circulation. 2006;113(2):280-5.
15. Petit CJ, Rome JR, Wernovsky G, Mason SE, Shera DM, Nicolson SC, et al. Preoperative brain injury in transposition of the great arteries is associated with oxygenation and time to surgery, not balloon atrial septostomy. Circulation. 2009;119(5):709-16.
16. Wells WJ, Blackstone E. Intermediate outcome after Mustard and Senning procedures: a study by the Congenital Heart Surgeons Society. Semin Thorac Cardiovasc Surg Pediatr Card Surg Annu. 2000;3:186-97.
17. Vejlstrup N, Sørensen K, Mattsson E, Thilén U, Kvidal P, Johansson B, et al. Long-term outcome of Mustard/Senning correction for transposition of the great arteries in Sweden and Denmark. Circulation. 2015;132(8):633-8.
18. Moons P, Gewillig M, Sluysmans T, Verhaaren H, Viart P, Massin M, et al. Long term outcome up to 30 yearsafter the Mustard or Senning operation: a nationwide multicentre study in Belgium. Heart. 2004;90(3):307-13.
19. Losay J, Touchot A, Serraf A, Litvinova A, Lambert V, Piot JD, et al. Late outcomes after arterial switch operation for transposition of the great arteries. Circulation. 2001;104(12 Suppl 1):1121-6.
20. Fricke TA, d'Udekem Y, Richardson M, Thuys C, Dronavalli M, Ramsay JM, et al. Outcomes of the arterial switch operation for transposition of the great arteries: 25 years of experience. Ann Thorac Surg. 2012;94:139-45.
21. Raju, V, Burkhart HM, Durham III LA, Eidem BW, Phillips SD, Li Z. Reoperation after arterial switch: a 27-year experience. Ann Thorac Surg. 2013;95(6):2105-13.
22. Sharma R, Bhan A, Choudhary SK, Kumar RP, Juneja R, Kothari SS, et al. Ten-year experience with the arterial switch operation. Indian Heart J. 2002;54(6):681-6.
23. Schidlow DN, Jenkins KJ, Gauvreau K, Croti UA, Giang DTC, Konda RK, et al. Transposition of the great arteries in the developing world - surgery and outcomes. J Am Coll Cardiol 2017;69(1):43-51.
24. Norwood WI, Dobell AR, Freed MD, Kirklin JW, Blackstone EH. Intermediate results of the arterial switch repair. A 20-institution study. J Thorac Cardiovasc Surg. 1988;96(6):854-63.
25. Foran JP, Sullivan ID, Elliott MJ, de Leval MR. Primary arterial switch operation for transposition of the great arteries with intact ventricular septum in infants older than 21 days. J Am Coll Cardiol. 1998;31(4):883-9.
26. Iyer KS, Sharma R, Kumar RK, Bhan A, Kothari SS, Saxena A, et al. Serial echocardiography for decision making in rapid two-stage arterial switch operation. Ann Thorac Surg. 1995;60(3):658-64.
27. Nakazawa M, Oyama K, Imai Y, Nojima K, Aotsuka H, Satomi G, et al. Criteria for two-stage arterial switch operation for transposition of the great arteries. Circulation. 1988;78(1):124-31.
28. Lacour-Gayet F, Piot D, Zoghbi J, Serraf A, Gruber P, Macé L, et al. Surgical management and indication of left ventricular retraining in arterial switch for transposition of the great arteries with intact ventricular septum. Eur J Cardiothorac Surg.2001;20(4):824-9.
29. Iyer PU, Moreno GE, Caneo FL, Faiz T, Shekerdemian LS, Iyer KS. Management of late presentation congenital heart disease. Cardiology in the Young. 2017;27(Suppl 6):S31-9.
30. Jonas RA, Giglia TM, Sanders SP, Wernovsky G, Nadal-Ginard B, Mayer Jr JE, et al. Rapid, two stage arterial switch for transposition of great arteries and intact ventricular septum beyond the neonatal period. Circulation. 1989;80(3):1203-08.

31. Bisoi AK, Ahmed T, Malankar DP, Chauhan S, Das S, Sharma P, et al. Midterm outcome of primary arterial switch operation beyond six weeks of life in children with transposition of great arteries and intact ventricular septum. World J Pediatr Congenit Heart Surg. 2014; 5(2):219-25.
32. Poirier NC, Yu JH, Brizard CP, Mee RB. Long term results of left ventricular reconditioning and anatomic correction for systemic right ventricular dysfunction after atrial switch procedures. J Thorac Cardiovasc Surg. 2004; 127(4):975-81.
33. Poirier NC, Mee RB. Left ventricular reconditioning and anatomical correction for systemic right ventricular dysfunction. Semin Thorac Cardiovasc Surg Pediatr Card Surg Annu. 2000;3:198-215.
34. Bellinger DC, Wypij D, Rivkin MJ, DeMaso DR, Robertson Jr RL, Dunbar-Masterson C, et al. Adolescents with d-transposition of great arteries corrected with arterial switch procedure: neuropsychological assessment and structural brain imaging. Circulation. 2011; 124(12):1361-9.
35. Fricke TA, Loyer BR, Huang L, Griffiths S, Yaftian N, Dalziel KM, et al. Long-term quality of life in adult survivors after the arterial switch operation. Eur J Cardiothorac Surg. 2018;54(6): 1001-3.
36. Kalfa D, Kasmi L, Geronikola N, Calderon J, Lambert V, Belli E, et al. Cognitive outcomes and health-related quality of life in adults two decades after the arterial switch operation for transposition of the great arteries. J Thorac Cardiovasc Surg. 2017;154(3):1028-35.
37. Kreutzer C, De Vive J, Oppido G, Kreutzer J, Gauvreau K, Freed M, et al. Twenty-five-year experience with Rastelli repair for transposition of the great arteries. J Thorac Cardiovasc Surg. 2000;120(2):211-23.
38. Dearani JA, Danielson GK, Puga FJ, Mair DD, Schleck CD. Late results of the Rastelli operation for transposition of great arteries. Semin Thorac Cardiovasc Surg Pediatr Cardiac Surg Annu. 2001;4:3-15.
39. Hazekamp MG, Nevvazhay T, Sojak V. Nikaidohvs Réparation à l'Etage Ventriculairevs Rastelli. Semin Thorac Cardiovasc Surg Pediatr Card Surg Annu. 2018;21:58-63.
40. Yeh T, Ramaciotti C, Leonard SR, Roy L, Nikaidoh H. The aortic translocation (Nikaidoh) procedure: midterm results superior to the Rastelli procedure. J Thorac Cardiovasc Surg. 2007;133(2): 461-9.
41. Hazekamp MG, Gomez AA, Koolbergen DR, Hraska V, Metras DR, Mattila IP, et al. Surgery for transposition of the great arteries, ventricular septal defect and left ventricular outflow tract obstruction: European Congenital Heart Surgeons Association multi-centre study. Eur J Cardiothorac Surg. 2010;38(6):699-706.

37 CHAPTER

Double Outlet Right Ventricle

KS Remadevi

INTRODUCTION

Double outlet right ventricle (DORV) is a type of ventriculoarterial connection in which both great vessels arise either entirely or predominantly from the right ventricle (RV).[1-3] Although the presence of aortic-mitral or pulmonary-mitral discontinuity and bilateral coni (infundibula) are important descriptors, these features are not considered absolute prerequisites for the diagnosis of DORV. This definition only describes the ventriculoarterial connection, but does not include morphology and relations which are essential components in segmental approach to congenital heart disease (CHD). The DORV spectrum encompasses extremely variable morphologic features and pathophysiologic disturbances. DORV can also be associated with discordant or univentricular atrioventricular (AV) connections, AV valve atresia, or atrial isomerism with complete atrioventricular septal defect (AVSD). This chapter is limited to DORV with usual atrial arrangements, concordant AV connections, and normal sized ventricles.

INCIDENCE

In a cross-sectional, observational study from North India, DORV accounted for 1.2% of significant CHDs.[4] The birth prevalence of DORV was 0.1 per 1,000 live births. The global prevalence was found to be similar (0.106 per 1,000 live births) in a recent meta-analysis of 260 studies.[5]

MORPHOLOGY AND TYPES OF DOUBLE OUTLET RIGHT VENTRICLE

The hearts in DORV have no phenotypical uniformity. In a recent study of 100 hearts, where each had at least 75% of arterial roots supported by RV, only 23% had bilateral infundibula.[2] Other previous series also have shown that there is fibrous continuity between the leaflets of an AV valve and an arterial valve in majority of hearts with DORV.[6,7] Infundibulum is the sleeve of musculature that lifts the arterial valves from the base of the heart (AV valves), thereby resulting in discontinuity. Thus, hearts do not need bilateral infundibula so as to fulfill the criteria of double outlet from the RV. When both arterial trunks arise predominantly or exclusively from RV, the muscular outlet septum invariably becomes a right ventricular structure (*see* **Figs. 3A and B**) rather than an interventricular structure as seen in hearts with one to one ventriculoarterial connection such as normal heart, tetralogy of Fallot (TOF), and transposition of the great arteries (TGA).[8,9] The channel between the ventricles or ventricular septal defect (VSD) is, therefore, roofed by the inner heart curvature or ventriculoinfundibular fold (*see* **Figs. 2A and B**) which can either be fibrous or muscular.[9] Overriding arterial valves exists in various patterns when the potential anatomical diagnosis is DORV.[8] Morphologically, the spectrum of DORV lies between VSD with aorta overriding the crest of muscular interventricular septum as in TOF at one end and, TGA with VSD where pulmonary artery (PA) overrides the crest of ventricular septum at the other end.[1,8]

Morphologic Modifiers of Double Outlet Right Ventricle

- *Location of VSD*: The VSD is the only outlet of the left ventricle (LV) in DORV. In majority of individuals with DORV, the defect is a typical conoventricular VSD located between the anterior and posterior limbs of the septomarginal trabeculation [trabecula septomarginalis (TSM)] or septal band.[1,7,8] It is the orientation and development of the conal septum that determines whether the defect is subpulmonic, subaortic, or doubly committed. In other words, VSD does not move around the interventricular septum, and the relationship of the VSD to the semilunar valve depends on the relationships of the great arteries to each other, which in turn depends on the conal septal development.[1,7] This relationship of VSD to semilunar valves has surgical significance.
- *Size of the VSD*: Majority of VSDs are unrestrictive. VSD is considered restrictive (*see* **Figs. 2A and B**), if its diameter is smaller than the age-matched diameter of the normal aortic valve.[10] Restrictive VSDs are reported in at least 10% of cases.[1] Rarely DORV can occur with intact

ventricular septum.[2] When there is no VSD, mitral valve and left ventricular hypoplasia usually coexist.[1]

- *Great artery relationships*: There are two basic patterns of great artery relationship in DORV: Spiraling around each other as in normal and parallel.[1] When the great arteries are parallel to each other, there can be any degree of anteroposterior variation of the aorta around the PA. Aorta can be rightward and side by side with the PA, rightward and anterior to the PA, directly anterior to the PA or aorta can be leftward, and anterior to the PA.
- *Ventricular outflow tract obstruction*: Pulmonary outflow tract obstruction is common in DORV with subaortic or doubly committed VSD. Subaortic obstruction with or without obstructive lesions of the aortic arch is common in DORV with a subpulmonary VSD.[1,11]
- *Conduction system*: In DORV with concordant AV connections, AV node lies in the usual position, i.e., subendocardially, within the triangle of Koch and adjacent to the right fibrous trigone (central fibrous body). In a perimembranous (conoventricular) VSD as in most DORVs, the bundle of His penetrates the right fibrous trigone and lies along the posteroinferior margin of VSD at or near the crest of the muscular interventricular septum, irrespective of whether the defect is subaortic, subpulmonic, or doubly committed.[1]
- *Coronary artery anatomy*: The coronary artery pattern depends on the position of the great arteries. In most cases of DORV, it is similar to normal except that the aortic sinuses and hence coronary artery orifices are rotated clockwise, so that left coronary artery arises more posteriorly and right coronary artery (RCA) arises more anteriorly.[1,11] With a right sided and anterior aorta, the coronary artery pattern is similar to that seen in TGA. In Wilcox[7] series, up to 30% of patients with DORV had coronary abnormalities with 3% having single coronary artery from anterior or posterior facing sinus. Occasional origin of left anterior descending from RCA with this vessel crossing RV outflow from right to left as in TOF is also seen.

CLASSIFICATION OF DOUBLE OUTLET RIGHT VENTRICLE (BOX 1)

In 1972, Lev and associates[3] classified DORV into four types based on the relation between the great arteries and VSD: DORV with subaortic VSD, DORV with subpulmonary VSD (Taussig-Bing heart), DORV with doubly-committed VSD, and DORV with noncommitted VSD. Despite major limitations, this widely used classification is still useful with physiological and surgical implications.

More recently, the Congenital Heart Surgery Nomenclature and Database Project classified DORV in a concise way as given here, which conveys a broad sense of the relational anatomy of the VSD, clinical presentation, and general approach to surgical repair.[1]

BOX 1: Classification of double outlet right ventricle

Based on the relationship of great arteries with VSD (Lev et al.)
- DORV with subaortic VSD
- DORV with subpulmonary VSD
- DORV with doubly committed VSD
- DORV with noncommitted VSD

Based on location of VSD, clinical presentation, and surgical approach (Nomenclature database, Walters et al.)
- DORV, VSD type
- DORV, TOF type
- DORV, TGA type
- DORV with noncommitted VSD

(DORV: double outlet right ventricle; VSD: ventricular septal defect; TGA: transposition of the great arteries; TOF: tetralogy of Fallot)

Tetralogy of Fallot Type

Double Outlet Right Ventricle with subaortic or doubly committed VSD and pulmonary outflow tract obstruction (**Figs. 1A and B**). This is the most common variant of DORV constituting approximately 33–36% of cases from surgical series.[12,13] VSDs are mostly subaortic as in TOF, but can also be doubly committed. Aorta overrides the interventricular septum by >50%. There is minimal or absent conus under the aorta with prominent subpulmonic conus, such that the great arteries are either normally related or side by side with aorta to the right in the majority. In about one-fourth of patients, aorta was found to be somewhat anterior to PA.[11] Though pulmonary outflow obstruction is most often infundibular, all types of pulmonary stenosis observed in hearts with TOF may be seen in DORV.[1,11]

Ventricular Septal Defect Type

Double Outlet Right Ventricle with subaortic or doubly committed VSD without pulmonary outflow obstruction (**Figs. 2A and B**). This variant constitutes 21–[illegible]% of surgical series of patients with DORV.[12,13] Morphologic features are similar to TOF type except that pulmonary outflow is unobstructed.

Transposition of the Great Arteries Type

Double Outlet Right Ventricle with subpulmonic VSD, also known as Taussig-Bing anomaly (**Figs. 3A and B**). This is also a common type of DORV constituting 18–32% of cases from surgical series.[12,13] VSDs are usually unrestrictive. There is a large conus beneath the aorta so that the aorta is relatively pushed anteriorly. Subpulmonic conus is small or absent with PA arising biventricularly over the VSD. Aorta is to the right (side by side or slightly anterior to) of PA. Subaortic stenosis due to infundibular narrowing and coarctation of aorta are commonly associated.[11]

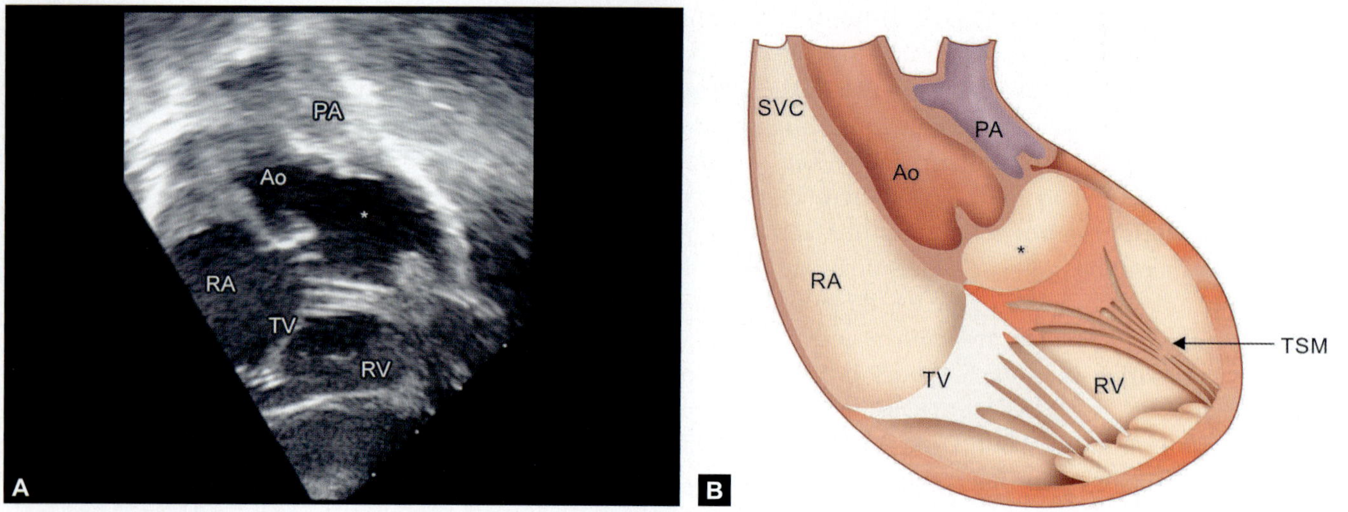

Figs. 1A and B: Subcostal long axis echocardiographic view of double outlet right ventricle (DORV), tetralogy of Fallot (TOF) type (A) and schematic drawing (B). Note that ventricular septal defect (VSD) is doubly committed with narrow pulmonary outflow.
(Ao: aorta; asterisk(*): ventricular septal defect; PA: pulmonary artery; RA: right atrium; RV: right ventricle; SVC: superior vena cava; TV: tricuspid valve; TSM: trabecula septomarginalis).

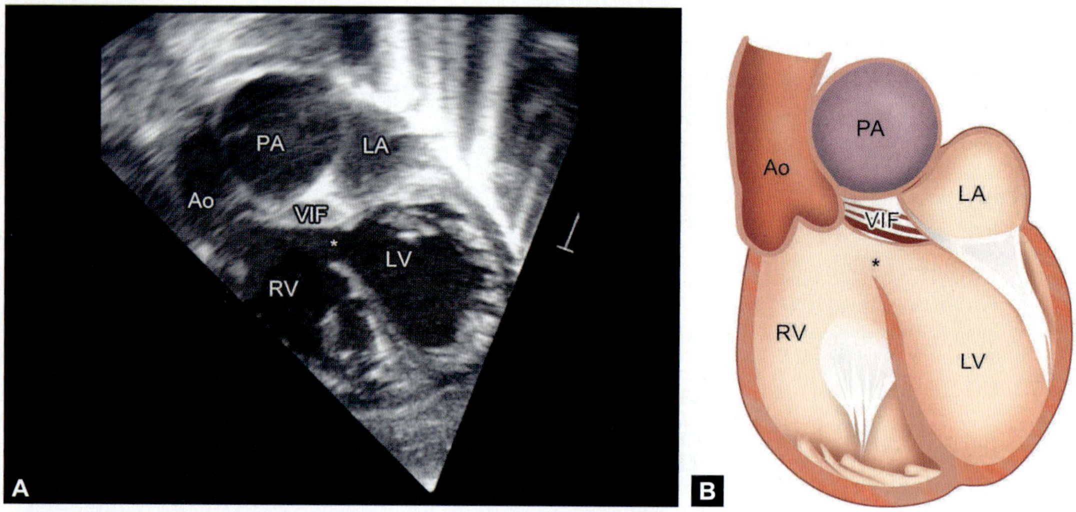

Figs. 2A and B: Subcostal short axis echocardiographic view of double outlet right ventricle (DORV), ventricular septal defect (VSD) type (A) with schematic drawing (B). Note that VSD is restrictive, i.e., obviously smaller than the aortic annulus.
(Ao: aorta; asterisk(*): subaortic ventricular septal defect; LA: left atrium; LV: left ventricle; PA: pulmonary artery; RV: right ventricle; VIF: ventriculoinfundibular fold)

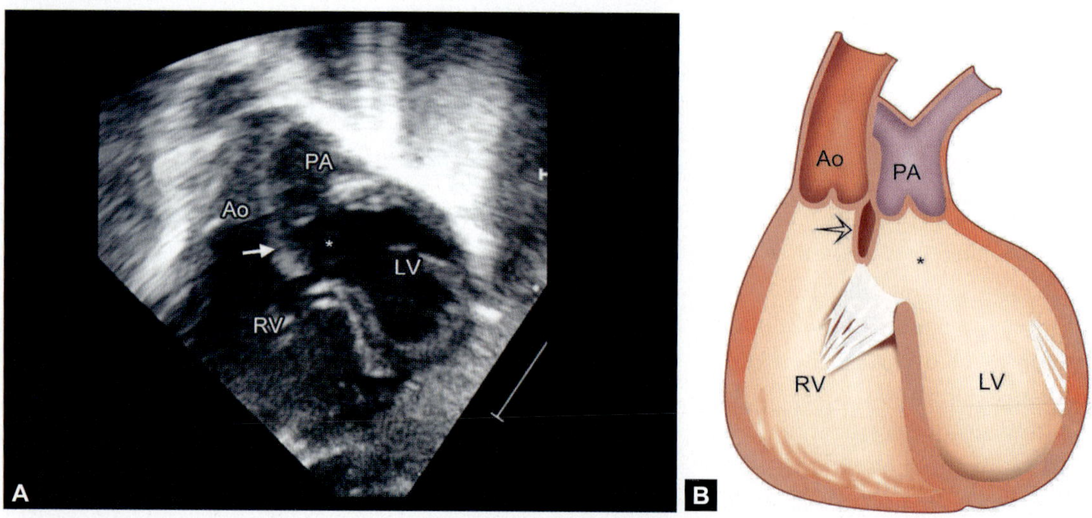

Figs. 3A and B: Subcostal short axis echocardiographic view of double outlet right ventricle (DORV), TGA type (A) with schematic drawing (B).
(Ao: aorta; asterisk(*): subaortic ventricular septal defect; LV: left ventricle; PA: pulmonary artery; RV: right ventricle; arrow: conal septum which is a right ventricular structure).

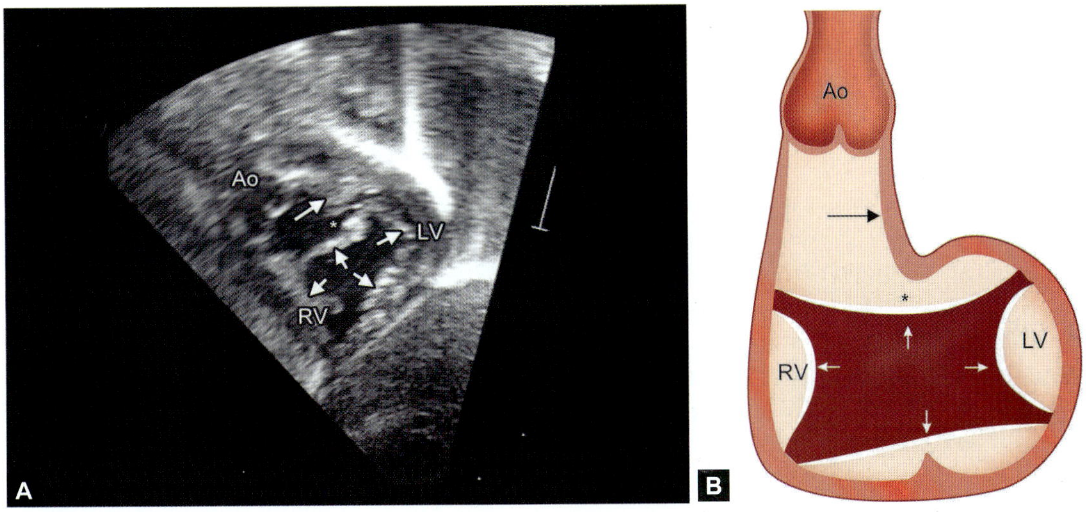

Figs. 4A and B: Subcostal short axis echocardiographic view of double outlet right ventricle (DORV), remote ventricular septal defect (VSD) type (A) with schematic drawing (B). Patient had complete atrioventricular septal defect, Rastelli Type C with attenuated right anterior leaflet of the common atrioventricular (AV) valve and pulmonary atresia. Though VSD has extension to the outlet septum, elongated subaortic conus makes the VSD remote. (Ao: aorta; asterisk(*): outlet extension of the inlet VSD; arrow: subaortic conus; arrowheads: open leaflets of common AV valve; LV: left ventricle; RV: right ventricle)

Noncommitted Ventricular Septal Defect Type (Figs. 4A and B)

Double Outlet Right Ventricle with noncommitted (remote) VSD was described in 5–22% of patients in surgical series.[13,14] Remoteness of the VSD to the arterial valves is one of the most controversial issues in DORV. Functionally, this implies that an unobstructed tunnel from LV to one of the arterial trunks can be created only with difficulty. Defects involving the inlet septum without perimembranous extension and trabecular interventricular septum are classified as remote. In addition, conoventricular VSD is also considered remote when the distance between the VSD and the arterial valves is greater than the aortic valve diameter.[10,12,15,16] In this type, neither great vessel is directly related to the VSD, being separated by bilateral conus and VSD opens into the body of RV. DORV with atrioventricular septal defect (AVSD) usually resembles AVSD with TOF having type C Rastelli anatomy with a large subaortic component of the VSD.[15] Hence, DORV/AVSD with remote inlet VSD is quite rare. Outflow obstruction [subaortic obstruction or pulmonary outflow tract obstruction (POTO), usually infundibular] may be associated with noncommitted VSD type.[15,16]

PATHOPHYSIOLOGY AND CLINICAL PRESENTATION

The clinical features are extremely variable depending on the subtype. It can mimic TOF, large VSD, or TGA with VSD depending on the anatomic subtype. Hence, pathophysiology and clinical features are described separately for each subtype.

Tetralogy Type (Tetralogy of Fallot Type)

As blood from the LV is directed to the aorta (subaortic VSD), presentation is similar to TOF with symptoms and saturation depending on the degree of pulmonary stenosis. Though most are asymptomatic at birth, pulmonary stenosis generally increases over time in infancy resulting in progressive symptoms and desaturation. Clinical findings are indistinguishable from TOF. Cyanotic spells can occur as in TOF. Chest radiograph and electrocardiogram (ECG) are similar to patients with TOF.

Ventricular Septal Defect Type

Physiology is like a large VSD with pulmonary overcirculation. Infants present at 4–6 weeks of age with congestive heart failure, as pulmonary vascular resistance falls after birth. Failure to thrive occurs if not operated early. Physical examination, chest radiograph, and ECG are indistinguishable from that of a large VSD with increased pulmonary blood flow.

Transposition of the Great Arteries Type

Oxygenated blood from LV passes through the VSD to PA as the VSD is subpulmonic, whereas deoxygenated blood from RV flows into the aorta. This unfavorable streaming results in pulmonary arterial oxygen saturation greater than that of aorta (TGA physiology). These patients present in the neonatal period with cyanosis and congestive heart failure due to increased pulmonary blood flow. The degree of cyanosis is determined by the degree of streaming and the presence and size of additional shunts such as atrial septal defect (ASD) and patent ductus arteriosus (PDA). Those with aortic arch hypoplasia and subaortic obstruction will develop symptoms earlier. ECG shows combined ventricular hypertrophy with right axis deviation of QRS as in other large post-tricuspid shunts. Chest radiograph demonstrates cardiomegaly with increased pulmonary vascularity.

Double Outlet Right Ventricle with Noncommitted Ventricular Septal Defect

Unlike the other types, clinical presentation is heterogeneous. Clinical presentation depends on a number of factors which include precise location of the VSD with possible favorable or unfavorable streaming of blood, presence of outflow tract stenosis, and other associated lesions. Findings in ECG and chest radiograph will also depend on the pathophysiology.

DIAGNOSIS

Clinical presentation, physical examination, and pulse oximetry followed by detailed transthoracic echocardiogram provides us in most cases with a comprehensive diagnosis and roadmap to management. Clinical evaluation, chest X-ray, and ECG can help identify one of the physiological subtypes but, the diagnosis of DORV and the anatomic subtype can only be made through meticulous echocardiography.

Echocardiography

A diagnosis of DORV is made on the basis of echocardiography either in utero or postnatally. It provides noninvasive anatomical and hemodynamic information. Echocardiographer needs to follow a systematic, segmental approach as in the evaluation of any CHD. Several anatomical features should be defined to reach an optimal surgical plan (**Box 2**). Multiple imaging planes are required to reach a comprehensive diagnosis. Sub-costal views are particularly useful.

Identifying DORV by echocardiography can be a difficult task. Plane of the long axis of the ventricular septum can vary during cardiac cycle making diagnostic confusion regarding the degree of override. Hence, arterial trunks should be assigned to the respective ventricles based on the proportion of their valves committed to and supported by each ventricle as imaged from the short axis plane.[9,17]

Once a diagnosis of DORV is made, the location of interventricular communication relative to the origin of the great arteries needs to be determined. Echocardiogram demonstrates the area that will be closed by the surgeon so as to connect one of the arterial trunks to LV, in other words, routability of the VSD to aorta or PA.[9,17] Subcostal sagittal, coronal, and oblique views (at an angle of 45° relative to the coronal and sagittal planes) and parasternal long axis views are particularly useful (*see* **Figs. 1A and B to 4A and B**). Once the position of VSD and routability are decided, adequacy of VSD to be the future LV outlet is assessed by comparing its diameter to the age-matched aortic annulus. Tricuspid-pulmonary annular distance should also be measured (should be equal to or more than aortic annulus) to ensure unobstructed LV to aorta tunnel without compromising RV outflow tract. This distance can be estimated from subxiphoid view.

Finally, biventricular repair of DORV requires adequate volumes of both ventricles after surgery. Long intraventricular tunnel compromises the right ventricular volume as a part of RV is incorporated into the left ventricular outflow tract (LVOT). Hence, it is important to estimate the cavity size of remaining RV after the intended surgery.[10]

BOX 2: Echocardiographic assessment of double outlet right ventricle.

- Position and adequacy (size) of the VSD
- Great artery relationship
- Aortomitral or pulmonary-mitral discontinuity
- Distance between the tricuspid valve and the pulmonary valve in subaortic VSDs
- Morphology of outflow tracts for potential obstruction
- Coronary artery anatomy
- Straddling of AV valves
- Right and left ventricular volumes
- Associated abnormalities: Additional VSDs, arch abnormalities, systemic and pulmonary venous abnormalities, atrial isomerism, etc.

(AV: atrioventricular; VSD: ventricular septal defect)

Role of Three-dimensional Imaging

In majority of cases, transthoracic echocardiography including three-dimensional (3D) displays provide sufficient information for surgical decision-making. When data is inadequate, contrast-enhanced computed tomography (CT) and magnetic resonance imaging (MRI) acquired in 3D volumes will reveal all the required anatomical data with precision, increasing our understanding of complex DORVs.[10] The commitment of an overriding outflow tract can be shown with better precision using 3D data set obtained by CT or MRI. In addition, the 3D data sets are now used to print 3D models which make the understanding of complex DORV better and aids in surgical planning. 3D print models can also be used for rehearsal of the intended procedure before the actual surgery on the patient so that the outcome of the procedure is precisely predicted with better surgical outcomes in complex cases.[18]

SURGICAL APPROACH AND OUTCOMES

Simple patch closure of VSD in DORV results in isolation of LV from the semilunar valves. Anatomic repair requires deliberate tunneling of VSD to one of the semilunar valves ensuring unobstructed LVOT. The first successful repair of DORV was performed by Kirklin and associates in 1957 at the Mayo Clinic in a patient with DORV and subaortic VSD.[19] Since then various surgical procedures have been described over time owing to the complexity and diversity of anatomy. Surgical decision-making in DORV requires careful assessment of multiple factors which include the following:

- Anatomy and physiology as discussed earlier
- Patient's age, body size, and clinical condition
- Surgeon's preferences.

Thus, each patient requires individualized approach and decision-making to have optimal outcome.

TABLE 1: Preferred surgical approach and timing in double outlet right ventricle (DORV).

Type of DORV	*Surgery*	*Timing*
VSD type	Intraventricular tunnel repair (IVR)	Young infant (3–6 months of age)
TOF type	IVR with relief of pulmonary outflow tract obstruction. Interim palliation if not suitable for early corrective surgery	Infant (6–12 months of age, earlier if symptomatic)
TGA type	IVR of VSD to PA with arterial switch operation	Neonatal period
Noncommitted VSD	Biventricular repair preferred. Interim palliation with PA band or aortopulmonary shunt may be required in early infancy Staged univentricular palliation if not suitable for biventricular repair	Corrective surgery deferred beyond infancy in most patients due to complex anatomy

(PA: pulmonary artery; TGA: transposition of the great arteries; TOF: tetralogy of Fallot; VSD: ventricular septal defect)

General Surgical Strategy and Timing based on the Type of Double Outlet Right Ventricle (Table 1)

Double Outlet Right Ventricle: Ventricular Septal Defect Type

Simple intraventricular baffling that directs the LV blood through the VSD to the aorta (intraventricular tunnel repair or IVR) is the preferred surgery, provided tricuspid–pulmonary annular distance is adequate.[1,11] If the VSD is restrictive (diameter less than that of the aortic valve), it needs enlargement which should be achieved without injuring the AV conduction axis. Surgery is done in young infancy by 3-6 months of age. Rarely in patients with refractory heart failure, who are not candidates for complete repair, an interim palliative PA band is required. Complications after surgery are rare.

Double Outlet Right Ventricle: Tetralogy of Fallot Type

Intraventricular tunnel repair with relief of pulmonary outflow tract obstruction in infancy is the preferred surgery.[1,11] Repair is essentially that for TOF except that the VSD is closed with the tunnel technique rather than with a straight patch. However, if there are additional concerns such as branch PA hypoplasia, requirement of extracardiac conduit, or the patient is too small, initial palliative procedure (aortopulmonary shunt or other transcatheter interventions such as stenting of patent ductus arteriosus or balloon pulmonary valvotomy) is preferred by many centers, followed by definitive repair later in life.[1,11]

Double Outlet Right Ventricle: Transposition of the Great Arteries Type (Taussig–Bing Malformation)

The preferred surgery is an arterial switch operation (ASO) combined with IVR of VSD to the PA in the neonatal period.[1,11] Arch hypoplasia, if present, also needs to be addressed surgically. Infundibular resection will also be required in those with substrate for future right ventricular outflow tract obstruction (RVOTO).

Intraventricular repair known by the name, Kawashima operation, was also done successfully in small series of patients with Taussig–Bing heart, when the great arteries are side by side with the aorta to the right of the pulmonary trunk and there is adequate tricuspid–pulmonary annular distance, as discussed earlier.[1,11,20] In patients with anteroposterior great arteries, tricuspid-pulmonary annular distance is likely to be inadequate to allow creation of the tunnel so that ASO must be employed.

Other surgical procedures employed for DORV, TGA type, when there is coexisting pulmonary outflow obstruction (LV outflow stenosis) so that IVR with ASO is not an option include the following:[1,11,21,22]

- *LeCompte intraventricular repair (REV or Reparation L'etage Ventriculaire)*: IVR is performed connecting LV to aorta. PA is transected and translocated anterior to aorta, to the right ventricular outflow tract. REV results in pulmonary regurgitation with resultant immediate and long-term issues.
- *Aortic and/or pulmonary root translocation*: A highly complex group of surgeries which includes aortic root translocation with right ventricular outflow tract reconstruction (Nikaidoh procedure). This operation results in a straight LVOT which does not compromise RV volume. Multiple modifications involving double root or pulmonary root translocations have been described in different anatomic situations.
- *Rastelli procedure*: Involves IVR with RV to PA conduit. This operation has the inherent need for multiple reoperations for conduit replacement as the child grows.

Double Outlet Right Ventricle with Noncommitted Ventricular Septal Defect

Biventricular repair is preferred in DORV with non-committed VSD, but remains technically challenging. Because of complexity, corrective surgery is often deferred beyond 6 months of age or later. Initial palliation with either an aortopulmonary shunt or PA band may be needed in symptomatic patients depending on the physiology. Techniques for correction are diverse depending on the anatomy and pathophysiology. These include the following:

- *Intraventricular tunnel repair:* Different techniques such as multiple patches or intraventricular conduit were employed to make long LV to aorta tunnel in DORV with noncommitted VSD.[23,24] In those with inlet VSD (AV canal type) without conoventricular extension, it is often necessary to enlarge the VSD anteriorly and superiorly to make an unobstructed tunnel from LV to aorta. If the tunnel obstructs pulmonary outflow tract, a valved extracardiac conduit is placed from RV to PA or REV is performed.[16] Mandatory presence of long tunnel increases the risk for subaortic obstruction in addition to creating an akinetic area in the LVOT that can impair the LV function.[15,16]
- *IVR with ASO*: Routing of VSD to the PA with ASO was successfully done in cases when VSD is closer to PA.[15] In such cases, this technique creates a shorter tunnel, which is not affected by the presence of tricuspid chordae, and is independent of the distance between the pulmonary and the tricuspid valve. Hence, the long-term risk of subaortic obstruction is also reduced.
- *Fontan operation*: In complex DORVs, where there is significant straddling of AV valves, ventricular hypoplasia, or in remote VSDs in which intraventricular tunnel connecting LV to aorta or PA is not an option, staged single ventricle strategy is generally advised.[1,11] However, there is controversy regarding the optimal treatment strategy for certain complex DORVs. Selection of single-ventricle palliation versus two-ventricle strategies in most complex of the DORVs remains a function of institutional bias and surgeon's preferences.[11]

Surgical Outcomes: Early and Late

Surgical outcome of DORV depends on the anatomic variant and associated anomalies. Overall early postoperative mortality for biventricular repair is favorable and ranges from 3.3 to 7.4% as per most recent series.[12,13,25,26] Risk factors associated with early mortality as per two recent large series were surgical strategy of IVR with ASO, DORV with noncommitted VSD, low weight at operation (<4,000 g), associated surgical procedure, and preoperative PA hypertension (pulmonary vascular disease).[13,25] Anatomic type of DORV influenced the outcomes. DORV with subaortic VSD was associated with excellent outcome even in an earlier era, with 99% early postoperative and 97% 10-year survival rates.[14] Reoperation for tunnel stenosis was rarely required (<2%).[14] On the contrary, early and late mortality and late reoperation rates were significantly higher in DORV with noncommitted VSD.[13] A major early complication following biventricular repair of DORV was complete heart block. In a recent series of 238 patients, 11% underwent pacemaker implantation for postoperative complete heart block and VSD enlargement significantly increased the risk.[26]

In a large series by Villemain et al.,[13] which included 433 patients who underwent biventricular repair between 1991 and 2013, survival at 10 years was 86.2%, and freedom from reoperation at 10 years was 61.4%. 80% of late mortality occurred within 1 year after the repair. In addition to the subtype of DORV with noncommitted VSD, other anatomic risk factors associated with significantly increased risk of late mortality were restrictive VSD, associated coronary artery abnormalities, and mitral valve cleft.

Late Complications and Risk of Reoperation after Biventricular Repair (Box 3)

In the previously mentioned series by Villemain et al.,[13] one-third of the patients had to undergo reoperation, with freedom at reoperation at 10 years being 61.4%. Major indications for reoperations were left ventricular outflow tract obstruction (LVOTO), RVOTO, valve repair, and residual VSD.[26] Acquired RVOTO was the main cause of reoperation in Taussig–Bing type.[13] LVOTO (subaortic obstruction related to baffle stenosis) was the major cause of reoperation after IVR for DORV with noncommitted VSD.[13,16,25] In a series of patients with DORV and noncommitted VSD who underwent biventricular repair, 26% underwent reoperation for LVOTO at a median follow-up of 5 years.[16] Risk factors for development of LVOTO other than noncommitted VSD were younger age at biventricular repair (<1 year) and subaortic conus.[26] The longer the tunnel, the greater the risk of subaortic obstruction.[15,16,25] It took approximately >3 years to develop LVOTO, suggesting that the development of LVOTO is related to somatic growth.[25] Incidence of LVOTO was reduced in DORV with noncommitted VSD, when IVR of VSD to PA with ASO was used as the surgical strategy instead of IVR of VSD to aorta, as this results in shorter LV to neoaorta tunnel.[15,16,25] Significant LVOTO was treated with modified Konno procedure with good outcome.[25]

Outcome: Comparing Biventricular Repair with Fontan Procedure

In a historical review of 124 patients by Brown et al.,[27] 25% underwent modified Fontan procedure for complex DORV and had a 15-year survival of 89%, statistically similar to biventricular repair. In a retrospective review of nearly 400 patients, Bradley et al.[28] found that biventricular repair, especially Rastelli-type reconstruction, is associated with higher late mortality and reintervention than Fontan procedure. They concluded that extending biventricular

BOX 3: Major postoperative complications in DORV after biventricular repair

- Left ventricular outflow tract obstruction due to baffle stenosis
- Right ventricular outflow tract obstruction and pulmonary regurgitation
- Postoperative complete heart block
- Residual ventricular septal defect
- Arrhythmias and sudden cardiac death
- Neoaortic valve regurgitation and coronary artery stenosis following arterial switch operation

repair to borderline anatomic candidates, especially with hypoplastic left-sided structures and a nonsubaortic VSD may be of questionable benefit. However, the inherent limitation of Fontan circulation with risk of late ventricular failure, arrhythmias, and other noncardiac complications resulting late morbidity and mortality remains a concern.[29]

CONCLUSION

- DORV encompasses a morphologically and physiologically diverse group of CHDs that can mimic a large VSD, TOF, or transposition of the great arteries (TGA) with VSD.
- Echocardiography provides the definitive diagnosis, supplemented by further 3D imaging in complex cases.
- Each patient requires an individualized approach to surgical correction. Surgical strategy is as variable and challenging as the disease itself, ranging from intraventricular tunnel repair in the simplest of the substrates to multiple-staged surgeries to achieve biventricular repair, or even univentricular palliation in those with complex anatomy.
- Despite the challenges, the outcomes are continuing to improve with evolution of better surgical strategies and advancements in perioperative care. Need for reoperations related to recurrent outflow obstructions after complex biventricular repair remains a concern, particularly in the subgroup of DORV with noncommitted VSD.

REFERENCES

1. Walters HL III, Mavroudis C, Tchervenkov CI, Jacobs JP, Lacour-Gayet F, Jacobs ML. Congenital heart surgery nomenclature and database project: double outlet right ventricle. Ann Thorac Surg. 2000;69(suppl 4):S249-63.
2. Ebadi A, Spicer DE, Backer CL, Fricker FJ, Anderson RH. Double outlet right ventricle revisited. J Thorac Cardiovasc Surg. 2017; 154(2):598-604.
3. Lev M, Bharati S, Meng CCL, Liberthson RR, Paul MH, Idriss F. A concept of double outlet right ventricle. J Thorac Cardiovasc Surg. [illegible]
4. Saxena A, Mehta A, Sharma M, Salhan S, Kalaivani M, Ramakrishnan S, et al. Birth prevalence of congenital heart disease: a cross sectional observational study from North India. Ann Pediatr Cardiol. 2016;9(3):205-9.
5. Liu Y, Chen S, Zu¨hlke L, Black GC, Choy M, Li N, et al. Global birth prevalence of congenital heart defects 1970–2017: updated systematic review and meta-analysis of 260 studies. Int J Epidemiol. 2019;48(2):455-63.
6. Howell CE, Ho SY, Anderson RH, Elliot MJ. Fibrous skeleton and ventricular outflow tract obstruction in double outlet right ventricle. Ann Thorac Surg. 1991;51(3):394-400.
7. Wilcox BR, Ho SY, Macartney FJ, Becker AE, Gelis LM, Anderson RH. Surgical anatomy of Double Outlet Right Ventricle with situs solitus and atrioventricular concordance. J Thorac Cardiovasc Surg. 1981;82(3):405-17.
8. Anderson RH, McCarthy K, Cook AC. Double outlet right ventricle. Cardiol Young. 2001; 11(3):329-44.
9. Bharucha T, Hlavacek AM, Spicer DE, Theocharis P, Anderson RH. How should we diagnose and differentiate hearts with double outlet right ventricle? Cardiol Young. 2017; 27(1);1-15.
10. Yim D, Dragulescu A, Ide H, Seed M, Grosse-Wortmann L, van Arsdell G, et al. Essential modifiers of double outlet right ventricle. Revisit with endocardial surface images and 3-dimensional print models. Circ Cardiovasc Imaging. 2018;11(3):e006891.
11. Kouchoukos NT, Blackstone EH, Hanley FL, Kirklin JK. Double outlet right ventricle. In: Kirklin/Barratt-Boyes Cardiac Surgery: Morphology, Diagnostic Criteria, Natural History, Techniques, Results and Indications, 4th edition. Philadelphia: Elsevier Saunders; 2013. pp. 1931-61.
12. Artrip JH, Sauer H, Campbell DN, Mitchell MB, Haun C, Almodovar MC, et al. Biventricular repair in double outlet right ventricle: surgical results based on the STS-EACTS International Nomenclature classification. Eur J Cardiothorac Surg. 2006; 29(4):545-50.
13. Villemain O, Belli E, Ladouceur M, Houyel L, Jalal Z, Lambert V, et al. Impact of anatomic characteristics and initial biventricular surgical strategy on outcomes in various forms of double outlet right ventricle. J Thorac Cardiovasc Surg. 2016;152(3):698-706.
14. Kirklin JW, Pacifico AD, Blackstone EH, Kirklin JK, Bargeron LM. Current risks and protocols for operations for Double Outlet Right Ventricle. J Thorac Cardiovasc Surg. 1986;92(5):913-30.
15. Lacour-Gayet F, Haun C, Ntalakouraa K, Belli E, Houyel L, Marcsek P, et al. Biventricular repair of double outlet right ventricle with non-committed ventricular septal defect (VSD) by VSD rerouting to the pulmonary artery and arterial switch. Eur J Cardiothorac Surg. 2002; 21(6):1042-8.
16. Belli E, Serraf A, Lacour-Gayet F, Hubler M, Zoghby J, Houyel L, et al. Double Outlet Right Ventricle with non-committed ventricular septal defect. Eur J Cardiothorac Surg. 1999;15(6):747-52.
17. Mahle WT, Martinez R, Silverman N, Cohen MS, Anderson RH. Anatomy, echocardiograpy, and surgical approach to double outlet right ventricle. Cardiol Young. 2008; 18(Suppl 3):39-51.
18. Yoo SJ, van Arsdell GS. 3D printing in surgical management of double outlet right ventricle. Front Pediatr. 2018;5:289.
19. Kirklin JW, Harp RA, McGoon DC. Surgical treatment of origin of both great vessels from right ventricle, including cases of pulmonary stenosis. J Thorac Cardivasc Surg. 1964;48:1026-36.
20. Mavroudis C, Backer CL, Muster AJ, Rocchini AP, Rees AH, Gevitz M. Taussig–Bing anomaly: arterial switch versus Kawashima intraventricular repair. Ann Thorac Surg. 1996;61(5):1331-8.
21. Sakata R, Lecompte Y, Batisse A, Borromee L, Durandy Y. Anatomic repair of anomalies of ventriculoarterial connection associated with ventricular septal defect. I. Criteria for surgical decision. J Thorac Cardiovasc Surg. 1988;95(1):90-5.
22. Marathe SP, Talwar S. The science and art of aortic and/or pulmonary root translocation. Ann Pediatr Cardiol. 2020;13(1): 56-66.
23. Lu T, Li J, Hu J, Huang C, Tan L, Wu Q, et al. Biventricular repair of double outlet right ventricle with noncommitted ventricular [illegible] conduit. J Thorac Cardiovasc Surg. 2020;159(6):2397-403.
24. Barbero-Marcial M, Tanamati C, Atik E, Ebaid M. Intraventricular repair of double outlet right ventricle with non-committed ventricular septal defect: advantages of multiple patches. J Thorac Cardiovasc Surg. 1999;118(6):1056-67.
25. Li S, Ma K, Hu S, Hua Z, Yang K, Yan J, et al. Surgical outcome of 380 patients with double outlet right ventricle who underwent biventricular repair. J Thorac Cardiovasc Surg. 2014; 148(3):817-24.
26. Oladunjoye O, Piekarski B, Baird C, Banka P, Marx G, del Nido PJ, et al. Repair of double outlet right ventricle: midterm outcomes. J Thorac Cardiovasc Surg. 2020;159(1):254-64.
27. Brown JW, Ruzmetov M, Okada Y, Vijay P, Turrentine MW. Surgical results in patients with double outlet right ventricle: a 20-year experience. Ann Thorac Surg. 2001;72(5):1630-5.
28. Bradley TJ, Karamlou T, Kulik A, Mitrovic B, Vigneswaran T, Jaffer S, et al. Determinants of repair type, reintervention, and mortality in 393 children with double outlet right ventricle. J Thorac Cardiovasc Surg. 2007;134(4):167-73.
29. Kutty S, Jacobs ML, Thompson R, Danford DA. Fontan circulation of the next generation. Why it's necessary and what it might look like. J Am Heart Assoc. 2020;9(1):e013691.

38
CHAPTER

Corrected Transposition

Nitin Rao, Suman Vyas

INTRODUCTION

Congenitally corrected transposition of the great arteries [atrioventricular (AV) discordance with ventriculoarterial discordance], or CCTGA or L-TGA, is an uncommon lesion with a prevalence of 0.03 per 1,000 live births—accounting for approximately 0.5% of congenital heart malformations.[1]

This defect was first described by Von Rokitansky in 1875 when he described two autopsies wherein transposition of the great arteries was functionally corrected by the position of the interventricular septum. Anderson in 1957 and Schiebler in 1961 described the clinical manifestations and added the word "Congenitally" to the term Corrected Transposition.[2]

This is a rare congenital heart disease with both AV and ventriculoarterial discordance (described further). This has been described by other names too—double discordance, physiologically corrected transposition, congenitally corrected transposition, or L-transposition; essentially, all are the same.

In CCTGA, the venous drainage is normal—the systemic veins drain to the right atrium and pulmonary veins to the left atrium. However, the atria are discordantly connected to the ventricles: the right atrium to the left ventricle (LV) and the left atrium to the right ventricle—the so-called AV discordance. In addition, the ventricles are inverted (right-to-left change in position) and are connected to the opposite great arteries—LV is connected to the pulmonary artery (PA) and right ventricle to the aorta—the ventriculoarterial discordance.[2] Thus, there is a double discordance at both, the AV and the ventriculoarterial levels. Therefore, the effects of ventricular inversion are "*corrected*" by the associated transposed great arteries. So, effectively, the systemic venous blood reaches the PA and the pulmonary venous blood reaches the aorta leading to physiological correction (**Fig. 1**).

However, despite this apparently normal physiology, natural history and hemodynamics are often far from normal. One of the main reasons is that the right ventricle (which is a weaker ventricle) is the systemic ventricle.[3] By default, ventricles are always accompanied by the ipsilateral AV valve, the ipsilateral conduction bundle, and the coronary artery. The right ventricle, therefore, carries with it the tricuspid valve, the right conduction bundle, and the right coronary artery. The right coronary artery is smaller than the left and has to perfuse an RV that is now the systemic ventricle. Associated cardiac conditions also impact long-term outcome [ventricular septal defects (VSDs), pulmonary stenosis (PS), and AV valve anomalies]. Besides, the conduction tissue has an unusual spatial arrangement that predisposes these patients to complete heart block.[4]

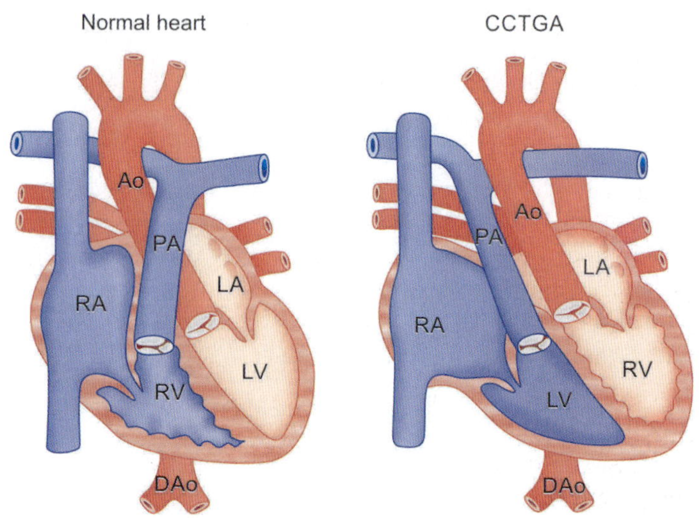

Fig. 1: Normal heart and corrected transposition.
(CCTGA: congenitally corrected transposition of the great arteries; Ao: aorta; LA: left atrium; LV: left ventricle; PA: pulmonary artery; RA: right atrium; RV: right ventricle)

MORPHOLOGY

Most patients will have a visceral situs solitus and about 25% cases will have an abnormal cardiac situs—either a dextrocardia or mesocardia.[5,6] Ventricular topology places the morphologic RV to the left of the morphologic LV.

The interventricular septum tends to be more horizontal or sagittal, resulting in a malalignment of the atrial and ventricular septae. The left AV valve has features of a tricuspid valve (three papillary muscles with insertion on the ventricular septum), while right-sided AV valve has the features of a mitral valve (two papillary muscles and no insertion onto the ventricular septum).

The great arteries are transposed with the aorta arising from the RV and the PA from the LV. The aortic valve is leftward and anterior to the pulmonary valve (L-transposition).

ASSOCIATED LESIONS/PROBLEMS

Associated lesions are seen in almost 90% of cases of CCTGA.

Ventricular Septal Defect

Approximately 80% of patients will have a VSD—mostly perimembranous and generally large in size, though subarterial and midmuscular defects may also be seen.

Pulmonic Stenosis

Congenitally corrected transposition of the great arteries may have varying degrees of pulmonic stenosis [effectively a left ventricular outflow tract (LVOT) obstruction]—the incidence ranges from 30 to 50%. This may rarely be isolated, valvar or infundibular, but is usually associated with a large VSD. In about 30% of cases with VSD and PS, there may be an abnormal left AV valve as well.[2] The obstruction may be *muscular* from the ventriculoinfundibular fold, *membranous* with tissue derived from the membranous septum, or due to *tissue tags* from the AV valves. *Malalignment of the conal septum* can be associated with a conoventricular septal defect and *subpulmonary stenosis*[2] (**Fig. 2**).

About 10–15% of patients have either a right ventricular (RV) inflow or outflow tract obstruction. Inflow obstruction may be due to an obstructing supratricuspid valvar stenosing ring (cor triatriatum) that is seen inferior to the left atrial appendage.

Left Atrioventricular Valve (Tricuspid) Anomalies

These are intrinsic to CCTGA. Tricuspid valve (left AV valve) regurgitation (TR) represents a major risk factor and RV dysfunction appears to be almost always secondary to long-standing TR. At autopsy, almost 90% hearts show some affliction but clinically, far less are manifest. The most common feature is a dysplasia of valve leaflets with or without a displacement of the septal and posterior leaflets of the tricuspid valve. Rarely, the AV valves may straddle the muscular inlet septum[6] and sometimes, the tricuspid valve may be Ebstenoid (12–13% of cases) resulting in severe regurgitation. This "Ebstenoid" variant differs from the usual Ebstein anomaly of the tricuspid valve in that the atrialized portion of the right ventricle is not thinned. Rarely, the septal leaflet can be absent, and this variant may be associated with a VSD and aortic arch obstruction. Tricuspid valve anomalies will influence modes of surgical repair. This left AV valve tends to deteriorate over time and paradoxically, worsening regurgitation is one of the long-term complications after surgical repair.

Other associated anomalies include a straddling and/or overriding left AV valve, superoinferior ventricles (criss-cross heart), coarctation of the aorta/aortic interruption, valvar or subvalvar aortic stenosis, hypoplasia of one ventricle, and a common arterial trunk.[6]

Rarely, the mitral valve (right AV valve) may be abnormal with some straddling or with abnormalities in cusp number and tension apparatus. This valve may also be dysplastic or stenotic or have a cleft leaflet.[6]

Coronary Artery Anatomy

Generally, the coronary arteries arise from the posterior facing sinuses of the aortic valve. They show a mirror image distribution with the right coronary artery bifurcating into circumflex and anterior descending arteries, while the left coronary artery runs in the left AV groove and gives rise to the infundibular and marginal branches.[5,7]

There have been a number of coronary artery variations reported including a single coronary artery, a sinus node

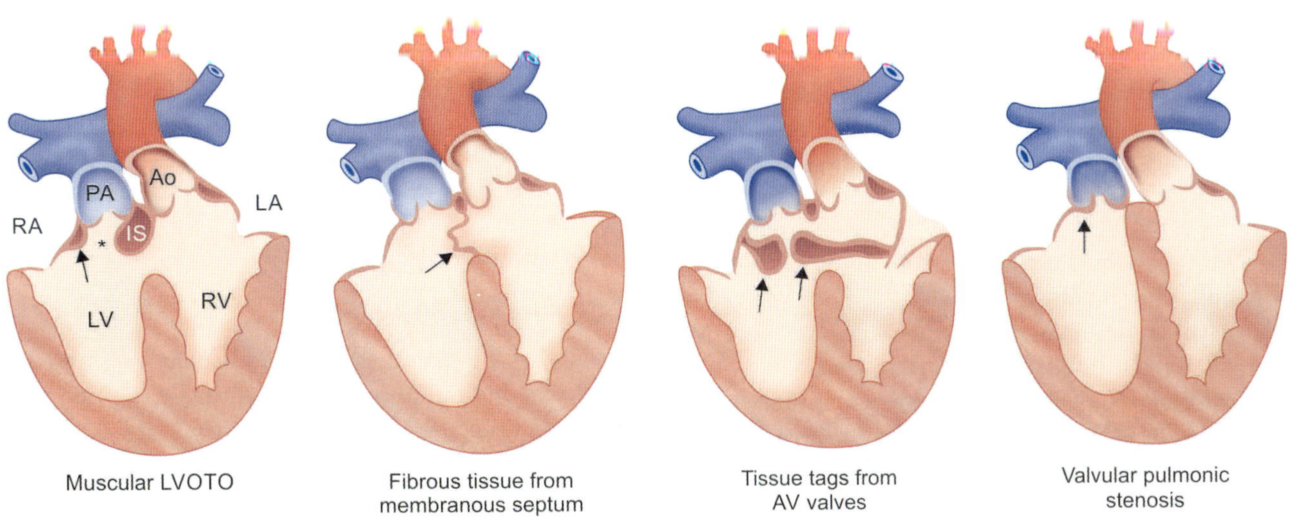

Fig. 2: Levels of left ventricular (LV) outflow obstruction in congenitally corrected transposition of the great arteries (CCTGA). (Ao: aorta; LA: left atrium; LV: left ventricle; RA: right atrium; RV: right ventricle; PA: pulmonary artery; LVOTO: left ventricular outflow tract obstruction)

artery arising from the circumflex artery and any major coronary artery crossing the RV outflow tract.[7]

Conduction Tissue

The conduction tissue in CCTGA is abnormal and is potentially problematic.[8] The sinoatrial (SA) node is normally located but the AV conduction tissue is abnormal. In CCTGA, there are two AV nodes—a normal posterior node without any AV bundle and an abnormal right AV node giving origin to the penetrating AV bundle. This is because the regular AV node located at the apex of the triangle of Koch cannot give origin to a penetrating conduction bundle—owing to the malaligned septae in CCTGA. Thus, an anomalous second AV node is present located beneath the opening of the right atrial appendage at the lateral margin and this node gives rise to the penetrating AV bundle which courses into the upper interventricular septum from where it descends and branches.[2] In CCTGA, the development of the normal AV bundle is hindered by the atrial and ventricular septal malalignment, which is related to the size of the LVOT and pulmonary trunk. Therefore, normal AV conduction is more likely with pulmonary stenosis or atresia, while heart blocks are more likely in patients with a normal LVOT.[9]

Complete Heart Block

About 10% of CCTGA patients may have complete heart block at initial presentation. In addition, the risk of natural onset AV block continues at a rate of approximately 2% per year after diagnosis.[9] AV block is more likely with an intact ventricular septum.

Right Ventricular Function

As age advances, RV (systemic ventricle) function starts deteriorating.[10] Bos et al. at the Mayo Clinic compared a few echocardiographic indices in CCTGA patients with normal subjects. All values were significantly lower in patients with CCTGA compared with control subjects. They concluded that patients with asymptomatic CCTGA have an RV dysfunction quantifiable by echocardiography.[6]

Congestive heart failure (CHF) is common as age advances, more so by the fourth and fifth decades of life. Tricuspid (systemic AV) valvular regurgitation is strongly associated with RV dysfunction (the systemic ventricle). By the age of 45 years, 67% of patients with associated lesions have CHF, while only 25% of patients without associated lesions have CHF.[11] Significant residual dysfunction of the right ventricle is common in patients operated late, especially in adults who may be referred late for surgery.[12]

The potential factors for systemic ventricular failure include significant associated cardiac lesions, a history of arrhythmia, pacemaker implantation, and prior surgery of any type, particularly tricuspid valvuloplasty or replacement. Aortic regurgitation is also relatively common in patients with CHF.

FETAL COURSE

The fetus with CCTGA may be diagnosed antenatally during a referral for cardiac screening, or because of hydrops fetalis. Hydrops fetalis may result from severe left AV valve regurgitation or complete AV block with bradycardia. CCTGA is usually compatible with normal prenatal growth and development and the short-term survival in some reported series is good.[13] However, the outcome is very guarded in the fetus with severe AV valve regurgitation.[14,15]

NATURAL HISTORY AND LONG-TERM OUTCOME

Natural history and long-term outcome in complex and unusual CHDs such as CCTGA are influenced by associated lesions namely, the systemic (right) ventricle, the left AV valve, and the occurrence of complete heart block.

The underlying problem is the issue of the RV as the systemic ventricle. Additionally, associated lesions also tend to affect this systemic RV function by way of volume overload (VSDs) and pressure overload (pulmonary outflow obstruction). TR will volume load the ventricle and reduce its afterload as well. The complex interactions of these anatomic and physiologic variables complicate outcome analysis.[2]

Unoperated Natural History

Although there have been case reports of long-term survival with age, this is probably unusual.[16] In one of the largest multi-institutional studies, Graham[11] reported on the long-term outcome of 182 adult patients with CCTGA from 19 institutions and compared 2 groups—those with associated cardiac conditions and those without lesions. CHF, significant RV dysfunction, and TR were commoner in patients with associated lesions. At 45 years of age, 67% patients with associated defects had heart failure compared to 25% of those without associated defects. Beauchesne et al. followed 44 unoperated patients for up to 144 months and found that the majority (59%) had grade 3 or greater systemic AV valve regurgitation and that many were symptomatic due to systemic RV dysfunction.[12] It has been reaffirmed, in subsequent studies, that systemic AV valve regurgitation and ventricular dysfunction are major long-term concerns.[17,18] *The only major variable correlating with decreased survival was left AV valve regurgitation.*

CLINICAL FEATURES

Patients with isolated CCTGA are usually asymptomatic in childhood and manifest later in adulthood.

In children, symptoms and severity are largely determined by the associated defects and patients may come to attention because of bradycardia or heart failure. CHF usually indicates a large VSD, left AV valve regurgitation, arch obstruction, or a combination.[2]

Occasionally, it is an abnormal heart sound or cardiomegaly on chest X-ray (possibly severe AV valve regurgitation) that prompts a cardiac evaluation. Characteristically, the second sound is single and accentuated—due to the anterior positioned aorta. Patients are usually acyanotic unless there is pulmonic stenosis/atresia. Other findings are reflective of associated lesions such as VSD and AV valve regurgitation.[2]

Electrocardiography

The three salient ECG features in CCTGA include the following:

1. Disturbances in conduction and rhythm
2. QRS and T wave patterns reflective of ventricular inversion
3. Change in P wave, QRS, ST segment, and T wave due to associated cardiac lesions.

In CCTGA, the ventricular conduction bundle branches are reversed and therefore the sequence of initial activation is from right to left and usually in a more anterior and superior direction. Consequently, q waves are absent in the left precordial leads and present in the right precordial leads with QS complexes in the right precordial leads, large Q waves in leads III and aVf, and also left axis deviation[8] (**Fig. 3**).

Atrioventricular conduction varies from PR prolongation to complete heart block.[9] More than 75% of patients with CCTGA exhibit some form of AV block and the overall incidence of complete heart block is almost 30%—across all age groups. The incidence of CHB may be as high as 10% at initial presentation with a long-term risk of about 2% per year[9] (**Fig. 4**).

Accelerated conduction across bypass tracts may occur in CCTGA with Ebsteinoid left AV valve. Supraventricular tachycardia, atrial fibrillation, and atrial flutter may all occur.

An upright P wave in lead I indicates a normal atrial situs and an absent R wave in lead V1 with Q waves in left precordial leads indicates a reversed septal depolarization due to ventricular inversion.

Chest X-ray

Radiological features vary as per the underlying associated cardiac defect, for example, cardiomegaly and pulmonary plethora or features of pulmonary edema are due to a large VSD or significant AV valve regurgitation. The most common great arterial relation in CCTGA is side by side or oblique with the aorta being left and anterior that results in a convex upper left heart border with a concavity in the pulmonary bay.

Echocardiography

Echocardiography is the mainstay of diagnosis. A sequential systematic segmental approach is of utmost importance (more specifically in CCTGA) to outline the anatomy and associated defects. Echocardiography is also vital in understanding the hemodynamics as surgical strategies evolve.

Although visceral situs solitus is the norm, 5% cases may have a situs inversus and inferior vena cava (IVC) interruption is commoner in this subset. With regard to cardiac situs, up to 25% of patients with CCTGA will demonstrate an abnormal situs (dextro or mesocardia).[2] A small proportion may show criss-cross AV connections or superoinferior ventricles.

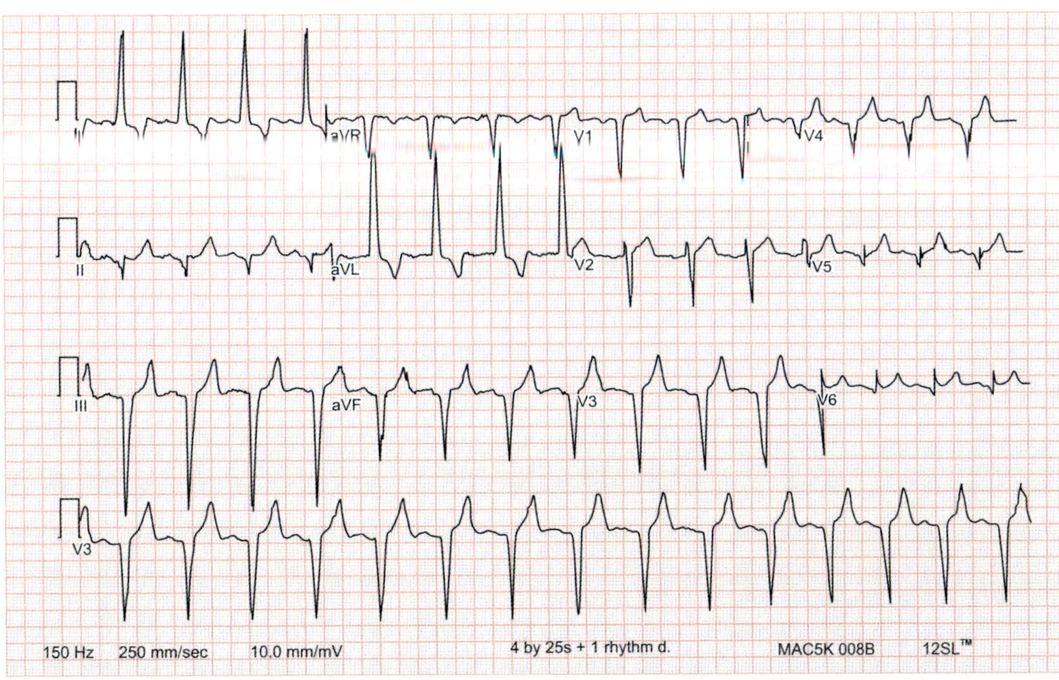

Fig. 3: Electrocardiogram (ECG) in congenitally corrected transposition of the great arteries (CCTGA) showing absent q waves in V6 and deep q in V1.

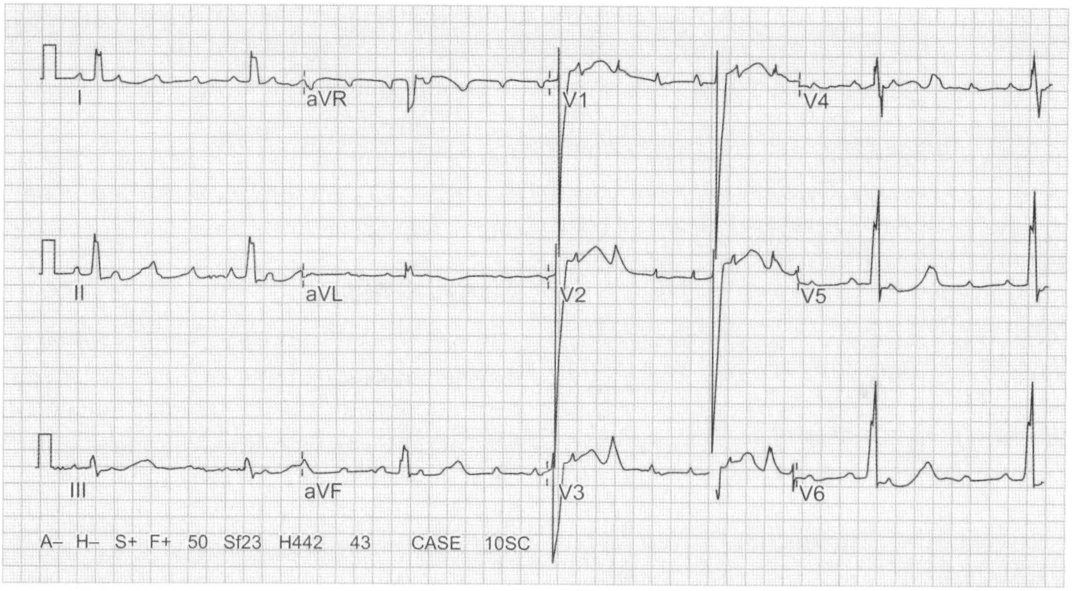

Fig. 4: Electrocardiogram (ECG) in congenitally corrected transposition of the great arteries (CCTGA) showing complete heart block.

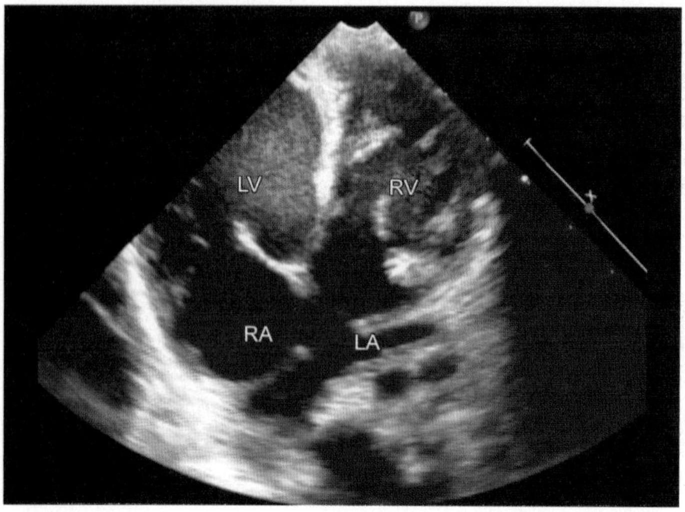

Fig. 5: Apical four-chamber view in congenitally corrected transposition of the great arteries (CCTGA) showing ventricular inversion.
(LA: left atrium; LV: left ventricle; RA: right atrium; RV: right ventricle)

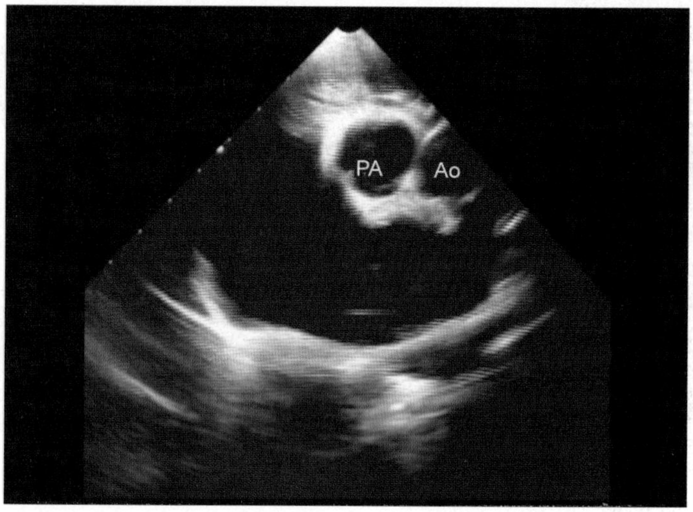

Fig. 6: Parasternal short axis view—congenitally corrected transposition of the great arteries (CCTGA) with side-to-side great arteries.
(Ao: aorta; PA: pulmonary artery)

Echocardiographically, *the subcostal view* demonstrates malalignment of both atrial + ventricular septae and helps differentiate the ventricles. The RV is characterized by the presence of a moderator band, an irregular and coarse endocardial surface of the morphologic RV relative to the smooth endocardial surface of the LV, and a round or triangular shape to the RV cavity versus an elongated or ellipsoidal shape to the left ventricular cavity.[2] Notably, the AV valves are differentiated by a more apically displaced valve in the RV relative to the LV (exaggerated in the presence of an Ebstein-like malformation and absent in the presence of an AV septal defect or a large perimembranous inlet VSD), a trileaflet (tricuspid) versus a bileaflet (mitral) AV valve, and chordal attachments of the AV valve of the RV directly to the septum (tricuspid valve).

The subcostal view also profiles the LVOT to the PA relation and outflow tract obstruction, if present (almost 30–50% of cases) may be outlined as well.

The *apical four-chamber* view profiles the AV discordance (**Fig. 5**), the usual perimembranous inlet VSD and also the AV valve anatomy with particular reference to the Ebsteinoid left AV (tricuspid) valve; while color-flow Doppler in this view helps quantify AV valve regurgitation.

The *parasternal long axis* view outlines the interventricular septum, the parallel outflow tracts, and any outflow obstruction, while the *parasternal short axis* view shows the great artery relation—the aorta being anterior and leftward (L transposed) to the PA. This is the usual arrangement; however, many exceptions are possible including a side-to-side orientation of the great arteries[19] (**Figs. 6 and 7**).

A VSD is present in >60% of patients with corrected TGA. Most defects are perimembranous and may be partially closed by the septal tricuspid leaflet. Sometimes, there may be straddling of the AV valve (commonly the tricuspid valve) associated with muscular inlet VSDs.[2]

A *right aortic arch* is seen in 15–18% of cases, while the incidence of an atrial septal defect is about 12%. The ASD is usually a secundum defect; however, it may occasionally be a part of an AV septal defect.[20]

The coronary arteries are usually imaged easily since the aorta is anterior. 76% patients will have a coronary distribution concordant with the ventricular anatomy. However, sometimes single coronary artery and other anomalies occur.[2]

Other abnormalities including an interrupted aortic arch or coarctation of aorta or Cor triatriatum can occur especially in the presence of subaortic stenosis or severe tricuspid valve regurgitation (**Fig. 8**).

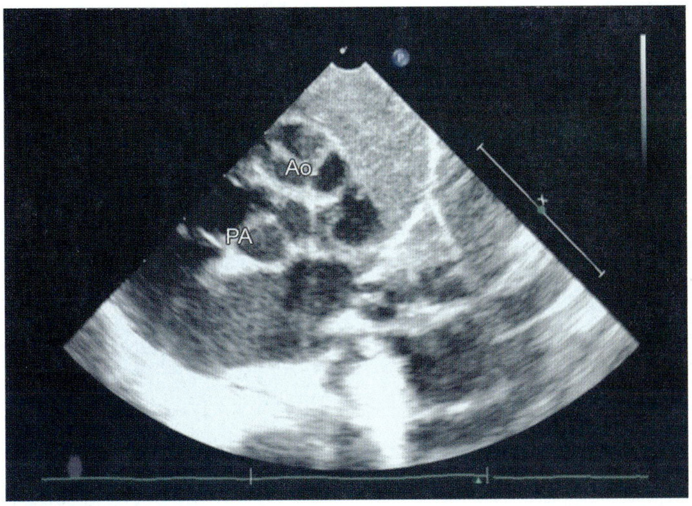

Fig. 7: Parasternal short axis view—congenitally corrected transposition of the great arteries (CCTGA) with L-Malposed great arteries.
(Ao: aorta; PA: pulmonary artery)

Transesophageal echocardiography and three-dimensional echocardiography are being increasingly useful to evaluate older patients or postoperative patients with poor transthoracic windows and also to assess the AV valve, the outflow tracts, etc.

CT Scan/MRI

Computed tomography/magnetic resonance imaging (CT/MRI) is complimentary to echocardiography and is helpful when echocardiographic images are suboptimal or in the diagnosis of extracardiac associations.

Computed tomography angiography (CTA) helps to identify anatomy especially abnormal AV and ventriculoarterial relationships and CT imaging also accurately profiles the malposed great arteries (**Figs. 9 to 11**). Cardiac-gated cine CT can additionally assess function.

Cardiac MRI allows both anatomic and physiologic assessment (including ventricular volumes), especially in evaluating the RV. MRI is also reliable in assessing the adequacy of LV retraining prior to a double-switch operation (**Fig. 12**).

Computed tomography/magnetic resonance imaging are vital in postoperative evaluation and follow-up in assessing outflow obstructions, ventricular dysfunction with regurgitant fraction and volumes (**Figs. 13 and 14**).

CARDIAC CATHETERIZATION

There is a limited role for cardiac catheterization since most anatomic and functional details are obtained by noninvasive imaging (echocardiography/CTA/MRI). There is a potential risk of developing heart block during catheterization, especially while trying to enter the PA and therefore, caution should be exercised.

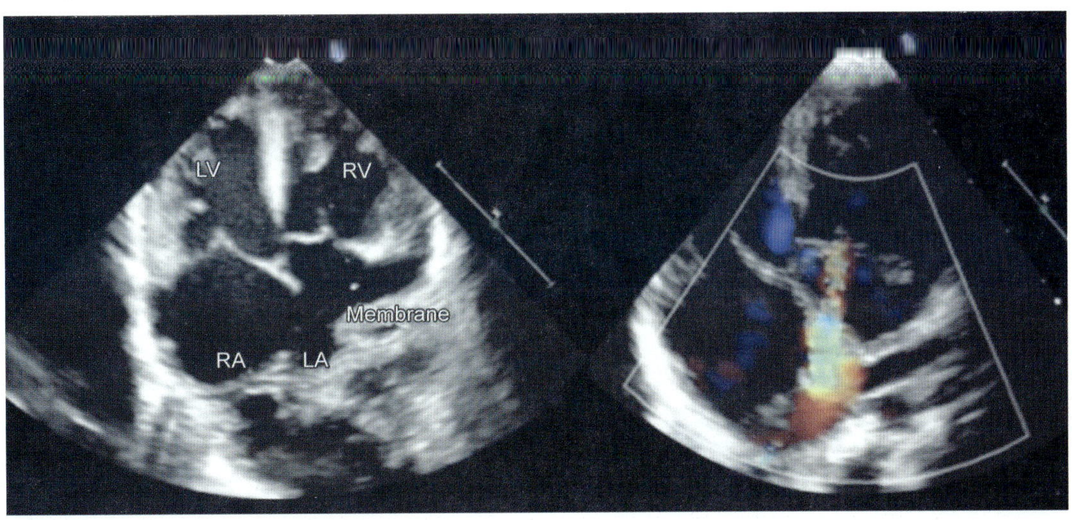

Fig. 8: Apical four-chamber view in 2D and color Doppler showing membrane in left atrium (LA)—congenitally corrected transposition of the great arteries (CCTGA) with cor triatriatum with turbulent flow across it.
(LA: left atrium; LV: left ventricle; RA: right atrium; RV: right ventricle)

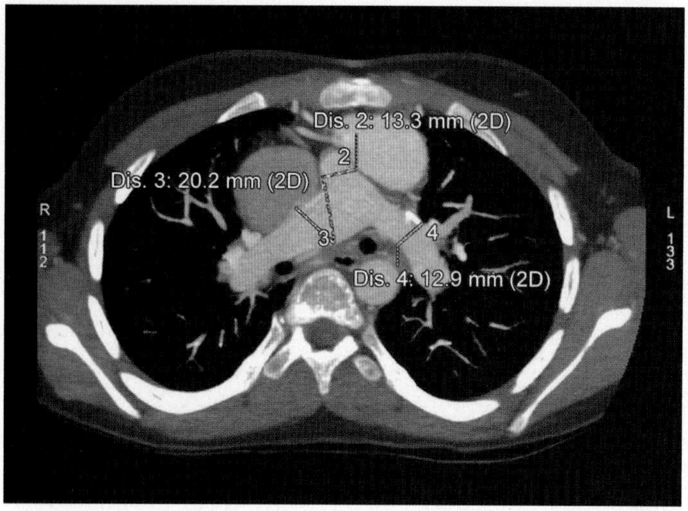

Fig. 9: Computed tomography (CT) angiography in congenitally corrected transposition of the great arteries (CCTGA) showing aorta anterior and to the left of pulmonary artery.

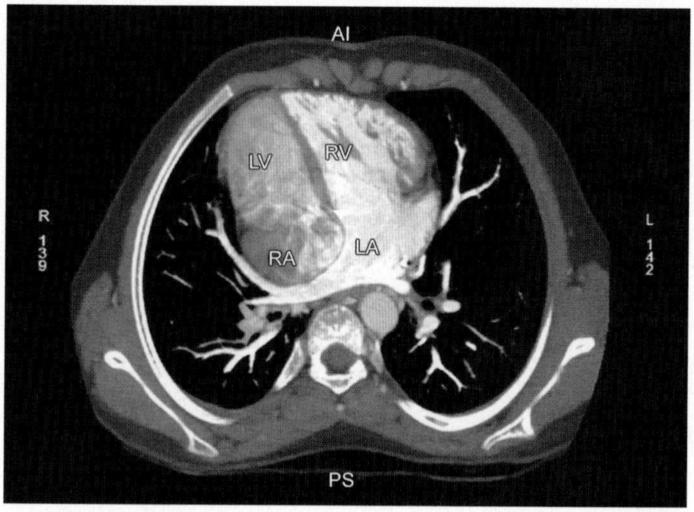

Fig. 10: Computed tomography (CT) angiography in congenitally corrected transposition of the great arteries (CCTGA) showing atrioventricular discordance.

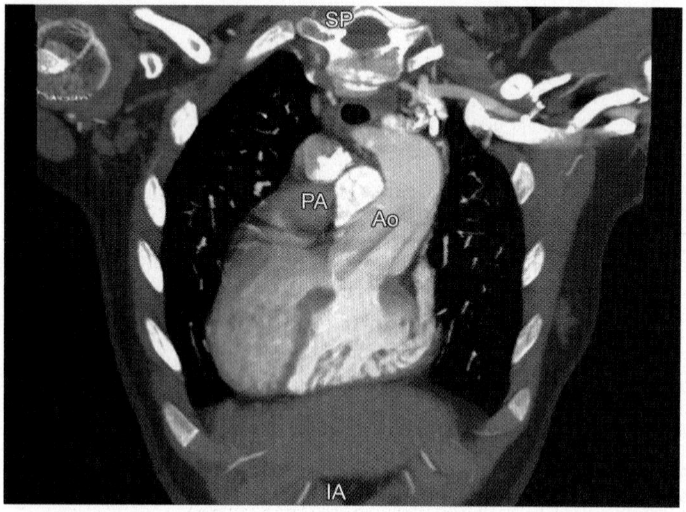

Fig. 11: Computed tomography (CT) angiography of congenitally corrected transposition of the great arteries (CCTGA) showing dextrocardia with ventriculoarterial discordance, large ventricular septal defect (VSD), dilated and L-malposed aorta.

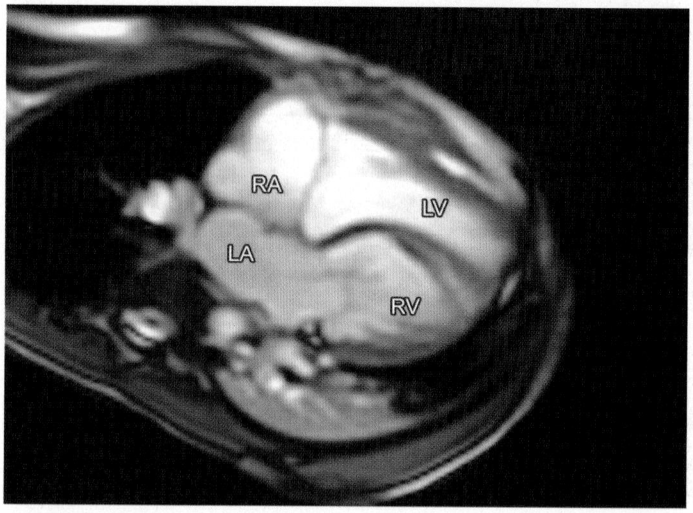

Fig. 12: Magnetic resonance imaging (MRI) of congenitally corrected transposition of the great arteries (CCTGA) showing atrioventricular discordance.

(LA: left atrium; LV: left ventricle; RA: right atrium; RV: right ventricle)

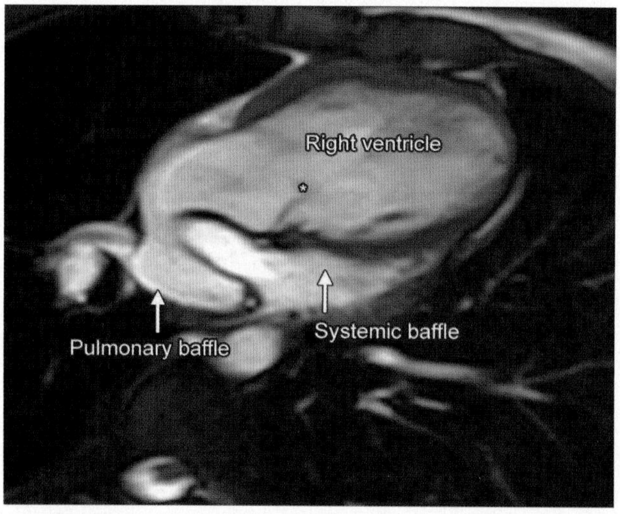

Fig. 13: Magnetic resonance imaging (MRI) showing venous baffles in a postoperative case—double switch for congenitally corrected transposition of the great arteries (CCTGA) + Ebstenoid tricuspid valve.

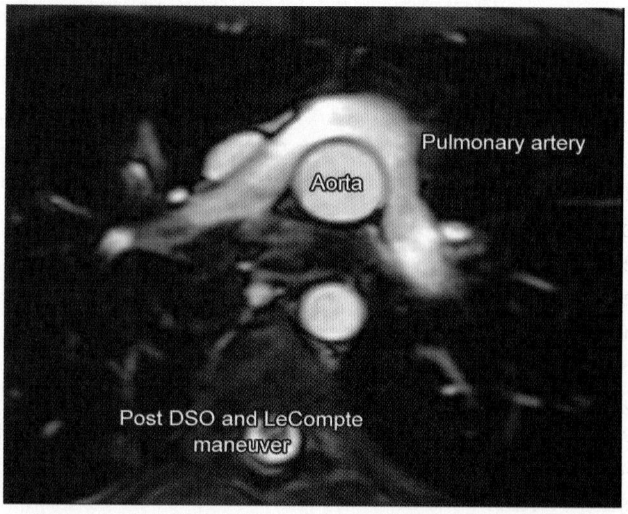

Fig. 14: Magnetic resonance imaging (MRI) of congenitally corrected transposition of the great arteries (CCTGA)—postdouble switch operation and LeCompte maneuver.

Common indications for cardiac catheterization include assessing the LVOT gradient, quantifying the left-to-right shunt or assessing pulmonary vascular resistance and reversibility prior to surgery, outlining aortopulmonary collaterals, and rarely to delineate the coronaries or to evaluate unexplained cyanosis.

Catheterization is necessary in the assessment of left ventricular hemodynamics in patients undergoing left ventricular retraining prior to an anatomic repair (AR) and also in patients undergoing a single ventricle palliation.

MANAGEMENT

Medical Management

Duct-dependent lesions in neonates with CCTGA (pulmonic atresia/severe stenosis or severe coarctation of the aorta/interruption of the aortic arch) will need initial stabilization and prostaglandin infusion to maintain ductal patency until further palliation [Blalock–Taussig (BT) shunt/patent ductus arteriosus (PDA) stent, etc.].[2]

Later, medical management is determined by associated lesions such as systemic AV valve regurgitation and heart failure. Diuretics, angiotensin-converting enzyme (ACE) inhibitors, and beta-blockers (to be used with caution because of the risk of developing complete heart block) may be prescribed when required.

Pacing

Complete heart block either spontaneous or postoperative, is a common complication in CCTGA. AV block is commoner in the presence of associated cardiac anomalies and may need permanent pacing. Pacing may be endocardial, epicardial, or a combination of the two depending on various factors, including the patient's age/weight/size/venous anatomy/intracardiac lesions and shunts, and type of surgical repair.

There is a role of biventricular pacing and cardiac resynchronization therapy (CRT) in CCTGA patients with significant heart failure and ventricular dyssynchrony.[21]

Surgical Management

The surgical treatment strategies have evolved over the decades varying from no intervention to physiological repair (PR), anatomical repair, or a single-ventricle palliation. Repair was initially focused on correction of the underlying aberrant physiology, but of late, the focus has shifted toward anatomic correction to avoid failure of the morphologic right ventricle.[22]

Physiological Repair

The conventional strategy had been physiological surgical repair which included VSD closure (single-stage VSD closure or staged-PA band initially followed by VSD closure later), with or without insertion of a LV to PA conduit (for pulmonic stenosis) and either repair or replacement of the regurgitant systemic AV valve. So effectively, the intracardiac defects were corrected but the double discordance persisted, namely, the morphologic RV in the systemic position.

The results of this physiologic repair were generally unsatisfactory, with a 10-year survival of approximately 60% and high rates of morphological right ventricle failure and perioperative heart block.[23] There is a risk of RV dysfunction and TR (the biggest drawbacks) in the long-term and survivors of physiologic repair have a markedly reduced exercise capacity.

Anatomic Repair

The failure of the nonanatomic repair due to RV failure and tricuspid valve insufficiency led to an interest in "anatomic" repair. In 1990, Ilbawi and colleagues developed the concept of double-switch or AR, which was attractive because it restored the mLV to the systemic circulation and possibly, better long-term results.[24] He carried out an atrial switch and combined it with a VSD closure and a Rastelli operation (so effectively creating a "double switch") in a case of CCTGA, VSD, and pulmonic stenosis. A few years later, Imai and colleagues combined an atrial switch with an arterial switch in a patient with CCTGA, without pulmonic stenosis, thus carrying out a "double switch".[25]

A double-switch procedure combines the (1) *Senning atrial baffle procedure*, which redirects blood flow at the atrial level, with (2) *the Arterial switch procedure*, where the great arteries are transected and reversed (**Fig. 15**).

A successful outcome after this procedure is dependent on the LV being adequately prepared for functioning at systemic arterial pressure.

Complications could be expected to include those due to atrial switch (sinus node dysfunction, atrial arrhythmias,

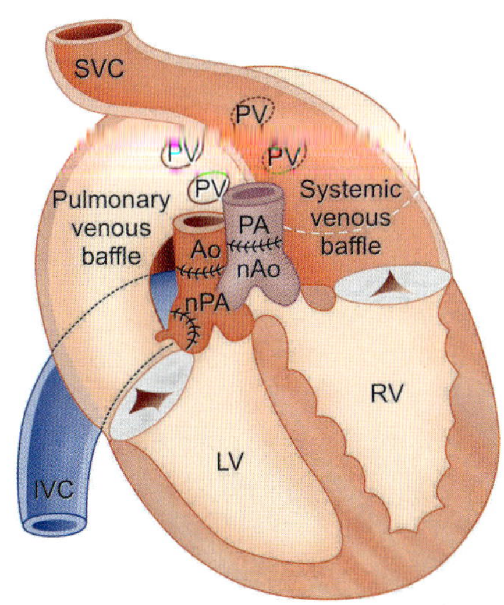

Fig. 15: Double switch → atrial switch and arterial switch in congenitally corrected transposition of the great arteries (CCTGA).

(IVC: inferior vena cava; LV: left ventricle; nAo: neoaorta; nPA: neopulmonary artery; PA: pulmonary artery; PV: pulmonary valve; RV: right ventricle; SVC: superior vena cava)

and baffle obstruction), problems inherent to a ventricular switch (subaortic obstruction or aortic regurgitation, conduit obstruction or regurgitation), and/or the arterial switch (coronary obstruction, aortic regurgitation/PA stenosis).

Several single centers have reported 10-year survivals of 78–100% for patients undergoing the atrial plus arterial switch and 60–96% for the atrial switch plus the Rastelli procedure.[23]

At least 4% of patients will require a pacemaker within 5 years of AR, and pacemaker implantation is strongly associated with LV dysfunction. The incidence of surgically acquired heart block is up to 20%, with freedom from pacemaker implantation of 70–80% at 15 years.[26] Also, sinus node dysfunction and tachyarrhythmias may occur in the long term. Baffle obstruction is another factor, with a reported risk of baffle complications of about 12% at 25 years.[27] The Double Switch Group (atrial + arterial switch) is at a significantly higher risk for late mLV dysfunction and aortic regurgitation than the Rastelli + Senning group.

Reinterventions

There is a high rate of reinterventions after AR. These include RV-pulmonary arterial conduit replacement/ballooning, aortic valve replacements, reinterventions on the Senning pathways (surgical/percutaneous) and interventions for mLV outflow tract obstruction.

A small subset of patients (representing approximately 15% of all patients with CCTGA) with an intact ventricular septum and absence of subpulmonary stenosis will have a nontrained or detrained LV incapable of sustaining the systemic pressures later. Such patients are not candidates for an arterial switch unless undertaken early. If undertaken later, these patients will need LV retraining before an anatomical repair can be carried out.

Left Ventricular Retraining Prior to Anatomical Repair

Since the morphologic LV has been working in the low-pressure pulmonary circuit, for quite some time, it may not be able to support the systemic circulation following an arterial switch and may require some preparation to cope and withstand this systemic circulation.

One of the approaches is an initial pulmonary artery banding (PAB) followed by a double switch operation 6–12 months (or more) later. Generally, a PAB is required in patients with an intact ventricular septum presenting beyond the third month of age. The PA band is placed around the main PA, to acutely raise the morphologic LV pressure to approximately 75–80% of the systemic pressure. Excessive PAB tightening may lead to mLV dysfunction and at times, sequential tightening of the PAB may result in an optimal retraining of the mLV. The upper age limit at which success can predictably be expected is 15–16 years.[28]

Left ventricular retraining produces good results in prepubescent patients but, in older patients, the response is less predictable and is associated with higher early and late mortality.[29] Despite a variety of strategies, LV retraining remains a risk factor for long-term outcome.

This strategy of PA banding also works well prophylactically for individuals without associated lesions wherein a PA band will decrease the degree of tricuspid valve insufficiency in most patients with a detrained LV. This improvement is clearly associated with the "septal shift" induced by increasing the LV pressures. Hanley and others from University of California San Francisco (UCSF) found that placement of a PAB resulted in a decrease in the degree of TR in 16 of the 24 patients, whether mild, moderate, or severe regurgitation.[30]

Tricuspid valve repair/replacement: Surgical options in managing TR at AR, especially when associated with Ebsteinoid dysplasia, are varied and challenging.[31] For significant TR, valvuloplasty (repair) should be considered and if unsatisfactory, valve replacement may be needed.[32]

Fontan Pathway (Univentricular Repair Strategy)

Finally, for those patients with difficulty in routing the VSD to the aorta or other technical complexities (such as unbalanced ventricles), the univentricular repair—*the Fontan pathway*—is an acceptable palliation.

The long-term mortality and morbidity also have been exceptionally low with actuarial survival at 10 years, reaching 91% and freedom from reoperations and arrhythmias being 87%. The Fontan procedure has been shown to have a better late survival over the PR. Marathe and others from Australia compared patients who underwent either an AR or a Fontan procedure and reported particularly good results following the Fontan surgery.[33]

TRANSPLANTATION

Despite all surgical options, some patients continue to present with severe heart failure, and no meaningful surgical options exist other than mechanical circulatory support and cardiac transplantation.

CONGENITALLY CORRECTED TRANSPOSITION OF THE GREAT ARTERIES AND PREGNANCY

Successful pregnancy can be achieved in most women with CCTGA. The rate of fetal loss and maternal cardiovascular morbidity is increased. However, the risk of congenital heart disease in offspring of women with CCTGA is uncertain since the reported number of births is very less. In one series of 22 women with 60 pregnancies, none of the 50 live offspring had been diagnosed with congenital heart disease.[34]

FOLLOW-UP

In the follow-up of these patients whether unoperated or operated with conventional surgical techniques, they must be monitored for the following issues:

- ECG changes for complete heart block and arrhythmia
- Biventricular function and function of the systemic AV valve
- The PA conduit and venous baffle for stenosis/regurgitation and also the development of aortic regurgitation
- PA branch stenosis (after previous shunt or conduit surgery).

CONCLUSION

Congenitally corrected transposition of the great arteries (CCTGA) has the following interesting features[6]:

- Patients with this entity should not be considered "corrected".
- The morphologically right ventricle supports the systemic circulation.
- Frequent coexisting anomalies include VSD, pulmonary outflow tract obstruction, and an Ebstein-like malformation of the morphologically tricuspid valve.
- There is an ever-present risk of complete heart block.
- Late RV dysfunction and TR occur in both operated and nonoperated individuals.
- The classic surgical operation confers a PR as the morphologically right ventricle retains its function as the systemic ventricle.
- An AR is more complicated, but advantageous as the morphologically LV becomes the systemic ventricle.
- *Patients with CCTGA, whether unoperated, operated with either a physiological or AR require life-long cardiac surveillance.*

REFERENCES

1. Van Praagh R, Van Praagh S. Morphologic anatomy. In: Fyler D, (Ed). Nadas' Pediatric Cardiology. Philadelphia, PA: Hanley and Bellus; 1992. pp. 17-25.
2. Atallah J, Rutledge J, Dyck JD. Congenitally corrected transposition of the great arteries. In: Allen HD, Gutgesell HP, Clark EB, Driscoll DJ, (Eds). Moss and Adams's Heart Disease in Infants Children and Adolescents, 8th edition. Philadelphia, PA: Lippincott Williams and Wilkins; 2013. pp. 1147-58.
3. Warnes CA. Congenitally corrected transposition: the uncorrected misnomer. J Am Coll Cardiol. 1996;27(5):1244-5.
4. Wilkinson JL, Anderson RH. Anatomy of discordant atrioventricular connections. World J Pediatr Congenit Heart Surg. 2010;2(1):43-53.
5. Losekoot TG, Becker AE. Discordant atrioventricular connexion and congenitally corrected transposition. In: Anderson RH, Macartney FJ, Shinebourne EA, Tynan M, (Eds). Paediatric Cardiology. Edinburgh: Churchill Livingstone; 1987. pp. 867-88.
6. Freedom R, Yoo SJ, Williams WG. Conditions with double discordance (congenitally corrected transposition of the great arteries) In: Freedom R, Yoo SJ, Mikailian H, Williams WG, (Eds). The Natural and Modified History of Congenital Heart Disease. Hoboken: Blackwell Publishing; 2004. pp. 356-65.
7. Chiu I-S, Wu S-J, Chen S-J, Wang J-K, Wu M-H, Lue H-C. Sequential diagnosis of coronary arterial anatomy in congenitally corrected transposition of the great arteries. Ann Thorac Surg. 2003;75(2):422-9.
8. Losekoot TG, Anderson RH, Becker AE, Danielson GK, Soto B. Congenitally Corrected Transposition. Edinburgh: Churchill Livingstone; 1983. pp. 3-190.
9. Huhta JC, Maloney JD, Ritter DG, Ilstrup DM, Feldt RH. Complete atrioventricular block in patients with atrioventricular discordance. Circulation. 1983;67(6):1374-7.
10. Dobson R, Danton M, Nicola W, Hamish W. The natural and unnatural history of the systemic right ventricle in adult survivors. J Thorac Cardiovasc Surg. 2013;145(6):1493-503.
11. Graham TP, Bernard YD, Mellen BG, Celermajer D, Baumgartner H, Cetta F, et al. Long-term outcome in congenitally corrected transposition of the great arteries: a multi-institutional study. J Am Coll Cardiol. 2000;36(1):255-61.
12. Beauchesne LM, Warnes CA, Connolly HM, Ammash NM, Tajik AJ, Danielson GK. Outcome of the unoperated adult who presents with congenitally corrected transposition of the great arteries. J Am Coll Cardiol. 2002;40(2):285-90.
13. Sharland G, Tingay R, Jones A, Simpson J. Atrioventricular and ventriculoarterial discordance (congenitally corrected transposition of the great arteries): echocardiographic features, associations, and outcome in 34 fetuses. Heart. 2005;91(11):1453-8.
14. Paladini D, Volpe P, Marasini M, Russo MG, Vassallo M, Gentile M, et al. Diagnosis, characterization and outcome of congenitally corrected transposition of the great arteries in the fetus: a multicenter series of 30 cases. Ultrasound Obstet Gynecol. 2006;27(3):281-5.
15. Allan L. Atrioventricular discordance. In: Allan L, Hornberger L, Sharland G, (Eds). Textbook of Fetal Cardiology. London: Greenwich Medical Media; 2000. pp. 183-93.
16. Shinbane JS, Shriki J, Hindoyan A, Ghosh B, Chang P, Farvid A, et al. Unoperated congenitally corrected transposition of the great arteries, non-restrictive ventricular septal defect, and pulmonary stenosis in middle adulthood: Do multiple wrongs make a right? World J Pediatr Congenit Heart Surg. 2012;3(1)123-9.
17. Presbitero P, Somerville J, Rabajoli F, Stone S, Conte MR. Corrected transposition of the great arteries without associated defects in adult patients: clinical profile and follow up. Br Heart J. 1995;74(1):57-9.
18. James H. The natural history of congenitally corrected transposition of the great arteries. World JPediatr Congenit Heart Surg. 2011; 2(1):59-63.
19. [illegible] Echocardiography. Baltimore: Williams and Wilkins; 1993. pp. 245-79.
20. Snider R, Serwer G, Ritter S. Abnormalities of Ventriculoarterial Connection. Echocardiography in Pediatric Heart Disease, 2nd edition. St Louis: Mosby; 1997. pp. 297-343.
21. Hofferberth SC, Alexander ME, Mah DY, Bautista-Hernandez V, del Nido PJ, Fynn-Thompson F. Impact of pacing on systemic ventricular function in L-transposition of the great arteries. J Thorac Cardiovasc Surg. 2016; 151(1):131-8.
22. Tweddell J. What do we really know about the management of patients with congenitally corrected transposition of the great arteries? J Thorac Cardiovasc Surg. 2017;154(3):1023-5.
23. Hraska V, Duncan BW, Mayer JE, Jr, Freed M, del Nido PJ, Jonas RA. Long-term outcome of surgically treated patients with corrected transposition of the great arteries. J Thorac Cardiovasc Surg. 2005;129(1):182-91.
24. Ilbawi MN, DeLeon SY, Backer CL, Duffy CE, Muster AJ, Zales VR, et al. An alternative approach to the surgical management of physiologically corrected transposition with ventricular septal

defect and pulmonary stenosis or atresia. J Thorac Cardiovasc Surg. 1990;100(3):410-15.

25. Yamagishi M, Imai Y, Hoshino S, Ishihara K, Koh Y, Nagatsu M, et al. Anatomic correction of atrioventricular discordance. J Thorac Cardiovasc Surg. 1993;105(6):1067-76.
26. Hraska V, Mitchell ME, Woods RK, Frommelt MA. What surgical improvementsare needed to prove that anatomical repair is superior to physiologic repair in the majority of patients with corrected transposition of great arteries? J Thorac Cardiovasc Surg. 2017;154(3):1019-22.
27. Brizard CP, Lee A, Zannino D, Davis AM, Fricke TA, d'Udekem Y, et al. Long-term results of anatomic correction for congenitally corrected transposition of the great arteries: a 19-year experience. J Thorac Cardiovasc Surg. 2017;154(1):258-65.
28. Myers PO, del Nido PJ, Geva T, Bautista-Hernandez V, Chen P, Mayer JE Jr, et al. Impact of age and duration of banding on left ventricular preparation before anatomic repair for congenitally corrected transposition of the great arteries. Ann Thorac Surg. 2013;96(2): 603-10.
29. Poirier NC, Mee RB. Left ventricular reconditioning and anatomical correction for systemic right ventricular dysfunction. Semin Thorac Cardiovasc Surg Ped Card Surf Annu. 2000;3: 198-215.
30. Ibrahimiye AN, Mainwaring RD, Patrick WL, Downey L, Yarlagadda V, Hanley FL. Left ventricular retraining and double switch in patients with congenitally corrected transposition of the great arteries. World J Pediatr Congenit Heart Surg. 2017;8(2): 203-9.
31. Myers PO, Bautista-Hernandez V, Baird CW, Emani SM, Marx GR, del Nido PJ. Tricuspid regurgitation or Ebsteinoid dysplasia of the tricuspid valve in congenitally corrected transposition: Is valvuloplasty necessary at anatomic repair? J Thorac Cardiovasc Surg. 2014;147(2):576-80.
32. Acar P, Sid D, Bonnet D, Aggoun Y, Bonhoeffer P, Kachaner J. Maintaining tricuspid valve competence in double discordance: a challenge for the pediatric cardiologist. Heart. 1998;80(5): 479-83.
33. Marathe SP, Jones MI, Winlaw DS, Ayer J, Sun J, Orr Y, et al. Congenitally corrected transposition: complex anatomic repair or Fontan pathway? Asian Cardiovasc Thorac Ann. 2017;25(6):432-9.
34. Connolly HM, Grogan M, Warnes CA. Pregnancy among women with congenitally corrected transposition of great arteries. J Am Coll Cardiol. 1999;33(6):1692-5.

39 CHAPTER

Univentricular Hearts

K Sivakumar

INTRODUCTION: WHAT IS A UNIVENTRICULAR HEART?

Univentricular heart refers to a group of cardiac anomalies characterized by a *single functional ventricle* (**Box 1**). Heart chambers are characterized by clear-cut anatomical boundaries between the atrial and ventricular myocardial masses by the anatomical atrioventricular (AV) junction. The ventriculoarterial junction provides similar demarcation between the ventricular mass and fibrous wall of the arterial roots. These anatomical boundaries divide the heart into segments. Each ventricle is tripartite with inlet, apical, and outlet components. When one or the other ventricle is insufficient in size to support either the systemic or pulmonary circulation, there is a functionally univentricular arrangement. Univentricular AV connection refers to connection of both atria to one ventricle either through two AV valve orifices (double-inlet), single AV valve orifice (one valve is atretic), and common orifice (common AV valve). Such hearts with *univentricular AV connections* are called as univentricular hearts.

BOX 1: Different types of univentricular hearts.

- Univentricular AV connections:
  - Single ventricle:
    - Single ventricle of LV morphology
    - Single ventricle of RV morphology
    - Single ventricle of mixed LV and RV morphology
    - Single ventricle of indeterminate morphology:
      - Double-inlet AV connection
      - Single-inlet (atresia of one valve)
      - Common-inlet (common AV valve)
  - Tricuspid atresia:
    - Associated with normally related great arteries:
      - With pulmonary atresia
      - With pulmonary stenosis
      - Without pulmonary stenosis
    - Associated with d-transposed great arteries:
      - With pulmonary atresia
      - With pulmonary stenosis
      - Without pulmonary stenosis
    - Associated with L-malposed great arteries
- Biventricular AV connections with hypoplastic or ineffective ventricles:
  - Hypoplastic ventricle:
    - Hypoplastic left heart:
      - Mitral atresia
      - Mitral hypoplasia
      - Aortic atresia
      - Aortic hypoplasia
    - Hypoplastic right heart:
      - PA-IVS
      - Small TV/RV
  - Ineffective ventricle:
    - Severe Ebstein anomaly of tricuspid valve
    - Uhl's anomaly of right ventricle
- Biventricular AV connection with well-formed ventricles:
  - Difficult surgical subset:
    - Tetralogy of Fallot with hypoplastic LV
    - TGA with hypoplastic LV
    - DORV with nonroutable VSD:
      - Inlet VSD
      - Remote trabecular VSD
      - Multiple Swiss cheese VSD

Contd...

Contd...

    - Superoinferior ventricles:
    - Criss-cross AV connections
  - Complex anatomy:
    - Right isomerism—heterotaxy
    - Left isomerism—heterotaxy
  - High-risk surgery:
    - AV discordance, VSD with PS
    - Straddling AV valve
    - Unbalanced AV canal defect

(AV: atrioventricular; DORV: double-outlet right ventricle; IVS: intact ventricular septum; LV: left ventricle; PA: pulmonary atresia; PS: pulmonary stenosis; RV: right ventricle; TGA: transposition of the great arteries; TV: tricuspid valve, VSD: ventricular septal defect)

Such hearts referred as "single ventricle" by Van Praagh or "univentricular AV connection" by Robert Anderson were uniformly associated with very poor survival.[1] These lesions along with tricuspid atresia and mitral atresia share similar hemodynamics. They remained anatomical and imaging curiosities till 50 years earlier, when Fontan surgery was introduced as a palliation for streamlining their circulation. This surgery allows children with a potentially lethal defect to survive to adulthood leading to a new cohort of adult congenital heart disease-palliated population. These patients are significantly different from people with two

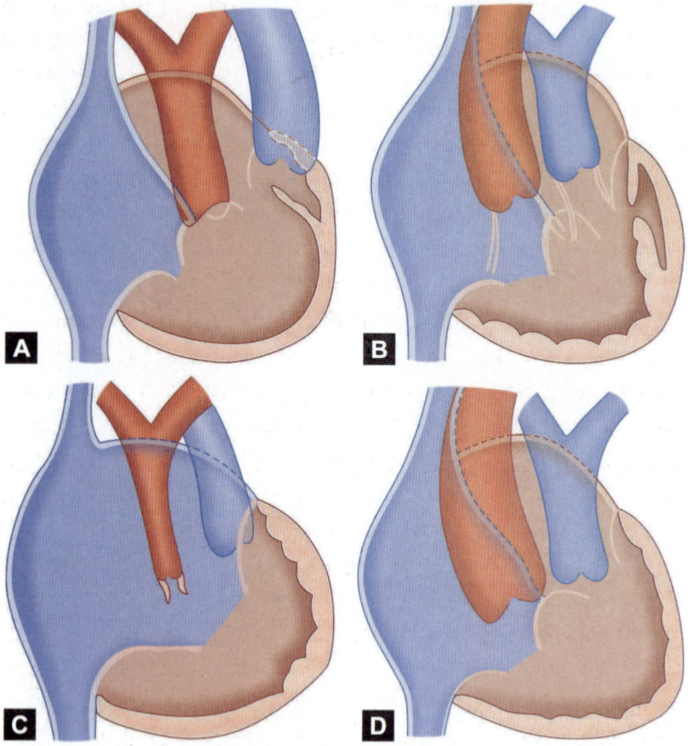

Figs. 1A to D: Univentricular atrioventricular (AV) connection-single ventricle. Single ventricles are grouped according to their morphology into left ventricular morphology (the most common type), right ventricular morphology (next common type), mixed morphology, and indeterminate morphology (both are rare). There can be two separate AV valves or valves.

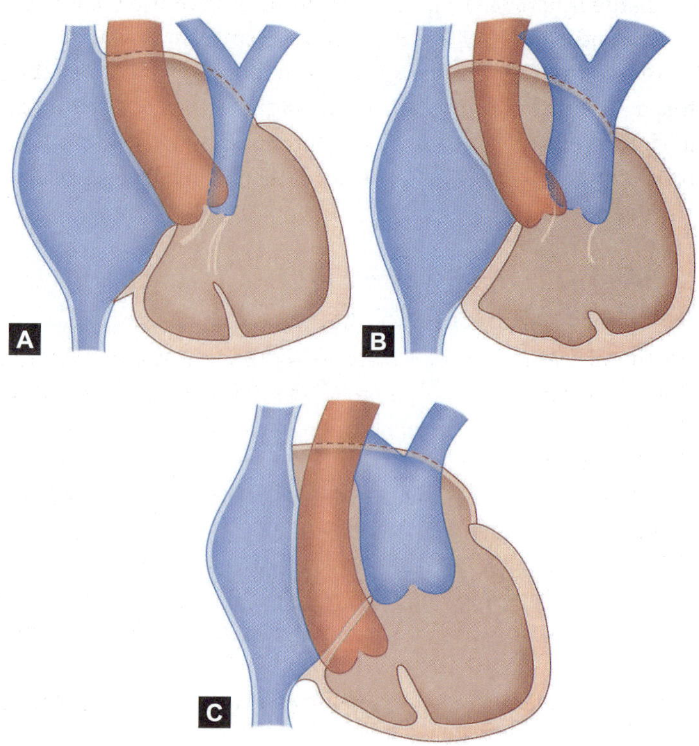

Figs. 2A to C: Univentricular atrioventricular (AV) connection-tricuspid atresia. Tricuspid atresia is grouped as type I with normal related great arteries and type II with transposed great arteries. They are further subgrouped as (A) Pulmonary atresia; (B) Pulmonary stenosis; (C) Unobstructed pulmonary outflow.

ventricles with unique clinical complications and natural history. Single ventricle (**Figs. 1A to D**) and tricuspid atresia (**Figs. 2A to C**) are the two common forms of univentricular hearts.

A second group of heart defects where there is a *biventricular AV connection but one of the ventricles is incapable* of supporting the systemic or pulmonary circulation also were palliated with this Fontan approach. A classic example is hypoplastic left heart syndrome with varying degrees of hypoplasia of inflow and outflow of the left ventricle. A similar situation arises in pulmonary atresia with intact ventricular septum with gross hypoplasia of tricuspid annulus and diminutive right ventricle that can no longer support pulmonary circulation. These hypoplastic right ventricles are often associated with extensive myocardial sinusoids that communicate to the epicardial coronaries, thereby preventing a biventricular surgical correction. Ineffective ventricles in such biventricular AV connections also include severe forms of Ebstein anomaly of tricuspid valve, Uhl's anomaly of the right ventricle with the absence of a contractile right ventricle.

A third group of heart defects with a *biventricular AV connection and reasonably well-formed two ventricles where repair is difficult* also are palliated in this univentricular approach. They include unbalanced AV canal defects where the septation of an asymmetric AV canal might lead to distorted ventricular inflow causing stenosis or regurgitation of the AV valve. Similarly, double-outlet right ventricles with ventricular septal defects (VSDs) that are not located in conotruncal septum are difficult for routing the left ventricle toward one of the great arteries and they are also often palliated in this method. The typical locations of VSD in such double-outlet right ventricles are inlet defects or multiple remote trabecular muscular defects.

The last category of lesions palliated by Fontan pathway includes complex *biventricular AV connections carrying high surgical risks* during a biventricular repair. They include various forms of heterotaxy syndromes that are associated with anomalies of systemic and pulmonary veins, AV connections, varying hypoplasia of one of the ventricles, and anomalies of the outflow tracts.

The other lesions in this category include patients with:

1. Atrioventricular septal defects in association with tetralogy of Fallot that carries risk of right ventricular failure and AV valve regurgitation after extensive surgery.
2. Atrioventricular discordance with VSD and pulmonary stenosis that needs combination of Senning and Rastelli surgery with risks of injury to conduction tissues.
3. Tetralogy of Fallot or transposition of great arteries with hypoplastic ventricles.

4. Large inlet VSD with marked straddling of the AV valves, and other similar complex morphologies.

Even though these lesions individually are amenable for a biventricular connection, such complex repairs of a deformed heart with multiple anomalies carry more mortality in institutions that have low volume of surgeries of similar nature.

PATHOPHYSIOLOGY OF UNIVENTRICULAR HEARTS

Postnatal circulation in normal hearts consists of blood flow in series that passes from the left ventricle through the systemic circulation to return to the right ventricle and finally to pulmonary circulation. The key pathophysiological features in univentricular hearts are highlighted in italics (**Box 2**). All forms of univentricular hearts have some degree of *parallel circulation* and *admixture*, where there is recirculation of venous blood in systemic circulation and oxygenated blood in the pulmonary circulation. This leads to inefficiency of heart and *volume overload* of the ventricles. Unlike low pressures in normal right ventricle in a structurally normal heart, most univentricular forms of hearts described above cause *pressure overload* of ventricles leading to *ventricular hypertrophy* and resultant *diastolic dysfunction* and restricted filling.

BOX 2: Pathophysiological effects in univentricular hearts.

- *Effects on pulmonary circulation*:
  - Minimal or no obstruction to outflow:
    - Overcirculation
    - Pulmonary hypertension
    - Heart failure
  - Severe obstruction and atresia:
    - Severe cyanosis
    - Duct dependency
- *Effects on systemic circulation*:
  - Obstructed aortic outflow:
    - Neonatal shock
    - Duct dependency
    - Suprasystemic ventricular pressures
  - Obstructed arch:
    - Reduced lower body perfusion
    - Systemic hypertension
    - Ventricular hypertrophy
- *Volume overload is caused by*:
  - Parallel circulation and admixture
  - Pulmonary overcirculation
  - AV valve regurgitation
- *Pressure overload* is caused by:
  - Outflow obstruction
  - Aortic arch obstruction
- *Systemic venous hypertension* is caused by:
  - AVV atresia, stenosis, leak
  - Systolic heart failure
  - Diastolic failure
  - Restrictive PFO
- *Pulmonary venous hypertension* is due to:
  - AVV atresia, stenosis, leak
  - Systolic heart failure
  - Diastolic failure
  - Restrictive PFO
  - Anomalous PV drainage
- *Admixture*:
  - Favorable streaming (Ao saturation > PA saturation)
  - Unfavorable streaming (PA saturation > Ao saturation)

(Ao: aorta; AV: atrioventricular; AVV: atrioventricular valve; PA: pulmonary atresia; PFO: patent foramen ovale; PV: pulmonary venous)

Excessive pulmonary blood flow in patients without pulmonary stenosis leads to *heart failure* but negligible hypoxia. If there is significant pulmonary stenosis or atresia, *cyanosis* is profound. Some neonates with pulmonary atresia present with *duct dependency*. If systemic outflow is obstructed, neonates present in *circulatory shock*, dependent on ductal patency to maintain circulation. Noncritical systemic outflow obstruction results in *suprasystemic ventricular pressures*, undue ventricular hypertrophy, and predisposes to *ventricular failure*.

Right AV valve atresia, stenosis, or regurgitation may lead to *systemic venous hypertension*, unless a large atrial septal communication decompresses the atrium. A similar left-sided pathology leads to *pulmonary venous hypertension*. Fetal pulmonary venous hypertension may lead to *lymphangiectasia of lungs* and lead to severe *pulmonary arterial hypertension*. Anomalous pulmonary venous drainage seen in heterotaxy syndromes may also lead to similar effects.

Admixture of blood in majority of these lesions may give a *favorable or unfavorable streaming* of blood in the outflow tracts. When aortic oxygen saturation is higher than that of pulmonary artery, it is called favorable streaming leading to minimal cyanosis. On the contrary, a higher oxygenation in pulmonary artery is called unfavorable streaming and leads to intense cyanosis due to transposition like physiology.

Fetal blood flow patterns in some univentricular hearts predispose to distal obstructions. Tricuspid atresia and transposed great arteries with restrictive VSD lead to subaortic stenosis, which predisposes to *aortic arch obstruction and coarctation*. A similar situation is seen in single ventricle of left ventricular morphology and restrictive bulboventricular foramen or unbalanced AV canal with subaortic stenosis. Another influence of fetal blood flow is seen in hearts with left AV valve stenosis or atresia, which is caused by restricted flows through the foramen ovale. These patients uniformly display thickened muscular atrial septum with very *restrictive or absent interatrial communications*.

CLINICAL FEATURES OF UNIVENTRICULAR HEARTS

Table 1 summarizes the clinical features. Neonatal presentation is seen in very critical forms of univentricular hearts.[2] Severe obstruction or atresia of pulmonary outflow leads to severe cyanosis and duct dependency, manifesting in the first week of life that is refractory to oxygen supplementation and fails hyperoxia-hyperventilation test. They need prostaglandin

TABLE 1: Clinical features of univentricular hearts.

Age	*Pathophysiology*	*Clinical syndrome*	*Symptoms*	*Clinical signs*	*Basic tests*
Newborn	Obstructed pulmonary flows	Duct-dependent hypoxia	Severe cyanosis in 1–7 days	No murmurs, single S2	Oligemic lungs in chest X-ray
	Obstructed systemic blood flows	Shock state; duct-dependent systemic flow	Pale, cold, "sepsis-like" features	Absent pulses, cold extremities	Acidosis on blood gases
	Excessive pulmonary flows	Congestive heart failure	Tachypnea, poor feeds, diaphoresis	Hyperkinetic precordium S3, apical diastolic murmur	Cardiomegaly plethora on chest X-ray
	Aortic arch obstruction	Duct-dependent systemic flow Oliguria, acidosis	Respiratory distress	Weak femoral pulse	Limb blood pressure
Infant and toddler	Excessive pulmonary flows	Congestive heart failure	Tachypnea, poor feeds, diaphoresis	Hyperkinetic precordium S3, apical diastolic murmur	Cardiomegaly plethora on chest X-ray
	Obstructed pulmonary flows	Hypoxic spells	Severe cyanosis	Faint outflow murmur	Oligemic lungs in chest X-ray
	Venous hypertension	Heart failure	Cyanosis, poor feeds	Large liver, distress	Ground-glass lungs in chest X-ray
Older child/adult	Optimal balance in circulation	Compensated heart failure	Fatigue, occult heart failure	Cyanosis, systolic or continuous murmurs	Cardiomegaly

E1 followed by aortopulmonary shunt or ductal stenting. Critical systemic outflow obstruction may lead to shock state with absent pulses, lactic acidosis, hypothermia, and hypoglycemia. Duct-dependent systemic circulation may improve with prostaglandin, inotropes, and permissive hypercapnia. Vigorous hyperventilation with high oxygen causes pulmonary vasodilatation and worsens heart failure and shock in hypoplastic left heart syndrome.

In the absence of pulmonary stenosis, postnatal fall in pulmonary vascular resistance leads to pulmonary overcirculation and heart failure in 2–6 weeks. They have hyperkinetic precordium, systolic outflow murmurs, flow diastolic apical murmurs, and third heart sounds. Presence of AV valve regurgitation or stenosis may worsen features of heart failure. Aortic arch obstruction may be missed if femoral pulses are not compared to arm pulses. A majority of these patients have malposed aorta leading to single aortic component of second sound and palpable aortic pulsations in left upper sternal border.

In the presence of pulmonary stenosis, cyanosis is progressive as duct closes and somatic growth of the child warrants higher oxygenation. Hypercyanotic spells may rarely occur, though not typical as in Fallot's tetralogy. Prominent jugular venous pulsations, cardiomegaly, left upper sternal border pulsations, abnormal right-sided precordial pulsations, and situs anomalies may be present in these patients and differentiate from tetralogy of Fallot.

The natural history is unfavorable in univentricular hearts and survival beyond infancy is limited to an extreme minority (<10%) of these patients. Clinical examination may show features of abnormal situs in heterotaxy, prominent atrial systolic pulsations on jugular veins, cardiomegaly, abnormal left parasternal pulsations, single second sound, outflow murmurs, and flow diastolic murmurs. Pulmonary vascular disease in advanced pulmonary hypertension may lead to severe cyanosis and disappearance of murmurs.

Rare anecdotal adult survivors owe their extended lifespan to a balanced circulation enabled by moderate levels of pulmonary stenosis without causing life-threatening hypoxia. The factors that help in this unusual adult survival include presence of aortopulmonary collaterals, persistent patency of arterial duct, compensatory ventricular hypertrophy, optimal levels of pulmonary stenosis, and combinations of anomalies that mutually nullify the effects of each other. An example of such a combination occurs in a complex heart in heterotaxy syndrome with transposition physiology where aortic saturation is lower than pulmonary circulation that is helped by an associated total anomalous pulmonary venous drainage that acts as a natural atrial switch to save the patient from hypoxia.

INVESTIGATING PATIENTS WITH UNIVENTRICULAR HEARTS

The key role of investigation in patients with univentricular hearts is to:

- Establish diagnosis—the morphological type according to the classification is done by echocardiography

- Identify adequacy of pulmonary blood flows—that can be either antegrade through the pulmonary valve or through other sources such as arterial duct or aortopulmonary collaterals
- Identify adequacy of systemic blood flows—includes flows across the aortic valve and across the aortic isthmus
- Rule out systemic venous congestion—congested inferior caval veins and hepatic veins that show flow reversals
- Rule out pulmonary venous hypertension—poor interatrial septal communications and identification of anomalous pulmonary venous drainage
- Assess ventricular volume overload, ventricular systolic function by objective criteria such as ejection fraction or speckle strain, which is used for longitudinal follow-up of patients with advancing age
- Assess pressure overload, ventricular hypertrophy, and diastolic dysfunction
- Assess AV valve anatomy, function, mechanism of regurgitation to plan surgical repairs
- Identify factors that favor survival such as aortopulmonary collaterals and arterial duct
- Diagnose extracardiac anomalies in heterotaxy and other syndromes.

Most information is obtained from a detailed echocardiography (**Figs. 3 to 5**). Additional information can be obtained from electrocardiogram (situs identification, sick sinus, AV nodal disturbances, pre-excitations, specific pattern identification), peripheral smear of blood (asplenia syndrome), ultrasound abdomen and cranium to identify anomalies and adverse effects, computed tomography for aortopulmonary collaterals and anomalous pulmonary veins, magnetic resonance imaging for ventricular function and volumes, nuclear imaging for spleen, and genetic testing (*see* Chapter 40).

PRINCIPLES OF MANAGEMENT IN UNIVENTRICULAR HEARTS

Initial Management in Newborns and Young Infants

The management of patients depends on their pathophysiology mentioned earlier and is explained in **Figure 6**. The surgical management is carried out in three stages; the first stage is carried out in neonatal period or early infancy.

Pulmonary oligemia due to severe pulmonary stenosis or atresia is managed in neonatal period with prostaglandin E1 to maintain ductal patency followed by stenting of ductus arteriosus or aortopulmonary shunt (**Figs. 7A to C**). The former is increasingly utilized to avoid neonatal surgery and its associated morbidity. Despite improvement of hypoxia, there is volume loading of the univentricular heart after shunts. Contrary to the postshunt management in Fallot's tetralogy where final correction is postponed to 6–12 months of age, children with univentricular heart are planned for second-stage palliation earlier within 3–6 months. Interval morbidity between first and second stage caused by stent or shunt occlusion is avoided by low-dose aspirin therapy. Iron therapy to prevent relative anemia is imperative in these patients.

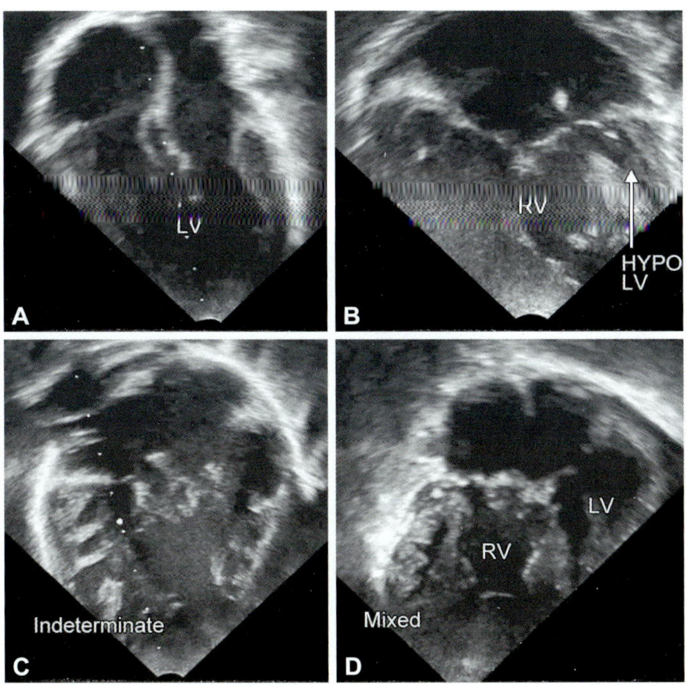

Figs. 3A to D: Echocardiographic view—single ventricle. (A) Left ventricular (LV) morphology; (B) Right ventricular (RV) morphology; (C) Indeterminate morphology; (D) Mixed morphology.

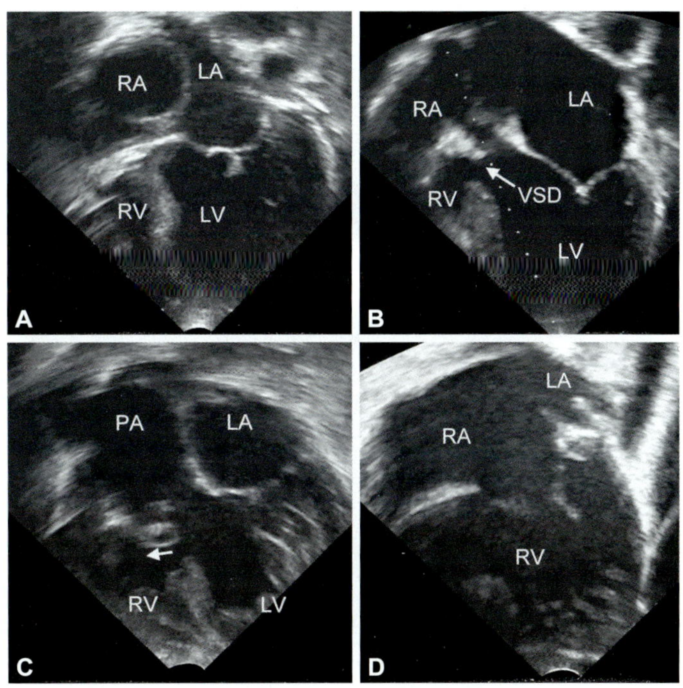

Figs. 4A to D: Echocardiographic view—tricuspid and mitral atresia. (A) Tricuspid atresia Kuhne Ia; (B) Tricuspid atresia Kuhne Ib; (C) Tricuspid atresia Kuhne IIc; (D) Mitral atresia.

(LA: left atrium; LV: left ventricle; PA: pulmonary artery; RA: right atrium; RV; right ventricle; VSD: ventricular septal defect)

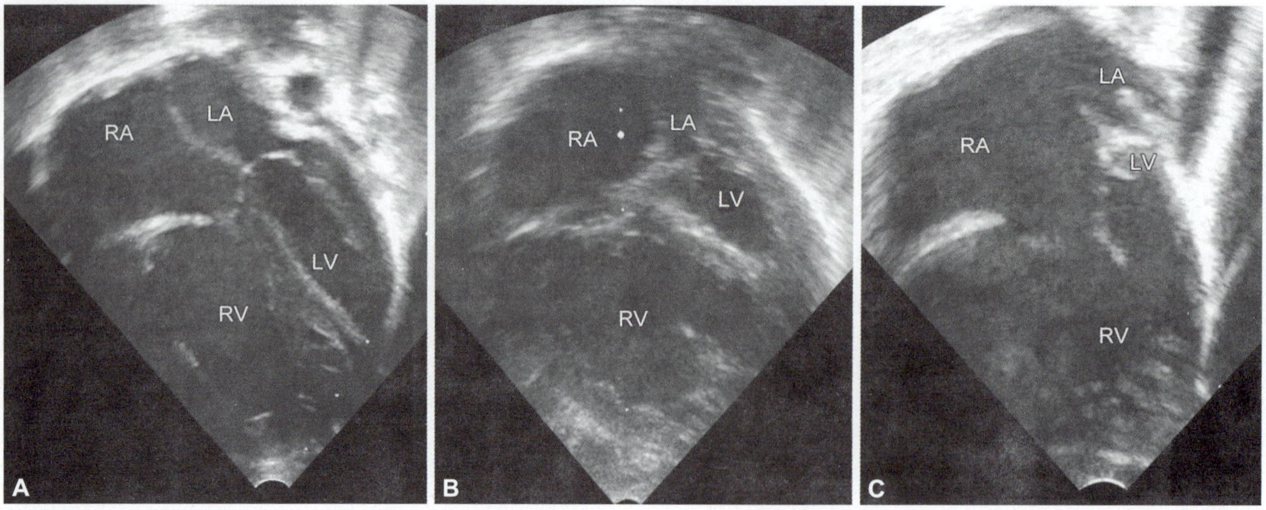

Figs. 5A to C: Echocardiographic view—hypoplastic left heart syndrome. (A) Mild hypoplasia; (B) Severe hypoplasia; (C) Very diminutive left ventricle (LV) with mitral atresia.

(LA: left atrium; LV: left ventricle; RA: right atrium; RV: right ventricle)

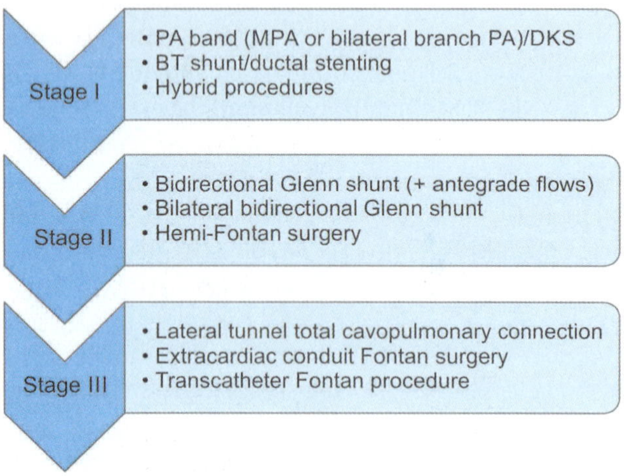

Fig. 6: Management plan in univentricular hearts. The surgical plan comprises an early neonatal first stage, followed by diversion of superior vena caval flows toward the pulmonary circulation in stage II that is performed at 3–12 months and then a final stage at 3–10 years where the inferior vena caval blood is also routed toward the pulmonary circulation.

(BT: Blalock–Taussig; DKS: Damus–Kaye–Stansel; MPA: main pulmonary artery; PA: pulmonary artery)

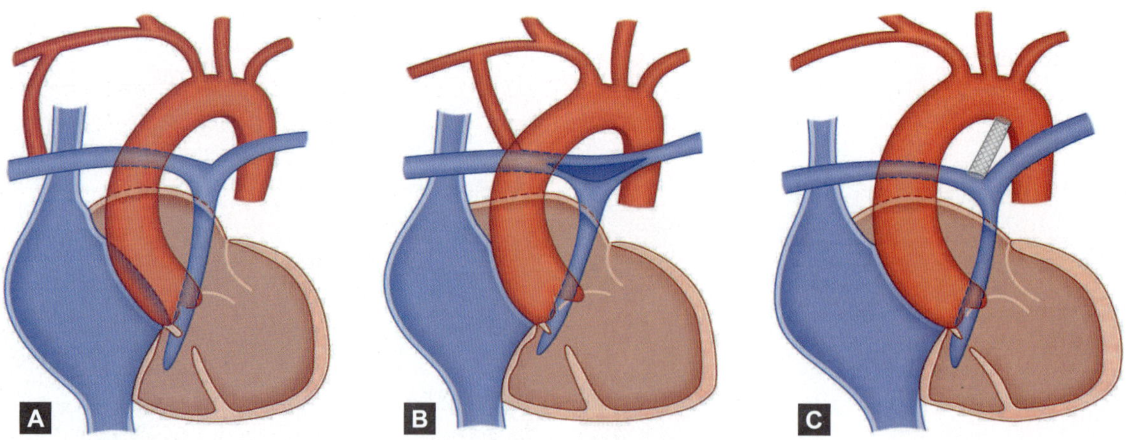

Figs. 7A to C: First stage palliation in oligemic lungs (A); Modified Blalock–Taussig shunt from subclavian artery to ipsilateral pulmonary artery through thoracotomy is largely replaced in recent times by central sternotomy (B); Another method of palliation is transcatheter stenting of the ductus arteriosus (C).

Banding the pulmonary arteries controls excessive pulmonary overflow (**Figs. 8A to C**). Ductal stents and aortopulmonary shunts improve pulmonary oligemia. Pulmonary venous hypertension is relieved by balloon atrial septostomy or surgical atrial septectomy. Heart failure is managed with diuretics. Ventricular systolic dysfunction

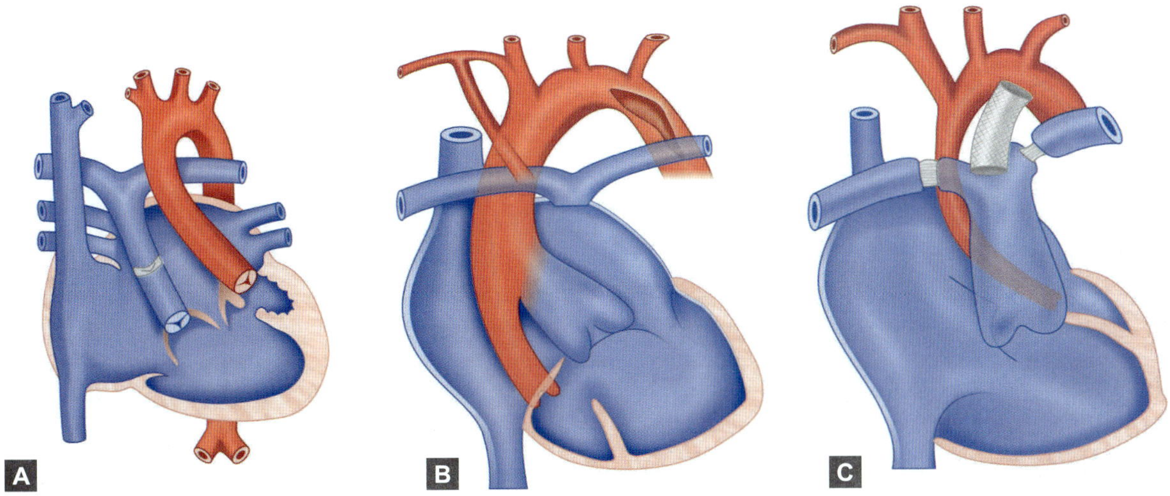

Figs. 8A to C: First-stage palliation in plethoric lungs. (A) Pulmonary artery banding is commonly performed within the first 6–8 weeks to prevent volume overload of the ventricles; (B) Patients at risk of subaortic stenosis or aortic arch obstruction are managed by Damus–Kaye–Stansel procedure where the main pulmonary artery is anastamosed to ascending aorta and pulmonary circulation is maintained through a modified Blalock–Taussig (BT) shunt; (C) A hybrid way of achieving a stage I palliation utilizes ductal stenting, balloon atrial septostomy, and bilateral pulmonary artery banding.

with or without AV valve regurgitation may need after load-reducing agents. Optimizing ventilation by allowing permissive hypercapnia is followed in hypoplastic left heart syndrome to avoid excessive pulmonary vasodilation. Associated hypothermia, sepsis, metabolic acidosis, and hypoglycemia will need routine neonatal intensive care. Antibiotic prophylaxis and special vaccines are warranted in asplenia. Inotropes are used in shock state.

Banding the main pulmonary artery controls pulmonary overcirculation. In patients with associated aortic arch obstruction and pulmonary venous hypertension due to restrictive foramen ovale, neonatal surgery addresses these additional problems too. Certain cardiac morphologies with substrate for subaortic narrowing (tricuspid atresia with transposition and restrictive VSD, unbalanced AV canal defect with subaortic narrowing, and single ventricle with restrictive bulboventricular foramen) may need more extensive surgery. Damus-Kaye-Stansel (DKS) procedure is performed in these patients, where main pulmonary artery is connected end-to-side to ascending aorta and the disconnected distal pulmonary artery is provided blood flow through an aortopulmonary shunt. Some patients with hypoplastic left heart may be palliated in first-stage by hybrid Norwood stage I procedure which comprises of bilateral branch pulmonary artery banding along with ductal stenting and balloon atrial septostomy. Unilateral banding may be needed if there is anomalous aortic origin of a disconnected pulmonary artery.

Stage II Palliation

The second stage comprises of interruption of aortopulmonary shunts, arterial duct, and aortopulmonary collaterals and performing a bidirectional cavopulmonary shunt—end-to-side from superior vena cava to pulmonary artery (**Figs. 9A and B**). This bidirectional Glenn shunt surgery will be

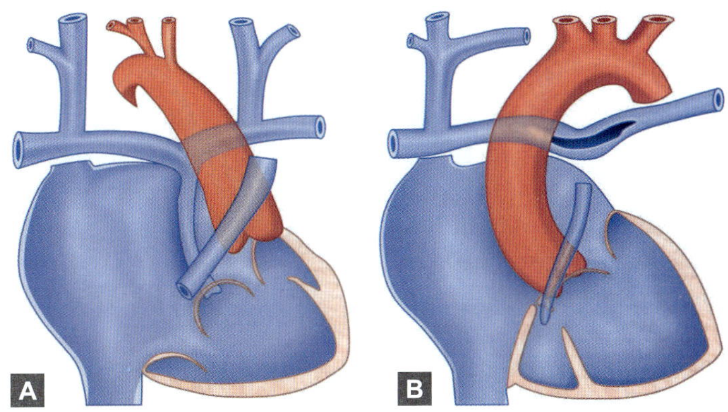

Figs. 9A and B: Second-stage palliation. Connecting the superior vena cava to pulmonary circulation forms the second-stage palliation. Antegrade pulmonary blood flow is either retained or interrupted in this stage (A). The anastomosis is completed bilaterally in patients with dual superior vena cava (B).

performed bilaterally in patients with bilateral superior vena cava and combined with repair of the narrowed confluence at ductal insertion site in patients with stenosis in this area. Unidirectional shunt connecting superior vena cava end-to-end to pulmonary artery is currently not performed. Pulmonary artery is interrupted during this surgery in all patients including those palliated with pulmonary artery banding to reduce pulmonary artery pressures and permit the passive flow. Preservation of antegrade blood flow from the ventricle into the pulmonary artery provides pulsatile blood flow that increases pulmonary artery growth, increases pulmonary arterial capacitance, recruits pulmonary arterioles and reduces pulmonary vascular resistance, delays hypoxia, provides "hepatic factor X" to delay development of arteriovenous malformations and rarely act as a final destination therapy in a few patients. The disadvantages include persistent ventricular volume overload, increased pulmonary artery pressures, lead to superior vena caval and

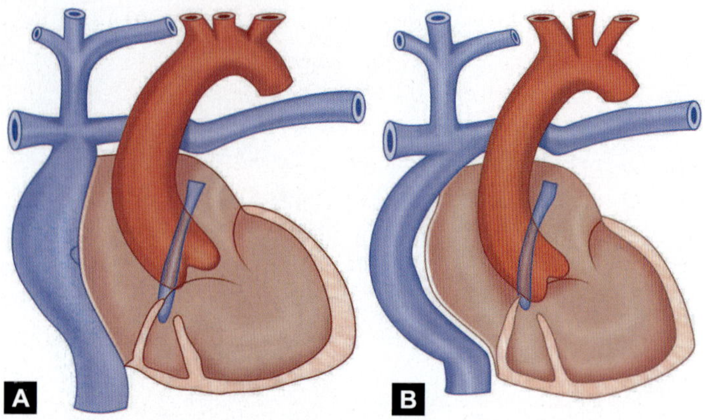

Figs. 10A and B: Final-stage palliation. Connecting the inferior vena cava to the pulmonary circulation is the final-stage palliation for univentricular hearts. The two common and recent forms of achieving this are lateral tunnel Fontan surgery (A) also called as total cavopulmonary connection and extracardiac conduit Fontan surgery (B).

cerebral congestion, increase pleural effusions, and render some patients unsuitable for third stage.

Stage III Palliation

The third stage, Fontan procedure is the final stage in the stepwise palliation of a functionally univentricular heart (**Figs. 10A and B**). Fontan and Baudet introduced this surgery in 1971 as a solution for tricuspid atresia by diverting systemic venous flows passively without an intervening ventricular pump directly into the pulmonary artery. The fundamental requisite for this passive flow is the low resistance pulmonary vascular bed that allows the pressure gradient between the two vascular bed (higher pressures in systemic vasculature and lower pressures in pulmonary vasculature) to allow flow through the lungs without an intervening ventricular pump. Apart from this pressure gradient that maintains this passive flow, the additional contributors are chest wall (diaphragmatic and thoracic cage) excursions, and peripheral skeletal muscles in the body that aid in systemic venous return toward the thorax. The resultant circulation places pulmonary and systemic vasculature in series with functional single ventricle as the only pump. This palliation is largely criticized as it only aims at oxygenating the systemic venous blood without providing a pulmonary circulatory pump.

ALTERED CIRCULATION AFTER FONTAN SURGERY

The new circulation after Fontan surgery is inherently characterized by decreased preload and increased afterload to the single ventricle, which prevents significant increase of cardiac output leaving these patients with little hemodynamic reserve. They become more dependent of their heart rate and AV nodal conduction for augmenting the cardiac output unlike normal biventricular hearts that utilize additional stroke volume and contractility reserves. The patients with Fontan circulation are additionally more dependent on respiration and skeletal muscles to augment venous return and cardiac output. Older types of Fontan surgery involved atriopulmonary anastomosis resulting in atrial enlargement, arrhythmias, thrombus formation, and poor mechanics. Recent modifications include lateral tunnel Fontan surgery and extracardiac conduit Fontan surgery with or without a fenestration to act as a pop-off for the systemic veins into the atrium. Survival is better with recent modifications of Fontan and systemic left ventricle.

HOW TO CARE FOR PATIENTS AFTER GLENN AND FONTAN SURGERIES

Univentricular hearts in developed economies are managed by stage I palliation in their early neonatal period to prevent significant hypoxia-related brain injury in oligemic patients and development of pulmonary arterial hypertension in patients with excessive pulmonary blood flow. The volume overload of ventricles is prevented in these patients by performance of stage II palliation within 3–6 months, when the pulmonary arteries and pulmonary vascular bed is relatively small due to the small weight of the patients at that age. The final palliation is completed between 2 and 4 years again to minimize the effects of continuing hypoxia that is not eliminated by the Glenn shunt.

The entire timeframe is shifted to later age in low-middle income countries. While stage I is performed in late neonatal or early infancy, Glenn shunt is done at 6–12 months and Fontan completion is performed at 4–10 years of age. The reasons behind this deferred treatment are to allow the caregivers to sort out the other associated neonatal morbidities such as sepsis, syndromic evaluations, detailed family counselling, and to overcome the challenges posed by a low bodyweight neonate in the pediatric cardiac intensive care unit. Additionally, economic constraints also contribute. A similar late age at second and third stages allows surgery on relatively larger sized pulmonary arteries and well-developed pulmonary vascular bed.

The fundamental differences between the early interventions followed in developed countries (focusing on preservation of ventricular function at the cost of challenging the small pulmonary vasculature to a passive venous flow) and later interventions in low-middle-income countries (focusing on surgery on a well-developed pulmonary vascular bed and allowing a permissive strategy on ventricular overload and hypertrophy) have found equal merits and demerits in their approaches. A passive cavopulmonary flow after second stage needs both a good functioning ventricle to pump the blood through both circulations and a good well-developed pulmonary vascular bed.

Role of pediatrician after first-stage correction comprises of aspirin to maintain patency of the shunt, guarded use of diuretics and afterload reducing agents after banding, vaccines and antibiotics for intercurrent infections, close monitoring of saturations, and growth to prevent inter-stage mortality and patient counselling. Following second stage, aspirin prevents thrombosis in passive venous flows, iron prevents relative anemia, respiratory physiotherapy and breathing exercises maintain healthy ventilatory mechanics, guarded use of diuretics and pulmonary or systemic vasodilators in appropriate situations. As there is a high incidence of thrombus formation in the first year after the third-stage Fontan surgery, it is common practice to give oral anticoagulation with warfarin monitored by prothrombin time evaluations and appropriate dietary restrictions of vitamin K-rich foods. Promotion of respiratory and skeletal muscle strength by regular monitored exercises, breathing exercises, yoga, avoidance of air pollution, healthy lifestyle avoiding active, and passive smoking will play a role in longevity of patients after third stage.

Drug therapy after Fontan surgery may include diuretics in patients with high venous pressures and effusions, pulmonary vasodilators such as sildenafil or bosentan in patients with evidence of high pulmonary vascular resistance, angiotensin-converting enzyme inhibitors in patients with significant AV valve regurgitations or ventricular systolic dysfunction, antiarrhythmic agents such as amiodarone for automatic or reentrant arrhythmias, beta-blockers to control ventricular rate in supraventricular arrhythmias and antibiotic prophylaxis in asplenia syndrome.

PROBLEMS ON LONG-TERM FOLLOW-UP AFTER THE FONTAN OPERATION

Post-Fontan patients may present with heart failure under four clinical groups: (1) systolic dysfunction, (2) diastolic dysfunction, (3) normal pressures, and (4) abnormal lymphatics. Arrhythmias occur in 13–16% of patients and increase with time after surgery. They can result from sick sinus syndrome, suture lines, atrial fibrillation, and progressive atrial dilatation. Some of these arrhythmias may need electrophysiological studies but results may be suboptimal and procedure may be challenging due to lack of access from venous lines. Despite 80% acute success after radiofrequency ablations, recurrences occur in 30–45% after 1 year (**Table 2**).

Liver fibrosis results from chronicity of venous congestion (less related to severity of venous congestion).[3] Hepatocellular carcinoma occurs in 1.3% of Fontan survivors. Protein-losing enteropathy is due to hypoperfusion leading to inflammation and venous congestion. The loss of mucosal integrity of gastrointestinal epithelium leaking immunoglobulins and clotting factors in the lumen. It is common in children, usually 3–8 years after surgery and occurs in 10% of Fontan patients. The treatment includes albumin infusions, enteral budesonide, heparin, diuretics, spironolactone, sildenafil, digoxin, rapid atrial pacing, and lymphatic interventions.[4,5]

Lymphatic insufficiency is caused by increased production and reduced drainage. In early days after surgery, it manifests as chylothorax and chylous ascites. After 1–2 years, they manifest with plastic bronchitis, where endobronchial leak of proteinaceous material leads to formation of viscid bronchial casts that lead to asphyxia. Thromboembolic events occur in one-third of Fontan patients. They occur due to nonpulsatile flow, venous congestion, low cardiac output, dilated atrium, arrhythmia, and protein-losing enteropathy. Asymptomatic pulmonary emboli, pulmonary infarctions, and slow elevation of pulmonary vascular resistance occur in patients with thromboembolism on pulmonary vasculature.[6,7] In patients with fenestrations and atrial arrhythmias, thromboembolism affects systemic vasculature too.

Renal dysfunction arises due to poor perfusion and venous congestion. In contrast to renal failure in usual clinical practice that is identified by elevation of creatinine levels, alternative markers such as cystatin C levels can better identify Fontan patients, who have low creatinine production. Cyanosis after Fontan surgery may result from fenestration, baffle leaks, pulmonary vein compression, venous collaterals, and pulmonary arteriovenous malformations. Pulmonary function tests show impaired exercise capacity, low vital capacity, high residual volume, skeletal muscle dysfunction, and poor performance on cardiopulmonary exercise testing. These abnormalities affect passive cavopulmonary flows and worsen Fontan failure. General health perception and psychological health are also affected due to the various somatic abnormalities.

Conception is not a common occurrence due to poor maternal health as fertility and ovulation are impaired. Early abortions and teratogenicity of various medications also contribute to fetal losses. Multidisciplinary team approach is needed in managing a pregnancy in these patients. Arrhythmias, thromboembolism, and heart failure are more common during pregnancy. Noncardiac perioperative care also needs vigilance. Anesthetics, hypoxia, atelectasis, thromboembolism, pneumonia, volume loss, and excess fluids may destabilize the precarious hemodynamics in a patient after Fontan surgery.

CURRENT STATUS OF FONTAN SURVIVAL

Perioperative mortality after Fontan surgery in carefully selected patients has reduced to 1% in current era. 10-year survival after Fontan surgery has improved to 97% with the current methods using lateral tunnels or extracardiac conduits. In best centers, current survival at 25 years is 76%, but these patients have older atriopulmonary Fontan circulations. Survival of patients operated in the last two decades is far better compared to older reports.

A number of factors have been shown to be associated with reduced survival after Fontan surgery. They include male gender, specific diagnostic categories such as hypoplastic

TABLE 2: Problems after Fontan surgery.

No.	Hemodynamic problem	Investigation	Management	Prognosis
1.	Heart failure from systolic or diastolic dysfunction	Echocardiogram Magnetic resonance	Diuretics ACEI AT blocker	May worsen despite therapy
2.	Arrhythmias – atrial reentrant or automatic	ECG Holter electrophysiological study	Antiarrhythmics RF cryoablation	Success in 80% but recurs
3.	Pleural effusions, chylothorax, and ascites	Fluid analysis, ultrasound, CXR	Diuretics, octreotide, TPN	subsides on therapy
4.	Liver fibrosis, cirrhosis, adenoma, and carcinoma	Elastography ultrasound, MRI	Diuretics, avoid hepatotoxic drugs	Slow progress in liver disease
5.	Protein losing enteropathy with hypocalcemia	Fecal alpha-1 antitrypsin, and albumin	Budesonide Heparin	Guarded prognosis
6.	Plastic bronchitis with asphyxia	Bronchoscopy, sputum examination	tPA inhalation, physiotherapy, lymphatic interventions	Often fatal outcome
7.	Lymphatic occlusions	Magnetic resonance lymphangiography	Lymphatic interventions	Guarded prognosis
8.	Pulmonary thromboembolism	CT lungs, CXR, pulmonary angiography	Heparin, oral anticoagulation	Early treatment is beneficial
9.	Systemic thromboembolism	Vascular Doppler, CT angiography	Heparin, oral anticoagulation	Early treatment is beneficial
10.	Renal dysfunction	Cystatin C, urea, creatinine	Optimize hemodynamics	Avoid nephrotoxic drugs
11.	Cyanosis due to baffle leaks and fenestrations	Contrast echocardiogram	Fenestration closure	Appropriate treatment feasible
12.	Pulmonary function abnormalities	Spirometry cardio-pulmonary exercise test	Physiotherapy, breathing exercise	Active treatment helps
13.	General health abnormalities	Quality of life index	Multidisciplinary team work	Support groups will help
14.	Psychological health due to repeated clinic visits	Psychometric assessment	Active counseling	Support groups will help
15.	Fertility and pregnancy related issues	Ultrasound and hormonal assays	Multidisciplinary approach	Counseling and adoption service
16.	Noncardiac surgical morbidity	Anesthetic risk assessment	Prevent hypoxia, lung complication	Usually manageable

(ACEI: angiotensin-converting-enzyme inhibitors; AT: angiotensin; CT: computed tomography; CXR: chest X-ray; ECG: electrocardiography; MRI: magnetic resonance imaging; RF: radiofrequency; tPA: tissue plasminogen activator; TPN: total parenteral nutrition)

left heart syndrome, older type of Fontan procedure, earlier surgical era, older age at procedure, and concomitant valve replacement. Prolonged pleural effusions, elevated venous pressures, lower oxygen saturation, low ventricular systolic function by echocardiography, larger end-diastolic volumes on magnetic resonance also correlate with poor survival. Additionally, low peak heart rate and oxygen uptake on exercise cardiopulmonary testing, low serum sodium, high pro-brain natriuretic peptide level, arrhythmias, presence of complications such as protein-losing enteropathy or plastic bronchitis, and multisystem problems also correlate with poor survival.

Catheter interventions that may be needed in patients following Fontan surgery include stent angioplasty of stenosed or occluded conduits, dilatation and stenting of anastomosis, recanalization and stent angioplasty of branch pulmonary arteries, aortic coarctation dilatation and stenting, lymphatic interventions, closure or creation of fenestrations, device closure of persistent antegrade flows from ventricles, closure of venovenous and aortopulmonary collaterals, electrophysiological studies, and radiofrequency ablation of arrhythmias.[8,9]

Fontan surgery offers hope to a large number of patients with a single functional ventricle and provides a long-term palliation extending to third or fourth decades. Despite the myriad of problems involving multiple organs, many patients maintain adequate quality of life, thanks to the multiple medical and interventional therapies performed in these survivors.

CONCLUSION

This chapter has looked to provide an overview on a diverse set of conditions that are unified by the fact that they can be managed through a staged palliative strategy that typically culminates in the Fontan operation. Essential concepts required in understanding their physiology and management have been presented here. With improvements in access to comprehensive pediatric heart care, it can be expected that an increasing number of patients will be offered palliative operations for univentricular hearts and there is a need for caregivers to be familiar with the concepts presented here.

REFERENCES

1. Khairy P, Fernandes SM, Mayer JE Jr, Triedman JK, Walsh EP, Lock JE, et al. Long-term survival, modes of death, and predictors of mortality in patients with Fontan surgery. Circulation. 2008;117(1):85-92.
2. Gatzoulis MA, Munk MD, Williams WG, Webb GD. Definitive palliation with cavopulmonary or aortopulmonary shunts for adults with single ventricle physiology. Heart. 2000;83(1):51-7.
3. Kiesewetter CH, Sheron N, Vettukattill JJ, Hacking N, Stedman B, Sadler HM, et al. Hepatic changes in the failing Fontan circulation. Heart. 2007;93(5):579-84.
4. Hebson CL, McCabe NM, Elder RW, Mahle WT, McConnell M, Kogon BE, et al. Hemodynamic phenotype of the failing Fontan in an adult population. Am J Cardiol. 2013;112(12):1943-7.
5. Hebert A, Mikkelsen UR, Thilen U, Idorn L, Jensen AS, Nagy E, et al. Bosentan improves exercise capacity in adolescents and adults after Fontan operation: the TEMPO (Treatment With Endothelin Receptor Antagonist in Fontan Patients, a Randomized, Placebo-Controlled, Double-Blind Study Measuring Peak Oxygen Consumption) study. Circulation. 2014;130(23):2021-30.
6. Giardini A, Balducci A, Specchia S, Gargiulo G, Bonvicini M, Picchio FM. Effect of sildenafil on haemodynamic response to exercise and exercise capacity in Fontan patients. Eur Heart J. 2008;29(13):1681-7.
7. Potter BJ, Leong-Sit P, Fernandes SM, Feifer A, Mayer Jr JE, Triedman JK, et al. Effect of aspirin and warfarin therapy on thromboembolic events in patients with univentricular hearts and Fontan palliation. Int J Cardiol. 2013; 168(4):3940-3.
8. John AS, Johnson JA, Khan M, Driscoll DJ, Warnes CA, Cetta F. Clinical outcomes and improved survival in patients with protein-losing enteropathy after the Fontan operation. J Am Coll Cardiol. 2014;64(1):54-62.
9. Sivakumar K. Physiology of Fontan operation; complication and management. In: Cardiology Update 2019 Textbook. Kanti M (Ed). New Delhi: Das Evangel Publication; 2019. pp 753-66.

40 CHAPTER

Isomerism (Aka Heterotaxy): What Does it Mean and What Does it Do?

Rohit S Loomba, Diane E Spicer, Robert Anderson

INTRODUCTION

Isomerism, also referred as heterotaxy, is a unique clinical entity that is characterized by disruption of normal left-right patterning in the body such that there is symmetry of structures bilaterally that are normally asymmetric.[1,2] For instance, in the setting of left isomerism, both the left- and right-sided lungs have two lobes, this being the morphologic feature of the left lung. Such anatomic abnormalities can be noted throughout the body, and may also be accompanied by organ dysfunction. While all organ systems can be affected, there is variability in the number of systems affected in each patient, and the degree to which the system is affected.[3] The isomeric features, furthermore, are confined to the heart and the lungs, with the abdominal organs tending to be "jumbled up."

Isomerism affects 1 in 10,000 live births, and is associated with increased morbidity and mortality.[4-7] Early clinical recognition can help guide evaluation for associated abnormalities, and allow for early intervention. We review here the clinical features, proposed mechanisms, and implications of isomerism. We start with details regarding isomerism, and then in the final section synthesize the data to provide the primary care provider with a template by which to evaluate and manage these patients.

TERMINOLOGY

The significance of isomerism was first emphasized by Ivemark in the 1950s, who pointed to "implications of agenesis of the spleen on the pathogenesis of conotruncus anomalies in childhood".[8] With subsequent identification of increasing numbers of cases, similar congenital cardiac malformations were identified in children who had multiple spleens. It then became customary to group the patients as demonstrating heterotaxy, with the overall group segregated further into those having asplenia as opposed to polysplenia.[9,10] This permitted recognition of the constellations of recurrent cardiac and noncardiac findings associated with either asplenia or polysplenia. The term heterotaxy, meaning a departure from the normal, continued to be used, although patients were recognized as fitting into one or other of the groups despite having a solitary spleen.

As advancements in medicine allowed for more sophisticated genetic studies to be performed, it was soon found that the findings of so-called "heterotaxy" could be reproduced by knocking out the genes responsible for laterality. Studies of the resulting knock-out mice led to the appreciation that, in these settings, the atrial appendages lost their asymmetry, becoming morphologically identical on both sides, in other words isomeric. It was then found, with time, that the other associated findings statistically clustered better, when the findings were segregated into the subsets of right as opposed to left isomerism, rather than in terms of asplenia or polysplenia.[11,12]

With these findings being based on the true morphology and genetic underpinning of the clinical entity, it is now appreciated that isomerism is, indeed, the more appropriate term. Necroscopy findings also demonstrate that findings tend to cluster better when classified as either being consistent with left or right isomerism.[1,13,14] This means that treatment of patients is better determined according to the presence of left or right isomerism, rather than the state of the spleen. This is not to ignore that significance of splenic structure, so it is important to appreciate that, in most patients, asplenia correlates with right isomerism while polysplenia correlates with left isomerism. For the remainder of this section, nonetheless, we will base our descriptions on the isomeric features.

Those who still have to be convinced of the value of this approach often cite the difficulties that currently exist in being able to image with accuracy the morphology of the atrial appendages. As some of the specific findings segregate very well between the two subsets, features more easily imaged can be used to classify the syndrome into the left or right isomeric subsets. Additionally, as computed tomography (CT) and magnetic resonance imaging (MRI) are improving rapidly, the atrial appendages can now be better evaluated by imaging.[15,16] With experience, it should also prove feasible to distinguish the appendages echocardiographically.

CARDIOVASCULAR SYSTEM (TABLE 1)

Atrial Appendages

The atrial appendages are morphologically distinct. They represent anatomic structures that are present bilaterally, but which are not usually symmetric. In the normal situation, the right atrial appendage is pyramidal in shape, has a broad junction with the venous component, and has pectinate muscles that encircle the entirety of the atrioventricular junction. The left atrial appendage, in contrast, is usually finger-like, has a narrow junction with the venous component, and has pectinate muscles that are confined with-in the appendage, the atrial vestibule being confluent with the smooth-walled atrial body.

The atrial appendages lose their asymmetry in the setting of isomerism. In those with left isomerism, both atrial appendages are finger-like, with smooth-walled atrial chambers inferiorly (**Fig. 1**). In those with right isomerism, both atrial appendages are pyramidal, with the pectinate muscles encircling the atrioventricular junctions to meet at the crux[3,16,17] (**Fig. 2**). Necroscopic evaluation of explanted hearts demonstrates that hemodynamic aberrations, and surgery, can alter the shape of the atrial appendage but not the extent of the pectinate muscles.[13] Thus, it is the extent of the pectinate muscles that is the final arbiter of recognition. Necroscopy, however, is obviously of no help when evaluating patients clinically. Imaging of the atrial appendages is often exceedingly difficult by transthoracic echocardiography, although this may be done in the fetus. Other imaging modalities perform better at this task. CT and MRI can now provide resolution ample enough to demonstrate the pectinate muscles and their extent.[16] As protocols for both modalities are improving, patients with complex congenital malformations of the heart are increasingly getting scanned with CT or MRI.

Systemic Veins

Systemic venous anomalies are the rule in the setting of isomerism, even if the venous drainage itself seems to be usual or mirror-imaged. Patients may have either a right- or left-sided superior caval vein, often with both being present. A right-sided superior caval vein is present in slightly over four-fifths of patients with isomerism, irrespective of the subtype as there is no difference between those with right or left isomerism. A left-sided superior caval vein is present in approximately two-thirds, once again with no difference between the subtypes. What does differ between the subsets, however, is the drainage of the left-sided superior caval vein if it is present. A coronary sinus is only present in the setting of left isomerism. Hence, a left-sided superior caval vein can only drain to the coronary sinus in the setting of left isomerism. The left-sided superior caval vein draining to the roof of the left-sided, morphologically right atrium, therefore, is more frequently noted in those with right isomerism.[13]

The inferior caval vein is also usually anomalous. In approximately four-fifths of those with left isomerism, its hepatic segment is interrupted, and venous drainage is

TABLE 1: Summary of cardiovascular system involvement in isomerism.

Affected structure	*Right isomerism*	*Left isomerism*	*Clinical implications*
Superior vena cava (SVC)	Bilateral SVC; left SVC draining directly to atrium with absent coronary sinus	Bilateral SVC may be present; left SVC generally drains to coronary sinus	Both SVCs will need to be anastomosed to the pulmonary artery during the Glenn shunt
Inferior vena cava (IVC)	Usually intact	Interrupted with azygous continuation in 80%	Interrupted IVC can make catheterization challenging; the Glenn shunt would divert IVC blood to the pulmonary arteries and therefore cannot be performed at an early age
Hepatic veins	Hepatic veins may not drain via the IVC and may drain to atria directly		Important during the final Fontan operations when all hepatic veins need to be included in the Fontan pathway
Pulmonary veins	Total anomalous drainage via an extracardiac pathway to SVC or portal vein is common	Drain anomalously to both the atria	Will need to be addressed during surgery. If obstructed, this will need to be addressed early; If not at the time of Glenn shunt
Atria	About a third have common atrium		No specific implications for single ventricle palliation; will need to be septated if two-ventricle repair is contemplated
Atrioventricular (AV) junction	Single AV valve orifice in majority (75%)	Two AV valve orifices in the majority (60%)	May complicate two-ventricle repair; valve regurgitation may develop or progress and can be an important consideration in single ventricle palliation
Ventriculoarterial connections	Pulmonary atresia common	Obstructions to either outflow tracts described; pulmonary atresia uncommon	Complicates palliative or corrective surgery Pulmonary atresia necessitates prostaglandin followed by neonatal intervention
Conduction system	Dual AV node and supraventricular tachycardia is common	Bradyarrhythmias, junctional rhythm, complete heart block commoner	Yearly Holter; special precautions in early postoperative period Potential need for pacemaker

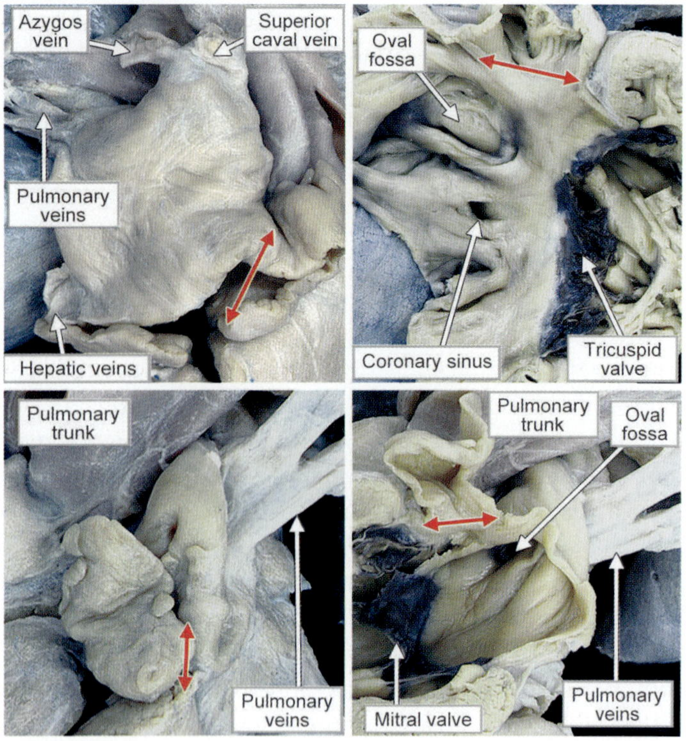

Fig. 1: In the left upper panel, there is a right-sided, morphologically left atrium and in the left lower panel, a left-sided morphologically left atrium, both with finger-like appendages that have a narrow junction (red arrows) with the venous component of the atrium. Note the large azygos vein in the left upper panel branching from the superior caval vein, this patient with interruption of the hepatic portion of the inferior caval vein and azygos continuation. The hepatic veins drain directly into the right-sided atrium. The right upper and lower panels demonstrate the internal anatomy of the atriums and atrial appendages in this heart with concordant atrioventricular and ventriculoarterial connections. Both atrial appendages have a narrow junction (red arrows) with the venous component and the pectinate muscles are confined to the appendage. The remainder of the atrial vestibule is smooth walled. In the right upper panel, note the well-formed coronary sinus. In this specimen, the pulmonary veins drain to the right-sided, morphologically left atrium and the atrial septum is intact.

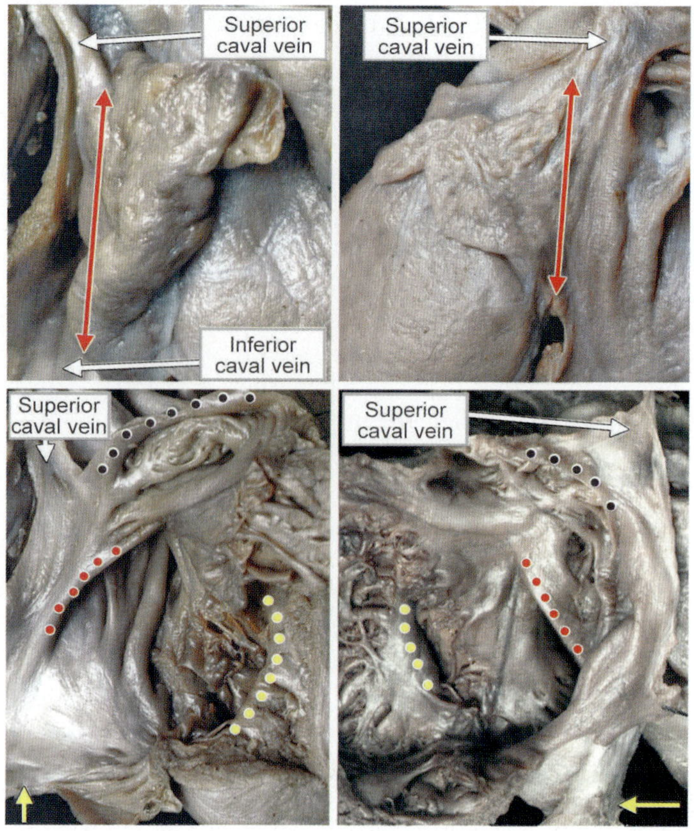

Fig. 2: The upper panels show the right-sided (left panel) and the left-sided (right panel) morphologically right atrial appendages. Both have a superior caval vein entering the roof of the atrium with an inferior caval vein joining the floor of the right-sided atrium in the left upper panel. The appendages have a pyramidal tip and a broad attachment (double-headed red arrows) with the venous component. The lower panels show the opened atrioventricular junctions of the right and left sides of the heart. There is an unbalanced atrioventricular septal defect that is left dominant, the red dots marking the leading edge of the atrial septum and the red dots the crest of the ventricular septum. The inferior caval vein opens to the right-sided atrium in the left lower panel and is marked with a yellow arrow in both panels. Note the prominent terminal crest (black dots) extending from the cavoatrial junction in both atriums and the pectinate muscles extending from this prominent muscle and around the atrioventricular junctions.

via the azygos or hemiazygos venous system (**Fig. 1**). The abdominal segment of the azygos venous system then enlarges along its length, and drains into the superior caval vein. This is important surgically, as construction of a Glenn procedure in this setting results in increased venous return going directly to the pulmonary arteries. If the inferior caval vein is intact in the setting of left isomerism, then it most frequently connects to the right-sided atrium, although in approximately 5% of patients with left isomerism, it may empty into the left-sided atrium.[13]

The inferior caval vein is almost always intact in the setting of right isomerism, connecting to the right-sided atrium in two-thirds, and to the left-sided atrium in the remainder, although in a small proportion, two inferior caval veins may be present[13] (**Fig. 2**).

Hepatic venous connections are also anomalous in the setting of isomerism. In the setting of left isomerism, the hepatic veins connect via a venous confluence to one or other atrium in a majority (~70%) of patients. In 15% of those with left isomerism, the hepatic veins connect to the right-sided atrium, while in 7%, the hepatic veins connect into the left-sided atrium, the remainder having bilateral hepatic venous drainage[13] (*see* **Fig. 1**).

In those with right isomerism, the hepatic veins connect to the inferior caval vein in two-thirds of patients, and then the right-sided atrium in approximately one-quarter of patients. The remainder have connection to the left-sided atrium or to both atriums.[13]

Pulmonary Veins

Pulmonary venous connections are also anomalous in both left and right isomerism. In the setting of left isomerism, the pulmonary veins nearly always connect to the atriums: pulmonary veins returning to the right-sided atrium (~40%), both atriums (~35%), and left-sided atrium (~25%) (*see* **Fig. 1**). This differs from those with right isomerism, in which three-fifths of patients have pulmonary veins connecting in an extracardiac fashion. In ~35% of those with right isomerism, the pulmonary veins will connect in a supracardiac fashion, ~25% will connect in an infradiaphragmatic fashion, and ~5% will connect in a mixed fashion. The remainder will have pulmonary venous connections to the atriums themselves, albeit in anatomically abnormal fashion.[13]

Atriums

Previously the entity known as isomerism was referred to as atrial isomerism. It is now acknowledged that the atriums themselves are not isomeric, merely their appendages. In most patients (~two-thirds), there is an interatrial communication. A common atrium is also seen in equal proportion (~36%) of those with left and right isomerism.[13]

Atrioventricular Junction

The atrioventricular connections in the setting of isomerism should be described as being biventricular and mixed, being sure to describe any abnormal ventricular relationships along with ventricular topology. Those hearts with left isomerism more often have biventricular and mixed connections, while univentricular atrioventricular connections are more common with right isomerism. While over half of those with isomerism have a common atrioventricular junction, this is more frequent in those with right isomerism (79% vs. 65%) (*see* **Figs. 1 and 2**). Two separate atrioventricular orifices, whether in the setting of a common atrioventricular junction or not, are most frequently seen in those with left isomerism (60% vs. 17%). In those with a common atrioventricular junction, there may be two separate orifices which are created by the presence of a tongue of tissue that connects the bridging leaflets.[13]

The atrioventricular connection itself is most often mixed (91% in left isomerism vs. 82% in right isomerism). The remainder in each group have either double inlet to a morphologically left or right ventricle or a solitary, indeterminate ventricle. Double-inlet left ventricle is almost exclusively seen in the setting of right isomerism.[13] Absence of an atrioventricular connection, whether right- or left-sided, is rare.

Ventriculoarterial Connections

The ventriculoarterial connections do differ in those with left versus right isomerism. Several additional variables must be described, including the type and mode of connection, arterial relationships, and infundibular morphology. In those with left isomerism, the ventriculoarterial connections are most often (~60%) concordant (*see* **Fig. 1**). In one-third of patients, there is a double-outlet from the morphologically right ventricle, with discordant connections present in one-tenth of patients. Aortic coarctation or atresia is more common in those patients with left isomerism. Double outlet from a solitary, indeterminate ventricle and single outlet from a solitary, indeterminate ventricle are seen in <1% of patients with left isomerism. Pulmonary atresia is more frequently noted in right isomerism (45% vs. 9%). In right isomerism, discordant ventriculoarterial connections are most common, present in slightly over half of patients. One-third of patients with right isomerism will have double outlet from a morphologically right ventricle. Approximately 5% of patients with right isomerism will have double or single outlet from a solitary, indeterminate ventricle. The remainder have concordant ventriculoarterial connections.[13]

The relationship of the aorta to the pulmonary artery also differs between those with left and right isomerism. In the setting of left isomerism, the most common relationship, which is noted in two-fifths, is a posterior, rightward aorta with usual spiraling of the great vessels. This is in contrast to those with right isomerism, in which the most common relationship, which is noted in one-third of patients, is an anterior and rightward aorta. Usual spiraling of the great vessels, nonetheless, is noted in a very small proportion of patients with right isomerism.[13]

Ventricular Topology

In those with both left and right isomerism, the ventricular topology is most frequently right-handed. Single indeterminate ventricles are mostly only seen in the setting of right isomerism.[13]

Aorta

In both left and right isomerism, the aortic arch is generally left-sided, although a right-sided aortic arch is noted in 25% of those with left isomerism and 37% of those with right isomerism. Interruption of the aortic arch is seen in small (~2%) but equal proportion of patients with left and right isomerism. Coarctation of the aorta is also noted in a similar proportion (~12%) of patients with left and right isomerism.[13]

Coronary Arteries

The coronary arteries have an abnormal branching pattern in two-thirds of patients with either left or right isomerism. In an equal proportion of those with left or right isomerism (one-third), there is a single coronary artery present.[13]

Conduction System

The conduction system is often abnormal in the setting of isomerism. Surface electrocardiogram analysis demonstrates a right-sided focus for atrial depolarization in half of both of those with left or right isomerism. Approximately a quarter in each subset have a left-sided focus, while the remaining quarter have multiple focuses of atrial depolarization.[18]

In respect to the atrioventricular node, a solitary posteriorly located node is noted in ~90% of those with left isomerism, compared to ~20% of patients with right isomerism. Twin atrioventricular nodes are often present (~80%) in those with right isomerism. Twin atrioventricular nodes are noted in ~15% of those with left isomerism.[18]

Arrhythmias are noted in both subsets of isomerism, with atrioventricular block being the most common arrhythmia in those with left isomerism and supraventricular tachycardia being the most common arrhythmia in those with right isomerism. Age of onset of arrhythmia is similar in both subsets, usually occurring between 3 and 4 years of age. Ablations can be successful in both subsets of patients, although the complex venous anatomy in these patients can make ablations technically difficult. Permanent pacemaker implantation is needed in ~10%, with no difference of need for pacemaker implantation between those with left and right isomerism.[19-21]

Junctional rhythms may be present in those with left isomerism with relatively low heart rates. This can present a challenging clinical dilemma as rates can be relatively low for age, but the cardiac output can be maintained. These patients need to be monitored closely with time for possible clinical symptoms associated with the junctional bradycardia and the need for pacemaker implantation needs to be regularly addressed. While it may be tempting in some patients to leave permanent pacemaker leads without pacemaker generator implantation, potential risks of this approach must be kept in mind. Magnetic resonance imaging, which may be helpful in the future, may not be feasible as there is a theoretic risk of burns secondary to pacemaker lead heating in the magnetic resonance field. While this is mostly based on ex-vivo studies, the presence of pacemaker leads without a pacemaker generator (so-called "jailed" leads) is a contraindication to MRI. Additionally, such wires may not be functional several months later if a pacemaker generator is eventually implanted.[19,20]

It is reasonable to perform at least annual Holter evaluations on patients with isomerism, regardless of their history of arrhythmia.[19,20]

PULMONARY SYSTEM

With respect to the airways and the lungs themselves, the most frequent anatomic anomaly noted in the setting of isomerism is the loss of asymmetry in the bronchi and the lungs. In left isomerism, both the bronchi generally (95%) are morphologically left. A morphologically left bronchus is one that is hyparterial (having no bronchial branching above the pulmonary artery that extends to the lower lobe) and generally has a longer length before bifurcation (**Fig. 3**). In right isomerism, both the bronchi generally (94%) are morphologically right. A morphologically right bronchus is one that is eparterial (having bronchial branching above the pulmonary artery that extends to the lower lobe) and has a shorter length before bifurcation (**Fig. 3**). The tracheobronchial angle also differs between a morphologically left and right bronchus. There have been cases in which the trachea gives rise to four bronchi, one pair that is superior with continuation of the trachea with another pair of bronchi that arise inferior. All of these bronchi are isomeric.[22-26] Computed tomographic angiography can help nicely delineate the bronchial anatomy (**Fig. 4**).

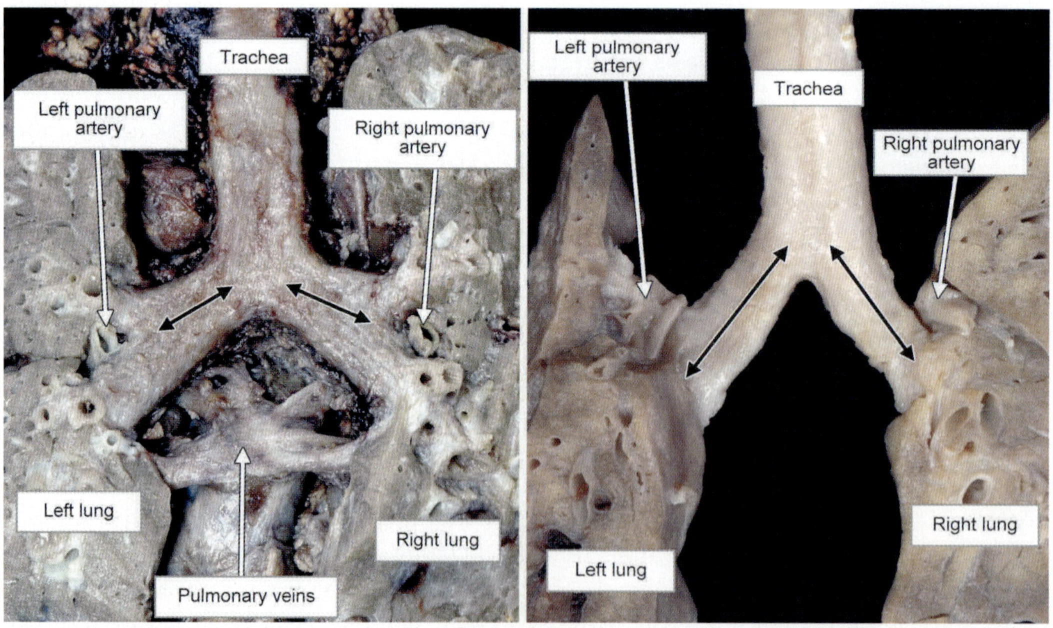

Fig. 3: The right and left panels are viewed posteriorly. The right panel demonstrates bilateral, morphologically right bronchi that are short (black arrows) and eparterial with the first bronchial branch lying above the pulmonary artery branch that extends to the lower lobe of the lung. The left panel demonstrates bilateral, morphologically left bronchi that are long (black arrows) and hyparterial or lying beneath the pulmonary artery that extends to the lower lobe of the lung.

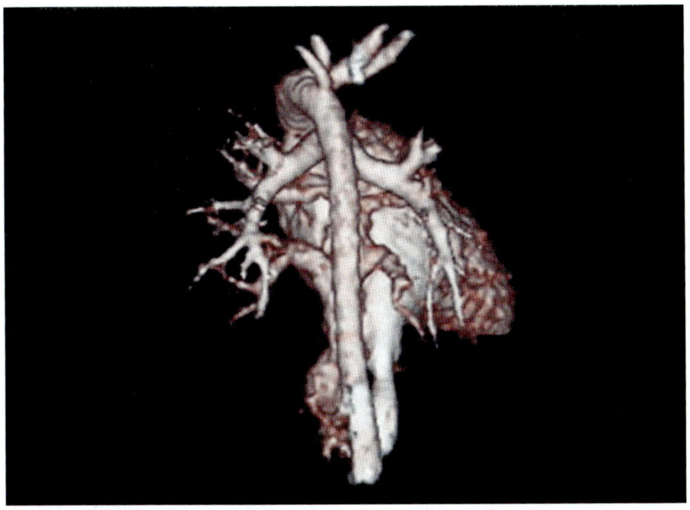

Fig. 4: Computed tomographic angiography in a patient with left isomerism. This three-dimensional reconstruction demonstrates the heart, the aorta, and the bronchi from the posterior aspect. The similarity of the tracheobronchial angles and length of the bronchi until the first branching demonstrates left isomerism.

While the bronchi are often isomeric in the setting of isomerism, so are the lungs. In a majority of cases of both left and right isomerism, the lungs are morphologically similar on both sides. As one would expect, in the setting of left isomerism, the lungs are most often (~80%) morphologically left. A morphologically left lung is bilobed. Intuitively, in the setting of right isomerism, the lungs are most often (~90%) morphologically right. A morphologically right lung is trilobed.[13]

While these anatomic findings are interesting, the question arises as to whether or not there are any functional differences. A study of sinopulmonary symptoms in those with isomerism demonstrated that those with left isomerism were more likely to have reactive airway disease requiring bronchodilators, were more likely to require supplemental oxygen at home, and were more likely to require tracheostomy. The precise mechanism of this is unclear.[27]

Pulmonary vascular resistance may also be impacted by the presence of isomerism. Studies in both children and adults with isomerism have demonstrated elevated pulmonary vascular resistance. Once again, the mechanism of this is unclear and the effect of pulmonary vasodilators has not been specifically characterized in this population.[28-32]

The findings in the pulmonary function may be secondary to ciliary dysfunction. This will be discussed later, but both sensory and motile cilia may play a role in pulmonary function. Ciliary dysfunction, known to be found in greater frequency in those with isomerism, thus may mediate some of the abnormalities in pulmonary function.[33]

A study comparing cardiopulmonary exercise testing in Fontan patients with isomerism, Fontan patients without isomerism, patients with primary ciliary dyskinesia but no congenital heart disease, and healthy controls demonstrated that Fontan patients with isomerism tended to have both a degree of restrictive and obstructive lung disease with the obstructive component being more similar to that of the primary ciliary dyskinesia group rather than Fontan patients without isomerism. There were limitations to the study, particularly selection bias. Further work must be done to characterize pulmonary function in patients with isomerism.[33]

Yearly cardiopulmonary exercise testing is advisable in patients whom this is tolerated starting at approximately 5–6 years of age.

CENTRAL NERVOUS SYSTEM

Central nervous system (CNS) anomalies are present in some children with isomerism. It appears that these are more frequent in those with right isomerism. Anatomic anomalies include agenesis of the corpus callosum, holoprosencephaly, myelomeningocele, and neural tube defects.[17,34,35]

Hydrocephalus has also been demonstrated to be more frequent in both children and adults with isomerism. This may be attributable to ciliary dysfunction as both motile and sensory cilia play a role in the regulation of cerebrospinal fluid.[36]

In the normal arrangement, synaptic arrangements are not symmetric about the midline in the brain. A study utilizing knockout mice demonstrated that in mice with right isomerism there was isomeric synaptic arrangement in the hippocampus. This was reproduced in another study at a later time as well. No autopsy study in humans has been conducted to determine whether or not this may be the case in humans with isomerism. The potential functional implications of such a finding also remain unclear.[37]

While neurodevelopmental abnormalities have been noted in a larger proportion of children with congenital heart disease when compared to the general population, specific comparisons of those with isomerism have not been published. Some, as of yet unpublished data does seem to indicate that isomerism may be associated with increased frequency of neurodevelopmental abnormalities and that this may be mediated by ciliary dysfunction.

GASTROINTESTINAL SYSTEM

Perhaps the most frequently noted gastrointestinal anomaly in those with isomerism is abnormal arrangement of the abdominal organs, most notably the stomach and the liver. While the stomach and liver may be abnormally located in the abdomen, this is not always noted in isomerism. A right-sided stomach is noted in about one-third of those with left isomerism and a similar proportion of those with right isomerism (**Figs. 5 and 6**). The liver is most frequently (~50%) midline in both left and right isomerism. An autopsy study did demonstrate fatty liver changes in a quarter of patients with right isomerism compared to no such findings in any

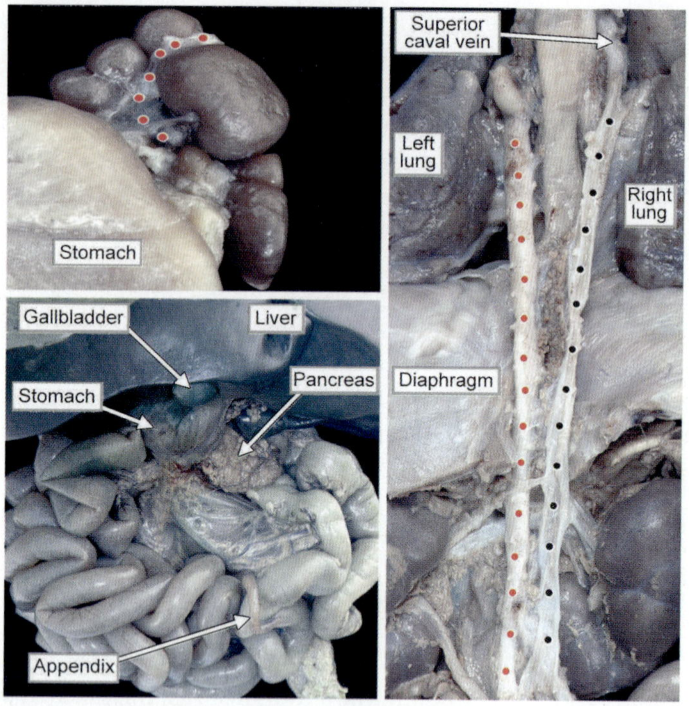

Fig. 5: The left upper panel shows an anterior view of multiple spleens along the lateral aspect of the stomach. There are splenules on both sides of the dorsal mesogastrium (red dots). In the left lower panel is an anterior view of the abdominal organs with the midline, roughly symmetric liver lifted off of the gastrointestinal tract. This patient's liver is green secondary to biliary atresia. The bowel is malrotated with the appendix in the left lower quadrant. The stomach was small and in the midline along with the gallbladder. The pancreas was just to the left of the midline and was ovoid rather than elongated. The right panel is a posterior view of the organ block removed at autopsy, demonstrating the large azygos vein (black dots) branching from the superior caval vein to the right of the midline with the aorta (red dots) running parallel to it and to the left of the midline. Both vessels extend inferior to the diaphragm, the azygos vein compensating for the interruption of the hepatic portion of the inferior caval vein.

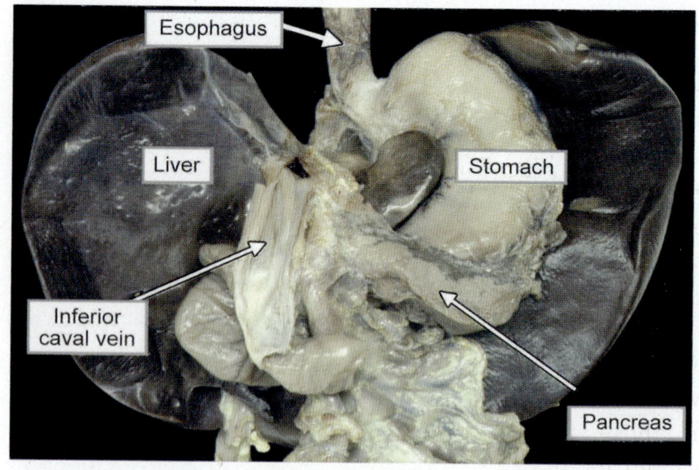

Fig. 6: This posterior view shows a symmetric, midline liver with a left-sided inferior caval vein, along with a right-sided stomach and pancreas in a patient with right atrial isomerism. Note the absence of the spleen.

patient with left isomerism. This same study demonstrated fibrosis of the liver in 20% of patients with left isomerism and 7% of those with right isomerism. The implications and mechanism of such findings was not assessable.[3]

It should also be noted that biliary atresia may be present in those with left isomerism. Approximately 5% of those with left isomerism will have findings consistent with biliary atresia (**Fig. 5**).

The gallbladder is on the right side in approximately half of patients with isomerism, midline in one-quarter, and on the left side in another quarter of patients (**Fig. 5**). The pancreas tends to be left-sided in approximately half of patients with isomerism and then right-sided in the other half. The pancreas may also demonstrate agenesis. Anatomic anomalies of the pancreas have not translated into functional abnormality of the pancreas with greater frequency in studies of those with isomerism.[3,38-40]

Intestinal malrotation is noted in a large proportion of patients with isomerism. The rate of malrotation appears to be equal in those with left and right isomerism, being seen in approximately three-fifths of patients. The risk of volvulus in those with isomerism and intestinal malrotation, however, is under 5%. Thus, it is now recommended not to undertake an upper gastrointestinal study unless there are clinical concerns for intestinal obstruction. If intestinal malrotation is incidentally detected, a prophylactic Ladd procedure should not be performed. Ladd procedure should only be done in a patient with documented intestinal malrotation who is symptomatic.[2,41-50]

IMMUNOLOGIC SYSTEM

The immune system may also be affected in the setting of isomerism. Indeed, it was splenic morphology that was used initially to segregate the subtypes of what was then referred to as heterotaxy. The spleen is often abnormal in those with isomerism.[3] A majority (~90%) of those with left isomerism will have multiple spleens, with the remainder either having a solitary spleen or an absent spleen (**Fig. 5**). A majority (~85%) of those with right isomerism will have an absent spleen with the remainder either having a solitary spleen or multiple spleens[3] (**Fig. 6**).

In respect to the spleen, anatomy is less important. It is function that is more important. It has now been demonstrated that, in those with isomerism, the spleen may be abnormal in function despite its anatomy.[51,52] Those with a single, solitary spleen or multiple spleens may have abnormal splenic function, which may still increase risk of infection with encapsulated organisms. It is still recommended to obtain a splenic ultrasound shortly after birth to document splenic anatomy. Splenic function testing by Howell–Jolly body assessment or by pitted red blood cell testing is not accurate until 2 years of age.[53-55]

All patients with isomerism should be started on prophylactic antibiotics (amoxicillin) early in life. Those with a solitary spleen or multiple spleens can have splenic function testing done at 2 years of age. If the function is normal, then antibiotics may be discontinued. Otherwise, antibiotics should be continued until 5 years of age. Those with an absent spleen should be kept on antibiotics until 5 years of age at which point, they may be discontinued.[56-60]

Vaccinations and immunizations are of utmost importance in this population due to their increased risk of infection as well. Local vaccination schedules should be adhered to closely. Those with isomerism should also receive a 23-valent polysaccharide pneumococcal vaccination after 2 years of age in addition to (not in place of) the 13-valent polysaccharide pneumococcal vaccination. Meningococcal vaccination should also be slightly altered in those with isomerism with Hib-MenCY-TT being administered at 2 months, 3 months, 5 months, and then 12 months of age.

As approximately one-third of those with isomerism may have documented bacteremia, it is important to be vigilant.[60] Studies have demonstrated that of those with isomerism and bacteremia have an increased risk of mortality. Febrile episodes in those with isomerism should lead to routine evaluation. Those with temperatures of 38.5°C or greater should be evaluated with a laboratory evaluation consisting of a complete blood count with manual differential, C-reactive protein, and blood culture. Chest radiographs and urine culture may be obtained if felt clinically indicated. All isomerism patients with a fever >38.5°C should receive one dose of intramuscular ceftriaxone if well-appearing. Those who are well appearing can then be discharged with close follow-up of the blood cultures. Those who are ill-appearing should be started on intravenous antibiotics and admitted with antibiotics being continued for at least 48 hours while blood cultures are closely monitored.[59]

GENITOURINARY SYSTEM

Genitourinary anomalies are noted more frequently in those with right isomerism, with approximately 15% of those with right isomerism having such an anomaly identified. These include horseshoe kidney, ectopic ureters, ureteral duplication, cystic kidney, solitary kidney, and cloacal duplications. What have yet to be delineated are the functional implications of isomerism on kidney function.[3,17]

MORBIDITY AND MORTALITY

The importance of any clinical entity is the effect it has on overall morbidity and mortality. Morbidity has been discussed earlier in this section. Morbidity and mortality are indeed greater in those with isomerism, even when underlying cardiac malformations are taken into consideration. This holds true for those with functionally univentricular and biventricular circulations.[21,61-76]

Mortality seems to be the highest in the first 3 years of life with 73% survival at 3 years of age when all patients with isomerism are considered together. Those with left isomerism seem to have lower early mortality compared to those with right isomerism who have greater early risk of mortality. However, at 14 years of age, those with left isomerism tend to have a greater risk of mortality. The reason behind this is not fully understood. For those with left isomerism, survival is 94% and 83% at 5 and 10 years of age, respectively. For right isomerism, survival is 76% and 64% at 5 and 10 years of age, respectively.[67,77]

Those with biventricular circulation have markedly greater survival when compared to those with functionally univentricular circulation at all ages.

GENETICS

The precise genetic underpinnings of isomerism are still unclear. What has been demonstrated is that knockout of particular genes in the mouse model leads to reproducible, isomeric atrial appendage morphology. It is the atrial appendage morphology that stays consistent with genetic perturbation, and not splenic anatomy. Several genes have been noted to be affected in humans with isomerism including, but not limited to *Nodal, SHH, ZIC3, PITX2, Lefty A, Lefty B, ACVR, CCDC, CDC, DNAAF, DNAH, FOXH1*, and *NKX*. Recent data demonstrate that certain genes being affected may alter the overall phenotype of isomerism, and may also be associated with different clinical courses.[12,48,78-91]

A mutation in one of the genes associated with isomerism is noted in approximately one-quarter of patients with isomerism. It is important to note that current ciliopathy and isomerism (aka heterotaxy) panels still have low overall yield. Obtaining such testing may be helpful in the future as more is delineated. Such testing should be performed if resources allow.

CILIARY DYSFUNCTION

Ciliary dysfunction has been noted in approximately half of patients with isomerism.[33] These have been relatively small studies to date. It is important to note that ciliary dysfunction is not the same as primary ciliary dyskinesia. In primary ciliary dyskinesia, the actual ultrastructure of the cilia is abnormal while in ciliary dysfunction, the actual ultrastructure of the cilia may be normal. What is abnormal in ciliary dysfunction is the actual function of the cilia themselves. This can be quantified by video microscopy to assess the ciliary beat frequency and other characteristics of the beat frequency itself. Electron microscopy is not the test of choice as it does not provide functional analysis of the cilia and normal ciliary ultrastructure does not portend normal ciliary function.

While cilia are most frequently thought of in their motile variety, most cells have at least a single, sensory cilium. These sensory cilia are still not very well understood, but disturbances in sensory ciliary function along with motile ciliary function may result in the anatomic and functional abnormalities noted in isomerism.

Nodal cilia present on the embryonic node are responsible for dictating nodal flow, which creates right-left patterning. Abnormal ciliary function at this stage can lead to a loss of normal nodal flow and thus can lead to a loss of normal right-left patterning. There is growing evidence that this is the underlying mechanism behind isomerism.[92-97]

PRACTICAL CONSIDERATIONS FOR THE PRIMARY CARE PROVIDER

It is not practical for the primary care provider to understand at length all the nuances of isomerism as outlined in this chapter. It is, however, important for the primary care provider to understand that isomerism can affect any of the organ systems, anatomically and/or functionally.

Isomerism should be suspected and intentionally ruled out when there are right-left patterning abnormalities, congenital heart disease consistent with isomerism (atrioventricular septal defect, double-outlet right ventricle, interrupted inferior caval vein, or bilateral superior caval veins), or absence of a spleen or multiple spleens, intestinal nonrotation, or malrotation. When a constellation of these findings occur together, then a diagnosis of isomerism should be made. There is no strict criteria for diagnosis and thus this is a clinical diagnosis. It should be kept in mind that making the diagnosis of isomerism is best to be done with erring on the side of caution and being more liberal with the diagnosis as the major implication will be initiation of empiric antibiotics, which would otherwise generally not be harmful.

Once a diagnosis of isomerism is made, it is important to identify the anatomic placement of the major organs: heart, lungs, stomach, liver, intestines, and spleen. Much of this can be delineated by radiographs (**Fig. 7**). Delineation of intestinal and splenic anatomy is not of the utmost importance, and can be deferred if there are no concerns of intestinal obstruction. If there are signs of intestinal obstruction, then an upper gastrointestinal series should be obtained.

Once the general organ placement is established, it is important to then ensure that the cardiac anatomy is entirely delineated, particularly if the suspicion of isomerism happens prior to complete cardiac evaluation. Referral to a pediatric cardiologist and echocardiography can aid in confirming the diagnosis.

The burden of arrhythmia is significant in isomerism and thus primary care providers should be alert for this. If possible, yearly ECG and/or Holter monitor evaluation should be obtained. Otherwise, there should be a low threshold to obtain such arrhythmia evaluation if symptoms of arrhythmia are described.

As some of these children will have ciliary dysfunction, they may have abnormal respiratory mechanics. For children who have had repeated issues with atelectasis parents can be taught how to provide mechanical chest physiotherapy at home as needed.

Once isomerism is suspected, the child should be started on amoxicillin until 5 years of age. If a spleen is present, as previously described, then functional testing can be done at 2 years of age, otherwise amoxicillin can be started and continued until 2 years of age.

Due to the high incidence of bacterial illness, and the increased morbidity and mortality of bacterial illnesses in those with isomerism, primary care providers need to have

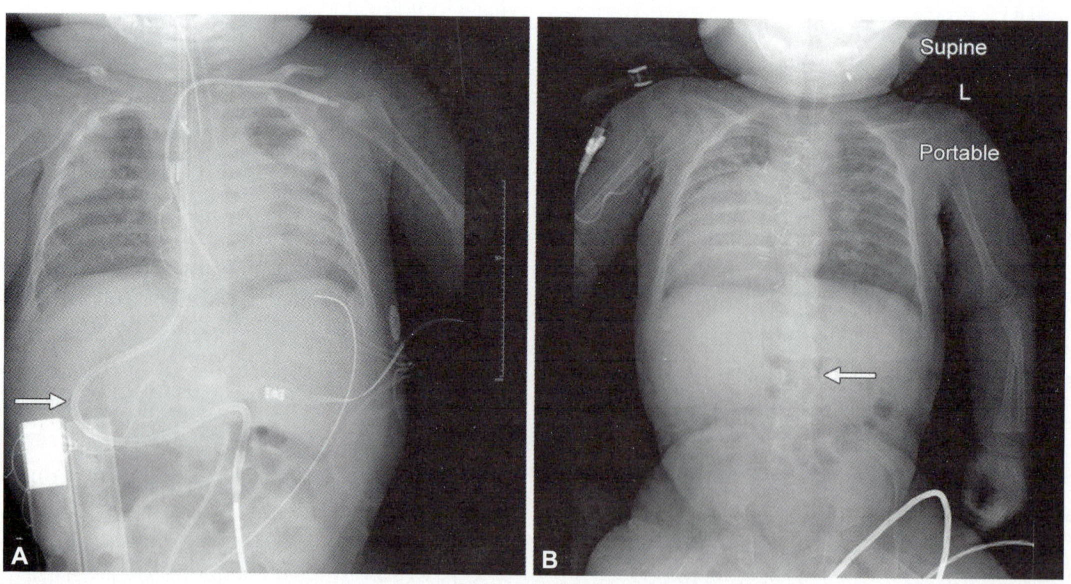

Figs. 7A and B: Radiographs of the chest and abdomen in two separate patients with isomerism with differing arrangement of the thoracoabdominal organs. (A) A patient with left isomerism in whom the cardiac apex is leftward and the heart lies predominantly in the left chest. The liver is midline and the stomach is on the right as demonstrated by the course of the nasojejunal tube which is delineated by an arrow; (B) A patient with right isomerism in whom the cardiac apex points rightward and the heart lies predominantly in the right chest. The liver is midline and the stomach is right sided as demonstrated by the nasogastric tube which is delineated by an arrow.

Flowchart 1: Some key evaluations and steps of management when caring for a child with isomerism.

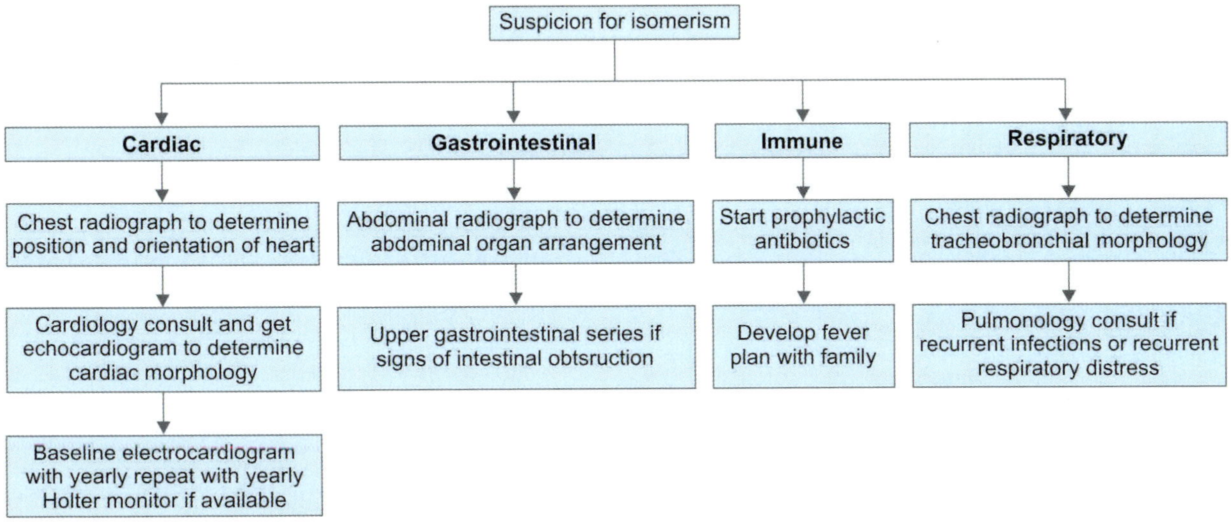

TABLE 2: A summary of extracardiac manifestations of isomerism (heterotaxy).

Organ/organ system	*Abnormality*	*Clinical implications*
Respiratory system	Abnormal ciliary motility; bilateral right- or left-sided lungs	Delayed recovery from cardiac surgery, frequent respiratory infections, reactive airway disease, potential worsening of pulmonary hypertension, may contribute to early Fontan failure
Nervous system	Agenesis of the corpus callosum, holoprosencephaly, myelomeningocele, and neural tube defects; abnormal ciliary motility of cells lining ventricles	Higher than usual incidence of hydrocephalus, Incremental adverse effect on neurodevelopment
Gastrointestinal system	Abnormal arrangements of abdominal viscera; Intestinal malrotation	Volvulus of the intestine or stomach; biliary atresia (5% of left isomerism); fatty liver
Immune system	Anatomical absence or poorly functional spleen	Vulnerability to infections with encapsulated organisms requires antibiotic prophylaxis and special attention to vaccination against *Pneumococcus, Meningococcus*, and *Haemophilus influenzae*

a fever protocol in place that is explained to the family. Such a fever protocol is outlined above and is meant to promote early evaluation if there is concern for, or confirmed, fever.

These are the most high-yield considerations to be kept in mind by primary care providers and are outlined in **Flowchart 1**. Other detailed considerations, while outlined above, are for reference in the event these situations arise. Subspecialty referral will likely be necessary in these events and access to care and availability of financial and technical resources may affect what can be done for some of these occurrences.

CONCLUSION

Isomerism represents a highly complex, multiorgan clinical entity. Data from the current era demonstrate that isomerism is likely a ciliopathy in which nodal cilia impact nodal flow and thus disrupt normal right-left patterning. Thus, internal asymmetry is lost anatomically, and organ function is also affected. Care of the patient with isomerism requires knowledge of the nuances of isomerism and the assistance of a multidisciplinary approach to try to achieve optimal outcomes. **Tables 1 and 2** present a summary of abnormalities seen in isomerism together with their clinical implications.

REFERENCES

1. Loomba RS, Hlavacek AM, Spicer DE, Anderson RH. Isomerism or heterotaxy: which term leads to better understanding? Cardiol Young. 2015; 25(6):1-7.
2. Jacobs JP, Anderson RH, Weinberg PM, Walters 3rd HL, Tchervenkov CI, Del Duca D, et al. The nomenclature, definition and classification of cardiac structures in the setting of heterotaxy. Cardiol Young. 2007;17 Suppl 2:1-28.
3. Loomba RS, Ahmed MM, Spicer DE, Backer CL, Anderson RH. Manifestations of bodily isomerism. Cardiovasc Pathol. 2016; 25(3):173-80.
4. Loomba RS. The prevalence of isomerism from a European registry: live births, fetal deaths, and terminations of pregnancy. Congenit Anom (Kyoto). 2016;56(6):256-7.
5. Evans WN, Acherman RJ, Restrepo H. Heterotaxy in southern Nevada: prenatal detection and epidemiology. Pediatr Cardiol. 2015;36(5):930-4.

6. Lopez KN, Marengo LK, Canfield MA, Belmont JW, Dickerson HA. Racial disparities in heterotaxy syndrome. Birth Defects Res A Clin Mol Teratol. 2015;103(11):941-50.
7. Lin AE, Krikov S, Riehle-Colarusso T, Frías JL, Belmont J, Anderka M, et al. Laterality defects in the national birth defects prevention study (1998-2007): birth prevalence and descriptive epidemiology. Am J Med Gen A. 2014;164A(10): 2581-91.
8. Ivemark BI. Implications of agenesis of the spleen on the pathogenesis of conotruncus anomalies in childhood; an analysis of the heart malformations in the splenic agenesis syndrome, with fourteen new cases. Acta Paediatr Suppl. 1955;44(Suppl 104):7-110.
9. Katcher AL. Familial asplenia, other malformations, and sudden death. Pediatrics. 1980; 65(3):633-5.
10. Van Went JJ, Van Went GF, Delleman JW, Becker AG. Spina bifida and so-called asplenia syndrome occurring separately in sibs. Teratology. 1977;15(2):195-8.
11. Bamforth SD, Braganca J, Farthing CR, Schneider JE, Broadbent C, Michell AC, et al. Cited2 controls left-right patterning and heart development through a Nodal-Pitx2c pathway. Nat Gen. 2004;36(11):1189-96.
12. Meno C, Shimono A, Saijoh Y, Yashiro K, Mochida K, Ohishi S, et al. Lefty-1 is required for left-right determination as a regulator of lefty-2 and nodal. Cell. 1998;94(3):287-97.
13. Tremblay C, Loomba RS, Frommelt PC, Perrin D, Spicer DE, Backer C, et al. Segregating bodily isomerism or heterotaxy: potential echocardiographic correlations of morphological findings. Cardiology in the young 2017:27(8):1-11.
14. Loomba RS, Anderson RH. Polysplenia or left isomerism? Intern Med. 2016;55(5):555.
15. Uemura H, Ho SY, Devine WA, Anderson RH. Analysis of visceral heterotaxy according to splenic status, appendage morphology, or both. Am J Cardiol. 1995;76(11):846-9.
16. Mori S, Anderson RH, Nishii T, Matsumoto K, Loomba RS. Isomerism in the setting of the so-called "heterotaxy": the usefulness of computed tomographic analysis. Ann Pediatr Cardiol. 2017;10(2):175-86.
17. Loomba R, Shah PH, Anderson RH. Fetal magnetic resonance imaging of malformations associated with heterotaxy. Cureus. 2015;7(5): e269.
18. Smith A, Ho SY, Anderson RH, Connell MG, Arnold R, Wilkinson JL, et al. The diverse cardiac morphology seen in hearts with isomerism of the atrial appendages with reference to the disposition of the specialised conduction system. Cardiol Young. 2006;16(5):437-54.
19. Loomba RS, Aggarwal S, Gupta N, Buelow M, Alla V, Arora RR, et al. Arrhythmias in adult congenital patients with bodily isomerism. Pediatr Cardiol. 2016;37(2):330-7.
20. Loomba RS, Willes RJ, Kovach JR, Anderson RH. Chronic arrhythmias in the setting of heterotaxy: differences between right and left isomerism. Congen Heart Dis. 2016;11(1):7-18.
21. Atz AM, Cohen MS, Sleeper LA, McCrindle BW, Lu M, Prakash A, et al. Functional state of patients with heterotaxy syndrome following the Fontan operation. Cardiol Young. 2007;17 Suppl 2:44-53.
22. Landing BH, Lawrence TY, Payne VC Jr, Wells TR. Bronchial anatomy in syndromes with abnormal visceral situs, abnormal spleen and congenital heart disease. Am J Cardiol. 1971; 28(4):456-62.
23. Loomba RS, Pelech AN, Shah PH, Anderson RH. Determining bronchial morphology for the purposes of segregating so-called heterotaxy. Cardiol Young. 2016;26(4):725-37.
24. Partridge J. The radiological evaluation of atrial situs. Clin Radiol. 1979;30(1):95-103.
25. Partridge JB, Scott O, Deverall PB, Macartney FJ. Visualization and measurement of the main bronchi by tomography as an objective indicator of thoracic situs in congenital heart disease. Circulation. 1975;51(1):188-96.
26. Van Mierop LH, Eisen S, Schiebler GL. The radiographic appearance of the tracheobronchial tree as an indicator of visceral situs. Am J Cardiol. 1970;26(4):432-5.
27. Loomba RP, Pelech AN, Anderson RH. Sinopulmonary complications in the setting of bodily isomerism. EC Paediatrics. 2016;2(5):228-36.
28. Krieger EV, Leary PJ, Opotowsky AR. Pulmonary hypertension in congenital heart disease: beyond Eisenmenger syndrome. Cardiol Clin. 2015;33(4):599-609.
29. Loomba R. Comment on pulmonary hypertension in a patient with congenital heart defects and heterotaxy syndrome. Ochsner J. 2015;15(4):401.
30. Loomba RS, Aggarwal S, Arora RR, Anderson R. Bodily isomerism is an independent risk factor for pulmonary hypertension in adults with congenital heart disease. Ther Adv Res Dis. 2016;10(3):194-9.
31. Nakanishi T. Pulmonary arterial hypertension associated with congenital heart disease. Personal perspectives. Int Heart J. 2015;56 Suppl:S1-3.
32. Yousuf T, Kramer K, Jones B, Keshmiri H, Muhyaldeen Dia M. Pulmonary hypertension in a patient with congenital heart defects and heterotaxy syndrome. The Oschner J. 2015; 15(3):1-3.
33. Nakhleh N, Francis R, Giese RA, Tian X, Li Y, Zariwala MA, et al. High prevalence of respiratory ciliary dysfunction in congenital heart disease patients with heterotaxy. Circulation. 2012;125(18):2232-42.
34. Bonneau D, Marechaud M, Odent S, Piegay I, Godard A, Amati P. Heterotaxy-neural tube defect and holoprosencephaly occuring independently in two sib fetuses. Am J Med Genet. 1999;84(4): 373-6.
35. Clouchoux C, du Plessis AJ, Bouyssi-Kobar M, Tworetzky W, McElhinney DB, Brown DW, et al. Delayed cortical development in fetuses with complex congenital heart disease. Cereb Cortex. 2013;23(12):2932-43.
36. Nijhawan K, Loomba RS. Increased risk of hydrocephalus in adults with isomerism. EC Paediatrics. 2016;2(6):250-8.
37. Kawakami R, Dobi A, Shigemoto R, Ito I. Right isomerism of the brain in inversus viscerum mutant mice. PloS One. 2008;3(4):e1945.
38. Adeyemi SD. Combination of annular pancreas and partial situs inversus: a multiple organ malrotation syndrome associated with duodenal obstruction. J Pediatr Surg. 1988;23(2):188-91.
39. Ben Ahmed Y, Ghorbel S, Chouikh T, Nouira F, Louati H, Charieg A, et al. Combination of partial situs inversus, polysplenia and annular pancreas with duodenal obstruction and intestinal malrotation. JBR-BTR. 2012;95(4):257-60.
40. Jeong JH, Kim GH, Song GA, Lee DG, Moon JY, Cheong JH, et al. Polysplenia syndrome with congenital agenesis of dorsal pancreas presenting as acute pancreatitis and the role of endoscopic ultrasonography in its diagnosis. Korean J Gastroenterol. 2012;60(1):47-51.
41. Choi M, Borenstein SH, Hornberger L, Langer JC. Heterotaxia syndrome: the role of screening for intestinal rotation abnormalities. Arch Dis Child. 2005;90(8):813-5.
42. Hill SJ, Heiss KF, Mittal R, Clabby ML, Durham MM, Ricketts R, et al. Heterotaxy syndrome and malrotation: does isomerism influence risk and decision to treat. J Pediatr Surg. 2014;49(6): 934-7; discussion 7.
43. Landisch R, Abdel-Hafeez AH, Massoumi R, Christensen M, Shillingford A, Wagner AJ. Observation versus prophylactic Ladd for asymptomatic intestinal rotational abnormalities in heterotaxy syndrome: a systematic review. J Pediatr Surg. 2015;50(11): 1971-4.
44. Landisch RM, Loomba RS, Salazar JH, Buelow MW, Frommelt M, Anderson RH, et al. Is isomerism a risk factor for intestinal volvulus? J Pediatr Surg. 2018;53(6):1118-22.

45. Newman B, Koppolu R, Murphy D, Sylvester K. Heterotaxy syndromes and abnormal bowel rotation. Pediatr Radiol. 2014;44(5):542-51.
46. Papillon S, Goodhue CJ, Zmora O, Sharma SS, Wells WJ, Ford HR, et al. Congenital heart disease and heterotaxy: upper gastrointestinal fluoroscopy can be misleading and surgery in an asymptomatic patient is not beneficial. J Pediatr Surg. 2013;48(1):164-9.
47. Pockett CR, Dicken B, Rebeyka IM, Ross DB, Ryerson LM. Heterotaxy syndrome: is a prophylactic Ladd procedure necessary in asymptomatic patients? Pediatr Cardiol. 2013; 34(1):59-63.
48. Prendiville TW, Barton LL, Thompson WR, Fink DL, Holmes KW. Heterotaxy syndrome: defining contemporary disease trends. Pediatr Cardiol. 2010;31(7):1052-8.
49. Tashjian DB, Weeks B, Brueckner M, Touloukian RJ. Outcomes after a Ladd procedure for intestinal malrotation with heterotaxia. J Pediatr Surg. 2007;42(3):528-31.
50. Yu DC, Thiagarajan RR, Laussen PC, Laussen JP, Jaksic T, Weldon CB. Outcomes after the Ladd procedure in patients with heterotaxy syndrome, congenital heart disease, and intestinal malrotation. J Pediatr Surg. 2009; 44(6):1089-95; discussion 95.
51. Nagel BH, Williams H, Stewart L, Paul J, Stumper O. Splenic state in surviving patients with visceral heterotaxy. Cardiol Young. 2005; 15(5):469-73.
52. Rodin AE, Sloane JA, Nghiem QX. Polysplenia with severe congenital heart disease and Howell-Jolly bodies. Am J Clin Pathol. 1972; 58(2):127-34.
53. Casper JT, Koethe S, Rodey GE, Thatcher LG. A new method for studying splenic reticuloendothelial dysfunction in sickle cell disease patients and its clinical application: a brief report. Blood. 1976;47(2):183-8.
54. Corazza GR, Ginaldi L, Zoli G, Frisoni M, Lalli G, Gasbarrini G, et al. Howell-Jolly body counting as a measure of splenic function. A reassessment. Clin Lab Haematol. 1990;12(3):269-75.
55. Chiu SN, Shao PL, Wang JK, Chen HC, Lin MT, Chang LY, et al. Severe bacterial infection in patients with heterotaxy syndrome. J Pediatr. 2014;164(1):99-104.e1.
56. Falletta JM, Woods GM, Verter JI, Buchanan GR, Pegelow CH, Iyer RV, et al. Discontinuing penicillin prophylaxis in children with sickle cell anemia. Prophylactic Penicillin Study II. J Pediatr. 1995;127(5):685-90.
57. Gaston MH, Verter JI, Woods G, Pegelow C, Kelleher J, Presbury G, et al. Prophylaxis with oral penicillin in children with sickle cell anemia. A randomized trial. N Engl J Med. 1986; 314(25):1593-9.
58. Loomba RS, Geddes GC, Shillingford AJ, Hehir DA. Practice variability in management of infectious issues in heterotaxy: a survey of pediatric cardiologists. Congen Heart Dis. 2017; 12(3):332-9.
59. Loomba RS, Geddes GC, Basel D, Benson DW, Leuthner SR, Hehir DA, et al. Bacteremia in patients with heterotaxy: a review and implications for management. Congen Heart Dis. 2016;11(6): 537-47.
60. Loomba RS, Pelech AN, Anderson RH. Factors influencing bacteraemia in patients with isomerism and CHD: the effects of functional splenic status and antibiotic prophylaxis. Cardiol Young. 2017:27(4):639-47.
61. Chen W, Ma L, Cui H, Yang S, Xia Y, Zou M, et al. Early- and middle-term surgical outcomes in patients with heterotaxy syndrome. Cardiology. 2015;133(3):141-6.
62. Cheung YF, Cheng VY, Chau AK, Chiu CS, Yung TC, Leung MP. Outcome of infants with right atrial isomerism: is prognosis better with normal pulmonary venous drainage? Heart. 2002;87(2): 146-52.
63. Cohen MS, Schultz AH, Tian ZY, Donaghue DD, Weinberg PM, Gaynor JW, et al. Heterotaxy syndrome with functional single ventricle: does prenatal diagnosis improve survival? Ann Thorac Surg. 2006;82(5):1629-36.
64. Foerster SR, Gauvreau K, McElhinney DB, Geva T. Importance of totally anomalous pulmonary venous connection and postoperative pulmonary vein stenosis in outcomes of heterotaxy syndrome. Pediatr Cardiol. 2008;29(3):536-44.
65. Gilljam T, McCrindle BW, Smallhorn JF, Williams WG, Freedom RM. Outcomes of left atrial isomerism over a 28-year period at a single institution. J Am Coll Cardiol. 2000;36(3):908-16.
66. Hashmi A, Abu-Sulaiman R, McCrindle BW, Smallhorn JF, Williams WG, Freedom RM. Management and outcomes of right atrial isomerism: a 26-year experience. J Am Coll Cardiol. 1998;31(5):1120-6.
67. Loomba RF, Frommelt PC, Anderson RH. Predictors of mortality in patients with isomerism. J Pediatr Care. 2016;2(15):1-6.
68. Aeba R, Katogi T, Takeuchi S, Kawada S. Long-term follow-up of surgical patients with single-ventricle physiology: prognostic anatomical determinants. Cardiovasc Surg. 1997;5(5):526-32.
69. Bartz PJ, Driscoll DJ, Dearani JA, Puga FJ, Danielson GK, O'Leary PW, et al. Early and late results of the modified fontan operation for heterotaxy syndrome 30 years of experience in 142 patients. J Am Coll Cardiol. 2006; 48(11):2301-5.
70. Berg C, Geipel A, Kamil D, Knüppel M, Breuer J, Krapp M, et al. The syndrome of left isomerism: sonographic findings and outcome in prenatally diagnosed cases. J Ultrasound Med. 2005;24(7): 921-31.
71. Escobar-Diaz MC, Friedman K, Salem Y, Marx GR, Kalish BT, Lafranchi T, et al. Perinatal and infant outcomes of prenatal diagnosis of heterotaxy syndrome (asplenia and polysplenia). Am J Cardiol. 2014;114(4):612-7.
72. Harden B, Tian X, Giese R, Nakhleh N, Kureshi S, Francis R, et al. Increased postoperative respiratory complications in heterotaxy congenital heart disease patients with respiratory ciliary dysfunction. J Thorac Cardiovasc Surg. 2014;147(4): 1291-8.e2.
73. Humes RA, Feldt RH, Porter CJ, Julsrud PR, Puga FJ, Danielson GK. The modified Fontan operation for asplenia and polysplenia syndromes. J Thorac Cardiovasc Surg. 1988; 96(2):212-8.
74. Kim SJ, Kim WH, Lim HG, Lee CH, Lee JY. Improving results of the Fontan procedure in patients with heterotaxy syndrome. Ann Thorac Surg. 2006;82(4):1245-51.
75. Knott-Craig CJ, Danielson GK, Schaff HV, Puga FJ, Weaver AL, Driscoll DD. The modified Fontan operation. An analysis of risk factors for early postoperative death or takedown in 702 consecutive patients from one institution. J Thorac Cardiovasc Surg. 1995;109(6):1237-43.
76. Koudieh M, McKenzie ED, Fraser CD Jr. Outcome of Glenn anastomosis for heterotaxy syndrome with single ventricle. Asian Cardiovasc Thorac Ann. 2006;14(3):235-8.
77. Loomba RS, Nijhawan K, Anderson R. Impact of era, type of isomerism, and ventricular morphology on survival in heterotaxy: implications for therapeutic management. World J Pediatr Congen Heart Surg. 2016;7(1):54-62.
78. Bartoloni L, Blouin JL, Pan Y, Gehrig C, Maiti AK, Scamuffa N, et al. Mutations in the DNAH11 (axonemal heavy chain dynein type 11) gene cause one form of situs inversus totalis and most likely primary ciliary dyskinesia. Proc Natl Acad Sci USA. 2002;99(16):10282-6.
79. Bedard JE, Haaning AM, Ware SM. Identification of a novel ZIC3 isoform and mutation screening in patients with heterotaxy and congenital heart disease. PloS One. 2011;6(8):e23755.
80. Belmont JW, Mohapatra B, Towbin JA, Ware SM. Molecular genetics of heterotaxy syndromes. Curr Opin Cardiol. 2004;19(3):216-20.
81. Cao R, Long F, Wang L, Xu Y, Guo Y, Li F, et al. Duplication and deletion of CFC1 associated with heterotaxy syndrome. DNA Cell Biol. 2015;34(2):101-6.

82. Catana A, Apostu AP. The determination factors of left-right asymmetry disorders- a short review. Clujul Med. 2017;90(2): 139-46.
83. Chhin B, Hatayama M, Bozon D, Ogawa M, Schön P, Tohmonda T, et al. Elucidation of penetrance variability of a ZIC3 mutation in a family with complex heart defects and functional analysis of ZIC3 mutations in the first zinc finger domain. Hum Mutat. 2007;28(6): 563-70.
84. D'Alessandro LC, Casey B, Siu VM. Situs inversus totalis and a novel ZIC3 mutation in a family with X-linked heterotaxy. Congenit Heart Dis. 2013;8(2):E36-40.
85. Davit-Spraul A, Baussan C, Hermeziu B, Bernard O, Jacquemin E. CFC1 gene involvement in biliary atresia with polysplenia syndrome. J Pediatr Gastroenterol Nutr. 2008;46(1):111-2.
86. Guimier A, Gabriel GC, Bajolle F, Tsang M, Liu J, Noll A, et al. MMP21 is mutated in human heterotaxy and is required for normal left-right asymmetry in vertebrates. Nat Genet. 2015;47(11):1260-3.
87. Izumi K, Noon S, Wilkens A, Krantz ID. NKX2.5 mutation identification on exome sequencing in a patient with heterotaxy. Eur J Med Genet. 2014;57(10):558-61.
88. Ma L, Selamet Tierney ES, Lee T, Lanzano P, Chung WK. Mutations in ZIC3 and ACVR2B are a common cause of heterotaxy and associated cardiovascular anomalies. Cardiol Young. 2012; 22(2):194-201.
89. Meno C, Saijoh Y, Fujii H, Ikeda M, Yokoyama T, Yokoyama M, et al. Left-right asymmetric expression of the TGF beta-family member lefty in mouse embryos. Nature 1996; 381(6578):151-5.
90. Shiraishi I, Ichikawa H. Human heterotaxy syndrome - from molecular genetics to clinical features, management, and prognosis. Circ J. 2012;76(9):2066-75.
91. Loomba RF, Frommelt PC, Anderson RH. Genetic disturbances in patients with bodily isomerism from a single center: clinical implications of affected genes and potential impact of ciliary dyskinesia. Cardiogenetics. 2016;6(1):15-21.
92. Blum M, Vick P. Left-right asymmetry: cilia and calcium revisited. Curr Biol. 2015;25(5):R205-7.
93. Hirokawa N, Tanaka Y, Okada Y, Takeda S. Nodal flow and the generation of left-right asymmetry. Cell. 2006;125(1):33-45.
94. Nonaka S, Shiratori H, Saijoh Y, Hamada H. Determination of left-right patterning of the mouse embryo by artificial nodal flow. Nature. 2002;418(6893):96-9.
95. Okada Y, Nonaka S, Tanaka Y, Saijoh Y, Hamada H, Hirokawa N. Abnormal nodal flow precedes situs inversus in iv and inv mice. Mol Cell. 1999;4(4):459-68.
96. Okada Y, Takeda S, Tanaka Y, Izpisua Belmonte JC, Hirokawa N. Mechanism of nodal flow: a conserved symmetry breaking event in left-right axis determination. Cell. 2005;121(4):633-44.
97. Tabin CJ, Vogan KJ. A two-cilia model for vertebrate left-right axis specification. Genes Dev. 2003;17(1):1-6.

41
CHAPTER

Infective Endocarditis

Ritchie Sharon Solomon

INTRODUCTION

Infective endocarditis (IE) occurs due to microbial infection on the endothelial surface of the heart. Though, there has been a significant advancement in the management of IE over the years, it is still associated with serious complications and morbidity. Native and prosthetic heart valves are common sites of IE. As the endothelial layers of cardiac chambers (atria and ventricles), arterial walls, and heart valves are in direct continuity, parts of mural endocardium may also be involved in IE. Predisposing factors for IE are uncorrected structural cardiac defects, intravenous catheters, implanted cardiac implants/devices, intracardiac patches, and palliative shunts done for complex cyanotic congenital heart diseases (CHDs) apart from immunocompromised hosts and IV substance abusers.

EPIDEMIOLOGY

The annual worldwide incidence of IE is about 3–10 per 100,000 population.[1] In the early antibiotic era, the pattern of disease in high-income countries and low middle-income countries was similar. Over the last three decades, the pattern of disease worldwide has changed. In developed countries such as USA before 1970s, most of the cases with IE had underlying rheumatic heart disease (RHD). As the prevalence of RHD has declined in developed countries over the past two decades, CHD has now become the predominant underlying cause for IE in those regions. Early surgical correction of CHD together with increase in palliative surgeries for complex CHD has enabled better long-term survival and has changed the substrate for IE. Postoperative IE is possible especially in children with palliative surgeries or in presence of residual shunts when prosthetic material is used.[2,3] Advanced neonatal and pediatric intensive care has increased IE in children with structurally normal heart. About 8–10% of children develop IE without any structural heart disease or other easily identifiable risk factors.[4] Degenerative valve disease, diabetes, intravenous drug abuse, and cancer are risk factors in the adult population.

The data on prevalence of IE from developing countries is scarce. Single-center studies in India had shown a decline in RHD being a predisposing factor for IE in children.[5,6] Overall incidence of IE in our country is high amongst the younger population (<40 years) compared to elderly population in developed nations.[7-10] Even in other low- and middle-income countries incidence of IE is high in younger people.[11,12] RHD is the predominant underlying condition for IE in our country[9,10,13] as in other developing countries.[14,15] More than two-thirds of patients have native valve endocarditis (NVE).[13,16] Published Indian data reveal blood culture positivity ranging between 40 and 60%.[9,10,13] Streptococci and staphylococci were the most common microbial organisms isolated.[7,13,16] *Staphylococcus aureus*, coagulase-negative *Staphylococcus* (CONS), *Streptococcus* species (*mitis*, *bovis*, *sanguinis*), and *Enterococcus* are among the most common microbes isolated. Prior antibiotic usage significantly increases the number of culture-negative endocarditis (CNE).[7,9]

RISK FACTORS FOR INFECTIVE ENDOCARDITIS IN CHILDREN

- Unoperated structural CHD:
  - Cyanotic CHD
  - Acyanotic CHD
- Postpalliative surgeries for complex CHD (univentricular heart):
  - Blalock–Taussig shunt
  - Glenn shunt
  - Fontan procedure
- Prosthetic material (postcardiac procedure):
  - Biological (animal heart valves)
  - Nonbiological (valves made of metal alloys/synthetic material)
  - Cardiovascular devices (pacemaker implants, intra-cardiac electrodes, and cardiac stents/conduits)
  - Intracardiac devices used for closure of left-to-right shunts such as atrial septal defect (before endothelialization)
- Residual defects following corrective surgeries for CHD
- Acquired heart disease:
  - RHD

TABLE 1: Risk stratification based on relative risk for endocarditis.

High-risk group	*Moderate-risk group*
Prosthetic valves	Uncorrected atrial septal defect (other than ostium secundum defect)
Complex cyanotic CHD	Uncorrected ventricular septal defect
Palliative systemic artery to pulmonary artery shunts (Blalock–Taussig shunt)	Uncorrected patent ductus arteriosus
Central venous catheters	Bicuspid aortic valve
Previous episode of IE	Rheumatic heart disease
Intravenous drug users	Hypertrophic cardiomyopathy

(CHD: congenital heart disease; IE: infective endocarditis)

Flowchart 1: Pathogenesis for infective endocarditis.

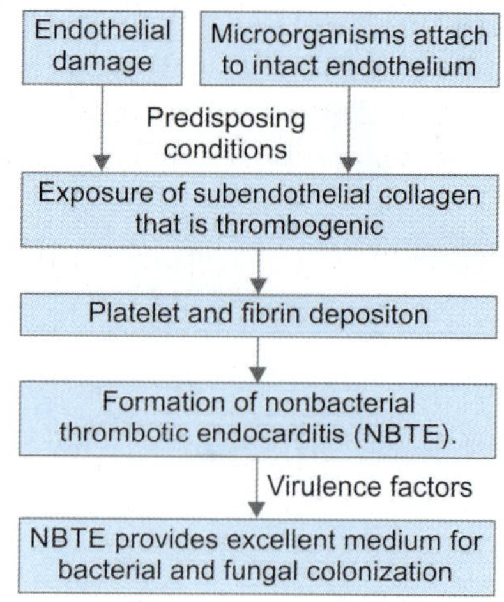

- Mitral valve prolapse
- Connective tissue disorders

- Previous history of IE
- Catheter-related bloodstream infections—central venous lines and umbilical lines
- Prematurity with immune compromise
- Heart transplantation.

The relative risk of having IE can be divided into high-risk and moderate-risk groups as given in **Table 1**. The incidence of IE in the high-risk group is about 300–2,160 cases per 100,000 person-years compared to the moderate risk group where it is about 50 to 440 cases per 100,000 person-year.

ETIOPATHOGENESIS

Formation of Nonbacterial Thrombotic Endocarditis (NBTE)

Pathogenesis of IE involves complex interactions between invading microbes and the host. Development of IE depends on various factors such as cardiac anatomy, immune system of host, vascular endothelium, virulence of microorganisms, and peripheral sources of bacteremia. The concomitant happening of several independent factors that leads to IE are:

- Exposed cardiac endothelium that provides a substrate for microbial adhesion and colonization
- Bacteremia by a microbe that has the qualities of adhesion and colonization in cardiac tissue
- Formation of an infected mass by aggregate of proliferating organism within a protective cover made of fibrin and platelets.

The endothelial layer inside the heart is generally resistant to infection by various microbes except for few virulent microorganisms. Formation of NBTE is the first step and it progresses into IE. The main inciting event is denudation or damage to endothelium, which leads to deposition of fibrin and platelets and subsequent formation of NBTE (**Flowchart 1**). Gross and Friedberg first described NBTE in 1936. Electron microscopic studies of damaged valves in experimental animals injected with bolus of bacteria reveal bacterial adherence to the surface of NBTE within 24 hours. Endothelial damage or interaction of microorganisms with intact endothelium leads to exposure of subendothelial valve collagen. Subsequent fibrin and platelet deposition over the exposed subendothelial area leads to NBTE formation. Endothelial damage may also be due to direct mechanical injury from intracardiac devices or intravascular catheters due to friction effect of the foreign body. Impingement of high velocity jet on the endothelium due to turbulence of blood flow across cardiac defects, stenotic or regurgitant valves leads to denuded endothelium. The combination of fibrin and platelet forms the vegetation. Adhesion of microorganisms to vegetation leads to formation of an infective vegetation. Colonization with bacteria triggers a vicious cycle of endothelial injury and thrombus deposition.

Pathogens causing IE may enter bloodstream from skin, mucosal surfaces, or from focal sites of infection. Entry of microbes through percutaneous cannula, catheters, and contaminated intravenous fluids can lead to bacteremia. IE can occur due to direct infection of an implanted valve or device.

Virulence Factors

Gram-positive cocci express multiple adhesins that enhance their capability to attach to host cell and hence serve as potent virulence factors. Gram-positive cocci also have affinity toward fibronectin in endothelial layer when it is exposed. Microbial surface components recognizing adhesive matrix molecules (MSCRAMMs) are surface adhesin molecules of *S. aureus* that are responsible for attachment of the microorganism to collagen, laminin, fibrinogen, fibronectin, and thrombospondin. These interactions with host proteins are important for adherence to denuded endothelium, bacterial persistence, and engulfment by host cell. *S. aureus* may bind directly or be internalized by endothelial cells. Specific surface proteins such as clumping factor and coagulase enhance binding of *S. aureus* to fibrinogen. There seems to exist a mutual cooperation between binding of fibronectin and fibrinogen in the early steps of pathogenesis in *S. aureus* IE. Proliferation and further persistence of bacteria within mature vegetation is because of another virulence factor called as α-toxin.

Formation of a multilayered aggregate of bacteria made up of proteinaceous matrix and polysaccharide is known as biofilm. Biofilm formation over prosthetic valve/devices enables microbial adherence to its surface, enhances bacterial persistence, and leads to antibiotic tolerance.[17] Biofilm also prevents penetration of host immune cells and antimicrobial agents, thereby reducing its ability to kill microbes.

Dextran, a bacteria-derived extracellular polysaccharide, mediates adherence of oral streptococci to NBTE. FimA (surface protein adhesin),[18] Hsa (sialic acid-binding adhesin), and a phage encoded bacterial adhesin that mediates interaction between platelets, fibrinogen, and bacteria are other virulence factors that probably play a role in streptococcal IE.

Evolution of Vegetation

The size of vegetation increases due to continued bacterial proliferation and platelet–fibrin deposition. Gram-positive cocci strains (staphylococci and streptococci) causing IE are potent stimulators of platelet aggregation and platelet degranulation. Platelet-derived von Willebrand factor (vWF) and vWF receptor play a role in enhancing binding of *S. aureus* to platelets. Bacterial surface antigens in *Streptococcus sanguinis* promote platelet aggregation.

Platelets play a crucial role in enhancing host defenses against proliferation of organisms within vegetation. Platelets engulf the staphylococci into vacuoles that fuse with α-granules that contain platelet microbicidal proteins (PMPs). These antibacterial PMPs are also released inside the vegetation that prevents bacterial proliferation. *S. aureus* virulence is also contributed by its resistance to PMPs. Bacteria that are deep inside the vegetation may have reduction in metabolic activity which may promote its survival against certain antibiotics.

Proinflammatory chemokine response is stimulated once the organisms enter endothelial cells, which causes increase in levels of monocyte chemotactic peptide, interleukin (IL)-6, and IL-8. Amplification of procoagulant cascade happens due to release of tissue thromboplastin once the monocytes enter endothelial cell. This cascade will lead to progression of vegetation and also enhances the antibacterial effects of platelets as mentioned above. Invasion of tissues and formation of abscess are characteristic of IE.

Immunological Response

Cellular and humoral immune responses are both activated in IE. There is production of agglutinating antibodies, complement fixing antibodies, opsonic antibodies, and macroglobulins by the host to combat the microorganism. Rheumatoid factor (RF) develops in many cases after 6 weeks of IE. RF blocks opsonizing activity of IgG, thereby contributing to pathogenesis and may lead to microvascular damage.

Immune complexes are responsible for glomerulonephritis and for some of the peripheral manifestations of IE such as Roth spots and Osler's nodes. These peripheral lesions are probably septic embolic-like phenomenon due to deposition of immune (antigen-antibody) complexes causing acute vasculitis. Response to IE management is characterized by decreasing immune complex titer.

ORAL FLORA IN CHILDREN

Oral mucosa in children contains both pathogenic and nonpathogenic microorganisms. The oral flora in children generally consists of Viridans group of streptococci (VGS), *Haemophilus* species, *Prevotella*, *Actinomyces* species, and *Staphylococcus* species. Periodontal disease causing organisms such as *Capnocytophaga* and *Aggregatibacter actinomycetem comitans* can be found along with others in older children. As the child enters adulthood, there is considerable increase in VGS. Soon after cleaning of tooth surface, there is formation of dental plaque biofilm. Poor dental hygiene leads to a more pathogenic bacterial flora entering the plaque. The plaque bacteria seen in subgingival (gingival cervice) space such as gram-negative and anaerobic species are also present in supragingival areas in children. Plaque formation leads to gingival inflammation. Gingivitis leads to increase in depth of the gingival crevice that is present between the tooth surface and gingival cervicular mucosa. Normally the gingival cervicular mucosa is a protective barrier to bacterial invasion. Routine tooth brushing or minor dental procedures cause transient bacteremia in children with gingivitis. Gingivitis causes thinning and ulceration that increases the possibility of bacteria to enter gingival capillary circulation. Hence, minimal gingival manipulation may lead to bacteremia in children.

Dental procedures are frequently the source for VGS bacteremia. Teeth cleaning, tooth extractions, manipulations of gingiva, and dental injections are associated with variable risks of bacteremia ranging from 0 to 97%.[19] Incidence of bacteremia from daily activities such as tooth brushing far exceeds that of dental office procedures. Children with IE are mostly due to low-grade bacteremia caused by frequent activities of daily living.

MICROBIOLOGICAL PROFILE

Majority of IE in children are caused by Gram-positive cocci (**Table 2**). The most common Gram-positive organisms are VGS group (*Strep. sanguinis*, *Strep. mutans*, and *Strep. mitis*), staphylococci (*S. aureus* and coagulase negative staphylococci—CONS), and β-hemolytic streptococci. *Enterococcus* species causing IE is rare in children.

TABLE 2: Microbes commonly associated with infective endocarditis.

	Microorganism	*Type*
A.	Bacteria	Gram-positive cocci · Staphylococci: – *Staphylococcus aureus* – Coagulase-negative staphylococci—*Staphylococcus epidermidis, Staphylococcus capitis* · Streptococci: – Viridans group - *Streptococcus sanguinis* - *Streptococcus oralis* - *Streptococcus mutans* - *Streptococcus mitis* – Beta-hemolytic streptococci – Nutritionally variant streptococci—Abiotrophia, *Granulicatella* species · *Enterococci*: – *Enterococcus faecalis* · Gram-negative: - *Pseudomonas aeruginosa* - *Escherichia coli* - *HACEK group: Haemophilus, Aggregatibacter, Cardiobacterium, Eikenella corrodens*, and *Kingella*
B.	Fungi	*Candida albicans*, aspergillosis, and histoplasmosis
C.	Atypical	*Coxiella burnetii, Bartonella* species, *Brucella* species, and *Tropheryma whipplei*

Staphylococcus aureus is the most common cause of IE in some series and is definitely the cause for acute endocarditis that is rapidly progressing. *S. aureus* or CONS are frequently associated with IE caused due to prosthetic valves, prosthetic material, and intravascular catheters. Postoperative endocarditis due to *S. aureus* usually manifests within 60 days after cardiac surgery. Postoperative IE due to CONS may present even more than a year after cardiac surgery.

Abiotrophia or *Granulicatella* species generally cause subacute endocarditis mostly in native valves or in postcardiac surgery (>60 days).

Infective endocarditis in neonates is predominantly due to *S. aureus*, CONS, and *Candida* species. Group B *Streptococcus*, *Streptococcus pneumoniae*, and Gram-negative bacilli are rare causes of neonatal IE.

Infective endocarditis in drug abusers in pediatric–adolescent age group is usually due to *S. aureus*.

Fungal endocarditis is quite common in infants and children especially due to central venous infusions with high glucose concentrations and is usually due to *Candida albicans*. Vegetation due to fungus is generally very large, friable, and has a higher propensity for embolization leading to complications.

CLINICAL FEATURES

The clinical presentation is generally acute or subacute/indolent. Acute or rapidly progressing fulminant IE is usually due to *S. aureus* or *Strep. pneumoniae*. In acute IE, children present with high-grade fever and rapidly changing symptoms requiring urgent intervention. Subacute IE is characterized by prolonged low-grade fever, fatigue, myalgia, weight loss, and rigor. Though many findings are nonspecific, presence of this cluster of symptoms should prompt us to evaluate carefully for IE. As the presentation for IE is very diverse and nonspecific, the diagnosis is frequently missed or delayed causing increased morbidity and mortality. IE should be considered as a differential diagnosis in all cases of sepsis or pyrexia of unknown origin in the presence of risk factors. Clinical assessment in suspected cases of IE should include evaluation of risk factors, detailed history, and search for clinical findings. The sensitivity and specificity of any single sign is low and IE should not be excluded on the basis of clinical examination alone.

Clinical findings are generally due to the following phenomena:

- *Bacteremia/fungemia*: Fever, chills, rigors, loss of appetite, fatigue, and malaise
- *Valvulitis*: Valvar regurgitation and congestive cardiac failure
- *Immunological responses*: Arthralgia, Roth spots, Osler's nodes, splinter hemorrhages, petechiae, and microscopic hematuria
- *Embolic phenomenon*: Hemiparesis, hematuria due to renal infarct, splenic infarct, pulmonary embolism, peripheral arterial embolism, and osteomyelitis. Dislodgement of part of vegetation may lead to its lodging in a vascular bed downstream from the heart causing septic embolic manifestation. Bacteria embedded inside the septic emboli can invade neighboring tissues and lead to formation of visceral abscess (e.g., lung abscess).

ORGAN-SPECIFIC MANIFESTATIONS

Cardiac Manifestations

Common sites for vegetation are on the atrial surface of atrioventricular valves, ventricular surface of semilunar

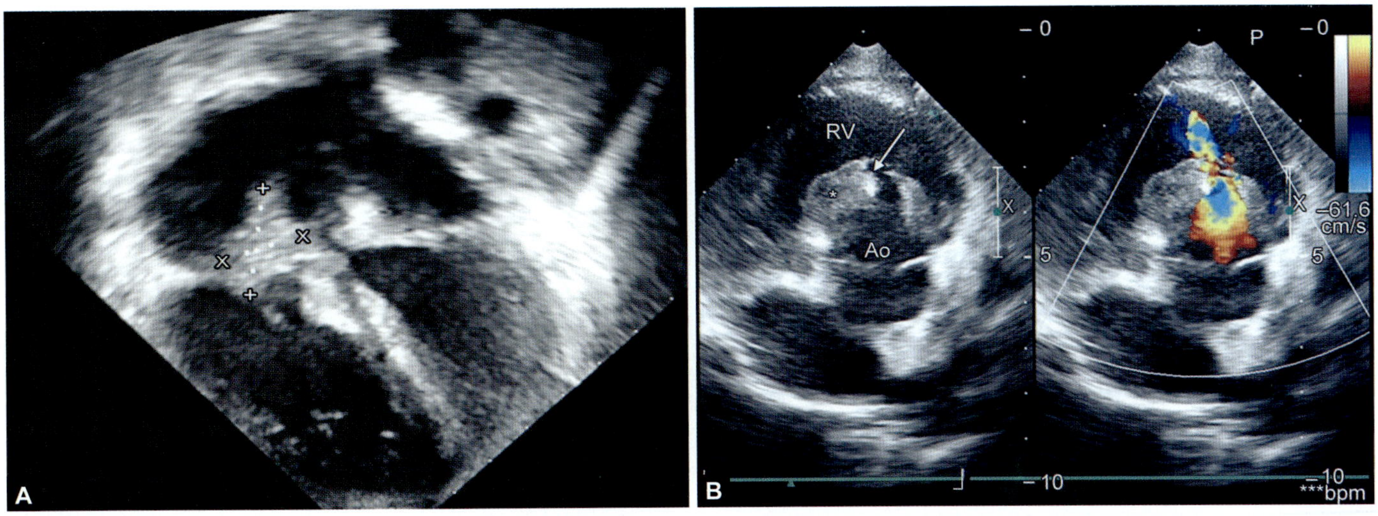

Figs. 1A and B: (A) Vegetation seen attached to tricuspid valve in a neonate with endocarditis. This is demarcated by the cross marks; (B) Infective endocarditis in a patient operated for tetralogy of Fallot. The vegetation (arrow) is on the surgical patch in the vicinity of a site of turbulence resulting from a residual ventricular septal defect.
(Ao: aorta; RV: right ventricle)

valves, and along the line of closure of valve leaflet. Vegetation attached to tricuspid valve in a neonate is seen in **Figure 1A**. Vegetation may lead to destruction and perforation of valve leaflet, rupture of chordae tendinae, or papillary muscle leading to severe valve regurgitation and acute cardiac failure. IE due to *S. aureus* may result in the formation of valve ring abscess with fistula formation into myocardium. Cardiac murmur (new onset) or changing murmur is a common finding and is due to new-onset valve regurgitation. Paravalvular or myocardial extension of infection causes new-onset conduction disease such as first-degree heart block, bundle branch block, or complete heart block. In cyanotic CHD children with a surgically created systemic to pulmonary artery shunt, change in murmur may not be well appreciated. Such children with palliative procedures will have a fall in oxygen saturation due to obstruction to shunt flow by vegetation.

Pulmonary Manifestations

Right-sided IE of tricuspid valve may lead to shower of septic emboli into lungs resulting in septic pulmonary emboli that may cause infarction. Usually, indwelling central venous catheters are the source of infection in right-sided IE. Empyema, pneumonia, and pleural effusion may also be present. Chest radiographs may show wedge-shaped densities in peripheral lung fields.

Neurovascular Manifestations

Infection of arterial wall leads to localized enlargement of arteries (mycotic aneurysm) and may be present in acute IE or may present long after successful treatment for IE. Various causes hypothesized for the formation of these aneurysms are:

- Occlusion of vasa vasorum due to emboli
- Immune complex deposition in arterial wall
- Direct bacterial invasion of arterial wall leading to abscess formation.

Mycotic aneurysms are common at bifurcation points of cerebral vessels and it can happen at any vascular bed. Cerebral aneurysms can be symptomatic, especially when bleeding complications arise. Cerebral emboli will cause stroke. Septic cerebral embolus leads to brain abscess and meningitis.

Splenic Manifestations

Splenomegaly is more commonly found in chronic cases of IE. Splenic infarct/abscess can occur. Splenic abscess tends to produce fever, pain, and leukocytosis.

Skin Manifestations

Various skin findings are as follows:

- Petechiae
- Cutaneous infarcts
- *Osler's nodes*: Characterized by small, raised lesions in pads of fingers and toes that are tender (arteriolar intimal proliferation with extension into venules and capillaries associated with thrombosis and necrosis). Perivascular infiltrates made of monocytes and neutrophils are seen around the dermal vessels. Immune complexes may be found inside the lesions
- *Janeway lesions*: Small, flat erythematous lesions on palms and soles which are nontender.

Ocular Manifestations

Roth spots are retinal hemorrhages with pale central white spot that may be seen. It is an immunological phenomenon seen on fundoscopic evaluation. Fibrin-platelet plugs or lymphocytes surrounded by edema and hemorrhage occur in the nerve fiber layer of retina.

Renal Manifestations

Renal involvement may be in the form of renal infarct due to emboli, renal abscess due to seeding by an embolus, or an immune complex deposit-mediated glomerulonephritis.

COMPLICATIONS OF INFECTIVE ENDOCARDITIS

Tissue disintegration and invasion due to enzymes and toxins released by microbes and the host response causes serious complications.

The children who are at higher risk for complications of IE are those with:

- *S. aureus* IE
- Fungal IE
- Presence of unoperated cyanotic CHD
- Presence of systemic-to-pulmonary shunts
- Left-sided IE
- Presence of prosthetic cardiac valve
- Prolonged clinical symptoms (>3 months)
- Children <2 years of age.

Cardiac Complications

Congestive cardiac failure due to worsening valvular regurgitation, ventricular dysfunction, periannular extension of infection, atrioventricular block, rupture of sinus of Valsalva, obstruction of intracardiac conduits, and pericardial effusion can happen in high-risk cases. Periannular extension of infection, especially of aortic valve IE, can result in the formation of fistulous tracts into pericardium, cardiac chambers, or vascular structures. The tissues destroyed will not regrow and the valvular regurgitation will persist if it is due to bacterial destruction of valve tissue.

Extracardiac Complications

- *Embolic complications*: Emboli in pulmonary, renal, cerebral, or peripheral arteries
- *Central nervous system (CNS)*: Brain abscess, stroke, seizures, and meningitis
- *Mycotic aneurysms*: In systemic or pulmonary arteries
- *Abdomen*: Splenic infarcts, renal infarcts, glomerulonephritis.

DIAGNOSIS

Combination of clinical, microbiological, and echocardiographic evidence is required to diagnose IE. In many resource-limited areas, diagnosis of IE is based on clinical diagnosis of cardiac murmur, embolic manifestation, and immunological vascular phenomenon along with positive blood culture. Presence of risk factors such as indwelling catheters, or prosthetic material in a febrile child should raise the possibility of IE. High index of clinical suspicion is needed especially in a febrile child with a new regurgitant murmur or in presence of CHD.

Blood Culture

It is the most important laboratory test in the diagnosis of IE. Identifying the microorganism responsible for IE is the key to diagnosis and to formulate a treatment plan. Blood cultures should be done before administration of antibiotics. The probability of isolating a microbe is as high as 90% when three sets of blood cultures are done. As bacteremia is continuous and low grade, timing of collection of blood with respect to fever cycle is not necessary. Amount of blood to be drawn depends on the blood culture detection system and is very important for good yield of a positive result.

- *Optimal amount*:
  - *Infants*: 1–3 mL
  - *Older children*: 5–7 mL
- *Number of cultures*:
  - Three blood cultures by separate venipunctures on the first day of admission (1–2 hours interval in severely ill child) and if there is no growth by day 2 of incubation, we should do two or three more blood cultures.
  - Generally there is no value in doing more than five blood cultures in 2 days unless child has previously received antibiotics in last 2 weeks.

In children who have negative blood cultures and not acutely ill, withholding antibiotics for 48 hours and then repeating blood cultures may be done to isolate the organism. Aerobic incubation is usually done, but BACTEC and newer molecular identification methods are more sensitive and yield faster results, compared to conventional methods. When antibiotic therapy has been started before blood collection for culture studies, the rate of obtaining a positive blood culture decreases considerably. The possibility of having fastidious organisms should be borne in mind when blood cultures are negative. Serological analysis and nucleic acid amplification tests (NAATs) should be considered in select cases when blood cultures continue to be negative.

Echocardiography

Echocardiography is the second most important investigation for the diagnosis of IE (*see* **Figs. 1A and B**). Echocardiography is considered the gold standard for assessment of cardiac manifestations of IE. Transthoracic echocardiography (TTE) is generally adequate for assessment in children weighing <60 kg. Transesophageal echocardiography (TEE) will be advantageous in imaging aortic root abscess, IE involving sinus of Valsalva, prosthetic valve endocarditis (PVE), and in paravalvular leak or dehiscence. When TTE images are not of good quality, especially in children with chest deformities or in the presence of intracardiac prosthetic material, TEE should be done. Serial echocardiography is recommended if initial echocardiography is negative but clinical suspicion of IE is high. Serial echocardiography is also important to detect intracardiac complications of vegetation and to plan timely surgical management if necessary, for a successful outcome.

Laboratory Investigations

Complete blood count with analysis of red blood cell indices will reveal anemia (anemia of chronic diseases). Leukocytosis may be present with predominance of immature forms, especially in acute IE. Neonates with IE may present with thrombocytopenia. Acute phase reactants (erythrocyte sedimentation rate and C-reactive protein) will be elevated. Urine microscopy can identify microscopic hematuria. When child has immune complex-mediated glomerulonephritis, renal parameters may be elevated with proteinuria and red blood cell casts in urine along with hematuria. Elevated RF and hypergammaglobulinemia may also occur. Electrocardiogram (ECG) may be useful to identify conduction disorders and ventricular ectopy that are life-threatening complications of IE.

MODIFIED DUKE CRITERIA

The major and minor criteria under Duke Criteria are mentioned in **Table 3**. The application of various criteria for diagnosis of IE is given further.

TABLE 3: Modified Duke criteria.

S. No	*Modified Duke criteria*
	Major criteria
1.	Positive blood culture
	• Typical microorganisms which are consistent for IE in two or more blood cultures taken separately – Viridans group of streptococci (VGS), *Streptococcus bovis*, HACEK group or – Community-acquired *Staphylococcus aureus* or enterococci (when there is no other primary focus) or • Microorganisms which are consistent with IE (persistently positive blood cultures) – At least two or more positive blood cultures (taken >12 hours apart) or – All of the three or majority of ≥4 blood cultures (irrespective of timing) – *Coxiella burnetii* identified in a single blood culture or IgG antiphase-1 antibody titer >1:800
2.	Evidence for endocardial involvement
	• Echocardiography is considered positive if the following are found: – Intracardiac mass on valves or supporting structure or in path of regurgitant jet or on implanted prosthetic material suggestive of vegetation (oscillating) or – Abscess or – Newly detected partial dehiscence of prosthetic valve • New valve regurgitation
	Minor criteria
1.	Predisposing cardiac condition, intravenous drug usage
2.	Fever ≥38°C
3.	*Vascular phenomenon*: Janeway lesions, arterial emboli, intracranial hemorrhage, conjunctival hemorrhage, and septic pulmonary infarcts
4.	*Immunological phenomenon*: Osler nodes, Roth spots, glomerulonephritis, and rheumatoid factor
5.	Positive blood culture that does not meet the major criterion listed above or serological evidence of infection by an organism consistent with IE

(IE: infective endocarditis; IgG: immunoglobulin G)

DEFINITE INFECTIVE ENDOCARDITIS

- *Clinical criteria*:
  - Two major criteria

  or
  - One major criterion + three minor criteria

  or
  - Five minor criteria
- *Pathological criteria*:
  - *Based on microorganisms*: Detected by culture or histology (vegetation/intracardiac abscess)
  - *Based on pathological lesions*: Histologically proven acute IE from vegetation or intracardiac abscess.

POSSIBLE INFECTIVE ENDOCARDITIS

Findings are consistent with IE but do not meet all criteria needed for "definite" IE and cannot come under "rejected" IE.

REJECTED INFECTIVE ENDOCARDITIS

- Resolution of features of IE within 4 days of antibiotic therapy.
- No pathological evidence (at surgery or autopsy) of IE after antibiotic therapy for ≤4 days.
- Firm alternative diagnosis is available for the present manifestations.

DIFFERENTIAL DIAGNOSIS FOR INFECTIVE ENDOCARDITIS

Rheumatic fever, Libman–Sacks endocarditis, and NBTE (marantic endocarditis) are close differential diagnosis for IE. In rheumatic fever, the major presenting features are polyarthritis, chorea, erythema marginatum, and subcutaneous nodules in addition to the presence of carditis. In patients with history suggestive of systemic lupus erythematosus, Libman–Sacks endocarditis may occur. Marantic endocarditis is a sterile vegetation in adults with cancerous growth involving pancreas, colon, or lung. Kawasaki disease may mimic IE. But the predominance of peripheral skin and eye manifestations favor Kawasaki disease. Fever of unknown origin caused by viruses (infectious mononucleosis and cytomegalovirus) and bacteria (*Mycobacterium tuberculosis*, *Listeria monocytogenes*, *Salmonella typhi*, and *Brucella* species) may need to be carefully ruled out whenever modified Duke Criteria are not satisfied in a particular child.

PRINCIPLES IN MANAGEMENT

The treatment of IE in children is similar to that of IE in adults. Multidisciplinary approach involving the pediatrician, infectious disease specialist, cardiologist, and cardiac surgeon is important for good outcomes. When suspicion for IE is high in children who are not severely ill and in whom the blood cultures are persistently negative or when the microorganism isolated is probably a contaminant, it is reasonable to withhold antibiotic therapy for ≥48 hours while blood cultures are repeated. Generally, the course of antimicrobial therapy is 4–6 weeks and bactericidal drugs are preferred. The microorganisms are in high concentration within the platelet-fibrin matrix with low metabolic activity and cell division rate. Due to this reason, there is low susceptibility to β-lactam and other cell wall active antibiotics. Compliance to treatment is very important for a successful outcome. Sometimes outpatient management is necessary due to socioeconomic reasons, but long-term parenteral therapy is always recommended. Antibiotic susceptibility testing will help us in deciding the best regimen of antibiotics. Minimum inhibitory concentrations (MICs) of antibiotics for the pathogen isolated should be known before starting treatment. The treatment protocol should concur with three basic principles namely:

1. Prolonged antibiotic therapy
2. Parenteral antibiotics for full duration of therapy
3. In case of antimicrobial resistance, combination therapy is advised so as to achieve a synergistic effect.

The choice of antimicrobial drug in IE is given in **Tables 4 and 5**. The duration of antimicrobial therapy for various categories is given in **Table 6**.

INDICATIONS FOR SURGERY

The decision toward surgery in IE is always a challenge due to the possibility of acute, life-threatening complications of the disease and comorbidity. Surgery can optimize source control when the infected tissue is removed and it reduces the possible morbidity due to embolic events. Though timely cardiac surgery may be life-saving, it is also associated with significant risk for the child as most of them are extremely sick with multiorgan dysfunction. In stable children, surgery is best delayed until antibiotics are completed to decrease the risk of perioperative complications and early PVE. Early surgical intervention in certain situations (patients with hemodynamic instability or perivalvular complications) will greatly improve the outcomes in IE. Surgery may have to be considered in the following conditions:

- *Vegetation*:
  - Persistent vegetation, especially in anterior mitral leaflet, measuring >10 mm
  - One or more embolic events during first 2 weeks of antimicrobial therapy
  - Increase in size of vegetation after 4 weeks of antibiotics
  - Fungal endocarditis
  - Infected prosthetic materials—Gor-Tex, Dacron, and homografts
- *Perivalvular extension*:
  - Valvular rupture and dehiscence
  - Acute-onset atrioventricular block
  - Large abscess or its extension
- *Valvular dysfunction*:
  - Severe aortic/mitral valve regurgitation
  - Congestive cardiac failure

Surgical mortality for IE in children is about 15%, with the risk factors for death being age <1 year, prematurity, and fungal IE.[20] Early surgical intervention in staphylococcal

TABLE 4: Empirical antibiotic therapy in infective endocarditis (IE).

Type of IE	*Antibiotic therapy*	*Alternative drug therapy*
Not severely ill child: Unknown microbe • Initial empirical therapy (blood culture report—not known) or • Culture-negative endocarditis after 48 hours of blood cultures		
Native valve IE *or* Late prosthetic valve IE (PVE)—1 year after surgery	Ampicillin/sulbactam (200–300 mg/kg/day divided every 4–6 hours) + Gentamicin (3–6 mg/kg/day divided every 8 hours) *with or without* Vancomycin (60 mg/kg/day divided every 6 hours) For PVE—add rifampicin (15–20 mg/kg/day divided every 12 hours)	Vancomycin (60 mg/kg/day divided every 6 hours) + Gentamicin (3–6 mg/kg/day divided every 8 hours)
Nosocomial IE associated with vascular cannulae *or* Early prosthetic valve IE (PVE)—≤1 year after surgery	Vancomycin (60 mg/kg/day divided every 6 hours) + Gentamicin (3–6 mg/kg/day divided every 8 hours) + Cefepime (100–150 mg/kg/day divided every 8–12 hours) *Or* Ceftazidime (100–150 mg/kg/day divided every 8 hours) Add rifampicin (20 mg/kg/day divided every 8 hours) if prosthetic material is present	

TABLE 5: Choice of antimicrobial therapy based on microorganisms causing infective endocarditis (IE).

Type of organism in IE	*Antibiotic therapy*	*Alternative drug therapy*
Streptococci		
Highly susceptible to penicillin G (MBC ≤0.1 μg/mL) Viridans streptococci, group A, B, C, G Group D streptococci (*Strep. bovis* and *Strep. equinus*)	Penicillin G (2–3 lakh U/kg/day divided every 4 hours) Or Ceftriaxone 100 mg/kg/day divided every 12 hours	Vancomycin (40 mg/kg/day divided every 8–12 hours) Or Cefazolin (100 mg/kg/day divided every 8 hours) Or Ceftriaxone (100 mg/kg/day divided every 12 hours)
Relatively resistant to penicillin (MBC ≥0.2 μg/mL Viridans streptococci (less susceptible) Enterococci	Penicillin G (2–3 lakh U/kg/day divided every 4 hours) Or Ampicillin (200–300 mg/kg/day divided every 4–6 hours) + Gentamicin (3–6 mg/kg/day divided every 8 hours) × 2 weeks (gentamicin—for whole course in enterococcal IE)	Enterococci: Vancomycin (40 mg/kg/day divided every 8–12 hours) + Gentamicin (3–6 mg/kg/day divided every 8 hours) Enterococci: Aminoglycoside-resistant/ contraindicated- Ampicillin (200–300 mg/kg/day divided every 4–6 hours) + Ceftriaxone (100 mg/kg/day divided every 12 hours) *Other than enterococcal IE:* Ceftriaxone (100 mg/kg/day divided every 12 hours) + Gentamicin (3–6 mg/kg/day divided every 8 hours)
**Staphylococci: S. aureus or coagulase-negative staphylococci*		
Susceptible to ≤1 μg/mL penicillin G (rare)	Penicillin G (2–3 lakh U/kg/day divided every 4 hours)	Oxacillin (200 mg/kg/day divided every 4–6 hours) Or Nafcillin (200 mg/kg/day divided every 4–6 hours) Or Cefazolin (100 mg/kg/day divided every 8 hours) Or Vancomycin (40 mg/kg/day divided every 8–12 hours)
Resistant to 0.1 μg/mL penicillin G	Oxacillin or nafcillin (200 mg/kg/day divided every 4–6 hours) +/– Gentamicin (3–6 mg/kg/day divided every 8 hours) × 3–5 days	Cefazolin (100 mg/kg/day divided every 8 hours) Or Vancomycin (40 mg/kg/day divided every 8–12 hours)—for those allergic to β-lactam antibiotics
Resistant to 4 μg/mL oxacillin (MRSA)	Vancomycin (40 mg/kg/day divided every 8–12 hours)	Daptomycin 6 mg/kg every 24 hours [illegible] mg/kg
Vancomycin resistant	Daptomycin 6 mg/kg every 24 hours <6 years: 10 mg/kg	
*When prosthetic material is present in staphylococcal IE, add rifampicin and gentamicin for initial 2 weeks.		
Gram-negative Enteric Bacilli		
	Ceftazidime (100–150 mg/kg/day divided every 8 hours) Or Cefotaxime (200 mg/kg/day divided every 6 hours Or Ceftriaxone100 mg/kg/day divided every 12 hours Or Cefepime (100–150 mg/kg/day divided every 8–12 hours) + Gentamicin (3–6 mg/kg/day divided every 8 hours) Or Tobramycin (3–6 mg/kg/day divided every 8 hours) Or Amikacin (15 mg/kg/day divided every 8–12 hours)	Piperacillin/Tazobactam 240 mg/kg/day divided every 8 hours) + Gentamicin (3–6 mg/kg/day divided every 8 hours) Or Tobramycin (3–6 mg/kg/day divided every 8 hours) Or Amikacin (15 mg/kg/day divided every 8–12 hours)

Contd...

Contd...

Type of organism in IE	*Antibiotic therapy*	*Alternative drug therapy*
HACEK Group		
	Ceftriaxone (100 mg/kg/day divided every 12 hours) Or Cefotaxime (200 mg/kg/day divided every 6 hours) Or Ampicillin–sulbactam (200–300 mg/kg/day divided every 4–6 hours)	Ampicillin (200–300 mg/kg/day divided every 4–6 hours)—if susceptible + Gentamicin (3–6 mg/kg/day divided every 8 hours) Or Tobramycin (3–6 mg/kg/day divided every 8 hours) Or Amikacin (15 mg/kg/day divided every 8–12 hours)
Fungal IE (Candida species and Aspergillus species)		
	Surgical resection + Amphotericin B (1 mg/kg/day) given over 3–4 hours Or Amphotericin liposomal/lipid associated (3–5 mg/kg/day in a single dose) +/- Flucytosine (150 mg/kg/day divided every 6 hours)	When surgery cannot be done - Amphotericin B followed by imidazole (e.g., itraconazole, fluconazole, voriconazole) for suppression Amphotericin B (1 mg/kg/day) given over 3–4 hours Or Amphotericin liposomal/lipid associated (3–5 mg/kg/day in a single dose)

HACEK group: *Haemophilus, Aggregatibacter, Cardiobacterium, Eikenella corrodens*, and *Kingella* species

MBC: Minimum bactericidal concentration

MRSA: Methicillin-resistant *Staphylococcus aureus*

- Therapy is generally for 4–6 weeks unless mentioned near the drug.
- Longer duration of therapy may be needed for PVE, recurrent IE, IE due to uncommon species, and fungal endocarditis. Dosages for neonates and infants are not included.

TABLE 6: Duration of antimicrobial therapy for infective endocarditis (IE).

Type of IE	*Duration (weeks)*
Native valve IE (oxacillin-susceptible staphylococci)	4–6
Native valve IE (oxacillin-resistant staphylococci)	6
Prosthetic valve IE (staphylococci)	6
Native valve IE (Highly susceptible streptococci)	4
Native valve IE (Relatively resistant streptococci)	4
Prosthetic material present and caused by Viridans streptococci or *Streptococcus bovis*	6
Native/prosthetic valve IE (*Enterococcus*)	4–6
Native/prosthetic valve IE (*Enterococcus*—treated with vancomycin)	6
Enteric Gram-negative endocarditis	6
Native/prosthetic valve IE (HACEK group)	4
Culture-negative endocarditis (Native valve)	4–6
Culture-negative endocarditis (Prosthetic valve)	6

(HACEK: *Haemophilus, Aggregatibacter, Cardiobacterium, Eikenella corrodens*, and *Kingella*)

IE may decrease the risk of abscess formation and embolization.[21] Surgery for IE in India is not that common due to scarce resources and lack of affordability for cardiac surgery.[22]

CHALLENGING SITUATIONS IN MANAGEMENT OF INFECTIVE ENDOCARDITIS

Partially-treated Infective Endocarditis

Antibiotic therapy initiated before obtaining blood culture reduces the recovery rate of the bacteria by 35–40%. It is one of the important causes for CNE. If the children are hemodynamically stable, stoppage of antibiotics for >48 hours may yield a positive blood culture report. Blood culture report is vital in rapid and accurate diagnosis of IE. Delayed diagnosis leads to delay in the initiation of therapy that may lead to progression of infection, complications, and bad outcomes. One-third of patients who subsequently have IE were labeled as possible IE due to doubtful or negative findings on echocardiography or blood cultures.

Culture-negative Endocarditis

Diagnosis of CNE is made when the blood cultures are persistently negative, though the child has clinical or echocardiographic features of IE. Incidence of CNE in developed countries is around 5%. The common causes for CNE are as follows:

- Recent antibiotic usage
- Organisms that grow poorly in vitro—HACEK (*Haemophilus, Aggregatibacter, Cardiobacterium, Eikenella corrodens*, and *Kingella*) group

- *Fastidious organisms*: *Granulicatella* and *Abiotrophia*
- *Other rare microbes*: *Coxiella burnetii*, *Tropheryma whipplei*, *Brucella* species, *Bartonella* species, and *Mycoplasma* species.

Diagnosis of fungal endocarditis by blood culture is difficult in many cases due to very low or no sensitivity for yeast and filamentous fungi, respectively.

How to proceed in CNE?

In children who are currently receiving antibiotics, if duration of antibiotic usage is for <4 days, stoppage of antibiotic therapy may be useful in yielding a positive blood culture after a few days. Other microbiological testing methodologies that can be tried in CNE are listed below.

- *Serological tests*: Detection of serum antibodies against specific pathogens.

  It is useful to diagnose IE due to *Coxiella burnetti*, *Bartonella* species, *Brucella* species, *Mycoplasma*, and *Legionella pneumophila*.
- *Histopathology*: Examination of resected vegetation or valves using special stains is beneficial in IE due to *T. whipplei*, *C. burnetii*, and *Bartonella* species.
- *Polymerase chain reaction (PCR)*: Amplification of 16S ribosomal DNA for bacteria or 18S ribosomal DNA for fungi and later sequencing will lead to pathogen identification. Pathogens that may be identified by this technique are streptococci, staphylococci, *T. whipplei*, and *C. burnetii*.
- *Immunohistology*: Specific monoclonal or polyclonal antibodies will help in detecting antigen in valve tissues. This technique is useful in IE caused by *Bartonella* species, *T. whipplei*, and *C. burnetii*.

Examination of surgical materials such as valves, vegetations by conventional culture techniques may yield false positive results in 13–55% cases. NAATs such as PCR may be helpful in such specimens. Better specificity of test results is obtained when culture based testing methods are supplemented by histological examination of tissues or molecular methods.

EARLY POSTOPERATIVE INFECTIVE ENDOCARDITIS

Prosthetic valve endocarditis is highest within 12 months of surgery and its incidence is around 1.4–3.1%.[23] Most of the studies consider that IE occurring within a year of surgery to be considered as early PVE. Some authors use 60 days as the cut off time to define early PVE. Early PVE is due to infection acquired in the perioperative period (inside the operating theater or in the postoperative intensive care period). Most of the PVE cases happen within 4 months of cardiac surgery. Late PVE (>1 year after surgery) is usually community acquired and the microbiological profile also is similar to NVE. CONS, *S. aureus*, and Gram-negative bacilli infections are the most common organisms causing early PVE. Current guidelines recommend empirical therapy for early PVE and culture-negative cases with a combination of vancomycin, gentamicin, rifampicin, and cefepime in view of the high possibility of methicillin-resistant *S. aureus*. Linezolid or quinupristin/dalfopristin may be used when vancomycin is not tolerated or in vancomycin-resistant enterococci. Though prolonged antibiotic therapy is needed in most of the cases, successful outcomes may need surgical removal of infected material. Rifampicin is considered mainly in staphylococcal PVE as it has good tissue penetration. Early valvular operations may be needed in the management of early PVE for improved survival. Mechanical prosthesis has higher risk of early PVE especially within 3 months of surgery compared to bioprosthesis. Infection of mechanical valves is usually in the junction between annulus and the sewing ring. Bioprosthetic valve infection usually is localized to the leaflets causing rupture or perforation. Allografts lack prosthetic material and incidence for early PVE is very low. Surgically created intracardiac conduits or shunts involve prosthetic material such as Dacron, Gore-Tex, or homografts and hence they have very high propensity for the development of IE. Presence of vegetation at these sites may lead to obstruction, dehiscence, or embolization distally. Removal of the infected patch/device/implant or pacemaker along with antibiotic therapy is preferred in cases of postoperative IE.

Cardiac Implantable Electronic Devices-related Infective Endocarditis

Infection of cardiac implantable electronic devices (CIEDs) is associated with high mortality. CIEDs include permanent pacemakers and implantable cardioverter defibrillators (ICDs). Local device infection is limited only to the pocket of the cardiac device and is suspected when there are local signs of inflammation. Cardiac device-related infective endocarditis (CDRIE) is said to be present when the infection extends into the electrode leads, cardiac valves, and endocardial surface. Pocket infection may extend along the electrodes to involve the intracardiac portion of pacemaker or ICD. Hematogenous seeding during bacteremia may also occur. *Staphylococci* and more specifically CONS are responsible for most of the cases. Management includes complete removal of hardware and prolonged antibiotic therapy.

Fungal Endocarditis

Management of fungal IE is difficult and mortality may be as high as 50%.[24] Except in neonates, medical therapy in fungal IE is usually unsuccessful and surgery is needed in most cases. Immunocompromised children, presence of indwelling central catheters, preterm babies, and children with prosthetic valves are predisposed to develop fungal IE. Nearly two-thirds of the cases are due to *Candida* species. The first-line antifungal agent is amphotericin B, though it

TABLE 7: Antibiotic regimens for endocarditis prophylaxis.

	Drug	Route	Dosage (single dose 30–60 minutes before procedure)
Standard oral prophylaxis	Amoxicillin	Oral	50 mg/kg
Unable to take orally	Ampicillin Or Cefazolin Or Ceftriaxone	IM/IV IM/IV IM/IV	50 mg/kg 50 mg/kg 50 mg/kg
Allergic to penicillin	Clindamycin Or Cephalexin Or Azithromycin/Clarithromycin	Oral Oral Oral	20 mg/kg 50 mg/kg 15 mg/kg
Allergic to penicillin and unable to take orally	Clindamycin Or Cefazolin	IV IM/IV	20 mg/kg 50 mg/kg

does not completely penetrate the vegetation. Imidazoles such as fluconazole have been recommended for suppressive therapy for a prolonged time period, extending for years if needed, whenever curative surgery is not done. Liposomal forms of amphotericin B may be used in children with renal impairment with serum potassium monitoring.

PREVENTION OF INFECTIVE ENDOCARDITIS AND PROPHYLAXIS RECOMMENDATIONS

As the morbidity and mortality associated with IE is quite high, any method that can prevent the disease from occurring is desirable. Corrective surgical procedures for cardiac defects and decreasing the possibility of bacteremia can prevent IE. Most instances of IE cannot be attributed to the antecedent invasive procedure. The likelihood of activities of daily living such as brushing of teeth and chewing causing bacteremia is quite common. Hence, American Heart Association (AHA), European Society of Cardiology (ESC), and National Institute for Health and Clinical Excellence (NICE) have recommended changes in previous existing IE prophylaxis guidelines for invasive procedures. AHA and ESC groups have recommended restricted recommendation for routine IE prophylaxis, whereas NICE group have completely eliminated routine IE prophylaxis. As per AHA guidelines, IE prophylaxis is to be given to individuals with cardiac conditions that are associated with the highest risk of adverse outcomes from IE. IE prophylaxis is recommended for following group of patients (AHA 2007 guidelines):

- Prosthetic cardiac valve
- Unoperated cyanotic CHD
- Surgeries done in complex cyanotic CHD (palliative shunts and conduits)
- Prosthetic material/device implanted inside heart (for 6 months postprocedure)
- Residual defects following corrective surgery for CHD
- Heart transplants
- Previous IE.

Infective endocarditis prophylaxis is to be given only for dental procedures that involve perforation of oral mucosa or manipulation of gingival tissue/periapical region of teeth. IE prophylaxis is not advised for removal of orthodontic appliances, placement of orthodontic brackets, bleeding from lips/oral mucosa, or shedding of deciduous teeth. Routine IE prophylaxis for procedures involving respiratory tract (upper/lower), gastrointestinal tract (upper/lower), or genitourinary tract is not recommended by any group. The recommended antibiotic prophylaxis as per AHA is given in **Table 7**.

Poor oral hygiene leading to periodontal or periapical infections may produce bacteremia even in the absence of dental procedures. Hence, caregivers of children who are susceptible for IE should be educated on the need to maintain good oral hygiene that will go a long way in preventing endocarditis.

CONCLUSION

Changes in epidemiological profile of IE in recent decades due to improved treatment outcomes for CHD has generated a new group of at-risk patients. With advanced pediatric and neonatal intensive care, strategies to minimize iatrogenic bacteremia will reduce the incidence of IE. As the classical signs of IE are often absent in children, a high index of suspicion is essential in children at high risk for early diagnosis and appropriate management.

REFERENCES

1. Murdoch DR, Corey GR, Hoen B, Miró JM, Fowler Jr VG, Bayer AS, et al. Clinical presentation, etiology, and outcome of infective endocarditis in the 21st century: the International Collaboration on Endocarditis-Prospective Cohort Study. Arch Intern Med. 2009; 169(5):463-73.

2. Morris CD, Reller MD, Menashe VD. Thirty-year incidence of infective endocarditis after surgery for congenital heart defect. JAMA. 1998;279(8):599-603.
3. Johnson JA, Boyce TG, Cetta F, Steckelberg JM, Johnson JN. Infective endocarditis in the pediatric patient: a 60-year single-institution review. Mayo Clin Proc. 2012;87(7):629-35.
4. Stockheim JA, Chadwick EG, Kessler S, Amer M, Abdel-Haq N, Dajani AS, et al. Are the Duke criteria superior to the Beth Israel criteria for the diagnosis of infective endocarditis in children? Clin Infect Dis. 1998;27(6):1451-6.
5. Dhawan A, Grover A, Marwaha RK, Khattri HN, Anand IS, Kumar L, et al. Infective endocarditis in children: profile in a developing country. Ann Trop Paediatr. 1993;13(2):189-94.
6. Bhandari S, Kaul U, Shrivastava S, Tandon R, Bhatia ML. Infective endocarditis in children. Indian J Pediatr. 1984;51:529-32.
7. Jain SR, Prajapati JS, Phasalkar MA, Roy BH, Jayram AA, Shah SR, et al. Clinical spectrum of infective endocarditis in a tertiary care centre in western India: a prospective study. IJCM 2014;5(5): 177-87.
8. Math RS, Sharma G, Kothari SS, Kalaivani M, Saxena A, Kumar AS, et al. Prospective study of infective endocarditis from a developing country. Am Heart J. 2011;162(4):633-8.
9. Garg N, Kandpal B, Garg N, Tewari S, Kapoor A, Goel P, et al. Characteristics of infective endocarditis in a developing country-clinical profile and outcome in 192 Indian patients, 1992–2001. Int J Cardiol 2005;98(2):253-60.
10. Choudhury R, Grover A, Varma J, Khattri HN, Anand IS, Bidwai PS, et al. Active infective endocarditis observed in an Indian hospital 1981-1991. Am J Cardiol 1992;70(18):1453-8.
11. Khan NU, Farman MT, Sial JA, Achakzai AS, Saghir T, Ishaq M. Changing trends of infective endocarditis. J Pak Med Assoc. 2010;60(1):24-7.
12. Tariq M, Alam M, Munir G, Khan MA, Smego RA. Infective endocarditis: a five Year experience at a tertiary care hospital in Pakistan. Int J Infect Dis. 2004;8(3):163-70.
13. Padmaja K, Sudhaharan S, Vemu L, Satish OS, Chavali P, Neeraja M. Clinicomicrobiological spectrum of infective endocarditis—from a tertiary care centre in south India. Iran J Microbiol. 2017;9(5):257-63.
14. Tuğcu A, Yildirimtürk O, Baytaroğlu C, Kurtoğlu H, Köse O, Sener M, et al. Clinical spectrum, presentation, and risk factors for mortality in infective endocarditis: a review of 68 cases at a tertiary care center in Turkey. Turk Kardiyol Dern Ars. 2009;37(1):9-18.
15. Nunes MC, Gelape CL, Ferrari TC. Profile of infective endocarditis at a tertiary care center in Brazil during a seven-year period: prognostic factors and in-hospital outcome. Int J Infect Dis. 2010;14(5):e394-8.
16. Gupta A, Gupta A, Kaul U, Varma A. Infective endocarditis in an Indian setup: Are we entering the 'modern' era? Indian J Crit Care Med. 2013;17(3):140-7.
17. Flemming HC, Wingender J. The biofilm matrix. Nat Rev Microbiol. 2010;8(9):623-33.
18. Burnette-Curley D, Wells V, Viscount H, Munro CL, Fenno JC, Fives-Taylor P, et al. FimA, a major virulence factor associated with Streptococcus parasanguis endocarditis. Infect Immun. 1995; 63(12):4669-74.
19. Baltimore RS, Gewitz M, Baddour LM, Beerman LB, Jackson MA, Lockhart PB, et al. Infective endocarditis in childhood: 2015 update: a scientific statement from the American Heart Association. Circulation. 2015;132(15):1487-515.
20. Russell HM, Johnson SL, Wurlitzer KC, Backer CL. Outcomes of surgical therapy for infective endocarditis in a pediatric population: a 21-year review. Ann Thorac Surg. 2013;96(1):171-5.
21. Shamszad P, Khan MS, Rossano JW, Fraser CD Jr. Early surgical therapy of infective endocarditis in children: a 15-year experience. J Thorac Cardiovasc Surg. 2013;146(3):506-11.
22. Kothari SS, Ramakrishnan S, Bahl VK. Infective endocarditis—an Indian perspective. Indian Heart J. 2005;57(4):289-94.
23. Chastre J, Trouillet JL. Early infective endocarditis on prosthetic valves. Eur Heart J. 1995;16 Suppl B:32-8.
24. Tissieres P, Jaeggi ET, Beghetti M, Gervaix A. Increase of fungal endocarditis in children. Infection. 2005;33:267–72.

42

CHAPTER

Rheumatic Fever and Rheumatic Heart Disease

M Zulfikar Ahamed

ACUTE RHEUMATIC FEVER

INTRODUCTION

Rheumatic fever (RF) is a disease of children which licks the joints, bites the heart and stings the brain. The bite on the heart may be very severe and that is what makes us afraid of RF. It is the delayed, nonsuppurative sequela of upper respiratory tract infection by group A beta-hemolytic streptococci (GABHS), which can be often recurrent.[1] It's link to the preceding streptococcal infection of the throat is well defined in the statement "*The chain that links the throat to heart*". The first episode of RF needs to be distinguished from episodes and relapses (**Box 1**).

Though its incidence has declined in many parts of the world, it still continues to remain as a major public health problem along with rheumatic heart disease (RHD) in India and other low- and middle-income nations, especially in the young.[2] Acute RF is also one of the challenging diseases where accurate diagnosis still eludes the clinician sometimes. This is particularly true recently when many trainees have less exposure to RF/RHD during their training years.

HISTORICAL PERSPECTIVE

The first description of RHD probably derives from Vieussens who did the first autopsies of valvular lesions in 1715. "*Rheumatism*" as a term was coined by Baillie in 1797. Pitcain in 18th century discerned a link between acute rheumatism and heart disease and in 1812 Wells published his treatise on "Rheumatism of the Heart". Latham in the early 19th century described rheumatic endocarditis and pericarditis.

BOX 1: Rheumatic fever: recurrence, relapse, and rebound.

- *Recurrence*: A new episode of RF following another group A beta-hemolytic streptococci (GABHS) infection occurring 8 weeks after stopping treatment
- *Rebound*: Manifestations of RF occurring within 4–6 weeks of stopping therapy or on tapering drugs
- *Relapse*: Worsening of RF while under treatment and often with carditis

The hallmark article, which clearly defined "pancarditis" concept in RF, was by Bouillard who is considered the father of RF/RHD.[3] In India, the first description of RF/RHD came in 1938 by Stolt. Sujoy Roy from India is credited with coining the term "juvenile mitral stenosis (MS)".[4]

History of RF/RHD in the 20th century is punctuated by experience from sanatoria treatment in the United States of America and the United Kingdom in the prepenicillin era and use of steroids and penicillin in the treatment in the 2nd half of the century (**Table 1**). The year 1944 saw the first T Duckett Jones criteria for diagnosis of RF, which was later adopted by the American Heart Association (AHA) and was revised several times, last of which was in 2015.[4] The year 2002 saw a new WHO perspective on RF and its diagnosis, which reinforced the application of 1992 Jones criteria. World Heart Federation (2012) has recently outlined the echocardiographic criteria of RF/RHD.[5] The recent revision of T Duckett Jones criteria by AHA appeared in 2015, and this has brought in important changes in how we make a diagnosis of RF.[6]

GENERAL EPIDEMIOLOGY OF ACUTE RHEUMATIC FEVER

Incidence of RF, Prevalence of RHD, and Disease Burden

It is estimated that 3 of 1000 children who get streptococcal throat infection will develop RF. During an epidemic, this attack rate may go up to 3/100, possibly due to increased virulence of bacteria. Global prevalence of RF/RHD varies appreciably and ranges from 14/1,000 to 0.04/1,000. In the USA, prevalence is 2/100,000. In India, it ranges from 0.9/1,000 to 6.4/1,000. Globally 500,000 children get RF annually and the total burden of RF/RHD is 15–20 million.[2] A conservative estimate puts the figure of total RF/RHD burden in India as 1–2 million and the incidence, approximately 50,000 per year.[7] In Kerala, the prevalence of RHD is approximately be

TABLE 1: Historical landmarks of rheumatic fever and rheumatic heart disease.

Year	*Landmark*	*Credit*
1797	"Rheumatism"	Baillie
1790s	Link between rheumatism and heart disease	Pitcain
1812	Treatise on rheumatism of the heart	Wells
1850s	Endocarditis/Pericarditis in acute rheumatism	Latham
1860s	Pancarditis in rheumatic fever	Bouillard
1886	Acute rheumatic fever	Cheadle
1904	Aschoff nodule	Aschoff
1931	Link between rheumatic fever and streptococcal infection	Coburn
1935	First clinical rheumatic fever in India	Wig
1938	First autopsy in rheumatic heart disease in India	Stolt
1938	Secondary prophylaxis with sulfadiazine	Coburn
1944	Jones Criteria	Duckett Jones
1949	Steroids in rheumatic carditis	Kendall, Hench, Reichstein
1951	Primary prophylaxis	Wannamaker
1951	Secondary prophylaxis	Stollerman
2015	Latest revision of the guidelines for diagnosis of rheumatic fever	American Heart Association

TABLE 2: Rheumatic heart disease prevalence studies in India.[7]

Year	*Agency*	*Rate*
1972	Berry	2/1,000
1972–75	Indian Council of Medical Research	2.2–11.0/1,000
1981	Koshy	4.9/1,000
1991	KS Reddy	1.8/1,000
1995	Padmavathi	1–5.4/1,000
2002	Amrita Institute of Medical Sciences	0.05/1,000

around 1/1,000 and there is a perception that the number of cases of RF reporting to hospitals is declining (**Table 2**). However, RF is second only to Kawasaki disease as the cause of acquired heart disease in children even in Kerala. Even after the near elimination of RF in the United States of America, there have been resurgences, which probably indicates that there may be a cyclic fall and rise in RF in developed nations also.[8]

The current Indian Council of Medical Research (ICMR) data collected from various parts of India during 2000–2010 suggests that the prevalence of RHD may range from 0.05/1,000 to 2.2/1,000.[7]

Epidemiological Triad of Rheumatic Fever

Agent

Only *GABHS* is responsible for RF even though group G and C can cause throat infection. While the basis of "rheumatogenicity" of GABHS is not clearly understood, some strains are thought to be capable of inducing RF and some are not.[1] Cardiac virulence may be related to the strain. Skin infection by streptococci generally does not cause RF. This could be due to:

- Low intensity antibody response
- Neutralization of streptococcal antibodies by skin lipids
- The skin pathogens may not be rheumatogenic.

However, repeated skin infection may amplify the immune response to GABHS infection of the throat, especially in tropical countries. Skin infection is not ruled out as a cause of RF in Australian studies.[9]

Host

Rheumatic fever occurs commonly between 5 and 15 years and is a disease of school children. It is rare before 5 years and virtually unheard of below 3 years. The first attack of RF may occur as late as 30 years and recurrence as late as 40 years. The male-female ratio is nearly equal even though there is a female predominance among RHD patients. RF bites the heart at a young age and maims it during young adulthood.

Familial clustering of RF may point to either an environmental factor or genetic factor. Many studies have shown that certain human leukocyte antigen (HLA) types have been linked to RF, e.g., DR4, DR3, DR1, and DW10. DR3 is the common antigen found in Indian children. The genetic susceptibility has also been highlighted by the presence of B-cell alloantigen in children with RF/RHD. Recently, genome-wide association studies (GWAS) suggest

HLA-DQA1 to HLA-DQB1 region, but also the immunoglobulin heavy chain locus, including the IGHV4-61 gene segment, on chromosome 14 as a possible basis for susceptibility to RF.[10]

Environment

Overcrowding, lack of sanitation, and poverty have been implicated as predisposing factors. Globally as well as in India RF still remains as a disease of the poorest and the marginalized.[7] Climatic and seasonal variations are not distinct in India unlike in the temperate regions, where RF is more common in the spring.

Disease Trends

The prevalence of RHD and incidence of RF have noticeably declined in many parts of the world. Much of the decline in RHD prevalence appears to have resulted from a general improvement in health care and human development indices[11] (**Box 2**). Indeed, like many other diseases such as tuberculosis, measles, malaria, RHD burden largely mirrors overall human development in any given region. Over the years, RHD is largely become confined to the poorest and most marginalized populations of the world.

PATHOGENESIS OF RHEUMATIC FEVER

The currently accepted theory of genesis of RF is that of immune mimicry, by which, it is proposed that certain streptococcal antigens share immunological properties of heart valves and cell membrane and antibodies produced against streptococcal antigens cross-react with cardiac and other tissues producing damage (**Flowchart 1**). Tissue inflammation occurs mostly in the heart, synovial membrane, and subcutaneous tissue and in brain. Both cell-mediated immunity and humoral-mediated immunity are involved. Initial valve insult could be antibody mediated. Both CD4 and CD8 cells participate. CD4 cells breach endothelial integrity and caused subendocardial damage. This leads to both carditis and RHD. In the heart, the inflammation essentially involves all the three layers: (1) endocardium, (2) myocardium, and (3) pericardium. This is called pancarditis. And yet the principal target is endocardium. Clinical evidence of myocardial element is rather scarce, cell necrosis is rare and troponin T is negative; however, interstitial myocarditis is found in endomyocardial biopsy.[1]

There are three phases of RF process. The first is the exudative phase that lasts 2–3 weeks. This is followed by the proliferative phase that lasts a few months. Finally, the fibrotic phase that happens over months to years. The exudative phase is influenced by nonsteroidal anti-inflammatory drugs (NSAIDs) and steroids and proliferative phase is possibly influenced by steroids. No drug influences the fibrotic/scarring phase. The biotransformation from exudative and proliferative phases to fibrotic phase may be helped by T-cell products. Hence, there is a belief that acute RF is predominantly caused by B-cell activity and RHD is possibly influenced and mediated by T-cell immunity.[1] In carditis, antiheart, antimyosin, antitropomyosin, and antilaminin antibodies are produced. Antisynovium and antivimentin antibodies are produced in arthritis. Skin and keratin antibodies are produced in erythema marginatum and subcutaneous nodules. In Chorea, antibodies are perhaps targeted against neuronal epitopes in the basal ganglia.

BOX 2: Rheumatic fever—possible causes of decline.

- Improved environmental and social conditions
- Increased antibiotic use in upper respiratory infections
- Better housing and easier access to medical care
- Possibly decreased virulence of bacteria
- Impact of secondary prophylaxis

PATHOLOGY OF RHEUMATIC FEVER

Pathology of RF can involve the following features:

- *Carditis*: Pathologically, it is a pancarditis involving endocardium, myocardium, and pericardium. *Endocardial* involvement is "sine qua non" of carditis and causes valvulitis. There are small valvular vegetations known as verrucae with a characteristic "MacCallum"

Flowchart 1: Etiopathogenesis of rheumatic fever and rheumatic heart disease.

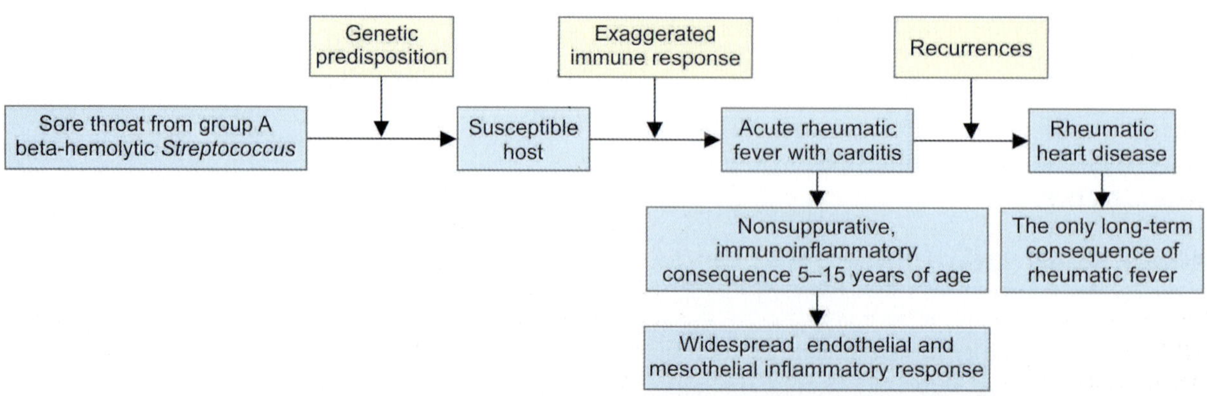

patch, situated on the posterior left atrium (LA) wall. The valve under highest closing pressure is maximally affected. The least affected is the valve which has the lowest closing pressure. Consequently, mitral valve is affected in almost all patients, aortic valve in about 50%, tricuspid valve in <10% and pulmonary valve is affected in <1%. Myocardial involvement is characterized by the characteristic "Aschoff" nodule. There is cellular infiltration and although autopsy reveals *myocardial* involvement is seen in 35–95%, ventricular function is not directly affected by RF. *Pericardial* involvement is nearly universal and is fibrinous. The pericarditis invariably resolves and does not lead to constrictive pericarditis.

- *Arthritis*: Joint involvement is early and causes exudative effusion with swelling. There is minimal synovial thickening. Arthritis resolves completely.
- *Chorea*: Cerebral cortex, cerebellum, and basal ganglia are involved. Aschoff body is absent.
- *Subcutaneous nodules*: Central fibrinoid necrosis is the hallmark with inflammatory cells.

CLINICAL FEATURES

The clinical picture can be dramatic and acute with fever, arthritis, carditis with congestive heart failure (CHF) or be relatively quiet with silent carditis. On an average, 70–80% children report a previous sore throat. The latent period can be from 7 days to 35 days (mean 2–3 weeks). In chorea, latency may be long (2–6 months).

Rheumatic fever is a disease with no diagnostic gold standard either clinically or by investigation. Hence in order to make the diagnosis easy and accurate, Duckett Jones proposed criteria in 1944. It has been modified several times and the last modification was in 2015.[6] It is to be remembered that the criteria are based on a construct rather than a gold standard. WHO proposed diagnostic criteria in 2003 (**Table 3**). Currently, the diagnosis of RF—both primary and recurrence, depends on a sound framework provided by 2015 Jones criteria (**Table 4**) and WHO 2004 criteria.[12] The revised 2015 criteria takes into account the background prevalence of RF and RHD in the region and accordingly adjusts the criteria to increase sensitivity in high-prevalence regions and improve specificity in low-prevalence regions.[6]

It is interesting to note that the clinical profile of RF has changed over the years in the following fashion:

- Severe polyarthritis is becoming less common.
- Clinical carditis is now the most commonly seen major criterion.
- Incidence of both chorea and subcutaneous nodules is diminishing.
- The throat infection preceding RF episodes is less severe and often barely noticeable.
- Subclinical carditis is now well-recognized and widely accepted.

Patients may present with polyarthritis (or with only polyarthralgia or monoarthritis) and with several (3 or more) other minor manifestations, together with evidence of recent group A streptococcal (GAS) infection. Some of these cases may later turnout to be RF. It is prudent to consider them as cases of "probable RF" (once other diagnoses are excluded) and advise regular secondary prophylaxis. Such patients require close follow-up and regular examination of the heart.

TABLE 3: 2002–2003 WHO criteria for the diagnosis of rheumatic fever (RF) and rheumatic heart disease (RHD) (based on the revised Jones criteria).

Category	*Criteria*
Primary episode of RF	Two major* or one major and two minor** manifestations plus evidence of a preceding group A streptococcal infection***
Recurrent attack of RF in a patient without established RHD	Two major or one major and two minor manifestations plus evidence of a preceding group A streptococcal infection
Recurrent attack of RF in a patient with established RHD	Two minor manifestations plus evidence of a preceding group A streptococcal infection
Rheumatic chorea, insidious onset rheumatic carditis	Other major manifestations or evidence of group A streptococcal infection not required
Chronic valve lesions of RHD	Patients do not require any other criteria to be presenting for the first time with pure diagnosed as having rheumatic heart mitral stenosis or mixed mitral valve disease and/or aortic valve disease[d]

*Major manifestations:
Carditis
Polyarthritis
Chorea
Erythema marginatum
Subcutaneous nodules

**Minor manifestations
Clinical: Fever, polyarthralgia
Laboratory: Elevated acute phase reactants (erythrocyte sedimentation rate or leukocyte count)
Electrocardiogram: Prolonged PR interval

***Supporting evidence of a preceding streptococcal infection within the last 45 days
Elevated or rising antistreptolysin-O or other streptococcal antibody, or a positive throat culture, or rapid antigen test for group A streptococci, or recent scarlet fever

[d]Congenital heart disease should be excluded.

TABLE 4: Revised Jones criteria (2015), American Heart Association and World Heart Federation.

Low-risk populations: Rheumatic fever incidence of <2/100,000 in school-going children; RHD prevalence <1/1,000	*Moderate or high-risk populations*: Rheumatic fever incidence of >2/100,000 in school-going children; RHD prevalence >1/1,000
Major criteria	
Carditis: Clinical or subclinical (echo evidence alone)	*Carditis*: Clinical or subclinical (echo evidence alone)
Arthritis: Polyarthritis only	*Arthritis*: Polyarthritis, or monoarthritis, polyarthralgia
Chorea	Chorea
Erythema marginatum	Erythema marginatum
Subcutaneous nodules	Subcutaneous nodules
Minor criteria	
Polyarthralgia	Monoarthralgia, or polyarthralgia
Fever (>38.5°C)	Fever (>38.0°C)
ESR ≥60 mm in the first hour and/or CRP ≥3.0 mg/dL	ESR ≥30 mm in the first hour and/or CRP ≥3.0 mg/dL
Prolonged PR interval	Prolonged PR interval

Initial rheumatic fever: 2 major criteria or 1 major plus 2 minor criteria, with evidence of previous GABHS infection.
Recurrence: 2 major criteria or 1 major plus 2 minor or 3 minor criteria, with evidence of previous GABHS infection.

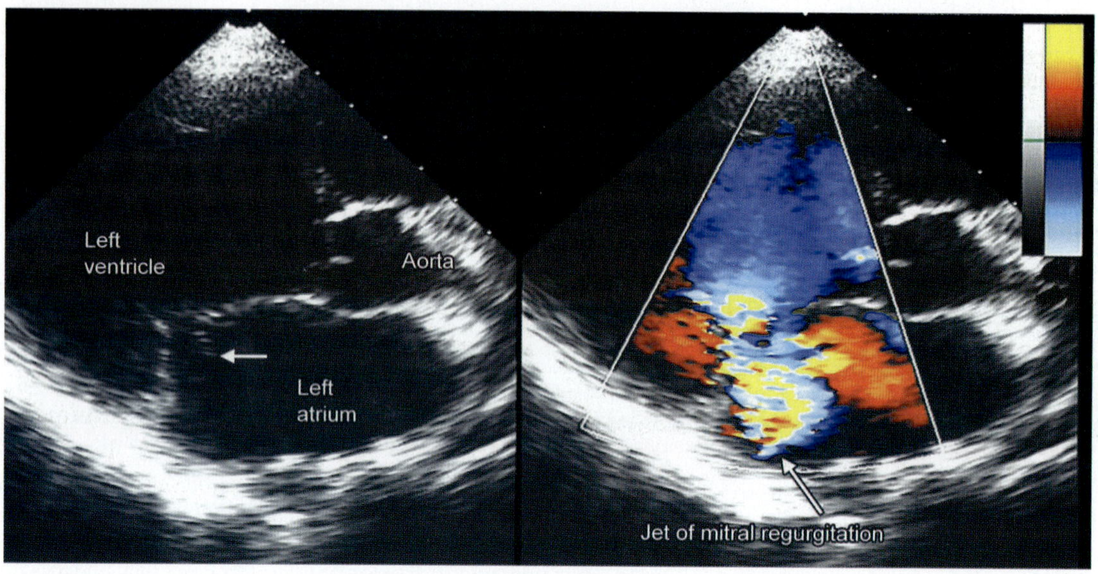

Fig. 1: Parasternal long-axis view of echocardiogram from a patient with acute rheumatic fever and severe mitral regurgitation resulting from flail mitral valve leaflet. The tip of the flail leaflet points toward the left atrium (white arrow in the left frame).

Carditis

Carditis is the most specific of all major criteria. The incidence is approximately 50–75% clinically and is an early presentation and is often asymptomatic. Being a pancarditis, it may present with varying combination of endocarditis, myocarditis, and pericarditis. Approximately 80% of carditis occurs within 2 weeks of the illness. Carditis happens to be the most common major criterion currently and can be clinical or subclinical. The major contribution to CHF is mechanical, mostly due to mitral regurgitation (MR) or added aortic regurgitation (AR) (**Fig. 1**). Myocarditis is a relatively minor contributor to heart failure, if at all.

The clinical features of carditis are summarized in **Table 5**. **Box 3** has some additional points of practical value.

In our experience at the Sree Avittom Thirunal (SAT) Hospital, Thiruvananthapuram, we found the following clinical features of rheumatic carditis (**Table 6**).

Subclinical Carditis

When there is evidence of regurgitation of the mitral valve by echocardiography with no accompanying murmur, a diagnosis of subclinical carditis should be considered. The overall incidence is 16–18%.[13] Isolated aortic valve regurgitation is rare but AR may accompany MR. In rheumatic chorea, clinical carditis may be present in one-third and additional subclinical carditis in one-third. Carditis is virtually universal in the presence of subcutaneous nodules.

TABLE 5: Clinical features of rheumatic carditis.

Affected structure	*Manifestation*
Pericarditis	Chest pain, pericardial rub, pericardial effusion
Myocarditis*	Disproportionate tachycardia, cardiomegaly, S3 gallop, soft S1
Endocarditis	Apical pansystolic murmur of mitral regurgitation that typically radiates to the axilla, early diastolic murmur of aortic regurgitation, mid-diastolic murmur resulting from flow acceleration across the mitral valve (Carey Coombs murmur); valve involvement can be clinically silent with echocardiographic evidence of mitral and/or aortic regurgitation with/without morphologic features of valve involvement; recurrence of rheumatic fever may be identified by the detection of a new murmur or a change in the existing murmurs

*It is quite controversial whether isolated myocarditis is clinically manifest in acute rheumatic fever. All features of "myocarditis" occur only in the presence of significant acute mitral regurgitation and do not occur in isolation.

BOX 3: Rheumatic carditis—practical points.

- Myocarditis without valvulitis is unlikely to be rheumatic
- Pericarditis without murmur of valvulitis unlikely to be rheumatic
- Carditis lasts for 8–12 weeks in 95% of cases
- Involvement of mitral valve is nearly 100%, aortic valve 20%, tricuspid under 5%, and pulmonary valve under 1%
- Isolated aortic regurgitation without mitral regurgitation is very uncommon in rheumatic fever

TABLE 6: Sree Avittom Thirunal (SAT) Hospital experience with acute rheumatic fever.

Clinical feature	*Percentage positive*
Soft first heart sound	100
Third heart sound (LVS3)	60
Cardiomegaly	50
Heart failure	30
Apical pansystolic murmur	95
Apical mid-diastolic murmur	50
Early diastolic murmur	10

Indolent Carditis

Chronic, insidious onset carditis can present with nonspecific symptoms, but will have murmurs of MR, often with heart failure. Nearly 10% of all carditis may be indolent in nature. Acute phase reactants are usually elevated but antistreptolysin-O (ASO) could be negative. Carditis lasting for >12 weeks can occur in 5% and this is sometimes referred to as chronic carditis.

Fulminant Carditis

Rarely, child presents with severe refractory CHF and in pulmonary edema. They usually have acute MR due to either chordal rupture or acute annular dilatation. These patients require intensive management and sometimes need emergency valve replacement.

Polyarthritis

Polyarthritis is expected to occur in 60–75% of acute RF. Polyarthritis in the context of diagnosis of RF is defined as swelling of more than or equal to two joints accompanied by two or more of the following: limitation of movement, warmth over the joint, and pain or tenderness. Tenderness can be out of proportion to the objective findings of local inflammation and often quite severe with excruciating pain on touch. Pain in the joint alone is referred to as arthralgia. The usual joints affected larger ones knee, ankle, elbow, shoulder, etc. Hip joint, spinal joints, and temporomandibular joint are seldom involved. The arthritis can be migratory or additive. In the SAT experience involving 100 consecutive patients with RF and arthritis, polyarthritis was seen in 60%, polyarthralgia in 25% and monoarthritis was seen in <10%.

Arthritic typically occurs early in RF and may the only major manifestation in older patients with RF. Rheumatic arthritis is often termed as migratory because of the sequential joint involvement. This is not as common as generally believed. Monoarthritis may occur, typically when anti-inflammatory therapy is initiated before RF is fully expressed. Frequently, several joints may be affected simultaneously, or the arthritis may be additive rather than migratory. Inflammation in a specific joint usually resolves inside of 2 weeks and the entire bout of polyarthritis in about a month if untreated.

Poststreptococcal Reactive Arthropathy

Poststreptococcal reactive arthropathy (PSRA) can be considered a distinct entity related to streptococcal infection. The arthropathy affects older children and adolescents, has a shorter latent period, generally nonmigratory and involving smaller joints also. The clinical response to aspirin is sluggish. It may persist longer. Even though considered benign, occasional reports have noted valve involvement on follow-up.

Chorea

Chorea is a delayed clinical manifestation of RF and is more common in girls. It is defined as a purposeless, involuntary movement involving both proximal and distal limbs. This may be associated with poor handwriting, poor scholastic performance, and emotional incontinence.

BOX 4: Differential diagnosis of chorea.

- Choreoathetoid cerebral palsy (CP)
- Juvenile Huntington's chorea
- Postencephalitic chorea
- Wilson's disease
- Hallervorden–Spatz disease
- Systemic lupus erythematosus
- Subacute sclerosing panencephalitis
- Oral contraceptive-induced chorea

The incidence is on a decline with an average of ≤10%. It has a latent period of 1–6 months and can last around 3 months (6–12 months). About two-thirds of patients with chorea have carditis which could be clinical or subclinical. Over a 20-year follow-up, RHD can be expected to occur in 27%.

The differential diagnosis of chorea is listed in **Box 4**.

Subcutaneous Nodules

Subcutaneous nodules are painless, 0.5–2 cm sized nodules found over extensor surfaces aspects of bony prominences, back, occiput, scapula, and mastoids (**Fig. 2**). They are best appreciated when child bends down. It is uncommon in young adults and adolescents.

The incidence is decreasing. It now accounts for <5% of all major criteria; >90% with subcutaneous nodules will have associated cardiac involvement. Majority of nodules disappear (70%) by 1 month and <5% may remain beyond 12 weeks.

Erythema Marginatum

It is the least common major criterion and it occurs as red macules with serpiginous margins. They are nonpruritic and often involve trunk and upper limbs. It has now become a clinical curiosity. The rash is very transient and often may be missed. Erythema marginatum like lesions can occur in poststreptococcal glomerulonephritis (PSGN) and drug reactions.

Other Manifestations

- *Fever*: Fever can be either high grade or low grade initially, later becoming high grade. It often responds well to aspirin.
- *Arthralgia*: It is increasingly found in children presenting with carditis. The revised Jones criteria recognizes polyarthralgia as a major criterion in high-prevalence regions.
- *Epistaxis*: Rarely, it can occur during acute episodes.
- *Abdominal pain*: Pain abdomen may occur. It has been varyingly attributed to either mesenteric adenitis or hepatic pain due to heart failure.
- *Rheumatic pneumonia*: It is of historical significance only and seldom observed now. The reason for the presentation is also debated.

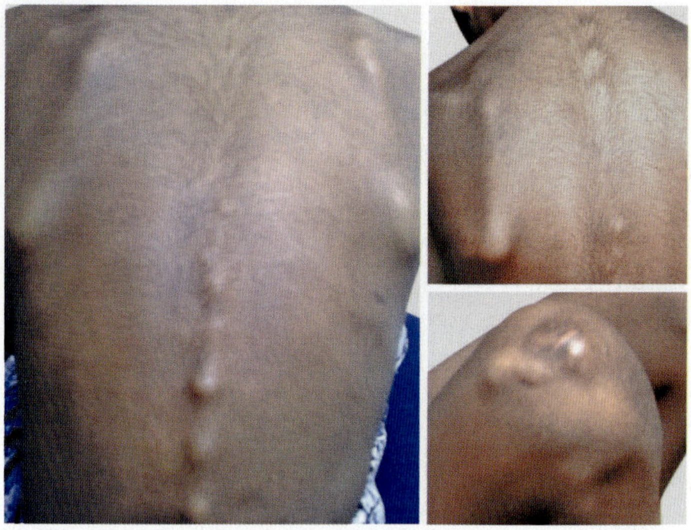

Fig. 2: Subcutaneous nodules over the external bony prominences of spine, knee, and scapulae in acute rheumatic fever.

CLINICAL DILEMMAS IN RHEUMATIC FEVER

Polyarthritis

- Juvenile idiopathic arthritis is an alternative diagnosis especially when smaller joints are involved. It may have reasonable response to aspirin, may have accompanying nodules also. It can have pericardial and valvular involvement. Resolution of the dilemma may be by the following means:
  - Younger age of involvement (often < 4 years)
  - Smaller joints are involved
  - Hip, spine and temporomandibular joint involvement
  - Nonresolution beyond 3 weeks
  - Deformity after one or more episodes
  - Sluggish response to aspirin
  - Associated eye involvement and presence of rashes
  - Echocardiography is also helpful. RF has characteristic manifestations.
- Other polyarthropathies like systemic lupus erythematosus, Henoch-Schönlein Purpura, and acute leukemia may mimic RF. Differentiating points include age, clinical accompaniments, laboratory evaluation, and echocardiography.
- Limb pains in young children can be confused with polyarthralgia and can mimic RF. Careful history and careful auscultation and, if needed, laboratory evaluation will settle the tissue.
- Polyarthralgia alone can be a vexing issue. This is given more importance in suspected recurrence. Careful clinical follow-up in children may be advisable.
- Poststreptococcal reactive arthritis can be a differential diagnosis. It may be responsible for future development of RHD and will require secondary prophylaxis.

Carditis

- Underdiagnosis can occur with a loud rub masking the faint murmur. Soft apical faint murmur may be missed in the presence of high ambient noise.
- Overdiagnosis is more common. An innocent murmur accompanied by nonspecific symptoms may be misinterpreted as carditis. Preexisting nonrheumatic mitral valve prolapse may cause a dilemma in diagnosis. Certain congenital heart defects present with an apical murmur. Echocardiography allows easy distinction between RF and other causes.
- Infective endocarditis (IE) can be an important differential diagnosis as many clinical and laboratory findings are shared by IE and rheumatic carditis, especially if rheumatic recurrence is suspected. A carefully recorded history, laboratory tests including blood culture and echocardiography enable distinction between the two conditions. IE may occur in RHD patients. Diligently performed echocardiography and blood cultures allow detection of IE in these patients.
- Indolent carditis can present with vague symptoms, heart failure, murmurs, and cardiomegaly. It can be confused with either myocarditis or IE. Here again, echocardiography is very helpful in identifying features suggesting rheumatic basis.

Chorea

Because of long latent period, acute phase reactants may be normal and ASO negative. Sometimes chorea need not be rheumatic.

Rheumatic Fever in Adults

Dominant feature is polyarthritis with lesser incidence of carditis. Chorea and nodules are extremely rare. PSRA can mimic RF in adults.

LABORATORY INVESTIGATIONS

Acute Phase Reactants

Both the commonly used phase reactants are nonspecific.

Erythrocyte sedimentation rate (ESR): It is almost always elevated in acute RF. The thresholds for diagnosis in the revised Jones criteria of 2015 are >30 mm/1st hour for high-risk populations and >60 mm/1st hour for low-risk populations. The levels of ESR can be influenced by anemia (high ESR), heart failure, and use of NSAID (reduced ESR).

C-reactive protein (CRP): It is not affected by CHF or anemia and may be suited in those clinical situations where diagnostic dilemma of acute rheumatic activity exists on account of nondiagnostic ESR. A value of >3 mg/dL is the threshold accepted for low- and high-risk populations using the revised Jones criteria.

Other: There can be mild polymorphonuclear leukocytosis. Anemia of mild severity exists which is due to depressed erythropoiesis and increased plasma volume in those with heart failure.

Antistreptococcal Antibodies

The antibodies generated against various components of the *Streptococcus* include ASO, anti-DNase B, antistreptodornase, anti-DPNase, antistreptokinase, and antihyaluronidase. Of these, the commonly employed ones are ASO that peaks at 3–6 weeks after streptococcal throat infection and remains elevated for 3–6 months and anti-DNase that peaks at 6–8 weeks after streptococcal throat infection. By the end of 6 months, only 20% of RF patients retain ASO positivity.

Usually, a single measurement of ASO is done during suspected RF. If single value is taken, the diagnostic value is >240 in adults and >320 in children. ASO is usually positive in 70–80% of children with acute RF. In rheumatic chorea, it is positive in 20–40%. ASO is influenced by prior antibiotic therapy and steroids. If the titer is not of diagnostic level, it can be repeated after 5 days and a rising titer is said to be diagnostic.

While the diagnostic yield of antistreptococcal antibodies can be increased to 95% by the combined use of ASO and anti-DNase, this is seldom undertaken in practice. In the SAT hospital, the positivity of ASO in RF was 73%, rheumatic carditis was 70%, and for chorea, it was 30%.

Serial ASO is not routinely indicated because it should be positive in the acute polyarthritis phase of acute RF. If serial titers are done, samples are taken at 2–4 weeks intervals and should demonstrate rising titers.

Identification of *Streptococcus*

Throat swab culture is positive in only in 20–30%. Even if positive, it may still mean only a carrier state as GAS carrier state can be as high as 15% in some populations. A rapid antigen detection using coagulation, latex agglutination, and enzyme-linked immunosorbent assay (ELISA) techniques is a good practical alternative to throat swab culture. These tests may be of more help in primary prevention of RF.

Electrocardiogram in Rheumatic Fever

First-degree atrioventricular (AV) block (prolonged PR interval) is a minor criterion in acute RF. It is present in about 30% of RF. It is essentially a functional abnormality and need not indicate carditis. AV block can occur uncommonly. Complete heart block occurs, but is quite exceptional.

Echocardiography in Acute Rheumatic Carditis

The role of echocardiography has become considerably important after the identification of subclinical carditis in RF and subclinical valve affliction in apparently normal

TABLE 7: Echocardiographic findings suggestive of rheumatic fever.

Structure	*Modality*	*Findings*
Mitral valve	Two-dimensional (2D) imaging	· Thickened leaflets · Limited mobility of posterior mitral leaflet (PML) · Nodules on leaflet margins (25%) · Flail anterior or posterior leaflet [typically associated with severe mitral regurgitation (MR)] · Evidence of established rheumatic heart valve disease: Thickened chordal apparatus, varying degrees of stenosis, limited mobility of anterior mitral leaflet (AML)
	Color Doppler	Posteriorly directed jet of MR that often courses along the wall of left atrium
Aortic valve	2D and color Doppler	· Thick leaflet margins · Varying grades of aortic regurgitation · Reduced leaflet mobility
Tricuspid valve	2D and color Doppler	Rarely affected in the initial episode; chronic RHD is associated with organic tricuspid valve involvement in up to 30% with leaflet thickening, and varying degrees of tricuspid regurgitation (TR) and less commonly, tricuspid stenosis. The pulmonary artery systolic pressure can be quantified if there is TR and this could be elevated in acute and severe MR
Atria	M-mode and 2D	Left atrial enlargement is an inevitable consequence of significant MR
Ventricles	M-mode and 2D	Left ventricle (LV) enlargement is a result of MR. Left ventricular (LV) function tends to be well preserved except in the presence of acute severe MR. LV dysfunction is therefore rare in the absence of significant MR
Pericardium	Two-dimensional	The presence of a pericardial effusion in the absence of heart failure may point toward pericarditis

individuals. Echocardiography provides several specific pointers to the diagnosis of RF (**Table 7**) and helps guide treatment. It is essential to follow recommended guidelines[5] to label valve regurgitation as significant and not label any color Doppler jets of physiologic MR as significant. **Table 7** summarizes the echocardiographic findings in acute RF. Echocardiography is valuable in ruling out conditions with similar clinical features such as IE (vegetations), viral myocarditis (absence of structural valve affliction).

TREATMENT OF RHEUMATIC FEVER

The algorithm for management of RF is shown in **Flowchart 2**.

General Measures

Hospitalization is generally advised for confirming diagnosis, starting treatment, and education of the family. The laboratory tests that should be initially ordered should include a complete blood count, ESR and CRP as well as ASO titers. It is often advisable to obtain a throat swab culture. An electrocardiogram (ECG), chest X-ray should be obtained. An echocardiogram should be undertaken and this should be done systematically and meticulously. A blood culture is sometimes indicated if endocarditis is suspected. Rest is recommended for variable periods of time and this is dictated by the clinical condition and extent of involvement. The presence of carditis often merits rest for 2–3 weeks and return to school is often avoided for 6 weeks. **Table 8** suggests practical guidelines for the duration of bed rest.

Elimination of Streptococcal Infection

It is wise to assume that *Streptococcus* is being harbored in the throat even though culture is often negative. The goal of eradicating streptococcal infection is to mitigate the effects of repeated exposure to streptococcal antigens and antibiotics are indicated for this purpose. A single dose of intramuscular long-acting penicillin (1,200,000 units for children >25 kg and 600,000 units for those <25 kg) is the best option. Alternatives include oral penicillin V (250 mg every 6 hours for 10 days) or azithromycin (12.5 mg/kg/day once daily for 5 days) for those with penicillin allergy.

Suppressing Inflammation

Anti-inflammatory treatment with salicylates or steroids provides symptom relief but may not prevent chronic heart valve disease. The optimal aspirin dose should ensure an adequate response but avoid toxicity. Aspirin, 75 mg/kg/day divided into four to six doses, is generally adequate for achieving a clinical response. After 2 weeks, the dose can be decreased to 50 mg/kg/day for an additional 3–6 weeks. Any other NSAID can be used as an alternative for those allergic to aspirin.

Steroids rapidly relieve symptoms in patients with carditis that is severe enough to result in heart failure. The duration of hospitalization can be shortened by steroids. Steroids are also administered for those with little or no response to salicylates. Prednisolone in 2 mg/kg/day in three divided doses is the typical starting dose. Intravenous (IV) methylprednisolone can be considered in life-threatening circumstances and when oral steroids are not tolerated. The dose is 30 mg/kg/dose IV infusion × 3 days (maximum dose—1 g/day).

After about 2 weeks, dosage may be decreased by 25% every week. A period of overlap with aspirin may mitigate

Flowchart 2: Management of rheumatic fever.

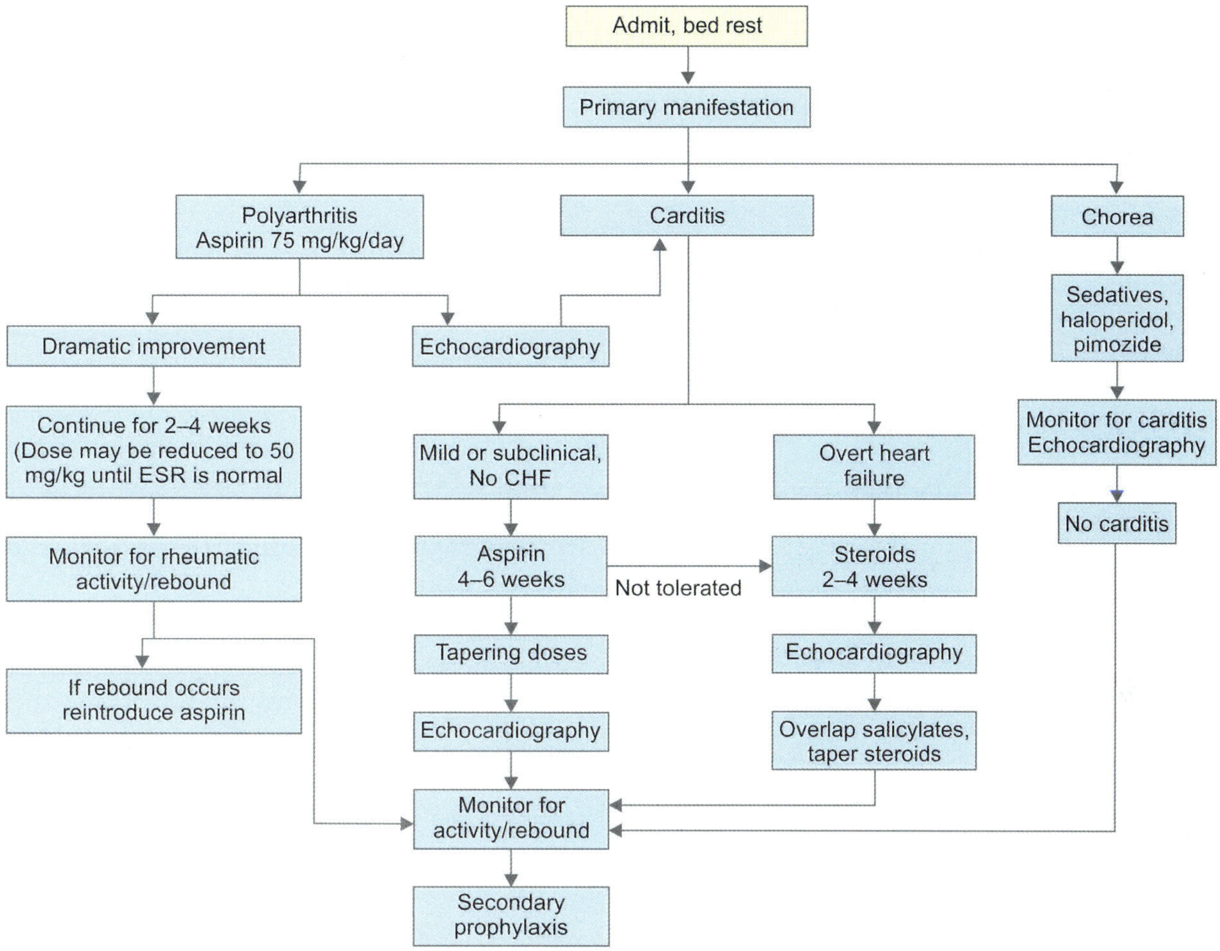

TABLE 8: Suggested guidelines for rest and activities in acute rheumatic fever.

Clinical	*Rest (weeks)*	*Ambulation (weeks)*	*Schooling (weeks)*
Polyarthritis	2	>2	6
Carditis—no heart failure of cardiac enlargement	4	>4	6–12
Carditis—no heart failure but cardiomegaly on X-ray	6	>6	12
Carditis—heart failure and cardiac enlargement	6	>6	4 weeks after subsidence

rebound resulting from steroid withdrawal. The total duration of treatment is determined by clinical recovery. Typically, 4-6 weeks of total treatment is advisable. It is reasonable to start tapering at the end of 2 weeks and do it over 2-3 weeks to avoid a rebound. Prednisolone is typically tapered by removing 5 mg from the total dose every third day. Aspirin 50 mg/kg/day to be added once the steroids are tapered off.

Heart Failure Management

Diuretics and angiotensin-converting enzyme inhibitors are often administered when a diagnosis of heart failure is made. Digoxin is also an option, although it is increasingly out of favor in recent times.

Management of Chorea

Chorea is often thought of as a self-limiting benign condition. Anti-inflammatory agents or steroids have little effect on chorea. Supportive measures and reassurance are important. Haloperidol (0.25–0.5 mg/kg/day), diazepam (0.25–0.5 mg/kg/day), valproic acid (15 mg/kg/day, in resistant cases) can all be given to alleviate symptoms. Pimozide (1–2 mg twice a day for children > 12 years) is a new agent that is potentially useful in rheumatic chorea.

Heart Valve Surgery in Rheumatic Fever

For patients with fulminant and refractory heart failure, valve replacement operation may be required for refractory heart failure from severe MR. Often either of the valve leaflets are flail. While valve repair can be considered for selected patients, the fear of recurrence often necessitates valve replacement.

NATURAL HISTORY OF RHEUMATIC FEVER

Once the acute inflammation resolves, MR may diminish over the subsequent months and in very rare instances, it may disappear. AR, however, tends to persist. Unfortunately, patients with RF are especially prone to recurrences after subsequent bouts of GABHS infection and with each recurrence there is scarring of the leaflets with progressive valve leakage and stenosis. The goal of secondary prophylaxis is to prevent these recurrences. It is increasingly recognized that valve lesions may progress without identifiable episodes of RF, especially in highly endemic regions.

Mortality in during acute episodes varies from 0.3 to 1.6%. Within 3–5 years, 30–40% of these children develop permanent cardiac lesions, mitral valve being the commonly involved (90%), the other valves to be involved are aortic (12%), tricuspid (5–8%), and pulmonary valve (<1%). The vast majority of carditis occurs within the first 2 weeks of the first attack of RF. If a child does not develop carditis by then it is unlikely to develop carditis later.[14] Chronic RHD develops due to recurring reactivation, chronic indolent rheumatic activity, and continuing hemodynamic stress on already damaged valve leaflets.

PREVENTION

Rheumatic fever and RHD are eminently preventable. The conventional framework for disease prevention can be applied to RHD prevention as well. This involves primordial, primary, and secondary prevention (**Flowchart 3**). Management of established heart valve disease requires tertiary care.

Primordial Prevention

Primordial prevention involves prevention of streptococcal pharyngeal and perhaps skin infection. This happens through improved living standards, access to primary healthcare services. An effective streptococcal vaccine would offer the ideal form of primary prevention but, in spite of several years of efforts, we do not as yet have an effective vaccine.[15]

Primary Prevention

This refers to prevention of occurrence of RF for the first time following an episode of streptococcal sore throat infection. Primary prophylaxis requires timely and effective management of streptococcal pharyngitis and perhaps skin infections as well. The antibiotic regimens are the same as they are for eliminating streptococci from the throat during an acute episode of RF. Diagnosis of streptococcal throat infection enables rational antibiotic administration. Clinical criteria are useful and are easy to follow (**Fig. 3**).

Secondary Prophylaxis (Prevention of Recurrences of RF)

Secondary prophylaxis is essentially to prevent recurrences of RF and is best achieved by 3 or 4 weekly injections of benzathine penicillin. Other alternatives such as oral penicillin V or G, sulfonamides are considerably less effective[16] (**Table 9**).

The recommendations on the duration of secondary prophylaxis are summarized in **Table 10**.

Among many health workers and patients, there is a reluctance to administer or receive injections respectively. This is due to factors such as a fear of anaphylaxis, pain, and unfamiliarity with its correct use and lack of preparedness with dealing with anaphylaxis. Deaths are reported after benzathine penicillin from a number of primary healthcare settings. They are almost entirely limited to patients with severe heart valve disease. The clinical features preceding these deaths are not well documented. Available information and anecdotes suggest

Flowchart 3: The prevailing paradigm for prevention of rheumatic fever and rheumatic heart disease. This Flowchart shows the sequence of events leading on to RHD and its consequences are shown here in blue boxes. The various interventions are shown in yellow boxes.

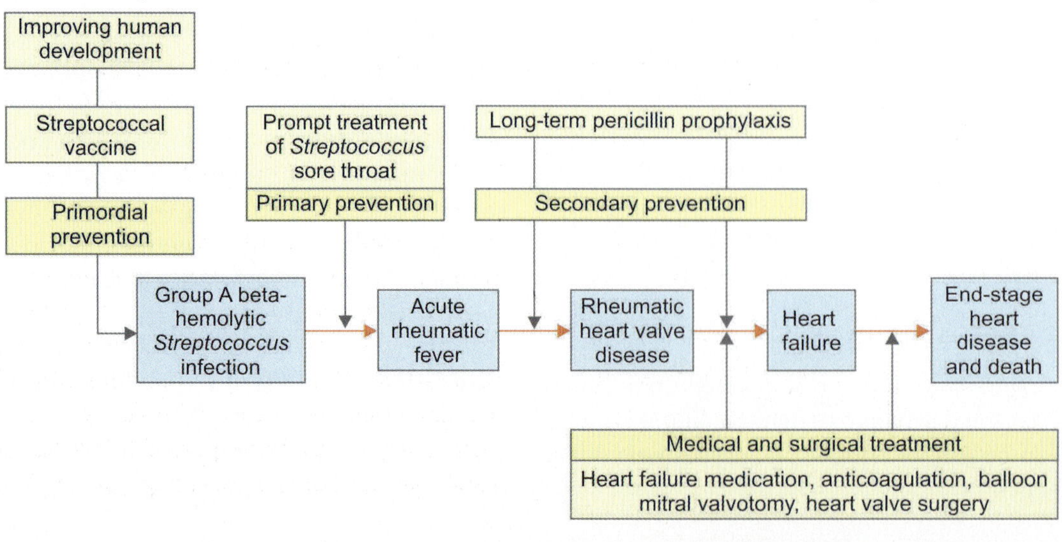

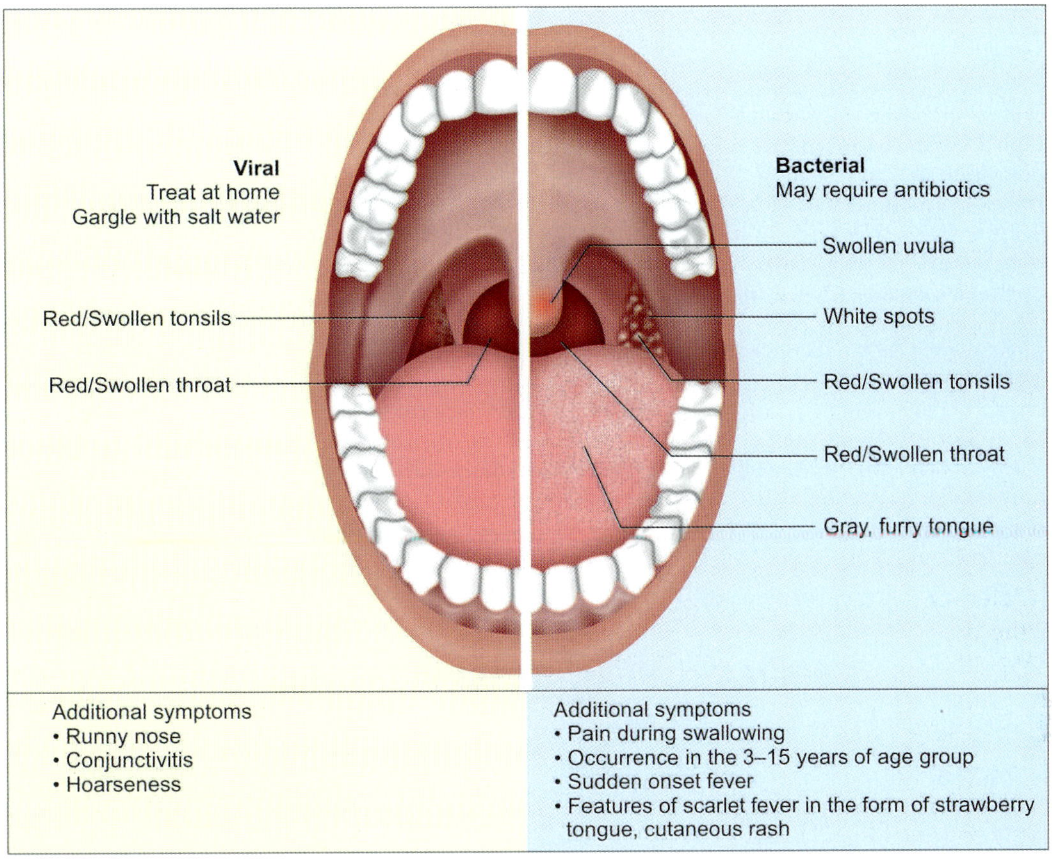

Fig. 3: Features that distinguish viral from bacterial sore throat.

TABLE 9: Secondary prophylaxis following an episode of rheumatic fever.

Antibiotic	*Mode of administration*	*Dose*
Benzathine penicillin	Single intramuscular injection every 3–4 weeks*	1,200,000 units for patients >25–30 kg; 600,000 units for patients <25 kg**
Penicillin V	Oral	250 mg twice daily
Sulfonamide# (sulfadiazine, sulfadoxine, sulfisoxazole)	Oral	1 g daily for patients >30 kg and 500 mg daily for patients <30 kg
Erythromycin (for those allergic to penicillin)	Oral	250 mg twice daily

*Three weekly injections are recommended for RF prophylaxis in high-prevalence regions.
**For patients <25 kg in high prevalence regions, 600,000 units can be administered every 2 weeks.
#Not recommended in pregnancy.

TABLE 10: Recommended schedule (duration) for secondary prophylaxis.

Category	*Subcategory*	*Recommendation*
Rheumatic fever	No carditis	5 years after the last attack or till 18 years of age (whichever is later)
Rheumatic fever	Carditis; no residual RHD	10 years after the last attack or till 25 years of age (whichever is later)
Rheumatic heart disease	Established rheumatic heart disease (RHD) and after heart valve surgery	Ideally lifelong; at least till 40 years of age

that these are not often a result of anaphylaxis. This happened not necessarily with the first injection, but could occur suddenly after any injection. These deaths are terrifying, and could cause a program to be stopped even when all other previous injections were administered without incident. Because of these incidents, it is perhaps reasonable in low-resource settings that are not prepared to deal with acute complications to administer oral penicillin V, especially to patients with severe disease. True anaphylaxis is exceedingly rare (1:10,000) and death from anaphylaxis is described in 1:30,000 injections. It is essential for centers that routinely administer benzathine penicillin to be prepared with a contingency plan to deal with anaphylaxis (**Box 5**).

BOX 5: Preparedness and protocol for anaphylaxis following penicillin administration.

Broad principles
- Key to successful resuscitation is anticipation and the preparedness for this eventuality
- It is life-threatening but is imminently reversible
- Success depends on the promptness in detection and instituting treatment
- The key drug is adrenaline and not steroids
- Occasional patient will need intubation for airway management

Outpatient facility
- Personnel: At least one nurse trained in cardiac resuscitation in addition to the physician
- Drugs: Adrenaline (1:1,000) loaded in 2-mL syringe; adrenaline (1:10,000) loaded in 10-mL syringe
- Venous access
- Volume replacement: Normal saline or plasma volume substitutes

Management protocol
- Administer adrenaline: Children: 0.1 mL/kg of 1:1,000 adrenaline—IM, 0.01 mL/kg of 1:10,000 adrenaline—IV; adults: 0.5 mL of 1:1,000 adrenaline—IM; 3–5 mL of 1:10,000 adrenaline—IM or IV; repeat dose can be given at 5-minute interval
- Administer volume: 1–2 L in adults and 20–40 mL/kg in children intravenously. Colloids are better than crystalloids in the setting of leaky capillaries
- CPR should be initiated as when necessary

RHEUMATIC HEART DISEASE IN CHILDREN

INTRODUCTION

Chronic RHD essentially involves the cardiac valves (rheumatic valvular heart disease). Most commonly affected are the mitral and aortic valves.[17] Rarely, tricuspid valve can be involved. Pulmonary valve involvement is quite rare.[18] Valvular heart disease can result in either stenosis or regurgitation or both, in varying proportion.

NORMAL MITRAL VALVE ANATOMY

Normal mitral valve apparatus has a complex anatomy and the following components:

1. *Leaflets*: Anterior mitral leaflet (AML) and posterior mitral leaflet (PML).
2. *Two commissures*: They are named medial commissure and lateral commissure.
3. *Two papillary muscles*: They are named posteromedial and anterolateral.
4. *Chordae tendineae*: There are approximately 120 chordae, both AML and PML being attached to both papillary muscles by 60 chordae each.

The normal mitral valve area (MVA) in adult is 4–6 cm^2 and in children 4 cm^2/m^2. No gradient exists across a normal mitral valve in diastole.

MITRAL STENOSIS

Hemodynamically significant MS is said to exist when valve area is <2.5 cm^2.[19] The vast majority of MS are rheumatic in origin especially in India. Rarely, congenital and exceptionally acquired nonrheumatic causes can result in MS[20,21] (**Box 6**).

BOX 6: Causes of left ventricular inflow obstruction in children.

Congenital

Mitral valve and tensor apparatus:
- Parachute mitral valve with single papillary muscle
- Funnel mitral valve

Mitral annulus:
- Supramitral membrane

Left atrium:
- Cor triatriatum

Acquired

Mitral valve:*
- Rheumatoid arthritis
- Systemic lupus erythematosus
- Mucopolysaccharidosis
- Carcinoid syndrome
- Fabry disease
- Whipple disease

Left atrium:
- Left atrial myxoma

*All causes of acquired mitral stenosis are exceedingly rare.

Pathogenesis of Rheumatic MS

Development of rheumatic MS could be explained by various mechanisms, including recurring RF with carditis, ongoing smoldering inflammation or due to a hemodynamic insult on an abnormally modified mitral valve after the first/initial carditis.[22] The usual latent period between acute RF and MS varies between 1 and 20 years. Rapid progression to juvenile MS is typically seen in regions with high disease prevalence. The term juvenile rheumatic MS (MS below 20 years of age) was a term coined by Sujoy Roy.[4] Pathologically, both valvular and subvalvular apparatus are involved, causing leaflet thickening, commissural fusion, and chordal shortening and fusion.

Pathophysiology

When MVA reaches <2.5 cm^2, a transmitral gradient develops to maintain a normal stroke volume. The fundamental changes in MS are:

- Increase in transmitral gradient in diastole and increased transmitral velocity across the mitral valve (**Fig. 4**).
- Left atrial (LA) pressure elevation and pulmonary venous hypertension (PVH). An elevated PVH is the fundamental reason for symptoms in MS.

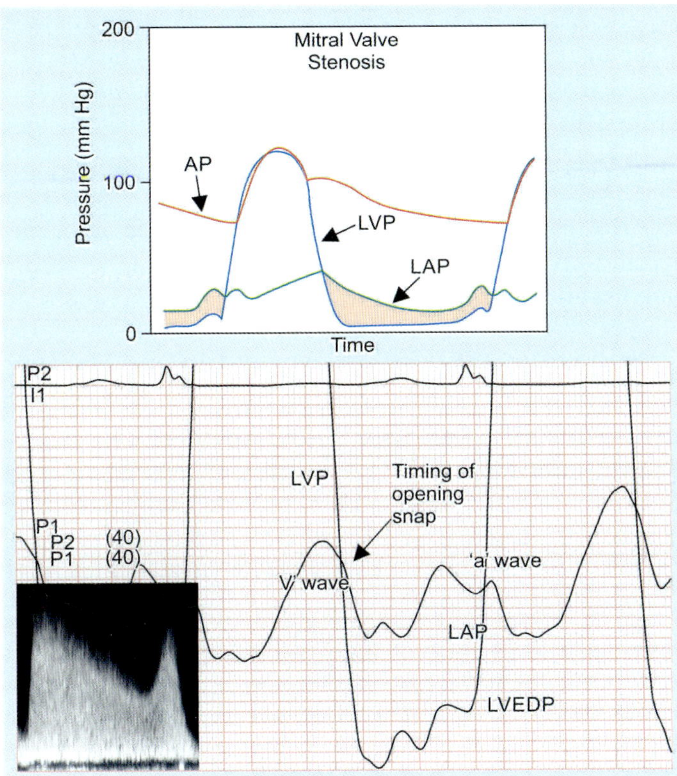

Fig. 4: Demonstrates the pathophysiology of mitral stenosis. The top panel shows the complete pressure tracings of left ventricle pressure (LVP), left atrial pressure (LAP), and aortic pressure (AP). The bottom panel shows an enlarged version recorded at low pressure scale to demonstrate the gradient between the LAP and LVP during diastole. The opening snap happens at the onset of LV filling as shown. The insert at bottom left is a Doppler echo tracing from the same patient showing the characteristic "M"-shaped flow acceleration across the stenotic valve that is seen in patient with MS and sinus rhythm. The second peak results from atrial contraction and is responsible for the presystolic accentuation of the mid-diastolic murmur.

- Elevated pulmonary venous pressure is passively transmitted to pulmonary artery, causing pulmonary hypertension. Dyspnea typically occurs when pulmonary venous pressure is beyond 15 mm Hg. Later vasoconstriction occurs and leads to further pulmonary arterial hypertension (PAH).[23] Much of this vasoconstriction is reversible with the rare exception of advanced long-standing MS.
- Eventually there is reduced filling of left ventricular (LV) and stroke volume and cardiac output declines. The systolic function and LV end-diastolic pressure (LVEDP) more or less remains normal.[23]
- Established PAH leads to right ventricular hypertrophy (RVH), which in turn can lead to right ventricular (RV) dysfunction and tricuspid regurgitation (TR).

Box 7 outlines the classification of MS based on severity.

Clinical Presentation

Trivial and mild MS could be asymptomatic. Moderate and severe MS are mostly symptomatic. The chief symptom is often dyspnea on exertion and much less commonly, palpitations. It progresses from exercise intolerance to orthopnea. Paroxysmal nocturnal dyspnea can punctuate the progression of symptoms.

Acute pulmonary edema presents catastrophically and occurs when mean LA pressure abruptly goes beyond 25–28 mm Hg. Less critical MS also could develop pulmonary edema, often precipitated by infection, anemia, thyrotoxicosis and pregnancy and atrial fibrillation (AF) in adults. Fatigue can occur, but is often overshadowed by dyspnea. Interestingly, gradual rise in PVH does not result in pulmonary edema even when pressures rise beyond 30 mm Hg. This is because of compensatory pulmonary vasoconstriction and efficient mobilization of pulmonary interstitial fluid by lymphatics.

Hemoptysis is a pulmonary venous symptom. It is almost always seen in advanced MS which is due to various reasons. Most often it is due to rupture of bronchial veins. It could also be due to pulmonary embolism, as a part of pulmonary edema, bronchitis which can accompany MS[24] and sometimes contributed to by use of anticoagulants.

BOX 7: Classification of severity of mitral stenosis (MS).

1. *Adults (based on valve area)*
   a. Severe MS : Mitral valve area (MVA) < 1 cm^2, significant symptoms (class II–IV)
   b. Moderate MS : MVA 1–1.5 cm^2, limitations in activity (class II–III)
   c. Mild MS : MVA 1.5–2.5 cm^2, exertional symptoms (class II)
   d. Trivial MS : MVA > 2.5 cm^2, usually no symptoms (class I)
2. *Association of pulmonary hypertension with severity of MS*
   a. Mild MS : Normal pulmonary artery (PA) pressure
   b. Moderate MS : Normal/mildly elevated PA pressure*
   c. Severe MS : Pulmonary arterial hypertension (PAH) always exists

*Increases on exercise.

Chest pain is mostly found in adults (15%), which is perhaps due to RV ischemia and PAH, as part of pulmonary embolism or, rarely, associated coronary artery disease. Hoarseness of voice, syncope, and edema are rare in children.

Complications of Mitral Stenosis

Box 8 lists the complications of MS. The most common complications include severe pulmonary hypertension and acute pulmonary edema. Stroke and embolism to other sites from LA clots that typically happens after AF. AF is a function of age and is extremely rare below 12 years and rare below 20 years. But, by 30 years age, the incidence increases to nearly 50%. AF can cause a decrease in cardiac output, worsen the symptoms, precipitate pulmonary edema and leads to thromboembolic episodes.

Systemic embolism is also a function of age and development of AF.[25] Infective endocarditis is rare in pure MS. It can occur with associated MR. Pulmonary embolism is uncommon in children.

BOX 8: Complications of mitral stenosis.

- Acute pulmonary edema
- Massive hemoptysis
- Pulmonary artery hypertension
- Atrial fibrillation
- Systemic thromboembolism
- Pulmonary embolism
- Infective endocarditis

Physical Findings

Signs of poor perfusion such as peripheral cyanosis are found only in the late phase of severe MS. Pulse can be of normal or of low volume. It is irregular in AF. The jugular venous pressure is elevated in severe MS with associated pulmonary hypertension. If elevated, either "a" or "v" waves can be prominent depending on the presence of PAH and TR. In AF, "a" wave is absent.

There is no cardiomegaly in isolated MS. Apex could be "tapping" because of the loud and palpable first heart sound and a diastolic thrill is often felt. Left parasternal heave, prominent epigastric pulsation, and palpable P_2 indicate PAH.

Auscultatory findings are summarized in **Figure 5**. The first heart sound is characteristically loud. It can be variable in AF. A relatively soft S1 in MS could indicate associated significant MR, AR, or heavily calcified valve. The second heart sound is closely split with loud P_2. Both S3 and S4 are absent.

The opening snap (OS) is quite characteristic of MS. It is sufficiently delayed after A2 (40–120 ms) to enable easy identification and results from doming of a pliable, noncalcific mitral valve. It is quite distinct, of medium pitch

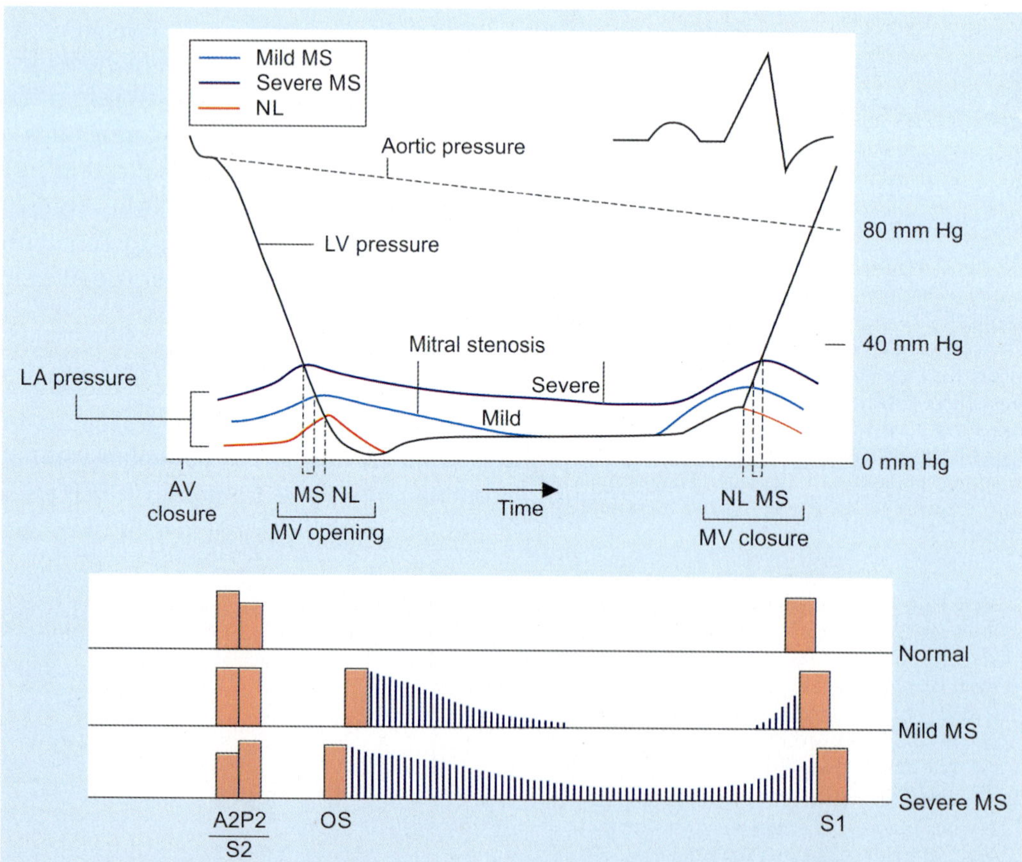

Fig. 5: Correlation between physical examination and severity of mitral stenosis (MS) in rheumatic heart disease.
(A2 P2: aortic and pulmonary components of second heart sound (S2); AV: aortic valve; LA: left atrium; LV: left ventricle; NL: normal; OS: opening snap; S1: first heart sound)

and is best heard medial to apex. The time interval between A2 and OS has an inverse relationship to severity of MS.[26] An ejection click could be heard at pulmonary area due to dilated pulmonary arteries as a consequence of PAH.

Mitral stenosis produces a low-pitched, rough and rumbling mid-diastolic murmur (MDM) which immediately follows OS. It has a presystolic accentuation in sinus rhythm. The murmur becomes prominent on left lateral position and exertion. It can also be heard at axilla and left lower sternal border.

Box 9 lists all the causes of the MDM in RHD in addition to MS.

Investigations

- Hemogram, acute phase reactants, ASO, international normalized ratio (INR), and renal and hepatic function tests are ordered according to the clinical circumstances.
- Chest X-ray will show no or minimal cardiomegaly. Cardiac enlargement is found in associated MR or AR. The enlargement of the pulmonary artery and LA appendage results in a characteristic straight left heart border. LA enlargement is common. Evidence of PVH is often seen as well (**Fig. 6**). Calcification of mitral valve is a late feature and this may be more easily identified through fluoroscopy.
- ECG in children is in sinus rhythm. LA enlargement and right atrial (RA) enlargement could be present. Right axis deviation and RVH are found in 50% of severe MS. LA enlargement is found in 90% of severe MS (**Fig. 7**).

Assessment of Severity

The practical points used to assess severity of MS are listed in **Box 10**.

BOX 9: Causes of mid-diastolic murmur in rheumatic heart disease.

- Severe AR—*Austin Flint* murmur
- Severe MR
- *Carey Coombs* murmur due to carditis
- Associated TS (at lower sternal border)

Echocardiography

This is the optimal mode of imaging in MS and is the most accurate one (**Figs. 8A and B**). It serves to assess the anatomy of mitral valve disease, severity of stenosis, associated involvement of other valves, hemodynamic consequences

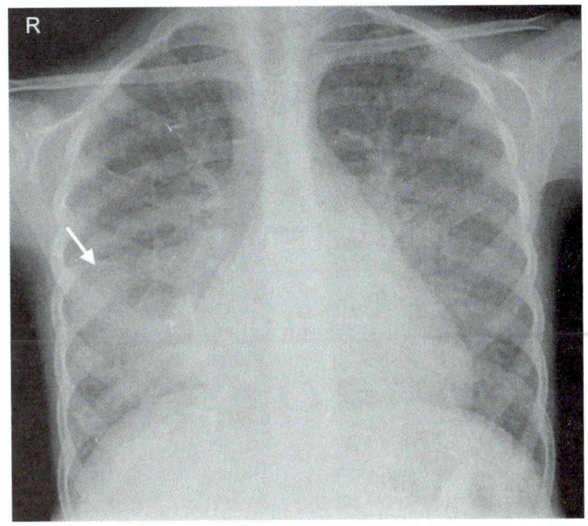

Fig. 6: Chest X-ray (posteroanterior view) from an 8-year-old patient with juvenile mitral stenosis as a result of rheumatic heart disease. There is evidence of severe pulmonary venous hypertension in the form of prominent upper lobe pulmonary veins (cephalization), interstitial haze and prominent interlobar fissures (arrow). Additionally, there is evidence of left atrial (lifting up of the left bronchus) and left atrial appendage (straightening of left heart border).

BOX 10: Clinical, X-ray, and ECG assessment of severity of mitral stenosis.

- Symptom status
- Low-volume pulse
- Elevated jugular venous pressure
- Presence of significant pulmonary hypertension clinically
- *Short A2-OS interval*: Inversely proportional to severity
- *Length of MDM*: Longer murmur associated with severe stenosis
- Loud first heart sound
- Left atrial enlargement and pulmonary venous hypertension (PVH) on X-ray
- Right axis deviation (>120%), right ventricular hypertrophy (RVH) and left atrial enlargement on ECG

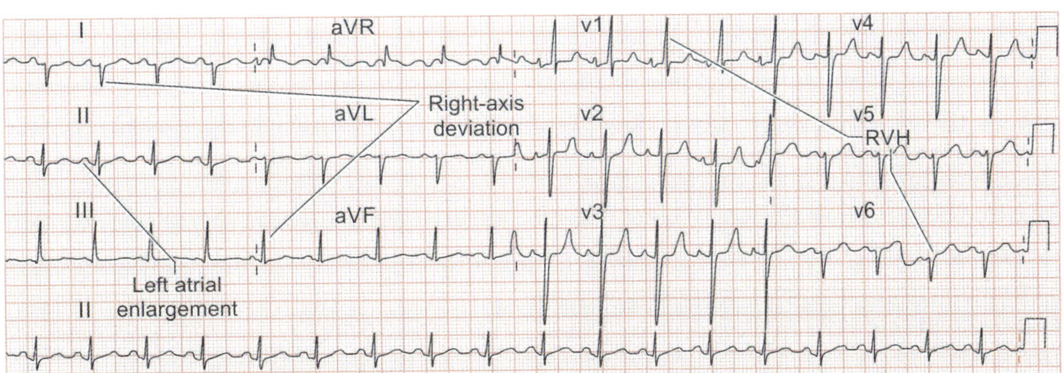

Fig. 7: Electrocardiogram from an 8-year-old child with rheumatic heart disease and severe mitral stenosis. There is evidence of right ventricular hypertrophy in the form of rightward deviation of the QRS axis, prominent "r" waves in V1 and persistent "s" waves in V5 and V6. Additionally, there is evidence of left atrial enlargement in the form of prominent broad "p" waves in lead II.

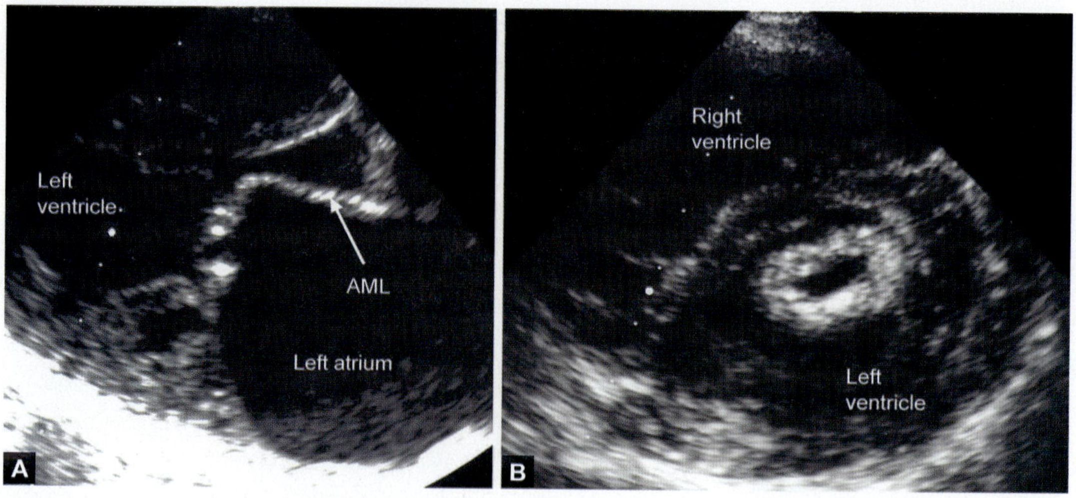

Figs. 8A and B: Two-dimensional echocardiography for rheumatic heart disease and mitral stenosis. (A) A diastolic frame from the parasternal long-axis view. The characteristic "dog-leg" or "elbow" deformity is shown in the anterior mitral valve leaflet (AML). The tips of the AML are thickened. The thick and shortened chordae attached to the posterior mitral leaflet are also shown in this frame; (B) A picture obtained from the parasternal short-axis view. This view captures the mitral valve orifice in mid-diastole and allows accurate estimation of the mitral valve area. This view is also very useful in planning balloon mitral valvotomy (BMV). In this patient, for instance, it can be anticipated that the commissures would split favorably after BMV.

TABLE 11: The general treatment measures and medical management for rheumatic mitral stenosis.

Treatment	*Rationale*
General measures	
Secondary rheumatic prophylaxis	Prevention of recurrences of rheumatic fever and disease progression
Supervision of physical activity	Unsupervised exertion can precipitate pulmonary edema
Correction of anemia	Anemia can significantly worsen symptom status
Salt restriction	Salt restriction can reduce intravascular volume and pulmonary venous congestion
Specific medications	
Diuretic	Reduce intravascular volume and pulmonary venous congestion
Beta-blocker	The gradient across the mitral valve is markedly worsened by tachycardia because of a disproportionate reduction in duration of diastole. Beta-blockers are very effective in reducing heart rate and mitigate symptoms in mitral stenosis. Beta-blockers can be used in both sinus rhythm as well as atrial fibrillation
Ivabradine[28]	Ivabradine reduces heart rate and has the same effect of beta-blockers with the added advantage of not provoking bronchospasm. Ivabradine is only effective in sinus rhythm
Oral anticoagulants	Prevention of development of left atrial clots and thromboembolism. Indicated when atrial fibrillation develops

that include LA enlargement, PAH, and RV status. The suitability for balloon mitral valvuloplasty (BMV) is assessed by Wilkins score.[27] Additional features that are identified by echo include the presence of LA and atrial appendage clots.

The MVA can be assessed by measuring the cross-sectional area (2D planimetry) or by Doppler-derived measurements (pressure half-time) and continuity equation.

Treatment

The general treatment measures and medical management for MS are summarized in **Table 11**.

Specific Treatment

Transcatheter balloon mitral valvotomy is the treatment of choice in isolated significant MS with a suitable valve anatomy.[29] Surgical closed mitral valvotomy is rarely performed even though it is a less expensive and equally effective alternative. Open surgical mitral commissurotomy under cardiopulmonary bypass is occasionally necessary when the valve anatomy does not permit safe BMV. A careful assessment of the valve anatomy by echocardiography is mandatory prior to BMV. Risk factors for a suboptimal result include the presence of calcification on the leaflet margin, MR that is more than mild or from one of the commissural edges and if there is severe subvalvular deformity. Additionally, the presence of a thrombus in the LA appendage requires anticoagulation and the procedure to be deferred until the clot resolves.

Balloon mitral valvotomy is indicated in all patients with severe rheumatic MS and symptomatic patients with moderate MS.

The results are dictated by valve anatomy and are excellent in those with predominant commissural fusion with doubling of existing valve area. The stroke volume improves by significantly and the gradient across the mitral valve and LA pressure declines dramatically. PAH often resolves over a few months after the procedure. In experienced hands, BMV has a success rate of >95%. Complications include thromboembolism, development of significant acute MR, cardiac perforation and tamponade. The procedural mortality is <1%.

During follow-up, the dilated valve may become narrow with time and repeat BMV may be needed if the valve is still suited for BMV. Eventually, the valve will need replacement or extensive open commissurotomy. Recurrence of symptoms after BMV situation could be due to restenosis, MR, aortic or tricuspid valve disease.

MITRAL REGURGITATION

Rheumatic MR is the most common heart valve affliction in RHD in children.[30] In the pathology of rheumatic MR, virtually all components of mitral valve tensor apparatus are involved—annulus, leaflets, and chordae tendineae. There is shortening, rigidity, deformity, and retraction of leaflets.

Other specific causes of chronic MR in children include mitral valve prolapse, IE, dilated cardiomyopathy, hypertrophic cardiomyopathy, collagen vascular disease, and endomyocardial fibrosis. Congenital causes of MR include cleft mitral valve, double orifice mitral valve, and mitral valve arcade. MR also occurs as a consequence of papillary muscle ischemia in anomalous left coronary artery from pulmonary artery and AV septal defect. The left-sided tricuspid valve is often incompetent in corrected transposition.

Pathophysiology

In chronic MR, left ventricle pumps blood both to aorta and LA. Functionally, the ejection into aorta and exists in parallel with regurgitation into LA. Hence, there is little resistance (afterload) to LV emptying. The MR starts before ejection during the isovolumetric contraction phase; this continues during ejection and continues even after ejection. The extent of MR depends upon regurgitant orifice in systole and systemic vascular resistance and pressure gradient between left ventricle and LA. The left ventricle initially compensates by Frank–Starling law that results in exaggerated contractility causing increased emptying. As a result, the end-systolic volume is often normal and sometimes lower than normal despite an increased end-diastolic volume (EDV). Some LV hypertrophy also occurs and this is referred to as eccentric hypertrophy because of the associated increased EDV. The stroke volume (across the aortic valve) remains normal. This is referred to as the compensated phase and may last several years during which the patient has minimal or no symptoms. However, with progressive LV dilation, the mitral annulus dilates and regurgitation worsens—MR begets more MR. Once decompensation occurs, end-systolic volume and ejection fraction first normalize and then decrease, stroke volume decreases and symptoms start to manifest with development of overt heart failure. The LA pressure increases leading to PVH that is a late feature of chronic severe MR. Pulmonary hypertension as a result of severe MR is a passive consequence of PVH. Right heart failure follows long-standing pulmonary hypertension. Long-standing atrial dilation results in AF. This is relatively rare in young children but quite common in adults. Acute MR is often associated with severe PVH and PAH because there is no time for compensation. Some children with chronic severe MR can have significant PAH as a result of an exaggerated vasoconstriction of the pulmonary arterioles.

Symptomatology

Most patients with mild or moderate MR are asymptomatic and, so are many severe MR in the initial stages. The asymptomatic phase can last several years. The most common symptoms are dyspnea and fatigue on effort that results from the effects of inadequate cardiac output. Later elevated LA pressures and pulmonary venous congestion also contribute to dyspnea. Palpitation is the result of cardiac enlargement and tachycardia. AF happens late as a result of chronic LA enlargement and results in wide fluctuations in heart rate that results in considerable discomfort. Chest pain and syncope are rare, as well as are hemoptysis and stroke. Features of right heart failure occur late.

Worsening of "stable MR" is often the result of one of the following events. They are:

- Development of AF
- Development of rheumatic reactivation
- Development of IE
- Reduction in LV function.

Physical Examination

Pulse can be normal or sometimes interpreted as "hyperkinetic". This is perhaps because of a rapid upstroke resulting from an initially forceful LV contraction. The jugular venous pressure is normal unless heart failure coexists. There is often cardiomegaly with forceful apex if MR is moderate or severe. A systolic thrill may be found by is often not felt in isolated MR. The precordium is often hyperkinetic. Evidence of PAH can be found in acute MR or chronic decompensated severe MR.

The first heart sound (S1) is typically soft due to failure to coaptation of the valve leaflets in isolated MR. However, in RHD, there is often some degree of associated MS and S1 may be normal or even loud. The second heart sound (S2) is often split wide due to early aortic valve closure (A2). The pulmonary component is loud if there is associated pulmonary hypertension. Moderate of severe MR usually has an accompanying LVS3.

The apical pansystolic murmur is quite typical in MR. It has a high and relatively uniform pitch, often described as blowing. It typically conducts to axilla and the back in RHD. Rarely, it may conduct to the front of chest. It increases on handgrip and expiration. A brief MDM without presystolic accentuation can occur in severe MR. It has been increasingly recognized that mild MR can be clinically silent.

Rheumatic MR needs to be sometimes distinguished from mitral valve prolapse, the other common cause for MR. The murmur of MVP is often late systolic and begins after a mid-systolic click. The MVP murmur characteristically begins earlier in systole and becomes louder in all maneuvers that reduce the LV filling such as standing. Additional details on the effect of various physiological maneuvers on murmurs are available in Chapter 5.

The severity of MR can be graded clinically. Severe MR is suggested by evidence of cardiomegaly, a mid-diastolic flow murmur, and associated PAH (loud P2). A systolic thrill at apex may also indicate severe MR but this is an insensitive sign.

Chest X-ray

In significant MR, cardiomegaly is expected and is variable with LV apex and LA enlargement is usual (**Fig. 9**). PVH is less prominent in chronic MR but is common in acute MR and in the decompensated state with LV dysfunction or when there is associated MS.

Electrocardiography

Severe MR is associated with LV volume overload pattern as suggested by prominent LV voltages and "q" waves in lateral chest leads. Features of LA enlargement are common but in general, "p" waves voltages and patterns are an insensitive indicator of LA enlargement.

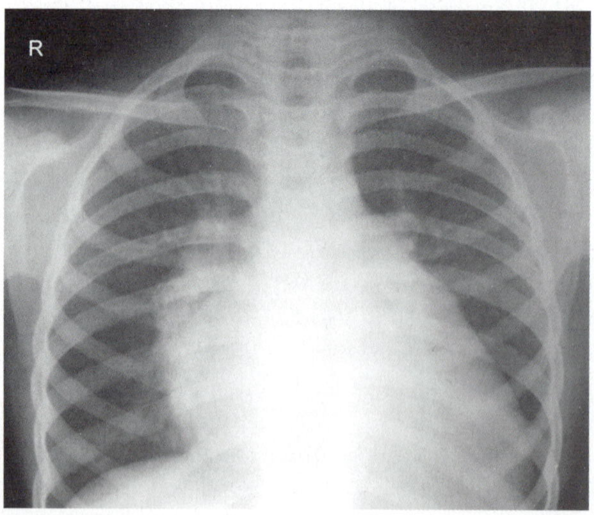

Fig. 9: Chest X-ray in mitral regurgitation showing cardiomegaly, pulmonary venous hypertension, left atrial and left ventricular enlargement.

Children with MR are generally in sinus rhythm despite significant LA enlargement. However, AF can occur in adolescents and young adults.

Echocardiography

It is the optimal and specific modality to assess MR. It establishes the diagnosis and etiology of MR and quantifies severity. Severity assessment is by LV and LA size measurement, color Doppler, quantitation of regurgitant fraction, regurgitant volume, and regurgitant orifice.[31]

The hemodynamic consequences of MR such as ventricular size and function, atrial enlargement, and pulmonary hypertension can be studied in detail (**Fig. 10**). Serial echocardiography is often used to guide decision regarding timing of surgery in asymptomatic severe MR. A detailed echocardiographic assessment of the valve and tensor apparatus is useful prior to mitral valve repair. Three-dimensional (3D) echo is increasingly utilized for delineation of MV anatomy prior to surgery. Transesophageal echocardiography is useful for children with poor windows, as a guide during surgical repair of the mitral valve and in careful evaluation of suspected endocarditis.

Natural History

Mild or moderate MR tends to remain stable for several years. While in mild MR, progression to severe MR is quite rare, a small proportion of moderate MR can progress. Progression is largely dictated by recurrences of RF and strict adherence to secondary prophylaxis is remarkably effective in preventing progression. Other events that result in progression to severe MR include IE and spontaneous chordal rupture.

Even severe MR can be stable for relatively long periods of time. They should be closely followed with serial

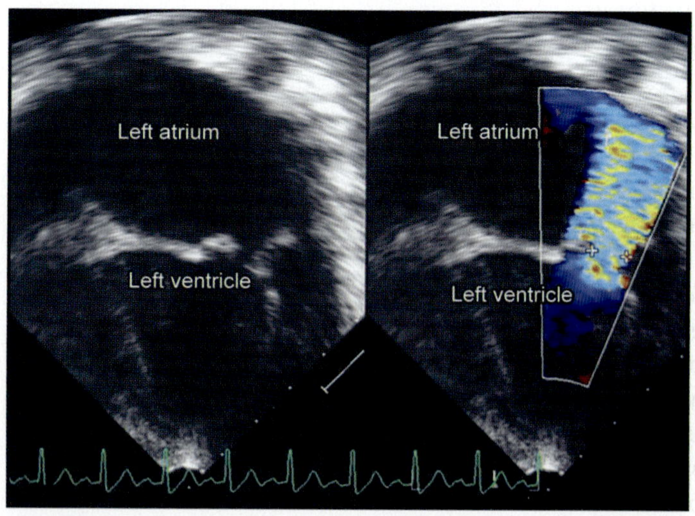

Fig. 10: Echocardiogram (apical four-chamber view) in a patient with severe mitral regurgitation showing left atrial and left ventricular enlargement with a posteriorly and laterally directed jet of mitral regurgitation into the left atrium. The mitral valve is thickened and there is poor coaptation between the mitral valve leaflets.

TABLE 12: Management of rheumatic mitral regurgitation.

Treatment	*Rationale and indications*
General measures	
Secondary rheumatic prophylaxis	Prevention of recurrences of rheumatic fever and disease progression
Infective endocarditis prophylaxis	Infective endocarditis prophylaxis is indicated in selected procedures where there is a perceived risk for transient bacteremia (*see* Chapter 41)
Supervision of isometric physical activity	Isometric exertion can precipitate clinical worsening
Specific medications	
Diuretic	Reduce intravascular volume and pulmonary venous congestion; indicated in those with decompensation and heart failure
Angiotensin-converting enzyme (ACE) inhibitor	The role of ACE inhibitor (enalapril) in chronic compensated MR is controversial. There is no physiologic benefit because the ventricle is already subject to very low afterload. However, it may be indicated in acute MR or as supportive therapy once LV dysfunction has set in
Surgical management	
Mitral valve repair	Preferred option in children because it avoids the need for long-term oral anticoagulation with its attendant risks and enables better preservation of ventricular function. The potential downsides are the need for surgical expertise and experience as well as the limited duration of benefit. Rheumatic recurrences are likely to result in worsening MR. Surgery is indicated in symptomatic patients with chronic severe MR and asymptomatic patients with evidence of ventricular dysfunction in the form of reduced left ventricular (LV) ejection fraction (<60%); or unacceptable LV dilation (LV end-systolic dimension of >28 mm/m^2)
Mitral valve replacement	Less preferred option to repair. Indicated when repair fails or is deemed not feasible because of unsuitable valve pathology

echocardiography and surgery is indicated whenever there is objective evidence of worsening LV function or development of symptoms. Surgery is typically needed within 5–10 years. Other complications that can develop during follow-up include AF that often results in dramatic worsening of symptoms, heart failure from decompensation.

Management

The management of rheumatic MR is summarized in **Table 12**.

Often, no medications other than secondary penicillin prophylaxis is necessary in asymptomatic patients with compensated chronic rheumatic MR. Medications are needed to relieve symptoms or when decompensation starts to set in (**Table 12**).

Patients with asymptomatic rheumatic MR should be followed closely with serial echocardiography. Surgery is generally indicated when there is early sign of ventricular dysfunction. It is important to recognize that the reduced afterload often results in a higher than normal ejection fraction in MR. Therefore, an ejection fraction of <60% may suggest the onset of ventricular dysfunction and surgery may be indicated. In older children and adults, LV end-systolic dimension of >28 mm/m^2 may mandate consideration for surgery. Surgical management should ideally be in the form of mitral valve repair.[16,32] The rationale and indications are summarized in **Table 12**. Prior to MV repair, it is essential to make a careful assessment of mitral valve pathology and discuss the nuances with the surgeon. In expert hands, the immediate results of MV repair are gratifying with success rates > 95%.

RHEUMATIC AORTIC VALVE DISEASE (AORTIC REGURGITATION)

The aortic valve is almost always affected in association with mitral valve affliction in RHD. AR is usual consequence of RHD. Rheumatic aortic stenosis is exceptional in children. This chapter will focus on AR. Rheumatic AR in children is second only to bicuspid aortic valve as cause of AR. It usually coexists with rheumatic mitral valve involvement.[16,30] Other pediatric causes of AR are IE, Marfan syndrome, collagen vascular diseases, and Takayasu arteritis. AR is also associated with congenital heart disease. The best example is ventricular septal defect (see Chapter 22) and aortic root dilation (aortopathy) that often happens late in a number of CHDs and late after selected operations such as the arterial switch operation.

Pathophysiology

The left ventricle pumps its entire output into aorta a portion of which returns back to the LV. This phenomenon causes and increases LV volume (LVEDV) leading to compensatory LV hypertrophy (LVH). This is termed as "eccentric LVH" because of the combination of increased LV volume as well as wall thickness. This enables compensation initially but later it leads to LV dysfunction and heart failure. LV dysfunction causes elevation of LVEDP which causes symptoms in the form of dyspnea because of elevation of LA and associated PVH.

Left ventricular hypertrophy increases increased oxygen demand and contributes to ischemia and LV dysfunction. Decrease in aortic diastolic pressure reduces coronary perfusion pressure and hence leads to coronary hypoperfusion and subsequent ischemia. Decrease in forward stroke volume (FSV) leads to reduction in forward cardiac output and also causes ischemia. Dyspnea in AR is due to elevated LVEDP and LV dysfunction. Chest pain has many causative factors such as reduced aortic diastolic pressure, increased LVEDP, myocardial supply or demand ischemia, and reduction in FSV.

Clinical Features

The clinical features are summarized in **Box 11**. Patients with AR are typically symptom free for long periods and may even have excellent exercise tolerance. Eventually symptoms develop. Dyspnea on effort is the most common symptom. Palpitations result from a large left ventricle that has significant volume changes that increase the perception of the heartbeat.

Physical Examination

The pulse is characteristically high volume and collapsing it can be "bisferiens", especially if there is an element of stenosis.

BOX 11: Symptoms of aortic regurgitation (AR).

- Patient with chronic AR can be asymptomatic for long periods
- Dyspnea on exertion is the most common symptom
- Anginal pain can occur
- Palpitation can occur due to hyperdynamic heart
- Fatigue could be a late feature
- Syncope is rare
- Nocturnal angina is characteristic in severe AR as during sleep, heart rate comes down, lengthening diastole and causing more of AR. Aortic diastolic pressure falls leading to reduction in coronary perfusion

As would be expected, the pulse pressure is widened with some elevation of systolic blood pressure (BP) and reduction of diastolic BP. A number of "peripheral" signs of severe AR have been described, all of which are the result of a widened pulse pressure and low diastolic pressure (**Table 13**). The most useful among them are collapsing pulse, Hill's sign, and Duroziez's murmur.

Precordial examination is characterized by cardiomegaly with hyperkinetic apex. Palpation may also reveal suprasternal pulsations and carotid shudder. The first heart sound (S1) is usually normal or soft. Soft S1 is due to increase in LVEDV with floating up of the mitral valve toward the orifice and can also be due to LV dysfunction. The second heart sound (S2) is normally split and A2 can be soft. S2 can also be single as P2 may be masked by early diastolic murmur (EDM). An LV third heart sound is ominous, indicating LV dysfunction.

The characteristic murmur of AR is high-pitched, blowing EDM heard over the left upper sternal edge in the 3rd or 2nd intercostal space. The EDM becomes longer with increasing severity. This is better heard with the bell of the stethoscope with the patient leaning forward. An MDM without presystolic accentuation is heard at apex (Austin Flint) in severe AR. This is due to floating up of the mitral valve at end-diastole causing a relative narrowing of mitral valve orifice or due to AR jet impinging on AML causing fluttering of the leaflet. It can be distinguished from an organic murmur of MS by the accompanying features (**Table 14**).

Investigations

X-ray shows cardiomegaly with LV apex (**Fig. 11**). The ascending aorta and aortic knuckle may be prominent in long-standing AR. The ECG shows features of LV volume overload with prominent LV forces and "q" waves in lateral leads.

Echocardiography is the optimal imaging as it serves to assess the aortic valve morphology, severity of AR, LV dimensions, and function as well as involvement of other valves (**Fig. 12**).

TABLE 13: Selected "peripheral" signs of severe aortic regurgitation.

Sign	*Description*
Hill sign	The measured lower limb BP can be normally up to 20 mm Hg higher than the upper limb BP. If the difference is >20 mm Hg, it is called a positive Hill sign. It can further be graded into mild (20–40), moderate (40–60), and severe (>60)
Quincke's sign	It is the capillary pulsation noted in the base of the nail bed when the examiner applies pressure over the distal end of the nail plate. This can be better appreciated by transmitting a light through the patient's fingertips
Corrigan's sign	It refers to the classical "waterhammer" pulse of AR
De Musset's sign	Head nodding with each heartbeat
Traube's sign	Pistol shot sound over the femoral artery
Duroziez's sign	Systolic murmur over femoral artery with proximal compression and diastolic murmur when compressed distally
Muller's sign	Systolic pulsations of the uvula

TABLE 14: Distinguishing Austin Flint murmur from organic mitral valve stenosis in rheumatic heart disease.

Feature	*Mitral valve stenosis*	*Austin Flint murmur*
Pulse volume	Normal/Low	High
Pulse pressure	Normal	High
Cardiomegaly	Absent	Present
Apex	Tapping	Forceful
First heart sound	Loud	Soft
Third heart sound	Never	Can be present
Opening snap	Present	Absent
Presystolic accentuation	Present	Absent

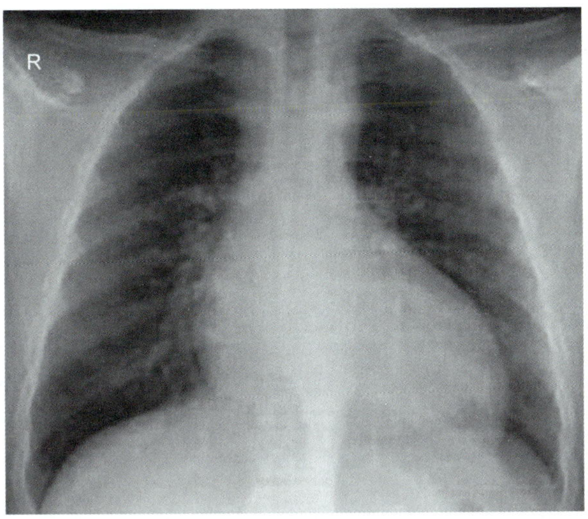

Fig. 11: Chest X-ray in aortic regurgitation showing left ventricular enlargement. Note the absence of significant pulmonary venous hypertension.

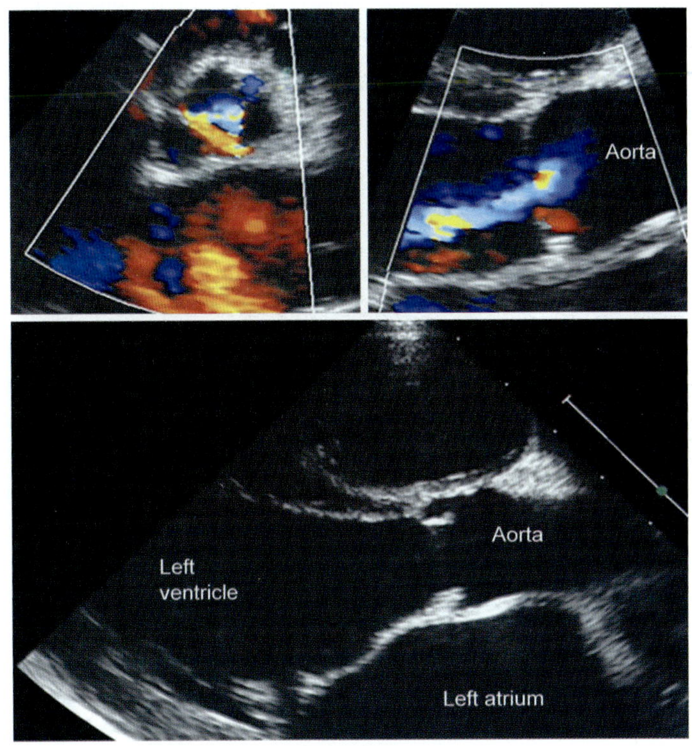

Fig. 12: Two-dimensional echocardiograms and color Doppler from a patient with rheumatic heart disease involving the aortic valve. The dominant lesion here is aortic regurgitation that is the result of fibrosis and shortening of the individual leaflet cusps. The jet is characteristically central (upper frames). The thickened cusps are seen in the lower systolic frame obtained in the parasternal short-axis view.

Natural History

Chronic severe AR can remain asymptomatic for a long period. Once symptoms develop, the clinical decline is often rapid. In the young, 10-year survival of severe asymptomatic AR is excellent, often > 90%. However, in either symptomatic AR or with LV dysfunction, survival at 10 years is <50%. Mild or moderate AR does not necessarily require valve replacement in patients undergoing severe mitral valve replacement.[33]

Treatment

The treatment of AR is summarized in **Table 15**.

The standard procedure is aortic valve replacement. Aortic valve repair is difficult to perform.[16,30] Additionally, the prosthetic valve in the aortic position is less vulnerable to thrombosis in the face of suboptimal anticoagulation.

TRICUSPID VALVE DISEASE

Tricuspid valve has three leaflets: (1) anterior, (2) septal, and (3) posterior. It has a valve area of 4–6 cm^2. Tricuspid valve in RHD can be affected functionally (due to PAH) or organically. Tricuspid valve disease can be either tricuspid stenosis (TS) or TR. It is almost always accompanied by mitral or aortic valve disease. Clinically apparent tricuspid valve disease occurs in 5%, echocardiographically 8%, and by autopsy approximately 15%.[34]

Tricuspid regurgitation in RHD is most often due to pulmonary hypertension and is associated with mitral valve disease. This is labeled as functional TR and often resolves with resolution of pulmonary hypertension once the mitral valve is managed successfully. On the other hand, organic involvement of the tricuspid valve results in disproportionately severe TR with RA and RV enlargement. This TR can be accompanied by varying degrees of stenosis. Jugular venous pressure is elevated with a prominent

TABLE 15: Management of rheumatic aortic regurgitation.

Treatment	*Rationale and indications*
General measures	
Secondary rheumatic prophylaxis	Prevention of recurrences of rheumatic fever and disease progression
Infective endocarditis prophylaxis	Infective endocarditis prophylaxis is indicated in selected procedures where there is a perceived risk for transient bacteremia (*see* Chapter 41)
Supervision of isometric physical activity	Isometric exertion can precipitate clinical worsening
Specific medications	
Vasodilators	Vasodilator therapy is not routinely recommended in chronic asymptomatic AR with normal LV systolic function. For patients with symptoms or with LV dysfunction, vasodilators may be used. Medical therapy is not a substitute for surgery in symptomatic patients with severe AR. ACE inhibitors, angiotensin receptor blockers, and calcium channel blockers may be used as vasodilators
Surgical management	
Aortic valve replacement (AVR)	The indications for AVR include: • Symptomatic severe AR regardless of LV systolic function • Asymptomatic chronic severe AR with LV systolic dysfunction (EF < 55%) or LV dilation with end-diastolic dimension > 38 mm/m^2 or end-systolic dimension > 28 mm/m^2 • Severe AR in a patient undergoing cardiac surgery for another indication (e.g., MVR)
Aortic valve repair	Aortic valve repair is seldom realistic in rheumatic heart disease

"v" wave. The TR murmur is pansystolic and heard best in the lower left sternal border and increases on expiration.

Predominant TS is a relatively uncommon manifestation and is seldom seen in children.[35] Obstruction to tricuspid valve flow is also be caused by carcinoid syndrome, RA myxoma, and some variants of Ebstein's anomaly. TS presents with progressive fatigue, dyspnea on exertion, and later frank right heart failure with edema. The jugular venous pressure is elevated with prominent "a" wave, S1 is either normal or loud. An OS is sometimes heard at tricuspid area will be followed by a MDM that is typically much softer than MS. A presystolic accentuation at lower left sternal border is sometimes identified. The murmur increases on inspiration.

The chest X-ray reveals cardiomegaly and RA enlargement and ECG often reveals RA enlargement and RVH. A "qR" pattern in V1 points to significant RA dilation. Echocardiography defines TV anatomy and physiology and enables quantification of pulmonary systolic pressures and severity of TS. In addition, involvement of other valvular is also defined.

Tricuspid regurgitation often resolves with resolution of PAH following management of left heart valve pathology. However, during surgery, surgeons often perform a tricuspid valve annuloplasty (De Vega Repair) to enable a faster and more predictable recovery. Significant dominant TS may require balloon valvotomy.

MULTIVALVE RHEUMATIC HEART DISEASE

In multivalve rheumatic disease, same valve can be involved with stenosis and regurgitation coexisting or different valves could be involved.[16,30] *A number of possible combinations are therefore possible.* It is important to precisely quantify the severity of involvement of the affected valves to ensure that correct decisions are taken regarding treatment. Clinical presentation is dictated by relative severity of individual lesions. There is also some degree of masking or neutralizing effect of some stenotic individual lesion on the downstream valve pathology. For example, MS is masked by TS and AR is masked by MS.

The combination of MS and MR is common in RHD. The dominant features of MS in the combination are loud S1, OS, and absence of LVS3. The dominant features of MR are an apical pansystolic murmur, soft S1, absent OS, and LVS3. Symptoms include dyspnea, palpitation, and fatigue. Both MDM and PSM are heard at apex. If significant MR and MS coexist, mitral valve repair may be a challenging option.

The combination of AR and MR is also common and it is surprisingly well tolerated. Over time, however, decompensation is inevitable from progressive LV enlargement.

The combined involvement of mitral and aortic valve may sometimes necessitate double valve replacement in children. This operation does not have a good long-term outcome.

CONCLUSION

This chapter has sought to present a comprehensive overview of acute RF and rheumatic heart valve disease. RF is a disease which licks the joints, bites the heart, and stings the brain. The bite on the heart may be very severe at times and the permanent scars are almost entirely limited to heart valves. While it is perhaps true that the incidence of RF and prevalence of RHD are on a decline in many parts of India and other low- and middle-income regions, there is still a substantial overall burden of RHD. Additionally, RF continues to affect the poorer and marginalized sections of the society. For these reasons, it is essential for every student of pediatrics to be familiar with the diagnosis and management of RF and RHD.

REFERENCES

1. Tandon R, Sharma M, Chandrashekhar Y, Kotb M, Yacoub MH, Narula J. Revisiting the pathogenesis of rheumatic fever and carditis. Nat Rev Cardiol. 2013;10:171-7.
2. Watkins DA, Johnson CO, Colquhoun SM, Karthikeyan G, Beaton A, Bukhman G, et al. Global, regional, and national burden of rheumatic heart disease, 1990-2015. N Engl J Med. 2017;377(8):713-22.
3. Hajar R. Rheumatic fever and rheumatic heart disease—a historical perspective. Heart Views. 2016;17:120-6.
4. Roy SB, Bhatia ML, Lazaro EJ, Ramalingaswami V. Juvenile mitral stenosis in India. Lancet. 1963;2:1193-5.
5. Remenyi B, Wilson N, Steer A, Ferreira B, Kado J, Kumar K, et al. World Heart Federation criteria for echocardiographic diagnosis of rheumatic heart disease—an evidence-based guideline. Nat Rev Cardiol. 2012;28:297-309.
6. Gewitz MH, Baltimore RS, Tani LY, Sable CA, Shulman ST, Carapetis J, et al. Revision of the Jones Criteria for the diagnosis of acute rheumatic fever in the era of Doppler echocardiography: a scientific statement from the American Heart Association. Circulation. 2015;131(20):1806-18.
7. Kumar RK, Tandon R. Rheumatic fever and rheumatic heart disease: the last 50 years. Indian J Med Res. 2013;137:643-58.
8. Veasy LG, Wiedmeier SE, Orsmond GS, Ruttenberg HD, Boucek MM, Roth SJ, et al. Resurgence of acute rheumatic fever in the intermountain area of the United States. N Engl J Med. 1987;316:421-7.
9. Davidson L, Knight J, Bowen AC. Skin infections in Australian Aboriginal children: a narrative review. Med J Aust. 2020;212: 231-7.
10. Muhamed B, Parks T, Sliwa K. Genetics of rheumatic fever and rheumatic heart disease. Nat Rev Cardiol. 2020;17:145-54.
11. Palafox B, Mocumbi AO, Kumar RK, Ali SK, Kennedy E, Haileamlak A, et al. The WHF roadmap for reducing CV morbidity and mortality through prevention and control of RHD. Glob Heart. 2017;12(1):47-62.
12. WHO Study Group on Rheumatic Fever and Rheumatic Heart Disease (2001: Geneva, Switzerland) and World Health Organization. (2004). Rheumatic fever and rheumatic heart disease: report of a WHO expert consultation, Geneva, 20 October - 1 November 2001. World Health Organization. [online] Available from: https://apps.who.int/iris/handle/10665/42898 [Last accessed July, 2021].
13. Tubridy-Clark M, Carapetis JR. Subclinical carditis in rheumatic fever: a systematic review. Int J Cardiol. 2007;119:54-8.
14. McCallum AH. Natural history of rheumatic fever and rheumatic heart disease. Ten-year report of a co-operative clinical trial of A.C.T.H., cortisone, and aspirin. Br Med J. 1965;2(5462):607-13.
15. Kumar RK, Paul M, Francis PT. Rheumatic heart disease in India: are we ready to shift from secondary prophylaxis to vaccinating high risk children. Curr Sci. 2009;97:397-404.
16. Kumar RK, Antunes MJ, Beaton A, Mirabel M, Nkomo VT, Okello E, et al. Contemporary diagnosis and management of rheumatic heart disease: implications for closing the gap: a scientific statement from the American Heart Association. Circulation. 2020;142(20):e337-57.
17. Chockalingam A, Gnanavelu G, Elangovan S, Chockalingam V. Clinical spectrum of chronic rheumatic heart disease in India. J Heart Valve Dis. 2003;12(5):577-81.
18. McCredie RM, Richards JG. Combined mitral and pulmonary valve stenosis. Br Heart J. 1966;28(1):139-42.
19. Krishnan MN. Mitral stenosis. In: Prabhakaran D, Kumar RK, Naik N, Kaul U (Eds). Tandon's Textbook of Cardiology. Gurugram, India: Wolters Kluwer India Pvt. Ltd.; 2019.
20. Thomas JD, Bonow RO. Mitral valve disease. In: Zipes D, Libby P, Bonow R, Mann D, Tomaselli G (Eds). Braunwald's Heart Disease. A Textbook of Cardiovascular Medicine, 11th edition. Gurugram, India: Elsevier India; 2019.
21. Maeder MT, Weber L, Buser M, Gerhard M, Haager PK, Maisano F, et al. Pulmonary hypertension in aortic and mitral valve disease. Front Cardiovasc Med. 2018;5:40.
22. Vasan RS, Selvaraj N. Natural history of acute rheumatic fever. In: Narula J, Virmani R, Reddy KS, Tandon R (Eds). Rheumatic Fever. Washington, DC: American Registry of Pathology Publication; 1999. pp. 347-58.
23. Gaasch WH, Folland ED. Left ventricular function in rheumatic mitral stenosis. Eur Heart J. 1991;12 Suppl B:66-9.
24. Wood P. An appreciation of mitral stenosis. I. Clinical features. Br Med J. 1954;1:1051-63.
25. Deverall PB, Olley PM, Smith DR, Watson DA, Whitaker W. Incidence of systemic embolism before and after mitral valvotomy. Thorax. 1968;23(5):530-6.
26. Delman AJ, Gordon GM, Stein E, Escher DJ. The second sound-mitral opening snap (A2-OS) interval during exercise in the evaluation of mitral stenosis. Circulation. 1966;33:399-403.
27. Wilkins GT, Weyman AE, Abascal VM, Block PC, Palacios IF. Percutaneous balloon dilatation of the mitral valve: an analysis of echocardiographic variables related to outcome and the mechanism of dilatation. Br Heart J. 1988;60:299-308.
28. Ramos JD, Cunanan EL, Abrahan LL 4th, Tiongson MD, Punzalan FE. Ivabradine versus beta-blockers in mitral stenosis in sinus rhythm: an updated meta-analysis of randomized controlled trials. Cardiol Res. 2018;9:224-30.
29. Carabello BA. Modern management of mitral stenosis. Circulation. 2005;112(3):432-7.
30. Wernovsky G, Anderson RH, Kumar K, Mussatto KA, Redington AN, Tweddell JS. Anderson's Pediatric Cardiology, 4th edition. Philadelphia, USA: Elsevier; 2019. pp. 1023-41.
31. Otto CM, Nishimura RA, Bonow RO, Carabello BA, Erwin JP 3rd, Gentile F, et al. 2020 ACC/AHA guideline for the management of patients with valvular heart disease: executive summary: a report of the American College of Cardiology/American Heart Association Joint Committee on clinical practice guidelines. Circulation. 2021;143(5):e35-71.
32. Remenyi B, Webb R, Gentles T, Russell P, Finucane K, Lee M, et al. Improved long-term survival for rheumatic mitral valve repair compared to replacement in the young. World J Pediatr Congenit Heart Surg. 2013;4:155-64.
33. Namboodiri N, Remash K, Tharakan JA, Shajeem O, Nair K, Titus T, et al. Natural history of aortic valve disease following intervention for rheumatic mitral valve disease. J Heart Valve Dis [illegible]
34. Yousof AM, Shafei MZ, Endrys G, Khan N, Simo M, Cherian G. Tricuspid stenosis and regurgitation in rheumatic heart disease: a prospective cardiac catheterization study in 525 patients. Am Heart J. 1985;110(1 Pt 1):60-4.
35. Goswami KC, Rao MB, Dev V, Shrivastava S. Juvenile tricuspid stenosis and rheumatic tricuspid valve disease: an echocardiographic study. Int J Cardiol. 1999;72(1):83-6.

SUGGESTED READING

1. Carapetis JR, MacDonald M, Wilson NJ. Acute rheumatic fever. Lancet. 2005;366(9480):155-68.
2. Dougherty S, Zuhlke L, Carapetis J, Wilson N. Acute Rheumatic Fever and Rheumatic Heart Disease. St Louis: Elsevier; 2019.
3. Narula J, Virmani R, Reddy KS, Tandon R. Rheumatic Fever. Washington, DC: American Registry of Pathology Publication; 1999.
4. Rheumatic fever and rheumatic heart disease: report of a WHO Expert Consultation. World Health Organization, Geneva, 2004 (Technical Report Series No. 923). [online] Available from: https://apps.who.int/iris/handle/10665/42898 [Last accessed July, 2021].

43

CHAPTER

Myocarditis

Navaneetha Sasikumar

DEFINITION AND EPIDEMIOLOGY

Myocarditis is an inflammatory disease of the myocardium and is diagnosed by established histological, immunological, and immunohistochemical criteria.[1]

The clinical presentation of myocarditis varies from an undiagnosed subclinical condition to sudden cardiac death. Coupled with the challenges in establishing a confirmed diagnosis, ascertaining the actual incidence of this disease is quite a difficult task. Nevertheless, biopsy-proven myocarditis accounted for 46% of dilated cardiomyopathies with an identified cause in children.[2] In adults, myocarditis is responsible for 10–50% of newly diagnosed dilated cardiomyopathies.[3] Autopsy series of sudden cardiac death in the young reports an incidence of myocarditis that varies from 2 to 4%.[4,5] Also, the incidence of myocarditis in autopsy series of children and young adults (0.6–1.8%) is higher when compared to the general population (0.05–0.1%).[6-8] A contemporary review of cardiovascular deaths in children of the United States attributed 4.6% of deaths to myocarditis.[9]

A bimodal age distribution has been classically described with peaks in infants and teenagers.[10] In recent pediatric data from Germany and Finland, the median age was found to be 13 and 14 years, respectively.[11,12] Though there is no gender predilection to myocarditis in children between 0 and 6 years of age, male sex has an higher incidence, with teenage boys and young adult men being considered most susceptible to the disease.[12]

CLASSIFICATION

Myocarditis can be classified according to various features. From a clinical perspective, it can be either uncomplicated or complicated (presence of ejection fraction <50% on first echocardiogram, sustained ventricular arrhythmias, heart failure, low cardiac output syndrome/hemodynamic instability on admission). In the Lombardy registry of adults presenting with acute myocarditis, despite having raised necrosis biomarkers and late gadolinium enhancement (LGE) on cardiac magnetic resonance (CMR), mortality and heart transplantation was 0% in the short term for the uncomplicated cases. This translated to 0% major adverse events at 5-year follow-up as well.[13] Myocarditis associated with ventricular dysfunction has also been termed "inflammatory cardiomyopathy".[1] Fulminant myocarditis is a distinct form of complicated myocarditis characterized by a sudden and severe inflammation of the myocardium resulting in myocyte necrosis, edema, and cardiogenic shock.[14]

According to the time of onset of symptoms, acute myocarditis is classically considered to have symptom onset within the previous 30 days of presentation without any previous history of heart failure or cardiomyopathy. This contrasts with later presentations, where the clinical differentiation of myocarditis from cardiomyopathy becomes increasingly difficult.

From a diagnostic/etiological perspective, myocarditis can be infectious or noninfectious. The former includes viral, bacterial, fungal, rickettsial, protozoal, and helminthic causes. Noninfectious myocarditis can be immune-mediated or toxin/drug-mediated (**Table 1**).

The pathological approach classifies myocarditis into lymphocytic, eosinophilic, neutrophilic, giant cell, and granulomatous varieties with major implications in management and prognosis.

ETIOLOGY

As mentioned in the etiological approach to classification, myocarditis can be caused by a variety of agents (**Table 1**). Acute myocarditis most commonly results from a recent viral infection in most geographic locations. Classically, enteroviruses such as coxsackie B and adenoviruses were implicated. A change in trend has been reported from North America and other developed countries, following the increase in utilization of polymerase chain reaction (PCR) to identify viral genome from myocardium. Parvovirus and human herpes virus 6 have been the major pathogens thus identified, along with hepatitis C, Epstein–Barr virus, and cytomegalovirus.[15] In a nationwide Japanese study, coxsackie A and B, influenza A and B, and adenovirus accounted for the

TABLE 1: Etiologic approach to classification of myocarditis.

Infectious		*Noninfectious*			
Bacterial	*Staphylococcus, Streptococcus, Pneumococcus, Meningococcus, Gonococcus, Salmonella, Corynebacterium diphtheriae, Haemophilus influenzae, Mycobacterium (tuberculosis), Mycoplasma pneumoniae*, and *Brucella*	Immune-mediated myocarditis		Toxic myocarditis	
Viral	• *RNA viruses*: Coxsackieviruses A and B, echoviruses, polioviruses, influenza A and B viruses, respiratory syncytial virus, mumps virus, measles virus, rubella virus, hepatitis C virus, dengue virus, yellow fever virus, Chikungunya virus, Junin virus, Lassa fever virus, rabies virus, human immunodeficiency virus-1, and SARS-CoV-2 • *DNA viruses*: adenoviruses, parvovirus B19, cytomegalovirus, human herpes virus-6, Epstein-Barr virus, varicella-zoster virus, herpes simplex virus, variola virus, vaccinia virus	Allergens	• Tetanus toxoid, vaccines, serum sickness • *Drugs*: penicillin, cefaclor, colchicine, furosemide, isoniazid, lidocaine, tetracycline, sulfonamides, phenytoin, phenyl-butazone, • Methyldopa, thiazide diuretics, and amitriptyline	Drugs	Amphetamines, anthracyclines, cocaine, cyclo-phosphamide, ethanol, fluorouracil, lithium, catecholamines, hematine, interleukin-2, trastuzumab, clozapine immune checkpoint inhibitors
Spirochetal	Borrelia (Lyme disease), Leptospira (Weil disease)	Allo-antigens	Heart transplant rejection	Heavy metals	Copper, iron, and lead
Protozoal	*Trypanosoma cruzi, Toxoplasma gondii, Entamoeba*, and *Leishmania*	Auto-antigens	• Infection-negative lymphocytic, infection-negative giant cell • Associated with autoimmune or immune-oriented disorders: systemic lupus erythematosus, rheumatoid arthritis, Churg–Strauss syndrome, Kawasaki disease, inflammatory bowel disease, scleroderma, polymyositis, myasthenia gravis, insulin-dependent diabetes mellitus, thyrotoxicosis, sarcoidosis, Wegener's granulomatosis, and rheumatic heart disease (rheumatic fever)	Miscellaneous	Scorpion sting, snake, and spider bites, bee and wasp stings, carbon monoxide, inhalants, phosphorus, arsenic, and sodium azide
Parasitic	*Trichinella spiralis, Echinococcus granulosus*, and *Taenia solium*	Hypereosi-nophilic syndromes	Idiopathic neoplastic reactive (parasitic, familial, Churg–Strauss)	Hormones	Pheochromocytoma, vitamins: beriberi
Rickettsial	*Coxiella burnetii* (Q fever), *Rickettsia rickettsii* (Rocky Mountain spotted fever), and *Rickettsia tsutsugamuschi*			Physical agents	Radiation and electric shock
Fungal	Aspergillus, Actinomyces, Blastomyces, Candida, Coccidioides, Cryptococcus, Histoplasma, Mucormycoses, Nocardia, Sporothrix				

majority of cases where a virus was identified.[16] Several cases were reported during the influenza A H1N1 pandemic in 2009 as well as with the ongoing SARS-CoV-2 pandemic.[17-19]

Similar to bacterial and fungal causes, parasitic infections are generally an uncommon cause of myocarditis. It is to be noted that *Trypanosoma cruzi* (Chagas disease) is responsible for a significant number of cases in Africa, Central, and South America. This is associated with an eosinophilic infiltrate on histology and often, peripheral eosinophilia. Helminthic infection, particularly toxocariasis has been reported to be responsible for eosinophilic myocarditis in Asia.[20]

Immune-mediated myocarditis results from allergens as in vaccines, associated with serum sickness, or related to hypersensitivity to drugs. Alloantigens can be responsible for immune-mediated myocarditis in postheart transplant cases. Myocarditis occurs due to autoimmune/immune-oriented diseases as well.

Drugs, notably amphetamines, cyclophosphamide, and catecholamines; heavy metals such as copper, lead, and iron; substances of abuse such as ethanol and cocaine; and toxins from scorpion sting, snake, and spider bites, bee and wasp stings have also been known to cause myocarditis (*see* **Table 1**). Of late, the newer anticancer drugs called immune checkpoint inhibitors have also been implicated as causative agents of myocarditis in adults.[21]

PATHOLOGY AND PATHOPHYSIOLOGY

Multiple mechanisms have been proposed as to how a pathogen/agent causes myocarditis. The major ones range either from direct invasion of the myocytes by an infectious agent or multiplication within the myocytes leading to necrosis or destruction of cardiac tissue by host cellular/humoral immune components (activated by an infectious agent), which have infiltrated the cardiac tissue or owing to the toxic effect of exogenous chemicals or an endotoxin produced by an infectious agent. Host immune response can be stimulated by foreign antigens or even autoantigens. Molecular mimicry has also been proposed, wherein the host immune response is initially directed toward a pathogen, which shares epitopes homologous with proteins in the cardiac myocytes, thus directing the host immune response to produce autoantibodies against own heart tissue.[22] The reaction of the immune system is the key factor, which determines the severity of myocarditis. Hence, balance between the protective and deleterious effects of the immune and inflammatory responses is extremely important.

Animal models have been the cornerstone in understanding the pathological processes underlying myocarditis as well as progression to dilated cardiomyopathy in some cases. The host response is considered to be influenced by genetic makeup as well as sex hormones. Three characteristic phases have been identified in the development of myocarditis and its progression to dilated cardiomyopathy. Phase 1 is the acute phase. Here, viral replication occurs in the blood and susceptible tissues including myocardium, where the virus enters using specific receptors. Cardiac myocytes are damaged during this phase either via direct viral-mediated injury or via inflammatory cytokines. Myocyte death in phase one can also be from direct injury by toxins/drugs. Myocyte death exposes the normally hidden antigens within myocytes to the immune system.[23]

Phase two is the subacute phase where there is active myocardial inflammation, when the host immune system is pressed into action. Natural killer cells and macrophages migrate to the area followed by further release of inflammatory cytokines and infiltration of B and T cells. Autoantibodies are produced in response to hidden antigens that are exposed or due to molecular mimicry. In this process, lysis of myocytes continues. The overall immune response is aimed at eliminating the virus, which is not always achieved. When the virus/toxin is eliminated and negative immune modulation occurs, inflammation subsides, with complete recovery or minimal long-term myocardial damage.[23]

Phase three is the chronic phase. This phase happens only when myocarditis is not healed. Viral persistence in the myocardium can lead to ongoing inflammation and progression to cardiomyopathy, but it is not always the case. Autoimmunity with or without viral persistence can also be responsible. Thus, any of the following patterns can emerge (1) chronic microbial myocarditis where microbial agents, ongoing inflammation, ongoing destruction, and remodeling of myocardium are present, but there are no autoantibodies, (2) chronic microbial and immune myocarditis where autoantibodies are also present, in addition to all features of chronic microbial myocarditis, (3) chronic autoreactive myocarditis where there are no microbial agents, but autoantibodies are present leading to ongoing inflammation, destruction, and remodeling, and (4) dilated cardiomyopathy where there is no florid inflammation, but there is ongoing destruction and remodeling. Microbes and autoantibodies may or may not be present in this phase. A large number of serum cardiac autoantibodies have been detected with varying frequency in autoimmune myocarditis and dilated cardiomyopathy.[23]

CLINICAL FEATURES

The clinical presentation of myocarditis in children is quite nonspecific and the disease onset is insidious. This makes a high index of suspicion imperative for the diagnosis. Frequently, there is recent history of a nonspecific viral illness with upper respiratory symptoms or with abdominal pain, nausea, and vomiting. Clinical evaluation might reveal irritability, and/or lethargy, poor appetite, pallor, orthopnea, tachypnea, tachycardia, hepatomegaly, decreased perfusion, and abnormal lung signs. The diagnosis in children has remained elusive. It is noteworthy that the symptoms and signs are similar to common childhood illnesses such as pneumonia/sepsis. Compared to adults, children with myocarditis are less likely to present with an S3 gallop or hepatomegaly. It is not surprising for the patients to be initially diagnosed as having a respiratory illness such as asthma, pneumonia or acute bronchitis, sepsis, or even gastritis or gastroenteritis.

Cardiac signs and symptoms in children could be subtle at presentation, like tachycardia, borderline blood pressure, and unexplained metabolic acidosis. This is because their robust physiology compensates for cardiac dysfunction. Largely, cardiac presentation falls into either of these four clinical syndromes: (1) acute heart failure, (2) subacute or chronic heart failure, (3) chest pain in older patients and adolescents which is frequently nonischemic, from associated pericarditis, although could be ischemic. An acute coronary syndrome such as presentation of acute myocarditis is well known in older children, adolescents, and adults, and (4) life-threatening events viz. shock or syncope or sudden cardiac death from arrhythmia or heart block or seizure from hypoxia.

Fulminant myocarditis is a subset where patients present with distinct clinical features and outcomes. Onset is sudden and severe, resulting in an exceptionally high risk of death caused by cardiogenic shock, fatal ventricular tachyarrhythmias, or bradyarrhythmia. By definition, shock is a part and parcel of fulminant myocarditis. It could be cardiogenic shock or mixed cardiogenic and distributive shock, which is often identified at presentation or soon thereafter. Major subtypes associated with the fulminant presentation include lymphocytic myocarditis, giant cell myocarditis, necrotizing eosinophilic myocarditis, and immune checkpoint inhibitor-related myocarditis.[14] An endomyocardial biopsy (EMB) and tissue diagnosis is considered must in these patients to direct specific therapy for specific subsets. Paradoxically, it has also been noted that if these patients survive the hemodynamic collapse, they have a higher chance at complete recovery. A fulminant course is supposed to result from a vigorous immune response, thus leading to more effective viral clearance and hence better chance at complete recovery, if supported adequately. Fulminant presentation requires an expert team for management to decrease morbidity and mortality. Along with other measures, the key step is mechanical circulatory support at the right time, before organ damage from hemodynamic collapse ensues.[14]

Acute myocarditis is one of the most common causes of sudden cardiac death in children with no previously diagnosed heart disease. Autopsy findings of acute viral myocarditis without clinical symptoms have been found in association with sudden and unexplained death during anesthesia for minor surgical procedures, drowning accidents in children who were competent swimmers, and sudden infant death syndrome.[4-8,24]

INVESTIGATIONS

Chest X-ray

Cardiomegaly, pulmonary edema, or pleural effusions can be identified frequently.

Electrocardiogram

Almost all patients have an abnormal electrocardiogram (ECG), making it a readily available and sensitive tool for diagnosis in the appropriate clinical setting. This is despite the lack of specificity. Nevertheless, a normal ECG does not rule out the diagnosis. ECG abnormalities are widely variable and no single finding is specific for myocarditis. These include low-voltage QRS complexes, ST-T wave abnormalities—even ST elevation, which is concave, compared to the convex pattern in myocardial infarction, abnormal Q waves, QT prolongation, atrial or ventricular conduction delays, sinus tachycardia, atria and ventricular premature contractions, atrial and ventricular tachyarrhythmias, and varying degrees of atrioventricular block. Sinus tachycardia is the most common abnormality. Tachyarrhythmias are more frequently seen compared to bradyarrhythmias. Atrioventricular block has been found more commonly when Lyme disease, Chagas disease, giant cell myocarditis, and sarcoidosis is the underlying cause.

Biomarkers

Inflammatory markers such as leukocyte count, C-reactive protein, and erythrocyte sedimentation rate are often elevated in myocarditis. Serum markers of myocardial necrosis/cardiomyocyte damage or death include creatine phosphokinase-MB (CPK-MB) and troponins. Troponin is more sensitive than CPK-MB. Both are nonspecific for myocarditis. B-type natriuretic peptide (BNP) and N-terminal pro-BNP (NT-proBNP) can be elevated in myocarditis. They are more useful in differentiating cardiac from respiratory cause of breathlessness. Normal values of any of these do not exclude myocarditis.

Assessment of Viral Infection

Viral serology has limited utility in the diagnosis of acute myocarditis. A positive serology does not mean an event in the heart is related to the virus. It only means that there was an interaction of the peripheral immune system with an infectious agent. The high prevalence of immunoglobulin G (IgG) antibodies to cardiotropic viruses in the general population, similar induction of IgG antibodies by noncardiotropic enteroviruses and lack of correlation between viral serology and EMB findings are some of the reasons why a positive viral serology is not helpful in a setting of acute myocarditis. Clinical situations where serology helps include hepatitis C, rickettsial infection, Lyme disease in endemic areas, and human immunodeficiency in high-risk patients. On the other hand, the gold standard for diagnosis of associated viral causes is detection of virus in the tissue sample obtained by EMB. Older techniques such as cell culture have been sidelined by newer techniques such as PCR. This has helped to improve detection of viruses from minimal quantities of tissue obtained during biopsy. Detection of virus/viral particles by PCR does not necessarily imply a diagnosis of acute myocarditis. Positivity has also been found in about one-third of patients diagnosed with dilated cardiomyopathy, as discussed in the section of pathogenesis.[25] It is recommended that a peripheral blood sample be analyzed simultaneously by PCR with EMB.[23] The utility of a standalone peripheral blood or nasopharyngeal sample PCR for viral detection in the setting of myocarditis has not been substantiated.

Echocardiography

The availability and ease of performing a study even at the bedside for these often sick children makes echocardiography the go-to investigation not only in diagnosis of myocarditis, but also in surveillance in hospital and for follow-up after an episode. It goes without saying that in any infant or child presenting with heart failure or shock, underlying structural abnormalities should be thoroughly ruled out before attributing the clinical problem to a primary abnormality in function. The characteristic finding is decreased left ventricular systolic function with hypokinesia being global.[15] Left ventricular dilation is frequently present, it is more a function of duration of the insult, later presentations showing ventricular dilation.[14] Accordingly, when the presentation is fulminant, ventricular dysfunction is severe but there is minimal if any ventricular dilation. Increased wall thickness, presumed to be from myocardial edema is also characteristic of fulminant presentation.[14] When the disease is less severe, left ventricular function could be less severely affected or even not affected. Other echocardiographic findings include pericardial effusion, segmental or regional wall motion abnormalities, left ventricular diastolic dysfunction, pulmonary hypertension, right ventricular dysfunction, and thrombus formation as a complication of decreased contractility. Tissue Doppler imaging and myocardial strain imaging are more sensitive in identifying decreased ventricular function. Abnormalities thus identified are not specific to myocarditis as similar findings are expected in cardiomyopathy as well. In acute necrotizing eosinophilic myocarditis, which is seen in adolescents and adults, restrictive physiology with thick, edematous walls, mural thrombus from eosinophilic inflammation of the myocardium, and decreased systolic function are seen.[14]

Echocardiography can also assist in prognostication. Severe left ventricular dysfunction, presence of right ventricular dysfunction, and persistent diastolic dysfunction are all associated with worse outcomes, while smaller left ventricular dimensions and greater wall thickness are associated with better outcomes in children.[26-30]

Endomyocardial Biopsy

The gold standard for diagnosis of myocarditis is EMB. The technique was developed for and is widely used to follow-up postheart transplant patients. The procedure is done in the cardiac catheterization laboratory under fluoroscopic guidance. A bioptome is passed generally from the right internal jugular vein into the right ventricle and tissue samples are taken out from the interventricular septum. Tissue samples from the left side are taken only in exceptional circumstances. In trained and experienced hands, the procedure is generally safe. The rate of complications is reported to be 1–2% at experienced centers but was around 8.9% when including low-volume centers.[31,32] Complication rates are expected to be worse in a sick patient with acute myocarditis, heart failure and hemodynamic compromise compared to a stable walk in postheart transplant patient.

Tissue samples obtained are analyzed and reported according to the Dallas Criteria.[33] By Dallas criteria, histologic diagnosis of myocarditis requires an inflammatory infiltrate and associated myocyte necrosis or damage not characteristic of an ischemic event or another cause. Borderline myocarditis is when there is inflammation but no myocyte necrosis. More than 5 lymphocytes per high power field is considered to be positive for inflammation by light microscopy.[34] Low overall sensitivity, high inter-observer variability, and inability to detect a noncellular inflammatory process are among the major drawbacks of the Dallas criteria. Patchy involvement of myocardium and obtaining samples from the right ventricular side of the interventricular septum, when in fact the left ventricle, particularly lateral walls are more involved (as per recent CMR findings) are also supposed to contribute to the low yield of EMB.

In 1995, immunological/immunohistochemical criteria were added to the definition of myocarditis by World Health Organization/International Society and Federation of Cardiology Task Force on the Definition and Classification of Cardiomyopathies.[1] In this method, the type of infiltrating cells is identified by antibodies specific for activated T and B cells, macrophages, major histocompatibility class 1 and class 2 antigens, adhesion molecules, and endothelial cells. Peroxidase double staining procedure demonstrates the specific binding of antibodies. Inflammation in EMB samples is diagnosed by the presence of ≥14 leukocytes/mm^2 including up to 4 monocytes/mm^2 with the presence of CD3 positive T-lymphocytes, >7 cells/mm^2 by immunohistochemistry.[35,36] This increases the sensitivity of EMB for diagnosis. Based on type of inflammatory cell infiltrate, myocarditis can be classified into lymphocytic, eosinophilic, polymorphic, giant cell myocarditis, and granulomatous myocarditis (cardiac sarcoidosis).[36] Lymphocytic myocarditis (mononuclear infiltrate) is the most common pattern, mostly from a viral infection. Giant cell myocarditis shows lymphocytes and multinucleated giant cells and is rare. Acute necrotizing eosinophilic myocarditis is a subset of eosinophilic myocarditis where perivascular interstitial inflammatory infiltrates with eosinophils and associated remarkable, diffuse cardiomyocyte necrosis is seen. The pathognomonic feature is necrotizing angiitis of small vessels with sparing of subepicardial arteries.[14]

Immunohistochemical methods can also identify viral proteins in the myocardium. Lately, both RNA and/or DNA viruses in the myocardium are identified with a higher sensitivity by molecular analysis with DNA–RNA extraction and real time-polymerase chain reaction (RT-PCR) amplification of the viral genome. Detection of active viral replication and viral load can add information from a diagnostic, prognostic as well as therapeutic point of view. For example, in myocarditis caused by human parvovirus B19, viral load thresholds that are necessary to maintain active ongoing inflammation, which leads to chronic myocarditis and later cardiomyopathy as well as those that are suggestive of active myocarditis have been identified.[37] In addition, transcriptomic biomarkers which identify differently expressed genes, which produce inflammation in myocarditis have been found to improve clinical detection of myocarditis.[38]

Endomyocardial biopsy is best indicated and utilized when the clinical presentation is complicated and certainly when fulminant, provided trained and experienced hands are available for both obtaining the sample and reporting. In uncomplicated cases, the risk–benefit ratio does not support an EMB. In this aspect, it is important to remember that uncomplicated, stable patients can undergo CMR imaging which can provide insights into diagnosis as well as prognosis as discussed in the following section.[39] EMB is also indicated when the clinical evaluation points to specific causes which are known to cause severe disease, requiring specific therapy, e.g., suspected autoimmune disorder, peripheral eosinophilia, and use of immune checkpoint inhibitors.[39]

Cardiac Catheterization

When the presentation mimics acute coronary syndrome, coronary angiogram is warranted to rule out coronary artery disease. All patients with a complicated/fulminant presentation will benefit from invasive assessment of hemodynamics at multiple points during the management.

Cardiac Magnetic Resonance Imaging

The ability of CMR imaging to characterize tissue abnormalities such as myocardial edema and/or fibrosis, in addition to assess biventricular function and pericardial involvement, makes it an attractive option for noninvasive diagnosis of myocarditis. Performing CMR in children has its own challenges in the technical aspect as well as the actual procedural aspect. Technically, the smaller heart size necessitates higher spatial resolution. The higher heart rates necessitate higher temporal resolution. The ability to compromise either for the other as done in adult CMR acquisition sequences is quite limited in children. In addition, MRI acquisition necessitates breath holds, which younger children and infants cannot do, requiring general anesthesia with intubation for CMR acquisition. Nevertheless, CMR imaging is routinely done for children, using modified sequences, which are targeted at a specific clinical question and techniques to manage them in the scanner such as parental presence, MRI compatible audio-visual aids, etc. With respect to myocarditis, patients with a complicated clinical course cannot be shifted out from intensive care into the CMR scanner. Also, they cannot be kept inside the scanner for the long acquisition times typically needed for evaluation of myocarditis. Hence, CMR is primarily utilized for uncomplicated cases. The sicker patients with complicated myocarditis are more benefitted by EMB as previously discussed.[39]

Myocarditis is diagnosed on CMR based on the updated Lake Louise criteria (**Table 2**).[40] Specific sequences need to be acquired for answering specific questions. CMR targets to detect myocardial edema, hyperemia/capillary leak, myocardial necrosis, and fibrosis, in addition to assessment of biventricular function and presence of pericardial inflammation. T1-based markers include late gadolinium enhancement (LGE), T1 mapping, and calculation of extracellular volume. LGE looks for high intensity signals from

TABLE 2: 2018 updated Lake Louise criteria.

Main criteria	Myocardial edema (Based on T2-weighted imaging)	Regional high T2 signal intensity or global T2 signal intensity ratio >2.0 in T2W CMR images or Regional or global increase of myocardial T2 relaxation time on T2 mapping
	Nonischemic myocardial injury (based on T1-weighted imaging)	Regional or global increase of native myocardial T1 relaxation time or extracellular volume or Areas with high signal intensity in a nonischemic distribution pattern in late gadolinium enhancement images
Supportive criteria	Pericardial inflammation	Pericardial effusion in cine CMR images or High signal intensity of the pericardium in late gadolinium enhancement images, T1-mapping or T2-mapping
	Left ventricular systolic dysfunction	Systolic left ventricular wall motion abnormality in cine CMR images

(CMR: cardiac magnetic resonance)

myocardium, 10 minutes after intravenous administration of a gadolinium-based contrast agent. Positive LGE indicates areas of focal fibrosis, scarring, and myocardial necrosis. Pattern of LGE is subepicardial/mid wall in myocarditis contrasting with subendocardial/transmural involvement in ischemic events. Intracellular or extracellular edema, hyperemia and capillary leak, areas of myocyte necrosis, and fibrosis prolongs native T1 relaxation time and increases extracellular volume in myocarditis. T2-based markers include regional increase in signal intensity on T2-weighted imaging, global T2-signal intensity ratio compared to skeletal muscle and T2 mapping. T1- and T2-weighted images rely on regional differences of signal to generate tissue contrast. These images give qualitative information, while mapping techniques provide quantification of myocardial tissue abnormalities and brings in the much needed objectivity. Quantification helps in assessing severity and acuity of disease, monitoring disease activity on follow-up, and assessing the effect of therapy. Of these, myocardial edema detected by high-signal intensity on T2-weighted imaging or increased T2 signal ratio from the myocardium (compared usually to skeletal muscle) or increased T2 relaxation values on T2 mapping is particularly suggestive of disease activity or an acute process. In myocarditis, abnormalities of tissue characterization are classically in a noncoronary distribution as opposed to ischemic cardiomyopathy which is a close differential diagnosis in adults.

The Lake Louise criteria is based on the fact that combining T2-based imaging which detects myocardial edema with T1-based tissue characteristic that detects nonischemic myocardial injury will improve the diagnostic accuracy of CMR for acute myocarditis. Accordingly, if one criterion is present from both T1- and T2-weighted imaging, it points to strong evidence of acute myocardial inflammation, in the appropriate clinical setting (*see* **Table 2**). In such a setting, having only one marker may still support the diagnosis, but with lesser specificity.[40] The updated Lake Louise Criteria has a sensitivity of 87.5% and a specificity of 96.2%.[41] for detecting acute myocarditis. To detect myocardial edema, CMR should be done sufficiently early in the course of the disease. A negative scan can simply be because of the timing of CMR. Nevertheless, a normal CMR indicates a good prognosis on follow up.[42] On the other hand, positive LGE is an independent predictor of mortality on long-term follow-up.[43]

DIAGNOSIS

Based on the overall evaluation, patients can be classified as having either "possible," "probable," or "definite" myocarditis. Asymptomatic patients with elevated biomarkers, ECG findings, and/or abnormal cardiac function by echocardiogram or CMR constitute the "possible" group. If there is heart failure along with the above, it is considered "probable." A "definite" diagnosis requires confirmation by EMB.[44] For the clinical diagnosis of myocarditis, at least one of the four symptom complexes (acute heart failure/subacute or chronic heart failure/chest pain syndrome/life-threatening events) plus one of the four diagnostic criteria should be positive (positive ECG/raised troponin/new-onset ventricular dysfunction/tissue characterization by CMR). If the patient is asymptomatic, at least two diagnostic criteria should be fulfilled. Other diagnosis which can explain the clinical picture like congenital heart disease/valvular heart disease/coronary artery disease/noncardiac illness like hypothyroidism should be investigated and excluded.[23]

TREATMENT

Treatment is best tailored to the clinical features at presentation and the course of illness. Patients with the uncomplicated presentation should also be admitted to hospital and monitored for worsening of clinical status as changes can be sudden.

Symptomatic and Supportive Measures

These are the mainstay of treatment for myocarditis. Arrhythmia should be watched for and managed promptly, all precipitating factors should be monitored and corrected as and when required. Heart failure should be managed with diuretics and angiotensin-converting enzyme inhibitors. Oxygen supplementation, noninvasive or invasive mechanical ventilation might be required to maintain adequate oxygenation in patients with heart failure. Aldosterone antagonists and beta-blockers should be introduced at the right time, all under usual diligent monitoring. Digoxin should be avoided in myocarditis. Inotropes (milrinone, levosimendan, and dobutamine) should be considered for severe heart failure presentations. Shock should be identified early and managed expeditiously with a combination of inotropes and vasopressors; started and uptitrated depending on the physiology (warm and dry/warm and wet/cold and dry/cold and wet). Mechanical circulatory support will be needed for intractable heart failure/shock. Hemodynamic data indicating severe biventricular failure, presence of intractable ventricular arrhythmias, persistent high-grade atrioventricular block can all be used as clinical pointers for the need of mechanical circulatory support. Venoarterial extracorporeal membrane oxygenation (ECMO) and left ventricular assist devices are commonly utilized. ECMO increases left ventricular after load and is hence used in conjunction with another unloading strategy (atrial septostomy/vent/intra-aortic balloon pump/percutaneously implanted device like IMPELLA). In lymphocytic myocarditis with a complicated or fulminant presentation, ventricular function generally recovers while mechanical circulatory support/inotrope is on. On the other hand, in giant cell myocarditis requiring mechanical circulatory support, recovery is rare and frequently results in transplantation.[14] When mechanical circulatory support is required as bridge to recovery or transplantation for a long time period, durable left ventricular assist devices are the better option. Of pediatric patients admitted to intensive care unit, 25–50% will require mechanical ventilation, and 45–70% inotropic support, 7–19% ECMO, and 2–4% ventricular assist devices.[29,38,45,46] Patients with complicated presentations, especially those with features of intractable heart failure and shock need to undergo an EMB and given a chance to benefit from specific therapy of underlying pathology.

Specific Therapy

This is best approached according to the findings on EMB.[47] When there is no evidence of inflammation or active viral replication, management is primarily supportive. When EMB shows inflammation, but no evidence of viral replication by PCR, specific pathologies such as giant cell myocarditis, eosinophilic myocarditis, cardiac sarcoidosis, and autoimmune myocarditis associated with other known extracardiac autoimmune disease should be looked for. Initiation or intensification of immunosuppression is recommended, provided there are no contraindications for same like active viral replication in the myocardium, active or latent malignancy or extracardiac infection.[48] Steroids are the mainstay of therapy for sarcoidosis and eosinophilic myocarditis.[23] Giant cell myocarditis is managed with a combination of steroids and immunosuppressant regimens (cyclosporine/azathioprine-based, recently tacrolimus/mycophenolate-based) following the lines for heart transplant rejection regimens.[14] Giant cell myocarditis and acute necrotizing eosinophilic myocarditis have a particularly dismal prognosis with very high rates of death and/or transplantation.[14] Immunosuppression (steroids alone or in combination with other agents) can also be considered in lymphocytic myocarditis refractory to standard therapy provided active infection can be ruled out.[23] Cardiac autoantibodies might be positive in the autoimmune varieties. In such cases, neutralization or immunoadsorption of disease-causing antibodies have also been considered.[23] It is important to note that there is no data for blanket use of anti-inflammatory/immunosuppressive therapies including corticosteroids in all patients with myocarditis. The quality of data available for same is poor and large scale randomized controlled trials are required to make this recommendation.

Also, immunosuppression can negatively impact the clinical course when there is active viral replication in the myocardium. Accordingly, when EMB shows inflammation and evidence of viral replication by PCR, immunosuppression is contraindicated. As increased cytokine production has been implicated in myocardial depression and pump failure, antitumor necrosis factor therapy has been tried, but with no significant benefit. Interferon-β administration has been documented to cause viral clearance in chronic cases of cardiomyopathy with virus positivity attributed to enterovirus and adenovirus, but not human parvovirus B19.[49-51] Immunoglobulins may have role when there is active replication of human parvovirus B19 virus.[47] The antiviral drug telbivudine has shown promise in early studies for the same virus.[52]

Specific therapy can also be considered based on the clinical picture in the absence of histological/molecular diagnosis. Regardless of histology, immunosuppression is recommended in myocarditis associated with systemic autoimmune disorders. Another strategy worth consideration is the crucial early initiation of immunosuppression (pulse steroid therapy) in complicated myocarditis, especially fulminant presentations where risk of death/heart transplant is very high (hemodynamic instability/low cardiac output syndrome, life-threatening arrhythmias, wide QRS complex, severe ventricular dysfunction) regardless of underlying histology. Once a biopsy is obtained, strategy is modified as discussed previously.[39]

Role of Intravenous Immunoglobulin

Intravenous immunoglobulin (IVIG) modulates the immune response by multiple mechanisms (immunomodulatory, anti-inflammatory, antiviral) and is commonly used in pediatric myocarditis at a dose of 2 g/kg. Small case series have reported improved left ventricular dimensions, function and improved survival compared to controls.[53,54] Registry data and a Cochrane review failed to show any significant bene-fit.[38,55] Serious adverse events are rare with IVIG.[56] Also, IVIG does not have a negative impact on disease course compared to steroids/immunosuppression. Hence, IVIG can be considered as an option in viral/autoimmune myocarditis not responding to heart failure therapy, although a strong recommendation would require a well-planned, large-scale randomized controlled trial.

PROGNOSIS AND FOLLOW-UP

In the recently published Lombardy registry including adult and pediatric patients with biopsy or CMR-proven acute myocarditis, cardiac mortality and transplant rates at 1, 3, and 5 years of follow-up were 11.3%, 12.5%, and 14.7%, respectively, in the group with complicated presentation, compared with 0% in those with uncomplicated presentation.[13] Also, another large multicenter data of EMB-proven myocarditis patients showed that those with fulminant presentation had significantly higher rates of cardiac death and heart transplantation compared with those with NFM at 60 days (28.0% vs. 1.8%, p <0.0001) and at 7-year follow-up (47.7% vs. 10.4%, p <0.0001).[57] In this study, QRS width >120 ms was also an independent predictor of worse outcomes.

In a pediatric data from Germany including 195 children presenting with heart failure, 14% needed mechanical circulatory support, in-hospital death or heart transplantation rate was 7.7%.[11] Requirement of mechanical circulatory support was more in the 0–2-year age group. Most of the normalization of ventricular function occurs in

1–4 months after the acute episode. Recovery of left ventricular function can continue for as long as 3 years with a recovery rate of 52–54%.[38] Continued treatment with heart failure medications is necessary till the left ventricular form and function recovers completely. Follow-up is warranted lifelong.

Activity Restriction

Physical activity should be restricted for athletes as well as nonathletes for 6 months after an episode of acute myocarditis.[23] Return to competitive sports is considered after 3–6 months, when the ventricular function and serum biomarkers have returned to normal and there are no clinically relevant arrhythmias.[58]

REFERENCES

1. Richardson P, McKenna W, Bristow M, Maisch B, Mautner B, O'Connell J, et al. Report of the 1995 World Health Organization/International Society and Federation of Cardiology Task Force on the definition and classification of cardiomyopathies. Circulation. 1996;93(5):841-2.
2. Towbin JA, Lowe AM, Colan SD, Sleeper LA, Orav EJ, Clunie S, et al. Incidence, causes, and outcomes of dilated cardiomyopathy in children. JAMA. 2006;296(15):1867-76.
3. Cooper Jr. LT, Keren A, Sliwa K, Matsumori A, Mensah GA. The global burden of myocarditis: part 1: a systematic literature review for the Global Burden of Diseases, Injuries, and Risk Factors 2010 study. Glob Heart. 2014;9(1):121-9.
4. Gore I, Saphir O. Myocarditis: a classification of 1402 cases. Am Heart J. 1947;34(6):827-30.
5. Basso C, Calabrese F, Corrado D, Thiene G. Postmortem diagnosis of sudden cardiac death victims. Cardiovasc Res. 2001;50(2): 290-300.
6. Wakafuji S, Okada R. Twenty year autopsy statistics of myocarditis incidence in Japan. Jpn Circ J. 1986;50(12):1288-93.
7. Kytö V, Saraste A, Voipio-Pulkki LM, Saukko P. Incidence of fatal myocarditis: a population-based study in Finland. Am J Epidemiol. 2007;165(5):570-4.
8. Puranik R, Chow CK, Duflou JA, Kilborn MJ, McGuire MA. Sudden death in the young. Heart Rhythm. 2005;2(12):1277-82.
9. Vetter VL, Covington TM, Dugan NP, Haley DM, Dykstra H, Overpeck M, et al. Cardiovascular deaths in children: general overview from the National Center for the Review and Prevention of Child Deaths. Am Heart J. 2015;169(3):426-37.e23.
10. Ghelani SJ, Spaeder MC, Pastor W, Spurney CF, Klugman D. Demographics, trends, and outcomes in pediatric acute myocarditis in the United States, 2006 to 2011. Circ Cardiovasc Qual Outcomes. 2012;5(5):622-7.
11. Schubert S, Opgen-Rhein B, Boehne M, Weigelt A, Wagner R, Muller G. Severe heart failure and the need for mechanical circulatory support and heart transplantation in pediatric patients with myocarditis: results from the prospective multicenter registry "MYKKE". Pediatr Transpl. 2019;23(7):e13548.
12. Arola A, Pikkarainen E, Sipilä JO, Pykäri J, Rautava P, Kytö V. Occurrence and features of childhood myocarditis: a nationwide study in Finland. J Am Heart Assoc. 2017;6(11):e005306.
13. Ammirati E, Cipriani M, Moro C, Raineri C, Pini D, Sormani P, et al. Clinical presentation and outcome in a contemporary cohort of patients with acute myocarditis: multicenter Lombardy Registry. Circulation. 2018;138(11):1088-99.
14. Kociol RD, Cooper LT, Fang JC, Moslehi JJ, Pang PS, Sabe MA, et al. Recognition and initial management of fulminant myocarditis: a scientific statement from the American Heart Association. Circulation. 2020;141(6):e69-92.
15. Canter CE, Simpson KE. Diagnosis and treatment of myocarditis in children in the current era. Circulation. 2014;129(1):115-28.
16. Matsuura H, Ichida F, Saji T, Ogawa S, Waki K, Kaneko M, et al. Clinical features of acute and fulminant myocarditis in children - 2nd nationwide survey by Japanese Society of Pediatric Cardiology and Cardiac Surgery. Circ J. 2016;80(11):2362-8.
17. Randolph AG, Vaughn F, Sullivan R, Rubinson L, Thompson T, Yoon G, et al. Critically ill children during the 2009-2010 influenza pandemic in the United States. Pediatrics. 2011;128(6):e1450-8.
18. Puntmann VO, Carerj ML, Wieters I, Fahim M, Arendt C, Hoffmann J, et al. Outcomes of cardiovascular magnetic resonance imaging in patients recently recovered from coronavirus disease 2019 (COVID-19). JAMA Cardiol. 2020;5(11):1265-73.
19. Dolhnikoff M, Ferreira Ferranti J, de Almeida Monteiro RA, Duarte-Neto AN, Gomes-Gouvêa MS, Degaspare NV, et al. SARS-CoV-2 in cardiac tissue of a child with COVID-19-related multisystem inflammatory syndrome. Lancet Child Adolesc Health. 2020;4(10):790-4.
20. Sohn KH, Song WJ, Kim BK, Kang MK, Lee SY, Suh JW, et al. Eosinophilic myocarditis: case series and literature review. Asia Pac Allergy. 2015;5(2):123-7.
21. Palaskas N, Lopez-Mattei J, Durand JB, Iliescu C, Deswal A. Immune checkpoint inhibitor myocarditis: pathophysiological characteristics, diagnosis, and treatment. J Am Heart Assoc. 2020;9(2):e013757.
22. Olinde KD, O'Connell JB. Inflammatory heart disease: pathogenesis, clinical manifestations, and treatment of myocarditis. Annu Rev Med. 1994;45:481-90.
23. Caforio AL, Pankuweit S, Arbustini E, Basso C, Gimeno-Blanes J, Felix SB, et al. Current state of knowledge on aetiology, diagnosis, management, and therapy of myocarditis: a position statement of the European Society of Cardiology Working Group on myocardial and pericardial diseases. Eur Heart J. 2013; 34(33):2636-48d.
24. Shekerdemian L, Bohn D. Acute viral myocarditis: epidemiology and pathophysiology. Pediatr Crit Care Med. 2006;7(6): S2-7.
25. Camargo PR, Okay TS, Yamamoto L, Del Negro GM, Lopes AA, Myocarditis in children and detection of viruses in myocardial tissue: implications for immunosuppressive therapy, Int J Cardiol. 2011;148(2): 204-8.
26. Skouri HN, Dec GW, Friedrich MG, Cooper LT. Noninvasive imaging in myocarditis. J Am Coll Cardiol. 2006;48(10):2085-93.
27. Kim G, Ban GH, Lee HD, Sung SC, Kim H, Choi KH. Left ventricular end-diastolic dimension as a predictive factor of outcomes in children with acute myocarditis. Cardiol Young. 2017;27(3): 443-51.
28. Foerster SR, Canter CE, Cinar A, Sleeper LA, Webber SA, Pahl E, et al. Ventricular remodeling and survival are more favorable for myocarditis than for idiopathic dilated cardiomyopathy in childhood: an outcomes study from the Pediatric Cardiomyopathy Registry. Circ Heart Fail. 2010;3(6):689-97.
29. Kim HJ, Yoo GH, Kil HR. Clinical outcome of acute myocarditis in children according to treatment modalities. Korean J Pediatr. 2010;53(7):745-52.
30. Sachdeva S, Song X, Dham N, Heath DM, DeBiasi RL. Analysis of clinical parameters and cardiac magnetic resonance imaging as predictors of outcome in pediatric myocarditis. Am J Cardiol. 2015;115(4):499-504.
31. Bennett MK, Gilotra NA, Harrington C, Rao S, Dunn JM, Freitag TB, et al. Evaluation of the role of endomyocardial biopsy in 851 patients with unexplained heart failure from 2000-2009. Circ Heart Fail. 2013;6(4):676-84.
32. Singh V, Mendirichaga R, Savani GT, Rodriguez A, Blumer V, Elmariah S, et al. Comparison of utilization trends, indications, and complications of endomyocardial biopsy in native versus

donor hearts (from the nationwide inpatient sample 2002 to 2014). Am J Cardiol. 2018;121(3):356-63.
33. Aretz HT, Billingham ME, Edwards WD, Factor SM, Fallon JT, Fenoglio Jr JJ, et al. Myocarditis. A histopathologic definition and classification. Am J Cardiovasc Pathol. 1987;1(1):3-14.
34. Edwards WD, Holmes RH, Reeder GS. Diagnosis of active lymphocytic myocarditis by endomyocardial biopsy: quantitative criteria for light microscopy. Mayo Clin Proc. 1982;57(7):419-25.
35. Maisch B, Pankuweit S. Inflammatory dilated cardiomyopathy: etiology and clinical management. Herz. 2020;45(3):221-9.
36. Hazebroek MR, Everaerts K, Heymans S. Diagnostic approach of myocarditis: strike the golden mean. Neth Heart J. 2014;22(2): 80-4.
37. Bock CT, Klingel K, Kandolf R. Human parvovirus B19-associated myocarditis. N Engl J Med. 2010;362(13):1248-9.
38. Heidecker B, Kittleson MM, Kasper EK, Wittstein IS, Champion HC, Russell SD, et al. Transcriptomic biomarkers for the accurate diagnosis of myocarditis. Circulation. 2011; 123(11):1174-84.
39. Ammirati E, Veronese G, Bottiroli M, Wang DW, Cipriani M, Garascia A, et al. Update on acute myocarditis. Trends Cardiovasc Med. 2020;S1050-1738(20)30079-7.
40. Ferreira VM, Schulz-Menger J, Holmvang G, Kramer CM, Carbone I, Sechtem U, et al. Cardiovascular magnetic resonance in nonischemic myocardial inflammation: expert recommendations. J Am Coll Cardiol. 2018; 72(24):3158-76.
41. Ammirati E, Moroni F, Sormani P, Peritore A, Milazzo A, Quattrocchi G, et al. Quantitative changes in late gadolinium enhancement at cardiac magnetic resonance in the early phase of acute myocarditis. Int J Cardiol. 2017;231:216-21.
42. Schumm J, Greulich S, Wagner A, Grun S, Ong P, Bentz K, et al. Cardiovascular magnetic resonance risk stratification in patients with clinically suspected myocarditis. J Cardiovasc Magn Resonan. 2014;16(1):14.
43. Grün S, Schumm J, Greulich S, Wagner A, Schneider S, Bruder O, et al. Long-term follow-up of biopsy-proven viral myocarditis: predictors of mortality and incomplete recovery. J Am Coll Cardiol. 2012;59(18):1604-15.
44. Sagar S, Liu PP, Cooper Jr. LT, Myocarditis. Lancet. 2012; 379(9817):738-47.
45. English RF, Janosky JE, Ettedgui JA, Webber SA. Outcomes for children with acute myocarditis. Cardiol Young. 2004;14(5): 488-93.
46. Klugman D, Berger JT, Sable CA, He J, Khandelwal SG, Slonim AD. Pediatric patients hospitalized with myocarditis: a multi-institutional analysis. Pediatr Cardiol. 2010;31(2): 222-8.
47. Tschöpe C, Cooper LT, Torre-Amione G, Van Linthout S. Management of myocarditis-related cardiomyopathy in adults. Circ Res. 2019; 124(11):1568-83.
48. Caforio ALP, Adler Y, Agostini C, Allanore Y, Anastasakis A, Arad M, et al. Diagnosis and management of myocardial involvement in systemic immune-mediated diseases: a position statement of the European Society of Cardiology Working Group on Myocardial and Pericardial Disease. Eur Heart J. 2017;38(35):2649-62.
49. Schultheiss HP, Piper C, Sowade O, Waagstein F, Kapp JF, Wegscheider K, et al. Betaferon in chronic viral cardiomyopathy (BICC) trial: Effects of interferon-β treatment in patients with chronic viral cardiomyopathy. Clin Res Cardiol. 2016;105(9): 763-73.
50. Kühl U, Lassner D, von Schlippenbach J, Poller W, Schultheiss HP. Interferon-Beta improves survival in enterovirus-associated cardiomyopathy. J Am Coll Cardiol. 2012;60(14): 1295-6.
51. Schmidt-Lucke C, Spillmann F, Bock T, Kühl U, Van Linthout S, Schultheiss HP, et al. Interferon beta modulates endothelial damage in patients with cardiac persistence of human parvovirus b19 infection. J Infect Dis. 2010;201(6):936-45.
52. Van Linthout S, Elsanhoury A, Klein O, Sosnowski M, Miteva K, Lassner D, et al. Telbivudine in chronic lymphocytic myocarditis and human parvovirus B19 transcriptional activity. ESC Heart Fail. 2018;5(5):818-29.
53. Haque A, Bhatti S, Siddiqui FJ. Intravenous immune globulin for severe acute myocarditis in children. Indian Pediatr. 2009;46(9):810-1.
54. Drucker NA, Colan SD, Lewis AB, Beiser AS, Wessel DL, Takahashi M, et al. Gamma-globulin treatment of acute myocarditis in the pediatric population. Circulation. 1994;89(1):252-7.
55. Robinson J, Hartling L, Vandermeer B, Klassen TP. Intravenous immunoglobulin for presumed viral myocarditis in children and adults. Cochrane Database Syst Rev. 2015;5:CD004370.
56. Guo Y, Tian X, Wang X, Xiao Z. Adverse effects of immunoglobulin therapy. Front Immunol. 2018;9:1299.
57. Ammirati E, Veronese G, Brambatti M, Merlo M, Cipriani M, Potena L, et al. Fulminant versus acute nonfulminant myocarditis in patients with left ventricular systolic dysfunction. J Am Coll Cardiol. 2019;74(3):299-311.
58. Maron BJ, Udelson JE, Bonow RO, Nishimura RA, Ackerman MJ, Mark Estes NA, et al. Eligibility and disqualification recommendations for competitive athletes with cardiovascular abnormalities: Task Force 3: hypertrophic cardiomyopathy, arrhythmogenic right ventricular cardiomyopathy and other cardiomyopathies, and myocarditis: a scientific statement from the American Heart Association and American College of Cardiology. J Am Coll Cardiol. 2015;66(21):2362-71.

44 CHAPTER

Kawasaki Disease

Saji Philip, M Zulfikar Ahamed, Priyankar Pal, Surjit Singh, R Krishna Kumar

INTRODUCTION

Kawasaki disease (KD) is an acute self-limiting systemic vasculitis of unknown origin. This was defined as mucocutaneous lymph node syndrome by Dr Tomisaku Kawasaki in Japan who published the first 50 cases in 1967. It is now the leading cause of acquired pediatric cardiac disease worldwide, especially in developed countries.[1,2] Coronary artery lesions (CALs) with aneurysmal dilation, thrombosis, and/or stenosis, leading to myocardial infarction (MI) and death, have been recognized as the most severe complication in children.[3,4] Circulating immune complexes (ICs), triggered by infectious agents, bacteria, or viral or other unknown cause, have been detected in the early phase of KD, implicating that immunopathologic mechanisms might be involved in the pathogenesis of vasculitis in KD.[5-8] Attempts to produce coronary vasculitis have been made in mice, weanling rabbits, and guinea pigs by injecting infectious agents, foreign proteins, horse serum, and *Lactobacillus casei* cell walls.[9,10] Among the animal models, swine may be the unique and promising animal for biomedical research, especially in the field of cardiovascular diseases.[11,12] Recent advances in genetic analysis contribute to our understanding of pathogenesis and newer modalities in the management of KD.

EPIDEMIOLOGY

Kawasaki disease is more prevalent in Asian children. According to recent epidemiologic studies, Asian populations also have a much higher incidence of KD.[13] Seasonal variations, chronological and geographic clustering have been the other salient observations. Approximately 80–90% of patients with KD are below 5 years of age. *Japan* has the highest annual incidence in the world (359/ 100,000 children <5 years of age between 2017 and 2018 which further increased to 330.2 in 2015, followed by *South Korea* with 199.7 per 100,000 children <5 years of age in 2014. *Taiwan* has the third highest numbers with an estimate of approximately 700 new cases being added each year (82.8 per 100,000 children <5 years of age in 2010). *Hawaii* has complex multiracial and multiethnic population with an overall annual incidence of about 50.4/100,000; whereas the rate is much higher (210) for the Japanese ethnic children in Hawaii. *Beijing* has reported an increased incidence, increasing from 55.1 in 2004to 110 per 100,000 persons in 2014. In *Shanghai*, it increased from 16.2 (1997) to 71.9 (2012) per 100,000 children.[13-17] In *Hong Kong*, the average annual incidence was 39 per 100,000 between 1994 and 2000. In Western countries, the incidence of KD is significantly lower. *Canada* reported an annual incidence of 20.6 per 100,000 for the period between 1998 and 2007. The *United States* had an annual incidence of 17.1 per 100,000, whereas 12,000 new cases are detected every year in Japan. CALs after 30 days of illness were seen in only 3% of cases in Japan, indicating that almost all KD cases had received intravenous immunoglobulin (IVIG) as first-line therapy. The ratio of male and female KD patients approximates 1.5:1 in most countries.

Kawasaki disease has striking age distribution, with almost 100% cases occurring in children, 80–90% in children <5 years, and 50% in those <2 years old. We must admit that we do not have sufficient data to present the epidemiology in India till today except regional data from individual medical colleges. KD incidence at *Chandigarh, North India* during 2009–2014 was 7/100,000 children below 15 years of age. The first case was diagnosed in 1994. The number of cases detected during 1994–2017 is 680 and the trend shows a two-fold rise of KD cases in last 4 years (2014–2017). Recurrent KD was seen in 0.98% with 2% of these occurring within 10 months of the first episode. Incomplete KD was more common during recurrence.[18,19] The recurrence rate is approximately 2% in Taiwan and 3.5% in Japan. The case fatality rate is <0.1% in both *Japan* and *Taiwan*. The peak seasons of KD are late spring and summer as noted in Taiwan.[19]

ETIOPATHOGENESIS

Etiology though is unclear, both epidemiological and clinical features of KD strongly suggest possible infectious agents. Superantigen (unconventional protein that leads to massive T-cell activation and cytokine production) from infectious agents such as beta-hemolytic streptococci can trigger the IC vasculitis evidenced by very high titer of antistreptolysin O (ASO). Some of the implicated pathogens are *Staphylococcus*, *Streptococcus*, *Yersinia*, adenovirus, human parvovirus, herpesvirus, etc. More recently severe acute respiratory syndrome coronavirus 2 (SARS-Cov-2) also manifested as KD like illness. The lack of responsiveness of KD patients to antibiotic therapy makes a viral etiology more likely than bacterial. The prevalence of CD8 T-cells in the inflammatory infiltrate and the upregulation of cytotoxic T-cell and interferon pathway genes in the coronaries of children who have died of KD are also suggestive of a possible viral etiology. Other noninfectious agents may also trigger IC vasculitis leading to the signs and symptoms manifested in KD. Rowley and Shulman proposed a possible pathogenesis, where unknown infectious agents (possibly viral) infect the ciliated bronchial epithelium cells in a small subset of genetically predisposed children. These agents enter the bloodstream via macrophages. The circulating antigens then attach to B cell-mediated plasma to generate antibodies. This results in circulating ICs that damage the endothelium of medium and small vessels, particularly coronary arteries. Further, neutrophil-mediated lysosomal enzymes and platelet aggregation eventually damage the vessel wall causing aneurysms.[17]

Dengue Fever Triggering Kawasaki Disease

Incidence of KD or clinical features resembling KD is notably significant in the later course of dengue fever in India. High viral load modulates the human microvascular endothelial barrier function and disrupts the function of interendothelial junctional proteins during early infection with organ-specific cytogenic production. High levels of cytokines, chemokines, and adhesion molecules were differentially produced in a modelling study, which showed that it can potentially cause arteritis (including coronary arteritis), which is the hallmark of KD.[20-23] The other virus commonly associated with KD is adenovirus. In a monozygotic twin boy had adenovirus type 3 infection and subsequently developed KD proved by laboratory investigation specific to adenovirus.[24]

Environmental Factors

Researchers focused on the microbiology of aerosols during their efforts to isolate the causative agents of KD. Studies by Burns et al. on environmental triggers have opened up new light on causative agents. They suggest that the triggers for KD could also be wind-borne.[25]A single, specific agent has not been identified as a cause for KD till date.[24]All research and isolation of circulating ICs from the sera of patients with KD suggest that KD is an IC vasculitis. This was further corroborated by the swine animal model in which similar manifestations were reproduced by injecting horse serum.[11,12]

Genetic Susceptibility

Recent advanced studies on gene analysis in KD were reviewed by Kei Takahashi and team, contributing not only to prediction of disease susceptibility but also to improving our understanding of the pathogenesis of KD and development of new improved therapies.[26]

HISTOPATHOLOGY

Coronary arteritis begins 6–8 days after the onset of KD and even earlier at times, with inflammation of all layers of the artery. It begins as an edematous dissociation of tunica media with infiltration of monocytes, lymphocytes, and neutrophils. Periarteritis further damages the elastic lamina and smooth muscle cells (SMCs), leading to intense damage and dilation of the artery. Inflammatory infiltration continues at least until day 25 of the disease and then gradually starts to decrease. Myocarditis has not received much attention in KD,[27] it is a well-recognized component of the condition with subtle left ventricular (LV) dysfunction occurring in more than half of the patients during the acute phase of the disease and may even be transient. In KD, myocarditis develops even earlier than epicardial coronary arteritis; it peaks by disease day 10 and then disappears gradually after day 20. Inflammatory cell infiltration, consisting mainly of lobulated leukocytes and large mononuclear cells, is seen in the myocardial interstitium in all cases.[27] It is well known that tumor necrosis factor-alpha (TNF-α) is a key inflammatory cytokine that is initially produced by T-lymphocytes, followed by a secondary TNF-α release from monocytes and macrophages. TNF-α mediates endothelial cell activation through increased expression of adhesion molecules and also upregulates expression of chemokines that are important in the orchestration of leukocyte–endothelial cell interactions. Hence, the increasing role of monoclonal antibodies such as infliximab in treating KD is perhaps justified.

ANIMAL MODELS IN RESEARCH

Various studies on animal models on vasculitis, induced by *Candida albicans* cell wall, *Lactobacillus casei*, serum albumin from horse serum in murine, and swine models, mimic almost all features of KD. These findings are consistent with the role of IC vasculitis in the pathogenesis. Recent publication on rabbit model of arteritis displayed histopathological and ultrastructural features similar to those of KD.[11,12] Weanling rabbits and swine models may serve as experimental models for IC vasculitis that mimics KD than a murine model. It is speculated that circulating ICs (triggered by infectious agents) and immunopathologic mechanisms might be involved in the pathogenesis of vasculitis in KD.[5-8] Changes in the coronary arteries after IC vasculitis have been studied and are listed in **Table 1** and **Figures 1A to D**. Histopathology in human KD coronary arteritis is very much similar to immune-complex vasculitis induced by horse serum.

TABLE 1: Histopathology of coronary artery in immune complex vasculitis animal model.

Days	*Features*
2–4	Leukocyte and lymphocytic cellular infiltrates in the myocardium, perivenular and periarterial infiltrates in the heart. Cellular infiltrates in the smooth muscle cells and around the vasa vasorum of the aorta and in the distal tubular areas of the kidney
5–13	Intimal thickening, inner smooth muscle cells proliferation (**Figs. 1A and B**), patchy edematous changes, and early SMC disorganization in coronary arteries. Cellular infiltrates are few. Iliac artery shows mild intimal thickening
14–24	Intima and inner SMC proliferations, moderate-to-severe disorientation of SMC (**Fig. 1C**), edematous separation of SMC (moth-eaten appearance), subintimal changes, such as coagulation of the cytoplasm, and disorientation, separation, cytolysis, vacuolization, degranulation, collagen deposition in coronary arteries. Intimal proliferation of intramural artery
25–60	Patchy areas of fibrosis within the SMC (**Fig. 1D**), resolving stages, no further progression of proliferation of SMC in the tunica media and intima

(SMC: smooth muscle cell)

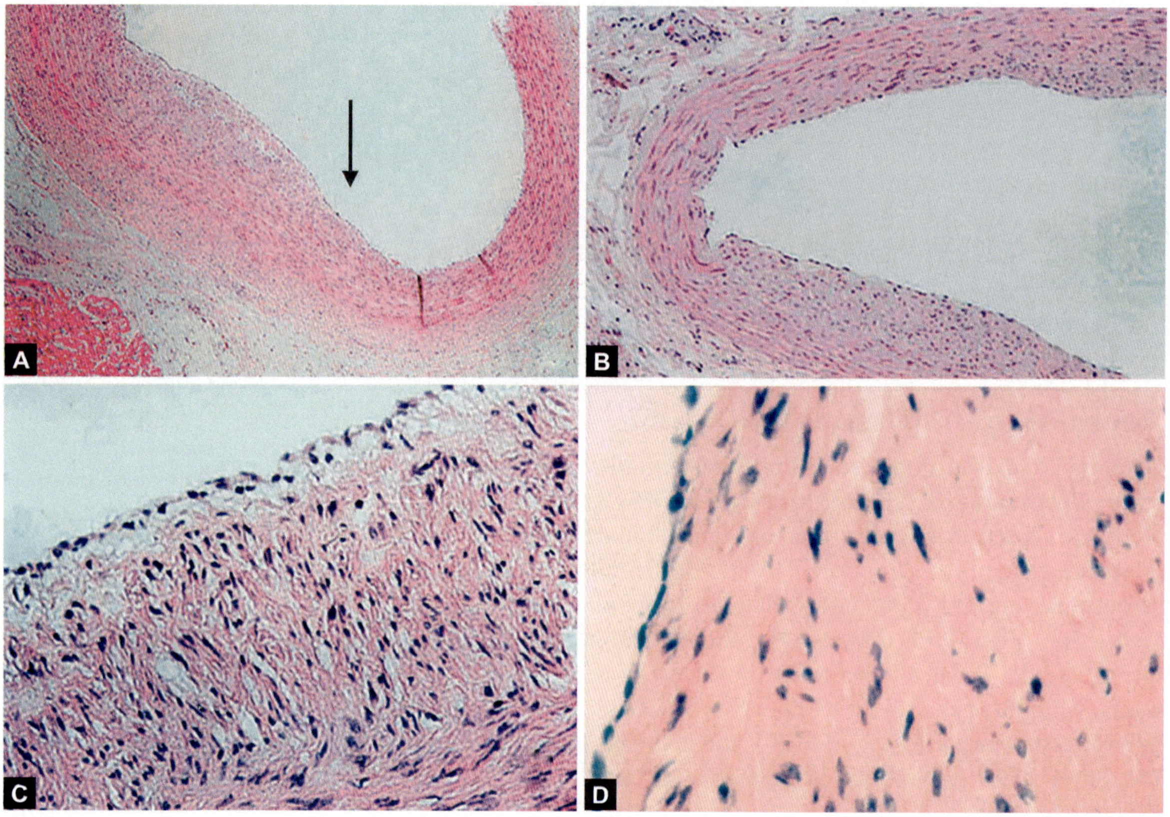

Figs. 1A to D: (A and B) Left anterior coronary artery showed intimal proliferation extending to media (5–13 days); (C) Disorientation of smooth muscles in vertical direction (14–24 days); (D) Fibrosis of the arterial wall (25–60 days).

CLINICAL SIGNS AND SYMPTOMS

Kawasaki disease is diagnosed on the basis of characteristic clinical signs and symptoms. There is no single diagnostic laboratory test.

General Feature and Diagnostic Criteria

The principal symptoms of KD are *fever persisting for 5 days or longer, bilateral conjunctival injection without exudate, changes in the lips and oral cavity, polymorphous exanthema, changes in the peripheral extremities, and acute nonpurulent cervical lymphadenopathy (>1.5 cm, usually unilateral, even >1 cm in infant is significant)*. At least five of those six principal signs and symptoms should be present for a diagnosis of KD[28,29] as per diagnostic guidelines of KD (MCLS: Infantile Acute Febrile Mucocutaneous Lymph Node Syndrome) adapted from Kawasaki Disease Study Group of the Ministry of Health, Labour and Welfare, Japan (**Box 1**).[28] High irritability and persisting fever in a child <6 months of age, erythema around the BCG (Bacillus Calmette-Guérin) scar (18–24%), perianal excoriation, "Beau's line" on nail bed, etc., are additional supporting evidence for the confirmation of KD. The KD

BOX 1: Diagnostic guidelines of Kawasaki disease (KD)* (MCLS: Infantile Acute Febrile Mucocutaneous Lymph Node Syndrome).

Principal symptoms

- Fever persisting for 5 days or more (inclusive of those cases in whom the fever has subsided before the 5th day in response to therapy)
- Bilateral conjunctival congestion
- *Changes of lips and oral cavity*: Redding of lips, strawberry tongue, diffuse injection of oral and pharyngeal mucosa
- Polymorphous exanthema
- Changes of peripheral extremities:
  - *Acute phase*: Reddening of palms and soles, indurative edema
  - *Convalescent phase*: Membranous desquamation from fingertips
- Acute nonpurulent cervical lymphadenopathy

At least five of the above six should be positive for diagnosis of KD by JMC and five of six with fever should be satisfied for AHA criteria. Further, one point less in JMC or 4/5 criteria is considered as incomplete KD.

However, patients with four of the principal symptoms can be diagnosed as KD, if 2D echocardiography or coronary angiography shows coronary aneurysm or dilatation.

Other significant symptoms or findings

The following symptoms and findings should be considered in the clinical evaluation of suspected patients:

- *Cardiovascular*: Auscultation (heart murmur, gallop rhythm, distant heart sounds), ECG changes (prolonged PR/QT intervals, abnormal Q wave, low-voltage QRS complexes, ST-T changes, arrhythmias), and chest X-ray findings (cardiomegaly)
- 2D echocardiographic findings (pericardial effusion, coronary aneurysms), aneurysm of peripheral arteries other than coronary (e.g., axillary), and angina pectoris or myocardial infarction
- *Gastrointestinal (GI) tract*: Diarrhea, vomiting, abdominal pain, hydrops of gallbladder, paralytic ileus, mild jaundice, slight increase of serum transaminase
- *Blood*: Leukocytosis with shift to the left, thrombocytosis, increased erythrocyte sedimentation rate (ESR), positive C-reactive protein (CRP), hypoalbuminemia, increased α2-globulin, slight decrease in erythrocyte and hemoglobin levels
- *Urine*: Proteinuria, increase of leukocytes in urine sediment
- *Skin*: Redness and crust at the site of BCG inoculation, small pustules, transverse furrows of the finger nails
- *Respiratory*: Cough, rhinorrhea, and abnormal shadow on chest X-ray
- *Joint*: Pain and swelling
- *Neurological*: Pleocytosis in cerebrospinal fluid (CSF), convulsion, unconsciousness, facial palsy, and paralysis of the extremities

*Guidelines for the diagnosis: The difference between JMC and American Heart Association KD criteria is that fever is included in the principal symptoms in JMC, whereas fever is an essential criteria to diagnose KD in AHA criteria

(AHA: American Heart Association; BCG: Bacillus Calmette–Guérin; ECG: electrocardiogram)

Adapted from: Kawasaki Disease Study Group of the Ministry of Health, Labour and Welfare, Japan.

cohort from Northern and Eastern India found that orange-brown chromonychia is a novel finding seen in 63% of patients.[29] Asymptomatic and sterile pyuria may be associated with coincidence of severe CAL, so it is necessary to look for pus cells on urine routine examination. Thrombocytosis or a rising trend of platelet count may be considered as an additional confirmatory diagnosis of KD. The only difference in American Heart Association (AHA) criteria is that fever is considered as a principal symptom and other five criteria were included as principal clinical findings. Few important diagnostic clues are irritability, rising trend of platelets, early periungual peeling, erythema around the BCG scar, nonexudative clean bulbar conjunctivitis, chromonychia, and Beau's lines. These signs enable further confirmation from other differential diagnosis overlapping with KD diagnosis (**Box 2 and Figs. 2A to E**). All cases of suspected KD must be evaluated for incomplete subset of KD and should be treated as KD once the criteria are fulfilled for incomplete KD to prevent coronary artery complications.

In fact, incomplete KD may be more prone for developing coronary artery complications than complete KD (**Box 3**). Other important diseases overlapping with the signs and symptoms of KD should be scrutinized for differential diagnosis (**Box 4**).

BOX 2: Few important striking signs in KD to confirm the diagnosis.

- Irritability with fever
- Early periungual and perianal excoriation often within 10 days in the acute phase of fever
- Rising trend of thrombocytosis
- Erythema around the BCG scar
- Orange-brown chromonychia (novel finding seen in 63%)
- Beau's line in 3rd to 4th week
- Clean bulbar conjunctivitis
- Sterile pyuria (>8–10 wbc/hpf)

(BCG: Bacillus Calmette–Guérin; KD: Kawasaki disease)

Cutaneous Manifestation in Kawasaki Disease

Kawasaki disease is the second common vasculitis in childhood following Henoch-Schönlein purpura. The most common cutaneous manifestation is the rash, which usually appears by the 5th febrile day. It is usually *erythematous, maculopapular* (**Fig. 3A**) present predominantly on the trunk. However, a variety of rashes have been described: *scarlatiniform, erythema multiforme-like, erythroderma*; and can sometimes be pruritic. A vesiculobullous or pustular rash is not consistent with KD, but erythema nodosum, ulcerative, or bullous lesion can rarely occur in association

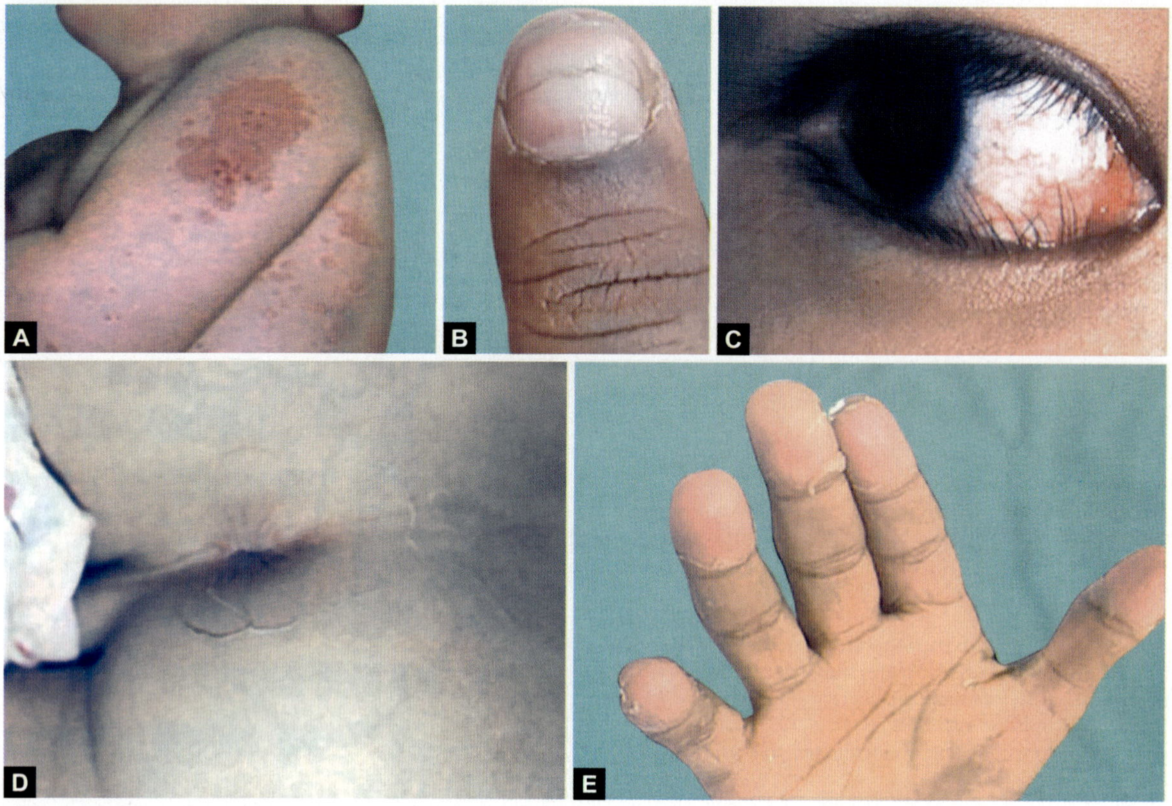

Figs. 2A to E: (A) Erythema around the BCG (Bacillus Calmette–Guérin) scar; (B) Beau's line—a transverse line or groove well seen over the thumb nail 3–4 weeks; (C) Nonpurulent conjunctivitis; (D) Perianal excoriation; (E) Typical periungual desquamation.

BOX 3: Evaluation of suspected case of incomplete Kawasaki disease (KD).

Children with fever >5 days with two or three fulfilled criteria Or infants with fever >7 days without explanation need laboratory test with CRP and ESR.

- If CRP <3 mg/dL and ESR <40 mm/hr, advise echocardiogram to see any coronary involvement, especially in presence of skin peeling. If coronaries are involved, treat as KD.
- If >3 mg/dL/or ESR >40 mm/hr, see for AHA special criteria* as given below:
  - Anemia for the age
  - Platelet count of >450,000 after the 7th day fever
  - Albumin <3 g/dL
  - Elevated ALT level
  - WBC count >15,000/mm^3
  - Urine >10 wbc/hpf (sterile pyuria)
  - Positive echocardiogram

*3 or >3 laboratory finding is significant and treat as KD
(AHA: American Heart Association; ALT: alanine aminotransferase; CRP: C-reactive protein; ESR: erythrocyte sedimentation rate; WBC: white blood cell)

BOX 4: Major differential diagnosis.

- Measles
- Scarlet fever
- Juvenile rheumatoid arthritis
- Stevens–Johnson syndrome
- Drug reactions
- Toxic shock syndrome
- Leptospirosis
- Staphylococcal scalded skin syndrome
- Mercury poisoning

with KD. Affection of the oral mucous membrane leads to erythema, *dry fissured lips*, and sometimes a *strawberry tongue*.

Extremity changes are one of the striking diagnostic features in KD. The erythema of the palms and soles together with edema of the hands and feet, which may occasionally be painful, often occur in the acute phase. The other classical finding is the periungual desquamation in the fingers and toes that starts around the end of the 2nd week (**Figs. 2E and 3B and E**). Though a consistent clinical finding, but because of the late appearance in the subacute phase, its clinical utility lies in only confirming the diagnosis retrospectively. The periungual desquamation (**Fig. 2E**) is however preceded by perineal desquamation (**Fig. 2D**) that may be present as early as end of the 1st week. Few patients may also have peri/supraorbital erythema followed by excoriations. Another well described albeit a bit rare sign are the transverse grooves called Beau's lines (**Fig. 2B**) on the nails, which may appear as late as 1–2 months after the disease onset. Beau's lines are better felt than visually appreciated.

An interesting finding, which is almost pathognomonic of KD, is reactivation of the BCG scar. Erythema around the scar may turn ulcerative in some cases (**Figs. 2A and 3C**) as observed in 10–15% of the children. A recently described

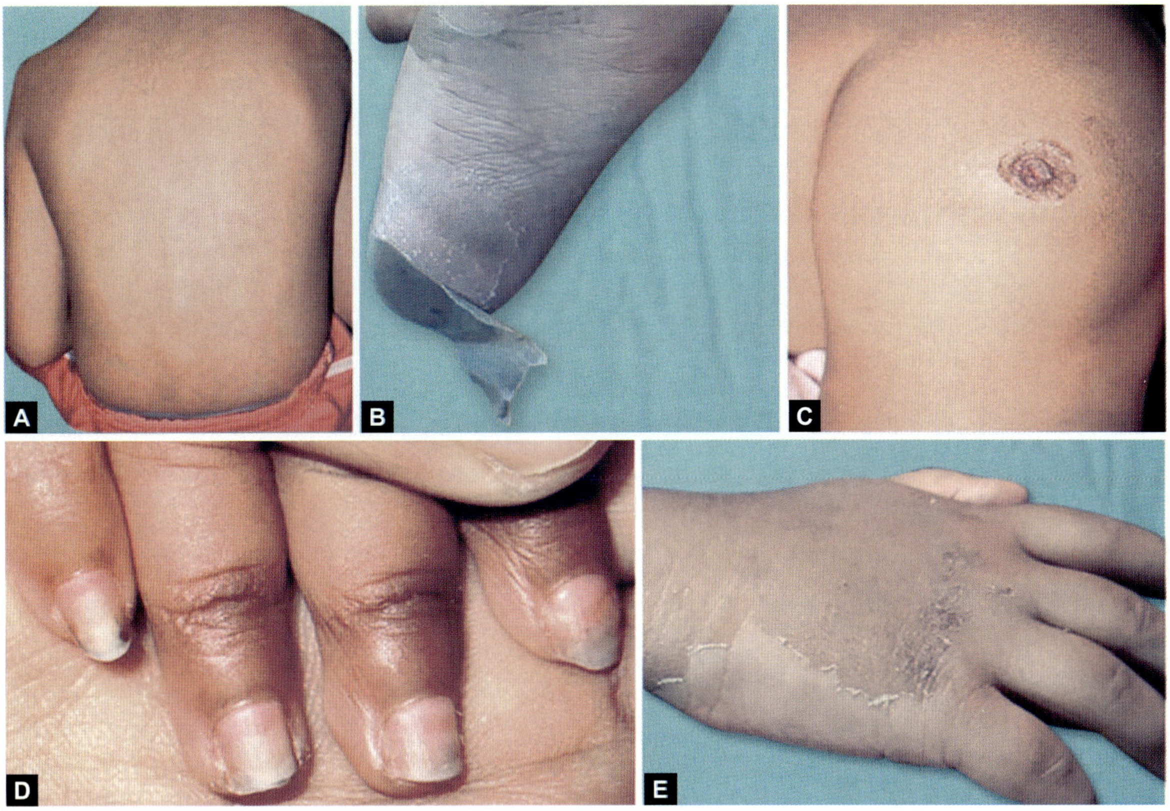

Figs. 3A to E: (A) Erythematous maculopapular rashes predominantly present on the trunk; (B) Exfoliation starts as periungual and then to entire sole and palm in severe cases; (C) Erythema around the BCG (Bacillus Calmette–Guérin) scar turning to mild ulcerative changes; (D) Chromonychia-striking brownish orange color change of nails in acute phase; (E) Exfoliation may extend to dorsum of hand in later phase.

clinical finding is orange-brown chromonychia, which means an abnormal reddish/orange brown change in color of the nail plates and/or subungual tissue. The colored lines start appearing usually around the 5th to 8th day of illness, though they may be noticed as early as the 4th day of fever mandating it as an early sign in the diagnosis.[30] Once it appears, the discoloration stays unchanged over the next 7–10 days. Better appreciated in the fingers (**Fig. 3D**) than toes, they start disappearing by the end of the 2nd week. Thus, on appearing, they are present throughout the acute phase of illness as opposed to most of the classical clinical signs in KD, which are known for their markedly temporary appearance.

Other than the chromonychia, few case reports describe some inconsistent nail changes following KD such as onycholysis, onychomadesis (spontaneous separation of the nail from the matrix), spontaneously resolving pincer nail deformity (transverse curling of the nail along its longitudinal axis), and leukonychia partialis (abnormally white proximal portion of the nail). However, all these nail abnormalities are nonspecific, may be associated with other systemic triggers and generally resolve spontaneously within 1–2 months.

Myocardial Involvement in Kawasaki Disease

Myocarditis is a well-recognized component of KD, with LV dysfunction occurring in more than half of the patients during the acute phase of the disease, and may be transient. In KD, myocarditis develops even earlier than epicardial coronary arteritis; it peaks by disease day 10 and then disappears gradually after day 20. Inflammatory cell infiltration, consisting mainly of lobulated leukocytes and large mononuclear cells, was seen in the myocardial interstitium in all cases.[27,30] Cardiac magnetic resonance imaging (MRI) is considered the gold standard noninvasive test for diagnosing myocarditis. Augmented inflammatory condition can be revealed by increased intensity of T2-weighted (T2W) images. Sensitivity of detecting edema in myocardium in acute phase of myocarditis is 84% with specificity of 75%. Multiple foci of hyperenhancement in the myocardium during early gadolinium enhancement (EGE) are consistent with myocarditis. Though MRI gives diagnostic confirmation, echocardiographic scan is sufficient to rule out myocarditis. Cardiovascular biomarkers for myocarditis in KD are creatine kinase-MB (CK-MB), cardiac troponin I (25-35% elevated in biopsy proved myocarditis). N-terminal pro-B-type natriuretic peptide (NT-proBNP) and soluble ST2 (sST2) were elevated in acute versus convalescent KD.[31] A titer of pro-BNP over 450 pg/mL and presence of an abnormal ECG (electrocardiogram) in a patient are more suggestive of myocarditis. Echocardiographic features of myocarditis are pericardial effusion, LV systolic dysfunction evidenced as low ejection fraction by strain echo or

Simpson method, and mitral regurgitation. The overall sensitivity of echocardiography in picking up CAL is 95%. Multidimensional computed tomography (MDCT) coronary angiography is more useful in identifying distal coronary lesions.

Rare Associations with Kawasaki Disease[32-35]

- A patient of KD may rarely present with hypotension, called Kawasaki shock syndrome. Hyponatremia is an important presenting symptom. Hence, checking for electrolytes during acute phase is justifiable.
- Papillary edema on Fundus examination.
- Bullae lesions, gangrene, jaundice, interstitial nephritis, cystic fibrosis, varicella infection, autoimmune hemolytic anemia, etc.
- KD may present as acute intestinal obstruction.
- KD may be complicated by macrophage activation syndrome (MAS). Also known as secondary hemophagocytic lymphohistiocytosis, MAS is a rare and potentially fatal complication of KD. The persistence of fever with splenomegaly, hyperferritinemia, thrombocytopenia, and elevated aspartate aminotransferase (AST) should prompt the consideration of MAS complicating KD.
- KD may be associated with hepatobiliary involvement.
- Adult-onset KD (mucocutaneous lymph node syndrome) and concurrent Coxsackievirus A4 infection.
- KD followed by Behçet's disease. Behçet's disease is a rare systemic vasculitis of unknown origin. HLA-B51 allele located on chromosome 6p has been the most strongly associated risk factor for Behçet's disease. HLA-B51 may be rarely associated with KD.
- Hemorrhagic pleural effusion.
- Meningococcal group-A sepsis associated with rare manifestations and complicated by Kawasaki-like disease.
- Laboratory investigations done from the day of suspicion of KD till discharge is essential for the appropriate treatment, follow-up, and evaluation for the treatment response (**Box 5**).

BOX 5: Laboratory investigations.

- Hemoglobin and complete blood count
- Platelet count to be repeated every 2–3 days to see the rising trend (thrombocytosis)
- ESR, CRP, ASO
- Sodium, potassium, and proBNP
- Liver function test; bilirubin, albumin, SGPT, SGOT
- NS1 antigen and dengue IgM, IgG serology (if fever persist for >5 days with profound thrombocytopenia)
- Serum ferritin
- Urine routine
- *Noninvasive tests*: Ultrasound abdomen, ECG, and 2D echocardiography
- First echocardiogram at 5–7 days of acute stage or as soon as you suspect or diagnose KD
- If baseline echocardiogram is normal, repeat after 5 days

(ASO: antistreptolysin O; CRP: C-reactive protein; ECG: electrocardiogram; ESR: erythrocyte sedimentation rate; Ig: immunoglobulin; proBNP: pro-B-type natriuretic peptide; SGOT: serum glutamic oxaloacetic transaminase; SGPT: serum glutamic pyruvic transaminase)

Serum Biomarkers for Kawasaki Disease

Current evidence suggests that NT-pro-BNP may be used as a diagnostic tool for KD. NT-pro-BNP has high diagnostic value for identifying KD in patients with protracted and undifferentiated febrile illness (NT-pro BNP values: 1 year >550 pg/mL, 1–2 years > 202 pg/mL; 2–3 years >189 Pg/mL; >3 years 152 pg/mL). ECG changes may also suggest early evidence of KD myocarditis.[36-38] Other laboratory investigations to be performed in all cases of suspected and diagnosed cases of KD are given in **Box 5**.

Coronary Aneurysms

The 2017 AHA guidelines emphasized the application of Z-scores for coronary artery evaluation and classified the severity of coronary abnormalities by using Z-scores. Coronary Z-scores of +2.5, +5.0, and +10.0 were recommended as the cut-off points for small, medium-sized, and giant coronary aneurysms, respectively (**Table 2**). These Z-scoring systems are usually applied for the right coronary artery (RCA), left main coronary artery (LMCA), and left anterior descending (LAD) (P-Sax view). Other coronary segments such as circumflex can be evaluated by comparing them to adjacent segments.[39]

Giant Aneurysm

Giant aneurysm can occur in 1% of CAL and is defined as diameter >8 mm or ≥ +10 Z score by coronary artery measurement (**Figs. 4A to C**). As per the echocardiographic follow-up, giant aneurysm will never resolve. In such cases, long-term antiplatelet and anticoagulant therapy are needed to keep the international normalized ratio (INR) around 2–2.2. Further follow-up is very essential and must be monitored every 4–6 months with ECG, echocardiography, and treadmill test (TMT).[39] Severe long-term complications can occur such as coronary artery stenosis resulting in early ischemic heart disease. Smooth muscle cells can migrate into intima producing myointimal proliferation; large amount of extracellular matrix and fibrosis results in calcification. Long-term follow-up studies done by Kato et al. showed calcification in 12% at 5 years, 44% at 10 years, and 94% at 20 years after diagnosis of KD.

Nongiant Coronary Aneurysm

Most coronary artery aneurysms (CAAs) from KD are small to medium sized. Regression of the aneurysms (by 50–60%) may occur within 1–2 years. The factors associated with early regression are: age (<1 year), shape (fusiform aneurysm gets resolved faster than saccular one), size (smaller), and position (distal CA involvement also has faster regression). Regression of aneurysm usually occurs by intimal proliferation.

TABLE 2: Coronary Z-score classification and timing of echocardiography.

Coronary artery	*Z-score/diameter*	*Timing of coronary 2D echocardiography involvement*
No involvement	<2	1-week interval till discharge, 1 month and 6 months, 2 years to see intimal dysfunction
Dilatation	>2 to <2.5	1–2-week interval, 1 month after treatment, 6 months, then till resolving to normal
Small aneurysm	>2.5 to <5	2-week interval till no progression 1 month, 6 months, and then till resolving to normal, after 2 years of stopping aspirin
Medium	>5 to <10/<8 mm	2-week interval till no progression 1 month, 6 months, and then till resolving to normal, after 2 years of stopping aspirin
Large/giant	>10/>8 mm	Weekly till 1 month and then monthly till 3 months, every 6 months to see for thrombus plus ECG/ TMT for older children
(if needed)/MDCT		

(ECG: electrocardiogram; MDCT: multidetector computed tomography; TMT: treadmill test)

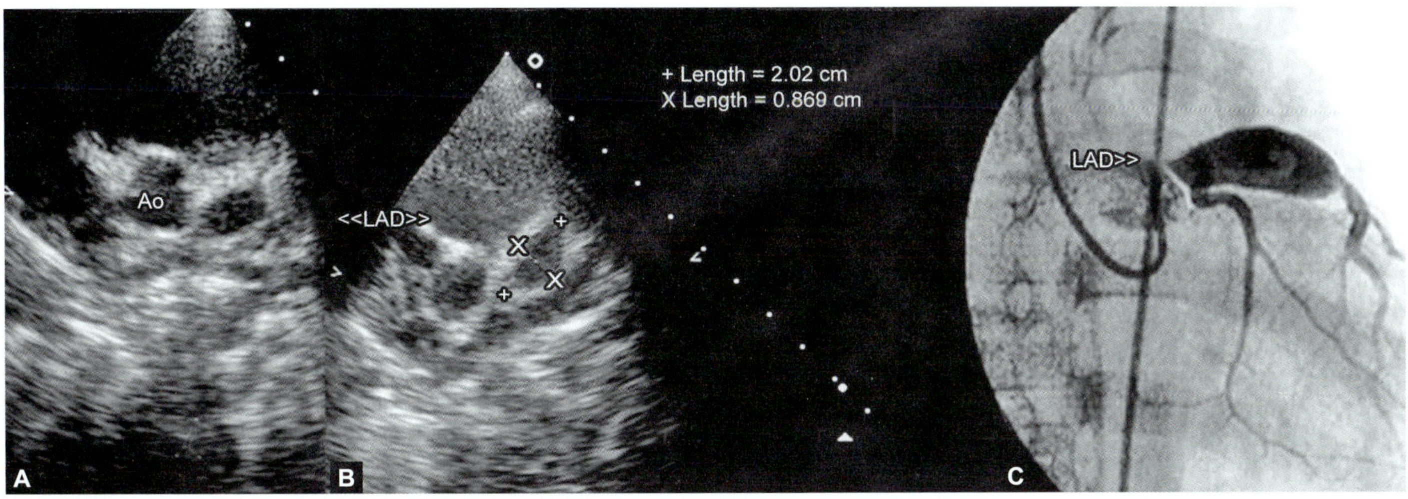

Figs. 4A to C: Giant coronary artery aneurysm (Z score >10). (A and B) Standard short axis view modified at the aortic valve level (Ao) in 2D echocardiogram; proximal segment of left anterior descending artery (LAD) with giant aneurysm marked (<<LAD>>) measuring 20 × 8.6 mm; (C) Coronary artery angiogram same case showed fusiform giant aneurysm of the proximal segment of LAD with normal left main and circumflex artery.

Accelerated Atherosclerosis

Persistent abnormal vascular wall morphology and dysfunction due to SMC proliferation and fibrosis of coronary walls may predispose to early atherosclerosis. A 10-year follow-up study of intravascular ultrasound (IVUS) showed various degrees of intimal thickening at the site of regression. Endothelial dysfunction was proved in the form of increased constriction with acetylcholine and poor dilatation with isosorbide dinitrate. Transient dilatation did not show any long-term ischemic findings. Atherosclerosis in children may occur only after 10–12 years and hence, fat-restricted diet should be advised in late-adolescent and middle-aged life.

MANAGEMENT OF KAWASAKI DISEASE[28,30]

Goal of initial therapies in the acute phase is preventing coronary artery abnormalities by reduction of inflammatory response to the endothelium. Hence, we should prevent inflammatory response by administering the well-accepted, gold standard regime such as single-dose IVIG (2 g/kg) and aspirin. IVIG should be administered as early as possible, preferably within 10 days of onset of fever. For children with a diagnosis of KD after 10 days of fever with symptoms of an ongoing inflammatory process such as high CRP and ESR, IVIG should nevertheless be administered as soon as possible (even up to 20 days). IVIG is not indicated for patients with low inflammatory markers, normalization of laboratory tests, and normal echocardiographic results in cases presenting after 10–12 days. IVIG exerts anti-inflammatory effects. Possible mechanisms of action of IVIG include the modulation of cytokine production; neutralization of toxins, pathogenic agents, and Fc receptors; augmentation of regulatory T-cell activity and suppression of antibody synthesis. Even with IVIG infusion, approximately 20% of patients may develop transient coronary dilatation, which resolves within 3–6 months of time. Around 5% of patients develop coronary aneurysms (1% of patients develop giant aneurysms) after 1 month of onset of the disease.

Acetylsalicylic acid (ASA) has been used in the treatment of KD for many years. Although ASA has important anti-inflammatory activity (at high doses) and antiplatelet activity (at low doses), it does not appear to lower the frequency of development of coronary abnormalities in children with KD. In acute phase, aspirin is given at a dosage of 60 mg/kg/day 6 hourly, though some countries use higher dosages till the child becomes afebrile for at least 48 hours. In order to avoid gastritis in children, aspirin must be given with sucralfate, antacids, or other proton pump inhibitors. Aspirin dosage is adjusted to low dose (3–5 mg /kg/day) as single dose, after the fever subsides for at least 48–72 hours of IVIG infusion. If there are no CALs, aspirin should be continued for 6–8 weeks. KD patients with coronary artery abnormalities must be administered medications for prevention of thrombosis. Low-dose aspirin is sufficient for prophylaxis in those with only coronary artery dilation or small aneurysms (Z scores 2.5–5). For patients with medium-sized coronary artery aneurysms (Z scores 5–10 and diameter <8 mm), dual antiplatelet agents use may be considered such as clopidogrel (dosage 0.2–1 mg/kg/day) or dipyridamole tablet (1 mg/kg/day). For KD patients with giant aneurysms (Z score >10 or diameter >8 mm), administering one anticoagulant, such as low-molecular-weight heparin (LMWH) or warfarin, is reasonable. The recommended therapeutic target in the United States is 0.5–1.0 of activated factor Xa level for LMWH or the INR of 2–2.2 for warfarin.[19,30]

Recent review on pathogenesis again prompts us to investigate *new drugs in KD* effectively; TNF-α is a pleiotropic inflammatory cytokine that has been strongly implicated in the development of aneurysm formation in patients with KD. *Infliximab* and *etanercept* are examples of these TNF-α receptor antagonists. Etanercept, although a TNF-α antagonist, has different mechanisms as compared to infliximab. Infliximab is a chimeric monoclonal immunoglobulin G (IgG) antibody that targets transmembrane TNF-α. This damages the cells, which express TNF-α, including cardiomyocytes.[40-42] On the other hand, etanercept is a soluble fusion-protein receptor that works more broadly on TNF (both TNF-α and lymphotoxin), and binds to only circulating TNF-α, thereby avoiding the adverse effect seen in infliximab. But we need more studies and both drugs play important role as pharmacological agents in recrudescent fever after first dose of IVIG or as a first-line therapy. Markedly activated neutrophils or high plasma neutrophil elastase in patients with KD have been implicated in poor response to IVIG. *Ulinastatin* is a urinary trypsin inhibitor and has a property to inhibit neutrophil elastase. Treated with ulinastatin as initial treatment for KD resulted in lower incidence of CAL (3% as opposed to 7% in control group). *Methotrexate* is a folic acid antagonist, which suppresses lymphocyte proliferation and has role in modulating cytokines, especially interleukin 6 (IL-6) that is highly expressed in KD. Inositol-trisphosphate 3-kinase C acts as a negative regulator of T-cell activation and activated T-cells may play a pivotal role in pathogenesis of KD. *Cyclosporine* also suppresses the activity of T-cell.

BOX 6: Treatment protocol of Kawasaki disease in acute phase.

- IVIG 2 g/kg as a single dose over a period of 10–12 hours [it can be given from the day of diagnosis (usually after 5 days of fever) and even up to 18 days in case of late diagnosis]. But presence of high inflammatory markers is mandatory.
- Aspirin 60 mg/kg/day in 6-hourly doses with sucralfate or antacids (ranitidine or other proton pump inhibitors) till child becomes afebrile for at least 48–72 hours.
  - Aspirin treatment should be changed to 3–5 mg/kg/day as single dose, once the fever subsides for 48–72 hours after IVIG infusion.
  - If no CALs, aspirin should continue till 6–8 weeks.
  - If coronary artery is involved, continue aspirin till CAL resolves, including intimal irregularities and thickening observed on 2D echocardiogram.
  - For the giant aneurysm, aspirin should be continued as lifelong therapy.
  - With CAL excluding simple ectasia, add clopidogrel 0.2–1 mg/kg/day maximum 75 mg/day till the resolution of CAL on2D echocardiographic follow-up.
- With giant aneurysm, add warfarin (keep INR 2.2)/coumadin/low molecular weight heparin (LMWH). LMWH is reasonable to administer in cases with Z score >10.
- Infliximab may also be considered as first line of therapy in cases admitted with diagnosis of severe CAL and in anticipated IVIG-resistant group. Infliximab will also be more economical in older children than IVIG.

(CAL: coronary artery lesion; IVIG: intravenous immunoglobulin; INR: international normalized ratio)

Studies have demonstrated the pivotal role of TNF-α-mediated matrix metalloproteinase (MMP)-9 activity, in modulating key pathogenic stages of the disease, leading to coronary artery damage and also in the pathogenesis of elastin breakdown in a murine model of KD with *L. casei* extract-induced coronary arteritis. *Doxycycline* inhibits T-cell activation and TNF-α production in peripheral immune cell and also directly inhibits MMP-9 enzymatic activity derived from TNF-α stimulated vascular SMCs. Therefore, doxycycline can mitigate TNF-α induced, MMP-9-mediated coronary elastin breakdown and improve coronary outcome. *Antioxidants* such as of vitamin A, C, and E have a greater role in mitigating CAL as an add-on drug therapy.[42] Additional dose of IVIG shows 71% response with 30% resistance. *Steroid pulse therapy (methyl prednisolone)* has been used in resistant IVIG cases with 100% response.

Treatment protocol with dosages of medications is given in **Box 6**.

RESISTANT KAWASAKI DISEASE

Studies with an additional dose of IVIG show 71% response and 30% resistance. In such cases, steroid pulse therapy (methylprednisolone) may give a 100% response. These studies recommend combination therapies in all IVIG-resistant cases, where steroid pulse therapy could be useful to prevent further damage of coronary arteries.[30,43]

TABLE 3: First-line therapy in resistant Kawasaki disease (KD).

Second dose of IVIG	2 g/kg
IVIG + Prednisolone	*IVIG*: 2 g/kg IV + oral prednisolone 2 mg/kg/day, divided every 8-hourly until afebrile, then prednisone orally until CRP normalizes, then taper over 2–3 weeks
IVMP	Not with IVIG, but can be given separately IVMP 30 mg/kg over 2–3 hours × 3 days, followed by oral for 2–4 weeks
or Infliximab*	5 mg/kg single infusion × 2 hours + IVMP
or Etanercept	0.8 mg/kg, subcutaneous/week + IVMP
or Ulinastatin	20,000–30,000 unit/kg OD IV × 3 days + IVMP
Cyclosporine A	3–8 mg/kg/day PO × 5–6 days depends on the febrile period (keep serum level 400–500 ng/mL).
Anakinra	2–6 mg/kg/day by subcutaneous injection

*Infliximab may be considered as preferred first-line therapy in resistant KD instead second dose of IVIG (desired drug of Indian Society of Kawasaki disease). Steroid may be added as per the severity of CAL.

(CAL: coronary artery lesion; IV: intravenous; IVIG: intravenous immunoglobulin; IVMP: intravenous methylprednisolone)

TABLE 4: Prediction scoring systems for IVIG-resistant cases.

1. Kobayashi score	(≥5 points; sensitivity 76%, specificity 80%)	
NA	≤133 mmol/L	2
AST	≥100 IU/L	2
Day of starting treatment (or diagnosis) day 4 after onset or earlier:		2
Neutrophils	≥80%	2
CRP	≥10 mg/dL	1
Platelets	≤300,000/μL	1
Age (months)	≤12 months	1
2. Egami score	(≥3 points; sensitivity 76%, specificity 80%)	
ALT	≥80 IU/L	2
Day of starting treatment (or diagnosis) day 4 after onset or earlier		1
CRP	≥8 mg/dL	1
Platelets	≤300,000/μL	1
Age (months)	≤6 months	1
3. Sano score	(≥2 points; sensitivity 77%, specificity 86%)	
AST	≥200 IU/L	1
Total bilirubin	≥0.9 mg/D	1
CRP	≥7 mg/dL	1
4. Satoshi Sato score	(3 or >3)	
Neutrophils	≥75%	2
IL6	>140 pg/ml	2
IL-6	70–140 pg/mL	1

(ALT: alanine aminotransferase; AST: aspartate aminotransferase; CRP: C-reactive protein; IL: interleukin; IVIG: intravenous immunoglobulin; Na: sodium)

Management protocol for IVIG-resistant group is given in **Table 3** as per personal experiences and may have institutional variations. CRP level of >8 mg/dL after initial IVIG is likely to fail additional dose of IVIG. In older children, plasma exchange may be considered as another mode of treatment if you have facility for plasmapheresis under an experienced hematologist to remove circulating ICs, thus we can save the cost of IVIG, especially in developing countries such as India. Younger children cannot undergo plasmapheresis due to various procedural reasons. Different scoring systems were developed by various authors as per their experiences (**Table 4**).

KAWASAKI DISEASE SHOCK SYNDROME

The incidence of Kawasaki disease shock syndrome (KDSS) is estimated to be 7%. KDSS can be defined as the presence of hypotension and shock requiring the initiation of volume expanders, the infusion of vasoactive agents, or transfer to intensive care units. Shock in KDSS is often moderate, with low lactate values and the need for treatment with inotropic and vasopressor agents. Although hemodynamic instability improves quickly on initiation of therapy with diuretic agents and vasopressor agents, a mild degree of ventricular diastolic dysfunction can persist after acute management. The causes of KDSS may involve the release of endogenous molecules that mediate a decrease in peripheral vascular resistance, myocardial dysfunction from myocarditis with or without myocardial ischemia, and capillary leakage, but the exact underlying mechanisms remain unclear. KDSS is often associated with more severe laboratory markers of inflammation and higher risk of coronary artery dilation. Such cases are also more likely to be resistant to IVIG therapy and often require additional anti-inflammatory treatment.[30]

LONG-TERM MANAGEMENT OF KAWASAKI DISEASE: IMPLICATIONS FOR THE ADULT PATIENT

Many scoring systems are available to predict unresponsiveness to IVIG therapy. Current long-term management protocols are calibrated to the degree of maximal and current coronary artery involvement reflecting the known likelihood of severe long-term cardiac complications. It has recently been suggested that all KD patients may be at potential risk of severe long-term cardiac complications. Based on the available evidence, patients with multiple large and/or giant CAA are at substantial risk of severe long-term cardiac complications and should have regular specialized follow-up. Patients with transient or no CAA have not been reported to be at risk of severe long-term cardiac complications. The influence of KD on the atherosclerotic process remains suboptimally defined and should be the focus of future studies. It is generally accepted that patients with no or transient coronary artery dilation during acute KD, comprising 95% of individuals diagnosed with KD in the past 25 years, live with long-term cardiovascular health comparable to the general population. An intermediate group of patients, those with small-to medium-sized CAA that may or may not have regressed, have an unclear long-term prognosis and, hence, must receive optimal follow-up that include TMT and ECG every 1–2 years. Crystal et al. found coronary artery Z-score regression in patients with normal acute-phase coronary arteries, suggesting that dilation is a common and spontaneously resolving characteristic of acute illness. As such, dilation is an acute-phase phenomenon of endothelial dysfunction and coronary artery deregulation, resulting in no permanent changes to the vasculature. However, endothelial dysfunction may persist in some patients with aneurysmal coronary artery dilatation.[42,44]

LONG-TERM FATE AND COMPLICATIONS OF GIANT CORONARY ARTERY ANEURYSM

Although rare, giant CAAs (8 mm or Z-score >10) are highly unlikely to resolve. They are associated with the most severe long-term complications, including progression to stenosis or occlusion, resulting in ischemic heart disease. Stenosis of persistent and regressed CAA may occur as a result of myointimal proliferation, an intrinsic process of postacute KD, in which SMCs migrate from the media to the intima, producing large amounts of extracellular matrix and fibrosis. This process may further result in calcification of the aneurysm site by a mechanism similar to arteriosclerosis, which may be accelerated with persistent inflammation in some patients. Calcification occurs primarily at the media-intimal or the subendothelial surface. Calcification is a prevalent and unique characteristic of giant CAA; affecting 12% of patients at 5 years, 44% at 10 years, and 94% at 20 years after diagnosis.[44,45] Thrombotic occlusions may also progress to calcification after the organization and recanalization of a nonocclusive mural thrombus. Myocardial infarction is the major cause of death from KD, resulting either from sudden thrombotic occlusion of a vessel, or gradual stenotic occlusion.[46] We should be careful in monitoring such high-risk cases with regular ECG, exercise test, and echocardiogram. In acute MI or ischemia, infants or children will present as severe irritability/incessant cry, vomiting, abdominal pain and at times, even shock. Older children may complain of chest pain. Symptoms in MI and findings in ECG are given in **Table 5**.

Routine investigations in such cases include troponin I and CK-MB like in adult cases of MI. Therapy with tissue-type plasminogen activator (tPA) is the most commonly administered therapeutic regimen for occlusive or near-occlusive coronary artery thrombosis in infants and children. A common regimen of tPA is 0.5 mg/kg/hr over 6 hours. An alternative regimen of tPA used in adult coronary artery thrombosis is 0.2 mg/kg intravenously (maximum 15 mg) stat, then 0.75 mg/kg over 30 minutes (maximum 50 mg) followed by 0.5 mg/kg over 60 minutes (maximum 35 mg). It should be administered together with low-dose ASA and low-dose intravenous heparin (10 U/kg/hr) with careful monitoring of

TABLE 5: Symptoms of myocardial infarction and ECG findings in children.

Symptoms	*ECG changes*
· Vomiting · Chest pain · Severe cry · Shock · Abdominal pain · Arrhythmia	· ST/T changes · T-wave invertion in ii, iii, aVF · q in ii, iii, aVF indicate infarction · Peaked J-point elevation indicate ischemia · Elevation/depression of ST-segment in V1-V3 · Wide QRS >35 ms, i AVL, V5, V6 · Prolonged QTC > 480 · Ventricular tachycardia

coagulation parameters to prevent bleeding, maintaining the fibrinogen level >100 mg/dL and platelet count of >50,000/ mm³. After completion of tPA, heparin dosage is increased as appropriate for age. The coronary artery thrombus should be reassessed with echocardiographic imaging after completion of the tPA infusion.[30]

Optimal definition of CAA is to be small if the Z-score is >2.5 to <5.0, large if the Z-score is > or 5.0 to <10.0, and giant if the Z-score is > or 10.0. This classification seems to appropriately apply to the circumflex branch despite a lack of normal values for this branch. The current AHA classification might not accurately classify CAAs in KD patients. Accurate classification is important for defining management and prognosis consistently across patient age and size. Based on studies reviewed in a meta-analysis, and the significant benefit in terms of reduced MI and death, long-term oral anticoagulation with warfarin together with aspirin appears to be the best management for children with giant coronary arteries.[43,45,46] All patients should be counseled in preventive care with regards to hyperlipidemia, hypertension, diabetes, obesity, and physical activities.

VACCINATIONS DURING THERAPY

For patients who have received high-dose IVIG, immunization with measles, mumps, rubella, and varicella vaccines should be delayed for 11 months after IVIG infusion. Reye syndrome is a risk in children who receive salicylates while they are experiencing active infection with varicella or influenza and has also been reported in patients taking high-dose ASA for a prolonged period of time after KD. The low-dose therapy used for antiplatelet effect has not been associated with the development of Reye syndrome. In the patient who presents with influenza and KD, administration of high-dose IVIG without aspirin and use of alternative antipyretic drugs (i.e., acetaminophen) as needed for fever should be considered. An alternative antiplatelet agent should be considered for a minimum of 2 weeks. All children ≥6 months should receive a seasonal influenza vaccine, as should their family members. Only inactivated vaccine should be administered to children on aspirin therapy.[30]

COVID-19 AND KAWASAKI DISEASE

Confirmatory rapid polymerase chain reaction (PCR) test was positive for SARS-CoV-2 in few children of KD cases during Covid-19 epidemic.[47] This RNA virus association had been observed with KD few years ago.[47-50] Circulating ICs, triggered by infectious agents, bacteria or viral or other unknown causes, have been detected in the early phase of KD already known to us, implicating that immunopathologic mechanisms might be involved in the pathogenesis of vasculitis in KD.[5-12] SARS-CoV-2 mimics the signs and symptoms of KD because the immune-pathogenic mechanism could be similar. Though this is not a particular causative agent to stress over etiopathogenesis of KD, it is worth considering it as one of the many triggering agents for circulating IC-producing vasculitis. CALs have been reported in cases with positive SARS-CoV-2. We do not know how and why a particular IC disease affecting coronary endothelium could trigger a host-immune response in genetically susceptible children. Also, there is not much work available yet on the genes implicated in susceptibility of an individual to KD with replication. Family linkage studies and genome-wide association studies with subsequent validation studies have implicated single-nucleotide polymorphisms in six genes or gene regions.[5,10] These polymorphisms likely vary across populations and results suggest that KD susceptibility and disease outcome, including aneurysm formation and response to IVIG, are influenced by variants in several different genes and signaling pathways.[30]

Many authors also noted that COVID-19 can produce myocarditis in children.[51,52] At the same time, all cases with myocarditis did not manifest signs and symptoms to fulfill the criteria for KD. Myocarditis in children can occur with many viral or bacterial diseases, and also will manifest in KD prior to the appearance of epicardial coronary arteritis. Published data indicate that myocardial inflammation can be documented in 50–70% of patients using gallium citrate Ga67 scans and technetium Tc99m-labeled white blood cell scans.[30] Acute LV dysfunction is generally transient and responds readily to anti-inflammatory treatment. The rapid improvement in LV function differs from that observed in other causes of myocarditis. Myocarditis in KD likely improves rapidly as the inflammatory process subsides because it results from interstitial edema and inflammation and only rarely from myocardial cell necrosis.[30] Hence, LV function study by routine Simpson method or global longitudinal strain (GLS) by 2D echocardiography in KD, and also in all other suspected viral illness including COVID-19 positive cases, is essential. In such cases, LV functions must be serially followed-up on 2D echocardiography to help in optimal and timely management.

D-dimer values in cases of myocarditis secondary to COVID-19 virus were investigated in one study and found to be within normal limits (D-dimer 3,285–7,180). In adult cases, many clotting issues and thrombosis occur in most of the organs including heart, resulting in stroke and MI. Thrombotic episodes have not yet been published in children with COVID-19. All such cases with positive SARS-CoV-2 responded well to IVIG and aspirin therapy. Hence, COVID-positive children, even without signs and symptoms of KD, may be given a trial of the same treatment protocol to prevent or mitigate myocarditis and thrombotic episodes. IVIG could be helpful in myocarditis. Role of hydroxychloroquine (HCQ) in children is yet to be proven. Possible mechanisms of IVIG include the modulation of cytokine production, neutralization of toxins, and pathogenic agents. Fc receptors, augmentation of regulatory T-cell activity, and suppression of antibody synthesis will certainly help in cases with SARS-CoV-2 even in the situation of myocarditis.

Finally, SARS-CoV-2 infection may be added as one of the differential diagnosis of KD. Once the criteria for KD are fulfilled in COVID-19 cases, treatment protocol remains the same as for KD.[47]

CONCLUSION

Kawasaki disease is a systemic vasculitis of unknown origin and can be caused by circulating ICs. These complexes are possibly triggered by infectious or non-infectious agents that have been detected in the early phase of KD, implicating that immune-pathogenic mechanisms might be involved in the vasculitis in KD. The timely diagnosis of KD may be difficult in patients aged <6 months because of atypical presentations. KD should always be considered in children with prolonged unexplained fever, thrombocytosis, skin-peeling, and with AHA special criteria. The role of the coronary Z scores has become increasingly crucial for managing and following up of CAL. Gold standard therapy for acute phase of KD is IVIG and aspirin, but add-on therapy will certainly mitigate the severity of coronary artery vasculitis. IVIG plus low-dose prednisolone are both reasonable choices of treatments for patients with refractory KD. But KD Society recommends infliximab as the first line and more economical choice in older kids in case of resistant KD. Giant aneurysm seldom resolves and needs lifelong antiplatelet and anticoagulant therapy. SARS-CoV-2 also may be considered as one of the differential diagnosis of KD. Timely diagnosis and an effective risk-stratified treatment regimen can reduce the incidence of coronary artery abnormalities. Long-term follow-up and parenteral counseling is most essential and crucial in coronary artery disease caused by Kawasaki disease.

REFERENCES

1. Kawasaki T. Acute febrile mucocutaneous syndrome with lymphoid involvement with specific desquamation of the fingers and toes in children: clinical observations of 50 cases. Arerugi (Jpn J Allergol). 1967;16(3):178-222.
2. Kawasaki T, Kosaki F, Okawa S, Shigematsu I, Yanagwa H. A new infantile acute febrile mucocutaneous lymph node syndrome (MLNS) prevailing in Japan. Pediatrics. 1974;54(3):271-6.
3. Fujiwara T, Fujiwara H, Ueda T, Nishioka K, Hamashima Y. Comparison of macroscopic, postmortem, angiographic findings of coronary aneurysms in children with Kawasaki disease. Am J Cardiol. 1986;57(10):761-4.
4. Imakita M, Sasaki Y, Misugi K, Miyazawa Y, Hyodo Y. Kawasaki disease complicated with mitral valve insufficiency. Autopsy findings with special reference to valvular lesion. Acta PatholJpn. 1984;34(3):605-16.
5. Takahashi K, Oharaseki T, Yokouchi Y. Update on etio and immunopathogenesis of Kawasaki disease. Current Opin Rheumatol. 2014;26(1): 31-6.
6. Naoe S, Shibuya K, Takahashi K, Wakayama M, Masuda H, Tanaka M. Pathological observations concerning the cardiovascular lesions in Kawasaki disease. Cardiol Young. 1991;1(3): 212-20.
7. Furuse A, Matsuda I. Circulating immune complex in the mucocutaneous lymph node syndrome. Eur J Pediatr. 1983; 141:50-1.
8. Mason WH, Jordan SC, Sakai R, Takahashi M, Bernstein B. Circulating immune complexes in Kawasaki syndrome. Pediatr Infect Dis. 1985; 4:48-51.
9. Lehman TJA, Walkwer SM, Mahanovsky V, McCurdy D. Coronary arteritis in mice following the systemic injection of group B Lactobacillus casei cell walls in aqueous suspension. Arthritis Rheum. 1985;28(6):652-9.
10. Onouchi Z, Ikuta K, Nagamatsu K, Tamiya H, Sakakibara Y, Ando M. Coronary artery aneurysms develop in weanling rabbits with serum sickness but not in mature rabbits: an experimental model for Kawasaki disease in humans. J Vasc Dis.1995;46(8):679-86.
11. Philip S, Lee WC, Liu SK, Wu MH, Lue HC. A swine model of horse serum-induced coronary vasculitis: an implication for Kawasaki disease. Pediatr Res. 2004;55(2):211-9.
12. Philip S, Lee WC, Wu MH, Cherian KM, Lue HC. Histopathological Evaluation of horse serum-induced immune complex vasculitis in swine: implication to coronary artery lesions in Kawasaki disease. PediatrNeonatol. 2014;55(4): 297-305.
13. Singh S, Vignesh P, Burgner D. The epidemiology of Kawasaki disease: a global update. Arch Dis Child. 2015;100(11):1084-8.
14. Ae R, Makino N, Kosami K, Kuwabara M, Matsubara Y, Nakamura Y. Epidemiology, treatments, and cardiac complications in patients with Kawasaki disease: the nationwide survey in Japan, 2017-2018. J Pediatr. 2020; 225:23-9.e2.
15. Kim GB, Han JW, Park YW, Song MS, Hong YM, Cha SH, et al. Epidemiologic features of Kawasaki disease in South Korea, data from nationwide survey, 2009-2011. Pediatr Infect Dis J. 2014;33(1):24-7.
16. Lin MC, Lai MS, Jan SL, Fu YC. Epidemiologic features of Kawasaki disease in acute stages in Taiwan, 1997-2010 effect of different case definitions in claims data analysis. J Chin Med Assoc. 2015;78(2):121-6.
17. Rowley AH, Shulman ST. The epidemiology and pathogenesis of KD. Frontiers in Pediatrics. 2018;6(374):1-3.
18. Singh S, Bhattad S. Kawasaki disease incidence at Chandigarh, North India, during 2009-2014. Rheumatol Int. 2016;36(10): 1391-7.
19. Liu YC, Lin MT, Wang JK, Wu MH. State-of-the art acute phase management of Kawasaki disease after 2017 scientific statement from the American Heart Association, Review. Pediatr Neonatol. 2018;59(6):543-52.
20. Soe HJ, Khan AM, Manikam R, Samudi Raju C, Vanhoutte P, Sekaran SD. High dengue virus load differentially modulates human microvascular endothelial barrier function during early efection. J Gen Virol. 2017;98(12):2993-3007.
21. Singh S, Jat KR, Suri D, Ratho RK. Dengue fever and Kawasaki disease: a clinical dilemma. Rheumatol Int. 2009;29(6):717-9.
22. Sopontammarak S, Preukprasert P. Concomitant dengue haemorrhagic fever with Kawasaki disease. South-east Asian J Trop Med Public Health. 2000;31(1):190-1.
23. Agarwal E, Shah D, Gupta P. Dengue fever triggering Kawasaki disease. Indian Pediatr. 2017;54(1):51-2.
24. Fukuda S, Ito S, Fujiwara M, Abe J, Hanaoka N, Fujimoto T, Katsumori H. Simultaneous development of Kawasaki disease following acute human adenovirus infection in monozygotic twins: a case report. Pediatric Rheumatol. 2017;15(1):39.
25. Rodó X, Curcoll R, Robinson M, Ballester J, Burns JC, Cayan DR, et al. Tropospheric winds from northeastern China carry the etiologic agent of Kawasaki disease from its source to Japan. Proc Natl Acad Sci U S A. 2014;111(22):7952-7.
26. Onouchi Y, Tamari M, Takahashi A, Tsunoda T, Yashiro M, Nakamura Y, et al. A genomewide linkage analysis of Kawasaki disease: evidence for linkage to chromosome 12. J Hum Genet. 2007:52(2):179-90.

27. Harada M, Yokouchi Y, Oharaseki T, Matsui K, Tobayama H, Tanaka N, et al. Histopathological characteristics of myocarditis in acute-phase Kawasaki disease. Histopathology. 2012;61(6): 1156-67.
28. JCS Joint Working Group. Guidelines for diagnosis and management of cardiovascular sequelae in Kawasaki disease. Digest version. Circ J. 2014;78(10):2521-62.
29. Pal P, Giri PP. Orange-brown chromonychia, a novel finding in Kawasaki disease. Rheumatol Int. 2013;33(5):1207-9.
30. McCrindle BW, Rowley AH, Newburger JW, Burns JC, Bolger AF, Gewitz M, et al. Diagnosis, treatment, and long-term management of Kawasaki disease. A scientific statement for health professionals from the American Heart Association. Circulation. 2017;135(17):e927-99.
31. Lin KH, Chang SS, Yu CW, Lin SC, Liu SC, Chao HY, et al. Usefulness of natriuretic peptide for the diagnosis of Kawasaki disease: a systematic review and meta-analysis. BMJ Open. 2015;5(4):e006703.
32. Lone YA, Menon J, Menon P, Vaiphei K, Rao KLN, Thapa B, et al. Kawasaki disease presenting as acute intestinal obstruction. J Indian Assoc Pediatr Surg. 2017;22(3):170-2.
33. García-Pavón S, Yamazaki-Nakashimada MA, Báez M, Borjas Aguilar KL, Murata C. Kawasaki disease complicated with macrophage activation syndrome: a systematic review. J Pediatr Hematol Oncol. 2017;39(6):445-51.
34. Keeling IM, Beran E, Dapunt OE. Kawasaki disease and hepatobiliary involvement: report of two cases. Ital J Pediatr. 2016;42:27.
35. Ueda Y, Kenzaka T, Noda A, Yamamoto Y, Matsumura M. Adult-onset Kawasaki disease (mucocutaneous lymph node syndrome) and concurrent Coxsackievirus A4 infection: a case report. Int Med Case Rep J. 2015;8:225-30.
36. Abe J, Matsuda A. Biomarkers associated with unresponsiveness to IVIG in children with Kawasaki disease. [Article in Japanese] Nihon Rinsho Meneki Gakkai Kaishi. 2013;36:27-34.
37. Kimura Y, Yanagimachi M, Ino Y, Aketagawa M, Matsuo M, Okayama A, et al. Identification of candidate diagnostic serum biomarkers for Kawasaki disease using proteomic analysis. Sci Rep. 2017;7:43732.
38. Qiu Y, Wu J, Fang XY, Lin Z, Wu BY, Cai RY, et al. Changes of P-selectin and E-selectin in children with Kawasaki disease [Article in Chinese]. Zhonghua Er Ke Za Zhi. 2004;42:688-92.
39. Manlhiot C, Millar K, Golding F, McCrindle BW. Improved classification of coronary artery abnormalities based only on coronary artery z-scores after Kawasaki disease. Pediatr Cardiol. 2010;31(2):242-9.
40. Ohashi R, Fukazawa R, Watanabe M, Tajima H, Nagi-Miura N, Ohno N, et.al. Etanercept suppresses arteritis in a murine model of Kawasaki disease: comparative study involving different biological agents. Int J Vasc Med. 2013; 2013:543141.
41. Manlhiot C, Niedra E, McCrindle BW. Long-term management of Kawasaki disease: implications for the adult patient. Pediatr Neonatol. 2013;54(1):12-21.
42. Philip S, Lee WC, Cherian KM, Wu MH, Lue HC. Role of antioxidants in horse serum mediated vasculitis in swine: potential relevance to early treatment in mitigation of coronary arteritis in Kawasaki disease. Pediatr Neonatol. 2017;58(4): 328-37.
43. Levin M, Burns JC, Gordon JB. Warfarin plus Aspirin or aspirin alone for patients with giant coronary artery aneurysms secondary to Kawasaki disease? Cardiology. 2014;129:174-7.
44. Tsuda E, Hamaoka K, Suzuki H, Sakazaki H, Murakami Y, Nakagawa M, et al. A survey of the 3-decade outcome for patients with giant aneurysms caused by Kawasaki disease. Am Heart J. 2014;167(2):249-58.
45. Kato H, Sugimura T, Akagi T, Sato N, Hashino K, Maeno Y, et al. Long-term consequences of Kawasaki disease. A 10 to 21-year follow-up study of 594 patients. Circulation. 1996;94(6): 1379-85.
46. Gordon JB, Kahn AM, Burns JC. When children with Kawasaki disease grow up. J Am Coll Cardiol. 209;54(21):1911-20.
47. Jones VG, Mills M, Suarez D, Hogan CA, Yeh D, Segal JB, et al. COVID-19 and Kawasaki disease: novel virus and novel case. Hosp Pediatr. 2020;10(6):537-40.
48. Shirato K, Imada Y, Kawase M, Nakagaki K, Matsuyama S, Taguchi F. Possible involvement of infection with human coronavirus 229E, but not NL63, in Kawasaki disease. J Med Virol. 2014; 86(12):2146-53.
49. Rowley AH, Baker SC, Shulman ST, Rand KH, Tretiakova MS, Perlman EJ, et al. Ultrastructural, immunofluorescence, and RNA evidence support the hypothesis of a "new" virus associated with Kawasaki disease. J Infect Dis. 2011;203(7):1021-30.
50. Belay ED, Erdman DD, Anderson LJ, Peret TC, Schrag SJ, Fields BS, et al. Kawasaki disease and human coronavirus. J Infect Dis. 2005;192(2): 352-3; author reply 353.
51. Dong N, Cai J, Zhou Y, Liu J, Li F. End-stage heart failure with COVID-19: strong evidence of myocardial injury by 2019-nCoV. JACC Heart Fail. 2020;8(6):515-7.
52. Kao CH, Hsieh KS, Wang YL, Wang SJ, Yeh SH. The detection of ventricular dysfunction and carditis in children with Kawasaki disease using equilibrium multigated blood pooling ventriculography and 99Tcm-HMPAO-labelled WBC heart scans. Nucl Med Commun. 1993; 14(7):539-43.

45 CHAPTER

Cardiomyopathy

Mani Ram Krishna

INTRODUCTION

Cardiomyopathies are less common in children compared to congenital heart diseases (CHDs). The estimated incidence from published data is around 1/100,000 children with a higher incidence in infants.[1] The cardiomyopathies may be primary when it is related to a genetic mutation (usually in one of the sarcomeric protein genes) or secondary. The secondary cardiomyopathies may be due to a more generalized genetic abnormality (e.g., mitochondrial abnormalities or Noonan syndrome), metabolic abnormality (ventricular dysfunction secondary to hypocalcemia), structural heart diseases [anomalous origin of left coronary artery from pulmonary artery (ALCAPA)], or cardiac arrhythmias (tachycardiomyopathy).

The cardiomyopathies are by definition "abnormalities of the ventricular myocardium not explained by abnormal loading conditions or congenital heart disease." A number of classifications have been proposed for cardiomyopathies and continue to be preferred by different workgroups. However, because of its simplicity and because of the broad etiological and genetic heterogenicity of the pediatric cardiomyopathies, the original morphological classification proposed by the World Health Organization (WHO) is preferred by most pediatric cardiologists. This classifies cardiomyopathy into three distinctive phenotypes[2]—dilated cardiomyopathy (DCM), hypertrophic cardiomyopathy (HCM), and restrictive cardiomyopathy (RCM) (**Flowchart 1**). Some experts consider left ventricular noncompaction cardiomyopathy (LVNC) to be a distinctive cardiomyopathy phenotype, but this continues to be disputed.

Flowchart 1: The original World Health Organization (WHO) classification of cardiomyopathy.

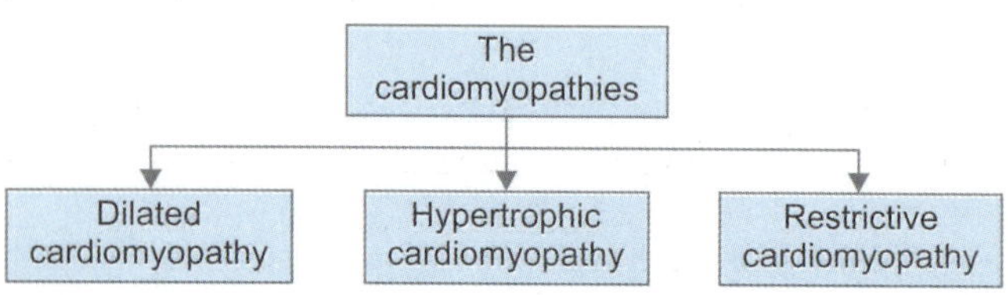

DILATED CARDIOMYOPATHY

Dilated cardiomyopathy is characterized by a dilated left ventricle (LV) and poor left ventricular contractility (**Fig. 1**). In children, LV dilatation is commonly defined as a left ventricle internal diameter in diastole (LVIDd) Z score of greater than +2. This is the most common form of cardiomyopathy in both children and adults. However, unlike the adult world where coronary artery disease is the most common cause of DCM, the etiology and clinical presentation in children are more heterogeneous and the outcomes of treatment are linked to the underlying cause rather than the severity of symptoms or ventricular dysfunction.

Epidemiology

There is very little data available on the incidence and prevalence of pediatric DCM. The three largest population-based studies from North America, Finland, and Australia suggested an incidence of between 0.5 and 1 per 100,000 population with a maximum incidence during infancy.[1,3,4] These estimates are likely to not accurately reflect the actual incidence because of the varying definitions used for cardiomyopathy in general and DCM in particular. The Finland registry did not include secondary causes of DCM

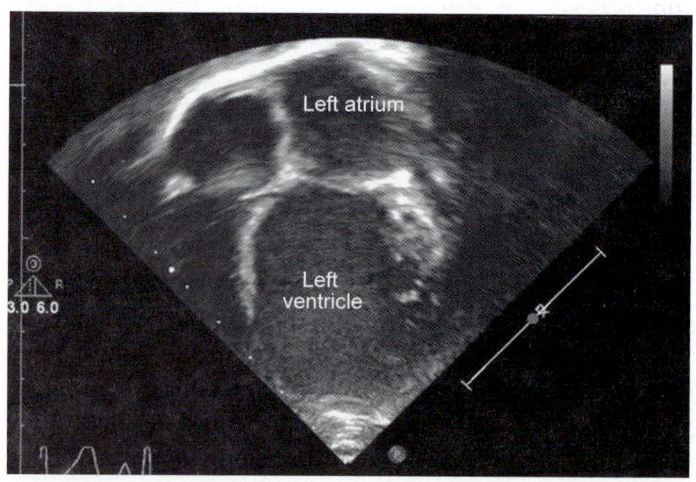

Fig. 1: Apical four-chamber echocardiography of a child with dilated cardiomyopathy demonstrating a dilated and thin-walled left ventricle.

TABLE 1: Classification of dilated cardiomyopathy in children.

Primary dilated cardiomyopathy	• Sarcomeric genes (actin, troponin T, beta myosin heavy chain) • Non-sarcomeric genes (laminopathies, muscular dystrophies, mitochondrial disorders)
Structural heart diseases	• Anomalous left coronary artery from pulmonary artery (ALCAPA) • Aortic stenosis • Coarctation of aorta
Arrhythmias	• Ectopic atrial tachycardia • Permanent junctional reciprocating tachycardia
Inflammatory conditions	• Viral myocarditis • Toxins
Nutritional conditions	• Thiamine deficiency • Selenium deficiency
Metabolic conditions	Storage disorders

including DCM secondary to structural heart diseases,[3] while the Australian registry did not include children older than 10 years.[4] There is no such epidemiological data available from our country, but the incidence is likely to be similar.

Etiology

The American Heart Association (AHA) classifies DCM into primary and secondary types[5] (**Table 1**). Primary DCM is due to a genetic mutation in one of the cardiac muscle proteins and includes sarcomeric gene mutations, mitochondrial gene mutations, neuromuscular disorders (such as Duchenne muscular dystrophy), and laminopathies. Secondary DCM is further classified into inflammatory (myocarditis), toxin-induced, metabolic (including lysosomal and glycogen storage disorders), nutritional, arrhythmias (tachycardiomyopathy), and structural heart disease.

The underlying etiology varies with age. The structural heart diseases and tachyarrhythmias associated with LV dysfunction present in infancy or early childhood. The primary DCM are likely to present in older children or in adolescence. An accurate etiology is not identified in 50% of the children with DCM and a vast majority are labeled as myocarditis. Viral myocarditis remains the most common cause of DCM[6] in children but with improvement in our understanding of genetic causes of DCM and increased access to next-generation genetic sequencing techniques, it is possible that a number of children wrongly labeled as viral myocarditis would be identified to have a genetic condition. It is hence imperative to obtain a detailed family history in every child diagnosed to have DCM.

It is important to recognize rare but potentially reversible causes of DCM caused by nutritional deficiencies.[5] Children with a severe form of protein energy malnutrition have been known to either present with heart failure or develop heart failure on institution of treatment. Although Kwashiorkor is now becoming uncommon due to improvements in infant and young child-feeding programs implemented on a nationwide scale, LV dysfunction can occur in the setting of micronutrient deficiency, particularly thiamine and selenium. Cultural feeding practices in certain parts of our countries have been shown to result in thiamine deficiency in breastfeeding infants[7] and it is hence important to pay attention to the dietary and cultural factors while obtaining clinical history.

TABLE 2: Ross classification of heart failure in infants.

Class I	Asymptomatic with no feeding difficulty and normal weight gain
Class II	Fast breathing and forehead sweating on feeding, normal feeding time and normal or marginally sub-optimal weight gain
Class III	Marked symptoms while feeding, prolonged feeding time and poor weight gain
Class IV	Fast breathing, sweating and grunting even when at rest

Clinical Features and Evaluation

The clinical presentation varies depending on the age of the child. In infants, the presentation is similar to other structural heart diseases. They present with feeding difficulty characterized by fast breathing, suck–rest–suck cycle, and forehead sweating. It is not unusual for the symptoms to be mistaken for a respiratory infection. This results in an inordinate delay in appropriate medical care. In acute conditions, the baby's weight is usually preserved, and this further misguides the pediatrician from a cardiac cause.

The clinical picture in children varies depending on the duration of illness. In acute conditions such as myocarditis, the presentation is more dramatic. Children present with acute-onset breathing difficulty, poor or no oral intake, altered sensorium, and cold clammy peripheries. There is often a history of preceding viral-like illness. Children with a more chronic etiology would have developed compensatory mechanisms. They hence present with controlled heart failure. The complaints in such cases include effort intolerance, inability to complete tasks performed comfortably in the past, excessive fatigue after returning from school, refusal to participate in physical activities, loss of appetite, and stunted growth.

The severity of symptoms is classified based on the New York Heart Association (NYHA) grading. In neonates and infants, the Ross modification of the NYHA grading is used (**Table 2**).

On clinical examination, all children with DCM irrespective of the cause have inappropriate tachycardia and tachypnea. Signs of poor peripheral perfusion include cold peripheries, thready pulses, hepatomegaly, and an increased capillary refill time. Their presence suggests a more severe circulatory compromise and children must be managed according to standard pediatric emergency management guidelines for a sick child.

Cardiovascular examination will show a displaced apical impulse denoting cardiomegaly. There may be increased precordial activity. A gallop rhythm is frequently heard on auscultation and the presence of a murmur may provide clues toward a structural heart disease.

When access to pediatric cardiac services is not readily available, a chest X-ray and electrocardiogram (ECG) should be obtained in all children with suspected DCM. There will be cardiomegaly on the chest X-ray (**Fig. 2**). The presence of pleural effusion should alert the pediatrician to a more severe cardiovascular compromise.

The ECG can be diagnostic in selected cases of DCM. The ECG changes are nonspecific in viral myocarditis. The most common ECG finding is sinus tachycardia with or without ST segment depression. However, a wide range of arrhythmias are known to occur in myocarditis including atrial tachycardia, junctional tachycardia, and rarely, ventricular arrhythmias. In a young infant with DCM, the presence of a deep q wave (**Fig. 3A**) in the anterolateral leads (Lead I, aVL, V5 and V6) is diagnostic of ALCAPA—a rare and potentially curable cause of DCM. The ECG also establishes the diagnosis in infants and children with tachycardia-induced cardiomyopathy (tachycardiomyopathy). Tachycardiomyopathies occur in the setting of incessant tachyarrhythmias where the tachyarrhythmia persists. The most common arrhythmias resulting in cardiomyopathy are ectopic atrial tachycardia (EAT) and permanent junctional reciprocating tachycardia (PJRT). In EAT, although every QRS axis is preceded by a P wave, the morphology of the P wave is different from a sinus rhythm with a change in axis (**Fig. 3B**). PJRT is a special type of reentrant tachyarrhythmia with a long R-P interval and a negative p wave in leads II, III, and aVF (**Fig. 3C**). The administration of adenosine helps differentiate these two types of tachyarrhythmias when the diagnosis is in doubt.

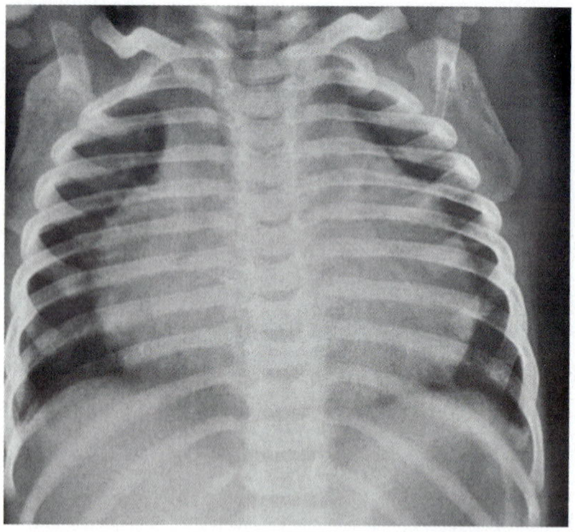

Fig. 2: Chest X-ray of a 1-year-old child with dilated cardiomyopathy and cardiomegaly.

The echocardiogram remains the most important investigation in the diagnosis of DCM. The severity of LV dysfunction is quantified based on the echocardiographic assessment of LV systolic function. The traditional mode of assessing LV function is based on quantification by motion mode ultrasound (M-mode) (**Fig. 4A**). This remains the common method of LV function quantification, although two-dimensional ultrasound quantification (**Figs. 4B and C**) is considered superior and is recommended. Newer modalities of LV function assessment like three-dimensional functional quantification (**Fig. 5**) and speckle-tracking echocardiography provide information about regional LV contractility and could provide important prognostic

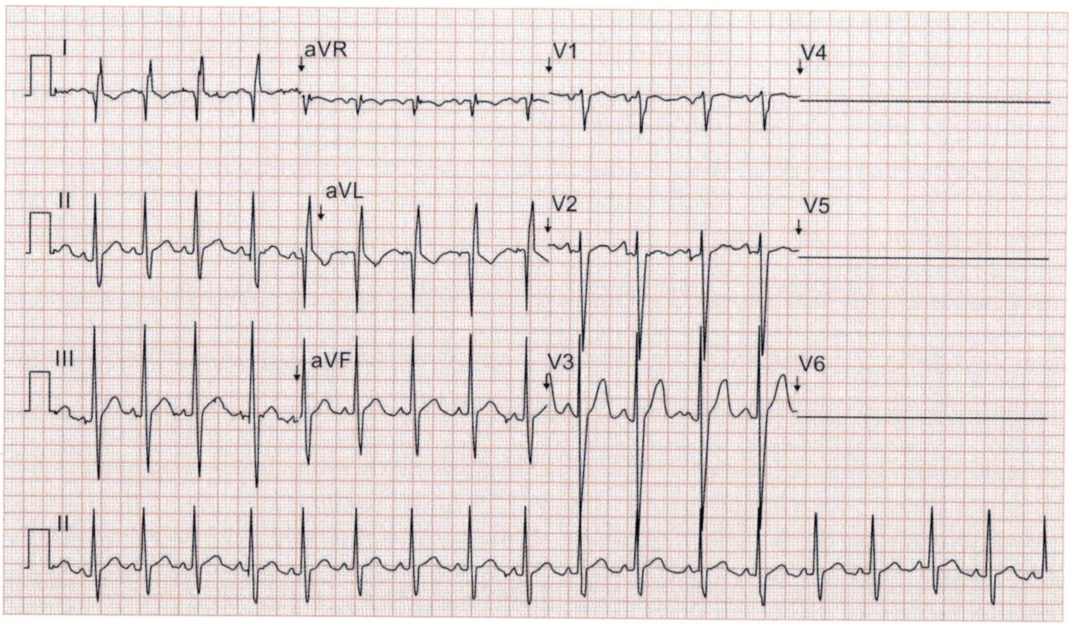

Fig. 3A: A standardized electrocardiogram (ECG) of a 3-month-old infant with anomalous left coronary artery from pulmonary artery in sinus rhythm showing deep Q waves in leads I and aVL.

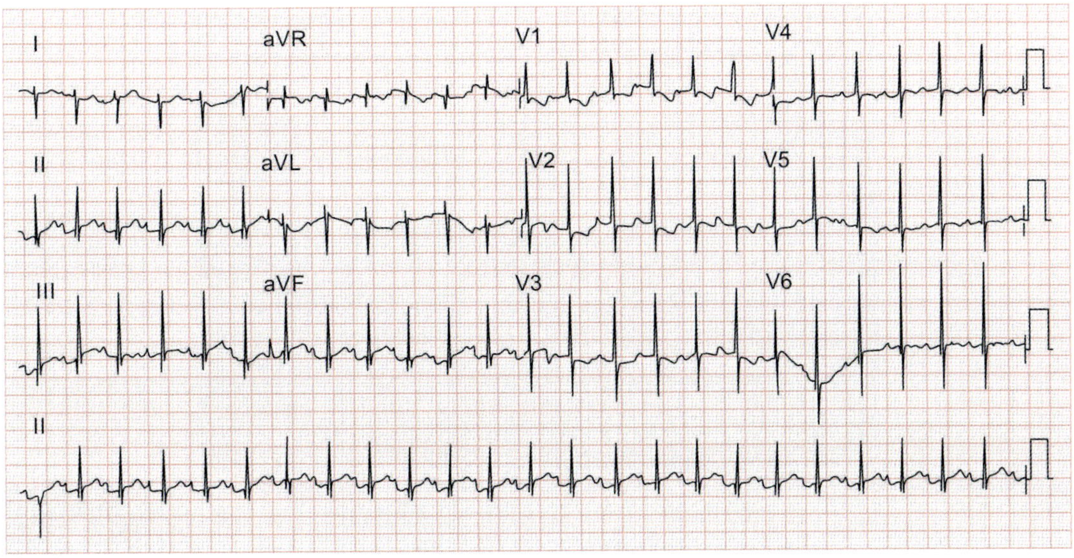

Fig. 3B: Standardized electrocardiogram (ECG) of an infant with tachyarrhythmia and ventricular dysfunction. The p wave is negative in aVL and positive in aVR suggesting an ectopic atrial rhythm.

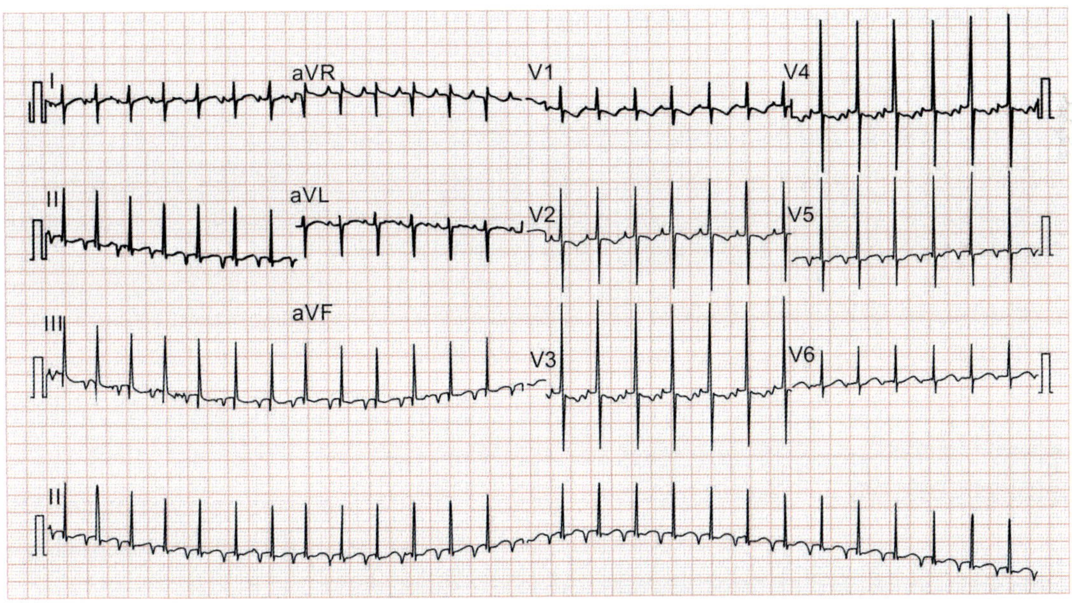

Fig. 3C: Standardized 12-lead ECG of a neonate with tachyarrhythmia and ventricular dysfunction. The p wave is negative in leads II, III and aVF suggesting permanent junctional reciprocation tachycardia (PJRT).

information for the cardiologist not available from traditional modalities of function assessment.[8] Structural heart diseases resulting in LV dysfunction can also be diagnosed by echocardiogram. ALCAPA should be suspected in every young infant with DCM and careful echocardiographic evaluation of the coronary artery origin performed (**Fig. 6**). The other structural heart diseases, which could result in LV dysfunction in young infants, include severe aortic stenosis (**Figs. 7A and B**) and coarctation of aorta.

The low cardiac output as a result of poor LV function results in hypoperfusion of all organ systems. It is hence important to obtain investigations to identify end-organ injury in all children with DCM. This includes liver function test, renal function evaluation as well as blood lactate levels to identify anaerobic metabolism. In selected cases, the blood levels of N-terminal B-type natriuretic peptide (NT pro-BNP) provide information about the severity and the long-term prognosis. BNP levels >4,500 pg/mL have been linked with poor clinical outcomes.[9]

An inborn error of metabolism should be suspected in children with DCM born out of a consanguineous marriage and in those with unexplained sibling deaths. When this is suspected, a quantitative blood and urine analysis of metabolites by tandem mass spectrometry (TMS) and gas chromatography-mass spectrometry (GC-MS) should be obtained. The traditional qualitative screening methods

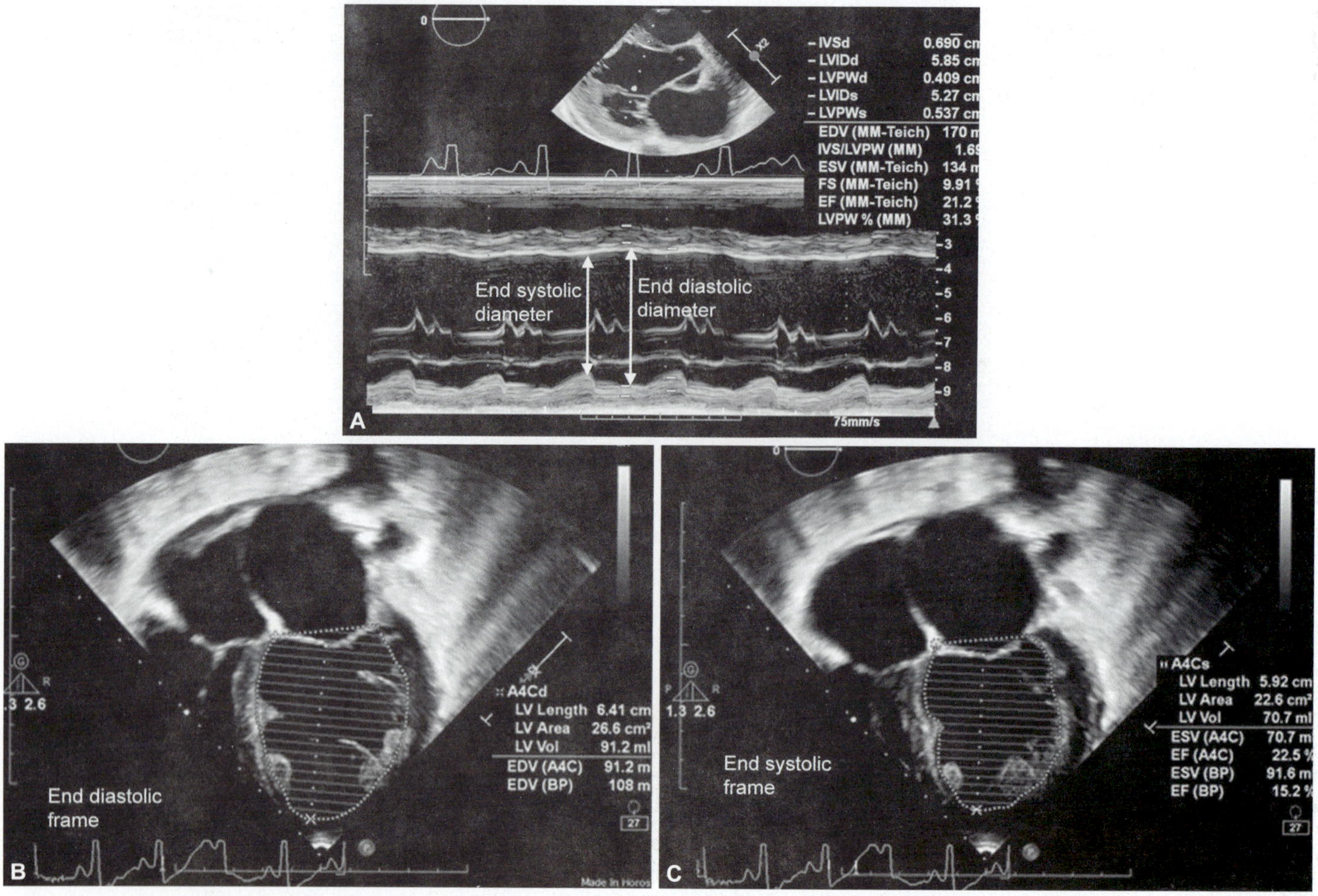

Figs. 4A to C: (A) M-mode echocardiography of a 5-year-old child with dilated cardiomyopathy depicting a dilated left ventricle with decreased systolic function. Assessment of left ventricle (LV) volumes in diastole (B) and systole (C) by two-dimensional echocardiography provides a more reliable assessment of LV function.

(EDV: end-diastolic volume; EF: ejection fraction; ESV: end-systolic volume)

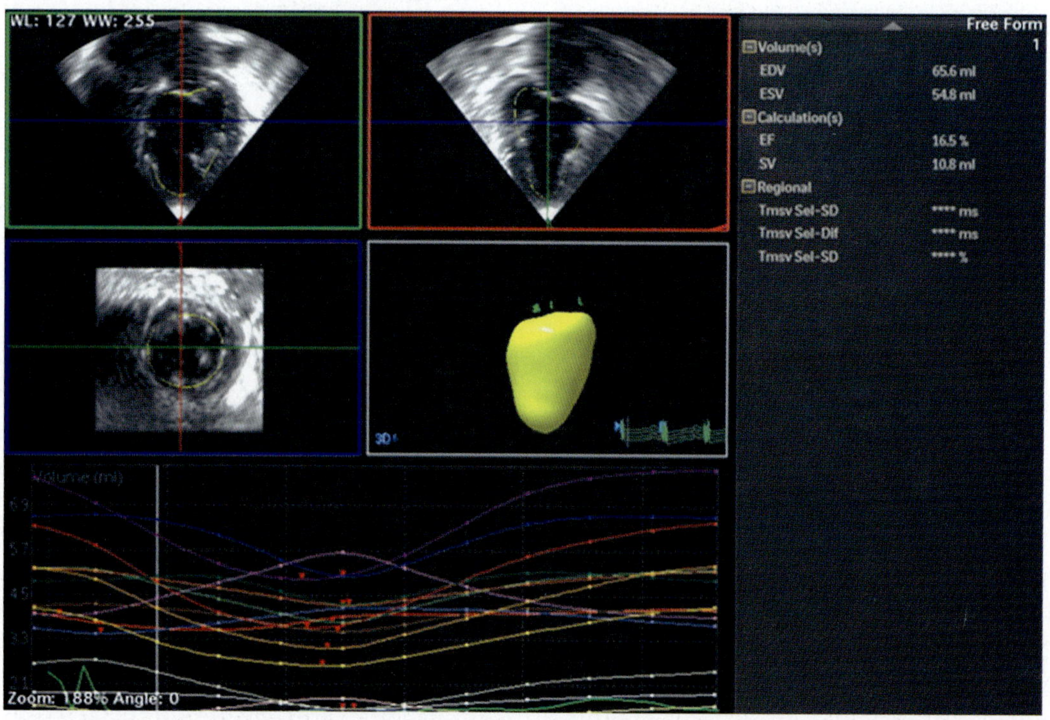

Fig. 5: Assessment of left ventricular function by three-dimensional echocardiography in the 5-year-old child with dilated cardiomyopathy (DCM) whose M-mode and two dimensional pictures are provided in Figure 4.

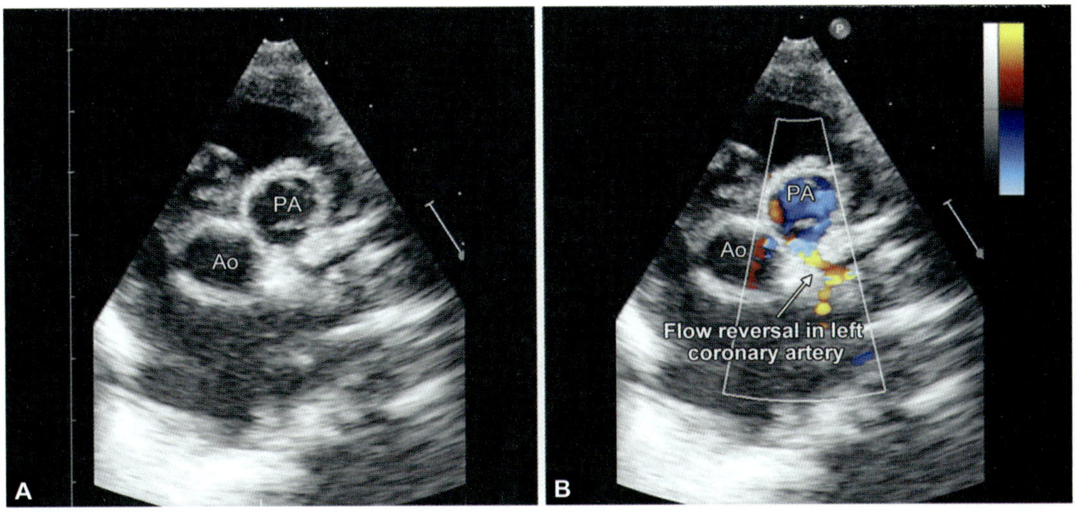

Figs. 6A and B: Simultaneous two-dimensional (A) and color Doppler echocardiography (B) of an infant with anomalous origin of the left coronary artery from the pulmonary artery (PA).
(Ao: aorta)

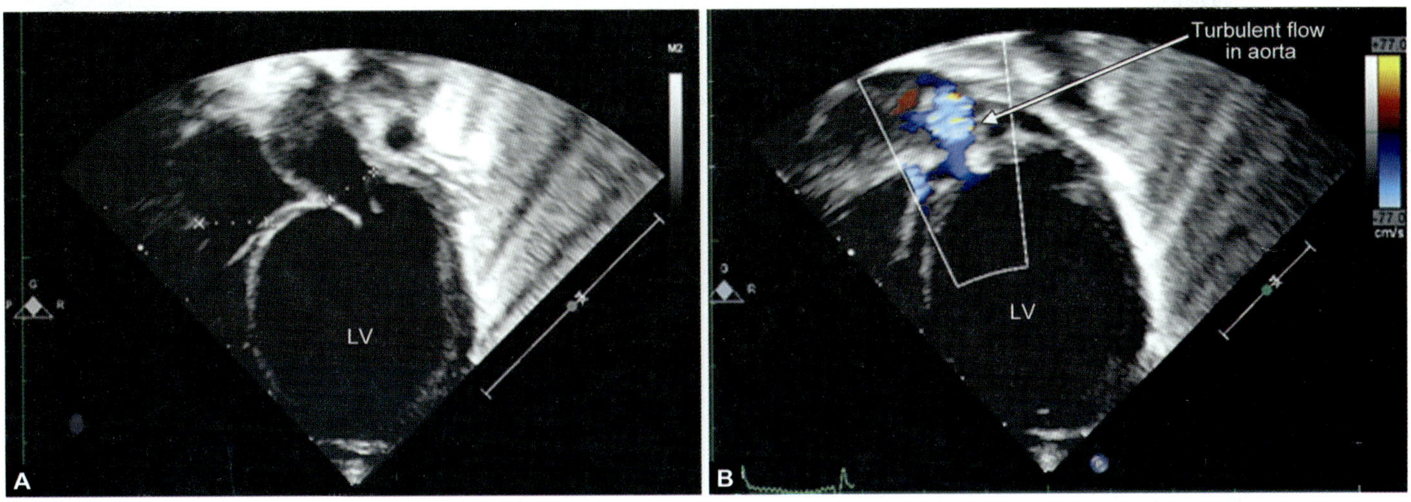

Figs. 7A and B: (A) Two-dimensional and (B) color Doppler of a neonate with severe left ventricular dysfunction and critical aortic stenosis.

lack sensitivity or specificity and provide no diagnostic information. They also have a very high false positive rate, which misleads the evaluation. These tests are best avoided in the current era.

When a primary or secondary genetic condition is suspected, genetic evaluation in consultation with a clinical geneticist should be offered as soon as the diagnosis is suspected. Genome-wide evaluation by massive parallel sequencing is more widely available at affordable costs in our country compared to the West. In addition to establishing an accurate diagnosis, genetic testing also provides an opportunity for cascade screening to identify relatives who might potentially be at risk for the disease. Interpretation of the results of genetic testing requires special expertise and this should be done in consultation with a clinical geneticist with experience in genetic cardiovascular diseases. Electronic connectivity has ensured that the expertise available in the West can be tapped remotely when not available locally.

Management

The management of secondary DCM involves treatment of the underlying cause. When structural heart diseases result in DCM, surgical or percutaneous interventions should be offered immediately. Timely detection and surgical repair of ALCAPA in a young infant result in normalization of LV function before the first birthday in a majority of cases. Severe aortic stenosis in a newborn can be relieved by balloon dilatation of the aortic valve (**Fig. 8**). Tachycardiomyopathies require specific antiarrhythmic pharmacological therapy to control the heart rate as well as to revert the abnormal rhythm. Correction of nutritional deficiencies results in a prompt improvement in LV function. In most cases, anti-failure therapy is required for a brief duration till the LV function recovers. The use of corticosteroids (prednisone) with angiotensin-converting enzyme (ACE) inhibitors has been shown to delay the progression of myocardial

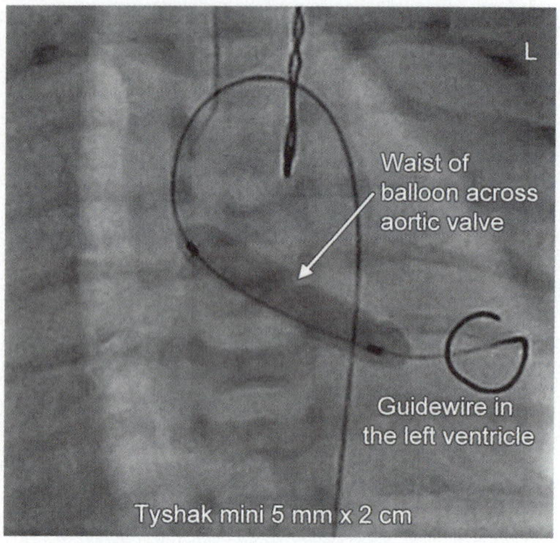

Fig. 8: A fluoroscopic image of balloon dilatation of the aortic valve in a newborn baby with severe aortic stenosis and left ventricular (LV) dysfunction.

dysfunction in children with muscular dystrophies. Children with underlying structural heart diseases which have been corrected by an intervention may not require long-term anti-failure management.

When no correctable secondary cause of DCM is identified, children will need to be managed depending on the severity of end-organ damage. When the baby or child presents with poor peripheral perfusion and tachypnea, it may be reasonable to provide ventilatory support by noninvasive ventilation or mechanical ventilation. A volume-controlled ventilation with low tidal volumes of 6–8 mL per kilogram is usually sufficient in these settings. The inotropes commonly used in DCM as well as their predominant mechanism of action is listed in **Table 3**. The use of intravenous immunoglobulin (IVIG) in children with presumed or proven myocarditis remains a subject of debate. Many pediatric cardiologists continue to prefer using IVIG despite the lack of robust evidence because of the lack of alternative effective therapies. A meta-analysis of available data showed no survival or recovery benefit with IVIG in children with myocarditis,[10] except in a small subset with a hyperacute clinical presentation.

Intensive care treatment will be required till peripheral perfusion improves and end-organ damage is reversed. Once this is achieved, children should be transitioned to oral anti-failure medications. The common anti-failure medications used in DCM are listed in **Table 4** and include a combination of diuretics (furosemide), afterload reduction agents (ACE inhibitors), cardiac remodeling agents (spironolactone), and agents to reduce heart rate (beta-blockers, carvedilol, and ivabradine). There are very few randomized controlled trials evaluating the efficacy of antifailure medications in children. Most of the medications used in clinical practice are based on the physiological action of the medication, anecdotal support of its use and the data available from large scale studies in adults with heart failure. Recently, a combination of angiotensin receptor and neprilysin inhibitor (sacubitril/valsartan) has been shown to be superior to conventional therapy with improved clinical outcomes in adults.[11] Early use in small-scale pediatric studies has been promising and the results of large-scale randomized controlled trials in varied ethnic groups are awaited.

TABLE 3: Inotropes used in the acute management of dilated cardiomyopathy.

Drug	*Dose*	*Mechanism of action*
Dobutamine	Adrenergic (β receptor) agonist	2.5–10 μg/kg/minute
Dopamine	Adrenergic and dopaminergic receptor agonist	2.5–10 μg/kg/minute
Milrinone	Phosphodiesterase inhibitor (inodilator)	0.3–0.7 μg/kg/minute
Levosimendan	Calcium sensitizer	12.5 μg/kg bolus followed by 0.1–0.2 μg/kg/minute
Adrenaline	Adrenergic agonist	0.04–0.2 μg/kg/minute

TABLE 4: Common anti-failure medications used in chronic treatment of pediatric dilated cardiomyopathy.

Agent	*Dose*
Decongestive therapy	
Furosemide (Lasix)	1 mg/kg/dose once to thrice daily depending on fluid overload
Anti-fibrotic therapy	
Spironolactone	1 mg/kg/dose once or twice daily
Cardiac re-modelling drugs	
Angiotensin converting enzyme inhibitors (ACEI)—enalapril	0.3–0.5 mg/kg/dose twice daily
Heart rate reduction agents	
Ivabradine	0.15–0.2 mg/kg/dose twice daily
Carvedilol	0.2–0.3 mg/kg/dose twice daily

Children who continue to worsen despite optimization of heart failure therapy will need to be considered for an orthotopic heart transplantation (OHT). OHT is not widely available in our country. The challenges facing OHT include the availability of donors of appropriate size, the very short cold ischemic time available to transplant the heart unlike other organs, and the high cost of the procedure as well as need for long-term immune-suppressive medications. Even in the West, many children listed for OHT deteriorate while on the waitlist. Such children may need support with a mechanical cardiac assist device such as the Berlin Heart. These devices are not widely available even in dedicated pediatric cardiac programs in our country.

It is important to provide attention to supportive care in addition to pharmacological therapy. This is usually done in consultation with the child's primary pediatrician. The nutrition of the child should be optimized with adequate calorie and protein intake and a balanced diet. Micronutrient supplementation should be provided in appropriate doses. Attention should be placed on ensuring immunization for all vaccine-preventable diseases. In addition to the vaccines recommended in the expanded immunization program, optional vaccines such as pneumococcal and yearly influenza vaccines should be administered after a detailed discussion with the parents about the likely benefits. During each clinic visit, the various growth parameters including weight, height, head circumference, and mid-arm circumference should be meticulously charted and children falling off the centile chart should be identified early and intervened.

Outcomes

The outcomes in pediatric DCM depend on the underlying cause.[6] Correctable causes of DCM, such as nutritional deficiencies, tachyarrhythmias, and structural heart diseases amenable to complete correction carry an excellent prognosis if identified and treated in a timely manner with a phased return of ventricular function to normal. Outcomes in children with genetic and metabolic conditions are usually disappointing despite early identification.

The outcomes in myocarditis and idiopathic DCM are variable. The age-old teaching of the rule of thirds with one-third showing complete recovery, 1/3rd partial recovery with controlled heart failure, and one-third progressing to end-stage heart failure resulting in death or heart transplantation still holds good based on recent data of long-term outcomes. There is no data available on long-term outcomes of pediatric heart transplantation in our country although short- and mid-term data is now emerging and appears promising.[12] The advantages of OHT will need to be balanced with the need for long-term immune-suppressive medications, structured follow-up including yearly catheterizations, and myocardial biopsies as well as need for a second transplantation at an older age.

HYPERTROPHIC CARDIOMYOPATHY

The AHA defines HCM as "a hypertrophied, nondilated ventricle (**Fig. 9**) in the absence of a hemodynamic cause."[5] The hemodynamic cause could include structural heart diseases such as aortic stenosis and coarctation of aorta as well as increased afterload, which can occur in the setting of systemic hypertension or aortoarteritis. In adults, a left ventricular septal thickness in diastole (IVSd) >15 mm is considered a definitive threshold and 13–15 mm considered probable disease. The diagnostic criteria for pediatric HCM based on Z scores have not been agreed upon but most authorities consider a septal thickness Z score of greater than +4 to indicate HCM.[5]

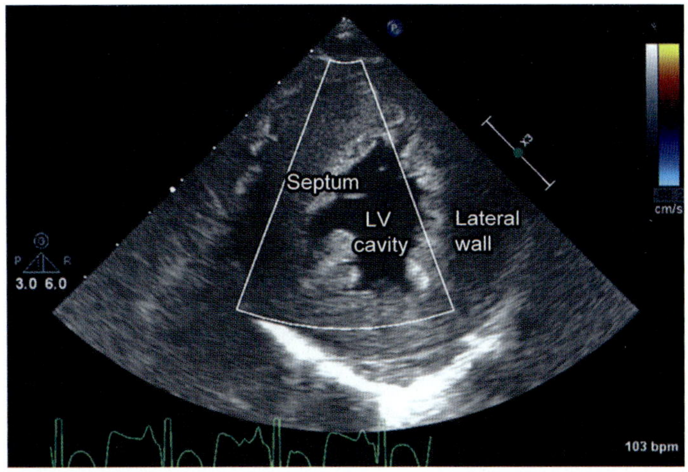

Fig. 9: Echocardiogram image in the parasternal view depicting a hypertrophied left ventricle (LV) with normal LV internal dimensions.

What is Different in Pediatric HCM?

In adults, a vast majority of HCM are related to mutations in the genes encoding for sarcomeric proteins. Of the sarcomeric proteins, the beta-myosin heavy chain (MYH7), myosin-binding protein C (MYBPC3), and cardiac troponin T (TnT) together account to >80% of the HCM cohort. However, the sarcomeric proteins constitute a minority in the pediatric age group. In >75% of children and 90% of infants with HCM, the etiology is not attributable to a sarcomeric gene mutation. The nomenclature of such non-sarcomeric HCM is debated. The AHA reserves the term HCM for hypertrophied hearts due to sarcomeric gene mutations while using the term HCM phenocopies for HCM due to other genetic causes.[5] The European Society of Cardiology (ESC) makes no such differentiation and uses the term HCM for all causes of ventricular hypertrophy.

Epidemiology

There is no data available on pediatric HCM in our country. The estimated incidence of HCM in adults is 1 in 500 based on studies from different geographical locations. The only data on pediatric HCM are from the population-based registries in Australia, Finland, and parts of North America.[1,3,4] These suggest an incidence of 0.25–0.5/100,000 population in children with the highest incidence in the first year of life.

Etiology

Unlike DCM, the majority of HCM is related to an underlying genetic condition. Recent registry-based reports have identified a genetic cause in 80% of pediatric HCM.[13] Recent improvements in massive parallel sequencing (next-generation sequencing or NGS) of DNA and the wider availability of advanced genetic testing methodologies would mean that the numbers are only likely to increase.

TABLE 5: Causes of hypertrophic cardiomyopathy in children.

Primary hypertrophic cardiomyopathy	Sarcomeric gene mutations
Syndromic hypertrophic cardiomyopathy	• Noonan syndrome • Noonan syndrome with multiple lentigines • Costello syndrome • Beckwith-Weifmann syndrome
Glycogen storage disorders	• Pompe disease • Danon disease • PRKAG2 mutations
Lysosomal storage disorders	• Mucopolysaccharidoses • Fabry disease
Other inborn errors of metabolism	• Fatty acid oxidation disorders • Mitochondrial disorders
Endocrine disorders	• Infant of diabetic mother • Acromegaly

The ESC classifies pediatric HCM into genetic and nongenetic/nonfamilial variants.[14] The genetic causes of HCM can be classified into four broad categories. These include:

1. Sarcomeric
2. Metabolic
3. Syndromic
4. Neuromuscular.

The individual causes in each subset are listed in **Table 5**. The sarcomeric mutations involved in pediatric HCM are the same as those described in the adult population. Among the syndromic causes of HCM, Noonan syndrome is the most common. Noonan syndrome was attributed to mutations only in the *PTPN1* gene. However, improvement in our understanding of molecular genetics as well as genotype-phenotype correlations has resulted in the identification of 12 different genes involved in the RAS-kinase pathway in which mutations can result in a Noonan's type phenotype.[15] The appropriate terminology for this subgroup is rasopathies.

Morphology

The striking morphological feature in HCM is the hypertrophy of the ventricles with increased ventricular mass. The involvement may be biventricular or restricted to the LV. Biventricular involvement is more common in nonsarcomeric genetic conditions. In these cases, LV involvement is usually circumferential. In contrast, sarcomeric HCM is usually limited to the LV with asymmetric septal hypertrophy. Asymmetric septal hypertrophy is also a hallmark in infants of diabetic mothers and is related to fetal hyperinsulinemia.

A subset of children with HCM may have features of left ventricular outflow tract (LVOT) obstruction. Earlier, this was believed to be a more severe form of disease and referred to as hypertrophic obstructive cardiomyopathy (HOCM). Our current understanding of the disease has enabled us to recognize that HOCM is not a separate pathological entity but only a morphological variant. Hence, the term HCM with an obstructive component is preferred. The obstruction is usually dynamic and is related to a Venturi effect pulling the anterior mitral leaflet toward the hypertrophied septum (termed systolic anterior motion or SAM).

Clinical Presentation and Evaluation

The clinical presentation of children with HCM varies with age. Infants with HCM often have severe disease and present with heart failure. The symptoms are indistinguishable from heart failure due to other causes. These include fast breathing, feeding difficulty, suck–rest–suck cycle and poor weight gain. The disease is often genetic and hence a previous sibling loss may alert the parents to present earlier for evaluation than would otherwise be the case.

Young children with HCM are often asymptomatic and present with an incidentally detected murmur or forceful apical impulse noted by an astute pediatrician. It is not uncommon in Western countries for children to be diagnosed with HCM after a parent or other first-degree relative is diagnosed with HCM, although this still remains unusual in our country.

Older children and adolescents with HCM present with heart failure or arrhythmias. Heart failure is related to diastolic dysfunction because of stiff, hypertrophied ventricles. Symptoms related to diastolic dysfunction include dyspnea on exertion, orthopnea, easy fatigability, and refusal to participate in physical activities. Arrhythmias related to HCM are generally ventricular in origin and more malignant. Syncope on exertion and sudden unexpected death are the common clinical presentations. HCM is the most common cause of sudden death in otherwise healthy young individuals worldwide. Rarely, older children may present with palpitation.

Clinical examination in infants reveals tachypnea, tachycardia, hepatomegaly, and crepitations. A murmur is unusual. In older children, a heaving type of apical impulse is often seen along with an ejection systolic murmur at the base of the heart. This is differentiated from valvar aortic stenosis by the absence of an ejection click.

The chest X-ray in infants usually has cardiomegaly with or without evidence of pulmonary venous congestion as well as hepatomegaly. The X-ray is often unremarkable in older children. The ECG may be diagnostic in some variants of HCM in children. The presence of a short P-R interval in a hypotonic infant with severe concentric left ventricular hypertrophy (LVH) is diagnostic of Pompe disease (**Fig. 10A**). A short P-R interval with evidence of ventricular pre-excitation is seen in two very specific glycogen storage disorders—Danon disease (caused by mutations in the *LAMP 2* gene) and mutations in the *PRKAG2* gene (**Fig. 10B**). Left axis deviation is noticeable in the ECG of children with some variants of Noonan syndrome (**Fig. 10C**). Conventional LVH

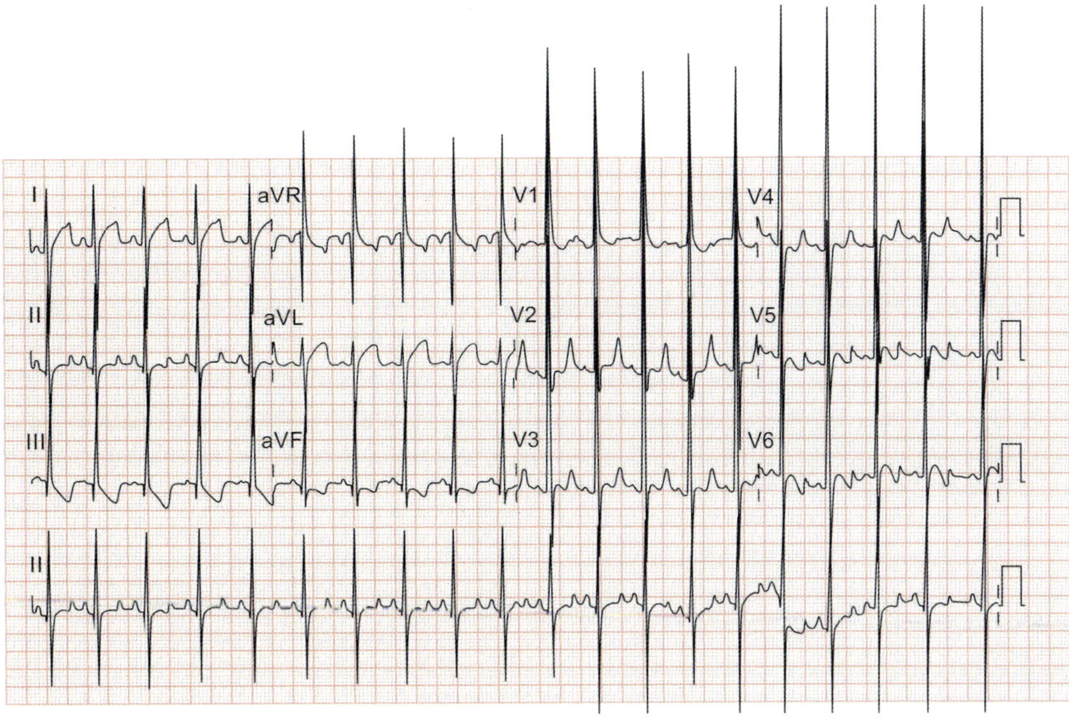

Fig. 10A: A 12-lead ECG of a neonate with Pompe disease demonstrating a short P-R interval and significant biventricular forces typical of the condition.

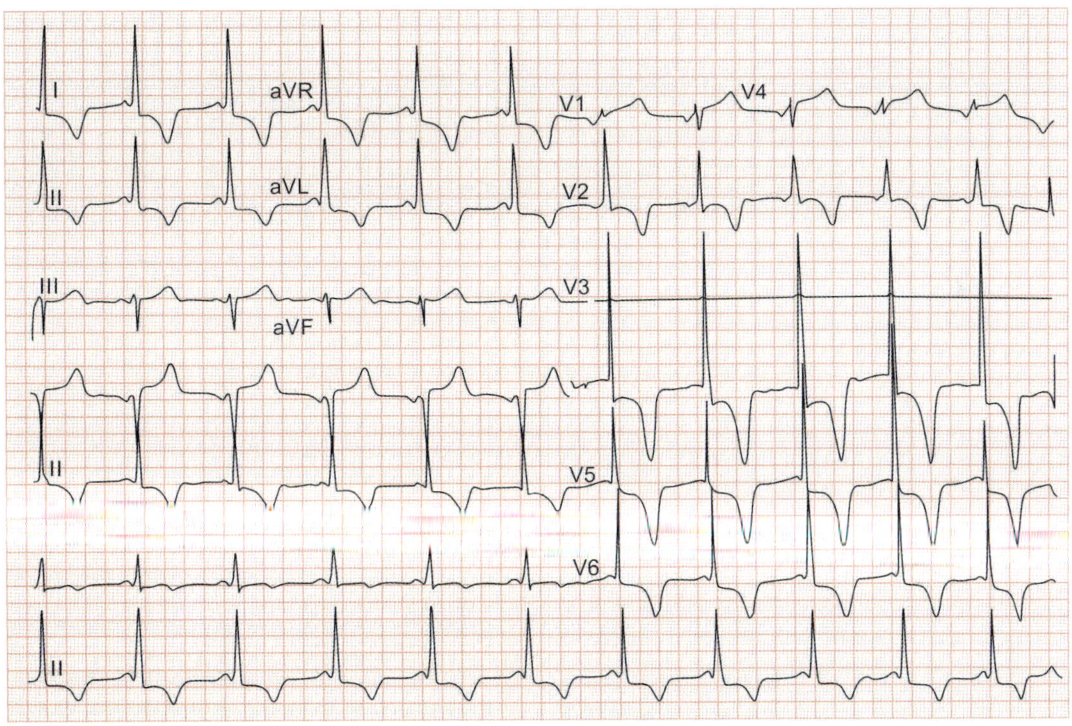

Fig. 10B: Electrocardiograph (ECG) of an 18-year-old boy with left ventricular hypertrophy (LVH). This shows LVH with a short P-R interval and relative bradycardia. The triad of short P-R interval, pre-excitation, and conduction abnormality is characteristic of PRKAG2 mutation.

voltage criteria have very poor specificity in older children who are thin and have compliant chest walls. The presence of an LV strain pattern is more useful in diagnosing severe LVH (**Fig. 10D**).

Echocardiogram is diagnostic in HCM. The echocardiographic calculation of septal wall thickness and LV mass is used to grade the severity of HCM. As mentioned earlier, children with sarcomeric HCM often have disproportionate septal involvement (**Fig. 11A**). Children with metabolic forms of HCM often have biventricular hypertrophy and circumferential LV involvement (**Fig. 11B**). This is often most striking in the infantile form of Pompe disease.

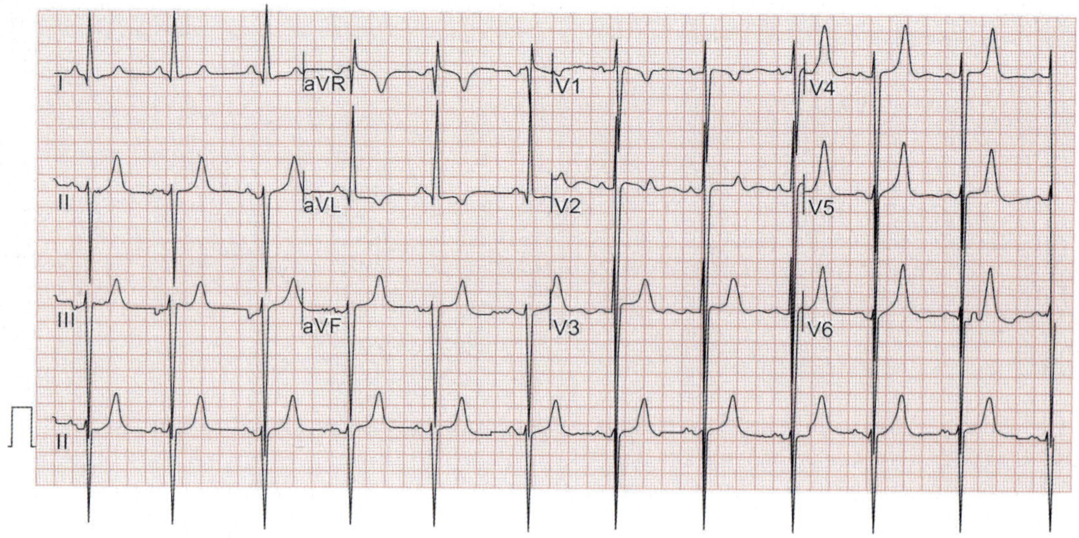

Fig. 10C: A 12-lead ECG of a 5-year-old child with left ventricular (LV) hypertrophy and dysmorphic features demonstrating left axis deviation typical of Noonan syndrome.

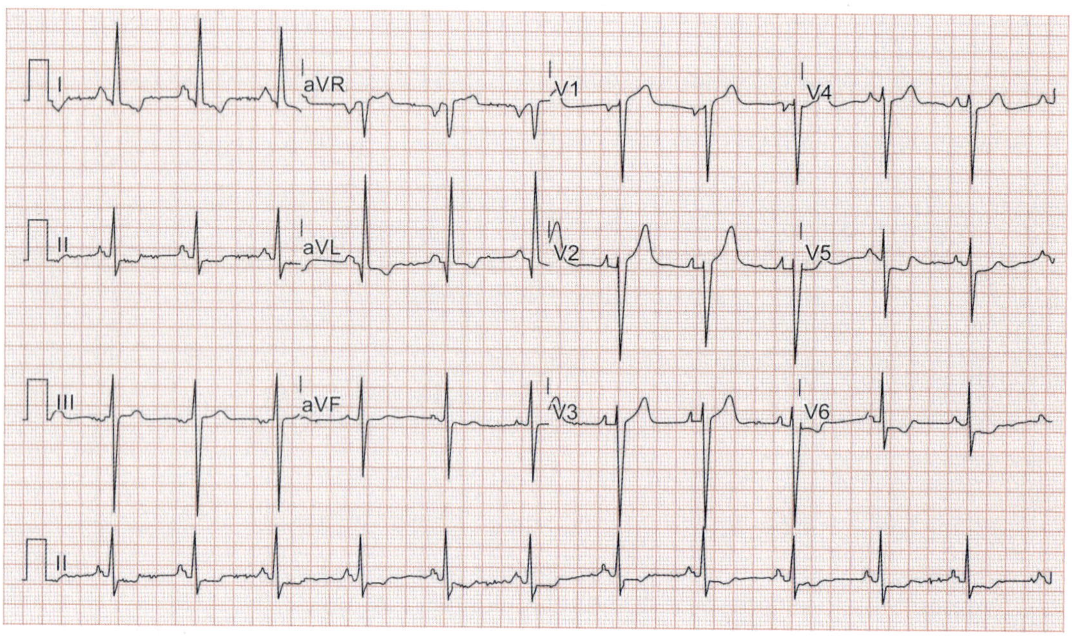

Fig. 10D: A 12-lead ECG of a 13-year-old with familial hypertrophic cardiomyopathy (HCM) demonstrating left ventricular hypertrophy (LVH) with ST-T changes in leads V5 and V6 suggestive of LV strain.

All children with HCM should undergo comprehensive evaluation of LV systolic and diastolic function by a pediatric cardiologist with expertise in cardiomyopathy evaluation. The LV is often hypercontractile in HCM; however, newer modalities of LV function evaluation such as speckle-tracking echocardiography can identify subclinical systolic dysfunction much earlier than conventional assessment. Echocardiography also helps identify LV outflow tract obstruction and the presence of SAM of the mitral valve.

Echocardiographic assessment of LVH is challenging in adolescents and those with high body mass index. Cardiologists are hence increasingly utilizing cardiac magnetic resonance (CMR) imaging in HCM assessment. In addition to the assessment of the LV thickness (**Fig. 12**), CMR helps detect subendocardial ischemia as well as myocardial fibrosis, which is not apparent on other imaging modalities.

Pediatric HCM is a genetic disease and genetic testing must be offered during the initial evaluation in all children with HCM. Given the heterogeneity of etiologies, a genome-wide assessment with or without mitochondrial sequencing should be preferred over specific HCM panels, which are often limited to sarcomeric genes and a few glycogen storage diseases which present in adults. This is best done in a specialized pediatric HCM clinic with cardiovascular genetic expertise. As in the case of DCM, expertise can be obtained remotely when not available locally.

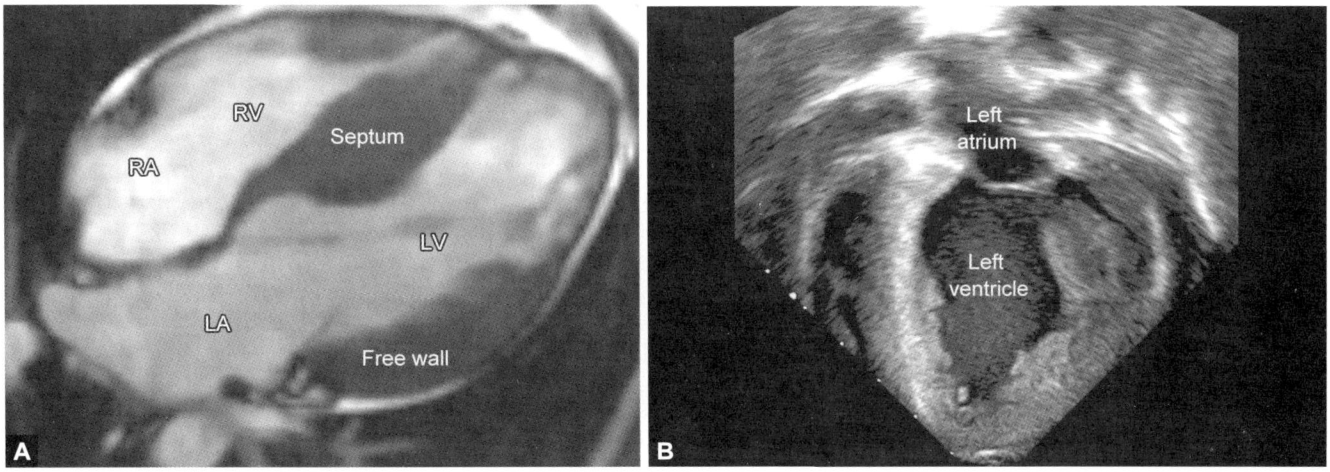

Figs. 11A and B: (A) Cardiac magnetic resonance (CMR) image of an adolescent with sarcomeric hypertrophic cardiomyopathy (HCM) with asymmetric septal involvement; (B) Echocardiographic image of a child with Pompe disease demonstrating severe concentric left ventricular hypertrophy.
(LA: left atrium; LV: left ventricle; RA: right atrium; RV: right ventricle)

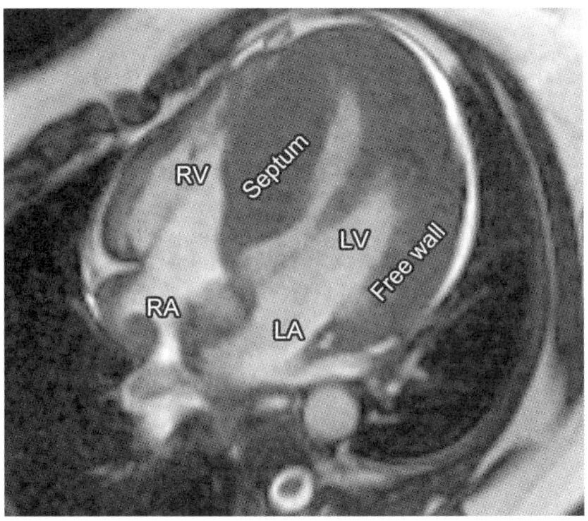

Fig. 12: Cardiac magnetic resonance (CMR) image in the apical four chamber of an adolescent with hypertrophic cardiomyopathy.
(LA: left atrium; LV: left ventricle; RA: right atrium; RV: right ventricle)

In children with Noonan syndrome, a detailed evaluation of hearing, vision, and growth in conjunction with a pediatrician should be performed.

Treatment

Pharmacological therapy in HCM is often disappointing. The drug group with the largest experience in pediatric HCM is beta-blockers. Nonselective beta blockade has been shown to be superior in HCM[16] with the best outcomes seen with propranolol and nadolol (not available currently in India). Beta-blockers are beneficial by multiple mechanisms. The heart rate reduction caused by beta-blockers is beneficial in children with LV diastolic dysfunction. Beta-blockers have been shown to reduce LV ejection acceleration ratio resulting in a drop in LVOT gradients in children who have an obstructive component. Beta-blockers also reduce myocardial oxygen consumption, which may be beneficial in HCM. Children with HCM often require high-dose beta-blocker therapy (>6 mg/kg/day of propranolol) and will require close monitoring for adverse effects of therapy. Other medications of potential benefit include disopyramide and verapamil.

Children with HCM and symptomatic LV outflow obstruction are often treated with beta-blockers and/or verapamil. When medical therapy prove insufficient, they often benefit from surgical septal myectomy, a surgical procedure where the excessive muscle in the LVOT is resected. The surgery when performed by a surgeon experienced with the procedure offers significant symptomatic relief but expertise in this surgery is often lacking because of the small pediatric subset of obstructive HCM. Additional therapies such as pacemaker insertion and alcohol septal ablation have only been reported anecdotally in children and should be reserved for special circumstances.

Beta-blockers remain the drug of choice for children with HCM and arrhythmias but are frequently insufficient. Most children with arrhythmias are at high risk for sudden death and will need insertion of an implantable cardioverter defibrillator (ICD). An electrophysiological study with radiofrequency ablation can be offered in selected children with arrhythmias.

Specific therapy is available for few genetic subsets of HCM. Enzyme replacement therapy in Pompe disease when initiated early in the disease course can reverse cardiac hypertrophy. Sirolimus has been shown to be effective in a certain form of rasopathy associated with multiple lentigines (referred to as LEOPARD syndrome).[17] With improvements in our understanding of the molecular mechanisms leading to LVH, individualized treatment should be possible in the future.

Prognosis

The prognosis in children with HCM depends on the underlying cause and the age at presentation.[18,19] An analysis of death in pediatric HCM reveals a very large peak in infancy and a smaller one in the teenage group. Infants with HCM often have severe disease and high mortality. The outcomes in HCM due to metabolic causes is invariably poor with >50% dying within 5 years of diagnosis. In contrast, those with neuromuscular disorders have a close to 100% 5-year survival. Adolescents and older children with HCM have a stable disease course with a death rate of 1 per 100 patient years. Risk factors for death include those with symptomatic heart failure and LV systolic dysfunction.[18]

RESTRICTIVE CARDIOMYOPATHY

Restrictive cardiomyopathy is a disease characterized by noncompliant ventricles with poor relaxation.[5] The ventricles have normal dimensions and systolic function but severe diastolic dysfunction. Biatrial dilatation and pulmonary arterial hypertension are present in almost all cases of RCM. RCM in the pediatric age group is almost always due to mutations in the sarcomeric or *desmin* genes. Rarely, it can be associated with lysosomal storage disorders, infiltrative disorders, or toxins. The causes of pediatric RCM are listed in **Table 6**.

The pathology of RCM is abnormal relaxation of the ventricles. This results in elevated filling pressure of both the ventricles. The atria hence need to pump blood into the ventricles actively as passive filling is limited. This results in distension of the atria and thinning of the atrial walls. The increased left atrial pressure results in pulmonary venous hypertension and reflex pulmonary arterial hypertension. The atrioventricular (AV) valves are usually normal in RCM. However, with disease progression, some degree of AV valve regurgitation is often present.

The clinical presentation of RCM is heart failure. The symptoms cannot be differentiated from heart failure of other causes. There is often biventricular failure with peripheral edema, abdominal distension, and painful hepatomegaly in addition to features of left heart failure. Other rare clinical presentations include syncope, thromboembolism, and sudden death. The ECG in RCM shows biatrial enlargement (**Fig. 13**). There may be AV conduction abnormalities in RCM due to infiltrative disorders.

Echocardiography is diagnostic in most cases of RCM. The echo is characterized by marked biatrial enlargement and diastolic dysfunction. The most useful echocardiographic indicator of diastolic dysfunction is tissue Doppler imaging of the medial and lateral annulus with very low "e" velocity indicating poor relaxation (**Fig. 14**). Echocardiographic differentiation from constrictive pericarditis may be challenging at times and may require additional imaging to document a thickened pericardium such as computed tomography (CT). The levels of serum NT pro-BNP are elevated in RCM but often normal in constrictive pericarditis. CMR may be useful to recognize myocardial fibrosis as well as infiltration.

TABLE 6: Causes of restrictive cardiomyopathy in children.

Primary restrictive cardiomyopathy—Genetic
Secondary restrictive cardiomyopathy
Lysosomal storage disorders
Iron overload due to hemolytic anemia treatment
Infiltrative disorders—Amyloidosis
Endomyocardial fibrosis

Drug therapy in RCM is seldom useful. Beta-blockers reduce heart rate and allow increased time for diastolic filling and are used invariably in all children with RCM. With progression of heart failure, most children with RCM will require heart transplantation.[20]

OTHER FORMS OF CARDIOMYOPATHY

Other rare forms of cardiomyopathy in children include LVNC and arrhythmogenic right ventricular cardiomyopathy (ARVC).

Left ventricular noncompaction cardiomyopathy is characterized by increased trabeculations in the LV (**Fig. 15**) with or without LV systolic dysfunction. LVNC is thought to be due to an embryonic arrest in maturation of the myocardium. Some authorities have doubted that LVNC is a separate disease entity but only a phenotype related to abnormal myocardial response.[21] The only well-documented variant of LVNC is due to Barth syndrome caused by mutation if the *Tafazzin* gene in the X chromosome. This is an X-linked recessive disorder characterized by LV dysfunction, neutropenia, and skeletal muscle involvement. The disease is malignant often resulting in death during infancy.[22]

Arrhythmogenic right ventricular cardiomyopathy is a genetic disease involving the right ventricle (RV). The disease is characterized by fibrofatty infiltration of the RV myocardium. Mutations in seven desmosome genes have

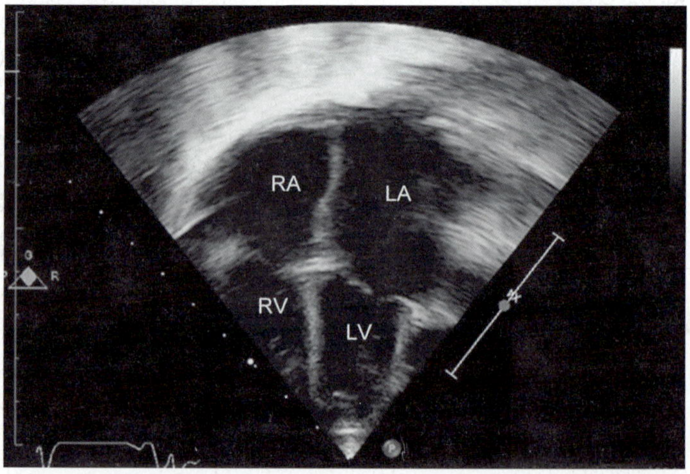

Fig. 13: Echocardiogram in the apical four-chamber view of a 5-month-old with restrictive cardiomyopathy showing significant dilatation of both the atria with normal ventricular dimensions.
(LA: left atrium; LV: left ventricle; RA: right atrium; RV: right ventricle)

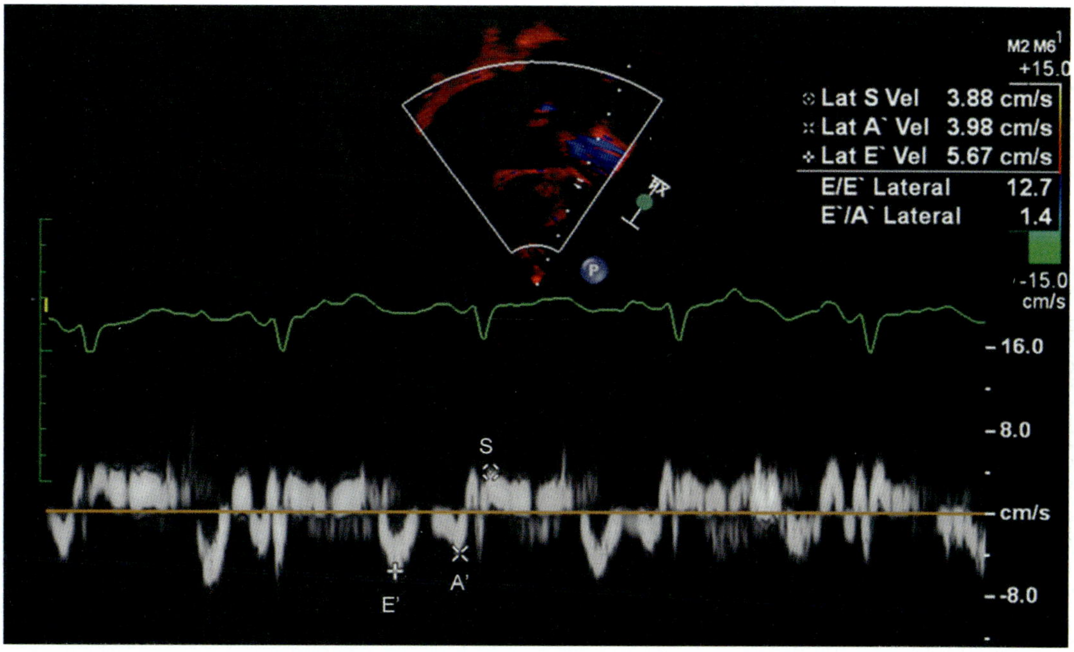

Fig. 14: Tissue Doppler imaging of the same infant in Figure 13 showing very low displacement of the lateral mitral annulus characteristic of restrictive cardiomyopathy.

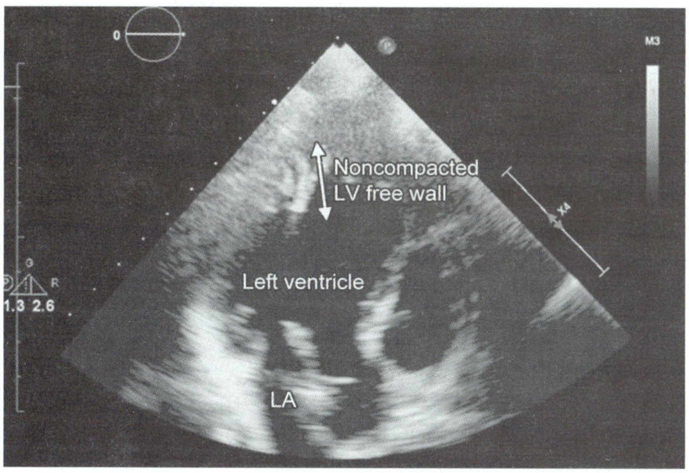

Fig. 15: Echocardiogram in the apical three-chamber view of a 5-year-old with heart failure. The apex of the left ventricle (LV) is hypertrabeculated. The child had familial left ventricular noncompaction cardiomyopathy (LVNC) due to an MYH7 mutation.

been linked to ARVC.[23] The disease is characterized by heart failure, ventricular arrhythmias, and sudden death. CMR is diagnostic and most children will require restriction of physical activities as well as implantation of an ICD.

REFERENCES

1. Lipshultz SE, Sleeper LA, Towbin JA, Lowe AM, Orav EJ, Cox GF, et al. The incidence of pediatric cardiomyopathy in two regions of the United States. N Engl J Med. 2003;348(17):1647-55.
2. Report of the WHO/ISFC task force on the definition and classification of cardiomyopathies. Br Heart J. 1980;44(6):672-3.
3. Arola A, Jokinen E, Ruuskanen O, Saraste M, Pesonen E, Kuusela AL, et al. Epidemiology of idiopathic cardiomyopathies in children and adolescents: a nationwide study in Finland. Am J Epidemiol. 1997;146(5):385-93.
4. Nugent AW, Daubeney PEF, Chondros P, Carlin JB, Cheung M, Wilkinson LC, et al. The epidemiology of childhood cardiomyopathy in Australia. N Engl J Med. 2003;348(17): 1639-46.
5. Lipshultz SE, Law YM, Asante-Korang A, Austin ED, Dipchand AI, Everitt MD, et al., on behalf of the American Heart Association Council on cardiovascular disease in the Young; Council on Clinical Cardiology; and Council on Genomic and Precision medicine. Cardiomyopathy in children: classification and diagnosis: a scientific statement from the American Heart Association. Circulation. 2019;140(1):e9-e68.
6. Towbin JA, Lowe AM, Colan SD, Sleeper LA, Orav EJ, Clunie S, et al. Incidence, causes and outcomes of dilated cardiomyopathy in children. JAMA. 2006;296(15):1867-76.
7. Sastry UMK, Jayranganath M, Kumar RK, Ghosh S, Bharath AP, Subramanian A, et al. Thiamine-responsive acute severe pulmonary hypertension in exclusively breastfeeding infants: a prospective observational study. Arch Dis Child. 2020;online ahead of print.
8. Balasubramanian S, Punn R, Smith SN, Houle H, Tacy TA. Left ventricular systolic myocardial deformation: a comparison of two- and three- dimensional echocardiography in children. J Am Soc Echocardiogr. 2017;30(10): 974-83.
9. Tigen K, Karaahmet T, Kahveci G, Tanalp AC, Bitigen A, Fotbolcu H, et al. N-terminal pro brain natriuretic peptide to predict prognosis in dilated cardiomyopathy with sinus rhythm. Heart Lung Circ. 2007;16(4): 290-4.
10. Yen C, Hung M, Wong Y, Chang CY, Lai CC, Wu KG. Role of intravenous immunoglobulin therapy in the survival of pediatric patients with acute myocarditis: a systematic review and meta-analysis. Sc Rep. 2019;9(1):10459.
11. Bohm M, Young R, Jhund PS, Solomon SD, Gong J, Lefkowitz MP, et al. Systolic blood pressure, cardiovascular outcomes and efficacy and safety of sacubitril/valsartan in patients with chronic heart failure and reduced ejection fraction: results from PARADIGM-HF. Eur Heart J. 2017;38(15):1132-43.
12. Garekar S, Meeran T, Patel V, Patil S, Dhake S, Mali S, et al. Early experience with pediatric cardiac transplantation in a limited resource setting. Ann Pediatr Cardiol. 2020;13(3):220-6.

13. Rupp S, Felimban M, Schanzer A, Schranz D, Marschall C, Zenker M, et al. Genetic basis of hypertrophic cardiomyopathy in children. Clin Res Cardiol. 2019;108(3):282-9.
14. Elliott P, Andersson B, Arbustini E, Bilinska Z, Cecch F, Charron P, et al. Classifications of the cardiomyopathies: a position statement from the European Society of Cardiology working group on myocardial and pericardial diseases. Eur Heart J. 2008;29(2): 270-6.
15. Carcavilla A, Suarez-Ortega L, Sanchez AR, Gonzalez-Casado I, Ramón-Krauel M, Labarta JI, et al. Noonan syndrome: genetic and clinical update and treatment options. Ann Pediatr (Barc). 2020;93(1):61.e1-61.e14.
16. Ostman-Smith I. Beta-blockers in pediatric hypertrophic cardiomyopathies. Rev Recent Clin Trials. 2014;9(2):82-5.
17. Marin TM, Keith K, Davies B, Conner DA, Guha P, Kalaitzidis D, et al. Rapamycin reverses hypertrophic cardiomyopathy in a mouse model of LEOPARD syndrome-associated with PTPN11 mutation. J Clin Invest. 2011;121(3): 1026-43.
18. Colan SD, Lipshultz SE, Lowe AM, Sleeper LA, Messere J, Cox GF, et al. Epidemiology and cause-specific outcome of hypertrophic cardiomyopathy in children: findings from the Pediatric Cardiomyopathy Registry. Circulation. 2007;115(6):773-81.
19. Moak JP, Kaksi JP. Hypertrophic cardiomyopathy in children. Heart. 2012;98(14):1044-54.
20. Webber SA, Lipshultz SE, Sleeper LA, Lu M, Wilkinson JD, Addonizio LJ, et al., on behalf of the Pediatric Cardiomyopathy Registry investigators. Outcomes of restrictive cardiomyopathy in childhood and the influence of phenotype: a report from the Pediatric Cardiomyopathy Registry. Circulation. 2012;126(10): 1237-44.
21. Anderson RH, Jensen B, Mohun TJ, Petersen SE, Aung N, Zemrak F, et al. Key questions relating to left ventricular non compaction cardiomyopathy: is the emperor still wearing any clothes? Can J Cardiol. 2017;33(6):747-57.
22. Kang SL, Forsey J, Dudley D, Steward CG, Tsai-Goodman B. Clinical characteristics and outcomes of cardiomyopathy in Barth syndrome: the UK experience. Pediatr Cardiol. 2015;37(1):167-76.
23. Bauce B, Nava A, Beffagna G, Basso C, Lorenzon A, Smaniotto G, et al. Multiple mutations in desmosomal proteins encoding genes in arrhythmogenic right ventricular cardiomyopathy/dysplasia. Heart Rhythm. 2010;7(1): 22-9.

46

CHAPTER

Pericardial Diseases in Children

Sakshi Sachdeva, Saurabh Kumar Gupta

INTRODUCTION

The pericardium is a protective layer around the heart and plays an important role in cardiac physiology. The pericardium is afflicted in a variety of diseases, both localized to the heart and as part of systemic illnesses. Pericardial diseases cause distinctive hemodynamic changes and some of the classic physical findings in cardiology. Although clinical overlap is common among various pericardial diseases, most cases can be categorized as having pericarditis, pericardial effusion with or without tamponade, and pericardial constriction. Other structural abnormalities such as the congenital absence of pericardium and pericardial cysts are rare. This chapter provides an overview of common pericardial diseases in children.[1]

ANATOMY OF PERICARDIUM

The pericardium comprises two layers namely parietal and visceral pericardium. The parietal layer is the outer layer consisting of elastin and collagen fibers, while the visceral layer composed of mesothelial cells, elastin, and collagen is located close to the epicardial surface of the heart. Both layers are separated from each other by pericardial space, which contains a small amount of serous pericardial fluid. Pericardium surrounds the entire heart and the base of the great arteries. The posterior aspect of the left atrium, however, lies outside the pericardium.[2]

FUNCTION OF PERICARDIUM

Although not essential for survival, the pericardium has some important functions. It acts as a barrier to prevent the spread of infections, inflammation, and neoplasia. The pericardial fluid permits free movement of the heart throughout the cardiac cycle, limits its acute distension, and helps in ventricular coupling. It is the parietal layer that provides pericardium its characteristic physical properties with a nonlinear pressure–volume curve (**Fig. 1**). At a low level of stretch, the pericardium is elastic but as the stretch increases, it stiffens abruptly resulting in an acute increase in pericardial pressure.[1,3]

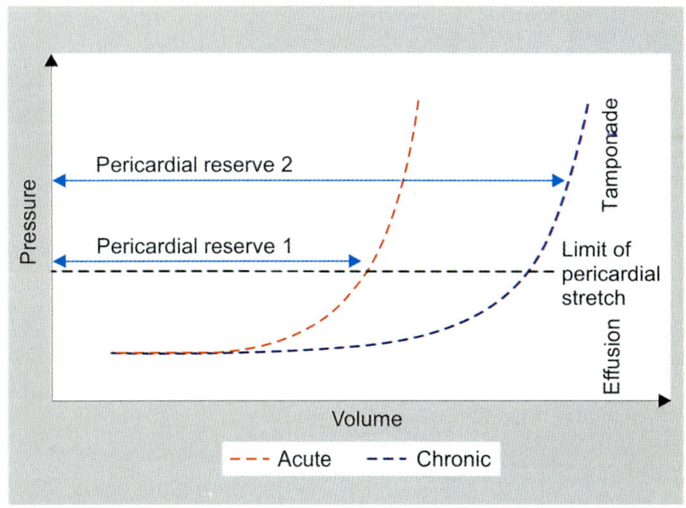

Fig. 1: Pressure volume curve of the pericardium.
(*Source*: Reproduced with permission from Gupta SK. Pericardial diseases in children. In: Wernovsky G, Anderson RH, Kumar K, Mussato KA, Redington A, Tweddell JS, Tretter J (Eds). Anderson's Pediatric Cardiology, 4th edition. Philadelphia: Elsevier; 2019. pp. 1063-75.)

PERICARDITIS

Pericarditis is the most common pericardial pathology encountered in clinical practice. It can be classified as acute, recurrent, or chronic, based on the duration of illness. Acute pericarditis is usually self-limiting, lasting [illegible] weeks. In some cases, the inflammation may continue up to 3 months, beyond which, it is labeled as chronic pericarditis.[4]

Acute Pericarditis

Acute pericarditis is an acute inflammation of the pericardium. The exact incidence of acute pericarditis in childhood is not known. Most cases are idiopathic or result from viral infections, although it is seen in other inflammatory and non-inflammatory conditions as well (**Table 1**). Older children and adolescents present with acute onset of sharp, substernal chest pain radiating to the trapezius ridge, which worsens with inspiration and on lying down and subsides with leaning forward. The pain in young children is variable, though postural and respiratory

TABLE 1: Common causes of pericarditis and pericardial effusion in children.

Infections	*Inflammatory*	*Iatrogenic*	*Miscellaneous*
Viral	Connective tissue disorders	Postcardiac intervention	Neoplasm
Bacterial	Post-pericadiotomy syndrome	Post-radiofrequency ablation	Radiation induced
Mycobacterial	Drug-induced		Trauma
HIV associated			Chronic renal failure
Fungal			Hypothyroidism

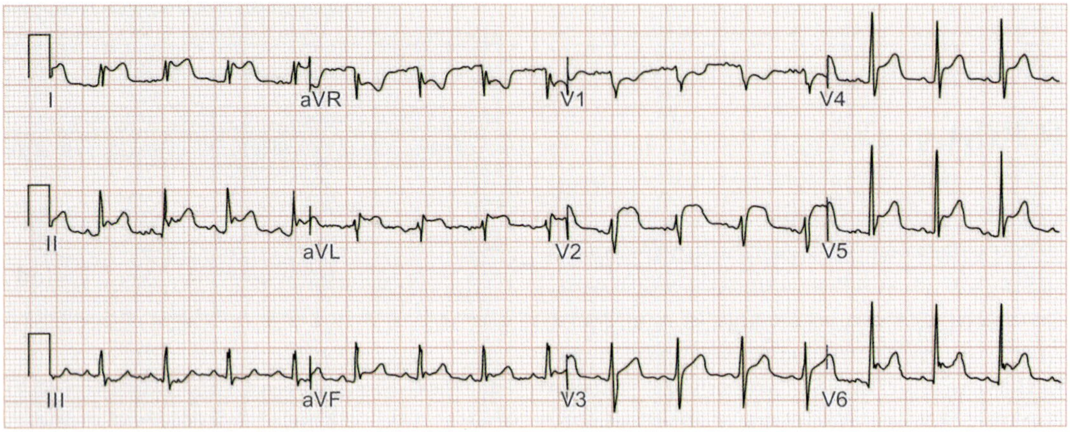

Fig. 2: A 12-lead electrocardiogram (ECG) from a patient with acute pericarditis showing coved up ST segment elevation in all the leads except leads V1 and aVR, which show ST depression. PR depression is seen in inferior leads. Lead aVR shows elevated PR segment.
(*Source*: Reproduced with permission from Gupta SK. Pericardial diseases in children. In: Wernovsky G, Anderson RH, Kumar K, Mussato KA, Redington A, Tweddell JS, Tretter J (Eds). Anderson's Pediatric Cardiology, 4th edition. Philadelphia: Elsevier; 2019. pp. 1063-75.)

variation is preserved. A pericardial friction rub is the most characteristic physical finding, which is a high-frequency, superficial scratching sound resulting from the friction between inflamed layers of the pericardium. The pericardial rub typically consists of three components corresponding to ventricular systole and early- and late-diastolic filling. It is best heard during inspiration, along the left sternal border, with the patient leaning forward. Frequent auscultation is required as the rub is often intermittent.[1] It disappears with the accumulation of significant pericardial fluid. Nonspecific symptoms and obvious difficulties in eliciting clinical signs make the diagnosis of acute pericarditis challenging in infants and young children.

Diagnostic Evaluation

Pericarditis should be suspected in children presenting with fever and characteristic chest pain. It should also be considered while investigating for fever of unknown origin.

Electrocardiogram

The electrocardiogram (ECG) is perhaps the most important diagnostic tool. It is useful in the diagnosis at an early stage of the disease. ECG shows sequential changes in ST and PR segments (**Fig. 2**). Based on ECG findings, four stages of acute pericarditis are described (**Table 2**), although each patient may not have this stage-wise transition.

TABLE 2: Sequential ECG changes according to the stage of pericarditis.

Stage of pericarditis	*ECG changes*
Stage 1	ST segment elevation, PR segment depression
Stage 2	ST segment normal, T wave flattening
Stage 3	T wave inversion
Stage 4	Normal ECG

In some patients, ST-segment changes are limited to only a few leads. Occasionally, PR-segment depression is the only ECG manifestation. The ECG may be completely normal in approximately 10% of patients with acute pericarditis. The ECG also sometimes provides clues toward the specific cause of acute pericarditis. For example, the presence of atrioventricular block may indicate Lyme disease, while low-voltage complexes and electrical alternans indicate significant pericardial effusion.

Chest Radiograph

The chest radiograph is essentially normal in an uncomplicated case of acute pericarditis. Cardiomegaly may be present if there is a significant amount of pericardial fluid.

Echocardiogram

The echocardiogram is done mainly to detect pericardial effusion. About two-thirds of patients with acute pericarditis

TABLE 3: Clinical diagnostic criteria for acute pericarditis.

Diagnosis made if any two of the following are present:
1. Pericarditic chest pain
2. Pericardial rub
3. New-onset ST-T changes on ECG
4. New-onset or worsening pericardial effusion
Besides, CRP, ESR, TLC count indicate the state of acute inflammation

have pericardial effusion. In the vast majority, the effusion is small and is of no concern. Large effusion is seen in about 3% of patients. New onset of left ventricular (LV) contractile dysfunction should alert the clinician to the possibility of myopericarditis.

Diagnostic Criteria

Clinical criteria for diagnosing pericarditis are given in **Table 3**. Elevated troponin and other markers of myocardial injury suggest concomitant myocarditis. Data from adults suggest that high-sensitivity C-reactive protein (hs-CRP) is elevated in three-fourths of patients with acute pericarditis and predict a higher rate of recurrence. In most cases, hs-CRP levels normalize within a week and in almost all cases by 4 weeks. The level of hs-CRP is useful in guiding the duration of therapy. Routine testing for detecting viral etiology is not recommended as the yield is low and it is not cost-effective.[4,5] A specific cause is identifiable in only 17% of patients and is more frequently found in cases having a subacute course with fever, large pericardial effusion, and poor response to nonsteroidal anti-inflammatory drugs (NSAIDs).

Treatment

Initial management should focus on screening for specific causes, prompt detection of pericardial effusion, and alleviation of symptoms. For symptomatic relief, the patient should receive NSAIDs. No studies have compared different NSAIDs for the treatment of acute pericarditis in children. Ibuprofen in a dose of 30–50 mg/kg per day in two to three divided doses is preferred considering its better side effect profile. Indomethacin, naproxen, and acetylsalicylic acid are other alternatives. Children with prompt response to NSAIDs and having mild pericardial effusion can be managed on an outpatient basis. Indications of hospitalization include children with severe symptoms, poor response to therapy, or those having large pericardial effusion.[1]

Patients with poor response to NSAIDs have traditionally been treated with corticosteroids. Their use, however, is associated with a higher rate of recurrence, particularly if steroid is used in a high dose for short duration. Therefore, a lower initial dose of 0.25–0.5 mg/kg/day of prednisolone with gradual tapering over 8–12 weeks is preferred. Colchicine is more effective than corticosteroids in reducing the risk of recurrences.[4,6] The recommended dose of colchicine is 0.5–1 mg/day for 3 months. These doses are generally well-tolerated. Gastrointestinal side effects result in withdrawal in approximately 10% of patients. Some authors recommend using both corticosteroid and colchicine in patients with poor response to NSAIDs. In such cases, NSAIDs are initially withheld and are resumed once corticosteroids are tapered.

Prognosis

Acute idiopathic pericarditis is usually self-limiting and complete resolution is expected within 2–3 weeks. Female gender, presence of large effusion, and failure of NSAIDs predict a higher risk of complications. In a large series of 453 adult patients with acute pericarditis, 3.1% developed cardiac tamponade and 1.5% developed pericardial constriction.[1]

Recurrent Pericarditis

Recurrent pericarditis is defined as the reappearance of pericardial inflammation after an initial attack of acute pericarditis with an asymptomatic period of 4 weeks or longer. While recurrent pericarditis is seen in 15–30% adults, it is uncommon among children. Symptoms are usually not as severe and findings of pericardial rub, ECG changes, and pericardial effusion are less frequent.

PERICARDIAL EFFUSION AND CARDIAC TAMPONADE

All causes of pericarditis can potentially result in pericardial effusion.[1,3,4,7] Pericardial effusions can be classified based on its onset (acute, subacute, or chronic), distribution (loculated or circumferential), composition (exudative, transudative, blood, or pus), and hemodynamic impact (none, cardiac tamponade, or effusive constrictive).

Pathophysiology

The hemodynamic consequences of pericardial effusion are determined by the amount of fluid and rapidity of accumulation. If there is a rapid accumulation of fluid, the pericardial pressure rises quickly. If the fluid accumulates gradually, during the initial phase, the intrapericardial pressure does not rise because of the compliant nature of pericardium. As a result, even large effusion may not have any compressive effect on cardiac chambers and consequently may remain asymptomatic.[3] But with continued accumulation, the stretching limit of the pericardium is reached and further accumulation of fluid tends to elevate the intrapericardial pressure. This nonlinear pressure–volume curve of pericardium results in an almost vertical rise in pericardial pressure after an initial slow ascent (*see* **Fig. 1**). This late steep rise in pressure is responsible for the rapid development of cardiac compression with additional accumulation of even a small amount of fluid. This is known as the "last drop" effect. This also explains the prompt improvement in the hemodynamic state with

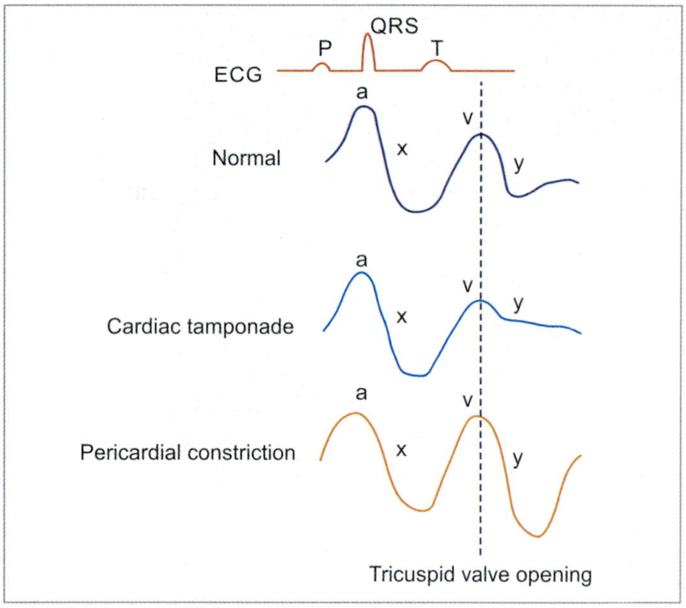

Fig. 3: The jugular venous pressure waveforms in normal state, in cardiac tamponade and pericardial constriction.
(ECG: electrocardiogram)

drainage of even a small amount of pericardial fluid in a child with cardiac tamponade.[1]

Cardiac tamponade, by limiting the space available for cardiac filling, presents with characteristic hemodynamic findings.[8] In the relatively fixed pericardial space, the cardiac chambers compete with the pericardial fluid, hence cardiac filling is impaired. The filling pressures in cardiac chambers are elevated and are equal to intrapericardial pressure. Due to fixed cardiac volume, the atria can fill only during ventricular systole when the blood exits the heart. These alterations in cardiac filling result in characteristic findings in jugular venous pulse and cardiac examination. The normal jugular venous waveform shows two descents, "x" descent during ventricular systole when atriums relax and "y" descent during early diastolic ventricular filling after the opening of the tricuspid valve. In patients with cardiac tamponade, elevated filling pressure limits early diastolic filling of the ventricles and manifests as a distinctive loss of "y" descent in jugular venous pressure (JVP) while "x" descent is preserved (**Fig. 3**).

Pericardial fluid allows normal transmission of thoracic pressure to cardiac chambers. As a result, during inspiration, the right ventricle is preferentially filled while constraints of fixed cardiac volume limit LV filling. The filling of the left and right ventricle, therefore, is 180° out of phase with each other and explains the exaggeration of ventricular interdependence. The LV systolic pressure falls when the systolic pressure in the right ventricle rises during inspiration and the reverse happens during expiration (ventricular discordance).[1]

Cardiac tamponade is not an "all-or-none" phenomenon. Instead, it represents a continuum from minimal hemodynamic impairment to a state of hemodynamic collapse.[8] Clinical examination is sufficient to recognize hemodynamic collapse but is inadequate in identifying milder hemodynamic compromise. Occasionally, cardiac tamponade may be regional, resulting from a localized clot or loculated effusion when typical physical, hemodynamic, and echocardiographic findings may be absent.

Clinical Presentation

The clinical presentation depends upon the speed of accumulation of pericardial fluid. In slowly accumulating pericardial effusion, the patient is often asymptomatic and effusion may be detected incidentally. Rapid accumulation of even small amounts of fluid, on the other hand, can cause symptoms. Initially, compensatory sympathetic stimulation causes tachycardia, diaphoresis, and peripheral vasoconstriction. With the progressive accumulation of fluid, compensatory mechanisms prove inadequate and cardiac output declines. Patients who are unable to mount a normal adrenergic response, such as those receiving β-blocking agents, are more susceptible to acute hemodynamic collapse.[1]

The JVP is markedly elevated with blunted "y" and preserved "x" descent. Unimpeded transmission of thoracic pressure to cardiac chambers and consequent preferential right ventricular filling during inspiration permits normal inspiratory fall in JVP (**Fig. 3**). Pulsus paradoxus, characterized by an abnormally large (>10 mm Hg) fall in blood pressure during inspiration, is another distinctive clinical feature. In reality, it only reflects exaggerated ventricular interdependence. Pulsus paradoxus is not unique to cardiac tamponade and may be present in pericardial constriction, pulmonary embolism, and other pulmonary diseases with wide respiratory variation in thoracic pressures.[9] Clinical recognition of pulsus paradoxus relies on respiratory variation in Korotkoff sounds. Unfortunately, this cannot be measured well by currently available oscillometric sphygmomanometers. As such, it is difficult to detect pulsus paradoxus in children due to high heart and respiratory rates. Nevertheless, respiratory variations in plethysmography waveform on pulse oximetry correlate well with invasive assessment of pulsus paradoxus and can be used at the bedside to ascertain the diagnosis and severity of tamponade in children.[10]

Investigations

Electrocardiogram shows sinus tachycardia, low QRS voltages, and electrical alternans. Low QRS voltage is a nonspecific sign. Electrical alternans reflecting to and fro movement of the heart with every beat, on the other hand, is specific for large effusion albeit with poor sensitivity. Nonspecific ST-T changes may be present in cases with coexisting pericarditis. The chest radiograph may be normal in patients with mild pericardial effusion. Large pericardial effusions present with a symmetrically enlarged cardiac

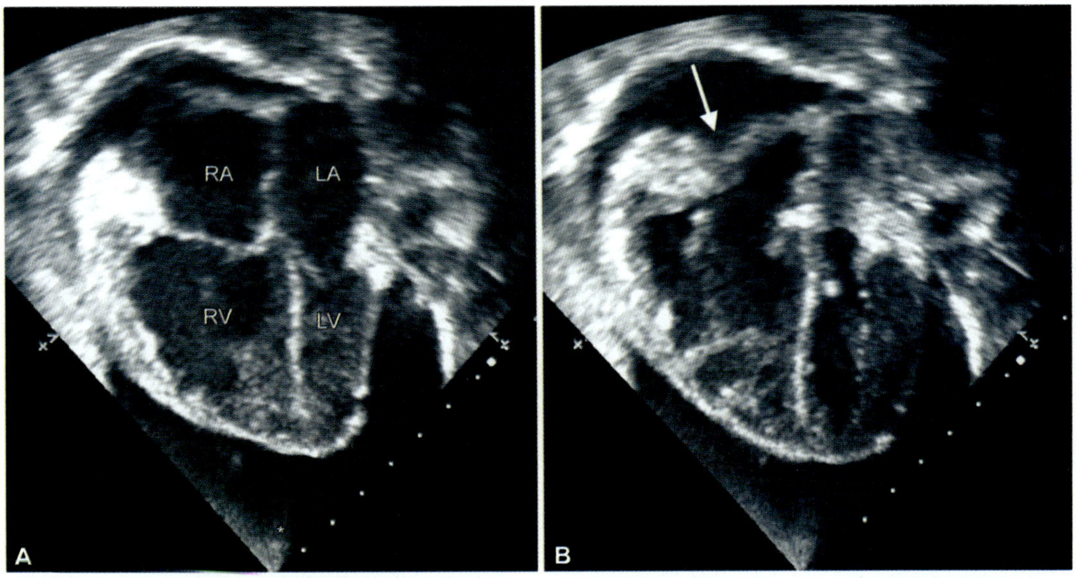

Figs. 4A and B: Two-dimensional echocardiogram in apical-four chamber view showing—(A) massive pericardial effusion (star); (B) with diastolic collapse (arrow) of the right atrium.
(LA: left atrium; LV: left ventricle; RA: right atrium; RV: right ventricle)

TABLE 4: Comparison of clinical and investigation findings in cardiac tamponade and pericardial constriction.

	Cardiac tamponade	*Pericardial constriction*
Clinical examination		
Plusus paradoxus	Present	Present in 1/3 cases
JVP Waveforms	Elevated Normal x descent Blunted y descent	Elevated Normal x descent Prominent y descent
Kussmaul sign	Absent	Present
Pericardial knock	Absent	Present
Echocardiography		
Atrial enlargement	Absent	Present
Cardiac chamber collapse	Present	Absent
Septal bounce	Present	Present
Mitral inflow respiratory variation >25%	Present	Present
Computed tomography		
Thickened pericardium	Absent	Present

silhouette with distinct margins assuming round, flask-like "water bottle" configuration.

Echocardiography detects pericardial effusion with very high accuracy. In adults and adolescents, based on the width of echo-free space between visceral and parietal pericardium at end-diastole, circumferential pericardial effusion is classified as small (<10 mm), moderate (10–20 mm), large (>20 mm), and very large (>25 mm). There is no such standard classification for children. Instead, the assessment of severity is based on a composite assessment of the width of effusion and its hemodynamic effect (**Figs. 4A and B**). Echocardiography also aids in assessing the hemodynamic impact of pericardial effusion. In appropriate clinical setting, a dilated inferior vena cava with <50% inspiratory collapse is highly suggestive of cardiac tamponade (**Table 4**). The echogenicity of pericardial fluid provides important information about the possible cause of the effusion. For example, fibrinous strands within the fluid suggest acute inflammation and are common with bacterial pericarditis.

Pericardial fluid compresses cardiac chambers when the pressure within the chamber falls below pericardial pressure. Hence, the cardiac chamber with the lowest pressure collapses first. Right atrial collapse exceeding one-third of the cardiac cycle is nearly 100% sensitive and specific for cardiac tamponade. There can be right ventricle collapse during early diastole. The duration of right ventricular collapse is proportionate to the severity of tamponade, initially occurring only during inspiration and extending to expiration at later stages. The collapse of right-sided chambers may be absent in conditions with elevated pressure in the right ventricle as in pulmonary hypertension, or pulmonary stenosis. Conversely, collapse may occur earlier in hypovolemia. A large pericardial effusion may cause beat-to-beat swinging of the heart.

Exaggerated ventricle interdependence is easily detected on Doppler echocardiography by marked respiratory variation in mitral and tricuspid inflow velocities. The mitral inflow velocity, measured at the peak of the E wave (early filling wave), increases >25% during expiration than during inspiration. In contrast, the tricuspid inflow velocity increases during inspiration.[1,3]

Management

Patients with established or impending tamponade present as an emergency with most requiring urgent pericardial drainage.[11] Intravenous hydration with normal saline should be started immediately. Inotropic agents should be started in those with hypotension, although their efficacy is limited in the absence of prompt pericardiocentesis. Patients with no or minimal symptoms can be managed medically. Pericardial effusion related to hypothyroidism responds quickly to thyroxine replacement therapy.

Close pericardiocentesis is done through a subxiphoid approach. It should be done under echocardiographic guidance, preferably in cardiac catheterization laboratory with fluoroscopic assistance. However, in emergency situations, it can be undertaken in intensive care unit (ICU) settings. A pigtail catheter is placed in the pericardial space for continuous drainage. The pericardial fluid analysis helps in finding out the etiology of pericardial effusion. In most clinical conditions with inflammation, infection, or injury, the pericardial fluid is exudative, while in cases with fluid overload and elevated systemic venous pressure, it is transudative. Drainage of pus confirms the diagnosis of bacterial pericarditis. Chylous effusion, rich in triglycerides, occurs after traumatic or surgical injury to the thoracic duct. Typical gold-paint cholesterol-rich effusion is seen in severe hypothyroidism. In addition to the routine measurement of cell counts, sugar, and protein, the pericardial fluid is subjected to special tests based on possible etiology. In cases with a high suspicion of tuberculosis, the analysis should include measurement of adenosine deaminase (ADA) level in the fluid and polymerase chain reaction (PCR) for *Mycobacterium*. In an appropriate clinical setting, measurement of tumor markers and malignant cells should also be done.

SPECIFIC PERICARDIAL DISEASES

Viral Pericarditis

Viral infection is the most common cause of pericarditis in children; Coxsackie virus being the most common causative agent. The clinical symptoms and course are similar to other viral illnesses. Patients generally appear less toxic than those with bacterial pericarditis, unless there is associated myocarditis. Pericardial effusion is common but tamponade is rare. The pericardial fluid is serous or serosanguinous with a lymphocytic predominance. PCR studies are useful in determining a specific viral etiology, although it is not routinely required.

Bacterial Pericarditis

Bacterial pericarditis is a serious and potentially life-threatening disease more common in children younger than 2 years.[12] The lung is the most common source of infection. Septic arthritis, osteomyelitis, meningitis, or other soft tissue infection may also cause hematogenous spread to the pericardium. Broad-spectrum antibiotics are mandatory and should be directed toward the most common causative organisms, *Staphylococcus aureus* and *Haemophilus influenzae*. In general, initial treatment should include intravenous penicillinase-resistant penicillin or vancomycin and a third-generation cephalosporin. An aminoglycoside may be added to sick and immunocompromised children. Antibiotics may be changed based on the culture and sensitivity pattern. All children should be treated with intravenous antibiotics for at least 3–4 weeks, irrespective of the initial response in clinical status. The penetration of antibiotics to the pericardial space is limited and, therefore, antibiotics alone may not be sufficient. An early pericardiocentesis and continuous drainage reduce pericardial inflammation and promptly resolve acute illness.

Most centers prefer pericardial window creation for purulent pericarditis. Others instill intrapericardial streptokinase (5,000 U/kg, not to exceed a total dose of 1 lakh unit) for liquefaction and better drainage of pericardial fluid.[13] This needs close monitoring and frequent aspiration to assess for pericardial hemorrhage. A duration of 8–10 days is generally sufficient and the pigtail catheter is removed when daily pericardial aspirate is <5–10 mL and there is no reaccumulation on echocardiography. If the fluid cannot be aspirated percutaneously, a surgical pericardial window or pericardiectomy is considered. The exact incidence of pericardial constriction following bacterial pericarditis is not known but is common with *S. aureus*, *H. influenzae*, and *Streptococcus pneumoniae* pericarditis.

Tubercular Pericarditis

Tubercular pericarditis is often due to direct extension of pulmonary tuberculosis but can also result from hematogenous spread from other foci. It typically presents with insidious onset of low-grade fever, night sweats, weight loss, malaise, dyspnea, and nonspecific chest pain. In an appropriate clinical setting, lymphocytic predominance, positive stain for acid-fast bacilli, and elevated ADA levels >50 U/L in the pericardial fluid are diagnostic of tubercular pericarditis and are sufficient to initiate antitubercular therapy.[14] There is no consensus about the use of corticosteroids in tubercular pericarditis but is generally preferred. The recommended dose of oral prednisolone is 1–2 mg/kg per day. It should be continued for 10–12 weeks with slow tapering after 4 weeks. Worldwide tubercular pericarditis remains one of the leading causes of pericardial constriction. In cases requiring pericardiectomy, the procedure should be deferred for at least 6 weeks after starting antitubercular therapy, allowing time for the development of a surgical cleavage plane.[15]

PERICARDIAL CONSTRICTION

Pericardial constriction is characterized by a thickened, inelastic, and noncompliant pericardium that limits the diastolic expansion of the ventricles. Constriction generally involves the entire pericardium, although localized constriction is occasionally seen. It is also known as chronic constrictive pericarditis, which is a misnomer as the constriction is not necessarily chronic and pericardium is hardly inflamed at the time of constriction. Tuberculosis is the most common cause worldwide. Other causes include idiopathic and viral pericarditis and radiation-induced pericardial constriction. Rarely, though counterintuitive, pericardial constriction can occur following cardiac surgery.[16]

Pathophysiology

In pericardial constriction, similar to tamponade physiology, the left and right ventricles compete for filling in a "fixed" and noncompliant space. As a result, filling pressures in all the cardiac chambers and in systemic as well as pulmonary veins are elevated. Early ventricular filling is exaggerated. In mid-diastole, stiff pericardium abruptly halts ventricular filling when the cardiac volume exceeds pericardial reserve volume.

In addition, thickened pericardium impedes the transmission of thoracic pressures to cardiac chambers. Hence, during inspiration, the pulmonary venous pressure falls without any simultaneous reduction in LV diastolic pressure. This leads to the reduced or completely abolished pressure gradient between pulmonary veins and the left ventricle. Thus, left ventricle filling is impaired in inspiration and the right ventricle fills preferentially. The reverse happens in expiration, causing exaggerated ventricular interdependence.

Severely restricted ventricular filling leads to elevated systemic venous pressure and a relatively fixed cardiac output. Simultaneous changes in the neurohormones also contribute to fluid retention.

Clinical Examination

Pericardial constriction typically presents with symptoms and signs of right-sided heart failure. Pedal edema is the rule with varying degrees of ascites and pleural effusion. The enlarged liver may be tender and may have systolic pulsations of tricuspid regurgitation. If left untreated, patients present with recurrent pleural effusion, ascites, and anasarca. Chronic malnutrition and high metabolic rate lead to muscle wasting and cachexia. In advance stages, cardiac cirrhosis may ensue.

Physical examination shows marked JVP elevation with prominent "y" descent due to rapid early diastolic filling of ventricles (*see* **Fig. 3**). JVP fails to fall or may paradoxically rise during inspiration (Kussmaul sign). One-third of patients may have pulsus paradoxus. Pericardial knock is the auscultatory hallmark, which is an early diastolic high-frequency sound coinciding with pericardial restrain during mid-diastolic filling.

Investigations

Electrocardiogram shows nonspecific T wave changes and reduced QRS voltage. Atrial fibrillation is seen in up to one-third of patients. Pericardial calcification is seen in a minority. It is commonly seen over the right atrium, atrioventricular groove, and diaphragmatic surface of the cardiac silhouette (*see* **Table 4**). Pleural effusion is common and pulmonary venous redistribution may be seen (**Fig. 5**).

Two-dimensional (2D) echocardiography shows an abrupt shift of ventricular septum during early diastole manifesting as "septal bounce". The septum is also shifted leftward during inspiration with the opposite happening during expiration. Systemic veins and hepatic veins

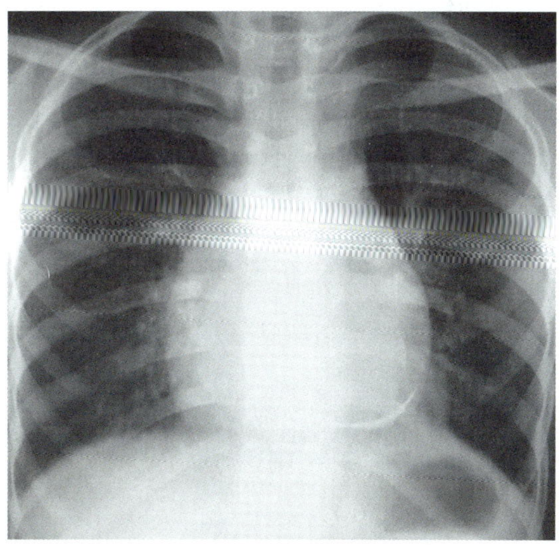

Fig. 5: Chest radiograph (posteroanterior view) from a child with pericardial constriction showing calcification of the diaphragmatic surface of the pericardium.

(*Source*: Reproduced with permission from Gupta SK. Pericardial diseases in children. In: Wernovsky G, Anderson RH, Kumar K, Mussato KA, Redington A, Tweddell JS, Tretter J (Eds). Anderson's Pediatric Cardiology, 4th edition. Philadelphia: Elsevier; 2019. pp. 1063-75.)

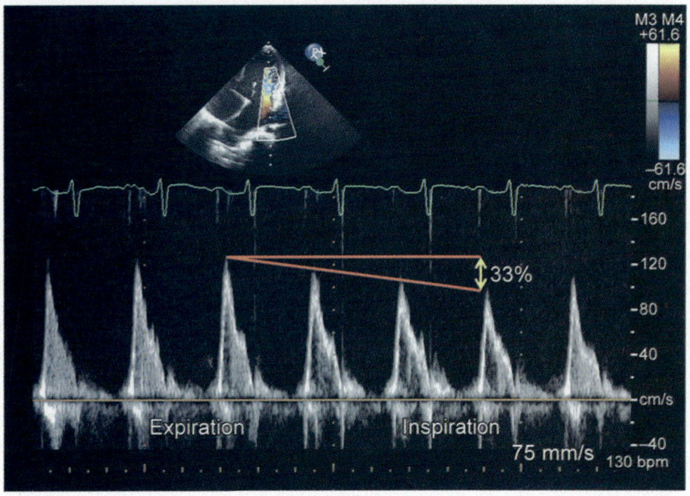

Fig. 6: Mitral valve Doppler showing exaggerated respiratory inflow variation.
(*Source*: Reproduced with permission from Gupta SK. Pericardial diseases in children. In: Wernovsky G, Anderson RH, Kumar K, Mussato KA, Redington A, Tweddell JS, Tretter J (Eds). Anderson's Pediatric Cardiology, 4th edition. Philadelphia: Elsevier; 2019. pp. 1063-75.)

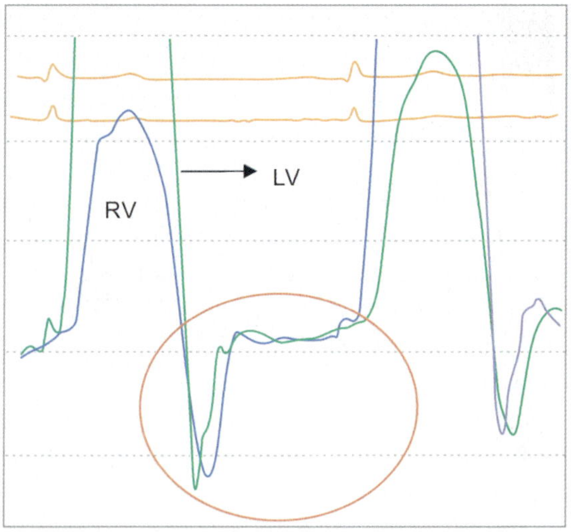

Fig. 7: Simultaneous left and right ventricular pressure traces showing dip and plateau or square root sign. Also, note that the diastolic pressures in both the ventricles are equal.
(*Source*: Reproduced with permission from Gupta SK. Pericardial diseases in children. In: Wernovsky G, Anderson RH, Kumar K, Mussato KA, Redington A, Tweddell JS, Tretter J (Eds). Anderson's Pediatric Cardiology, 4th edition. Philadelphia: Elsevier; 2019. pp. 1063-75.)

are dilated. Doppler interrogation reveals exaggerated respiratory variation in both mitral (>25%) and tricuspid (>40%) inflow velocities (**Fig. 6**).[17] Pericardial thickening cannot be commented well on echocardiography.

Cardiac catheterization is the gold standard for the diagnosis of constrictive physiology.[18] The diastolic pressure in all the cardiac chambers and systemic and pulmonary veins is elevated (>20 mm Hg) and equal (<5 mm Hg difference). Pressure tracings from the right and left ventricle demonstrate early diastolic dip, matching an exaggerated early diastolic filling, followed by a plateau (dip and plateau or square root sign) (**Fig. 7**).

The pericardial thickness of >2 mm on computed tomography (CT) and >4 mm on magnetic resonance imaging (MRI) is highly suggestive of pericardial constriction. In addition, MRI provide information about hemodynamic alterations unique to pericardial constriction.

Management

A carefully optimized regimen of diuretics and fluid restriction helps in symptomatic relief. Tachycardia is a compensatory mechanism to maintain cardiac output, therefore, beta-blockers, calcium channel blockers, and other rate-reducing drugs should be avoided. In patients with atrial fibrillation with a fast ventricular rate, digoxin is preferred for heart rate control. Surgical pericardiectomy, performed through a median sternotomy, is the definitive treatment and should be considered in all symptomatic patients. It is not recommended if the constriction is mild.[19] If the pericardium is densely adherent with difficult debridement, the waffle procedure is performed by making multiple transverse and longitudinal incisions in the percardium. Video-assisted partial pericardiectomy is an option in select cases with no adhesions.

PERICARDIAL DISEASES IN THE PRESENCE OF EXISTING CONGENITAL HEART DISEASE

Rarely, pericardial constriction can occur in a patient with pre-existing congenital heart disease (CHD). The combination of pericardial constriction and CHD poses a challenging clinical scenario with each lesion affecting the hemodynamics and clinical presentation of the other.[20,21] Intuitively, the presence of a large defect in the atrial or the ventricular septum abolishes exaggerated ventricular interdependence. A stepwise assessment may lead to successful management.[21] A poor understanding of this complex hemodynamic interaction, on the other hand, may result in an erroneous clinical decision. Therefore, caution must be exercised while evaluating such a patient.

CONGENITAL ABSENCE OF PERICARDIUM

It is a rare congenital anomaly. The absence of pericardium can be complete or partial. The pericardial defect may be left-sided or right-sided or rarely bilateral. Left-sided absence of the pericardium is the most common variant. A total absence of pericardium is much more common than partial defects. Most cases are asymptomatic or minimally symptomatic.[22] Cardiac chambers, most commonly the left atrial appendage, can rarely herniate through the defect with subsequent strangulation. Ventricular herniation, myocardial necrosis, and torsion of great vessels are other potential complications. These complications are more common in small partial defects. In complete absence,

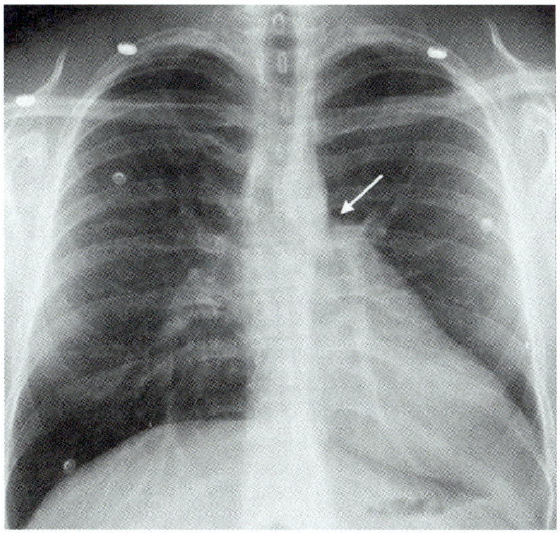

Fig. 8: Chest radiograph in anteroposterior view from an adolescent boy with absent pericardium. Cardiomegaly with inconspicuous right heart border is evident. Lung tissue (arrow) is interposed in prominent space between the aorta and the main pulmonary artery. The left heart border is straight and elongated (Snoopy sign).

(*Source*: Reproduced with permission from Gupta SK. Pericardial diseases in children. In: Wernovsky G, Anderson RH, Kumar K, Mussato KA, Redington A, Tweddell JS, Tretter J (Eds). Anderson's Pediatric Cardiology, 4th edition. Philadelphia: Elsevier; 2019. pp. 1063-75.)

excessive mobility of the heart can shift the cardiac impulse leftward.

Electrocardiogram shows nonspecific changes, most common being poor R wave progression and right bundle branch block. The chest radiograph shows a leftward shift of cardiac silhouette and the absence of the right heart border. The left cardiac border is straightened and elongated (Snoopy sign). In addition, the area between the aorta and the main pulmonary artery is prominent with the interposition of lung tissue (**Fig. 8**). Echocardiography shows distorted cardiac anatomy causing an apparent dilatation of the right ventricle and abnormal septal motion. Surgical repair, by patch closure of the defect, is indicated in cases with active or impending cardiac chamber herniation. The complete absence of pericardium is rarely symptomatic and usually requires no treatment.

REFERENCES

1. Gupta SK. Pericardial diseases in children. In: Wernovsky G, Anderson RH, Kumar K, Mussato KA, Redington A, Tweddell JS, Tretter J. (Eds). Anderson's Pediatric Cardiology, 4th edition. Philadelphia: Elsevier; 2019. pp. 1063-75.
2. Holt JP. The normal pericardium. Am J Cardiol. 1970;26(5): 455-65.
3. LeWinter MM, Imazio M. Pericardial diseases. In: Bonow RO, Zipes DP, Libby P, (Eds). Braunwald's Heart Disease: A Textbook of Cardiovascular Medicine, 11th edition. Philadelphia: Elsevier Saunders; 2018. pp. 1662-80.
4. Imazio M, Brucato M, Trinchero R, Adler Y. Diagnosis and management of pericardial diseases. Nat Rev Cardiol. 2009;6(12):743-51.
5. Abu FR, Banai S, Chorin U, Rogowski O, Keren G, Roth A. Diagnostic yield of extensive infectious panel testing in acute pericarditis. Cardiology. 2011;119(3):134-9.
6. Alabed S, Perez-Gaxiola G, Burls A. Colchicine for children with pericarditis: systematic review of clinical studies. Arch Dis Child. 2016; 101(10):953-6.
7. Bagri NK, Yadav DK, Agarwal S, Aier T, Gupta V. Pericardial effusion in children: experience from tertiary care center in Northern India. Indian Pediatr. 2014;51(3):211-3.
8. Reddy PS, Curtiss EI, Uretsky BF. Spectrum of hemodynamic changes in cardiac tamponade. Am J Cardiol. 1990;66(20): 1487-91.
9. Shabetai R, Fowler NO, Fenton JC, Masangkay M. Pulsus paradoxus. J Clin Invest. 1965;44(11): 1882-98.
10. Amoozgar H, Ghodsi H, Borzoee M, Amirghofran AA, Ajami G, Serati Z. Detection of pulsus paradoxus by pulse oximetry in pediatric patients after cardiac surgery. Pediatr Cardiol. 2009;30(1):41-5.
11. Sagrista-Sauleda J, Merce AS, Soler-Soler J. Diagnosis and management of pericardial effusion. World J Cardiol. 2011;3(5):135-43.
12. Feldman WE. Bacterial etiology and mortality of purulent pericarditis in pediatric patients: review of 162 cases. Am J Dis Child. 1979;133(6): 641-4.
13. Juneja R, Kothari SS, Saxena A, Sharma R, Joshi A. Intrapericardial streptokinase in purulent pericarditis. Arch Dis Child. 1999; 80(3):275-7.
14. Mayosi BM, Burgess LJ, Doubell AF. Tubercular pericarditis. Circulation. 2005;112(23):3608-16.
15. Talwar S, Nair VV, Choudhary SK, Sreeniwas V, Saxena A, Juneja R, et al. Pericardiectomy in children < 15 years of age. Cardiol Young. 2014;24(4):616-22.
16. Deepti S, Gupta SK, Ramakrishnan S, Talwar S, Kothari SS. Constrictive pericarditis following open-heart surgery in a child. Ann Pediatr Cardiol. 2016;9(1):68-71.
17. Oh JK, Hatle LK, Seward JB, Danielson GK, Schaff HV, Reeder GS, et al. Diagnostic role of Doppler echocardiography in constrictive pericarditis. J Am Coll Cardiol. 1994;23(1):154-62.
18. Doshi S, Ramakrishnan S, Gupta SK. Invasive hemodynamics of constrictive pericarditis. Indian Heart J. 2015;67(2):175-82.
19. Chowdhury UK, Subramaniam GK, Kumar AS, Airan B, Singh R, Talwar S, et al. Pericardiectomy for constrictive pericarditis: a clinical, echocardiographic, and hemodynamic evaluation of two surgical techniques. Ann Thorac Surg. 2006;81(2):522-9.
20. Gupta SK, Saxena A, Talwar S. Chronic constrictive pericarditis: unique cause of heart failure in a child with tetralogy of Fallot. Pediatr Cardiol. 2012;33(1):165-7.
21. Gupta SK, Ramakrishnan S, Kothari SS, Saxena A, Airan B. Hemodynamics of large ventricular septal defect and coexisting chronic constrictive pericarditis masquerading as Eisenmenger's syndrome. Catheter Cardiovasc Interv. 2014;83(2):263-9.
22. Abbas AE, Appleton CP, Liu PT, Sweeney JP. Congenital absence of pericardium: case presentation and review of literature. Int J Cardiol. 2005;98(1):21-5.

47 CHAPTER

Fetal Cardiology

Balu Vaidyanathan, Balaganesh Karmegaraj

INTRODUCTION

The availability of fetal echocardiography has provided a very unique opportunity to diagnose and understand various forms of congenital heart disease (CHD) from early gestation.[1] Prenatal diagnosis offers much wider options for management of the CHD to the expectant family, especially in low-resource settings. Prenatal diagnosis may reduce the burden of very complex forms of CHD and has the potential to significantly improve outcomes of infants with critical, correctable heart defects by planned perinatal care. A multidisciplinary team approach is required to provide an adequate counseling about the treatment options, survey for comorbid extracardiac and genetic anomalies, and to plan perinatal care.

In this chapter, we discuss the role of fetal echocardiography in the contemporary management of CHD, with a specific focus on low- and middle-income countries (LMICs).

INDICATIONS AND TIMING FOR FETAL ECHOCARDIOGRAPHY

Since most forms of CHD occurs in low-risk pregnancies, it is important to perform a basic screening of the fetal heart in all pregnancies.[2] A combination of the four-chamber view, outflow tracts, and three-vessel view enables accurate screening of the fetal heart and most cardiac anomalies can be suspected using these three views. In high-risk pregnancies, referral for a detailed fetal echocardiography may be considered.

Table 1 summarizes the indications for fetal echocardiography (high-risk subsets).

A pyramid-based approach is recommended for fetal heart screening during pregnancy in the current era. The initial evaluation of the fetal heart (four-chamber and outflows) can be done as a part of the first trimester evaluation at 11–13 weeks. This examination can be a part of the first trimester fetal evaluation protocol including nuchal translucency (NT) assessment, first trimester genetic markers, and a basic evaluation for major fetal anomalies. Most complex forms of CHD, especially those with abnormal four-chamber view, can be suspected during this stage. In suspected cases, a referral for an early fetal echocardiography can be considered. In routine situations, a more detailed evaluation of the fetal heart is done as a part of the mid-trimester anomaly scan at 18–22 weeks of gestation. During the latter part of the pregnancy (third trimester), evaluation of the fetal heart should be done to evaluate fetal heart rate and rhythm and cardiac function in high-risk cases or as follow-up evaluation in suspected cases of CHD.

PROTOCOL FOR FETAL ECHOCARDIOGRAPHY

Detailed guidelines have been established for the practice of fetal echocardiography by various clinical societies.

TABLE 1: Indications for fetal echocardiography.

Fetal	*Maternal*	*Familial*
• Abnormal 4-chamber view • Extracardiac anomalies—GIT, spina bifida • Chromosomal anomalies—VACTERL, trisomies, DiGeorge • Increased first trimester NT • Nonimmune hydrops • Irregular heart beat—tachy/bradyarrhythmias • Abnormal cardiac axis • IVF/ICSI	• Maternal CHD • Teratogen exposure • Metabolic disorders—diabetes mellitus • Maternal autoimmune disease • Intrauterine infections	• Previous child with CHD • Paternal CHD • Mendelian syndromes—TS, Noonan, DiGeorgeaa

(CHD: congenital heart disease; GIT: gastrointestinal tract; ICSI: intracytoplasmic sperm injection; IVF: in vitro fertilization; NT: nuchal translucency; TS: Tourette syndrome; VACTERL: vertebral defects, anal atresia, cardiac defects, tracheoesophageal fistula, renal anomalies, and limb abnormalities)

Originally, only the four-chamber view was included in screening protocols. However, this resulted in most of the outflow tract and aortic arch anomalies getting missed. Hence, in the current guidelines, the outflow tracts also have been included in the screening views for the fetal heart. In the extended basic scan guidelines laid down by the International Society for Ultrasound in Obstetrics and Gynecology (ISUOG), a transverse sweep of the fetal heart from caudal to cranial direction including the abdominal situs, four-chamber view, both outflow tracts, three-vessel view, and the three-vessel tracheal view is recommended.[3] **Figures 1A to F** summarize the views of the fetal heart recommend in the extended basic guidelines. For a more detailed evaluation, additional views in the sagittal plane (bicaval view, ductal, and aortic arches), parasagittal views (ventricular septum and outflows), evaluation of fetal heart rate, and rhythm and fetal cardiac function may be performed. Newer techniques such as 3D/4D spatiotemporal image correlation (STIC) enable precise anatomic diagnosis in cases with complex anatomy and enable postprocessing of the acquired datasets. **Figure 2** demonstrates the use of 3D/4D STIC technology in displaying images of normal fetal heart structures.

COMMON CONGENITAL HEART DISEASES WHICH CAN BE DIAGNOSED BY FETAL ECHOCARDIOGRAPHY

Almost all forms of major CHDs can be diagnosed in utero with a diagnostic accuracy of nearly 100% (**Table 2**). Abnormalities of the four-chamber view (typically complex CHD) are relatively easy to detect. Most forms of CHD of the univentricular heart morphology (e.g., hypoplastic left and right heart and tricuspid atresia), valvular anomalies such as Ebstein anomaly and atrioventricular septal defect, ventricular dysfunction, cardiac tumors, and pericardial effusion can be picked up by four-chamber view alone. A combination of the outflow and three-vessel views will enable diagnosis of abnormalities of outflow tracts [tetralogy of Fallot, transposition of great arteries, double-outlet right ventricle (RV), coarctation of aorta, and anomalies of arch sidedness]. Anomalies of pulmonary veins, mild forms of valvular defects (bicuspid aortic valve), peripheral pulmonary stenosis, and coronary abnormalities are difficult to diagnose in utero and the presence of an atrial septal defect and patent ductus arteriosus are physiological in the fetus.

Figures 3 and 4 summarize the common cardiac anomalies which can be diagnosed using the four-chamber and outflow tract/three-vessel views, respectively.

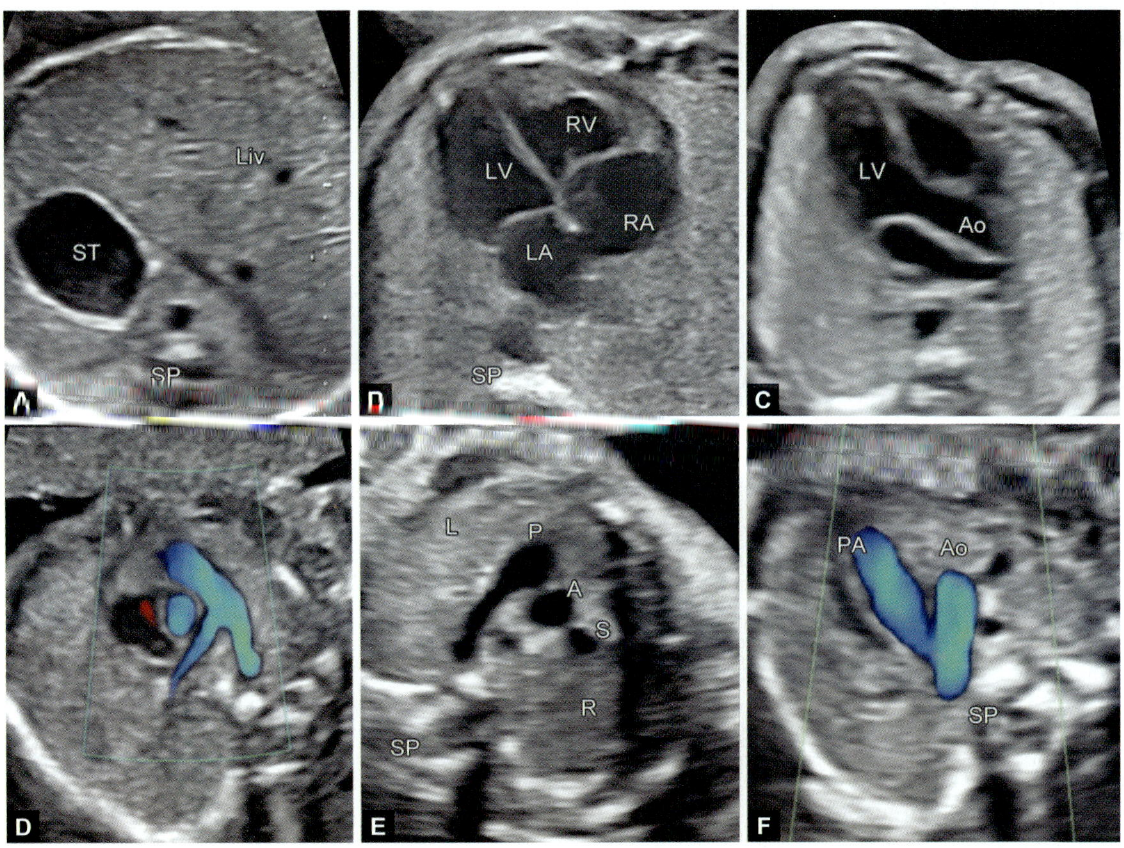

Figs. 1A to F: Protocol for evaluation of fetal heart in midtrimester anomaly scans—recommended views. (A) Transverse sweep of the fetal heart showing abdominal situs; (B) Four-chamber view; (C) Left ventricular outflow tract; (D) Right ventricular outflow tract and pulmonary artery bifurcation; (E) Three-vessel view with pulmonary artery anterior, aorta in middle, and superior vena cava posterior; (F) Three-vessel tracheal view with joining of the ductal and aortic arches in a V-shaped formation to the left of the spine.

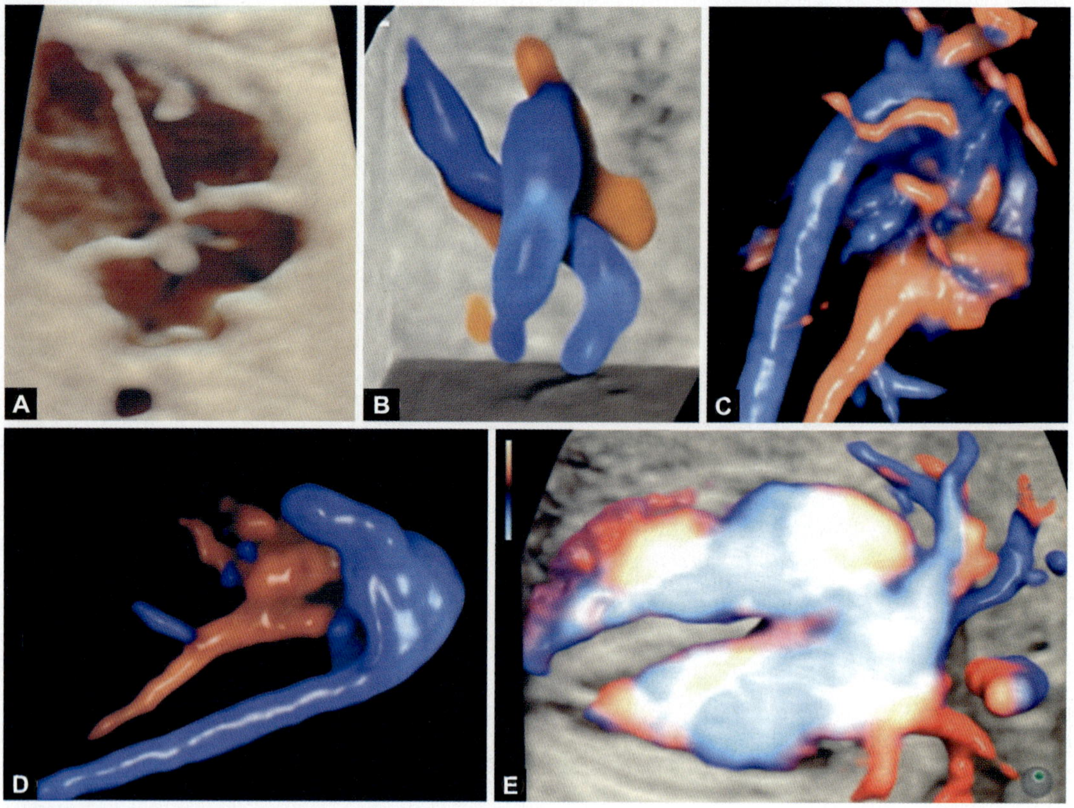

Figs. 2A to E: 3D/4D spatio-temporal image correlation (STIC) in evaluation of fetal heart—display of normal cardiac anatomy. 3D/4D spatio-temporal image correlation (STIC) rendering to display normal cardiac anatomy. The sequence shows a normal four-chamber view (A), crossing of outflow tracts (B), aortic arch with branches (C), ductal arch (D), and pulmonary veins draining to the left atrium (E).

TABLE 2: Cardiac conditions which can be diagnosed by fetal echocardiography.

Four-chamber view	*Outflow tracts and three-vessel view*
· Major septation defects (AVSD) · Significant chamber hypoplasia (HLHS/PA-IVS) · Major valve lesions · Ventricular dysfunction · Rhythm problems · Pericardial effusion	· Tetralogy of Fallot · Double outlet RV · Transposition of great arteries · Truncus arteriosus · Aortic arch anomalies

(AVSD: atrioventricular septal defect; HLHS: hypoplastic left heart syndrome; PA-IVS: pulmonary atresia with intact ventricular septum; RV: right ventricle)

COUNSELING AND MANAGEMENT AFTER PRENATAL DIAGNOSIS OF CONGENITAL HEART DISEASE IN THE FETUS

The principal role of a pediatric/fetal cardiologist comes after the diagnosis of a CHD has been made in utero.[1,2,4] The following aspects need to be considered when one counsels the family about the diagnosis and subsequent management.

- Natural history of the lesion—both in utero and in postnatal life
- What are the treatment options available?
- When should the treatment be instituted—in utero or after birth?
- What are the predicted outcomes with treatment for the condition diagnosed?
- Which are the centers where such treatment may be undertaken along with knowledge of the institutional outcomes?
- Financial considerations and availability of funding support by government schemes or nongovernment agencies.

The counseling plan has to be individualized and a different strategy may need to be followed for various families depending upon their financial and social background. Several centers in India are now undertaking complex surgical procedures in very tender hearts with excellent short-term and intermediate outcomes.[5] Most forms of CHD can be effectively corrected or palliated in early life with very good outcomes. However, it is generally agreed that the prognosis even after palliation is suboptimal for very complex forms of CHD (typically the single ventricle heart). The prognosis is also significantly affected if the CHD is associated with genetic or extracardiac anomalies.

The potential impact of fetal echocardiography on management of CHD may be considered under the following categories:

Termination of Pregnancy

This option may be discussed as a possible management option with families in situations where the CHD is very

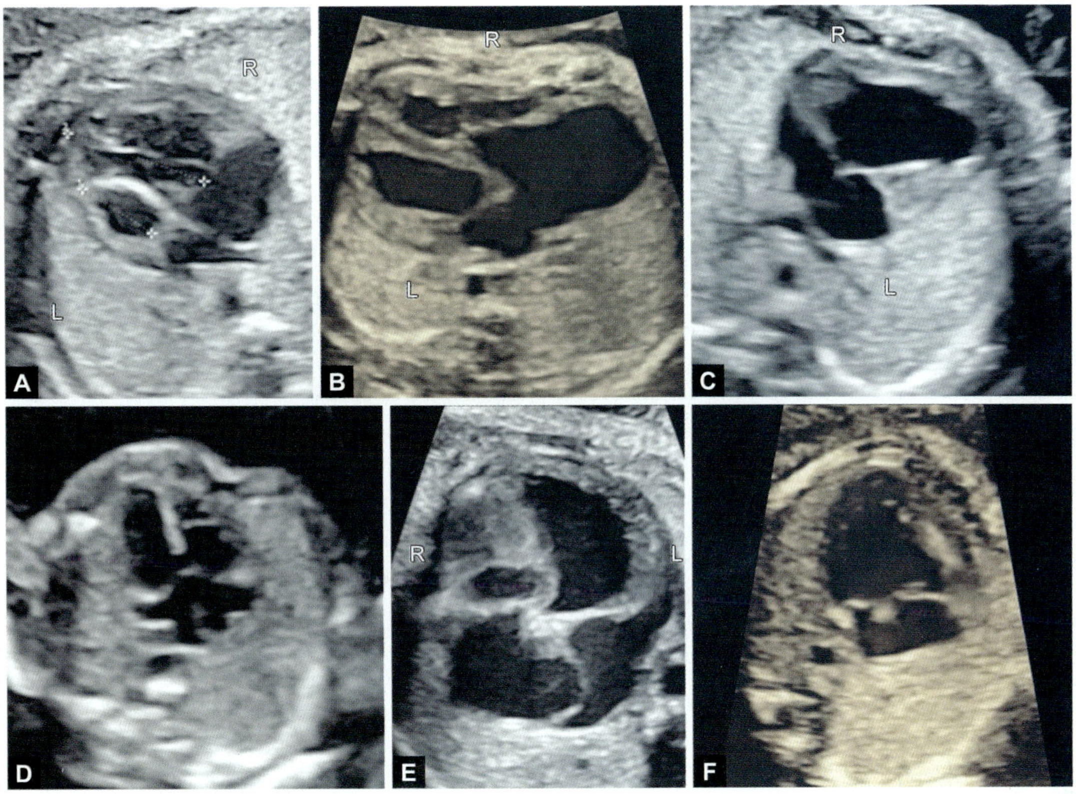

Figs. 3A to F: Common anomalies of the four-chamber view. Common abnormalities of four-chamber view showing hypoplastic left heart syndrome (A), Ebstein anomaly (B), unbalanced atrioventricular septal defect in right isomerism (C), complete atrioventricular septal defect, balanced type (D), pulmonary atresia with intact septum and hypoplastic right ventricle (RV) (E), and double-inlet left ventricle type of single ventricle (F).

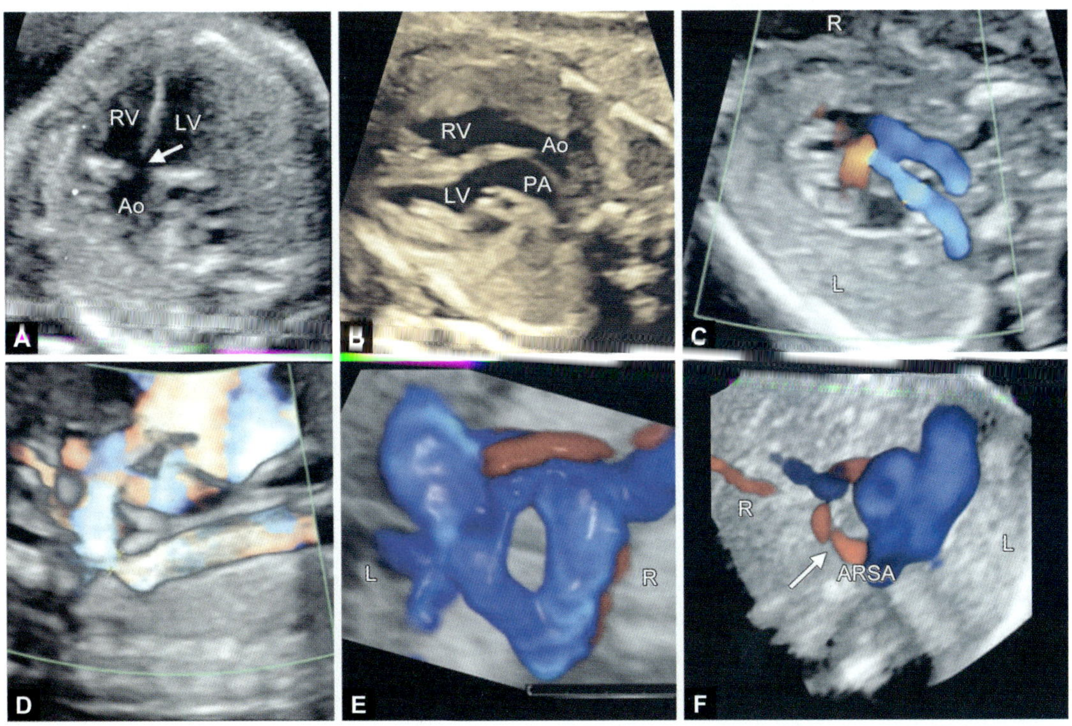

Figs. 4A to F: Common anomalies of the outflow tracts and three-vessel views. Common abnormalities of outflow tracts and aortic arches showing tetralogy of Fallot with ventricular septal defect with aortic override (A), transposition of the great arteries with intact ventricular septum (B), double-outlet right ventricle (RV) (C), coarctation of aorta (D), double aortic arch with dominant right arch (E), and left aortic arch with aberrant right subclavian artery (ARSA) (white arrow) (F).

complex and can be offered only palliative forms of surgery with guarded long-term prognosis.[6] Most of these patients require multiple palliative surgeries in the first decade of life in the single ventricle pathway. There is significant interstage mortality and morbidity [especially in CHD such as hypoplastic left heart syndrome (HLHS)]. A large proportion of these patients face significant medical and psychosocial issues in adolescent life due to long-term complications associated with the Fontan circulation. These challenges make long-term management of patients with complex forms of single ventricle very challenging in LMICs. The role of the fetal cardiologist is to provide a realistic prognosis about the underlying CHD and management options to the expectant family. The final decision to continue the pregnancy or consider termination of pregnancy needs to be made by the respective families in accordance to the local and regional laws concerning medical termination of pregnancy. In India, the legal limit for medical termination of pregnancy is up to 20 weeks of gestation.

Examples of very complex CHD with guarded long-term prognosis include the following:

- Hypoplastic left heart syndrome (HLHS)
- Complex forms of single ventricle physiology (often associated with abnormalities of pulmonary veins, pulmonary atresia, and abdominal situs). These conditions are often classified under the category of "heterotaxy" anomalies or isomeric hearts
- Complex form of tetralogy of Fallot with pulmonary atresia with nonconfluent pulmonary arteries and aortopulmonary collaterals
- Severe regurgitation of atrioventricular valves with hydrops—classical examples include Ebstein anomaly of tricuspid valve, pulmonary atresia-intact ventricular septum with severe tricuspid regurgitation, and right ventricular dysfunction
- Complex heart disease associated with major rhythm abnormalities such as complete heart block (typically seen in left isomerism).

Planned Peripartum Care

This scenario applies to those cardiac conditions that are potentially lethal in the neonatal period without intervention and where corrective surgery offers excellent long-term outcomes. In most of these conditions, the survival of the infant depends on the continued patency of the arterial duct after birth to maintain pulmonary or systemic blood flow. This is accomplished by starting an infusion of prostaglandin E1 when indicated. Once the duct starts to close, these babies can present with severe cyanosis or shock. It may be extremely hazardous to transport such sick babies to a tertiary care pediatric cardiac facility after they have started showing symptoms of decompensation.

Studies have shown that the major determinant of outcomes after corrective intervention in such patients is the preoperative status of the baby.[7] Hence, in such conditions, the best possible option after prenatal diagnosis would be to plan delivery in a center with pediatric cardiac facility so that immediate care can be delivered to the baby after birth.

The timing of delivery is based on obstetric indications and is preferably as close to term, if possible. Premature delivery before 37 weeks is associated with significantly increased mortality and morbidity (length of hospital stay) in neonates undergoing cardiac surgery. The mode of delivery is based on obstetric indications. A planned cesarean section is advised only in situations where the CHD is associated with hemodynamic compromise (e.g., CHD associated with hydrops fetalis) or uncontrolled fetal arrhythmias.

Examples of cardiac conditions where planned peripartum may be considered include the following:

- Transposition of the great arteries (especially with intact ventricular septum)—baby may require an emergency postnatal intervention called balloon atrial septostomy to correct hypoxemia followed by the corrective arterial switch operation
- Critical obstruction to right ventricular outflow tract resulting in duct-dependent pulmonary circulation—this includes conditions such as critical pulmonary stenosis/pulmonary atresia, tetralogy of Fallot, and allied physiologies
- Critical obstruction to left ventricular outflow tract resulting in duct-dependent systemic circulation—this includes conditions such as critical aortic stenosis, severe coarctation of aorta, and interrupted aortic arch
- Obstructed form of total anomalous pulmonary venous connection (TAPVC).

Studies from LMICs such as India have shown that a strategy of prenatal diagnosis and planned peripartum care can have significant benefits for neonates with critical forms of CHD.[8,9]

These include:

- *Improved preoperative status*: This is reflected in lower California modification of transport risk index of physiological stability (Ca-TRIPS) score, better clinical and laboratory parameters, and earlier conduct of a definitive cardiac intervention.[9]
- *Improved outcomes after intervention/surgery*: Studies from the developed countries have shown that prenatal diagnosis is associated with reduced mortality for critical CHD such as transposition of the great arteries and coarctation of aorta.
- *Reduced duration of hospital stay and lower in-hospital costs*: The improved preoperative status associated with prenatal diagnosis enables the earlier conduct of the definitive procedure and reduced consumption of ICU resources spent on preoperative stabilization. Studies have shown that the postoperative recovery may be expedited in such situations. Thus, the overall direct

costs of in-hospital care can be reduced by prenatal diagnosis and planned peripartum care for these critical CHD. This is particularly relevant in the setting of LMICs with resource constraints to treat neonates with critical CHD. Prenatal diagnosis thus can emerge as an attractive alternative strategy to improve perinatal outcomes, with an added cost advantage.

- *Impact on long-term neurodevelopmental issues*: Neurodevelopmental concerns constitute one of the most significant long-term morbidity in survivors of CHD.[10] It is possible that avoidance of neonatal transport, lesser hemodynamic instability prior to initiation of medical stabilization, and improved preoperative clinical status may offer neurological protection in these neonates with critical CHD. Future studies are needed to understand the possible benefits of prenatal diagnosis on long-term neurodevelopmental issues in these infants.

The counseling in these patients should include detailed information about the cardiac diagnosis, expected timing of interventions after birth, nature of the postnatal interventions including the costs, and the expected outcomes in a given institution. An excellent coordination between all concerned specialties (fetal and pediatric cardiology, obstetrics, cardiac surgery, neonatology, anesthesia, nursing, and counselor) is required to ensure that there is a smooth transition of care for these critically ill infants.

Multisystem Evaluation for Associated Anomalies

Genetic Syndromes

Around 30% of fetuses with CHD have associated genetic syndromes (**Table 3**). The most common genetic syndromes associated with CHD include various types of aneuploidies, deletion syndromes, and single-gene disorders. In particular, conotruncal anomalies, anomalies of aortic arch sidedness, and atrioventricular septal defects have a higher chance of associated genetic defects. In such cases, it is important to do a detailed anomaly scan to look for associated anomalies and review the results of first trimester screening (abnormal NT and triple marker test). If indicated, an amniocentesis and genetic testing by appropriate methods [karyotyping, fluorescence in situ hybridization (FISH) or micro-array deletion] should be undertaken. Consultation with specialists such as pediatric genetics is advised based on the results of the genetic evaluation. The prognosis of CHD associated with genetic anomalies is considerably worse compared to isolated CHD and this aspect needs to be considered in counseling and pregnancy management of such cases.

TABLE 3: Common genetic syndromes and associated congenital heart diseases.

Genetic syndrome	*Associated congenital heart disease*
Trisomy 21 (Down syndrome)	Atrioventricular septal defect and VSD
Trisomy 18	VSD, TOF
Trisomy 13	ASD, VSD, TOF
CATCH 22 (22q deletion) syndrome	Conotruncal anomalies (TOF, pulmonary atresias), interrupted aortic arch type B
Williams syndrome	Supravalvar AS and peripheral PS
Holt–Oram syndrome	Familial ASD
Ellis Van Creveld syndrome	Common atrium

(ASD: atrial septal defect; AS: aortic stenosis; PS: pulmonic stenosis; TOF: tetralogy of Fallot; VSD: ventricular septal defect)

Extracardiac Anomalies

About 20–30% of fetuses with CHD are associated with extracardiac anomalies. In many cases, CHD is detected as a part of the multisystem evaluation for associated anomalies when a structural anomaly is detected. The most common extracardiac anomalies associated with CHD include anomalies of gastrointestinal tract, kidneys, musculoskeletal system, and central nervous system anomalies. Of these, anomalies of the CNS are being increasingly recognized in recent studies and they include structural anomalies, variations in brain volume, cerebral metabolism, and cerebral blood flow. It is postulated that the in utero hemodynamic consequences of the CHD may result in significant variations in brain volume, metabolism, and cerebral blood flow and thus may contribute to long-term neurodevelopmental issues. Thus, in any fetus with major CHD, it is very important to do a detailed survey for associated anomalies and a detailed evaluation of the brain structure and function. Newer techniques such as 3D ultrasound, fetal brain magnetic resonance imaging (MRI), and magnetic resonance (MR) spectroscopy enable a detailed evaluation of these associated anomalies in the prenatal stage. Such patients will require detailed multidisciplinary counseling involving all concerned specialists in order to plan the peripartum care.

In Utero Treatment

There are limited situations where in utero therapy can be offered when a diagnosis of heart disease is made by fetal echocardiography. This includes the following:

- Fetal arrhythmias, including tachycardia and bradyarrhythmias
- Selected structural heart disease—fetal interventions.

Rhythm Disorders

Tachycardias: The most common forms of tachyarrhythmias in the fetus include supraventricular tachycardia (SVT) and atrial flutter. Most of these arrhythmias are diagnosed around the third trimester (28–32 weeks). Fetal SVTs include re-entry tachycardias, ectopic atrial tachycardia, and permanent junctional re-entry tachycardia (PJRT). Fetal tachycardias have a high-risk for progression to hydrops fetalis and in utero fetal compromise if the diagnosis and treatment is delayed. Diagnosis of these cases involves a detailed assessment of fetal heart rate and rhythm, associated CHD, and assessment of fetal cardiac function and features of fetal heart failure and hydrops fetalis. Associated hydrops fetalis significantly increases the risk of in utero fetal compromise.

Many of these tachyarrhythmias can be effectively managed using transplacental therapy.[11] The various drugs used for transplacental therapy include digoxin, flecainide, and sotalol. Often, a much higher dose of these antiarrhythmic medications are required in pregnancy and hence the treatment has to be initiated in-hospital with frequent monitoring of both the mother and the fetus. In refractory cases and in those with hydrops, direct administration of antiarrhythmic drugs such as digoxin to the fetus (intramuscular injection to the fetal thigh) is considered. Once sinus rhythm and cardiac function is restored, gradual tapering of the medications is done. In most cases, it is possible to effectively control the tachycardia in utero and continue pregnancy till near term. Peripartum management such as timing of delivery and type of delivery is decided on the basis of factors such as tachycardia control and overall fetal well-being. Most infants require continued medications after birth, typically for around a year.

Figures 5A to F demonstrate a classic case of fetal tachycardia (atrial flutter) which responded to combined transplacental and direct fetal therapy.

Bradycardias: The most significant bradyarrhythmia that requires treatment in utero is congenital complete heart block (CHB). This may be isolated or associated with CHD such as left isomerism or corrected transposition of the great arteries. Most cases of isolated CHB are associated with maternal autoimmune disease due to anti-SSA and anti-SSB antibodies. Since transplacental transfer of these antibodies typically occurs after 18 weeks, most of these cases manifest by around 20–24 weeks. The overall prognosis of fetuses with CHB in the absence of high-risk features and associated structural heart disease is good and the majority survives till term without need for any intervention.

Studies have identified high-risk features associated with fetal demise and in such fetuses targeted transplacental therapy with maternal steroids (dexamethasone) in conjunction with beta-agonists may improve outcomes.[12] The high-risk features for suboptimal outcomes include early onset of heart block (<20 weeks), associated CHD, severe valve regurgitation, ventricular dysfunction, and hydrops fetalis. A careful follow-up of the fetal heart rate, cardiac function, and fetal well-being is advised at 2–4 weekly intervals till near term. In stable cases, the pregnancy can be continued to near term and peripartum care can be based on obstetric indications. Fetuses with CHB and hemodynamic compromise may need earlier delivery and planned cesarean section. Most infants with fetal CHB will

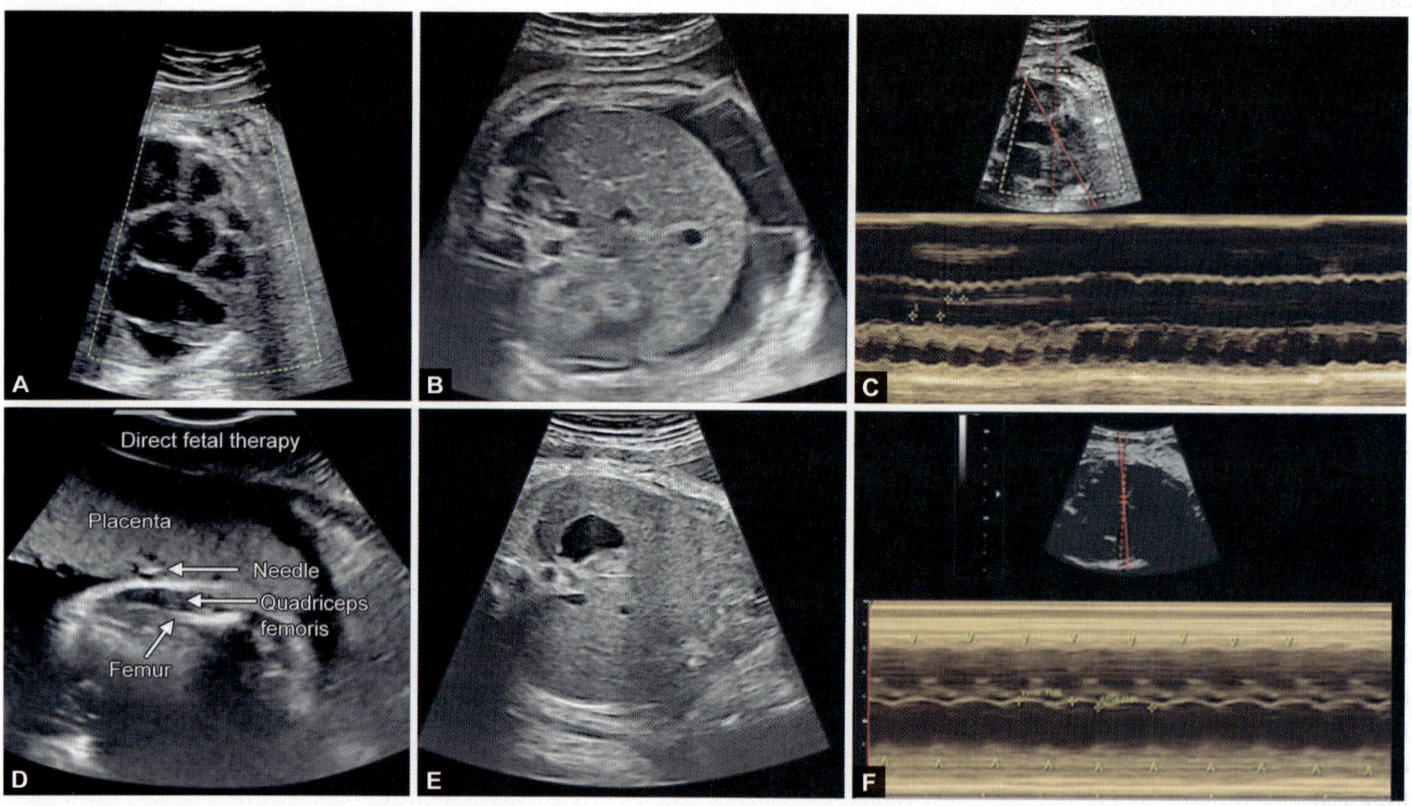

Figs. 5A to F: Fetal tachycardia—evaluation and management. Fetus with atrial flutter with hydrops fetalis at 30 weeks. Four-chamber view (A) and abdominal situs view (B) show significant pericardial effusion and ascites. M-Mode evaluation for cardiac rhythm shows diagnosis of atrial flutter with fast atrial rate and atrioventricular block (C). This fetus was managed by direct intramuscular injection of digoxin (D) and maternal transplacental therapy with sotalol and digoxin. Hydrops fetalis resolved in a weeks' time with resolution of ascites (E) with restoration of sinus rhythm (F).

require a permanent pacemaker implantation within the first year of life.

FETAL INTERVENTIONS FOR STRUCTURAL HEART DEFECTS

At present, the scope of fetal interventions is limited to very few conditions, especially severe obstruction to the outflow tracts.[13] The most common fetal intervention reported is fetal balloon aortic valvuloplasty for critical aortic stenosis with left ventricular dysfunction. Preliminary data suggest that this intervention may prevent progression of aortic stenosis into a more ominous form of heart disease, HLHS. Fetal balloon pulmonary valvuloplasty also has been successfully performed for fetuses with critical pulmonary stenosis. The third fetal cardiac intervention reported is balloon atrial septostomy (enlargement of the restrictive atrial septal communication) in fetuses with HLHS and restrictive patent foramen ovale in order to decompress the left atrium. Needless to say, these interventions are extremely resource intense and require a multidisciplinary team approach. At present, the scope of fetal cardiac interventions in developing countries is very limited.

HYDROPS FETALIS AND FETAL HEART DEFECTS

Hydrops fetalis refers to collection of fluid in ≥2 body cavities of the fetus. In the context of heart defects, presence of hydrops is often a sign of fetal heart failure and is often associated with a guarded prognosis. Fetal heart defects are one of the important causes of nonimmune hydrops fetalis. Some of the important fetal heart defects which can lead to hydrops fetalis include:

- Severe valvular regurgitation (Ebstein anomaly and atrioventricular septal defect)
- Uncontrolled fetal arrhythmias (both tachycardia and CHB)
- Myocardial disorders–fetal myocarditis and cardiomyopathy
- In utero restriction of foramen ovale and ductus arteriosus—isolated or associated with CHD
- Recipient twin in settings like twin-to-twin transfusion syndrome (TTTS)
- Arteriovenous fistulas with high output heart failure (e.g., vein of Galen malformation)
- Some forms of congenital portosystemic shunts.

A careful survey for these anomalies is mandatory as a part of evaluation of any fetus with hydrops fetalis. In particular, assessment of the fetal heart rate and rhythm is extremely important because fetal arrhythmias are a correctable cause of hydrops fetalis. A detailed assessment of cardiac function is also required in these cases using a combination of techniques for systolic and diastolic function. In addition, assessment of the fetal well-being and fetal biophysical profile using Doppler assessment (umbilical artery and vein, ductus venosus, middle cerebral artery) is crucial, both in initial evaluation and follow-up. Management is based on the underlying cause and hence it is very important to exclude a treatable cause such as tachyarrhythmia. Peripartum care and timing of delivery needs to be individualized based on the underlying diagnosis and response to in utero treatment.

PRENATAL DIAGNOSIS OF CONGENITAL HEART DISEASE: IMPLICATIONS TO PEDIATRICIANS AND NEONATOLOGISTS

Pediatricians form an integral component in the management algorithm of a patient with CHD. Neonates with critical forms of CHD form a clinical challenge to pediatricians and neonatologists. Clinical evaluation alone has very low sensitivity in neonates with critical CHD. The availability of pulse oximetry screening has enhanced early suspicion of cyanotic CHD. However, some critical forms of CHD such as transposition of the great arteries may present before the recommended timing of pulse oximetry screening. Pulse oximetry has an overall lower sensitivity for detecting critical left heart obstructions. The diagnostic confirmation of CHD requires echocardiography, especially to distinguish between various CHDs which may have a similar mode of presentation (e.g., HLHS and coarctation of aorta can both present with cardiogenic shock). Neonatal echocardiography requires expertise and often may not be available round the clock, especially in primary and secondary healthcare facilities. Thus, the pediatrician faces significant challenges with respect to diagnostic confirmation, prognostication, and planning the neonatal care in infants with critical CHD.

Prenatal diagnosis and counseling enable planning of the neonatal care in accordance to the family's preferences. Critical CHDs which can be offered corrective intervention or surgery with good long-term outcomes (e.g., transposition of the great arteries, critical aortic or pulmonary stenosis, and coarctation of aorta) may be offered a directed delivery in a center with pediatric cardiac facilities. The benefits of such a strategy have been already discussed in detail in a previous section. In situations of very complex CHDs or CHDs-associated multisystem anomalies where the prognosis is expected to be guarded, the information obtained from prenatal evaluation will help both the clinicians and families in planning the postnatal care. If the family's preference in such cases is not to pursue specialized cardiac care after birth, an informed decision to provide basic neonatal care (comfort care) may be taken with appropriate informed consent of the parents. This will avoid unnecessary escalation of intensive care in very complex CHDs and also reduces the need for transport to tertiary pediatric cardiac facilities. Further, it may also help the obstetrician in planning the timing and nature of delivery with emphasis more focused on the mother in such cases. This strategy may have significant benefits to the patient families as well as healthcare systems in limited resource settings.

CONCLUSION

Prenatal diagnosis offers a much wider options to the expectant family, especially in the setting of developing countries with limited resources to treat complex heart defects. Prenatal diagnosis and planned peripartum care offer an attractive alternative cost-effective strategy to improve perinatal outcomes for critical correctable forms of CHD. Hence, in the current era, it is very important to screen the fetus in all pregnancies and refer suspected cases for a more expert evaluation. A multidisciplinary approach is required once a CHD is diagnosed during pregnancy to provide a detailed family-centric counseling and management options during pregnancy and peripartum period.[14]

REFERENCES

1. Donofrio MT, Moon-Grady AJ, Hornberger LK, Copel JA, Sklansky MS, Abuhamad A, et al. Diagnosis and treatment of fetal cardiac disease: a scientific statement from the American Heart Association. Circulation. 2014;129(21):2183-242.
2. Allan L, Dangel J, Fesslova V, Marek J, Mellander M, Oberhansli I, et al. Recommendations for the practice of fetal cardiology in Europe. Cardio Young. 2004;14(1):109-14.
3. Carvalho JS, Allan LD, Chaoui R, Copel JA, DeVore GR, Hecher K, et al. ISUOG practice guidelines (updated): sonographic screening examination of the fetal heart. Ultrasound Obstet Gynecol. 2013;41(3):348-59.
4. Simpson JM. Impact of fetal echocardiography. Ann Pediatr Card. 2009;2(1):41-50.
5. Bakshi K, Vaidyanathan B, Sundaram KR, Roth SJ, Shivaprakasha K, Rao SG, et al. Determinants of early outcome after neonatal heart surgery in a developing country. J Thorac Cardiovasc Surg. 2007;134(3):765-71.
6. Moons P, Bovijn L, Budts W, Belmans A, Gewillig M. Temporal trends in survival to adulthood among patients born with congenital heart disease from 1970 to 1992 in Belgium. Circulation. 2010;122(22):2264-72.
7. Reddy NS, Kappanayil M, Balachandran R, Jenkins KJ, Sudhakar A, Sunil GS, et al. Preoperative determinants of outcomes of infant heart surgery in a limited-resource setting. Seminars Thoracic Surg. 2015;27(3):331-8.
8. Changlani TD, Jose A, Sudhakar A, Rojal R, Kunjikutty R, Vaidyanathan B. Outcomes of infants with prenatally diagnosed congenital heart disease delivered in a pediatric cardiac facility. Indian Pediatr. 2015;52(10):852-6.
9. Vijayaraghavan A, Sudhakar A, Sundaram KR, Kumar RK, Vaidyanathan B. Prenatal diagnosis and planned peripartum care as a strategy to improve pre-operative status in neonates with critical CHDs in low-resource settings: a prospective study. Cardiol Young. 2019;29(12):1481-8.
10. Marino BS, Lipkin PH, Newburger JW, Peacock G, Gerdes M, Gaynor JW, et al. Neurodevelopmental outcomes in children with congenital heart disease: evaluation and management. A Scientific statement from the American Heart Association. Circulation. 2012;126(9):1143-72.
11. Karmegeraj B, Namdeo S, Sudhakar A, Krishnan V, Kunjukutty R, Vaidyanathan B. Clinical presentation, management, and postnatal outcomes of fetal tachyarrhythmias: a 10-year single-center experience. Ann Pediatr Cardiol. 2018;11(1):34-9.
12. Eliasson H, Sonesson SE, Sharland G, Granath F, Simpson JM, Carvalho J, et al. Isolated atrioventricular block in the fetus. A retrospective, multinational, multicentric study of 175 patients. Circulation. 2011;124(18):1919-26.
13. McElhinney DB, Tworetzky W, Lock JE. Current status of fetal cardiac intervention. Circulation. 2010;121(10):1256-63.
14. Donaghue D, Rychik J. The fetal heart program: a multidisciplinary practice model for the fetus with congenital heart disease. Prog Pediatr Cardiol. 2006;22(1):129-33.

48

CHAPTER

Neonatal Cardiology

Sushil Azad

INTRODUCTION

Congenital heart disease (CHD) is the most common encountered congenital anomaly in neonatal age group accounting for around one-third of all anomalies. One-third to one-fourth of these lesions are potentially fatal during the neonatal age group. Overall prevalence of CHDs is estimated to be around 9 per 1,000 live births.[1] Chapter 1 discusses the epidemiology of heart disease with special reference to the Indian context.

The presentation of CHD in the newborn age varies from totally asymptomatic to life-threatening hypoxia or complete cardiovascular collapse. For CHD to manifest early in the neonatal period with symptoms, the lesions have to be at the severe end of the spectrum. Relatively milder lesions present later in life. The three cardinal signs of all symptomatic CHD in this period are (1) cyanosis, (2) tachypnea, and (3) hypoperfusion (inadequate systemic perfusion) that manifest variably with poor feeding, listlessness, and lethargy. Most of the symptomatic CHD present in neonatal age or early infancy either during transition from fetal to neonatal circulation due to closure of ductus arteriosus or after the fall in pulmonary vascular resistance (PVR) which occurs over 4–6 weeks. While early recognition and diagnosis of these babies are vital, the time "window" between onset of symptoms and a life-threatening situation is often short. For this reason, routine screening with pulse oximeter is now widely recommended for all neonates in many healthcare environments. The rationale and specifics of newborn screening are dealt with in considerable detail in Chapter 6.

TRANSITION FROM FETAL TO POSTNATAL CIRCULATION: NORMAL RESPONSE AND IMPLICATIONS IN PRESENCE OF CONGENITAL HEART DISEASE

Fetal hemodynamics is unique and much different from a postnatal circulation. Clinical manifestations of CHD are intimately related to postnatal changes in the circulation. At birth, dramatic changes occur as the gas exchange function is transferred from the placenta to the lungs. These differences are attributed to the site of gaseous exchange, which occurs at the lungs in newborn, whereas in the fetal life, placenta serves for gaseous exchange and nutrients. The presence of congenital heart lesions can affect the alterations in the circulation necessary and thus affect the postnatal survival.[2]

In the fetus, the gas exchange organ is the placenta, and its vascular connections are in a parallel arrangement with the other systemic organs, remote from the pulmonary circulation. In order to supply deoxygenated blood to the placenta and return oxygenated blood to the systemic organs, a series of extracardiac shunts (ductus venosus and ductus arteriosus) and an intracardiac communication (foramen ovale) are necessary (**Fig. 1**). Also, the presence of these shunts allows the fetal circulation to function in the presence of many critical congenital heart defects without affecting in utero survival. For a variable period of time, neonatal survival is also enabled by the fetal shunts that stay open transiently.[3]

With birth, the function of gas exchange is transferred from the placenta to the lungs, and therefore from the systemic circulation to the pulmonary circulation. The process of ventilation involving physical expansion of the lung with air and removal of the fluid in the airways, as well as an increase in alveolar oxygen concentration and circulatory adjustments associated with birth are largely the result of ventilation-induced decrease in PVR allowing increase in pulmonary blood flow to provide for oxygen uptake and carbon dioxide removal when the umbilical–placental circulation is abolished. The separation of the systemic and pulmonary circulation, characteristic of the postnatal circulation, is achieved by closure of the ductus arteriosus and foramen ovale.

Closure of the foramen ovale results from the rise in the left atrial pressure due to increase in pulmonary blood flow and pulmonary venous return to the left atrium. The decrease in umbilical venous return associated with

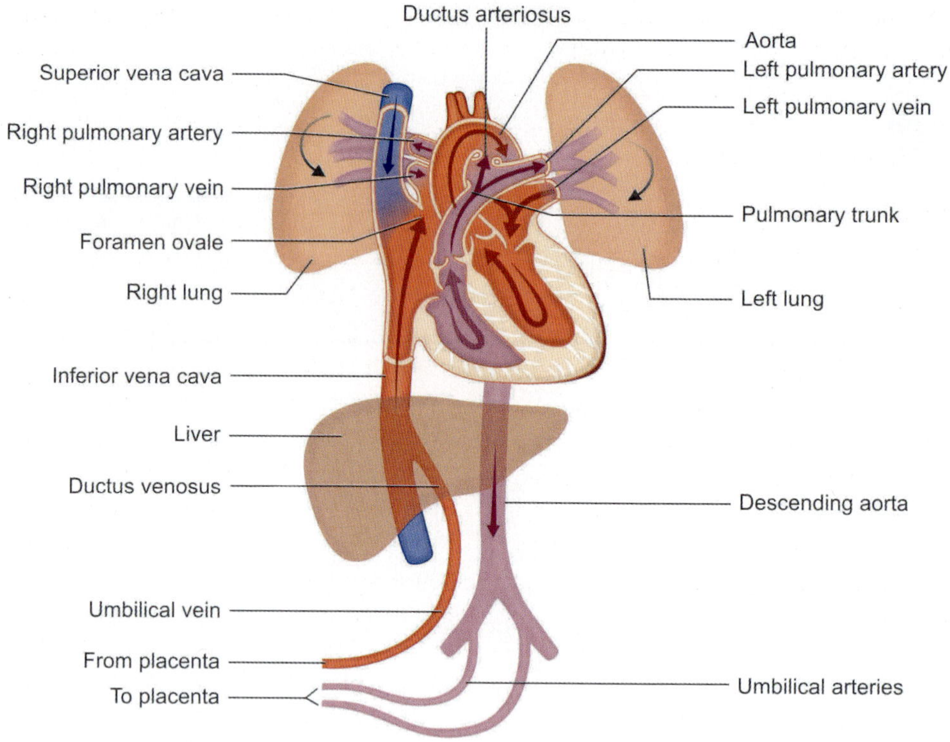

Fig. 1: The fetal circulation elaborating blood flow patterns through cardiac chambers and central blood with more oxygen traversing through the left side of the heart to the brain. Vessels with blood with low oxygen traversing through the right ventricle to lower body and placenta.

elimination of the placental circulation is not necessary for functional closure of the foramen ovale. Closure of the ductus arteriosus proceeds slowly and during the early neonatal period, small shunts through the ductus may occur before it closes completely. The vast majority of ducts almost close completely in the first 48 hours after birth. Apart from these changes, important alterations occur in the cardiac output and oxygen consumption. After initial increase in cardiac output and oxygen consumption in the immediate postnatal period, both decrease. These changes can be partly explained on the basis of the changes in surface area relative to body weight and changes in sympathetic nerve activity.

Another important aspect is understanding of changes in cardiac output. In comparing postnatal cardiac output with fetal cardiac output, it should be appreciated that cardiac output in the fetus is usually expressed as combined ventricular output, whereas postnatal cardiac output represents the output of one of the two ventricles. Also there is an increase in the ventricular output as the metabolic requirements increase after birth. These changes are required for a smooth transition and healthy survival of neonates with structurally normal heart, whereas they are potentially detrimental in those with critical congenital heart disease (CCHD).

With the separation of venous and arterial circulations presence of fetal shunts becomes unnecessary and their persistence may be undesirable.

Decline in the PVR occurs with the expansion of lungs, leading to increase blood flow in lung and reversal of flow in ductus arteriosus.[4] While a rapid decline occurs in the initial 48–96 hours, a slower decline continues up to 4–6 weeks of extrauterine life. The initial decline results from expansion of alveoli with air and immediate recruitment of lung vasculature, the later decline is from increase in the number of vessels with an increase in the net cross-sectional area of pulmonary arteriolar and capillary bed.

For most congenital structural heart disease, the fetal shunt pathways allow redistribution of ventricular blood flows so that systemic blood flow is adequate and fetal growth and development are usually not overtly affected. Uncomplicated ventricular septal defects (VSDs) do not alter the circulation significantly in either the fetus or immediate newborn period, with the important exception of premature infants. With severe left heart obstruction, the burden of systemic and pulmonary blood flow is transferred to the fetal right ventricle, with reversal of blood flow at the foramen ovale, and systemic blood flow almost entirely from the right ventricle via the ductus arteriosus. This "ductal-dependent" systemic circulation is poorly tolerated in the newborn, because normal closure of the ductus arteriosus progressively decreases systemic blood flow and progresses to circulatory failure and shock. Similarly severe right heart obstruction is also well tolerated in the fetus, because the combined fetal cardiac output can be transferred to the aorta, with the ductus arteriosus supplying predominantly lung blood flow. After birth, such "ductal-dependent" pulmonary blood flow can lead to critically low levels of pulmonary blood flow and severe hypoxia with closure of the ductus arteriosus.

An understanding of fetal hemodynamics and the acute and chronic changes that occur with transition to the newborn circulation are important for the care of normal newborns and are crucial to the recognition, diagnosis, and management of the newborn with significant CHD.

INITIAL ASSESSMENT OF A NEONATE WITH SUSPECTED CONGENITAL HEART DISEASE

Critical congenital heart diseases are those which if unrecognized and untreated can lead to death or severe morbidity in immediate newborn period. Included in the list of neonatal critical heart disease are duct-dependent lesions which could be either a duct-dependent systemic circulation presenting as heart failure or duct-dependent pulmonary circulation presenting as severe cyanosis on the closure of ductus and transposition of the great arteries with intact ventricular septum. Ideally, critical CHD should be diagnosed prenatally or identified through routine newborn pulse oximeter screening, but unfortunately majority of these conditions goes unrecognized in initial 24–48 hours and they present with sudden cardiovascular compromise after the closure of ductus arteriosus or the foramen ovale (in transposition). It is therefore essential to diagnose these problems early for optimum outcome.

Initial Presentation

Initial evaluation in all neonates should focus on three cardinal features which are cyanosis, tachypnea, and peripheral perfusion. Differential diagnosis of each include the following described here.

Cyanosis

- *Decreased pulmonary blood flow*: This can result from severely obstructed flow into the pulmonary arteries and a closing ductus arteriosus. Cyanosis can also result from [illegible] obstruction of pulmonary venous return such as in obstructed total anomalous pulmonary venous drainage which results in eventual reduction in pulmonary blood flow.
- Normal to increased pulmonary blood flow but with parallel circulation resulting from transposition of great arteries.

Decreased Systemic Perfusion

- Obstruction of the left heart (left ventricular outflow obstruction or mitral inflow obstruction)
- Cardiac dysfunction (without outflow obstruction).

Tachypnea

- Left-to-right shunts
- Admixture lesions, cyanotic congenital heart diseases with increased pulmonary blood flow such as total anomalous pulmonary venous connection (TAPVC) and truncus arteriosus.

Some lesions are complex with overlapping manifestations (e.g., an infant with hypoplastic left heart syndrome (HLHS) who has decreased systemic perfusion may also be tachypneic and mildly cyanotic). However, even in the most complex cases, one of the major signs usually predominates.

The neonate with cyanotic congenital disease often has a benign birth history with a normal or a nearly normal Apgar score. The ductus arteriosus usually maintains adequate blood flow and mixing immediately after birth, and cyanosis may not be apparent until hours or days after birth that the infant becomes cyanotic as duct closes or flow from duct becomes insufficient and child becomes cyanosed frequently during feeding or crying. Majority are not tachypneic or at most mildly tachypneic. Pulse oximeter screening enables identification of these conditions. The recent addition of routine pulse oximetry screening in many hospitals should greatly enhance our ability to diagnose such infants before discharge. Neonates with left heart obstructive lesions such as aortic stenosis (AS) or coarctation also have usually a benign perinatal history. These infants typically are stable during the first hours of life, but eventually develop poor feeding, pallor, diaphoresis, and tachypnea with respiratory distress. This may occur as late as 3–4 weeks after birth, so it is extremely important for every infant to be carefully assessed at the time of discharge and at subsequent visits during the first month of life. Tachypnea is often a subtle finding that develops over days or weeks, as PVR falls during the first 6 weeks of life. However, some patients with shunts at multiple levels or with VSD and associated left ventricular outflow obstruction or those with specific genetic syndromes can present with tachypnea in first few days of life.

Physical Examination

The principles of cardiovascular examination are enunciated in Chapter 5. General physical examination should include assessment for dysmorphic features of syndromes associated with cardiovascular disease, such as Down syndrome, trisomy 13 and 18, 22q11 deletion (DiGeorge) syndrome, Turner syndrome, Noonan syndrome, Williams syndrome, and trisomy 21.

All vital signs such as assessment of temperature, heart rate, respiratory rate, and blood pressure are measured in conjunction with respiratory status, perfusion, and color. The estimation of oxygen saturation should also be considered a vital sign in the infant and should not only be performed as part of the initial screen. Pulses should be carefully felt in all four extremities. Whenever there is a doubt, a four extremity blood pressure must be obtained. Weight, length, and head circumference are measured and plotted on growth charts to aid in identifying growth impairment. Peripheral cyanosis (acrocyanosis) is common in newborn infants and reflects their normally unstable peripheral vasomotor tone. Central cyanosis, which is indicative of arterial oxygen desaturation, is the important sign to recognize. Since it is difficult to appreciate cyanosis if saturations are >85%, so oxygen saturation should simultaneously be measured in the right hand and a lower extremity. A difference in oxygen saturation of 3–5% may be significant. Respiratory system should be evaluated to look for signs of respiratory distress that include tachypnea and presence of labored efforts in the form of intercostal and/or subcostal retractions, nasal flaring, and grunting.

Cardiac examination is of limited value. The limited sensitivity and specificity of physical examination is well documented. Nonetheless, physical examination of the cardiovascular system must be carried out because there are instances when it is of value. The cardiac examination begins with palpation of the precordium. Unlike the older patient, the normal neonate with thin sternum can have parasternal impulse. The left ventricular apical impulse is not usually palpable in a normal newborn infant because the dominant right ventricle displaces the left ventricle posteriorly. A palpable left ventricular impulse usually indicates increased left ventricular volume load as the ventricular cavity dilates and extends anteriorly and laterally. Auscultation should be performed in a systematic manner. In CHD, the splitting of the second heart sound provides important diagnostic information but in newborns with fast heart rates, it is difficult to assess second heart sound. If a splitting of the second heart sound is discernible, it is actually reassuring because most serious CHDs can then be ruled out. The location and frequency of murmur may help in possible differential diagnosis, especially in obstructive lesions but in case of many large left-to-right shunts, there may not be any murmur in immediate newborn period and murmur only appears as PVR falls. Additionally, in many critical CHDs, no murmurs may be audible.

In the rare instances when a diastolic murmur is heard in a newborn, it is of considerable value. The conditions associated with an early diastolic murmur include persistent truncus arteriosus with a regurgitant truncal valve, tetralogy of Fallot with absent pulmonary valve syndrome, and aorta to left ventricular tunnel.

Evaluation of Other Systems

Abnormalities of other organ systems are present in about 25–30% of newborns with congenital cardiovascular disease, and the frequency is higher in newborns with critical congenital cardiovascular disease so it is essential to perform a thorough head-to-toe examination. Some signs can be quite subtle. A submucous cleft palate may be missed if not specifically looked for. Cutaneous manifestations of conditions such as tuberous sclerosis can be of considerable diagnostic value.

Electrocardiogram

Electrocardiogram in a normal neonate has right ventricular dominance and thus a pattern of right ventricular hypertrophy is present with right axis deviation, prominent R waves, and upright T waves in the right precordium. T waves become inverted after 5–10 days in the precordial leads (**Fig. 2**). Presence of left ventricular forces is always abnormal. Electrocardiogram has limited specificity and sensitivity in the diagnosis of CHD in the neonate. However, in settings where echocardiography is not readily available, it is sometimes useful in ruling out the presence of significant heart disease particularly if combined with a physical examination, a postductal pulse oximeter, and chest X-ray. A detailed description on interpretation of the ECG (electrocardiogram) in the neonate is provided in Chapter 7.

Chest X-ray

The chest radiograph provides information about the heart size and contour, pulmonary blood flow, and the

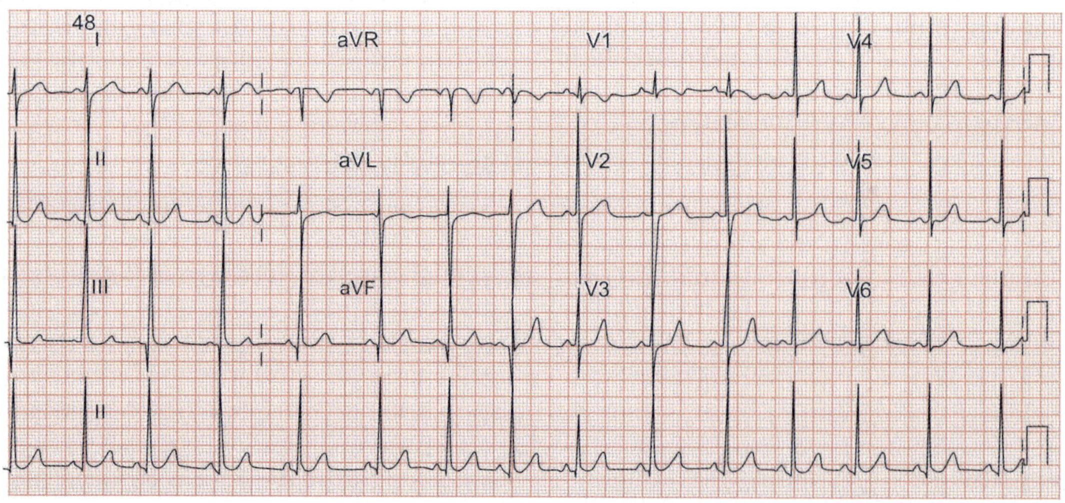

Fig. 2: Normal electrocardiogram (ECG) in a neonate with q waves in inferior leads, right QRS axis and prominent RV forces, and inverted T waves inverted in V1.

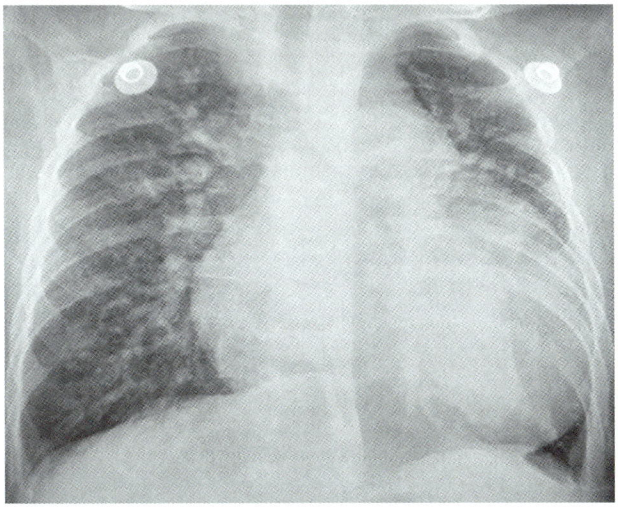

Fig. 3: Chest radiograph of a neonate with obstructed total anomalous pulmonary venous return, showing dilated right atrium, and right ventricle with pulmonary venous congestion.

lung parenchyma. Absence of a thymic shadow may point to the diagnosis of 22q11 deletion (DiGeorge). Increased pulmonary blood flow is often difficult to assess by conventional chest radiography at birth. Conversely, pulmonary venous congestion can be appreciated very soon after birth, as pulmonary blood flow increases dramatically and rapidly increases pulmonary venous pressures when the left side of the heart is critically obstructed. Lesions such as TAPVC with obstruction show increased venous markings and pulmonary edema within hours of birth (**Fig. 3**). Pulmonary oligemia is suggested by dark lung fields. This X-ray finding is of value in a hypoxic neonate when echocardiography is not available. A combination of significant desaturation with a dark lung fields (blue baby-black lungs) justifies starting prostaglandin even in the absence of a confirmed echocardiographic diagnosis.

Echocardiogram

Echocardiography is the mainstay of the diagnosis of the newborn with symptomatic cardiovascular disease. It is important to follow systematic and comprehensive approach to reach a conclusive diagnosis.

GENERAL PRINCIPLES OF MANAGEMENT OF NEONATE WITH CONGENITAL HEART DISEASE

The general approach to a neonate with CHD should follow the usual guidelines for management of a critically ill neonate. More detailed information regarding specific medical and surgical care on specific CHDs is provided in the chapters that describe individual defects (*see* Chapters 21–40) and postoperative care (*see* Chapter 13).

Use of Oxygen Supplementation

Although supplemental oxygen is often administered to infants with known or suspected CHD but rationale to use should be guided by underlying cardiovascular pathophysiology. Oxygen can sometimes have potentially detrimental effect in selected situations. The pulmonary vasculature responds to oxygen administration by vasodilation. This is detrimental in neonates with CHD and unobstructed pulmonary blood flow because pulmonary vasodilation results in pulmonary overcirculation and systemic hypoperfusion. Examples of such conditions include persistent truncus arteriosus and all examples of single ventricle physiology with no pulmonic stenosis. Additionally, in duct-dependent systemic circulation (e.g., HLHS, severe coarctation, and VSD with aortic arch interruption), there is the added concern of severe gut and visceral hypoperfusion from duct steal with resultant necrotizing enterocolitis, liver, and kidney injury. For this reason, in all neonates with CHD where a reduction in PVR is deleterious, oxygen administration should be avoided as far as possible or used with utmost caution. It is usually far better to have some resting desaturation (~80%) than have a newborn with pulmonary overcirculation.

An additional concern about oxygen administration is the potential for closure of the ductus arteriosus in duct-dependent situations, including duct-dependent pulmonary blood flow. This is a matter of some concern but perhaps is overcome by administration of prostaglandin.

Role of Mechanical Ventilation

Mechanical ventilation is often beneficial to the infant with heart failure with decreased systemic perfusion and inadequate systemic oxygen delivery because decreasing the work of breathing decreases oxygen consumption. It is also particularly helpful when there is pulmonary congestion from pulmonary venous obstruction (such as in obstructed total anomalous pulmonary venous return). However, in neonates with CHD presenting primarily with cyanosis, mechanical ventilation may not be needed particularly if the baby is comfortable and hypoxia is not severe (saturations in excess of 70%). Unfortunately, mechanical ventilations are often instituted because of low saturations alone. The failure of mechanical ventilation to restore normal oxygen saturations is often a clear indicator of underlying cyanotic CHD.

Use of Prostaglandins

Many neonates with CCHD present when ductus arteriosus starts to close soon after birth. Use of prostaglandin E1 (PGE1) is the initial therapy in most instances and the decision to initiate therapy with PGE1 is usually straightforward.

In deeply cyanotic neonates with a suspicion of heart disease, it is reasonable to initiate prostaglandin without confirmation of the exact CHD. Opening of the patent ductus arteriosus (PDA) promptly improves saturation when the pulmonary blood flow is duct-dependent (all forms of pulmonary atresia and critical pulmonary stenosis). In transposition with intact ventricular septum, the opening

BOX 1: Prostaglandin E1 administration guidelines.

Dosage

- Recommended starting dose: 0.05 μg/kg/min;
  - Increase to 0.1 μg/kg/min if desired effect not seen within 10–15 min
  - Reduce to 0.02 μg/kg/min 1–2 hours after the desired response is obtained

Preparation

- 1 amp = 1 mL = 500 μg
- So, 0.1 mL = 50 μg
- Now take 0.1 mL and dilute with 49.9 mL 10% Dextrose to make total solution of 50 mL
- Therefore 50 mL = 50 μg, i.e., 1 mL = 1 μg

Example: Suppose required dose is 0.01 μg/kg/min for 2 kg baby

= (0.01 × body wt × 60)

= μg/hr = (0.01 × 2 × 60)

= 1.2 μg/hr

= 1.2 mL/hr [1 μg = 1 mL]

BOX 2: Communication checklist for transportation for newborns with suspected heart disease.

Communication checklist for transportation

- *Prenatal background*: Term or preterm, birth order, age of mother, important maternal conditions
- *Birth*: Mode of delivery, relevant antenatal issues, Apgar scores, birth weight, significant postnatal events, if any?
- *Clinical presentation*: Why was heart disease suspected? Are there associated anomalies or abnormal facies?
- *Current condition*: Vitals (heart rate, respiratory rate, oxygen saturation, peripheral circulation), laboratory tests (a baseline arterial blood gas analysis report is valuable, if available), and feeding
- *Preliminary diagnosis of the cardiovascular condition*: Results of the physical examination, chest X-ray, ECG, and echocardiogram
- *What has been done so far to resuscitate the newborn?* What access has been obtained? Is the child ventilated or breathing spontaneously? What medications have been given (specifically, inotropes, and prostaglandin)?
- *Relevant socioeconomic issues*: What is the social and economic background of the family? Which family members are likely to accompany the child? How much has been communicated to them?
- *Logistics*: Transport distance, mode of transport, and transporting personnel? Expected time of departure and arrival?

of the PDA enables better mixing between the parallel circulations. However, PGE1 works best in transposition if there is a communication at atrial level. If the atrial septum is intact, PGE1 may not improve saturations significantly.

The second major category for PGE1 administration is duct-dependent systemic blood flow. This results from a critically obstructed aortic flow and presents with inadequate systemic perfusion. Included in the list of conditions with duct-dependent systemic circulation are critical AS and HLHS where the entire systemic blood flow is compromised as well as conditions such as interrupted aortic arch and critically severe coarctation where blood flow to the descending aorta is compromised. A number of specific considerations dictate the use of PGE1 (**Box 1**).

It is generally advisable to initiate PGE1 therapy for an infant with suspected cardiovascular disease before transporting to a tertiary care center for more definitive diagnosis and treatment. Confirmation of the diagnosis should not delay initiation of therapy. The main challenges with PGE1 include apnea and hypotension. Apnea is often transient and dose dependent. The initial dose of PGE1 reduced once the duct is usually 0.05 μg/kg/min. This can be reduced to as low as 0.01 μg/kg/min once the PDA is opened. In many instances, the apnea can be managed through bag and mask ventilation; however, it is sometimes necessary to intubate the baby. Many referring institutions prefer endotracheal intubation and mechanical ventilation for babies on PGE1 to ensure safety during transportation. Hypotension results from vasodilation and is usually responsive to fluid boluses. Other side effects of PGE1 include bradycardia, flushing, tachycardia, hypotension, and fever. Relatively rare side effects include seizures, diarrhea (2%), and gastric distension (1%). Leukocytosis and thrombocytopenia can be seen in babies receiving PGE1. Administration over days and weeks may result in capillary leak and tissue edema that may be noticeable during cardiac surgery. Long-standing usage can result in gastric outlet obstruction and cortical hyperostosis.

Transportation of a Newborn with Suspected Heart Disease

Newborns are typically born in facilities that do not have a pediatric cardiac program and need to be transported to tertiary programs that are often located at a considerable distance. Transport of sick neonates between facilities is a critical component of neonatal care and is well known to impact clinical outcomes. Regionalized systems of transport have been developed in advanced economies and they allow for minimum disruption in care for the newborn. The situation is strikingly different in India. Here, transport usually involves road transport over large distances to the few specialized neonatal facilities, in poorly equipped ambulances, often without appropriately trained medical personnel. Systems for effective communication or in-transit monitoring or management are poorly developed. These factors are especially important for neonates with heart disease. The critical elements in transportation of a neonate with suspected or proven to a tertiary are summarized here.

Comprehensive and accurate communication of information helps mitigate challenges during transport. Additionally, it is essential in ensuring adequate preparation in the receiving pediatric heart center.

The checklist in **Box 2** can serve as a guideline for communication between the referring pediatrician or neonatologist and the pediatric cardiology program before transportation is undertaken.

TABLE 1: Cyanotic congenital heart defects in newborns.

Physiologic category	*Conditions*	*Manifestations*
Reduced pulmonary blood flow	*Intact ventricular septum*: Pulmonary atresia, critical pulmonary stenosis, Ebstein anomaly, and severe congenital tricuspid regurgitation *Interventricular communication*: Pulmonary atresia or severe pulmonic stenosis in association with tetralogy of Fallot, double-outlet right ventricle, transposition with VSD, corrected transposition, single ventricle, and tricuspid atresia	Cyanosis, hypoxia as soon as the duct starts to close often in the first 48–72 hours after birth. Those with pulmonary stenosis will have variable degrees of cyanosis depending on severity of pulmonary stenosis. Milder forms of pulmonary stenosis can have minimal hypoxia. Chest X-ray shows dark lungs. Heart size is normal except for those with tricuspid valve disease
Increased pulmonary blood flow	Persistent truncus arteriosus, unobstructed total anomalous pulmonary venous return (TAPVR), transposition with VSD*, double-outlet right ventricle with subpulmonic VSD (Taussig–Bing anomaly)*, single ventricle with increased blood flow, and hypoplastic left heart syndrome	Cyanosis is often mild, heart failure is the dominant symptom. Chest X-ray shows increased pulmonary blood flow with cardiac enlargement
Obstruction of pulmonary venous return	Obstructed TAPVR, mitral atresia with a restrictive patent foramen ovale; hypoplastic left heart syndrome with restrictive patent foramen ovale	Cyanosis, hypoxia, and heart failure. Chest X-ray shows hazy lungs (ground glass appearance)
Parallel circulation with poor mixing	D transposition with intact ventricular septum	Cyanosis, hypoxia dominates symptoms in spite of there being an overall increase in pulmonary blood flow. Chest X-ray shows increased lung vasculature

*These conditions can potentially be classified in more than one category parallel circulation that contributes to reduced saturations.

It is essential to pay attention to every element of the transportation process. This includes accompanying personnel, monitoring vitals, and general care of the neonate. Specific concerns in babies with heart disease relate to apnea with prostaglandin that often necessitates endotracheal intubation and mechanical ventilation, the need to avoid excessive oxygenation and ventilation as mentioned previously in this chapter. It is important to also emphasize here that sepsis is common in newborns with heart disease and it can significantly worsen eventual outcomes. The potential for nosocomial sepsis is particularly high for sick newborns that are being transported. Meticulous attention to aseptic precautions is extremely important.

THE NEONATE WITH CYANOSIS

Cyanosis refers to visible duskiness of skin resulting from hypoxia and generally requires the presence of 3–5 g of deoxygenated hemoglobin. In a neonate, milder levels of desaturation (>85–90%) may be difficult to identify clinically. In the presence of anemia, it may be impossible to identify even greater degrees of desaturation. Because of these considerations, measurement of oxygen saturation is almost universally adopted. The pulse oximeter is sensitive and accurate especially in saturation ranges of 70–100%. At lower saturations, the numbers displayed on the oximeter may not be an accurate representation of the actual saturation.

Cyanosis in the absence of significant respiratory distress is almost always caused by structural heart disease because pulmonary disease as a cause of cyanosis is usually associated with severe respiratory distress. If the cyanosis is not recognized early, the child can rapidly decompensate. Neonates with hypoxemia can also be tachypneic but respiratory distress is rarely associated with features such as retractions and nasal flaring. The hyperoxia test can help identify the cause of desaturation. However, in practice, an echocardiogram is obtained and the hyperoxia test is rarely required. In hyperoxia test, 100% oxygen given to for 10 minutes and arterial blood gas is performed from a postductal artery (one of the femoral arteries of the umbilical artery). If the partial pressure of oxygen (PaO_2) remains low (<100 mm Hg), it suggests heart disease.[5] PaO_2 in excess of 200 mm Hg makes CHD quite unlikely and values between 100 and 200 constitute a gray zone. Selected patients with persistent truncus arteriosus and duct-dependent pulmonary circulation (e.g., VSD with arch interruption) may have postductal PaO_2 in excess of 100 mm Hg after oxygen.[6] There is insufficient validation of the hyperoxia test and in practice, an echocardiogram allows a rapid and accurate diagnosis and avoids the need for obtaining an arterial blood gas sample.

Cyanosis in cyanotic CHD results from mixing of systemic and pulmonary venous return which can occur at atrial, ventricular, or great vessels level.

Cyanotic CHDs are broadly subclassified according to the amount of pulmonary blood flow.[7] A more complete classification is presented in **Table 1**.

The first category of defects is conditions with reduced pulmonary blood flow. The main manifestations are that of cyanosis. There is no evidence of heart failure in most situations with the exception of severe tricuspid regurgitation and neonatal Ebstein anomaly. If the pulmonary blood flow is severely restricted, then pulmonary blood flow is maintained by aortic flow through ductus arteriosus. These lesions present with profound cyanosis after closure of ductus. Milder forms of the lesions may manifest at later age in life. On the other hand, defects with no restriction to pulmonary blood flow present with features of cyanosis, failure to thrive, and congestive heart failure after postnatal fall in PVR. Echocardiography is crucial for accurate diagnosis of the lesion, which helps in planning the further management.

In the second category, cyanotic CHD with increased pulmonary blood flow, cyanosis is mild and features of heart failure dominate. Included in this list are a number of conditions with a large interventricular communication and absence of pulmonary stenosis. Also included here is total anomalous pulmonary venous return and persistent truncus arteriosus that has communications at the great vessel level in addition to a large VSD. This is a group of conditions where oxygen administration is potentially deleterious because reductions in PVR results in increased pulmonary blood flow at the cost of systemic blood flow.

The third physiological category in **Table 1** is parallel circulation with little intercirculatory mixing. The classic example here is transposition of the great arteries with intact ventricular septum. Here, deoxygenated systemic venous blood is returned to the aorta and oxygen-rich pulmonary venous blood is pumped into pulmonary arteries. Survival requires mixing between the two circulations that best happens at the level of atrial septum.

Finally, obstruction of pulmonary venous return results in marked elevation of PVR that essentially serves to reduce the pulmonary blood flow and results in deep cyanosis. Examples include obstructed total anomalous pulmonary venous return, mitral atresia, or HLHS with restrictive atrial septal communication.

While echocardiography is essential for accurate anatomic and physiologic diagnosis, the chest X-ray can provide useful clues (*see* Chapter 8). In neonates with decreased pulmonary blood flow, the X-ray usually shows normal cardiac silhouette with pulmonary oligemia (**Fig. 4**). Exceptions are neonates with Ebstein anomaly, severe tricuspid regurgitation, and severe right ventricular dysplasia (Uhl's anomaly). A ground glass haze in a hypoxic neonate should raise the suspicion of obstructed total anomalous pulmonary venous return. Cyanotic heart disease with increased pulmonary blood flow has evidence of pulmonary plethora and increased heart size may be noted. While the egg on side appearance is considered diagnostic, it is only seen in a third of neonates with transposition (**Fig. 5**).

The electrocardiogram is also helpful. In general, any deviation from the age-appropriate neonatal ECG pattern (*see* Chapter 7) should raise the suspicion of CHD. Absent or decreased right ventricular forces are characteristically seen in pulmonary atresia with intact ventricular septum and tricuspid atresia. In the former, the axis is normal (**Fig. 6**) but the latter shows left axis deviation (**Fig. 7**). Right atrial enlargement may be seen but this is an insensitive sign.

THE NEONATE WITH SYSTEMIC HYPOPERFUSION

Reduced systemic perfusion is also a common presentation in neonates with CCHD and represents an important cause of mortality. Although this clinical scenario is usually of noncardiac etiology (most commonly sepsis), cardiac lesions should always be excluded. Hypoperfusion due to noncardiac causes is either by reducing systemic vascular resistance (SVR) or decrease in left ventricular function. Low SVR causes pooling of blood in various vascular beds, diminishing the effective circulating volume to a critical level.

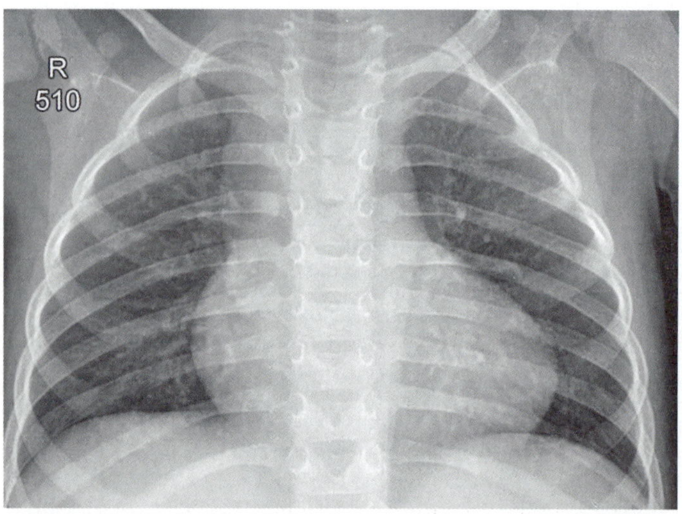

Fig. 4: Chest radiograph of a neonate with tetralogy of Fallot, showing normal cardiac silhouette with concave main pulmonary segment and reduced pulmonary vascularity.

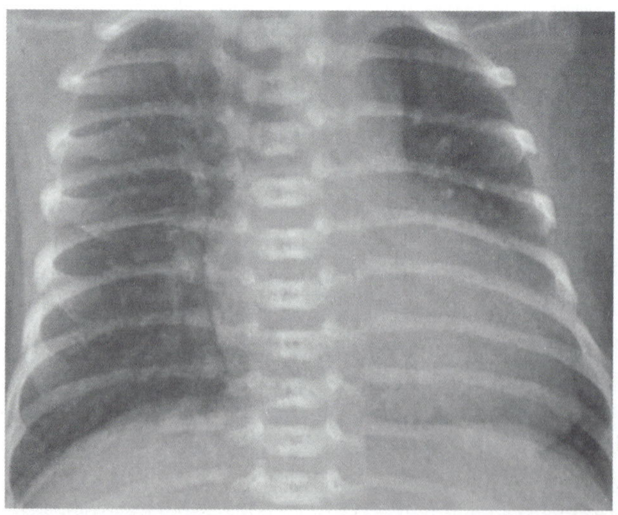

Fig. 5: Chest radiograph of a neonate with transposition with intact septum, showing mild cardiomegaly with narrow vascular pedicle and increased pulmonary vascularity.

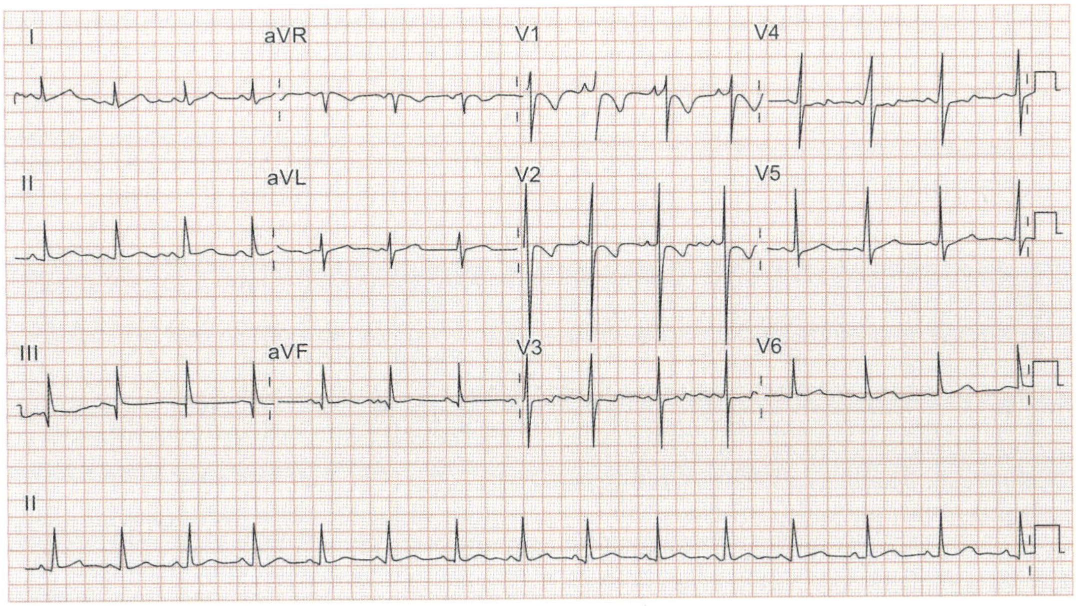

Fig. 6: Electrocardiogram (ECG) of a child with pulmonary atresia intact ventricular septum. Note the presence of right QRS axis and absent of right ventricular forces in precordial leads.

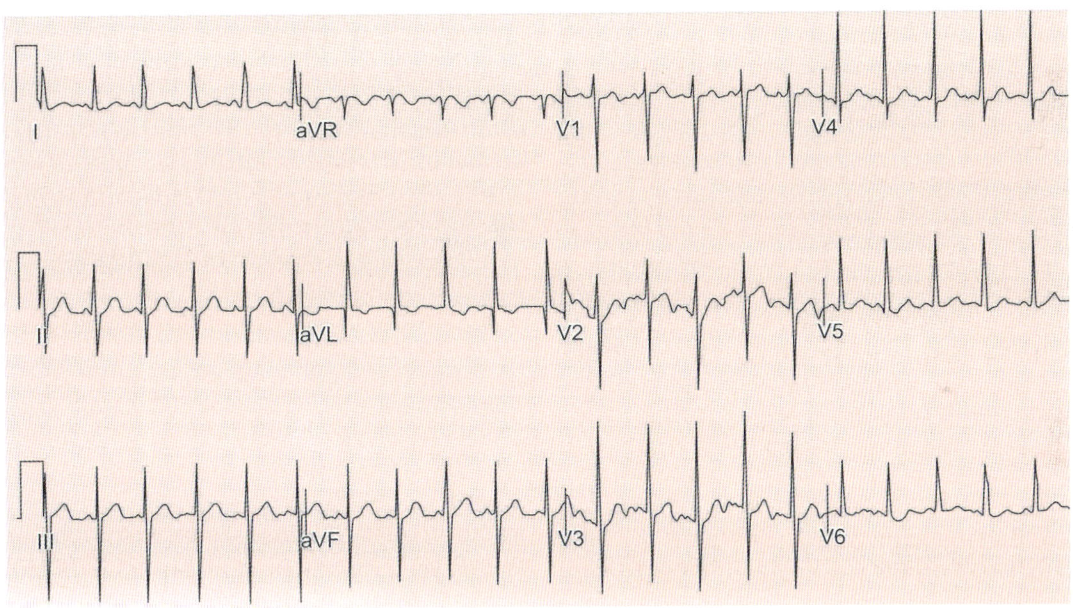

Fig. 7: Electrocardiogram (ECG) of patient with tricuspid atresia. Note the presence of left axis deviation, counter clockwise looping and absence of right ventricular forces in right precordial leads.

The signs of reduced perfusion include listlessness and lethargy, failure to accept feeds, cold extremities, and diminished capillary refill. Tachypnea with labored respiratory efforts is a common accompanying feature. This clinical presentation is not unique to heart disease and a diagnosis of neonatal sepsis is often considered as the likely cause. If heart disease is not considered as a possibility, it is likely to be missed. A low postductal saturation can point toward a duct-dependent circulation. Alternatively, a postductal blood gas sample obtained after oxygen administration can also point toward heart disease. It is wise to obtain echocardiograms at a low threshold for neonates labeled as "sepsis" when the response to initial treatment does not result in the expected degree of improvement.

The two hemodynamic categories of cardiovascular lesions that cause systemic hypoperfusion are as follows:

- *Left-sided obstructive lesions*: These include HLHS, critical AS, interruption of the aortic arch, and severe coarctation (**Table 2**; *See* details in Chapter 28).
- *Severe systemic ventricle dysfunction without obstruction*:[8] A variety of conditions can result in neonatal left ventricular dysfunction. They include myocarditis, metabolic causes, cardiomyopathies, and persistent tachyarrhythmias (tachycardiomyopathy).

TABLE 2: Left ventricular inflow and outflow obstructions.

Anatomic level	*Cardiac lesion*	*Manifestations*
Left atrium and mitral valve	· Cor triatriatum · Supravalvar mitral ring · Mitral atresia · Congenital mitral stenosis	Cor triatriatum is rare and results in pulmonary venous hypertension with pulmonary edema. Mitral atresia typically occurs in the context of hypoplastic left heart syndrome; it can also occur in association with other heart defects and manifests dramatically if there is a restrictive atrial communication. Supramitral ring and congenital mitral stenosis typically manifests later in infancy or childhood and is often associated with obstructions at multiple levels (Shone complex)
Left ventricular cavity	· Hypoplastic left heart syndrome (HLHS) · Endocardial fibroelastosis (EFE)	While HLHS manifests dramatically as a duct-dependent systemic lesion, EFE tends to present in association with critical aortic stenosis
Left ventricular outflow	· Subvalvar aortic stenosis · Aortic valve stenosis · Aortic atresia · Supravalvular aortic stenosis	Only severe aortic valve stenosis manifests during the neonatal period. Subvalvar narrowing and supravalvar narrowing tend to present later
Aortic arch	· Coarctation of aorta · Hypoplastic aortic arch · Interrupted aortic arch	Coarctation has a wide spectrum and often the relatively severe lesions present early. Coarctation is also associated with a wide variety of CHDs with increased pulmonary blood flow. Interrupted arch is often associated with VSD; details are discussed in Chapter 29

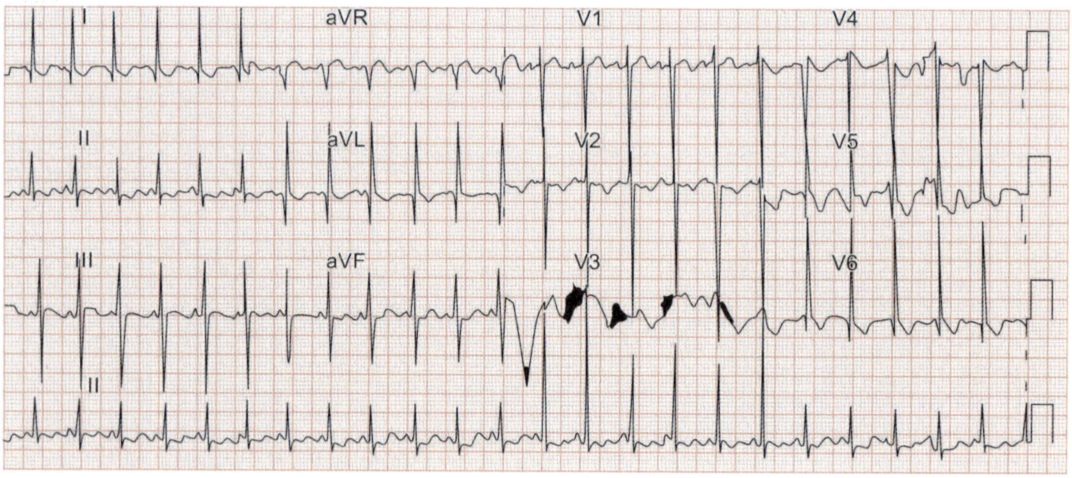

Fig. 8: Electrocardiogram (ECG) of patient with anomalous origin of left coronary artery from pulmonary artery (ALCAPA). Note the presence of deep Q waves in lead 1 and avL, V5 and V6 with ST depression and T wave inversion in these leads.

Obstructive lesions may remain asymptomatic in early neonatal period (typically first 24–72 hours) because of the presence of PDA, which maintains the forward flow to descending aorta or retrograde filling of ascending aorta.[9] On physical examination, peripheral pulses will be feeble in critical AS and HLHS, whereas those with severe coarctation of aorta (CoA) and interrupted aortic arch (IAA) will have feeble or absent femoral pulses. A gallop rhythm can be appreciated in ventricular dysfunction from conditions such as myocarditis together with muffled heart sounds. Chest X-ray may reveal cardiomegaly with features of pulmonary venous hypertension. Electrocardiogram shows right ventricular hypertrophy in severe coarctation or arch interruption. Left ventricular hypertrophy with strain pattern may be seen in critical AS. Absence of left ventricular forces is seen in HLHS. The ECG may show signs apicolateral ischemia suggesting anomalous left coronary artery from pulmonary artery (**Fig. 8**) in the occasional cases that present in the neonatal period. A consistent difference of >10 mm Hg between right upper and lower extremity blood pressure is suggestive of coarctation. Echocardiography is crucial to establish accurate anatomic and physiologic diagnosis.

Among these cardiac defects, HLHS is often the first to be noticed within hours of birth, as PDA is the sole systemic supply and even its slightest constriction leads to decreased systemic blood supply. Critical AS and interrupted aortic arch become symptomatic slightly later as some forward output across the aortic valve prevents onset of symptoms. Severe coarctation in most infants manifests with signs of hypoperfusion at 7–10 days of life and less severe forms may not be discovered until months or years after the neonatal period. Decreased femoral pulses can be appreciated well before features of low systemic output and this highlights the importance of complete physical examination including upper and lower limb blood pressure before discharge.

Irrespective of the etiology, initial management of neonates with cardiovascular collapse must consist of stabilization of the airway and correction of hypotension, electrolyte abnormalities, and metabolic acidosis. Early intubation and mechanical ventilation is imperative. Patients with a presumptive diagnosis of PDA-dependent systemic circulation should be started on prostaglandin E1 (PGE1) infusion.[9] The initial dose is often higher in neonates with duct-dependent systemic circulation because the duct needs to open fully (>5 mm) to enable systemic circulation. This is unlike duct-dependent pulmonary circulation where even a small degree of patency (2–3 mm) may be adequate to sustain the pulmonary blood flow. The typical starting dose is 0.05 μg/kg/min and this may be increased to 0.1 μg/kg/min if desired effect is not achieved. Once the desired effect is obtained, the dose can be reduced gradually to as low as 0.01 μg/kg/min. It is imperative to be mindful of ventilation. The FiO_2 should be as low as possible (<25%), ventilation should be gentle to keep PCO_2 in the 40s. A systemic saturation in the low 80s is acceptable because this usually enables adequate systemic perfusion. A lot of damage can result from pulmonary vasodilation and systemic hypoperfusion from overzealous hyperventilation and oxygenation. Definitive treatment depends on the type of cardiac defect and is discussed in the chapter on left-sided outflow tract obstructions (*see* Chapter 28).

THE NEONATE WITH RESPIRATORY DISTRESS

Respiratory distress with no cyanosis and normal peripheral perfusion are also one of the manifestations of neonate with symptomatic CHD. Particularly in the absence of a murmur, the diagnosis of heart disease is often delayed or missed entirely because respiratory distress alone in an acyanotic infant is commonly associated with pulmonary cause than with cardiac cause. Furthermore, symptoms usually develop gradually over the first few days or weeks of life, and the respiratory symptoms, such as tachypnea with feeding, are often subtle. It may take several weeks or more to recognize that the infant is growing poorly and could possibly have structural heart disease.

A cardiac etiology is suggested by the fact that the baby is often unperturbed by the tachypnea or because of abnormal cardiovascular examination or in the event oxygen saturation is low. An abnormal cardiac silhouette and vascular markings on chest X-ray may also suggest heart disease. Echocardiography should be performed in suspected cardiac disease. A common feature of this group of cardiac lesion is excessive pulmonary blood, where symptomatic neonates present with respiratory distress or failure to thrive without overt cyanosis. Symptoms are rather subtle and usually develop gradually over the first few days or weeks of life. Development of symptoms coincides with the timing of the drop in PVR except in neonates with very large arteriovenous malformations (rarely with hydrops fetalis) and preterm PDA, where they can present in early days of life. In addition to tachypnea, these neonates also exhibit signs and symptoms of congestive heart failure including failure to gain weight.[10] Excessive pulmonary blood flow results in increased precapillary pressures leading to excessive lymphatic flow. Lymphatics are unable to drain this excessive interstitial fluid production, causing accumulation of interstitial fluid. Interstitial edema leads to activation of J (juxtacapillary) receptors, which increase the respiratory rate. In addition, accumulation of interstitial fluid impairs bronchial function.

Table 3 lists the common left-to-right shunts that manifest in the neonatal period. At birth, the pressures in the left and right chambers and arteries are almost identical. Neonatal right ventricle and left ventricle are of equal thickness and stiffness. As a result, even in the presence of communication, left-to-right shunt across the defect, at birth is small or nonexistent. Although PVR begins to fall immediately at birth, it takes 4–6 weeks fall sufficiently to enable significant increases in pulmonary blood flow. In defects at ventricular and arterial level with the fall in PVR allows the left-to-right shunt to manifest early because the pressure head of the left side is directly communicated across

TABLE 3: Left-to-right shunts that manifest in the newborn period.

Anatomic level	*Cardiac lesion*	*Comments*
Atrioventricular (AV) septum	AV septal septum defect	Early presentation often results from severe associated AV valve regurgitation
Ventricular septum	Ventricular septal defect (VSD)	Isolated VSD seldom presents in the neonatal period; Early heart failure in neonates with VSD should point toward associated coarctation or arch interruption. In preterm infants, a premature fall in pulmonary vascular resistance (PVR) can result in early presentation
Aortopulmonary (AP) septum	AP window Anomalous origin of pulmonary artery branch from ascending aorta	AP window often presents in the neonatal period because the shunt is very large. Anomalous origin of one pulmonary artery from the aorta (hemitruncus) often manifests early with heart failure
Ductus arteriosus	Patent ductus arteriosus	Preterm newborns with PDA manifest early because of early fall in PVR

the defect. Clinically, this coincides with the appearance of shunt murmur. In atrial septal defects, a thick-walled and poorly distensible right ventricle prevents a large left-to-right shunt. It takes several months for the right ventricle to remodel and accept and enable an increase in pulmonary blood flow (*see* Chapter 21).

PERSISTENT PULMONARY HYPERTENSION OF THE NEWBORN

In normal neonatal circulatory transition, there is a rapid fall in PVR with the first breath and a marked increase in SVR with removal of placental circulation after clamping of umbilical cord. Persistent pulmonary hypertension of the newborn (PPHN) is characterized by sustained elevation in PVR with normal or low SVR and is also called as persistent fetal circulation, i.e., unsuccessful transition of fetal circulation at birth. Factors associated with high vascular tone in fetus are fluid-filled alveoli compressing pulmonary arteries, low alveolar and arteriolar PaO_2, and lack of pulmonary vasodilators such as prostaglandin I2 (PGI2) and nitric oxide (NO), the production of which is low in fetus and increases as gestational age increases. It is associated with significant mortality and adverse long-term sequelae among survivors. It is associated with a multitude of prenatal, perinatal, lung, and cardiac disorders.[11] The importance of PPHN in the context of heart disease lies in the fact that it figures in the differential diagnosis of CHD presenting at birth. Additionally, it is important to rule out specific conditions that are often mislabeled as isolated pulmonary hypertension (*see* Chapter 18). **Box 3** lists the etiology of PPHN.

Maternal factors include asthma, diabetes, or maternal use of nonsteroidal anti-inflammatory drugs with in utero constriction of the ductus arteriosus and use of selective serotonin reuptake inhibitors also contributes to PPHN. Ventricular dysfunction, myocarditis, premature ductal constriction, and left- or right-sided obstructive lesions can also lead to PPHN.

BOX 3: Etiology of persistent pulmonary hypertension in the newborn (PPHN).

- Idiopathic or "back lung" (10%):
  - Abnormal muscularization of pulmonary arteries
- Secondary causes:
  - Congenital diaphragmatic hernia
  - Parenchymal diseases of lung:
    - Respiratory distress syndrome
    - Pneumonia
  - Meconium aspiration syndrome:
    - Meconium stained fluid—5–24%
  - Birth asphyxia:
    - 20–25% of asphyxiated neonates can have pulmonary arterial hypertension
  - Transient tachypnea of the newborn
  - Pulmonary hypertension in premature infants
    - Bronchopulmonary dysplasia

Perturbations in NO-cyclic guanosine monophosphate (cGMP), prostacyclin-cyclic adenosine monophosphate (cAMP), and endothelin signaling pathways are considered to play an important role in the pathogenesis of PPHN.[11] It presents with cyanosis and respiratory distress within hours of birth, most commonly in term or near term neonates. However, it should also be considered in preterm infants presenting with cyanosis which is out of proportion to lung parenchymal disease.

Diagnosis

As the majority of cases of PPHN have a secondary etiology, a detailed history and thorough clinical examination may provide important etiology clues. On examination, the neonates have labile hypoxemia. Measuring preductal and postductal saturations gives important clue. A difference of >5–10% in saturations if noted is an important diagnostic clue. However, other important differential to be considered in this situations include obstructed total anomalous pulmonary venous return, CoA, and absence or aortic origin of one pulmonary artery. Also, we need to keep in mind important limitation of saturation difference which may not be seen if duct is closed. Another important term is reverse differential cyanosis which is seen in transposition of the great arteries with low saturations in upper limb as compared to lower limbs.

The cardiac examination reveals a prominent precordial impulse, loud second heart sound, and systolic murmur of tricuspid regurgitation (if present). Radiological findings depend on the primary etiology. It is also often helpful to assess response to changes with ventilatory parameters. Echocardiography is considered the gold standard for diagnosis and ruling out structural heart disease.[12,13] The diagnosis of PPHN should be considered on echocardiography in the presence of bidirectional or predominantly right-to-left shunting across the foramen ovale or ductus arteriosus. In the absence of foramen ovale or ductus arteriosus, other signs such as flattening or deviation of the interventricular septum toward left ventricle, tricuspid regurgitation velocity, and increased right ventricular dilation point toward the diagnosis of PPHN. Echocardiography is also critical for the evaluation of right and left ventricular function and monitoring the therapy.

Management

Management starts in delivery room, includes maintaining normothermia, euglycemia, electrolytes, and euvolemic state in the neonate. Alveolar hypoxemia is a potent pulmonary vasoconstrictor.[13] Oxygen being pulmonary vasodilator is the mainstay of treatment to reduce elevated PVR in the initial period but subsequently causes increase in pulmonary arterial contractility and reduces the response to NO. Therefore, the aim is to achieve "normoxia" (PaO_2

between 50 and 80 mm Hg). Acidosis along with hypoxemia is also a potent vasoconstrictor, hence a pH above 7.3 should always be maintained.

Mechanical ventilation needs to be instituted in neonates showing no improvement despite adequate supportive therapy and supplemental oxygen. Gentle ventilation should be approached with a target PaO_2 of 50–70 mm Hg and $PaCO_2$ of 40–60 mm Hg. Inadequate lung recruitment leads to treatment failure, hence strategies including use of optimal positive-end expiration pressure and high frequency ventilation (HFV) should be employed. Regarding mode of ventilation whether to use conventional or HFV, primary idea is to reduce ventilation perfusion mismatch and neither mode is effective in preventing the need of extracorporeal membrane oxygenation (ECMO). With use of HFV with inhaled NO, greatest improvement is seen in cases with respiratory distress syndrome and meconium aspiration syndrome. Hyperventilation and alkali infusion are no longer used as there are definite concerns regarding cerebral perfusion and sensorineural hearing loss with these.

Systemic hypotension is common in PPHN and it impairs oxygen delivery to tissues, worsens right-to-left shunting and gas exchange in parenchymal lung disorders. Adequate volume augmentation along with use of inotropes is aimed at optimizing cardiac output, reducing PVR and improving tissue oxygenation. Use of milrinone has an advantage as it also causes pulmonary vasodilatation but can cause systemic hypotension. It is more effective if left ventricular dysfunction is present.

Monitoring of Ventilation

Oxygenation index (OI) is an important index used for monitoring ventilation therapy. It is calculated by using formula.[13]

OI = Mean airway pressure (MAP) in cm of $H_2O \times 100/PaO_2$ in mm Hg

OI > 20–25 consider HFV

OI >25 consider inhaled nitric oxide (iNO)

OI > 40 consider ECMO

Specific Management

Inhaled Nitric Oxide

Inhaled nitric oxide is a rapid and selective pulmonary vasodilator and decreases the need for ECMO support in newborns. iNO diffuses into smooth muscle cells, increases levels of intracellular cGMP, and relaxes the vascular smooth muscle leading to pulmonary vasodilation. Current indications are OI > 15–25 with echocardiographic evidence of pulmonary arterial hypertension, or OI > 25 with or without evidence of right-to-left shunting on echocardiography. iNO should be used after achieving adequate ventilator alveolar recruitment with the usual starting dose of 20 ppm delivered via ventilator circuit.[14] It is important to measure nitric dioxide and methemoglobin daily during treatment. Failure to respond to this therapy is seen in 40% of cases cause could be inadequate lung expansion that can be managed by increasing positive end-expiratory pressure. In some cases, response can be achieved if used along with HFV. Once stabilized, weaning can be commenced within 4–5 days. Weaning has to be gradual. Other side effects apart from methemoglobinemia that need to be monitored are platelet dysfunction and pulmonary edema (in presence of left ventricular dysfunction).

Other inhaled pulmonary vasodilators such as prostacyclins (PGI2) such as epoprostenol have been used in certain cases.

Other Selective Pulmonary Vasodilators (*see* Chapter 18)

Sildenafil

Cyclic mononucleotides (cGMP and cAMP) via which iNO acts are degraded by phosphodiesterase (PDE) enzymes in the pulmonary artery smooth muscle cells. Sildenafil is a phosphodiesterase-5 inhibitor that increases endogenous NO by inhibiting its metabolism. It can be administered both by the enteral and intravenous routes. Sildenafil can be used alone or in combination with iNO. Currently, it is approved for only adults with pulmonary arterial hypertension. Oral dose is 1–3 mg/kg/day and IV dose is 0.4 mg loading followed by infusion 0.07 mg/kg/hour.

Endothelin 1 Receptor Blockers

Bosentan is a nonselective endothelin receptor blocker. Its use is off label with only case reports.

Other Therapies

In neonates, failing maximal conventional therapy even with iNO, ECMO remains the mainstay of treatment of neonates failing iNO and other therapies. Current indications are if OI >40. However, it is an expensive and invasive technique with significant potential sequelae that is only available in highly selected centers.

ARRHYTHMIAS

Chapter 52 presents a detailed overview on pediatric rhythm disorders. This section will present a brief overview on rhythm disorders in neonates. Disorders of cardiac rhythm can occur at any stage of life including fetal stage. The incidence of arrhythmia among infants is reported to be 24 per 100,000 live births.[15] Amongst these, only a small fraction has associated structural heart defects.[15] Although certain arrhythmias are more frequent in neonates, any type can occur. Re-entrant supraventricular tachycardia (SVT) involving atrioventricular (AV) bypass tracts (AVRTs) account for the majority (about 84%) of tachyarrhythmias encountered during neonatal age.[16,17] Almost 10–15% of these

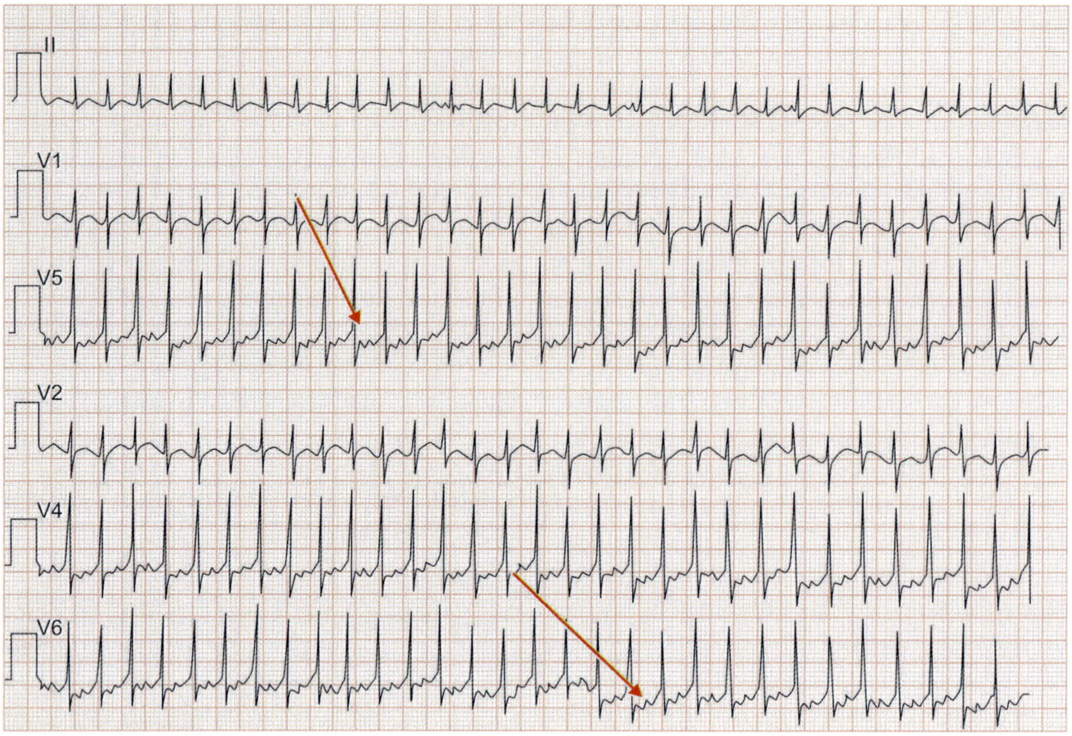

Fig. 9: Neonatal supraventricular tachycardia due to orthodromic atrioventricular (AV) re-entry. The QRS is normal. Red arrows highlight the retrograde P waves.

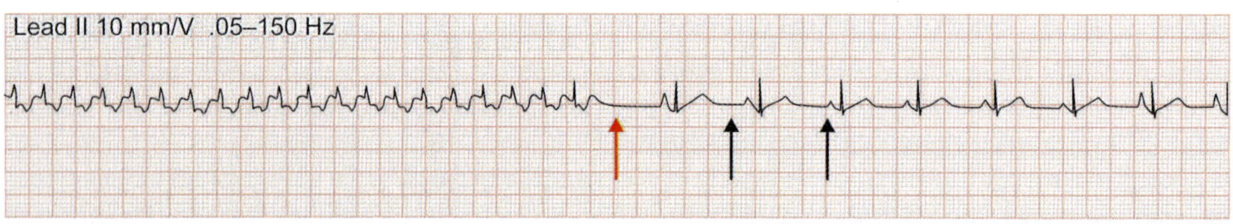

Fig. 10: Electrocardiogram showing termination of orthodromic atrioventricular (AV) re-entry tachycardia after adenosine. Red arrow shows the adenosine response and black arrows highlight sinus rhythm.

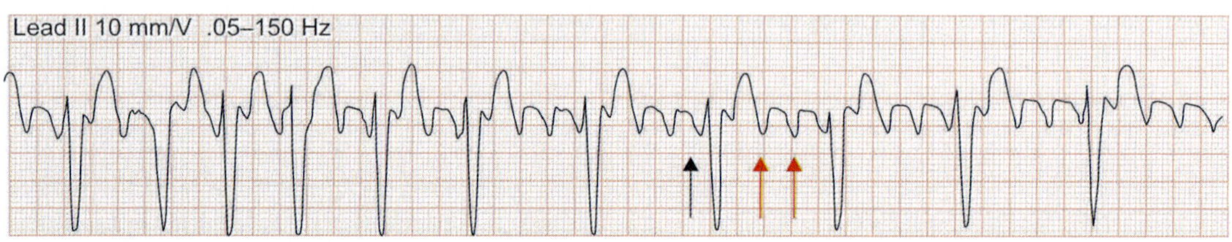

Fig. 11: Electrocardiogram showing atrial flutter with 3:1 conduction. Flutter waves are well seen (arrows). Black arrow highlights conducted P waves, whereas red arrows show nonconducted P waves.

neonates have associated structural heart disease. The ECG shows a typically narrow, regular QRS tachycardia (rates 230–300 beats/min). The P waves may not be easily discernible (**Fig. 9**) or may be seen as a deflection soon after the QRS complexes that are suggestive of retrograde conduction. It is characterized by abrupt onset and termination.

The accessory pathway may be visible during sinus rhythm in the form of a delta wave on ECG in a minority of cases. The AV node is required for the maintenance of re-entrant circuit in ORT, maneuvers blocking AV node (adenosine) will terminate tachycardia.[16,17] (**Fig. 10**). Another important category unique to the neonatal period is atrial flutter where the re-entrant circuit is the confined to the atrium only. It is conducted variably across the AV node at a rate of 1:1, 2:1, or 3:1. It is distinguished by the presence of saw tooth flutter P waves (**Fig. 11**). Adenosine administration results in transiently slowed AV conduction and unmasking of flutter waves on ECG. Atrial flutter in neonates is converted to sinus rhythm via overdrive pacing or low energy synchronized direct-current (DC) cardioversion.[17] In the absence of structural heart disease, atrial fibrillation (AF) in neonates is often self-limiting and therapy after initial conversion generally may not be required but occasionally it may recur. Another rare cause of tachyarrhythmia in neonates is ectopic

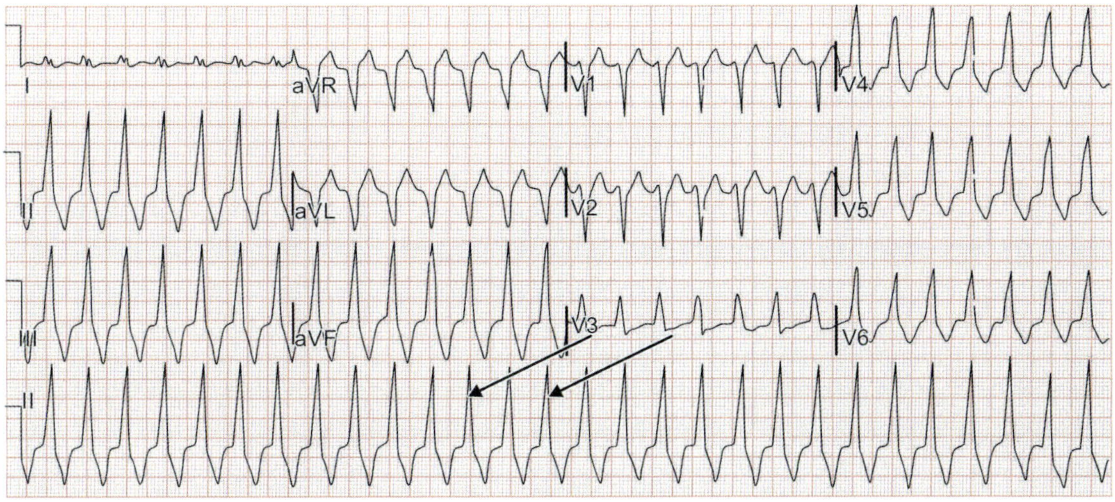

Fig. 12: Electrocardiogram showing wide complex QRS (arrows) ventricular tachycardia.

atrial tachycardia (EAT), which is distinguished by the abnormal P wave axis, normal QRS axis, and variable rate. In contrast to re-entrant SVT, the onset of EAT is gradual. EAT may occur during fetal life and may cause hydrops fetalis. EAT is generally more difficult to treat, intravenous β blockers might be used to acutely decrease heart rate which can then be switched to oral form. Flecainide or amiodarone is used in refractory cases only.[17]

Ventricular tachycardia (VT) is rare in the neonatal period. It is characterized by wide QRS complex and presence of AV dissociation during the tachycardia. Presence of VT is usually associated presence of myocarditis, cardiac rhabdomyomas, structural heart disease, medication, and ion channelopathies.[17] It is crucial to distinguish VT from SVT conducted with aberrancy, which sometimes is difficult. The presence of AV dissociation, fusion, and sinus capture beats usually confirms the ventricular origin of the tachycardia[17] (**Fig. 12**). Adenosine administration terminates SVT with aberrancy. If hemodynamically unstable VT develops, DC cardioversion should be performed. The occurrence of a VT merits careful work up under the supervision of an electrophysiologist.

Although bradycardia is relatively uncommon among neonates, it merits attention because it can be life-threatening. Most healthy newborns experience transient bradycardia, including sinus bradycardia, sinus pauses, and junctional escape beat, which resolves within 48–72 hours of life. Persistent sinus bradycardia is a sinus rate slower than normal for age which is mostly associated with hypoxia, acidosis, hypoglycemia, hypothyroidism, and increased intracranial pressure.[16]

Atrioventricular block is defined as a conduction disturbance of an impulse from the atria to the ventricle classified as, first-, second-, and third-degree block defined by the relationship of the atrium to the ventricle (*see* Chapter 52). First-degree AV block is the prolongation of the PR interval for age and may be caused by increased vagal tone and drugs that prolong the PR interval. Second-degree AV block refers to intermittent failure of conduction of the atrial impulse to the ventricles. In Mobitz type I second-degree AV block (Wenckebach), there is progressive PR prolongation prior to a single-blocked atrial impulse. Wenckebach conduction occurs occasionally in healthy neonates and may represent changes in autonomic tone. Mobitz type II second-degree AV block describes abrupt failure of AV conduction of an atrial impulse without prior PR prolongation. This is called high-grade second-degree AV block and may progress to complete AV block.

In third-degree AV block, no conduction occurs from the atria to the ventricles, and the RR interval is fixed. The atrial rate is normal for age and QRS complexes are regular and the heart rate, is usually 60–80 beats/min in neonates (**Fig. 13**). About 90% of congenital complete AV block in the absence of structural heart defect usually occurs in infants born to mothers with connective tissue disorders such as systemic lupus erythematosus, rest 10% are idiopathic. Maternal anti-Ro and anti-La antibodies are transmitted across the placenta which cross react with fetal cardiac tissue disrupting formation of the normal conduction system. The onset of complete AV block in neonates is usually during the intrauterine life. Most patients who have congenital complete AV block require a pacemaker at some point during life. Indications include a ventricular rate of <55 beats/min or in those with structural heart defect and a ventricular rate of <70 beats/min.

An additional cause for bradycardia and AV blocks is prolonged QT syndrome. The specific type associated with high-grade AV block is type III long QT syndrome. The ventricular repolarization is considerably prolonged and results in failure of the next impulse to conduct. This is a potentially life-threatening condition that requires specialized management (*see* Chapter 52).

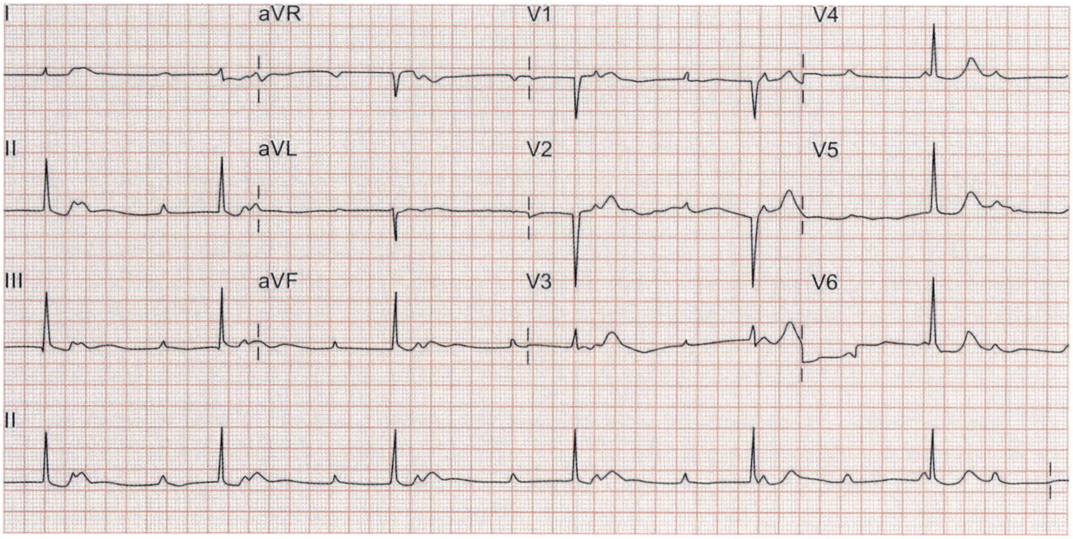

Fig. 13: Electrocardiogram of a neonate with 3rd degree atrioventricular (AV) block, showing AV dissociation and constant RR interval.

REFERENCES

1. Van der Linde D, Konings EE, Slager MA, Witsenburg M, Helbing WA, Takkenberg JJ, et al. Birth prevalence of congenital heart disease worldwide: a systematic review and meta-analysis. J Am Coll Cardiol. 2011;58(21):2241-7.
2. Rudolph AM. Congenital Diseases of the Heart: Clinical-Physiological Considerations. Chichester: Wiley-Blackwell; 2009.
3. Keane JF. Fetal and transitional circulation. In: Keane JF, Lock JE, Fyler DC, (Eds). Nadas' Pediatric Cardiology, 2nd edition. USA: Elsevier; 2006. pp. 75-9.
4. Mahle WT, Martin GR, Beekman RH 3rd, Morrow WR. Section on Cardiology and Cardiac Surgery Executive Committee. Endorsement of Health and Human Services recommendation for pulse oximetry screening for critical congenital heart disease. Pediatrics. 2012;129(1):190-2.
5. Gardner TH. Cardiac emergencies in the newborn period. Radiol Clin North Am. 1971;9(3):385-96.
6. Lees MH, King DH. Cyanosis in the newborn. Pediatr Rev. 1987;9(2):36-42.
7. Alboliras ET. The cyanotic newborn. In: Alboliras E, Hijazi ZM, Lopez L, Hagler DJ, (Eds). Visual Guide to Neonatal Cardiology. Hoboken: John Wiley & Sons; 2018.
8. Bhat, D. (2018). The hypoperfused newborn. In: Alboliras E, Hijazi ZM, Lopez L, Hagler DJ, (Eds). Visual Guide to Neonatal Cardiology. Hoboken: John Wiley & Sons; 2018.
9. Kabbani N, Kabbani MS, Al Taweel H. Cardiac emergencies in neonates and young infants. Avicenna J Med. 2017;7(1):1-6.
10. Alboliras ET. The tachypneic newborn. In: Alboliras E, Hijazi ZM, Lopez L, Hagler DJ, (Eds). Visual Guide to Neonatal Cardiology. Hoboken: John Wiley & Sons; 2018.
11. Jain A, McNamara PJ. Persistent pulmonary hypertension of the newborn: advances in diagnosis and treatment. Semin Fetal Neonatal Med. 2015;20(4):262-71.
12. Lakshminrusimha S, Keszler M. Persistent pulmonary hypertension of the newborn. Neoreviews. 2015;16(12):e680-92.
13. D'Alto M, Romeo E, Argiento P, Di Salvo G, Badagliacca R, Cirillo AP, et al. Pulmonary arterial hypertension: the key role of echocardiography. Echocardiography. 2015;32 Suppl 1:S23-37.
14. Sharma V, Berkelhamer S, Lakshminrusimha S. Persistent pulmonary hypertension of the newborn. Matern Health Neonatol Perinatol. 2015;1:14.
15. Turner CJ, Wren C. The epidemiology of arrhythmia in infants: a population-based study. J Paediatr Child Health. 2013;49(4): 278-81.
16. Ban JE. Neonatal arrhythmias: diagnosis, treatment, and clinical outcome. Korean J Pediatr. 2017;60(11):344-52.
17. Stacy AS, Killen M, Frank A, Fish M. Fetal and neonatal arrhythmias. Neoreviews. 2008;9:e242-52.

49

CHAPTER

Systemic Hypertension in Children

Alpana Ohri, Shakuntala S Prabhu

INTRODUCTION

Systemic hypertension is not uncommon in children. Its prevalence in developed countries has increased from 1 to 3.5% in recent times partly related to the obesity epidemic which increases the risk for adult hypertension and cardiovascular disease. Even youth with hypertension have evidence of accelerated vascular aging. It is mostly silent except when severe and hence likely to be missed unless measuring blood pressure (BP) becomes part of routine pediatric practice. In 2017, American Academy of Pediatrics (AAP) updated the clinical practice guidelines for screening and management of high BP in children and adolescents.[1]

DEFINITIONS, STAGING, AND CATEGORIZATION OF HYPERTENSION

In adults, definition of BP is based on approximate level of BP that marks an increase in cardiovascular events and death. However, in children, the definition continues to be based on the upper segment of the normal BP distribution and not on outcome data.[2] The recent AAP guidelines issued new BP reference standards for children between 1 and 13 years of age (**Flowchart 1**), which incorporates height in inches/centimeter and obviates the need for separate height percentile charts. These new BP normative tables (based on screening of BP in 50,000 healthy nonobese children) are thus more representative and easier to use than the previous ones. The recommendations for infants are to continue to use the earlier second task force tables. The tables by Dionne et al. must be used for neonates (26–44 weeks postmenstrual age).[3] Hypertension in adolescents ≥13 years should be defined as per adult thresholds of outcome data rather than percentile-based definitions.[4]

The AAP guidelines have revised the BP classification. “Elevated BP” has replaced the term “prehypertension” for BPs between 90th and 95th centile. Cut-offs for stages 1 and 2 hypertension have also been redefined (**Table 1**). The new BP charts now include height in centimeter rather percentile.

Severe hypertension has not been as rigorously defined but usually denotes BP ≥30 mm Hg above 95th percentile for children <13 years and >180/120 if the patient is ≥13 years. Severe hypertension has been traditionally divided into hypertensive emergencies and hypertensive urgencies. The former are associated with life-threatening symptoms and/or target-organ damage (encephalopathy, seizures, renal failure, and congestive heart failure). Hypertensive urgencies are defined as severe hypertension without acute target organ injury but with a high risk of developing the same.

SCREENING FOR HYPERTENSION

Awareness that essential hypertension has its origin in childhood lays emphasis on screening. AAP guidelines recommend annual BP measurement for all children ≥3 years. Children <3 years warrant regular measurements if they have congenital heart disease, recurrent urinary tract infection (UTI), urological malformation, solid organ transplant, bone marrow transplant, malignancy, neurofibromatosis, tuberous sclerosis, or sickle cell disease. Subgroups needing more frequent checks have been identified and include those who are obese, on medications known to increase BP, renal disease, history of coarctation, or diabetes, small for

TABLE 1: Updated definition of blood pressure (BP) categories and stages.

HTN classification	*Children aged 1–13 years (percentile based)*	*For children >13 years of age*
Normotensive	<90th percentile	<120/<80 mm Hg
Elevated BP	≥90th percentile or ≥120/80 mm Hg (lower) to <95th percentile	120–129/<80 mm Hg
Stage 1 hypertension	≥95th percentile to <95th percentile + 12 mm Hg or 130/80 to 139/89 (whichever is lower)	130–139/80–89 mm Hg
Stage 2 hypertension	≥95th percentile + 12 mm Hg or ≥140/90 (whichever is lower)	≥140/90 mm Hg

TABLE 2: Simplified screening table and blood pressure (BP) values requiring further evaluation.

Age (years)	BP (mm Hg)			
	Boys		Girls	
	Systolic	Diastolic	Systolic	Diastolic
1	98	52	98	54
2	100	55	101	58
3	101	58	102	60
4	102	60	103	62
5	103	63	104	64
6	105	66	105	67
7	106	68	106	68
8	107	69	107	69
9	107	70	108	71
10	108	72	109	72
11	110	74	111	74
12	113	75	114	75
>13	120	80	120	80

gestational age (SGA), pre-terms (<32 weeks), very low birth weight (VLBW) babies, neonatal intensive care unit (NICU) graduates, and those with umbilical arterial catheterization. To encourage BP screening, AAP guidelines provided a simplified BP table for initial screening by health workers. This table is based on 90th BP percentile values of children at 5th height percentile (**Table 2**). However, for establishing diagnosis, detailed BP charts as available in AAP guidelines are recommended.[1]

MEASURING BLOOD PRESSURE

Devices

Devices for recording office BP include mercury and aneroid sphygmomanometers, both of which rely on auscultation of Korotkoff sounds. Automatic oscillometric devices [noninvasive blood pressure (NIBP)] which measure mean arterial BP and indirectly calculate systolic and diastolic BP have also become very popular. Mercury devices are still considered the gold standard but carry an environment risk. Aneroid devices are fairly accurate but need to be calibrated regularly. Automated oscillometric BP monitors are ease of use, are less operator-dependent, but tend to overestimate BP. AAP recommends that NIBP be used only as a screening tool and in neonatal setups. All high BP values by NIBP must be counterchecked by auscultatory devices.

Procedure

A standardized procedure is recommended for measurement of BP in office practice. This includes the following:

- Child seated for 3–5 minutes with uncrossed legs in a quiet room
- BP to be measured in right arm at heart level
- Length of the bladder cuff should be 80–100% of arm circumference, width at least 40% with lower end of cuff 2–3 cm above antecubital fossa.

Diagnosis

Diagnosis requires BP readings ≥95th percentile at three different visits in the office setting by a trained healthcare professional using auscultatory method. Home BP measurements, finger/forearm recordings, oscillometric devices-based high readings are not sufficient to establish hypertension. In case, child has no symptoms related to high BP and values are in stage 1 or lower category, additional second and third BP measurements can be taken at weekly intervals. However, if symptomatic or stage II hypertension is recorded, the second and third readings should be taken at the same visit for quick diagnosis and emergency care.

Concept of White Coat Hypertension and Masked Hypertension

Hypertension may sometimes be detected intermittently and may not appear to be a sustained feature. White coat hypertension (WCH) is defined as casual/office BP levels that are ≥95th percentile but normal outside of a clinical setting. Diagnosis is best established by ambulatory blood pressure monitoring (ABPM) which shows <95th percentile mean ABPM values and <25% ambulatory blood pressure (ABP) load.[4] Masked hypertension (MH) also called reverse white-coat hypertension exists when BP measured in the clinic is not high but is high in the patient's usual surroundings. This too can be confirmed by ABPM, which shows mean BP ≥95th percentile and ≥25% BP load. WCH and MH are not innocuous and represent a prehypertensive state [associated with left ventricular hypertrophy (LVH)/other signs of target organ damage] predictive of cardiovascular morbidity.

Ambulatory Blood Pressure Monitoring

Ambulatory blood pressure monitoring is being increasingly recognized as a valuable tool in the investigation of pediatric hypertension. The updated guidelines recommend its routine use as it avoids many of the pitfalls of BP measurement, reflects true BP more accurately, and correlates better with target organ damage. It is a useful tool for identifying WCH/MH/isolated nocturnal hypertension, characterizing BP patterns, and assessing response to therapeutic interventions. It is particularly useful for children with chronic kidney disease (CKD), secondary hypertension, type 1 or 2 diabetes mellitus, obstructive sleep apnea syndrome, children born prematurely, and patients who have undergone solid-organ transplant or coarctation repair.

Ambulatory blood pressure monitoring involves repetitive (every 20–30 minutes) NIBP measurements in the nondominant hand (age appropriate cuff) using portable

TABLE 3: Suggested classification of ambulatory blood pressure monitoring (ABPM) in children.

Sr. no	*Category*	*Office BP*	*Mean ABPM*	*Ambulatory BP load*
1.	Normal	<90th percentile	<95th percentile	<25%
2.	Elevated HT	≥90th percentile	<95th percentile	≥25%
3.	Ambulatory HT	≥95th percentile	≥95th percentile	25–50%
4.	Severe ambulatory HT	≥95th percentile	≥95th percentile	≥50%
5.	White coat HT	≥95th percentile	<95th percentile	<25%
6.	Masked HT	<95th percentile	≥95th percentile	≥25%

(BP: blood pressure; HT: hypertension)

devices over an entire day on outpatient department (OPD) basis. Simultaneously, patient maintains a diary to account for times of physical activity, sleep, and drug intake. The results (need at least 40–50 readings) are interpreted as—mean BP (over 24 hours), BP load (percentage of measurements ≥95th percentile limit), and BP patterns (nocturnal dip—percentage drop from mean daytime to mean night time levels). These are compared with values from pediatric normative ABPM tables (**Table 3**). It is important to discard highly deviant values [outside range of systolic blood pressure (SBP) 60–220 mm Hg, diastolic blood pressure (DBP) 35–120 mm Hg, heart rate 40–180, pulse pressure 40–120 mm Hg] for correct interpretation.[5]

Mean BP values ≥95th percentile, BP loads in excess of 25%, and absence of nocturnal dipping are generally considered abnormal and predictive of target organ damage.

However, due to limited availability of pediatric instruments, normative standards being available only for children ≥120 cm, ABPM is yet to attain its rightful place in management of pediatric hypertension.

ETIOLOGY OF HYPERTENSION IN CHILDREN

Primary Hypertension/Essential Hypertension

Recent studies report a change in epidemiology of HT with increasing proportion of primary hypertension. This is likely to be due to genetic influences modified by body habitus and lifestyle of the individual. Compared with all other risk factors, the most substantial effect on the age-related increase in BP is due to body mass index (BMI). Obese adolescent girls have a six-fold increase in the prevalence of hypertension compared to their nonobese counterparts. Other lifestyle attributes such as high salt and poor potassium intake, decreased physical activity, smoking, stress, and alcoholism may be important contributory factors. Low birth weight and administration of antenatal steroids for fetal lung maturation to prevent respiratory distress syndrome are considered as important risk factors.[5] Essential hypertension often tracks into adulthood and is an important contributor to increased cardiovascular morbidity.[6,7]

TABLE 4: Causes of secondary hypertension.

Renal parenchymal Glomerulonephritis Reflux nephropathy Vasculitis Polycystic kidney diseases Chronic renal failure	*Endocrine* *Catecholamine excess* Pheochromocytoma Neuroblastoma Paraganglioma *Exogenous steroids* Cushing syndrome/disease *Congenital adrenal hyperplasia* 11-β hydroxylase deficiency 17-α hydroxylase deficiency *Primary hyperaldosteronism* *Monogenic defects* Apparent mineralocorticoid excess Liddle syndrome Glucocorticoid remediable aldosteronism Gordon syndrome
Renovascular Renal artery stenosis Fibromuscular dysplasia Aortoarteritis/Takayasu's arteritis	
Cardiac cause Coarctation of aorta	

Given the changing epidemiology of hypertension in youth, the 2017 AAP guidelines state that extensive workup for secondary cause of hypertension is not required for children ≥6 years of age who are obese, have a positive family history, and lack physical examination findings suggestive of secondary hypertension.

Secondary Hypertension

Many of the young children (below 6 years of age) especially with a lean habitus, negative family history and stage 2 hypertension are still likely to have secondary hypertension. Among these, renal and renovascular etiologies predominate. Cardiac and endocrine diseases form a smaller but significant subgroup with distinct therapeutic implications (**Table 4**).

Renal (34–76%)

These include renal parenchymal disease such as glomerulonephritis, hemolytic uremic syndrome (HUS), and systemic vasculitis. Another subgroup is of congenital abnormalities of the kidneys and urinary tract, especially reflux nephropathy and polycystic kidney disease. CKD constitutes another common cause. Children with glomerular disorders present often with oliguria, hematuria, and systemic features. On evaluation, they show deranged biochemistry and abnormal urinary sediment. Atypical HUS patients exhibit microangiopathic hemolytic anemia, thrombocytopenia, azotemia, and deranged complement levels. Patients with reflux nephropathy may have a past history of recurrent UTI in the form of fever, vomiting, loin pain, and dysuria. It is known that CKD and reflux nephropathy may present with only hypertension in the absence of any signs and symptoms. The former is diagnosed by deranged renal functions coupled with ultrasonography (USG) and the latter by dimercaptosuccinic acid (DMSA) scan.

Renovascular Disease (12–13%)

This refers to obstruction of the main renal arteries/veins or their branches. Some etiologies include aortoarteritis, fibromuscular dysplasia, vasculitis, and extrinsic compression of the renal vasculature. Renal vein thrombosis and renal artery thrombosis are important causes in neonates and may be sequelae of umbilical vessel cannulation. Presence of neurocutaneous markers typical of neurofibromatosis or Williams syndrome may be a clue toward underlying renovascular cause. Other important pointers of renovascular hypertension in children include stage 2 hypertension, significant diastolic hypertension, discrepant kidney sizes on ultrasound, hypokalemia, or an epigastric and/or upper abdominal bruit on physical examination. For suspected renovascular hypertension, Doppler USG is reliable in nonobese cooperative children ≥8 years when done by experienced hands (27–92% sensitivity).[8,9] Although renal angiography remains the gold standard, both CT angiography (64–94% sensitivity) and magnetic resonance angiography (62–98% sensitivity) are reasonable noninvasive imaging alternatives. Both plasma renin levels and captopril renograms have poor sensitivity and specificity.[9] Percutaneous digital subtraction angiography (DSA) remains the cornerstone for accurate diagnosis and can be transitioned to a therapeutic intervention (angioplasty).

Endocrine Forms of Secondary Hypertension

Endocrinopathies are a rare but important cause of secondary hypertension. Accurate diagnosis has the potential to provide curative treatment. Most forms of endocrine hypertension involve the adrenal gland, either cortex or medulla. Dysregulation in production of mineralocorticoids, glucocorticoids, or sex steroids leads to hypertension in case of former and excessive production of catecholamines in the latter.

Two forms of congenital adrenal hyperplasia (CAH) can present with hypertension. Out of these, 11β hydroxylase defect is more common than 17-α hydroxylase defect.[10] Children with 17-α hydroxylase deficiency are not virilized and hence go unrecognized till an older age when hypertension and hypogonadism may be the clinical features. Boys may have external genitalia of the female phenotype. Diagnosis requires hormonal studies on serum and urinary samples.

Acquired causes such as tumors—pheochromocytomas and paragangliomas—are among the most common endocrine causes of hypertension. These tumors produce excess amounts of catecholamines leading to severe, episodic/sustained secondary hypertension with associated symptoms of diaphoresis, headaches, palpitations, and tremors. Diagnosis requires plasma metanephrine and 24-hour urine catecholamines and metanephrine, metaiodobenzylguanidine (MIBG) scan.

Other causes include primary aldosteronism characterized by early-onset hypertension, hypokalemia, metabolic alkalosis coupled with a low-renin activity level and high aldosterone levels. It may develop secondary to adrenocortical adenoma or hyperplasia.

Rare monogenic causes of early-onset hypertension include four different conditions—apparent mineralocorticoid excess, Liddle syndrome, glucocorticoid remediable aldosteronism, and Gordon syndrome. AAP guidelines recommend additional genetic work-up in cases of suppressed plasma renin activity or elevated aldosterone renin ratio (ng/dL and ng/mL per hour, respectively) >10, especially in the presence of family history of early-onset hypertension or associated hypokalemia.

Causes of transient hypertension include the following:

- Acute glomerulonephritis, Henoch-Schönlein nephritis, hemolytic uremic syndrome, other causes of acute renal failure
- Posturologic surgery or renal transplantation
- Acute hypovolemia (nephrotic relapse, burns, adrenal + GI saline depletion)
- Acute hypervolemia (excessive administration of blood, saline, or plasma)
- Central nervous system (CNS) disease (tumor, infection, seizures, and injury)
- Guillain-Barré syndrome
- Hypercalcemia
- Lead poisoning
- Medications (steroids and sympathomimetic drugs).

EVALUATION OF HYPERTENSION IN CHILDREN AND ADOLESCENTS

First step in diagnosis of hypertension is to rule out associated target organ damage, especially if BP values are in stage 2 hypertension range. Subsequently, detailed evaluation can be done to identify underlying etiology and simultaneous comorbidities such as diabetes and dyslipidemia, which have cardiovascular implications.

History

Symptoms of target organ damage (left ventricular failure, encephalopathy, and renal failure) include history of

Flowchart 1: Diagnostic algorithm for investigations in hypertension.

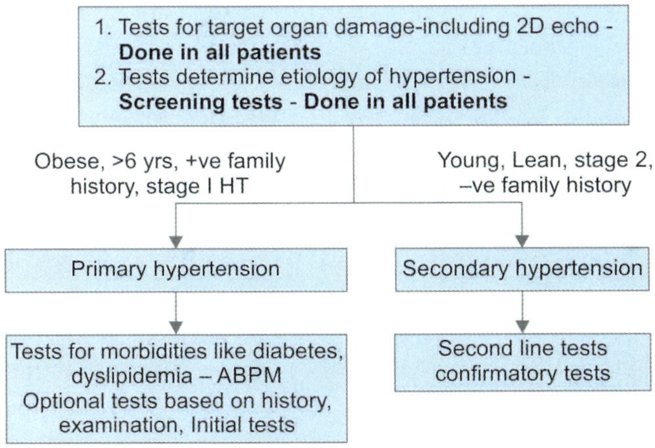

(ABPM: ambulatory blood pressure monitoring; HT: hypertension; 2D: two-dimensional)

shortness of breath, edema, headache, diminished vision, seizures, and poor urine output. Their presence necessitates urgent management. If patient has no acute symptoms and BP is stage 1 or lower, stepwise assessment for etiology and comorbid conditions should be obtained. History suggestive of secondary hypertension includes oliguria, hematuria, swelling, sweating, weight loss, palpitations, limb claudication, etc. History must include family history of hypertension, perinatal history such as birth weight and maternal pregnancy-induced hypertension (PIH). Detailed nutritional history should be taken to assess dietary intake including intake of high caffeine, alcohol, drugs, and junk food. It is crucial to take physical activity history, especially duration of outdoor activity and psychological history including mental stress and duration of sleep.

Physical Examination

Although the physical examination is often normal in hypertensive children, the focus is to identify evidence of end-organ damage and elicit clues to the etiology. Findings suggestive of hypertensive end-organ damage include altered sensorium, focal neurological deficit, retinal changes, apical heave with LVH, and respiratory distress with crepitations and edema.[11] Clues to secondary etiology include asymmetrical pulse volume, BP in aortic coarctation/renovascular hypertension, abdominal mass or palpable kidneys in polycystic kidney disease, acne, hirsutism, and/or ambiguous or virilized genitalia in CAH or hypercortisolism, café-au-lait spots in patients with neurofibromatosis often associated with renovascular hypertension.

CLINICAL FEATURES

Most hypertension is clinically silent. Nonspecific features in younger children include irritability, excessive sweating, feeding problems, and failure to thrive. Infants may present with cardiac failure. Severe or sudden rise of hypertension may manifest with headache, vomiting, altered sensorium, convulsions, facial palsy, or hemiparesis. Presentation as dilated cardiomyopathy is encountered occasionally. The cardiac dysfunction leads to a fall in BP that may sometimes lead to a missed diagnosis or underestimation of the severity of the hypertension. Examination for stigmata of collagen vascular disease and neurocutaneous syndromes should be done in all children with hypertension. Taking BP in all four limbs and palpation of all peripheral pulses should be always done. Abdominal auscultation for bruit should not be forgotten. Anthropometric evaluation including calculation of BMI is an important part of clinical examination. Children with BMI >95th centile for age are more likely to have higher BPs (*see* **Table 1**).

Investigations

The choice of tests as well as the rapidity of evaluation is entirely dependent on the age of the child, the clinical clues, the severity of hypertension, and the presence or absence of target organ damage. A practical stepwise approach that should be followed in a newly diagnosed patient is elucidated in **Flowchart 1**.[1] Detailed investigations are outlined in **Table 5**.

American Academy of Pediatrics guidelines recommend echocardiography for all patients to assess left ventricular mass, geometry, and function at the time of pharmacotherapy. Definition of LVH has been updated as left ventricular (LV) mass >115 g/body surface area (BSA) in boys, >95 g/BSA in girls.[1] Electrocardiogram (ECG), carotid intimal medial thickness (cIMT), and ambulatory arterial stiffness index (AASI) are not routinely needed in children. Renal function tests including urine routine must be done.

TREATMENT

Severe Hypertension

Approach to severe hypertension is outlined in **Flowchart 2**.

Hypertensive Emergencies

Severe hypertension that occurs acutely may lead to end-organ injury and manifest as emergencies in the form of hypertensive encephalopathy, left ventricular failure, retinopathy, or renal failure. The severity of the hypertension as well as the rate of rise of BP determine the occurrence of the damage. This requires emergency reduction of BP in a controlled manner. The goal should be to reduce the BP by 25% over 1 hour and then lower it gradually to 95th centile for age by 24 hours. Levels <95th centile should be achieved by 48 hours.[11] Rapid reduction to normal levels may cause hypoperfusion and ischemic damage to brain, retina, myocardium, and kidney.[12] When managing patients with hypertensive emergencies, two intravenous (IV) lines should be maintained, one for infusion of antihypertensive and the other for saline infusion (if the BP were to fall precipitously). Loss of pupillary reflex to light is an early indicator of retinal

TABLE 5: Investigations in a child with hypertension.

Screening tests Urinalysis BUN, Serum creatinine Serum electrolytes Lipid profile USG of kidneys	*For target organ damage* Ophthalmic evaluation Echocardiography Microalbuminuria
When primary hypertension is suspected *Mandatory tests* HBA1c (accepted screening for diabetes) SGOT, SGPT (to screen for steatohepatitis) Fasting lipid profile (screen for dyslipidemia) complete blood count *Optional tests* Thyroid function tests Drug screen Sleep study as indicated	*When secondary hypertension is suspected* *Second line investigations* DMSA renal scan Serology for ANA, ANCA, C3, C4 Doppler evaluation of renal vasculature Urinary VMA, catecholamines *Confirmatory tests* CT scan for tumors Renal biopsy for glomerular disease MCU for VUR MR angiography RAS Spiral CT renal angiography RAS Selective renal arteriography for RAS *Special tests for endocrine hypertension* Hormonal profile Serum cortisol, catecholamines, peripheral renin activity, aldosterone

(ANA: antinuclear antibodies; ANCA: antineutrophil cytoplasmic antibodies; BUN: blood urea nitrogen; CT: computed tomography; DMSA: dimercaptosuccinic acid; HBA1c: glycosylated hemoglobin, MCU: micturating cystourethrogram; MRI: magnetic resonance imaging; RAS: renal artery stenosis; SGOT: serum glutamic oxaloacetic transaminase; SGPT: serum glutamic pyruvic transaminase; USG: ultrasonography; VMA: vanillylmandelic acid; VUR: vescicoureteral reflux)

Flowchart 2: Proposed algorithm for initial management of children with severe hypertension.

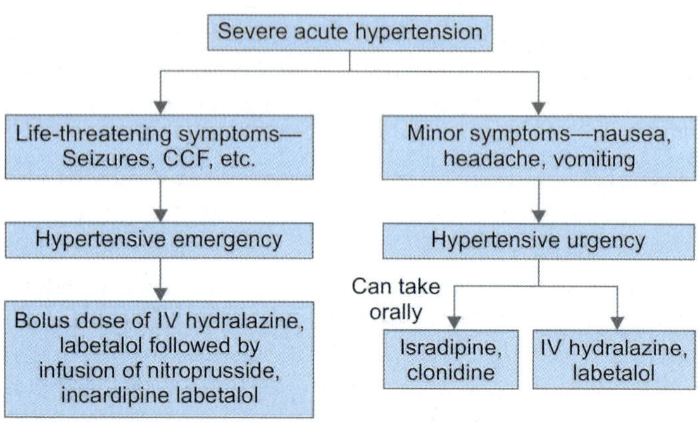

(CCF: congestive cardiac failure; IV: intravenous)

vascular ischemia, requiring immediate infusion of normal saline. Long-acting oral medications should be started early so that they may become effective when parenteral therapy is being tapered. Prolonged use of IV antihypertensive agents is avoided because it may result in sodium and water retention and tachyphylaxis.

Intravenous nitroprusside is the most widely used drug for hypertensive emergencies in children (**Table 6**). It acts rapidly and the dose can be titrated every few minutes to achieve the desired fall in BP but needs to be protected from light as it is photosensitive. It is both an arterial and venodilator, reduces preload and afterload and useful in congestive cardiac failure (CCF) induced by hypertensive crisis. Use of the drug for >24–48 hours can lead to accumulation of thiocyanate, especially in presence of renal and hepatic insufficiency. Thiocyanate poisoning can cause methemoglobinemia, metabolic acidosis, altered mental status, and seizures.

Intravenous hydralazine has been used in certain situations, particularly in neonates and pregnant teenagers, to control severe hypertension. In very sick and low-birth-weight neonates for whom enteral administration of medications is not possible, IV hydralazine is a good therapeutic option. It is a potent arterial vasodilator with an onset of action within 10 minutes, and its effect lasts for 2–4 hours. It can be administered intramuscularly when immediate IV access is not available. The side effects of hydralazine are tachycardia and sodium retention.

Labetalol is a combined α-1 and β-adrenergic blocking agent that can be administered either orally or intravenously. Intravenous labetalol can be administered as a continuous infusion or by bolus injection, which can be advantageous when an infusion cannot be started quickly. Adverse reactions are those expected from a beta-adrenergic blocker, including bradycardia, bronchospasm, and hyperkalemia, especially in presence of renal insufficiency. It is contraindicated in patients with acute left ventricular failure.

Severe hypertension from fluid overload in children with end-stage renal disease (ESRD) requires emergent ultrafiltration and dialysis. However, if the child is in CCF, inotropic agents with vasodilator properties will need to be used to stabilize the patient.

TABLE 6: Drugs for hypertensive emergencies.

Drug	Route	Dosage	Class	Comments
Nitroprusside	IV infusion	0.5–8 µg/kg/min	Vasodilator	Monitor for cyanide toxicity if used for >72 hours in patient in renal failure
Nicardipine	IV infusion	1–3 µg/kg/min	Calcium channel blocker	Avoid in asthma and heart failure
Labetalol	IV bolus	0.2–1 mg/kg/dose (max 40 mg/dose)	Alpha- and beta-blocker	Can cause reflex tachycardia
	IV infusion	0.25–3 mg/kg/hour		
Esmolol	IV bolus	100–500 µg over 1 minute; then 25–100 µg/kg/min; Increase to 500 µg/kg/min	Beta-blocker	Can cause heart failure, bradycardia, bronchospasm contraindicated in cocaine toxicity
Hydralazine	IV bolus	0.1–0.5 mg/kg/dose 4–6 hours	Vasodilator	Tachycardia, flushing, lupus-like syndrome

(IV: intravenous)

Diuretics can be effective in severe hypertension caused by acute glomerulonephritis. IV or transdermal nitroglycerin is generally not used as first line of therapy and has not been used in children. It is a venodilator and therefore reduces preload and cardiac output. It can cause methemoglobinemia, hypoxemia, reflex tachycardia, and tachyphylaxis. It is usually considered in adults as adjunctive therapy for acute coronary syndromes.

Sublingual nifedipine has been widely used in setups where hypertensive emergencies occur in the absence of intensive care unit (ICU) access. It is an effective drug to lower the BP but does so in an uncontrolled fashion. Despite the very real dangers of rapid acute reduction in BP, it has been widely used with a fair safety profile in children.[13,14]

Other therapeutic options available abroad for hypertensive crisis are IV infusions of nicardipine, esmolol, fenoldopam, clevidipine, etc. Intravenous nicardipine is a dihydropyridine calcium channel blocker that is considered first line of therapy in children with hypertensive crisis abroad. It is a very effective antihypertensive, lacks the negative inotropic effect of other calcium channel blockers, can be used for a longer period of time without the fear of cyanide toxicity, and is safe even in patients with renal and hepatic failure. However, it is not available in India.

The list of various drugs, routes, and doses are outlined in **Table 6**.

Hypertensive Urgencies

Hypertensive urgencies differ from emergencies in having no evidence of acute target organ damage. Children with hypertensive urgency do not need IV medications; can be treated with oral drugs but controlled reduction of BP over several hours is desirable. However, they need to be under close medical supervision as they have the potential to progress into an emergency.

Effective oral agents include nifedipine, clonidine, enalapril, isradipine, and labetalol. The onset of action of nifedipine (0.2 mg/kg, maximum 10 mg) administered orally is within 5–10 minutes, peaks at 30–60 minutes, and lasts for 2–6 hours. While children show reflex tachycardia, the occurrence of serious complications with the use of oral nifedipine in this situation is rare. Oral administration of clonidine (0.05–0.1 mg) is also effective, although the onset of action (30–60 minutes) and peak effect (2–4 hours) are delayed. Sedation and orthostatic hypotension occurs in many patients. Sublingual or oral administration of captopril (6.25–25 mg) also shows a rapid onset (10–30 minutes) and peak (1–2 hours), and relatively prolonged duration of action (4–8 hours). Minoxidil is a direct vasodilator that has been shown to be effective in children with severe chronic hypertension refractory to other oral agents, and also in children with chronic hypertension experiencing acute BP elevations. It has well-known side effects of hirsutism and fluid retention that are primarily seen with chronic use.

Isradipine is a second-generation dihydropyridine calcium channel blocker that has a rapid onset of action, usually reducing BP within 1 hour of administration, with its peak effect occurring in 2–3 hours. A liquid formulation is available abroad facilitating precise dosing even in infants and small children. In many centers across the world, isradipine has become the drug of choice for oral therapy of severe hypertension.

Sustained Hypertension

Target Blood Pressure

The target BP has been revised to <90th percentile and for those with CKD, BP targets were revised to below 50th percentile.

Nonpharmacological Interventions

In children with elevated BP and stage I hypertension without target organ damage, the initial therapy consists of nonpharmacological interventions. These consist of lifestyle changes that include dietary modifications, weight reduction, regular exercise, and reduction in stress. The Dietary Approaches to Stop Hypertension diet (DASH), which emphasizes increased fresh fruits and vegetables, fiber, and low-fat dairy, and decreased sodium intake, has been associated with lower BP in children and adolescents. Fruits and nuts are rich in potassium and magnesium and are known to have a beneficial effect in lowering the BP. Sodium intake should be reduced to <1.2 g per day in children below 10 years of age and to <1.5 g per day in older children. Reduction in sedentary habits such as watching TV, video and computer games and encouraging an increase in regular aerobic and vigorous exercise in the form of play, dancing, swimming, etc., for 30–60 minutes at least three to four times a week is most beneficial. For all children who are overweight, weight reduction is an important aspect of management as exercise causes a reduction of BP by producing vasodilatation as well as reducing peripheral insulin resistance. Cessation of smoking is an important consideration in adolescents. There are growing data that complementary medicine techniques for stress reduction (e.g., breathing awareness meditation, yoga) may decrease BP in children and adolescents. Family-based interventions involving the family in counseling on diet and exercise to make changes for the entire household has been shown to improve control of hypertension.

Children with well-controlled hypertension without target organ damage can participate in competitive sports but need BP monitoring at 2-monthly intervals to see the effect of participation on the BP. Children with target organ damage or poorly controlled hypertension should avoid competitive sports.

Pharmacological Treatment for Sustained Hypertension

Indications to initiate pharmacological treatment include the following:

- In hypertensive children and adolescents who have failed lifestyle modifications for 3–6 months
- Those with target organ damage such as LVH
- Symptomatic hypertension or stage 2 hypertension without a clearly modifiable factor (e.g., obesity).

The common initial drugs consist of either angiotensin-converting enzyme inhibitors (ACEI), angiotensin receptor blockers (ARBs) and long-acting calcium channel blockers (CCB), or thiazide diuretic (**Table 7**). Beta-blocker should

TABLE 7: Drugs used in the treatment of childhood hypertension.

Agents	*Dose and frequency*	*Comments*
ACE inhibitors		• Use cautiously if GFR <30 mL/min/1.73 m²; avoid in renal artery stenosis • Avoid in neonates. Monitor serum potassium, creatinine • Side effects: Hyperkalemia, impaired renal functions; anemia, neutropenia • Dry cough • Dose modification is needed in renal failure
Captopril	0.3–0.6 mg/kg/day; tid	
Enalapril	0.1–0.6 mg/kg/day; qd	
Lisinopril	0.06–0.6 mg/kg/day; qd	
Ramipril	6 mg/kg/day	
Angiotensin receptor blockers		Same as ACE inhibitors except that cough is not seen and dose modification is not needed in renal failure
Losartan	0.7–1.4 mg/kg/day; qd-bid	
Irbesartan	4–5 mg/kg/day	
Calcium channel blockers		• Extended release nifedipine must be swallowed as a whole • Side effects: Headache, flushing, dizziness, tachycardia; at higher doses: Lower extremity edema, erythema • Liquid formulation is available abroad
Nifedipine	0.25–3 mg/kg/day; qd-bid	
Amlodipine	0.05–0.5 mg/kg/day	
Isradipine	0.15–0.8 mg/kg/day	
Beta-blockers		• Avoid in asthma, heart failure; sleep disturbances, hyperlipidemia • Atenolol: Decrease dose by 50% at GFR <50 mL/min/1.73 m² • Metoprolol is not dialyzed. Preferred beta-blocker for patients on hemodialysis
Atenolol	0.5–2 mg/kg/day	
Metoprolol	1–6 mg/kg/day	
Propranolol	1–4 mg/kg/day	
Labetalol	1–40 mg/kg/day	
Central alpha agonist		Abrupt cessation may cause rebound hypertension; sedation
Clonidine	5–25 µg/kg/day; tid-qid	
Peripheral alpha antagonist		May cause "first dose" hypotension, syncope
Prazosin	0.05–0.5 mg/kg/day; bid-tid	
Vasodilators		• For hypertension refractory to other drugs • Side effects: Headache, palpitation, fluid retention, congestive heart failure, pericardial effusions, hypertrichosis with minoxidil
Hydralazine	1–8 mg/kg/day; qid	
Minoxidil	0.1–1 mg/kg/day; qd-bid	
Diuretics		• Monitor electrolytes, fluid status periodically • Loop diuretics: Metabolic alkalosis, hypokalemia, hypercalciuria • Thiazides: Dyslipidemia, hyperglycemia, hyperuricemia, hypokalemia • Hypomagnesemia • Amiloride, spironolactone—use cautiously with ACEI, angiotensin receptor blockers
Furosemide	0.5–6 mg/kg/day; qd-bid	
Metolazone	0.2–0.4 mg/kg/day; qd	
Hydrochlorothiazide	1–3 mg/kg/day; qd	
Amiloride	0.4–0.6 mg/kg/day; qd	
Spironolactone	1–3 mg/kg/day; qd-bid	

(ACEI: angiotensin-converting enzyme inhibitor; GFR: glomerular filtration rate)

TABLE 8: Choice of drugs in different conditions causing hypertension.

Condition	*Predominant cause of hypertension*	*Drug of choice*
End-stage renal disease	Fluid overload	Dialysis
Acute glomerulonephritis Acute kidney injury	Fluid overload	Furosemide, if fails—dialysis
Cocaine, amphetamine abuse	Transient sympathetic vasoconstriction and cardiac stimulation	Phentolamine and benzodiazepine
Catecholamine-secreting tumor	Sympathetic overactivity	Surgical resection. Prior preparation with liberating fluid to expand contracted intravascular volume, then prazosin. Later beta-blocker. Great care needed to manage hypertension intraoperatively
Hyperaldosteronism/monogenic causes of HTN	Excess aldosterone, cortisol, excess ENac activity	Aldosterone antagonists or potassium-sparing diuretics

(ENac: epithelial sodium channel; HTN: hypertension)

not be used as initial antihypertensive. ACEIs block the conversion of angiotensin I to angiotensin II—the most potent vasoconstrictor in the body and ARBs are direct receptor blockers. ACEI/ARBs have a beneficial effect on proteinuria and renoprotective and cardioprotective effects. They are the preferred drugs for children with CKD and those with cardiac dysfunction. Patients on ACEI/ARBs require glomerular filtration rate (GFR) and K monitoring. They should not be used in children with suspected bilateral renal artery stenosis and in children with GFR <30 mL/min. A 30% increase in serum creatinine from the baseline requires discontinuation or lowering of the drug dosage. Captopril and enalapril are the two most widely used drugs among ACEI and losartan most often used ARB.

Calcium channel blockers are good first-line antihypertensives. They inhibit cellular influx of calcium and produce vascular smooth muscle relaxation. The most widely used drug in this category is nifedipine. Amlodipine has the advantage of a longer duration of action and lends itself well to once daily dosing.

Diuretics may serve as first-line drugs when salt and water retention in the form of edema forms an important component of the hypertensive child or in a patient with postinfectious glomerulonephritis. When hypertension remains suboptimally controlled despite maximal doses of one drug, a second antihypertensive that is complementary to the first may be added.

CONDITION SPECIFIC TREATMENT

In situations in which the underlying condition causing hypertension has been identified, treatment should be targeted to the underlying pathophysiology of hypertension (*see* **Flowchart 1**). Drugs of choice in different conditions causing hypertension are elucidated in **Table 8**.[15]

NEONATAL HYPERTENSION

Normal BP in neonates depends on a variety of factors, including gestational age, postnatal age, and birth weight. Hypertension is reported in about 0.8% neonates, especially those with concurrent conditions, such as bronchopulmonary dysplasia (BPD), those who have history of umbilical arterial catheterization. We must know that oscillometric devices tend to overestimate BP, especially the first value. Average of second and third value must be taken. Also, BP must never be recorded while feeding (overestimates BP by 20 mm Hg) or on a pacifier (overestimates BP by 10%). Renovascular (renal artery or venous thrombosis) and renal parenchymal disorders are important causes of hypertension in this age group.[8] Treatment decisions should be tailored to the severity of the hypertension, and may include intravenous (when >99 percentile or symptomatic) and/or oral therapy. Newborns with severe hypertension are managed with continuous IV infusion of nitroprusside, labetalol, nicardipine, or esmolol. Effective oral agents include calcium channel blockers such as amlodipine or propranolol (except BPD), isradipine, hydralazine, and minoxidil. Both sublingual nifedipine and ACE inhibitors should be avoided. The sublingual nifedipine because of unpredictable magnitude of antihypertensive and the ACE inhibitors because of propensity to cause acute renal shutdown and adverse effects on nephron development.

CONCLUSION

This chapter has presented an overview of pediatric hypertension and outlined basic concepts and practical guidelines that should enable initial diagnostic evaluation and basic management. Because much of hypertension is clinically silent, considerable diligence is needed on part of the pediatrician when it comes to screening, performing diagnostic work-up, and motivating the patients and their families toward regular follow-up and adherence to nonpharmacological and pharmacological therapy.

REFERENCES

1. Flynn JT, Kaelber DC, Baker-Smith CM, Blowey D, Carroll AE, Daniels SR, et al. AAP Subcommittee on Screening and Management of High Blood Pressure in Children. Clinical practice

guideline for screening and management of high blood pressure in children and adolescents. Pediatrics. 2017;140(3): e20171904.
2. Guzman-Limon M, Samuels J. Pediatric hypertension: diagnosis, evaluation, and treatment. Pediatr Clin North Am. 2019; 66(1): 45-57.
3. Dionne JM, Harris KC, Benoit G, Feber J, Poirier L, Cloutier L, et al. Hypertension Canada's 2017 guidelines for the diagnosis, assessment, prevention, and treatment of pediatric hypertension. Can J Cardiol. 2017;33(5):577-85.
4. Sinha R, Saha A, Samuel J. American Academy of Pediatrics Clinical Practice Guidelines for screening and management of high blood pressure in children and adolescents: what is new? Indian Pediatr. 2019;56(4):317-21.
5. Flynn JT, Daniels SR. Update: ambulatory blood pressure monitoring in children and adolescents—a scientific statement from the American Heart Association. Hypertension. 2014;63(5):1116-35.
6. Flynn JT, Alderman MH. Characteristics of children with primary hypertension seen at a referral center. Pediatr Nephrol. 2005;20(7):961-6.
7. Lurbe E, Agabiti-Rosei E, Cruickshank JK, Dominiczak A, Erdine S, Hirth A, et al. European Society of Hypertension Guidelines for the management of high blood pressure in children and adolescents. J Hypertens. 2016;34(10): 1887-920.
8. Kanitkar M. Renovascular hypertension. Indian Pediatr. 2005; 42:47-54.
9. Villegas L, Cahill AM, Meyers K. Pediatric renovascular hypertension: manifestations and management. Indian Pediatr. 2020;15;57(5): 443-51.
10. Rodd CJ, Sockalosky JJ. Endocrine causes of hypertension in children. Pediatr Clin North Am. 1993;40(1):149-64.
11. Bagga A, Jain R, Vijayakumar M, Kanitkar M, Ali U. Evaluation and management of hypertension. Indian Pediatr. 2007;44(2):103-21.
12. Chandar J, Zilleruelo G. Hypertensive crisis in children. Pediatr Nephrol. 2012;27(5):741-51.
13. Calvetta A, Martino S, von Vigier RO, Schmidtko J, Fossali E, Bianchetti MG. What goes up must immediately come down! Which indication for short-acting nifedipine in children with arterial hypertension? Pediatr Nephrol. 2003;18(1):1-2.
14. Yiu V, Orrbine E, Rosychuk RJ, MacLaine P, Goodyer P, Girardin C, et al. The safety and use of short-acting nifedipine in hospitalized hypertensive children. Pediatr Nephrol. 2004; 19(6):644-50.
15. Baracco R. A practical guide to the management of severe hypertension in children. Pediatric Drugs. 2020;22(1):13-20.

50 CHAPTER

Lifestyle Diseases and Related Conditions: Childhood Obesity, Dyslipidemias, and Cardiovascular Risk Reduction during Childhood and Adolescence

Manu Raj

INTRODUCTION

This chapter discusses an important set of conditions that have a bearing on future risk of chronic cardiovascular disease (CVD). Globally noncommunicable diseases, specifically CVD and diabetes, have emerged as leading causes of deaths among the adult population. This is now true in all parts of the world including most low- and middle-income countries. It is increasingly apparent that the roots of adult CVD can be traced back to childhood. Lifestyle changes in childhood translate into risk for adult CVD. It is vitally necessary for pediatricians to understand the principles of preventing CVD later in life. While they need to offer advice to healthy adolescents and children, they now have to contend with a rapidly growing population of overweight and obese children in whom the need to make important changes in lifestyle are more immediately felt. This chapter is divided into three sections. The first deals with obesity in children and adolescents, the second relates to dyslipidemias in children, and the third examines principles of future CVD prevention.

OBESITY IN CHILDREN AND ADOLESCENTS

Introduction

Obesity in children and adolescents is growing at a rapid pace in most countries across the globe. Obesity among children aged 5–19 years increased eightfold between 1975 and 2016.[1] Across the globe, age-standardized prevalence of obesity increased from 0·7% (0·4–1·2) in 1975 to 5·6% (4·8–6·5) in 2016 among girls, and from 0·9% (0·5–1·3) in 1975 to 7·8% (6·7–9·1) in 2016 among boys.[1] Obesity rates in children aged 2–4 years had a much slower rise and between 1980 and 2015, the rates approximately doubled for this age group.[2] The estimated prevalence of obesity among children below 5 years of age in South Asia during 1980 was 2.4% for boys and 2.8% for girls. In 2015, this rose to 4.5% and 4%, respectively.[2]

The prevalence of overweight and obesity among children and adolescents in developing countries showed an increasing trend from 1980 to 2013. The figures rose from 8.1% in 1980 to 12.9% in 2013 for boys and from 8.4 to 13.4% in girls.[3] A large survey done in Kerala, India (2007) covering 25,000 school children (5–16 years) puts the prevalence of overweight and obesity at 6.57% (boys 7.33%, girls 5.87%) and 1.89% (boys 2.47%, girls 1.34%), respectively.[4]

Definition of Childhood Obesity and Overweight

The definition of obesity and overweight during the periods of childhood and adolescence is done using age and sex-specific nomograms for body mass index (BMI). Any child or adolescent with BMI equal to or more than the age-gender-specific 95th percentile is defined as obese. Children and adolescents with BMI equal to or exceeding the 85th but are below 95th percentiles are defined overweight and are at risk for obesity related comorbidities.[5]

Etiology of Obesity during Adolescence and Childhood

The fundamental basis of the current epidemic of childhood/adolescent overweight and obesity is a derangement of the energy balance equation. Basically, it is a simple imbalance between calories consumed and calories expended. Any leftover calories that are not consumed for daily functioning or physical movement is seen as a surplus and stored by the body in the form of adipose tissue resulting in increased adiposity.

Two significant trends are seen to dominate the current scene of childhood/adolescent obesity. The first is a global shift in the diet landscape toward increased intake of foods with high energy density. These high energy items are usually high in fat and/or sugars but low in several vitamins, minerals, and other useful micronutrients, often qualifying to be categorized as junk foods. The second is the worrying trend of global decline in physical activity. This decline can be attributed to the increasingly sedentary nature of currently popular recreation options available to the young such as watching TV and playing computer/video games. This decline is further augmented by the constantly

TABLE 1: Adverse outcomes in childhood obesity.[6]

Cardiovascular	• High blood pressure • Early onset of atherosclerosis • Left ventricular hypertrophy
Endocrine	• Insulin resistance • Diabetes mellitus [noninsulin-dependent diabetes mellitus (NIDDM)] • Menstrual abnormalities • Polycystic ovarian syndrome (PCOS)
Gastrointestinal	• Gallstones • Nonalcoholic steatohepatitis (NASH) • Hepatic fibrosis and cirrhosis
Neurological	Pseudotumor cerebri
Orthopedic	• Slipped capital femoral epiphysis • Tibia vara • Osteoarthritis
Psychosocial	• Obsessive concern about body image • Expectation of rejection • Progressive withdrawal • Low self-esteem and depression
Pulmonary	• Increased bronchial hyperactivity • Asthma exacerbation • Obstructive sleep apnea • Pickwickian syndrome • Pulmonary embolism
Renal	• Increased sensitivity to sodium • Decreased natriuresis and proteinuria

changing modes of transportation as well as by increasing urbanization. A minor subset of childhood adolescent obesity is due to non-nutritional reasons.

Clinical Manifestation of Obesity during Childhood and Adolescence

The clinical manifestations of childhood and adolescent obesity are summarized in **Table 1**.

Obesity in Childhood and Future Cardiovascular Health

Several large cohort studies have reinforced the impact of childhood BMI on future cardiovascular health. A recent systematic review reported that higher BMI in childhood (7 to <18 years) increased the risk of coronary heart disease (CHD) risk during adulthood [relative risk (RR) 1.09].[7] The Norwegian Health Surveys that followed up 227,000 adolescents for more than three decades reported a strong association between adolescent BMI and ischemic heart disease (IHD).[8]

In this study, the RR of IHD mortality at the end of follow-up (mean: 35 years) was 2.9 for males and 3.7 for females in the highest BMI category (i.e., BMI >85th percentile) compared with the reference BMI category (BMI 25th–74th percentile). These two studies are solid proof that obesity in childhood and adolescence increases the individual's susceptibility to future CHD during adulthood as well as the risk of dying from IHD.[7,8]

Cardiovascular Risk Profile in Obese Children

Obesity during childhood as well as adolescence is well known to result in significant increases in morbidity and mortality in adult life. Atherosclerotic cardiovascular disease (ASCVD) is a long process that begins early in childhood. The evolution of this process is heavily influenced over the life course. This influence is from a combination of nonmodifiable (genetic) factors and potentially modifiable risk factors. Childhood and adolescent obesity can be considered as the lead one among the modifiable risk factors that influence future CVD. Current research studies suggest that cardiovascular risk becomes abnormal around the 85th percentile of body weight. This is the point above which cardiovascular system changes are observed. In addition, lower high-density lipoprotein (HDL)-cholesterol, higher triglycerides (TGs), and elevated levels of other known CVD risk factors appear above this cutoff.

Prospective cohort studies have confirmed the association of childhood BMI on adolescent cardiovascular risk profile. The AVON longitudinal study reported that higher childhood BMI was associated with significant increases in systolic blood pressure (SBP), low-density lipoprotein (LDL) cholesterol, TGs, insulin levels along with lower values for HDL cholesterol in late adolescence (15–16 years).[9] In girls, a 1 SD increase over mean BMI during 9–12 years presented an odds ratio (OR) of 1.23 for high SBP (≥130 mm Hg); 1.19 for high low-density lipoprotein cholesterol (LDL-C) (≥2.79 mmol/L); 1.43 for high TGs (≥1.7 mmol/L); 1.25 for low high-density lipoprotein-cholesterol (HDL-C) (<1.03 mmol/L); and 1.45 for high levels of insulin (≥16.95 IU/L). The values in boys were 1.24 for SBP, 1.30 for LDL-C, 1.96 for TGs; 1.39 for HDL-C, and 1.84 for high insulin levels, respectively.[9] These findings suggest the strong adverse influence of obesity in childhood on cardiovascular health profile in adolescence.

Obesity-related Hypertension

The relationship of childhood obesity with BP is well known and confirmed by a multitude of studies done in the past. High BP (BP >95th percentile) was seen in more than a third of overweight children in the European pediatric cohort.[10] Among 26,008 children (age 12.6 ± 2.9 years, 56% females) who presented with overweight (BMI >90th percentile) or obesity (>97th percentile) in 98 specialized centers across Europe, high BP was seen in 35.4%.[10] Similar data was shown by an Indian study covering 25,000 school children in the age group of 5–16 years.[4] In this study, first instance hypertension was seen in 10.10% of normal weight children and adolescents. The corresponding figures for overweight and obese participants were 17.3% and 18.3%, respectively.[4] The rate of change in BMI seems to be more dominant than the absolute values of the same. This observation is based on a prospective cohort of over 12,000 school children from South India.[11] The cohort reported higher BP levels in children/adolescents with rapidly increasing BMI compared to the rest of the study population. Probable mechanisms that can result in elevated BP among obese children/adolescents include insulin resistance, amplified sympathetic nervous system activity, excessive activation of renin-angiotensin-aldosterone, sodium retention and derangement of vascular functions.[12,13] Among all the attributed reasons for obesity-related hypertension, insulin resistance requires more attention. The attributed reasons by which this condition increase BP are many and the major ones include an antinatriuretic effect of insulin, increased sympathetic activity, increased responses to endogenous vasoconstrictors, and deficient endothelium-dependent vasodilatation.[12] Among all possible risk factors associated with childhood/adolescent obesity, high BP remains the most popular adverse cardiovascular manifestation.

Insulin Resistance and Type II Diabetes Mellitus

Insulin resistance is strongly associated with childhood obesity. Approximately one in three obese children/adolescents will have insulin resistance during the prepubertal period. The prevalence doubles to two out of three in the pubertal period. In addition, glucose intolerance is seen in approximately 5% of obese children/adolescents.[14] Insulin resistance significantly alters glucose metabolism, resulting in increased secretion of insulin and leads to a state of chronic hyperinsulinemia. This scenario frequently leads to the development of type 2 diabetes in a subset of obese children/adolescents with insulin resistance. One in five obese children and adolescents will have prediabetes.[15] Approximately half of the prediabetic obese children will have dyslipidemia. In addition, one in five of those prediabetic children will have hypertension suggesting the clustering of risk factors in childhood/adolescent obesity.[15]

Atherogenic Dyslipidemia and Atherosclerosis

Obesity has a strong association with atherogenic dyslipidemia. Approximately one in three obese children/adolescents will have some form of dyslipidemia. Obesity during this age is also associated with higher values for total cholesterol (TC) levels (15%), LDL-C levels (15%), and TG levels (14%). Low HDL-C levels (11%) are also seen.[10]

Atherosclerosis is known to start in the very first years of life as suggested by landmark autopsy studies such as the Bogalusa Heart Study.[16] Autopsies done on young individuals in the first four decades of life suggest that the severity of lesions in the aorta and coronary arteries are associated with several risk factors known to be elevated in childhood/adolescent obesity.[16] These include BMI, BP, TC, TGs, LDL-C, and HDL-C.[16] Aortic intima media thickness (aIMT) and carotid intima media thickness (CIMT) are well-known surrogate markers of atherosclerosis and future cardiovascular risk.[17] In the Muscatine offspring study, both aIMT and CIMT were associated with adiposity during childhood and adolescence.[17] In adolescents (age 11–17 years), aIMT was also associated with TGs, SBP, diastolic blood pressure (DBP), and waist/hip ratio in addition to BMI.[17]

Cardiac Structural Changes Seen with Childhood Obesity

The hemodynamic changes that are seen with obesity during childhood and adolescence can impact the cardiac structural design. Adolescents with BMI in the overweight/obese range have larger left ventricular (LV) diameter and increased LV mass compared to normal weight counterparts.[13] LV hypertrophy is more prevalent in overweight and obese adolescents, largely compensating for the increased cardiac workload seen among such subjects.[13]

Sleep-disordered Breathing and Obstructive Sleep Apnea

Obesity during childhood and adolescence is associated with five times higher likelihood of exhibiting sleep-disordered breathing (SDB).[18] SDB is classically defined as an apnea hypopnea index (AHI) of >10. The pathophysiology of cardiovascular risk modification in obstructive sleep apnea syndrome (OSAS) among children is multifactorial. The probable reasons include oxidative stress, altered sympathovagal balance, elevated levels of inflammatory cytokines, vascular remodeling, and endothelial cell dysfunction.[19]

Evaluation of the Child/Adolescent with Obesity

All children/adolescents should be assessed for healthy eating and active living behaviors during routine pediatric consultations. Their height and weight should be measured accurately and BMI plotted on reference charts to determine the percentiles. Children/adolescents irrespective of BMI status should be further assessed by a family history, physical examination, and review of all systems. For children/adolescents in the overweight category without any risk factors, a lipid profile is desirable. Additional laboratory work is only advised for overweight children/adolescents with risk factors or those in the obese range (BMI ≥ 95 percentile). All such children/adolescents should have a fasting blood work that includes a fasting glucose and fasting lipid profile along with alanine aminotransferase (ALT) and aspartate aminotransferase (AST) measurement. In those children/adolescents with elevated fasting glucose in the prediabetes range, additional measurements such as hemoglobin A1C (HbA1C) or oral glucose tolerance tests may be done. A detailed work-up is advisable for overweight/obese children/adolescents with certain obesity-related conditions categorized under dermatological (acanthosis nigricans, hirsutism, and intertrigo), endocrinological (polycystic ovarian syndrome, precocious puberty, premature adrenarche, prediabetes, and type II diabetes), and gastrointestinal [cholelithiasis, constipation, gastroesophageal reflux disease (GERD), nonalcoholic fatty liver disease] issues. Special evaluation is also required for those with psychological/behavioral issues (anxiety, binge eating disorder, depression, and teasing/bullying experiences).

Management of Child and Adolescent Overweight and Obesity

Treatment of child/adolescent overweight and obesity requires a multidisciplinary team and should ideally include a pediatrician, nutritional specialist, physical instructor, and a behavioral therapist.[6] A motivated team of parents and caretakers is essential for the success of this multidisciplinary approach. The short-term goal of this treatment approach is to slow down the rate of weight gain initially, leading to a second state of weight maintenance and finally to a state of weight reduction. Weight reduction is attempted till BMI is within desirable range appropriate for age and gender. The long-term goal focuses to improve the health-related quality of life as well as to reduce the morbidity and mortality seen in association with excess adiposity.

Targets for Obesity Treatment

There are no targets identified for overweight/obese children younger than 2 years.[20] Such children are kept on regular follow-up without any active intervention. In the age group of 2–5 years, weight maintenance is recommended for overweight children and a minimal weight reduction (0.5 kg/month) is attempted for obese children. The same targets apply for children in the age group of 6–11 years. In those with BMI >99 percentile, a moderate weight reduction (up to 1 kg/week) may be attempted. In the next age group (12–18 years), weight maintenance is recommended for overweight and a moderate weight reduction (up to 1 kg/week) is recommended for obese subjects.[20]

Phases and Components of Obesity Treatment

The expert committee recommends a multiphased, graded approach for the treatment of childhood/adolescent overweight/obesity. The four phases are placed in ascending order of treatment intensity and include (1) prevention-plus, (2) structured weight management, (3) comprehensive multidisciplinary intervention, and (4) tertiary care intervention.[20] All patients should ideally start at the least intensive stage and then advance to higher stages based upon the response to treatment, age, BMI, health risks, and motivation. In addition, an empathetic and empowering counseling style is recommended to support patient and family behavior change. The first two phases can be attempted at regular pediatric practice clinics. The third and fourth phases should be attempted in specialized pediatric weight management clinics and tertiary care centers, respectively.

The five components of pediatric overweight/obesity treatment include dietary management, enhancement of physical activity, reduction of sedentary behavior, pharmacological therapy, and bariatric surgery.[20]

Dietary Management

The overall aim of dietary management is to establish weight maintenance or weight reduction without compromising normal nutrition. Initiation and maintenance of healthy eating patterns is the mainstay of this component. Recommended diet composition includes a fat intake equivalent of 30–40% of daily calorie requirement in children aged 1–3 years, with a reduction to 25–35% in those aged 4–18 years.[21] The recommendation for carbohydrate intake is 45–65% of daily calorie requirement in all children and adolescents. The same for protein intake is 5–20% of daily calorie requirement in children 1–3 years, gradually increasing to 10–30% for those aged 4–18 years.[21] The Dietary Intervention Study in Children (DISC) diet can be introduced in obese subjects who are 8 years or older.[22] DISC diet specifies 58% of total calorie intake from carbohydrates, 28% from fats (11% mono, 9% poly, and 8% or less from saturates) and 14% from proteins. This diet is safer and will not interfere with normal growth, development, and puberty. The intake of cholesterol should be restricted to a maximum of 75 mg/1,000 kilocalories and should not exceed 150 mg/day.[22] The recommendations also suggest adequate amounts of dietary fiber (age in years + 5 g/day).

Special emphasis is recommended for reducing the frequency of eat-outs and consumption of high energy, high fat, and high sugar food items popular at those outlets. Additional efforts should focus on planning of healthy snacks, providing balanced diet, and regular consumption of fruits and vegetables.

Enhancement of Physical Activity

Existing recommendations suggest that all children/adolescents should perform 60 minutes or more of moderate/vigorous physical activity to achieve ideal cardiovascular health.[23] Children/adolescents with BMI in the overweight/obese levels should perform at higher levels compared to the regular recommendation mentioned above to achieve weight maintenance or weight reduction. A feasible recommendation is to start at the recommended 60 minutes per day and slowly increase both the duration and intensity to levels comfortable to the child/adolescent. Prolonged periods of moderate intensity (e.g., brisk walking) are known to burn body fat more efficiently.[24] The providers should ensure that the prescribed activity is safe and developmentally appropriate. Regular supervision of activity and involvement of family members will aid in better compliance to physical activity interventions. Educating the child/caregivers about the additional benefits of physical activity will also increase the compliance to such interventions.

Reduction of Sedentary Behavior

Existing recommendations suggest that all children/adolescents should limit their daily screen time to less than 2 hours per day. This is based on the fact that every additional hour of sedentary activity substantially increases the risk of obesity and obesity-related health issues. Excess screen time is associated with higher failure rates for weight reduction attempts in adolescents and children and needs to be avoided at any cost.

Previous studies have documented that excessive TV viewing is associated with increased consumption of energy rich, fat, sweet, and salty snack foods as well as sugar sweetened beverages.[25] In addition, excessive TV viewing has a negative association with consumption of fruits and vegetables.[25] A reasonable recommendation will be to limit daily screen time to 60 minutes or less per day for children/adolescents with overweight/obesity.

Pharmacological Treatment

The two drugs currently in use among obese children and adolescents are orlistat and metformin. The only Food and Drug Administration (FDA)-approved drug to be used among obese children/adolescents (aged 12 years or older) now is orlistat.[26] This drug is a pancreatic lipase inhibitor and acts by increasing fecal fat loss. Side effects include flatulence, diarrhea, gallbladder diseases, and malabsorptive stools. All patients should be monitored regularly while on this drug and supplementation of fat-soluble vitamins should be done.[26] The drug is less useful in those populations where the fat composition is low. Metformin is a reasonable add-on in the treatment of obese adolescents who have impaired glucose tolerance, severe insulin resistance, or polycystic ovary syndrome (PCOS).[27] The drug appears to have similar minimal weight loss effects as seen in adults. Metformin should only be used in children aged ≥10 years. Pharmacotherapy should ideally be reserved as a second line of management and should be prescribed only when additional obesity-related issues are present.[6] This is attempted when such issues such as impaired glucose tolerance, insulin resistance, hepatic steatosis, lipid abnormalities, or significant menstrual dysfunction persist in spite of an adequate dose/duration of lifestyle interventions.[6]

Surgical Treatment

Surgical treatment of obesity is restricted to a subset of adolescents with severe obesity.

Candidates for such interventions should be (1) severely obese as defined by BMI > 40, (2) of reasonable skeletal maturity (age >13 years for girls and >15 years for boys), and (3) having obesity-related comorbidities that may improve with weight loss.[28] In extreme adolescent obesity (BMI > 50 kg/m^2), surgical treatment may be advised even with minor levels of comorbidities.

Three procedures are listed under surgical options to treat severe adolescent obesity, which are Roux-en-Y gastric bypass (RYGB), vertical sleeve gastrectomy (VSG), and laparoscopic adjustable gastric band (LAGB).[29] RYGB is often referred to as the standard-of-care for surgical management of severe obesity in adolescents. RYGB is performed via minimally invasive, laparoscopic techniques. This option results in significant weight loss via its effects on appetite, satiety, and regulation of energy balance. VSG leads to weight loss through similar effects mentioned above for RYGB.VSG reduces appetite via delayed gastric emptying and by altering neurohormonal feedback mechanisms. This procedure is becoming more common as an option for adolescent obesity management. At present, LAGB is approved only for obese people 18 years or older.

Late complications of these surgical options include obstruction of small-bowel, incisional hernias, and regaining of body weight. They can also result in vitamin and micronutrient deficiencies, which may require lifelong supplements. In addition, these patients should be meticulously followed up at regular intervals for the rest of their lives.[6]

Conclusion

Obesity during childhood and adolescence is a complex medical scenario. This condition evolves from the interplay of physical and environmental factors and the intensity of the same is dependent on individual drivers. The notable contributors to the global obesity drive include the unhealthy evolution of food choices, degrading activity environments, and the ever-increasing inclination to sedentariness during childhood/adolescence. All these have placed children and adolescents at a higher risk for obesity and associated health problems than they ever have been before. The management of obesity at this age includes a multifaceted approach that includes lifestyle modifications, behavioral counseling, pharmacotherapy, and surgical options. Interventions at the level of the family/pediatric physicians, school managements, government bodies, community organizations, and family should be widely promoted to aid in the prevention of obesity during this age.

PEDIATRIC DYSLIPIDEMIAS

Currently, adult CVD mortality has been curtailed due to significant improvements in treatment. The majority of this improvement in mortality is primarily from improvements in atherosclerotic risk factor treatment. There is a worrisome dominating trend that has the potential to upset these gains that happened in the last few decades. The trio of obesity,

TABLE 2: Acceptable, borderline-high, and high plasma lipid, lipoprotein, and apolipoprotein concentrations for children and adolescents.

Category	Low, mg/dL	Acceptable, mg/dL	Borderline-high, mg/dL	High, mg/dL
Total cholesterol	–	<170	170–199	≥200
LDL cholesterol	–	<110	110–129	≥130
Non-HDL cholesterol	–	<120	120–144	≥145
Apolipoprotein B	–	<90	90–109	≥110
Triglycerides	–			
0–9 years	–	<75	75–99	≥100
10–19 years	–	<90	90–129	≥130
HDL cholesterol	<40	<45	40–45	–
Apolipoprotein A-1	<115	<120	115–120	–

[*Source:* Adapted with modification from Expert Panel on Integrated Guidelines for Cardiovascular Health and Risk Reduction in Children and Adolescents: Summary report (2011)][30]
(HDL: high-density lipoprotein, LDL: low-density lipoprotein)

obesity-related dyslipidemia, and type 2 diabetes is having an epidemic level growth that can dominate the current and future scenarios of CVD. Both childhood and adolescence offer a prime opportunity to continue CVD risk factor reduction and address the emerging trend of pediatric and adolescent dyslipidemia.

The acceptable, borderline, and high values of lipids and lipoproteins in children and adolescents are presented in **Table 2**.

Pediatric dyslipidemias can be either primary or secondary to lifestyle factors, medical conditions, or medications. The major primary dyslipidemias are presented in **Table 3**.

TABLE 3: Summary of major primary lipid disorders in children and adolescents.

Primary lipid disorders	Lipid/lipoprotein abnormality
Familial hypercholesterolemia	
Homozygous	↑↑ LDL cholesterol
Heterozygous	↑ LDL cholesterol
Familial defective apolipoprotein B	↑ LDL cholesterol
Familial combined hyperlipidemia[a]	
Type IIa	↑ LDL cholesterol
Type IV	↑ VLDL cholesterol, ↑ triglycerides
Type IIb	↑ LDL cholesterol, VLDL cholesterol, triglycerides
Types IIb and IV	↓ HDL cholesterol (often)
Polygenic hypercholesterolemia	↑ LDL cholesterol
Familial hypertriglyceridemia (200–1,000 mg/dL)	↑ VLDL cholesterol, glyceridemia
Severe hypertriglyceridemia (≤1,000 mg/dL)	↑ Chylomicrons, VLDL cholesterol, ↑↑ triglycerides
Familial hypoalpha-lipoproteinemia	↓ HDL cholesterol
Dysbetalipoproteinemia (TC: 250–500 mg/dL; triglycerides: 250–600 mg/dL)	↑ IDL cholesterol, 50–600 mg/dL, 50–500 m

[a]These are the two lipid and lipoprotein disorders seen most frequently in childhood and adolescence; the latter most often manifests with obesity
[*Source:* Adapted with modification from Expert Panel on Integrated Guidelines for Cardiovascular Health and Risk Reduction in Children and Adolescents: Summary report (2011)][30]
(HDL: high-density lipoprotein; IDL: intermediate-density lipoprotein; LDL: low-density lipoprotein, VLDL: very low-density lipoprotein)

Familial Hypercholesterolemia

Familial hypercholesterolemia (FH) is a common genetic cause of premature CHD.[31] The majority of variations of FH are inherited as autosomal dominant conditions. Heterozygous familial hypercholesterolemia (HeFH) is common and is present in ~1 per 200–250 of the general population. Familial hypercholesterolemia in its homozygous form (HoFH) is a rare disease with an estimated prevalence of 1 per 160,000–300,000. Children with untreated HeFH have a dramatic increase in the risk of premature CHD after age 20 years. Individuals with HoFH are at extremely high risk and, if untreated, many will manifest coronary or other CVD in childhood or adolescence.[31]

Familial hypercholesterolemia is predominantly seen from mutations in the *LDLR* gene on chromosome 19. Approximately, 5–30% of cases of phenotypic FH are known to arise from mutations in unidentified genes, or have a polygenic origin. All the monogenic defects linked to FH will lead to reduced efficiency of LDL uptake and clearance in hepatocytes. This will then lead to increased serum levels of TC and LDL-C. The inheritance of a mutation in the gene from one parent is known to result in the heterozygous variant (HeFH). Inheritance of a mutation from each parent causes the homozygous FH (HoFH). In FH, there is attenuation of the clearance of plasma LDL-C by the LDL receptor. This defect leads to increased numbers of circulating

LDL particles. These can penetrate the arterial wall and can start accumulating in these walls. In due course, the LDL particles get oxidatively modified and can later trigger an inflammatory response. This inflammatory response can lead to vascular injury and formation of atherosclerotic plaque.[31,32]

Diagnosis

Familial hypercholesterolemia is usually diagnosed during childhood/adolescence by the presence of elevated LDL-C consistent with that seen in FH plus a history of premature CHD in their family and/or baseline elevated cholesterol in one parent and/or an FH-causing mutation. Any child with an LDL-C level ≥5 mmol/L (190 mg/dL) even after a trial of dietary intervention has a high probability of genetically based FH. In the presence of a family history of premature CHD in close relatives and/or a baseline high cholesterol in one parent, an LDL-C ≥4 mmol/L (160 mg/dL) is also suggestive of a high probability of the same condition.[31]

The gold standard for diagnosis of genetically defined FH is the detection of a pathogenic mutation, usually in the *LDLR* gene. The specific diagnostic cut-offs for LDL-C in the childhood age can be derived from the Simon Broome criteria. The threshold is 4 mmol/L (160 mg/dL) in children with FH aged <10 years.[33,34] Any LDL-C measurement should be repeated at least twice over 3 months before confirming the diagnosis of FH. It should be noted that an LDL-C level >13 mmol/L (500 mg/dL) is consistent with phenotypic HoFH. Secondary causes of elevated LDL-C (*see* **Box 1**) should be ruled out in the clinical workup for FH.

Management of Familial Hypercholesterolemia

Diet and lifestyle are critical elements in the management of FH in children. A fat-modified diet is currently recommended. This diet should have <30% of calories from total fat, <7% of calories from saturated fat, and <200 mg of cholesterol/day.[31] Due emphasis should be given to promote the intake of fruit and vegetables, wholegrain-based foods, low-fat dairy products, plant protein sources, fish and lean meats.[31] All children/adolescents with FH should be subjected to growth and developmental monitoring every 6 months. Pediatric physicians should strive hard to encourage physical activity and discourage smoking in patients with FH. The overall cardiovascular risk profile should be kept in the ideal range if possible.

Pharmacotherapy for Heterozygous Familial Hypercholesterolemia

The mainstay of pharmacotherapy in FH is statins. Currently, several statins including simvastatin, lovastatin, atorvastatin, fluvastatin, and rosuvastatin are approved for use in children older than 10 years with FH.[31] Pharmacological treatment for FH in children/adolescents should be initiated at the lowest recommended dose and slowly titrated up based on response to treatment.

In patients older than 10 years of age, a target LDL-C level <3.5 mmol/L (130 mg/dL) may be attempted. In those aged 8–10 years, a 50% reduction from pretreatment levels can be attempted.[31] Addition of ezetimibe or a bile-acid sequestrant may be required in a small subset of children/adolescents to attain target LDL-C goal. Such children/adolescents should be under long-term supplementation with fat-soluble vitamins. If initiated early on statins, children/adolescents may reach up to 100% CHD free survival at the end of the third decade of life. A small subset of pediatric/adolescent patients may remain with severely elevated LDL-C levels. Anyone with such persistent elevations should be referred to a specialist care involving a pediatric cardiologist. Patients with multiple cardiovascular risk factors or complications of pharmacologic therapy, or those with HoFH should only be treated in specialist care involving a pediatric cardiologist.[31]

Homozygous Familial Hypercholesterolemia

Children with HoFH usually have LDL-C levels >13 mmol/L (500 mg/dL). Occasionally, affected individuals with lower levels have been identified with genetic testing.[31]

These children may present with xanthomas as early as in the first few months of life and usually before 10 years of age. Any child with suspected HoFH should be referred promptly to specialized centers mentioned earlier. In children with HoFH, cardiovascular symptoms and signs are usually due to aortic stenosis and regurgitation. Both these conditions result from massive accumulation of cholesterol in the valvular and supravalvular regions of the aortic valve.[35] In addition, such deposits can also lead to coronary ostial stenosis. Several reports of affected children experiencing angina pectoris, myocardial infarction, and even death in early childhood have been published earlier. Usually, the timing of the first major cardiovascular events is during adolescence.[35]

In children with a high suspicion of HoFH, an extensive cardiovascular evaluation is recommended. A coronary computed tomography (CT) angiography is recommended to evaluate the aorta and coronary arteries. In addition, magnetic resonance imaging should also be done to evaluate the aorta. Coronary angiography is usually done depending on the clinical status as well as the outcome of noninvasive workup. All these children should be on regular, strict follow-up.[31]

A very aggressive cholesterol-lowering approach should be initiated at the time of the diagnosis using a combination of a statin and ezetimibe.[36] Lipoprotein apheresis should be started as soon as possible in centers where such facility is available. A new agent, injectable mipomersen, an antisense RNA (ribonucleic acid) therapy, which targets hepatic production of atherogenic apoB-containing lipoproteins, was recently approved as adjunct therapy for HoFH in patients aged ≥12 years.[31] Data related to this drug is currently in the evolving stage.

Liver transplantation is currently evolving as a new curative treatment option in HoFH patients who either fail to reach the treatment targets or cannot tolerate conventional treatment options.[36] Liver transplantation leads to the introduction of new functional LDLRs in those with HoFH. This increases the receptor activity close to 60% and can lead to reduction of LDL plasma levels by 80%.[37] Additionally, by restoring receptor activity to moderate levels, the liver transplant makes it easier for statins to control LDL levels in these patients.[37]A recently published study reported that pediatric HoFH patients (n = 8) who underwent orthotopic liver transplantation documented excellent reductions in TC, LDL, lipoprotein(a) [Lp(a)], and apolipoprotein B (ApoB)/ apolipoprotein A-I (ApoAI) ratio. These beneficial lipid levels were maintained when followed up after 2–6 years.[38]

The timing of diagnosing FH is critical to prevention of atherosclerosis. Statin treatment significantly improves cardiovascular outcomes. Early treatment initiation together with regular and meticulously planned follow-up is essential for ensuring better outcomes among children/adolescents with FH.[31]

Hereditary Hypertriglyceridemia

Children/adolescents usually present with hypertriglyceridemia from secondary causes. Any child/adolescent presenting with very high TG level (>500 mg/dL) should be investigated for genetic causes of hypertriglyceridemia. Monogenic hyperchylomicronemia can result from abnormalities in function of lipoprotein lipase (LPL), apolipoprotein C2 (ApoC2), and apolipoprotein A-5 (ApoA5).[39] Familial chylomicronemia syndrome (FCS) is a rare genetic disorder presenting during childhood/ adolescence with extreme hypertriglyceridemia.[40] FCS is characterized by LPL deficiency which leads to excessive accumulation of chylomicrons. These subjects may present with fasting plasma TG levels in excess of 1,000 mg/dL.[40] They usually present with nausea, vomiting, recurrent abdominal pain, and failure to thrive. Clinical examination may reveal eruptive xanthomas, lipemia retinalis, and hepatosplenomegaly. They may also present with acute pancreatitis. Apolipoprotein E (ApoE) mutations can result in a condition called dysbetalipoproteinemia. Such patients present with an orange discoloration in palmar skin creases. Clinical examination may reveal palmar tuberoeruptive xanthomas. The TG levels could be in the range of 500 to 2,000 mg/dL.

Two common polygenic primary hypertriglyceridemias seen are familial hypertriglyceridemia (1% prevalence) and familial combined hyperlipidemia (1–2% prevalence). These two conditions result in moderate TG elevations compared to FCS. In familial hypertriglyceridemia, TG elevations are in the range of 250–1,000 mg/dL.[41] Familial combined hyperlipidemia presents with high LDL-C and TGs.[41] This condition confers CVD risks in the range similar to that seen in those with FH.

BOX 1: Causes of secondary dyslipidemias.

Exogenous
- Alcohol
- *Drug therapy*: Corticosteroids
- Isotretinoin
- β-blockers
- Some oral contraceptives
- Select chemotherapeutic agents
- Select antiretroviral agents

Endocrine/metabolic
- Hypothyroidism/hypopituitarism
- T1DM and T2DM
- Pregnancy
- Polycystic ovary syndrome
- Lipodystrophy
- Acute intermittent porphyria

Renal
- Chronic renal disease
- Hemolytic uremic syndrome
- Nephrotic syndrome

Infectious
- Acute viral/bacterial infections
- HIV
- Hepatitis

Hepatic
- Obstructive liver disease/cholestatic conditions
- Biliary cirrhosis
- Alagille syndrome

Inflammatory disease
- Systemic lupus erythematosus
- Juvenile rheumatoid arthritis

Storage disease
- Glycogen-storage disease
- Gaucher disease
- Cystine-storage disease
- Juvenile Tay–Sachs disease
- Niemann–Pick disease

Other
- Kawasaki disease
- Anorexia nervosa
- Post solid organ transplantation
- Childhood cancer survivor
- Progeria
- Idiopathic hypercalcemia
- Klinefelter syndrome
- Werner syndrome

[*Source:* Adapted with modification from Expert Panel on Integrated Guidelines for Cardiovascular Health and Risk Reduction in Children and Adolescents: Summary report (2011)][30]

(HIV: human immunodeficiency virus; T1DM: type 1 diabetes mellitus; T2DM: type 2 diabetes mellitus)

Secondary Dyslipidemias

In several occasions, dyslipidemia in children/adolescents could be from secondary causes. These are listed in **Box 1**. Several medications can also lead to dyslipidemia in this age group.

Every child/adolescent presenting with dyslipidemia should be promptly evaluated to rule out secondary causes of dyslipidemia before initiating treatment strategies. In the majority of such cases, prompt management of the causative condition can bring back the lipid levels to within normal range.

Screening for Pediatric Dyslipidemias

Two approaches are currently being promoted for the screening for pediatric dyslipidemia, which are selective screening and universal screening. Selective screening can be of two types—target screening and cascade screening.[39] Target screening basically enables primary prevention of CVD. Under this approach, all children/adolescents (2–21 years) with unknown/positive family history results, a positive diagnosis of diseases associated with high risk for future CVD, and the presence of CVD risk factors are screened for dyslipidemias via a fasting lipid profile. The CVD risk factors mentioned for target screening are obesity, hypertension, diabetes, smoking, unhealthy dietary habits, and sedentary lifestyle. One worrisome point to note here is that selective screening based on family history and risk factors alone misses a third to two-third of children/adolescents with dyslipidemia.[30] The other option is cascade screening. Under this approach, all children 2 years or older with a first- or second-degree relative with a recorded history of early CVD (before 55 years in men and 65 years in women) should be screened by a fasting lipid profile. The NHLBI Expert Panel (2011) recommends universal screening for dyslipidemia between the ages of 9 and 11 years and between 17 and 21 years.[30] The goal of this testing is to reduce morbidity and mortality from heart disease in pediatric patients with FH. Universal screening in this age group will enable early diagnosis and effective disease management of FH.

Management of Pediatric Dyslipidemias

The management of pediatric dyslipidemias can be grossly divided into lifestyle interventions and pharmacological therapy.

Lifestyle Modifications

Any child or adolescent presenting with an LDL-C level of 130 mg/dL or greater should be selected for appropriate lifestyle modifications.[42] The initial strategy should focus on three items—dietary changes, physical activity, and weight loss (overweight/obese subjects). Any intervention that has the potential to improve BMI to the healthy range will also shift lipid levels to the desirable range. All children/adolescents with elevated lipid levels should have a minimum of 60 minutes of moderate/vigorous physical activity per day. This should be clubbed with reducing screen time to <2 hours/day. These subjects should have adequate sleep as well. Parents can be role models for active living. Children/adolescents show more compliance to exercise interventions when these are attempted together with a motivated parent/sibling.[30]

Dietary Intake

Dietary modifications have a significant role in improving dyslipidemia. The recommendations are to reduce total and saturated fat along with reduction of cholesterol sources.[30] This needs to be coupled with increased intake of dietary fiber from fruits, vegetables, and whole grains. A good start would be to follow a diet that provides <30% of total calories from fats. The energy from saturated fat should be in the range of 7–10% and TC intake should be kept below 300 mg/day.[42] These children/adolescents should be assessed at the end of 3 months. If the lipid level exceeds the therapeutic target, a more restrictive diet that provides 25% or less of total calories from fat, saturated fat to <7% of total calories, and cholesterol intake of <200 mg/day should be attempted.[30]

Two critical components of dietary interventions to tackle dyslipidemia are the availability of healthy snacks as well as unhealthy food items at home/community/school premises. Families should strive to present healthy snack options such as fresh fruits, nuts, and salads at home. Reducing home availability of unhealthy snacks such as junk foods and sweetened beverages are well known to result in better dietary patterns and improvements in BMI, lipids, and glucose metabolism among children/adolescents. Counseling parents about the need for strict dietary as well as physical activity interventions and their resultant long-term benefits is essential for involving them in the treatment strategy. Physicians/counselors should encourage eating together and group exercises in families. Healthy eating at home and exercising parents will enhance similar behavior in children/adolescents.

Pharmacologic Therapy

Pharmacologic therapy is added when lifestyle modifications fail to sufficiently mitigate the risks of ASCVD.[39] Even when pharmacologic therapy is added, lifestyle modifications should be continued as an adjuvant to the same. This add-on will enhance the efficacy of drugs and may also reduce the dose required for optimal control. Pharmacologic therapy can be instituted in any indicated child above the age of 8 years. The decision to start drug therapy is based on average lipid levels (at least two separate readings) and the presence/absence of other risk factors.[30]

Elevated LDLC: Statins (3-hydroxy-3- methyl-glutaryl-coenzyme A reductase inhibitors) are the first line of therapy for elevated levels of LDL-C during childhood/adolescence. Treatment with statins results in upregulation of LDL receptors, which leads to reduced plasma LDL-C. Initiation of statin therapy reduces risk of ASCVD. Six of the seven commercially available statins (excluding pitavastatin) are approved for pediatric patients (**Table 4**).

The treating physician should aim to bring down the LDL to below 130 mg/dL (ideally <100 mg/dL) or should try for a 50% or greater reduction from pretreatment levels.[44] If these targets are not achieved by the starting dose, dose escalation can be attempted till a maximum dose is reached. Physicians should note that doubling of the dose of statin will only result in an additional reduction in the

TABLE 4: Lipid lowering drugs for pediatric use.

Drug	*Age*	*Dose range*	*Indication*
Rosuvastatin	8–9 years	5–10 mg	HeFH
	10–17 years	5–20 mg	
Pravastatin	8–13 years	20 mg	HeFH
	14–18 years	40 mg	
Atorvastatin	10–17 years	10–20 mg	HeFH
	≥ 10 years	10–80 mg	HoFH
Fluvastatin	10–16 years	20–80 mg	HeFH
Simvastatin	10–17 years	10–40 mg	HeFH
Lovastatin	10–17 years	10–40 mg	HeFH
Colesevelam	10–17 years	3,750 mg	HeFH
Cholestyramine	6–12 years	80 mg/kg TID; maximum dose, 8 g/day	hypercholesterolemia
	adolescents	4 g BID	
Ezetimibe	10–17 years	10 mg	HeFH

(*Source*: Bays HE, Jones PH, Orringer CE, Brown WV, Jacobson TA. National Lipid Association Annual Summary of Clinical Lipidology 2016. J Clin Lipidol. 2016;10(1 Suppl):S1-43.)[43]

(HeFH: heterozygous familial hypercholesterolemia; HoFH: homozygous familial hypercholesterolemia; TID: ter in die)

range of 6%. In those children/adolescents whom the combination of lifestyle intervention and statins (in maximal dose) fails to bring the LDL-C levels to target range, add-on drugs should be considered.[43] These include bile-acid sequestrants (cholestyramine and colesevelam) or cholesterol absorption inhibitors (ezetimibe). Cholestyramine can be given to children older than 6 years while colesevelam and ezetimibe can be given to those aged 10 years or more.

Elevated triglycerides: Children/adolescents who present with TG levels of 500 mg/dL or greater are known to have high risk for secondary pancreatitis. TG levels should ideally be kept below this range to prevent this complication. Fibric acid derivatives (fibrates) and omega-3 fatty acids can decrease hepatic TG production and can be prescribed to treat high levels of TG in children/adolescents.[44] Orlistat (pancreatic lipase inhibitor) can increase circulatory clearance of TG and thereby decrease the risk of pancreatitis. Orlistat can be given in adolescents older than 12 years.

Monitoring of treatment and side effects: Children/adolescents on statins can have muscle-related symptoms, hepatic dysfunction, and hyperglycemia. Children/adolescents on BAS may experience gastrointestinal adverse effects (constipation and bloating) which can be reduced in incidence and intensity by increased dietary fiber and adequate fluid consumption. BAS may increase plasma TGs and should be used with caution in children/adolescents with TG levels >250 mg/dL. BAS should not be prescribed to those with TG levels >500 mg/dL. Children/adolescents on fibrate therapy may experience myopathy, cholelithiasis, and elevations in creatinine. Myopathy is more common in concomitant therapy with statins.

Any child/adolescent who is under pharmacotherapy for high LDL or TG should be under frequent follow-up to monitor compliance as well as to identify drug-related side effects.[44] All patients should have a complete workup [fasting lipids and liver function test (LFT)] at baseline, 1 month, 2 months, and then every 3 months on follow-up. Similarly, creatine kinase (CK) levels should be monitored in those taking statins, especially if patients report myalgia. Hepatic enzymes should be kept at levels below three times the upper limit of normal. In addition, a physical examination with anthropometric evaluation and BP monitoring should also be done during these visits.

The majority of pediatric/adolescent dyslipidemias will be identified and can be managed by the pediatric physician. The NHLBI Expert Panel Recommendations (2011) state that all children/adolescents with LDL-C levels of 250 mg/dL or greater and/or TG levels of 500 mg/dL or greater should be referred to a lipid specialist and be worked up as per guideline recommendations.[30] Those with persistently high levels and/or those with complex lipid abnormalities should be referred to a specialist care center involving a pediatric cardiologist.

CARDIOVASCULAR RISK REDUCTION DURING CHILDHOOD AND ADOLESCENCE

Atherosclerotic cardiovascular disease is the leading cause of mortality for majority of countries across the world. The classic risk factors for this group of diseases include older age, male sex, family history of ASCVD, high BP, dyslipidemia, smoking, diabetes mellitus, and excess body weight.

Two landmark studies, The Bogalusa Heart Study and the Pathobiological Determinants of Atherosclerosis in Youth (PDAY), shed light into the timing of the origin of ASCVD.[16,45] These studies are noted for two important findings. The first is that advanced levels of atherosclerosis including fibrous plaques can be present as early as adolescence. The second is that the coverage and advancement of these plaques show a strong association with BMI, high BP, high LDL-C, low HDL-C, diabetes mellitus, and cigarette smoking even during adolescence and early adulthood.[16,45]

Several measures of subclinical atherosclerosis have evolved in the last two decades and are quite popular now in assessing CVD risk in children and adolescents.[30] They include demonstration of coronary calcium on electron beam CT, increased CIMT assessed by ultrasonography (USG), endothelial dysfunction (reduced arterial dilation) with brachial USG, and increased LV mass with cardiac ultrasound. In adolescents with very high LDL (e.g., FH), associations with coronary calcium, CIMT, and endothelial function have been noted in several studies. Similarly, those children/adolescents with hypertension have shown associations with CIMT and LV mass. Diabetes and smoking too have shown associations with endothelial function and CIMT during childhood/adolescence.[30] Together, these studies confirm that atherosclerosis starts during childhood and the risk factors under play are the same for children and adults.Modifications in the three primary lifestyle components including diet, physical activity, and smoking attempted during childhood and adolescence will definitely enable us to mitigate the risk of future ASCVD.

Diet

Diet along with physical activity remains the two solid pillars of cardiovascular health promotion during childhood and adolescence just like in adulthood. A healthy eating pattern established during childhood and adolescence goes a long way in supporting both primordial and primary prevention of classic ASCVD risk factors such as obesity, high BP, and cholesterol abnormalities. The evidence for the benefit of these interventions during childhood and adolescence is limited and evolving. Early signals suggest that these can have significant benefits in the long term. An additional benefit in this regard is the fact that healthy eating behavior established during childhood and adolescence can track into adulthood with accompanying benefits. The Cardiovascular Risk in Young Finns Study suggests that healthful dietary patterns established in childhood/adolescence and their accompanying cardiovascular benefits track into adulthood.[46]

Two major cardiovascular risk factors—obesity and cholesterol levels—have shown strong associations with dietary patterns during childhood/adolescence. Adiposity is strongly linked to dietary fat intake, total energy consumption, consumption of energy dense food items, and intake of sugar sweetened beverages. Children/adolescents with consistently larger than required calorie intake are likely to increase body fat with accompanying increase in risk for ASCVD. Children/adolescents who report regular consumption of a proper breakfast are at lower risk for overweight/obesity and are more likely to consume a balanced diet.

Several clinical trials have suggested that diets low in total fat (<30% of energy), saturated fat (8–10% of energy), and cholesterol (200–300 mg/day) significantly reduce the TC and LDL cholesterol levels.

In those with adiposity in the range of overweight/obesity, the DISC diet can be introduced (≥8 years of age).[22] DISC diet specifies 58% of total calorie intake from carbohydrates, 28% from fats (11% mono, 9% poly, and 8% or less from saturates), and 14% from proteins. The intake of cholesterol should be restricted to a maximum of 75 mg/1,000 kilocalories and should not exceed 150 mg/day. Those with high BP, the DASH diet can be attempted and this diet has a reasonable efficacy in lowering BP.[47] In children/adolescents with abnormal cholesterol levels, the CHILD 1 (Cardiovascular Health Integrated Lifestyle Diet-1) or CHILD 2 diets can be attempted.[30]

All physicians at the primary care level as well as pediatric physicians should find time to counsel pediatric patients/caretakers to follow recommended dietary patterns in line with the evidence from clinical trials mentioned above. Children/adolescents should also be encouraged to consume daily fruits/vegetables as well as fiber rich foods as per recommendations. They should also be encouraged to limit their salt and added sugar intake. In addition, parents/children should be advised to be mindful of portion sizes and unhealthy dietary items that are rich in fat/sugar/salt while at home, in school canteens and during eat outs.

Physical Activity

Several clinical and epidemiological studies have confirmed the health-related benefits of regular physical activity beyond doubt. Increased levels of moderate-to-vigorous physical activity during childhood/adolescence are associated with reductions in SBP and DBP, reduced body fat percentage, lower BMI, improved fitness measures, lower levels of total and LDL-C level, lower TG level, higher levels of HDL cholesterol, and reductions in insulin resistance.[30]

Currently, evidence is accumulating regarding the harms of increased time spend in sedentary activities during childhood/adolescence. The major ones include decreased physical activity levels as well increased risk for several cardiovascular risk factors including obesity, hypertension, and insulin resistance.[30]

Two landmark studies, the Cardiovascular Risk in Young Finns Study and the Muscatine Study, report the strong association of optimal cardiovascular risk profiles with regular physical activity during childhood/adolescence.[46,48] In addition, several studies have documented the strong tracking of physical activity from childhood/adolescence to adulthood. This tracking is stronger for physical activity engagements during adolescence.

Children/adolescents who are physically active on a regular basis are more likely to adopt other health promoting actions including healthy eating and are less likely to engage in actions that compromise health compared to their counterparts reporting low levels of physical activity.

Several intervention studies published earlier have focused on the benefits of increasing physical activity as well as reduction of sedentary time during childhood/adolescence. The dominant ones among the benefits include reductions in both SBP and DBP, reductions in body fat and BMI, and increments for cardiorespiratory fitness. In addition, the cardiometabolic profiles also showed significant improvement.

These beneficial results are not consistent across studies and there is a lack of clarity for the dose and duration of physical activity required to achieve these benefits.

Current guidelines recommend that children (>6 years of age) and adolescents should engage in at least 60 minutes/day of moderate-to-vigorous physical activity. In addition, vigorous intensity physical activity along with muscle and bone strengthening activities need to be done at least 3 days per week.[30] The intensity of physical activity is quantified by metabolic equivalents (METs). One MET is the energy a person spends in an idle state. An activity of two METs means it is burning twice the energy compared to that burned at rest. Any activity below three METs (<3.5 Kcal/min) is classified as mild, three to six METs as moderate (3.5–7 Kcal/min), and more than six (>7 Kcal/min) as vigorous for children/adolescents. The recommendations also guide us to limit screen time of children/adolescents to >2 hours/day.

The majority of adolescents do not meet current physical activity guidelines as per a recently published systematic review (2020) that looked at 1.6 million school children aged 11–17 years from 146 countries.[49] This review reinforces the fact that strategies are needed to improve levels of physical activity in children and adolescents as well as to attenuate the decline in physical activity from childhood to adolescence.

All pediatric consultations should also add physical activity assessments at regular intervals. Self-reported physical activity levels are grossly over-reported and are quite unreliable. Newer technologies such as wearable low-cost activity monitors as well as those embedded in smart phones can be used to improve the accuracy of these assessments. In addition, assessment of average time spent for sedentary activities should also be documented.

All recommendations for increasing physical activity during childhood/adolescence should be age appropriate and feasible. For children, <6 years unlimited active playtime is recommended along with zero screen time till 2 years of age and <1 hour for 2–5 years of age. Children older than this age should be advised to follow the recommendations mentioned above for activity and sedentary time. Children/adolescents are encouraged by parental physical activity and those children/adolescents with regularly exercising parents report higher physical activity levels. Engaging in physical activity as a family assignment is known to improve compliance to physical activity interventions and this option should be advised to families during consultations.

Obesity

Childhood as well as adolescent obesity is associated with several adverse health conditions including a worsening of cardiovascular health profile. Several risk factors that are linked to cardiovascular health are known to be accelerated in the presence of obesity during childhood/adolescence. The major ones that show an increase include hypertension, type 2 diabetes mellitus, metabolic syndrome, sleep disorders including sleep apnea, LV hypertrophy, and abnormal lipid profiles (high levels of LDL-C and TGs, and low levels of HDL-C).[6,13]

Prevention of obesity in childhood and adolescence is the main pillar of cardiovascular health promotion during this phase of life. This is confirmed scientifically by the improvements in several CVD risk factor levels that accompany successful weight reduction among children/adolescents with overweight/obesity. The notable improvements include declines in SBP and DBP, improvement of blood lipids (reduction of TC, LDL-C, and TGs along with increases for HDL cholesterol), and reduced levels of inflammatory markers.[50] Those with insulin resistance also show a significant reduction of the same with weight loss.[50] A recommended approach to the management of overweight and obesity during childhood and adolescence is detailed in the previous section.

The tracking of obesity from childhood/adolescence to adulthood is also another issue that merits attention. Approximately, four out of five children who are overweight at 10–15 years of age will remain obese adults at 25 years of age.[51] In addition, one in four obese adults report being overweight during childhood.[51]

Regular pediatric consultation charts should include sections for weight, height, and BMI to be entered at every visit. It would be more beneficial if reference graphs applicable to the local settings are embedded in such charts for identification of obesity levels at every visit. In addition to documenting the BMI trajectories, data related to obesity status of parents as well as parental status of cardiovascular risk factors/ASCVD should be documented. Children/adolescents with obesity who also have a positive history of obesity/CVD in their family should be counseled as to the special need to tackle obesity for future cardiovascular health.

Blood Pressure

In children and adolescents, BP is labeled as elevated if measured values exceed 90th percentile based on studies in normal populations.[52] This status is defined by taking into account age, sex, and height of the child/adolescent.

Prehypertension during childhood/adolescence is defined as BP falling between the 90th and 95th percentiles for age, sex, and height or crossing 120/80 mm Hg, whichever is lower.[52] Recommendations to tackle prehypertension in this age group includes lifestyle intervention to improve BMI, diet restrictions to lower dietary sodium, and approaches to increase the level of physical activity.

Hypertension during childhood/adolescence is defined by SBP or DBP above the 95th percentile on at least three consecutive occasions.[52] Hypertension is categorized into stages I and II depending on the severity of BP elevation. Stage I hypertension is defined as BP above the 95th percentile but below the 99th percentile plus 5 mm Hg (12 mm Hg above the 95th percentile). Stage II hypertension is defined as BP above the 99th percentile plus 5 mm Hg.[52]

Stage I hypertension should be addressed by lifestyle changes aimed at improvement of BMI. Pharmacological intervention may be indicated if the BP stays elevated despite lifestyle interventions or if there is evidence of target organ damage. Stage II hypertension may also require earlier intervention with pharmacological therapy.

Previous research suggests that adolescents with elevated BP are highly likely to be hypertensive during adulthood.[53,54] The factors that increase the likelihood of BP remaining high during adulthood include excess weight gain over time, cigarette smoking, low physical activity, and unhealthy dietary patterns.[54]

Autopsy studies suggest that BP elevation in children and adolescents is associated with early atherosclerosis and is also related to increased LV mass.[55,56] 1 in 12 of children and adolescents with hypertension show increased LV mass index, a marker of high cardiovascular risk during adulthood.[57] The levels seen are in line with a four-fold increase in the risk of CVD during adulthood.

Clinicians should be aware that measurement of BP is an integral part of cardiovascular risk assessment among children and adolescents. Regular monitoring of BP after the age of 3 years and appropriate interventions to tackle elevated BP early in life will help us to significantly reduce the cardiovascular risk among children and adolescents.

Lipids and Lipoproteins

Over the past five decades, studies have accumulated data linking adverse levels of lipids and lipoproteins to the initiation and progression of the atherosclerotic process in children and adolescents.[58] Previously published research (postmortem studies) reinforces the strong link between atherosclerosis and abnormal levels of lipids/lipoproteins.[16,56] Findings suggest that early atherosclerotic lesions (fatty streaks) and advanced lesions (fibrous plaques) are significantly related to elevations in TC, LDL-C, and non-HDL-C, and low levels of HDL-C. The same studies also confirm the link between atherosclerosis and the presence as well as intensity of other potentially modifiable risk factors.[16,56,59] These modifiable factors include obesity, hypertension, and cigarette smoking.

Results of several recent imaging studies that attempted to assess subclinical atherosclerosis reaffirm the findings of earlier autopsy studies. These imaging studies indicate that abnormal levels of lipids and lipoproteins in childhood and adolescence are associated with several surrogate markers of cardiovascular risk.[58] These markers include endothelial dysfunction, coronary artery calcium, and increased CIMT.[58]

The combined results of studies mentioned above indicate that adverse levels of lipids and lipoproteins and their complex interactions with several modifiable risk factors can result in accelerated atherosclerotic processes in childhood and adulthood. These results also point to the significant importance of early life prevention of atherosclerosis.

Table 5 presents cut points recommended by National Cholesterol Education Program (NCEP) and American

TABLE 5: Lipids and lipoprotein distributions in children and adolescents ages 5–19 years.

	Males			*Females*		
	5–9 years	*10–14 years*	*15–19 years*	*5–9 years*	*10–14 years*	*15–19 years*
Total cholesterol, (mg/dL)						
50th P	153	161	152	164	159	157
75th P	168	173	168	177	171	176
90th P	183	191	183	189	191	198
95th P	186	201	191	197	205	208
Triglycerides, (mg/dL)						
50th P	40	50	68	57	68	64
75th P	58	74	88	74	85	85
90th P	70	94	125	103	104	112
95th P	85	111	143	120	120	126
LDL cholesterol, (mg/dL)						
50th P	90	94	93	98	94	93
75th P	103	109	109	115	110	110
90th P	117	123	123	125	126	129
95th P	129	133	130	140	136	137
HDL cholesterol, (mg/dL)						
5th P	38	37	30	36	37	35
10th P	43	40	34	38	40	38
25th P	49	46	39	48	45	43
50th P	55	55	46	52	52	51

(HDL: high-density lipoprotein; LDL: low-density lipoprotein)

(*Source*: Hickman TB, Briefel RR, Carroll MD, Rifkind BM, Cleeman JI, Maurer KR, et al. Distributions and trends of serum lipid levels among United States children and adolescents ages 4-19 years: data from the Third National Health and Nutrition Examination Survey. Prev Med. 1998;27(6):879-90.)[60]

Academy of Pediatrics (AAP) used to identify children and adolescents with abnormal lipid and lipoprotein levels. In addition, American Heart Association (AHA) recommends that TG levels of ≥150 mg/dL and HDL-C levels of ≤35 mg/dL be considered abnormal for children and adolescents.

Lipid levels in children/adolescents too exhibit tracking to adulthood similar to that seen for BP and obesity. Two landmark studies—Muscatine Study and the Bogalusa Heart Study—confirm the presence of tracking of lipid levels from childhood to adolescence.[61-63] The Muscatine Study reported that three-fourths of who were 5–18 years of age at baseline and had TC levels above the 90th percentile had elevated TC (≥200 mg/dL) when assessed in the third decade of their life.[61,62] The Bogalusa Heart Study reported that two-thirds of children with elevated TC in childhood persisted with elevated levels when assessed later during adulthood.[63]

Dyslipidemia in children and adolescents should be tackled by a dual approach—one that combines a population-based approach and an individual/high-risk approach.

The population-based approach should aim at promoting optimal lipid levels in all children and youth and should accomplish this by encouraging favorable lifestyle changes known to result in such changes.

The safety and efficacy of a restricted diet that consists of total fat of <30% of the caloric intake, saturated fat of <10% of the intake, and cholesterol intake of <200 mg/dL per day, with 1.5% cow's milk after 12 months of age has been confirmed earlier in the STRIP (Special Turku Coronary Risk Factor Intervention Project) Study.[64]

American Heart Association recommends that a balanced caloric intake with sufficient physical activity (60 min/day) should be promoted among children/adolescents.[65] The dietary changes suggested include increased consumption of fruits, vegetables, whole grains, fish, and low fat dairy products. AHA also recommends to limit intake of trans fats to <1% of total calories.[65]

The individual approach to tackle dyslipidemia among children and adolescents focuses on those at risk because of a positive family history of CVD and/or those who present with elevated levels of LDL-C or other major risk factors. These subjects are prescribed a therapeutic lifestyle change which is a combination of diet restrictions mentioned above supplemented with regular physical activity of not <60 minutes of moderate-to-vigorous intensity per day. Previous studies suggest that good adherence to a saturated fat- and cholesterol-restricted diet (<7% and <200 mg/day, respectively) can significantly reduce LDL-C levels by 10–15% from the baseline.[66]

American Academy of Pediatrics recommends that pharmacological interventions should be considered in children >8 years of age if LDL-C levels persist at ≥190 mg/dL when no risk factors are present. If risk factors are present, the cut-off for intervention is at ≥160 mg/dL.[58] The risk factors mentioned above include obesity, hypertension, positive family history of CVD, and/or cigarette smoking. For those with diabetes mellitus, this cut-off is at ≥130 mg/dL.[58] The details of pharmacotherapy is discussed under pediatric dyslipidemias.

Smoking and Tobacco Consumption

Tobacco use is undoubtedly the leading preventable cause of death globally. Globally, the age-standardized prevalence of daily smoking was 15.2% (14.7 and 15.7) in 2015.[67] There were 933.1 (901.5 and 966.5) million people who smoked tobacco daily.[67] The highest age-standardized rates of mortality were for smoked tobacco as a risk factor at 110.7 (101.0 and 120.3) per 100,000 deaths, compared to 33.0 (28.0 and 37.7), and 6.9 deaths (6.1 and 7.6) per 100,000 people in 2015 for alcohol and illicit drugs, respectively.[67] Four out of five adult smokers begin smoking either during childhood or adolescence. In view of this, prevention of smoking initiation and cessation interventions should be integrated with approaches to cardiovascular health promotion during childhood and adolescence.

The approach to tackle tobacco use during childhood/adolescence should be a double pronged one with individual and public health strategies similar to that used for lipid control in this age group.[58]

Government machineries should focus on curbing advertising/promoting tobacco products, and blocking the availability of tobacco products to children and adolescents. These two should be combined with large scale comprehensive tobacco control policies.

Behavioral interventions for the prevention of initiation and smoking cessation among children/adolescents were attempted by researchers earlier with mixed results. A systematic review of smoking prevention interventions delivered by healthcare providers by Christakis et al. showed a significant positive effect on the prevention of smoking initiation.[68] Another, recent Cochrane review looked at the efficacy of family-based programs to prevent initiation of smoking by adolescents and children.[69] Family-based interventions appear to have a positive effect on preventing children and adolescents from starting to smoke. The evidence was strongest for high-intensity programs used independently of school-based interventions. The review suggests that family interventions might reduce uptake or experimentation with smoking by between 16 and 32%.[69]

Pediatric physicians as well as physicians in family practice should emphasize a developmental approach incorporating the assessment of smoking status at every well-child visit.[58] Parents and caretakers should be encouraged and motivated to maintain a smoke-free home environment. Additional efforts should focus on avoiding exposure to second-hand smoke. Approaches for infants and young children should target parents/caretakers. Those who smoke in the household should be advised about the immediate as well as long-term impact of this behavior on children/

adolescents living with them. Such tobacco users should be motivated to quit and referred to smoking cessation programs.[58]

Assessment of smoking status along with health education sessions about the importance of remaining smoke-free should be attempted at schools. A combination of five strategies should be adopted here by the pediatric healthcare providers.[70] These strategies include (1) encouraging children to avoid environmental smoke exposure, (2) emphasizing the importance of not experimenting with smoking, (3) health education related to the health consequences of smoking and the risk of addiction, (4) presenting information to counter media influences, and (5) delivering nonsmoking messages during clinical encounters.

In the case of adolescents who started smoking, support and counseling either personally by the clinician/counselor or through enrolment in community-based smoking cessation programs should be attempted.[58] Research suggests that such approaches will yield positive outcomes in the majority of adolescent smokers. Adolescent smokers should also be given information related to quit-line numbers and community-based cessation programs.[58]

CONCLUSION

The risk factors for atherosclerotic CVD can develop during childhood and adolescence and is often a result of complex interactions between genetic and environmental factors. The roots of CVD are deeply embedded in families. All approaches to CVD prevention during childhood/adolescence must be directed at improving the family environment of young subjects. All attempts to prevent risk factor development (primordial prevention) and to delay/avoid the development of atherosclerotic lesions (primary prevention) should be encouraged by pediatric physicians, family members, school authorities, and government agencies. An integrated approach to prevention of atherosclerotic CVD during childhood/adolescence will definitely improve the likelihood of young subjects maintaining low-risk status into adulthood.

REFERENCES

1. NCD Risk Factor Collaboration (NCD-RisC). Worldwide trends in body-mass index, underweight, overweight, and obesity from 1975 to 2016: a pooled analysis of 2416 population-based measurement studies in 128·9 million children, adolescents, and adults. Lancet. 2017; 390(10113):2627-42.
2. Di Cesare M, Sorić M, Bovet P, Miranda JJ, Bhutta Z, Stevens GA, et al. The epidemiological burden of obesity in childhood: a worldwide epidemic requiring urgent action. BMC Med. 2019;17(1):212.
3. Ng M, Fleming T, Robinson M, Thomson B, Graetz N, Margono C, et al. Global, regional, and national prevalence of overweight and obesity in children and adults during 1980-2013: a systematic analysis for the Global Burden of Disease Study 2013. Lancet. 2014;384(9945): 766-81.
4. Raj M, Sundaram KR, Paul M, Deepa AS, Kumar RK. Obesity in Indian children: time trends and relationship with hypertension. Natl Med J India. 2007;20(6):288-93.
5. Donohoue PA. Obesity. In: Behrman RE, Kleigman RM, Jenson HB (Eds). Nelson Textbook of Pediatrics, 17th edition. Philadelphia: WB Saunders; 2004. pp. 173-7.
6. Raj M, Kumar RK. Obesity in children and adolescents. Indian J Med Res. 2010;132(5):598-607.
7. Owen CG, Whincup PH, Orfei L, Chou QA, Rudnicka AR, Wathern AK, et al. Is body mass index before middle age related to coronary heart disease risk in later life? Evidence from observational studies. Int J Obes (Lond). 2009; 33(8):866-77.
8. Bjørge T, Engeland A, Tverdal A, Smith GD. Body mass index in adolescence in relation to cause-specific mortality: a follow-up of 230,000 Norwegian adolescents. Am J Epidemiol. 2008;168(1): 30-7.
9. Lawlor DA, Benfield L, Logue J, Tilling K, Howe LD, Fraser A, et al. Association between general and central adiposity in childhood, and change in these, with cardiovascular risk factors in adolescence: prospective cohort study. BMJ. 2010;341:c6224.
10. I'Allemand D, Wiegand S, Reinehr T, Müller J, Wabitsch M, Widhalm K, et al. Cardiovascular risk in 26,008 European overweight children as established by a multicenter database. Obesity (Silver Spring). 2008;16(7):1672-9.
11. Raj M, Sundaram KR, Paul M, Sudhakar A, Kumar RK. Dynamics of growth and weight transitions in a pediatric cohort from India. Nutr J. 2009;8:55.
12. Kotchen TA. Obesity-related hypertension: epidemiology, pathophysiology, and clinical management. Am J Hypertens. 2010;23(11): 1170-8.
13. Raj M. Obesity and cardiovascular risk in children and adolescents. Indian J Endocrinol Metab. 2012;16(1):13-9.
14. Invitti C, Guzzaloni G, Gilardini L, Morabito F, Viberti G. Prevalence and concomitants of glucose intolerance in European obese children and adolescents. Diabetes Care. 2003;26(1):118-24.
15. Jin YY, Liang L, Fu JF, Wang XM. The prevalence of type 2 diabetes mellitus and prediabetes in children. Zhongguo Dang Dai Er Ke Za Zhi. 2011;13(2):138-40.
16. Berenson GS, Srinivasan SR, Bao W, Newman WP 3rd, Tracy RE, Wattigney WA. Association between multiple cardiovascular risk factors and atherosclerosis in children and young adults. The Bogalusa Heart Study. N Engl J Med. 1998;338(23):1650-6.
17. Dawson JD, Sonka M, Blecha MB, Lin W, Davis PH. Risk factors associated with aortic and carotid intima-media thickness in adolescents and young adults: the Muscatine Offspring Study. J Am CollCardiol. 2009;53(24):2273-9.
18. Sánchez T, Rojas C, Casals M, Bennett JT, Gálvez C, Betancur C, et al. Trastornosrespiratorios del sueñoenniñosescolares-chilenos: prevalencia y factores de riesgo [Prevalence and risk factors for sleep-disordered breathing in chilean schoolchildren]. Rev ChilPediatr. 2018;89(6): 718-25.
19. Katz ES, D'Ambrosio CM. Pediatric obstructive sleep apnea syndrome. Clin Chest Med. 2010; 31(2):221-34.
20. Spear BA, Barlow SE, Ervin C, Ludwig DS, Saelens BE, Schetzina KE, et al. Recommendations for treatment of child and adolescent overweight and obesity. Pediatrics. 2007;120Suppl 4:S254-88.
21. Dietary reference intakes for energy, carbohydrate, fiber, fat, fatty acids, cholesterol, protein, and amino acids (macronutrients). Washington, DC: National Academies Press; 2002.
22. Van Horn L, Obarzanek E, Friedman LA, Gernhofer N, Barton B. Children's adaptations to a fat-reduced diet: the Dietary Intervention Study in Children (DISC). Pediatrics. 2005; 115(6):1723-33.
23. Strong WB, Malina RM, Blimkie CJ, Daniels SR, Dishman RK, Gutin B, et al. Evidence based physical activity for school-age youth. J Pediatr. 2005;146(6):732-7.
24. Poirier P, Després JP. Exercise in weight management of obesity. Cardiol Clin. 2001; 19(3):459-70.

25. Coon KA, Tucker KL. Television and children's consumption patterns. A review of the literature. Minerva Pediatr. 2002;54(5):423-36.
26. Styne DM, Arslanian SA, Connor EL, Farooqi IS, Murad MH, Silverstein JH, et al. Pediatric obesity-assessment, treatment, and prevention: an Endocrine Society Clinical Practice Guideline. J Clin Endocrinol Metab. 2017; 102(3):709-57.
27. Freemark M. Pharmacotherapy of childhood obesity: an evidence-based, conceptual approach. Diabetes Care. 2007;30(2):395-402.
28. Inge TH, Krebs NF, Garcia VF, Skelton JA, Guice KS, Strauss RS, et al. Bariatric surgery for severely overweight adolescents: concerns and recommendations. Pediatrics. 2004;114(1):217-23.
29. Paulus GF, de Vaan LE, Verdam FJ, Bouvy ND, Ambergen TA, van Heurn LW. Bariatric surgery in morbidly obese adolescents: a systematic review and meta-analysis. Obes Surg. 2015; 25(5): 860-78.
30. de Jesus JM. Expert panel on integrated guidelines for cardiovascular health and risk reduction in children and adolescents: summary report. Pediatrics. 2011;128(Suppl 5): S213-56.
31. Wiegman A, Gidding SS, Watts GF, Chapman MJ, Ginsberg HN, Cuchel M, et al. Familial hypercholesterolaemia in children and adolescents: gaining decades of life by optimizing detection and treatment. Eur Heart J. 2015; 36(36):2425-37.
32. Stocker R, Keaney JF Jr. Role of oxidative modifications in atherosclerosis. Physiol Rev. 2004;84(4):1381-478.
33. van der Graaf A, Avis HJ, Kusters DM, Vissers MN, Hutten BA, Defesche JC, et al. Molecular basis of autosomal dominant hypercholesterolemia: assessment in a large cohort of hypercholesterolemic children. Circulation. 2011;123(11):1167-73.
34. Wald DS, Bestwick JP, Wald NJ. Child-parent screening for familial hypercholesterolaemia: screening strategy based on a meta-analysis. BMJ. 2007;335(7620):599.
35. Kolansky DM, Cuchel M, Clark BJ, Paridon S, McCrindle BW, Wiegers SE, et al. Longitudinal evaluation and assessment of cardiovascular disease in patients with homozygous familial hypercholesterolemia. Am J Cardiol. 2008; 102(11):1438-43.
36. Cuchel M, Bruckert E, Ginsberg HN, Raal FJ, Santos RD, Hegele RA, et al. Homozygous familial hypercholesterolaemia: new insights and guidance for clinicians to improve detection and clinical management. Eur Heart J. 2014;35(32):2146-57.
37. Mytilinaiou M, Kyrou I, Khan M, Grammatopoulos DK, Randeva HS. Familial hypercholesterolemia: new horizons for diagnosis and effective management. Front Pharmacol. 2018;9:707.
38. Martinez M, Brodlie S, Griesemer A, Kato T, Harren P, Gordon B, et al. Effects of liver transplantation on lipids and cardiovascular disease in children with homozygous familial hypercholesterolemia. Am J Cardiol. 2016; 118(4):504-10.
39. Elkins C, Fruh S, Jones L, Bydalek K. Clinical practice recommendations for pediatric dyslipidemia. J Pediatr Health Care. 2019;33(4): 494-504.
40. Davidson M, Stevenson M, Hsieh A, Ahmad Z, van Lennep JR, Crowson C, et al. The burden of familial chylomicronemia syndrome: results from the global IN-FOCUS study. J ClinLipidol. 2018;12(4):898-907.
41. Hegele RA, Ginsberg HN, Chapman MJ, Nordestgaard BG, Kuivenhoven JA, Averna M, et al. The polygenic nature of hypertriglyceridaemia: implications for definition, diagnosis, and management. Lancet Diabetes Endocrinol. 2014;2(8):655-66.
42. Jacobson TA, Maki KC, Orringer CE, Jones PH, Kris-Etherton P, Sikand G, et al. National Lipid Association Recommendations for patient-centered management of dyslipidemia: Part 2. J Clin Lipidol. 2015;9(6 Suppl):S1-122.e1.
43. Bays HE, Jones PH, Orringer CE, Brown WV, Jacobson TA. National Lipid Association Annual Summary of Clinical Lipidology 2016. J Clin Lipidol. 2016;10(1 Suppl):S1-43.
44. Wilson DP, McNeal C, Blackett P. Pediatric dyslipidemia: recommendations for clinical management. South Med J. 2015;108(1):7-14.
45. Strong JP, Malcom GT, McMahan CA, Tracy RE, Newman 3rd WP, Herderick EE, et al. Prevalence and extent of atherosclerosis in adolescents and young adults: implications for prevention from the Pathobiological Determinants of Atherosclerosis in Youth Study. JAMA. 1999; 281(8):727-35.
46. Raitakari OT, Juonala M, Kähönen M, Taittonen L, Laitinen T, Mäki-Torkko N, et al. Cardiovascular risk factors in childhood and carotid artery intima-media thickness in adulthood: the Cardiovascular Risk in Young Finns Study. JAMA. 2003;290(17):2277-83.
47. Couch SC, Saelens BE, Levin L, Dart K, Falciglia G, Daniels SR. The efficacy of a clinic-based behavioral nutrition intervention emphasizing a DASH-type diet for adolescents with elevated blood pressure. J Pediatr. 2008; 152(4):494-501.
48. Janz KF, Dawson JD, Mahoney LT. Increases in physical fitness during childhood improve cardiovascular health during adolescence: the Muscatine Study. Int J Sports Med. 2002;23Suppl 1:S15-21.
49. Guthold R, Stevens GA, Riley LM, Bull FC. Global trends in insufficient physical activity among adolescents: a pooled analysis of 298 population-based surveys with 1·6 million participants. Lancet Child Adolesc Health. 2020;4(1):23-35.
50. Hayman LL, Meininger JC, Daniels SR, McCrindle BW, Helden L, Ross J, et al. Primary prevention of cardiovascular disease in nursing practice: focus on children and youth: a scientific statement from the American Heart Association Committee on Atherosclerosis, Hypertension, and Obesity in Youth. Circulation. 2007;116(3):344-57.
51. Whitaker RC, Wright JA, Pepe MS, Seidel KD, Dietz WH. Predicting obesity in young adulthood from childhood and parental obesity. N Engl J Med. 1997;337(13):869-73.
52. National High Blood Pressure Education Program Working Group on High Blood Pressure in Children and Adolescents. The fourth report on the diagnosis, evaluation, and treatment of high blood pressure in children and adolescents. Pediatrics. 2004;114(2 Suppl 4th Report):555-76.
53. Chen X, Wang Y. Tracking of blood pressure from childhood to adulthood: a systematic review and meta-regression analysis. Circulation. 2008;117(25):3171-80.
54. Lauer RM, Clarke WR. Childhood risk factors for high adult blood pressure: the Muscatine Study. Pediatrics. 1989;84(4):633-41.
55. Newman WP 3rd, Freedman DS, Voors AW, Gard PD, Srinivasan SR, Cresanta JL, et al. Relation of serum lipoprotein levels and systolic blood pressure to early atherosclerosis. The Bogalusa Heart Study. N Engl J Med. 1986;314(3):138-44.
56. McGill HC Jr, McMahan CA, Zieske AW, Malcom GT, Tracy RE, Strong JP. Effects of nonlipid risk factors on atherosclerosis in youth with a favorable lipoprotein profile. Circulation. 2001;103(11):1546-50.
57. Daniels SR, Loggie JM, Khoury P, Kimball TR. Left ventricular geometry and severe left ventricular hypertrophy in children and adolescents with essential hypertension. Circulation. 1998;97(19):1907-11.
58. Daniels SR, Pratt CA, Hayman LL. Reduction of risk for cardiovascular disease in children and adolescents. Circulation. 2011;124(15):1673-86.
59. McGill HC Jr, McMahan CA, Zieske AW, Sloop GD, Walcott JV, Troxclair DA, et al. Associations of coronary heart disease risk factors with the intermediate lesion of atherosclerosis in youth. The Pathobiological Determinants of Atherosclerosis in Youth (PDAY) Research Group. Arterioscler Thromb Vasc Biol. 2000; 20(8):1998-2004.

60. Hickman TB, Briefel RR, Carroll MD, Rifkind BM, Cleeman JI, Maurer KR, et al. Distributions and trends of serum lipid levels among United States children and adolescents ages 4-19 years: data from the Third National Health and Nutrition Examination Survey. Prev Med. 1998;27(6):879-90.
61. Lauer RM, Lee J, Clarke WR. Factors affecting the relationship between childhood and adult cholesterol levels: the Muscatine Study. Pediatrics. 1988;82(3):309-18.
62. Lauer RM, Clarke WR. Use of cholesterol measurements in childhood for the prediction of adult hypercholesterolemia. The Muscatine Study. JAMA. 1990;264(23):3034-8.
63. Webber LS, Srinivasan SR, Wattigney WA, Berenson GS. Tracking of serum lipids and lipoproteins from childhood to adulthood. The Bogalusa Heart Study. Am J Epidemiol. 1991; 133(9):884-99.
64. Hakanen M, Lagström H, Kaitosaari T, Niinikoski H, Näntö-Salonen K, Jokinen E, et al. Development of overweight in an atherosclerosis prevention trial starting in early childhood. The STRIP study. Int J Obes (Lond). 2006;30(4):618-26.
65. Gidding SS, Dennison BA, Birch LL, Daniels SR, Gillman MW, Lichtenstein AH, et al. Dietary recommendations for children and adolescents: a guide for practitioners: consensus statement from the American Heart Association. Circulation. 2005;112(13): 2061-75.
66. American Academy of Pediatrics. National Cholesterol Education Program: Report of the Expert Panel on Blood Cholesterol Levels in Children and Adolescents. Pediatrics. 1992;89(3 Pt 2):525-84.
67. Peacock A, Leung J, Larney S, Colledge S, Hickman M, Rehm J, et al. Global statistics on alcohol, tobacco and illicit drug use: 2017 status report. Addiction. 2018;113(10):1905-26.
68. Christakis DA, Garrison MM, Ebel BE, Wiehe SE, Rivara FP. Pediatric smoking prevention interventions delivered by care providers: a systematic review. Am J Prev Med. 2003;25(4):358-62.
69. Thomas RE, Baker PR, Thomas BC, Lorenzetti DL. Family-based programmes for preventing smoking by children and adolescents. Cochrane Database Syst Rev. 2015;2015(2):CD004493. Published 2015 Feb 27.
70. Williams CL, Hayman LL, Daniels SR, Robinson TN, Steinberger J, Paridon S, et al. Cardiovascular health in childhood: a statement for health professionals from the Committee on Atherosclerosis, Hypertension, and Obesity in the Young (AHOY) of the Council on Cardiovascular Disease in the Young, American Heart Association. Circulation. 2002;106(1):143-60.

51 CHAPTER

Stroke in the Young

Shilpa Kulkarni, Bharat Dalvi, Sonam Kothari t

INTRODUCTION

Pediatric stroke ranks among top 10 causes of death. Approximately 10–25% of children with stroke will die, while around 66% of children will be left with lifetime disability that incurs a great cost to the family, society, and most importantly the child's future.[1-3] The incidence of stroke in children over 1 month of age in developed countries ranges from 1.2–13 per 100,000 per year. The risk is much higher in neonates and preterm occurring 1 in every 2,500–4,000 live births.[4-6] Average age-independent annual incidence in India also is in the same range of 13–33 cases per 100,000 per year.[7]

Stroke was described long back in 400 BC by Hippocrates using a term Apoplexy (Greek word) meaning "struck down with violence," a phenomenon of sudden paralysis that is often associated with ischemia.[8] Then over 2,000 years physicians struggled to define stroke. William Cole introduced the word stroke in 1689 in his essay on paralysis due to vascular origin.

The current World Health Organization definition of stroke (1970) is "rapidly developing clinical signs of focal (or global) disturbance of cerebral function, lasting >24 hours or leading to death with no apparent cause other than that of vascular origin."[9] But this definition has many flaws as time factor of 24 hours is misleading and permanent injury may occur well before 24 hours. Transient ischemic attacks are often associated with cerebral infarction and may occur without overt symptoms. Global disturbance of cerebral function as in watershed infarcts due to hypotension has a different pathophysiology, treatment, and prognosis as compared to other stokes. Thus, neurologists gave the working definition of stroke: it is characterized by a neurologic deficit attributed to an acute focal injury of the central nervous system by a vascular cause resulting in cerebral infarction, intracranial hemorrhage, or subarachnoid hemorrhage.[10]

CLASSIFICATION OF STROKE

A pediatric stroke can be classified by stroke type, the age at which it occurred and the vessels involved.[4]

- *Based on the stroke type*:
  - The three primary types are: Arterial ischemic stroke (AIS), cerebral sinovenous thrombosis (CST), and hemorrhagic stroke (HS).
    - AIS occurs due to sudden occlusion of one or more cerebral arteries. The underlying mechanism could be thrombosis or embolism. In adults, ischemic strokes are most common and account for 75–85% of strokes. In children also, AIS is the most common subtype, accounting for just over half of all strokes.
    - CST occurs in the superficial or deep venous system of the brain and accounts for approximately one in four pediatric stroke cases.
    - HS results from bleeding through a ruptured cerebral artery or bleeding into the site of an acute ischemic stroke. HSs include intracerebral hemorrhage and less commonly subarachnoid or intraventricular hemorrhage. In children, HSs are more common than in adults and account for under half of all childhood strokes.
- *Based on the time of occurrence*:
  - Perinatal stroke, where the stroke is presumed to have occurred between 28 weeks of gestation and 28 days of life
  - Childhood stroke is the one occurring between 29 days and 18 years of age
- *Based on the vessels involved*: Pediatric stroke is also classified by the number of vessels and type of arterial territory involved (anterior, posterior circulation stroke).

RISK FACTORS OF PEDIATRIC STROKE

Pediatric stroke is multifactorial and often multiple factors are responsible in around 25% of children with stroke.[11,12] The early recognition of these risk factors is necessary to prevent recurrent strokes and reduce the morbidity and mortality. The major categories of risk factors described by International Pediatric Stroke Study (IPSS) registry are vasculopathies, hematologic, cardiac, hematological, metabolic, and infectious with no etiology found in >20% of patients (**Table 1**).[14]

TABLE 1: Risk factors for childhood stroke.

Etiology	*Clinical conditions*
Vasculopathy	• Inflammatory and postinfectious: Postvaricella angiopathy, focal cerebral arteriopathy, and primary CNS angiitis • Arteriovenous malformations, Moyamoya disease, and craniocervical arterial dissection
Cardiac disorders	• Congenital heart disease • Bacterial endocarditis • Cardiomyopathies and prosthetic valves
Infection	Upper respiratory tract infections (Mycoplasma, Chlamydia, influenza A, parvovirus 19, etc.), herpes group of viruses, acute otitis media, bacterial or tuberculous meningitis, and HIV
Head/neck trauma	• Post-traumatic dissection and intracranial trauma • Mineralizing angiopathy with subcortical strokes secondary to trivial trauma
Hematologic	• Protein C, protein S, antithrombin III deficiency, factor V Leiden, prothrombin 20210, MTHFR mutations, and antiphospholipid antibodies • Sickle cell disease • Iron deficiency anemia
Metabolic	Homocystinuria, dyslipidemias, mitochondrial encephalopathy with lactic acidosis and stroke-like syndrome (MELAS), Fabry disease

(*Source*: Swaiman's Pediatric Neurology 2017[14])

(CNS: central nervous system; HIV: human immunodeficiency virus; MTHFR: methylenetetrahydrofolate reductase)

STROKE IN CHILDREN WITH HEART DISEASE

Cardiac disease is one of the most common causes of pediatric strokes. Congenital heart defects increase a child's risk of stroke 19-fold [odds ratio (OR), 19; 95% confidence interval (CI), 4.2–83].[15] Infants with congenital heart disease make up to 25% of the total pediatric stroke population. Preoperative stroke and white matter injury are common in neonates with congenital heart disease. In mixed congenital heart disease cohort studies, between 10 and 40% of infants have been diagnosed with preoperative stroke.[16]

Cardiac disorders are a major risk factor for AIS in infancy and childhood and present in 12–28% of cases.[11,12] Abnormalities in cardiac structure, ventricular function, flow pattern, rhythm disturbance, endothelial abnormality, valve structure, blood viscosity, and other factors may contribute to thrombus generation and subsequent cerebral embolization. Multiple AISs in multiple vascular territories (e.g., left and right) suggest a cardiac cause of stroke. Complex congenital heart diseases, particularly cyanotic lesions, carry the highest stroke risk. In a single-center Australian study, infants with cyanotic congenital heart defects undergoing palliative surgery had the highest risk of developing AIS during the periprocedural period; stroke occurred in 22 out of 2,256 cardiac surgeries (1%).[15]

Of all cardiac operations, single ventricle palliation carries the highest risk. Risk is particularly high in infants after the cavopulmonary anastomosis (Glenn shunt) where cerebral venous pressures are acutely elevated for a variable period of time after surgery. It is important to follow these patients carefully as risk persists for several months to years after the surgery. Traditionally, aspirin and iron supplements are administered to mitigate the problem but there is no evidence to support this practice.[17]

Cardiac catheterization is also an independent risk factor. Risk of symptomatic stroke after cardiac catheterization is estimated at 1:600-700. Interventional catheterization is more risky than diagnostic catheterization. Balloon atrial septostomy, in patients with transposition of the great arteries (TGA), prior to arterial switch surgery carries a stroke risk approaching 50%.[18]

A single-center case-control study of >5,500 children undergoing cardiac surgery documented a symptomatic AIS risk of 5.4/1,000 (1:185). Reoperation is an independent risk factor for occurrence of postoperative stroke.[19] The risk of stroke varies with type of surgery, e.g., the risk estimates of immediate or delayed stroke, following Fontan operation, range from 3% to 19%.[20-22] There are ongoing studies into neuroprotective measures during surgery (e.g., surgical strategies, bypass strategies, anesthetic agents, therapeutic hypothermia, and the use of erythropoietin and regenerative treatments) to reduce the incidence of postoperative stroke.[22]

In the acute care setting, all patients with a right-to-left shunt are vulnerable to iatrogenic strokes that result from air or particulate embolism from venous sources and it is necessary to be extremely careful and vigilant about the use of peripheral intravenous access, particularly in small infants.

Paradoxical embolism occurs when an abnormal communication exists between the right and the left side of the heart at the level of the interatrial septum—the persistence of patent foramen ovale (PFO). The embolic material arising in the systemic veins, mainly those of the lower extremities and pelvis bypass pulmonary circulation and reach cerebral vessels across the PFO resulting in stroke. Several studies indicate that the presence of PFO has a significantly higher relative risk in the occurrence of stroke in the young. The size of PFO, magnitude of right-to-left shunt, presence of shunt at rest, and associated aneurysm of the interatrial septum are some of the incremental risk factors for PFO-related strokes.

Another group of patients vulnerable to strokes are infants with tetralogy of Fallot and related physiology who have relative anemia. These babies are prone to strokes that result from altered rheology of red cells that clog the microcirculation. For this reason, prophylactic iron is often routinely administered to all infants with cyanotic heart disease.

CLINICAL FEATURES

Strokes generally present with focal neurologic deficits. Clinical presentation of stroke varies depending on stroke type, vessels involved, and the child's age. In a collective review, focal weakness was the most common presentation (hemi/monopoiesis) 16–94%, followed by headaches in 22–76%, altered mental state in 28–88%, and seizures in 16–48% of children.[6,11,23] Localization of the stroke can be done based on the functional deficits, especially in AIS, e.g., aphasia-dominant middle cerebral artery (MCA) stroke, dense hemiplegia-internal capsular involvement, visual deficits, ataxia, and/or brainstem dysfunction—posterior circulation stroke. Thrombotic strokes usually have a stuttering course as against embolic presenting with hyperacute onset.

Children with CST present with diverse and nonfocal symptoms without any localizing signs such as headache, seizures, lethargy, nausea, vomiting, or signs of increased intracranial pressure. HSs have catastrophic presentation with headaches, altered sensorium, vomiting, seizures, and focal neurological deficit.

DIFFERENTIAL DIAGNOSIS

There are many conditions which can mimic childhood stroke, e.g., migraine, focal seizures followed by transient postictal paralysis (Todd's paresis), acute raised intracranial pressure, traumatic brain injury, central nervous system infections, and demyelinating disorders.

MANAGEMENT

Pediatric strokes are far more common than it is thought of. Significant delays exist in the diagnosis of childhood stroke and factors contributing to the delays include the low incidence of stroke in pediatrics, varying clinical presentations, limited access to diagnostic neuroimaging, and poor awareness of pediatric stroke among pediatricians. Multiple studies have reported, both pre-hospital and in-hospital, delays from symptom onset to stroke diagnosis ranging from 6 to more than 24 hours.[24,25]

Imaging and Laboratory Testing

Noncontrast head computed tomography (CT) is sensitive for acute bleeding and should be obtained emergently to exclude a hemorrhagic cause of stroke. If a hemorrhagic stroke is identified, magnetic resonance venography (MRV) should follow as 10% of hemorrhages in children are due to cerebral venous sinus thrombosis (CVST).[26]

Noncontrast CT is also the initial study for diagnosing AIS in emergency situation or with no availability of MRI. Bland infarcts appear as low-density lesions within vascular territories, and CVST may present as linear densities in the deep and cortical veins. CT imaging after an AIS may be normal for the first 12 hours after the onset of symptoms. CT scan involves radiation exposure but it is quick and easily available as compared to MRI and does not require anesthesia.[26,27]

Role of Magnetic Resonance Imaging

Magnetic resonance imaging (MRI) is a more sensitive test for early detection of an infarction.[26-28] The diffusion-weighted imaging (DWI) can diagnose a stroke within 24 hours. The sequences required for the diagnosis include, (1) MRI with diffusion-weighted imaging/apparent diffusion coefficient (DWI/ADC), (2) axial gradient echo [e.g., susceptibility-weighted imaging (SWI)], (3) axial T2, (4) fluid-attenuated inversion recovery (FLAIR) if greater than 1 year of age, (5) 3D volumetric T1, and (vi) time-of-flight (TOF) magnetic resonance arteriography (MRA), and consideration of perfusion imaging is recommended as first choice.

Magnetic resonance arteriography and MRV should also be carried out to confirm vessel patency and define the vascular anatomy. MRA will yield further information about blood flow, and MRV will more reliably identify CVST.[27] However, MRI has a much longer acquisition time as compared to CT. This has a great significance in pediatric population because the children need to be given general anesthesia (GA) to remain steady for the prolonged time of data acquisition. This has logistic implications apart from higher costs. Of all the imaging modalities, catheter angiography (CA) yields the most precise details of vascular anatomy and is superior to MRA and computed tomography angiography (CTA) for visualization of tertiary branches and small cerebral arteries. It is considered as a gold standard for the diagnosis of vasculitis, vasculopathies, and dissection.[29]

Neuroimaging confirms the diagnosis of stroke and may point to an etiology but thorough laboratory work up, comprising hematological, biochemical and immunological tests, for etiology is recommended. This includes complete blood count with differential count, erythrocyte sedimentation rate (ESR), C-reactive protein (CRP), liver functions, renal functions, electrolytes, glucose, and a coagulation screen comprising international normalized ratio (INR)/prothrombin time (PT), activated partial thromboplastin time (aPTT), fibrinogen, antinuclear antibody (ANA), anti-double stranded deoxyribonucleic acid (anti-ds-DNA), lupus anticoagulant, antiphospholipid and anti-cardiolipin antibodies, homocysteine levels, lipid profile, hemoglobin electrophoresis, protein C, S, AT III, activated protein C resistance, factor V Leiden mutation, prothrombin gene mutation, and MTHFR (methylenetetrahydrofolate reductase) allele. Infective work-up for tuberculosis (TB), human immunodeficiency virus (HIV), and varicella should be considered depending on the clinical presentation and information obtained from laboratory investigations and imaging.[10]

Cardiac work-up includes comprehensive echocardiography as a routine work-up for all patients with stroke in the pediatric age group. Most of the children have excellent window for transthoracic imaging and therefore transesophageal imaging is rarely required. However, in adolescents and young adults or children with poor transthoracic imaging, transesophageal echocardiography should be obtained to look for a PFO, left atrial appendage, and atrioventricular valves—either native or prosthetic. In little older children, contrast echocardiography should be done to detect right-to-left shunt across the PFO or pulmonary arteriovenous malformation. The presence of desaturation also supports pulmonary arteriovenous malformation. It certainly increases the sensitivity of the test.[10] A bubble contrast study with appearance of contrast bubbles after three cardiac cycles heightens suspicion of pulmonary arteriovenous malformation and a contrast-enhanced chest CT allows precise definition and planning of treatment.

Treatment

The emergency management includes general supportive measures and specific stroke treatment. Unlike adult stroke, there are a lot of controversies in specific stroke treatment in children but the initial supportive measures are universal and include fever control, normalization of glucose, correction of dehydration, anemia and electrolyte abnormalities, maintenance of normal oxygenation, blood pressure control, and management of raised intracranial pressure. There is no role of prophylactic anticonvulsants except in HS.[10]

The specific treatment depends on the etiology of stroke. HSs may require surgical management, although controversial.[28] Prevention of rebleeding including correction of coagulation abnormalities and management of vascular malformations by surgical or endovascular treatment.[23]

In case of AIS, the goal-specific management involves reduction in the size of salvageable brain by thrombolysis. There are anecdotal reports of IV/IA recombinant tissue plasminogen activator (tPA) in children but there is a paucity of evidence in terms of its efficacy.[30] On the other hand, there is high-risk of hemorrhage in children with the use of these agents. An international study [TIPS (thrombolysis in pediatric stroke)] was started but had to be prematurely stopped due to inability to recruit adequate number of patients. According to few case reports, intra-arterial recombinant tissue plasminogen activator (rtPA) within 6 hours and intravenous within 3 hours of onset of stroke may be beneficial.

Second goal-specific management in AIS is prevention of further ischemia by using low-molecular weight heparin (LMWH) or unfractionated heparin (UFH). Although LMWH has reproducible pharmacokinetics and requires fewer monitoring tests, it cannot be reliably reversed with protamine, such as UFH, so if there is suspicion of hemorrhagic complications, UFH is preferred to LMWH. The practice of short-term anticoagulation is more prevalent in children than in adults as the underlying risk factors in pediatrics are dissection, vasculopathy, cardiac disorders, and coagulopathy than in adults with atherosclerosis and hypertension. Anticoagulation is continued for 3–6 months in children with proven dissection, sinus thrombosis, cardiac cases with high-risk of embolization.[31] The long-term anticoagulation could be in form of antiplatelets such as aspirin, clopidogrel, oral vitamin-K antagonist such as warfarin or subcutaneous LMWH injections. These measures need to be initiated in consultation with appropriate specialists after initial management and stabilization.

NEUROLOGICAL OUTCOME

In a study, among young adult survivors of childhood stroke, 37% had a normal modified Rankin score, 42% had mild deficits, 8% had moderate deficits, and 15% had severe deficits. Concomitant involvement of the basal ganglia, cerebral cortex, and posterior limb of the internal capsule predicts a persistent hemiparesis.[15] Survivors of childhood AIS have low-normal cognitive performance, with poorest performance in visual-constructive skills, short-term memory, and processing speed.[32,33] Younger age at stroke and seizures, but not laterality of stroke (left versus right), predicts worse cognitive outcome.[2] Despite advances in treatment, at least 1 of 10 children with ischemic or HS will have a recurrence within 5 years.[34,35] The cumulative stroke recurrence rate is 6.8% (95% CI, 4.6–10%) at 1 month and 12% (CI, 8.5–15%) at 1 year in a study of 355 children with stroke followed up for a median period of 2 years.[22] The recurrence is higher in arteriopathy. The recurrence risk after perinatal stroke, however, is negligible. More than 25% of survivors of perinatal ischemic stroke developed delayed seizures within 3 years.[36]

CONCLUSION

Pediatric stroke, a common disorder with huge morbidity, is a well described syndrome with various risk factors, especially cardiac. But specific protocols for treatment as in adults are lagging for the want of evidence. Issues for getting robust evidence are multifactorial etiologies, abundant stroke mimics, low index of suspicion, and less aggressive diagnostic work-up. Randomized controlled trials (RCTs) specific to children are clearly needed to better establish the safety and efficacy of both acute and preventative treatments.

REFERENCES

1. DeVeber G. In pursuit of evidence-based treatments for paediatric stroke: the UK and Chest guidelines. Lancet Neurol. 2005;4(7):432-6.
2. deVeber GA, MacGregor D, Curtis R, Mayank S. Neurologic outcome in survivors of childhood arterial ischemic stroke and sinovenous thrombosis. J Child Neurol. 2000;15(5):316-24.
3. Lanthier S, Carmant L, David M, Larbrisseau A, de Veber G. Stroke in children: the coexistence of multiple risk factors predicts poor outcome. Neurology. 2000;54(2):371-8.
4. Ferriero DM, Fullerton HJ, Bernard TJ, Billinghurst L, Daniels SR, DeBaun MR, et al. Management of stroke in neonates and children: a scientific statement from the American Heart Association/American Stroke Association. Stroke. 2019;50(3):e51-96.
5. Chung B, Wong V. Pediatric stroke among Hong Kong Chinese subjects. Pediatrics. 2004; 114(2):e206-12.

6. Earley CJ, Kittner SJ, Feeser BR, Gardner J, Epstein A, Wozniak MA, et al. Stroke in children and sickle-cell disease: Baltimore-Washington Cooperative Young Stroke Study. Neurology. 1998;51(1):169-76.
7. Kalra SGaV. Stroke in child. Indian J Pediatr. 2003;70:639-48.
8. Sacco RL, Kasner SE, Broderick JP, Caplan LR, Connors JJB, Culebras A, et al. An Updated Definition of Stroke for the 21st Century: A Statement for Healthcare Professionals from the American Heart Association/American Stroke Association. Stroke. 2013;44(7):1-26.
9. The World Health Organization MONICA Project (monitoring trends and determinants in cardiovascular disease): a major international collaboration. WHO MONICA Project Principal Investigators. J Clin Epidemiol. 1988;41(2):105-14.
10. Tsze DS, Valente JH. Pediatric stroke: a review. Emerg Med Intern. 2011;2011:734506.
11. deVeber G, Roach ES, Riela AR, Wiznitzer M. Stroke in children: recognition, treatment, and future directions. Seminars in pediatric neurology. 2000;7(4):309-17.
12. Ganesan V, Prengler M, McShane MA, Wade AM, Kirkham FJ. Investigation of risk factors in children with arterial ischemic stroke. Ann Neurol. 2003;53(2):167-73.
13. Dowling MM, Hynan LS, Lo W, Licht DJ, McClure C, Yager JY, et al. International Paediatric Stroke Study: stroke associated with cardiac disorders. International Journal of Stroke. 2013;8 Suppl A100:39-44.
14. Swaiman K, Ashwal S, Ferriero D, Schor N, Finkel R, Gropman A, et al. Swaiman's Pediatric Neurology, 6th edition. Philadelphia: Elsevier; 2017.
15. Benjamin EJ, Virani SS, Callaway CW, Chamberlain AM, Chang AR, Cheng S, et al. Heart Disease and Stroke Statistics-2018 Update: a report from the American Heart Association. Circulation. 2018;137(12):e67-492.
16. Medley TL, Miteff C, Andrews I, Ware T, Cheung M, Monagle P, et al. Australian Clinical Consensus Guideline: the diagnosis and acute management of childhood stroke. Int J Stroke. 2019;14(1):94-106.
17. Agarwal A, Firdouse M, Brar N, Yang A, Lambiris P, Chan AK, et al. Incidence and management of thrombotic and thromboembolic complications following the superior cavopulmonary anastomosis procedure: a literature review. Clin Appl Thromb Hemost. 2018;24(3):405-15.
18. McQuillen PS, Hamrick SE, Perez MJ, Barkovich AJ, Glidden DV, Karl TR, et al. Balloon atrial septostomy is associated with preoperative stroke in neonates with transposition of the great arteries. Circulation. 2006;113(2):280-5.
19. Domi T, Edgell DS, McCrindle BW, Williams WG, Chan AK, MacGregor DL, et al. Frequency, predictors, and neurologic outcomes of vaso-occlusive strokes associated with cardiac surgery in children. Pediatrics. 2008;122(6):1292-8.
20. Barker PC, Nowak C, King K, Mosca RS, Bove EL, Goldberg CS. Risk factors for cerebrovascular events following fontan palliation in patients with a functional single ventricle. Am J Cardiol. 2005;96(4):587-91.
21. Monagle P, Karl TR. Thromboembolic problems after the Fontan operation. Seminars in thoracic and cardiovascular surgery Pediatric cardiac surgery annual. 2002;5(1):36-47.
22. Sinclair AJ, Fox CK, Ichord RN, Almond CS, Bernard TJ, Beslow LA, et al. Stroke in children with cardiac disease: report from the International Pediatric Stroke Study Group Symposium. Pediatric neurology. 2015;52(1):5-15.
23. Mayer SA, Brun NC, Begtrup K, Broderick J, Davis S, Diringer MN, et al. Efficacy and safety of recombinant activated factor VII for acute intracerebral hemorrhage. New Engl J Med. 2008;358(20):2127-37.
24. Braun KP, Kappelle LJ, Kirkham FJ, Deveber G. Diagnostic pitfalls in paediatric ischaemic stroke. Dev Med Child Neurol. 2006;48(12):985-90.
25. Gabis LV, Yangala R, Lenn NJ. Time lag to diagnosis of stroke in children. Pediatrics. 2002; 110(5):924-8.
26. Roach ES, Golomb MR, Adams R, Biller J, Daniels S, Deveber G, et al. Management of stroke in infants and children: a scientific statement from a Special Writing Group of the American Heart Association Stroke Council and the Council on Cardiovascular Disease in the Young. Stroke. 2008;39(9):2644-91.
27. Younkin DP. Diagnosis and treatment of ischemic pediatric stroke. Current neurology and neuroscience reports. 2002;2(1):18-24.
28. deVeber G. Arterial ischemic strokes in infants and children: an overview of current approaches. Semin Thromb Hemost. 2003;29(6):567-73.
29. Husson B, Lasjaunias P. Radiological approach to disorders of arterial brain vessels associated with childhood arterial stroke—a comparison between MRA and contrast angiography. Pediatr Radiol. 2004;34(1):10-5.
30. Jain SV, Morton LD. Ischemic stroke and excellent recovery after administration of intravenous tissue plasminogen activator. Pediatr Neurol. 2008;38(2):126-9.
31. Firozvi K, Deveras RA, Kessler CM. Reversal of low-molecular-weight heparin-induced bleeding in patients with pre-existing hypercoagulable states with human recombinant activated factor VII concentrate. Am J Hematol. 2006;81(8):582-9.
32. Hajek CA, Yeates KO, Anderson V, Mackay M, Greenham M, Gomes A, et al. Cognitive outcomes following arterial ischemic stroke in infants and children. J Child Neurol. 2014;29(7):887-94.
33. Studer M, Boltshauser E, Capone Mori A, Datta A, Fluss J, Mercati D, et al. Factors affecting cognitive outcome in early pediatric stroke. Neurology. 2014;82(9):784-92.
34. Danchaivijitr N, Cox TC, Saunders DE, Ganesan V. Evolution of cerebral arteriopathies in childhood arterial ischemic stroke. Ann Neurol. 2006;59(4):620-6.
35. Tuppin P, Samson S, Woimant F, Chabrier S. Management and 2-year follow-up of children aged 29 days to 17 years hospitalized for a first stroke in France (2009-2010). Arch Pediatr. 2014;21(12):1305-15.
36. Wusthoff CJ, Kessler SK, Vossough A, Ichord R, Zelonis S, Halperin A, et al. Risk of later seizure after perinatal arterial ischemic stroke: a prospective cohort study. Pediatrics. 2011; 127(6):e1550-7.

52
CHAPTER

Rhythm Disorders in Children

Mani Ram Krishna

INTRODUCTION

The normal cardiac rhythm is initiated at the sinus node and traverses both atria before passing down to the ventricles through the atrioventricular (AV) node. This is termed as a sinus rhythm. The normal conduction pathway is illustrated in **Figure 1**. Any aberration in this normal conduction is termed an arrhythmia. These may include an abnormally fast heart rate (tachyarrhythmia) or slow heart rate (bradyarrhythmia). These could be occasional (transient) or prolonged (sustained). There is very little data on the incidence of arrhythmias in the pediatric population. Most published studies are based on the emergency department (ED) visits of large tertiary care centers. It is estimated that 55/100,000 pediatric ED visits are due to arrhythmias.[1] However, arrhythmias are much less frequent in the pediatric population compared to adults. Hence, pediatricians are much less comfortable in interpreting electrocardiograms (ECGs) as well as treating children with arrhythmias. In this chapter, we will attempt to define an approach toward the diagnosis of the common arrhythmia problems in childhood and their emergency management.

TACHYARRHYTHMIAS

Tachyarrhythmias can be initiated from anywhere along the conduction system. They are broadly classified into supraventricular tachycardia (SVT) and ventricular tachycardia (VT). SVT originates above the bundle of His. They are more common in children and in general cause less hemodynamic instability. VT, as the name implies, originate from the ventricle. These have a higher propensity to cause hemodynamic instability and are more difficult to treat. VT fortunately is less frequent in children compared to adults. A significant number of tachyarrhythmias occur in the early postoperative period after surgery for congenital heart disease (CHD). Such arrhythmias are usually not managed by the pediatrician and are not discussed in this chapter. We present a clinical approach toward a child presenting with tachyarrhythmia in this section.

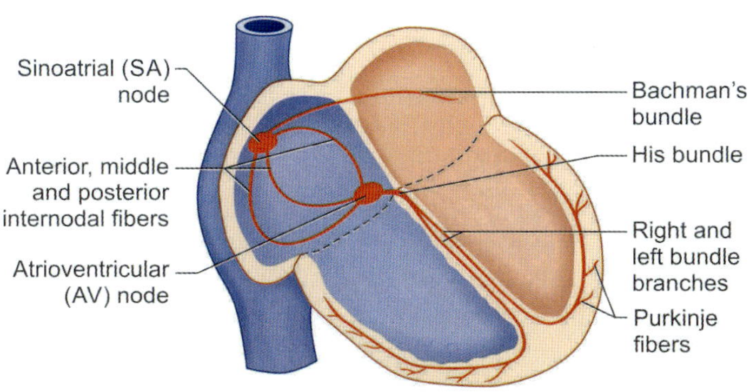

Fig. 1: Schematic diagram of the normal cardiac conduction pathway demonstrating the sinoatrial (SA) node, atrial conduction pathway, atrioventricular (AV) node, and the ventricular conduction pathways.

Etiopathogenesis

The common tachyarrhythmias in children are shown in **Flowchart 1**. Among the arrhythmias, atrioventricular re-entrant tachycardia (AVRT) and atrioventricular nodal re-entrant tachycardia (AVNRT) are the most common in children.[2] These arrhythmias occur as paroxysmal events and are frequently termed as paroxysmal supraventricular tachycardia (PSVT). The mechanism of arrhythmia in these tachycardia is re-entry. The AV groove is electrically insulated and cannot conduct electrical signals. These signals can pass to the ventricle through the AV node. Rarely, accessory pathways (APs) may exist between the atria and ventricle capable of conducting signals. These pathways are present in a subepicardial location (AVRT) or within the AV node (AVNRT). These pathways exhibit the ability to transmit retrograde (ventricle to atrium), antegrade (atrium to ventricle), or both. An AP capable of transmitting antegrade is evident on the ECG as a delta wave. The AP conducts faster than the AV node but has a longer refractory period. The SVT is usually triggered by an isolated early atrial beat (ectopic). The ectopic is conducted along the AV node as the AP is refractory and depolarizes the ventricle. It is then conducted retrograde through the AP into the atrium and is transmitted back to the ventricles setting up a circus movement (**Fig. 2A**). Localized re-entry within the atrium or the ventricles results in atrial flutter (**Fig. 2B**) and outflow tract tachycardia.

Flowchart 1: Classification of the common tachyarrhythmias in children based on their origin and mechanism.

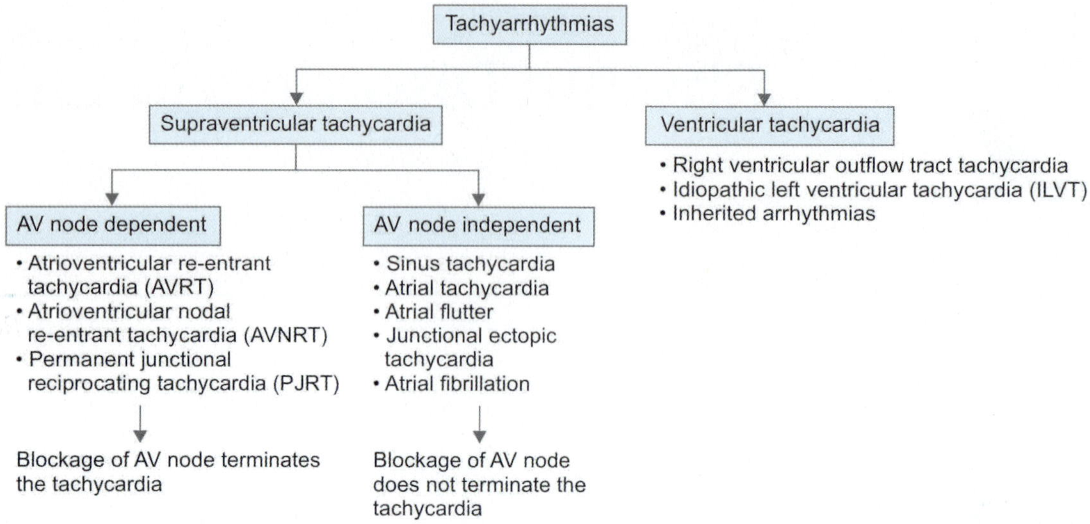

Permanent junctional reciprocating tachycardia (PJRT) occurs through a special type of AP close to the tricuspid valve annulus (**Fig. 2C**). Unlike PSVT, this results in an incessant arrhythmia. Re-entrant arrhythmias usually have a fixed heart rate and can be terminated by direct current (DC) cardioversion. AVRT is the most common tachyarrhythmia in neonates and infants. There is a bimodal age distribution of presentation with a peak in neonates and a later peak in the school-going age. In contrast, AVNRT is almost never seen in infancy. Although the dual AV node physiology exists from birth, symptomatic arrhythmias first occur in adolescence or young adulthood. Atrial flutter is more commonly associated with other structural heart disease but a lone form of atrial flutter rarely occurs in neonates. The clinical presentation is similar to other tachyarrhythmias but it has a low rate of recurrence and an excellent long-term outcome.

Another arrhythmia which is more common in children than adults is atrial tachycardia. The mechanism in atrial tachycardia is one of enhanced automaticity. Pacemaker cells are present in the sinus node, atria, AV node as well as the bundle branches.[3] Sinus node discharges at rates >60/minute while other subsidiary pacemakers discharge at a lower rate and it is by virtue of this nature that it serves as "the pacemaker" of the heart. Should a focus from a different part of the atrium develop the ability to "fire" at a rate higher than the sinus node it results in atrial tachycardia (**Fig. 2D**). A similar mechanism is responsible for junctional ectopic tachycardia (JET) (**Fig. 2E**) and some forms of idiopathic VT (**Fig. 2F**). Such automatic tachycardia have variation in the heart rate and a "warm-up" phase characterized by a slow increase in the heart rate during initiation of the abnormal rhythm (**Fig. 3**). They do not respond to cardioversion. Unlike PSVT, atrial tachycardia is "incessant." If the tachycardia persists beyond a few days, it could lead to ventricular dysfunction—a condition termed tachycardia-induced cardiomyopathy or tachycardiomyopathy.

A third mechanism of tachyarrhythmia is triggered activity during the diastole. Spontaneous depolarization can occur during diastole.[4] They are classified as early after-depolarization (phase 3) or late after-depolarization (phase 4). If the depolarization is of sufficient amplitude, it triggers the next wave of depolarization. This mechanism contributes to the ventricular arrhythmias in the inherited arrhythmias.

Clinical Features

The presentation of the tachyarrhythmia varies depending on the age of the child and the duration of the abnormal rhythm.

Infants with tachyarrhythmia have a lower reserve potential than older children and are hence more vulnerable to ventricular dysfunction even after a relatively short duration of tachycardia. The clinical features include irritability, fast breathing, feeding difficulty, and excessive sweatiness.[1] It is virtually impossible to distinguish symptoms of tachyarrhythmia from other causes of heart failure. However, the onset of heart failure is more rapid and new-onset symptoms in a previously well child should raise the suspicion of tachyarrhythmia. Infants with PSVT which last for a brief duration are usually asymptomatic. If recognized, it is usually when a parent notices rapid heartbeat while holding the infant or increased neck pulsations.

Older children experience PSVT as palpitation. Some children may not be able to express the symptom and may complain of chest pain or discomfort. With rapid heart rates, some children complain of unease and nausea. Frequent short-lasting episodes can be brought to notice because the parents notice episodic pallor or lethargy. Less frequent presentations include syncope and seizures. In children with pre-existing heart disease, sudden worsening of heart failure symptoms should raise the suspicion of a tachyarrhythmia.

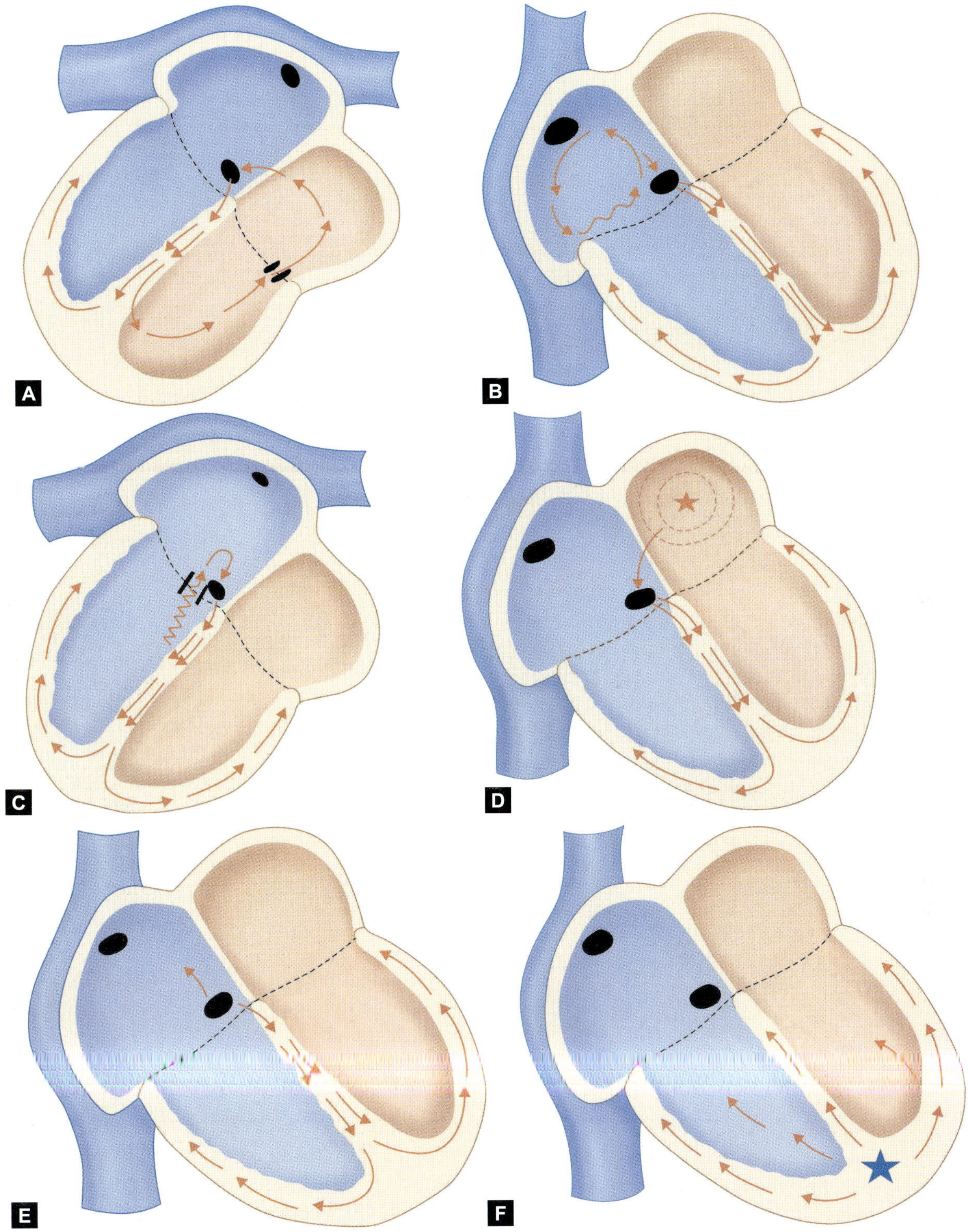

Figs. 2A to F: Schematic diagram of the mechanism of common childhood tachyarrhythmias. (A) Atrioventricular re-entrant tachycardia (AVRT): The signal originating from the sinus node is conducted antegrade across the atrioventricular (AV) node to the ventricles and then travels retrograde via the subepicardial accessory pathway to depolarize the atria again resulting in a circus movement; (B) Atrial flutter: This arrhythmia originates from a re-entrant pathway within the atrial tissue at a rate of approximately 300 beats per minute before being conducted to the ventricles through the atrioventricular (AV) node. The common form of flutter originates from the right atrium close to the tricuspid valve; (C) Permanent junctional reciprocating tachycardia: The mechanism of tachyarrhythmia is similar to atrioventricular re-entrant tachycardia (AVRT) but occurs through an accessory pathway close to the tricuspid valve. This pathway has a relatively slow conduction (indicated by wavy line) that contributes to the incessant nature of the tachycardia; (D) Atrial tachycardia: The signal arises from an ectopic atrial focus before depolarizing the ventricles through the atrioventricular (AV) node. The tachycardia can be a result of enhanced automaticity of the ectopic foci; (E) Junctional ectopic tachycardia: This is an automatic arrhythmia originating from the atrioventricular (AV) node region; (F) Ventricular tachycardia. This is an automatic tachyarrhythmia originating from an ectopic focus within the ventricle.

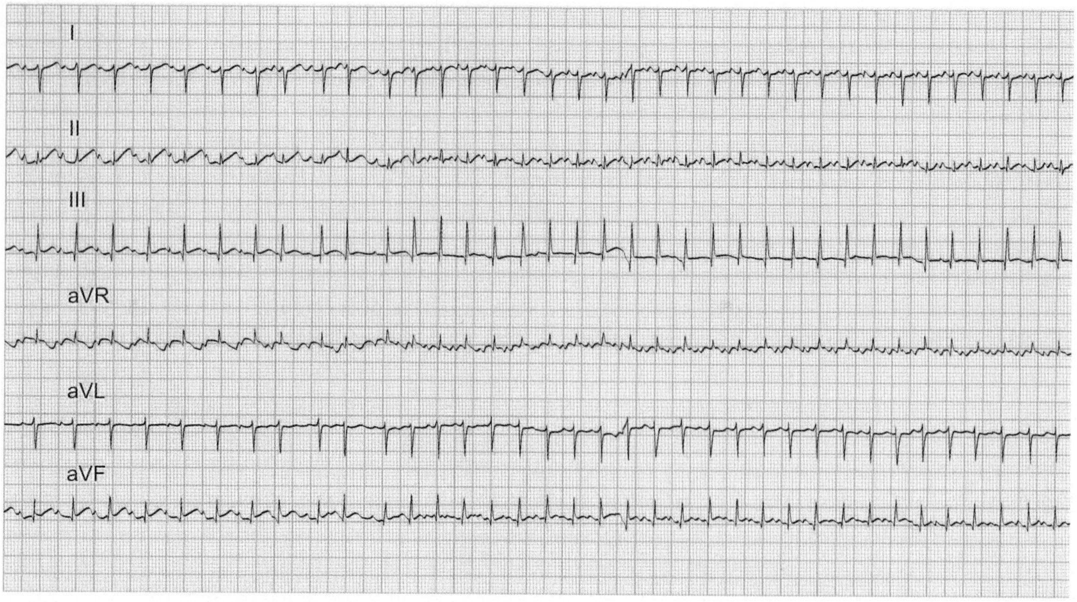

Fig. 3: Initiation of tachycardia in automatic arrhythmias demonstrating a warm up phase during which the heart rate increases slowly to the maximum rate seen at the right side of the strip.

Physical Examination

The pediatrician should focus on ensuring hemodynamic stability. If there are signs of hemodynamic instability, management should be according to standard pediatric advanced life support guidelines.[5] In children who are hemodynamically stable, a quick examination should be performed for signs of heart failure. This should include recording of pulse, blood pressure and respiratory rate, cardiomegaly, gallop rhythm, and liver enlargement. An ECG should then be obtained emergently.

Evaluation

An ECG should be obtained to confirm tachycardia and deduce the mechanism of arrhythmia. Efforts should be made to answer the following questions:

- *Is the heart rate regular or irregular?* There will be no irregularity in any of the AV node-dependent tachyarrhythmias (**Fig. 4A**). Irregularity may be noted in any of the AV node-independent tachyarrhythmias. In VT, irregularities in the form of a capture beat (**Fig. 4B**) (a QRS complex which is normally conducted from the sinus node) or a fusion beat (a fused complex of ventricular rhythm and sinus conducted rhythm) are diagnostic.
- *Are the QRS complexes narrow or wide?* A narrow complex QRS suggests supraventricular origin of the tachycardia (**Fig. 4A**). A broad QRS can be due to VT (**Fig. 4B and 5A**) or an SVT with aberrant conduction. In general, VTs are more likely to result in hemodynamic instability. Hence, a broad complex tachycardia in an unstable patient should be considered a VT. A QRS complex of >90 ms duration is considered broad complex. It is important to compare the ECG with previous available ECG. Children with corrected CHD have a broad QRS complex at baseline and a similar complex will be seen even during SVT. Based on the QRS morphology, broad QRS tachyarrhythmias are classified into monomorphic (where all QRS complexes are similar; **Fig. 5A**) and polymorphic (where there are more than one morphology of QRS complexes; **Fig. 5B**). Identifying the QRS morphology is important in understanding whether adenosine can be administered to a child presenting with a tachyarrhythmia.
- *Are P waves visible?* In AVNRT, the atrium is activated retrograde from the ventricle and the P wave is almost always buried in the QRS complex and not visible. A similar atrial activation occurs in AVRT. Here, the p wave may be visible or buried in the QRS complex. A regular narrow complex tachycardia without a clear p wave should be considered as PSVT. A typical sawtooth pattern of P wave is seen in atrial flutter (**Fig. 6A**). The absence of a P wave in an irregularly irregular rhythm is suggestive of atrial fibrillation (**Fig. 6B**).
- *What is the relation of the P wave to the QRS?* The pediatrician should attempt to answer two questions regarding the relation between the P and QRS relationship. Is there a consistent relationship between the P and the QRS:
  - Is there a constant relationship between the P wave and QRS complex? If every P wave is followed by a QRS complex, there is a 1:1 AV association. Such a relationship is apparent in PSVT, atrial tachycardia, and JET. In atrial flutter, the atrial rate is usually higher than the ventricular rate. Although the AV relationship in flutter may be variable, the most common form is a 2:1 AV relationship where QRS alternate P waves are followed by a QRS complex. If there is no consistent

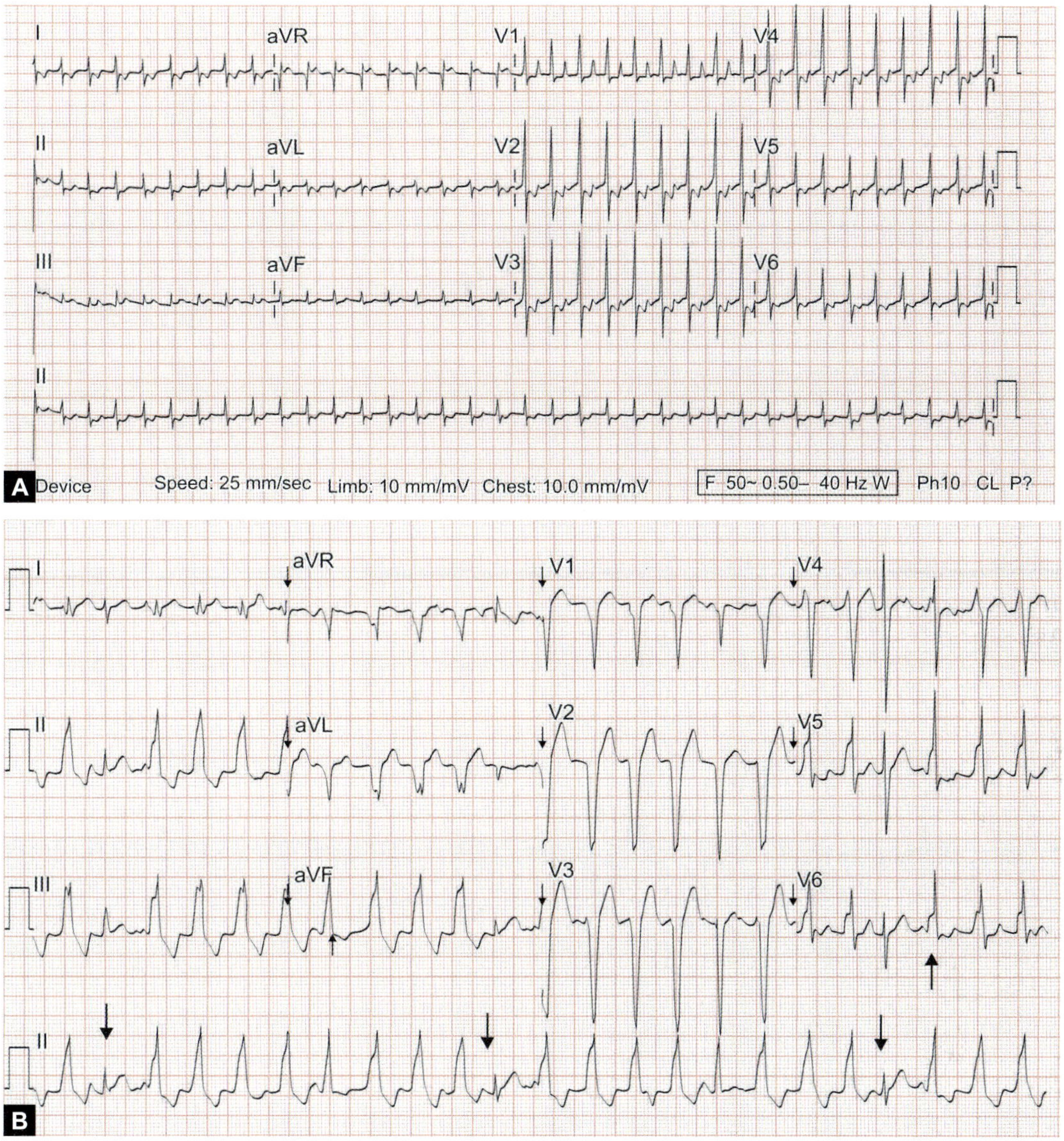

Figs. 4A and B: (A) A 12-lead ECG demonstrating a regular narrow QRS complex which is suggestive of a supraventricular origin. Re-entrant tachyarrhythmias tend to be regular while automatic tachycardias demonstrate a warm-up and slow down as in Figure 3; (B) A 12-lead ECG demonstrating a broad QRS complex. The causes include ventricular tachycardia or supraventricular tachycardia with an aberrant conduction. The downward arrows point to a normally conducted capture beat and the upward arrows point to a fusion beat.

relationship between the P wave and the QRS, there is said to be AV disassociation. AV disassociation is characteristic of VT and certain forms of JET.

- When there is 1:1 AV relationship, SVT is further classified based on the relationship of the P wave to the QRS as short RP tachycardia and long RP tachycardia. A tachycardia is considered to be a short R-P tachycardia if the P wave is closer to the previous QRS complex (**Fig. 7A**) and long R-P tachycardia if the P wave is closer to the next QRS complex (**Fig. 7B**). The atrium is activated from the ventricle in PSVT and JET. Hence, the P wave occurs after the QRS complex and these are short RP tachycardia. The long RP tachycardia includes atrial tachycardia and PJRT.

- *The adenosine response*: Frequently, the diagnosis may not be apparent even after a stepwise evaluation. A "P" wave at the end of the QRS complex or hidden in the T wave may be apparent to a trained eye but may be difficult for a pediatrician. In such situations, the diagnosis may be made apparent by the use of adenosine. The therapeutic use of adenosine in the treatment of PSVT is well known. However, adenosine is also an important diagnostic tool in determining the mechanism of tachyarrhythmias.

Adenosine is a naturally occurring substance. It acts on the sinus node and the AV node through the A1 receptors.[6] By increasing the refractoriness of the AV node, it blocks AV conduction. It also has a secondary negative chronotropic action on the sinus node.[7]

The most important antiarrhythmic action is blockage of the AV node. It does not have any effect on atrial or ventricular conduction. It hence effectively separates the atrium from the ventricle. The mechanism of the various

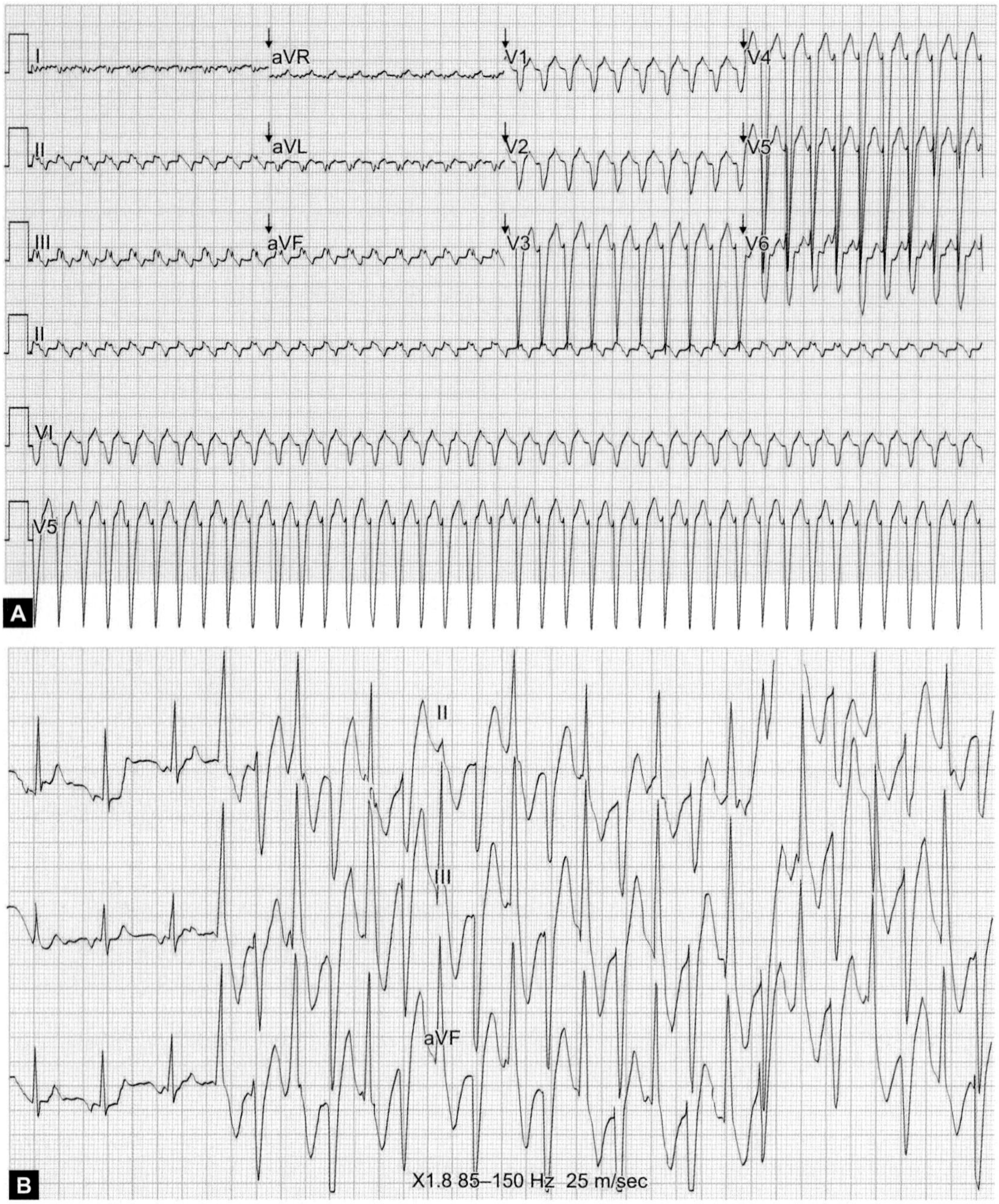

Figs. 5A and B: (A) A 12-lead electrocardiogram (ECG) of a monomorphic broad QRS tachycardia. The most likely underlying cause is a ventricular tachycardia although selected supraventricular tachycardias also can have a broad QRS because of abnormal atrioventricular (AV) conduction; (B) A 12-lead ECG of a polymorphic tachyarrhythmia where there are more than one morphology of QRS complexes.

arrhythmias is depicted in **Figure 2**. In PSVT, the AV node is an integral part of the circus movement. By blocking the AV node, adenosine terminates the arrhythmia (**Fig. 8**). Since this is a paroxysmal arrhythmia, it does not reappear once the adenosine effect wears off. In atrial flutter, adenosine has no effect on the flutter pathway. However, by reducing AV conduction and hence the ventricular rate, it may make the flutter waves more apparent (**Figs. 9A and B**). A similar effect is seen in atrial tachycardia. Frequently, the P wave is hidden in the preceding T wave. When AV conduction is blocked, the ectopic P wave is easily recognized (**Figs. 10A and B**). PJRT is also an AV re-entrant arrhythmia similar to PSVT and is hence terminated by adenosine. However, as it is an incessant pathway, the arrhythmia reappears as soon as the effect of adenosine on the AV node ceases. Adenosine however has no effect on JET. The effect of adenosine on various arrhythmias is mentioned in **Table 1**.

Adenosine can only be administered intravenously as the drug has no oral absorption. Adenosine is rapidly deaminated to inosine and inactivated in the red blood cells as well as vascular endothelium.[7] The half-life is only about 6 seconds. As adenosine is metabolized in the blood, deactivation begins as soon as it is injected. Hence, it should be administered through the largest bore cannula possible

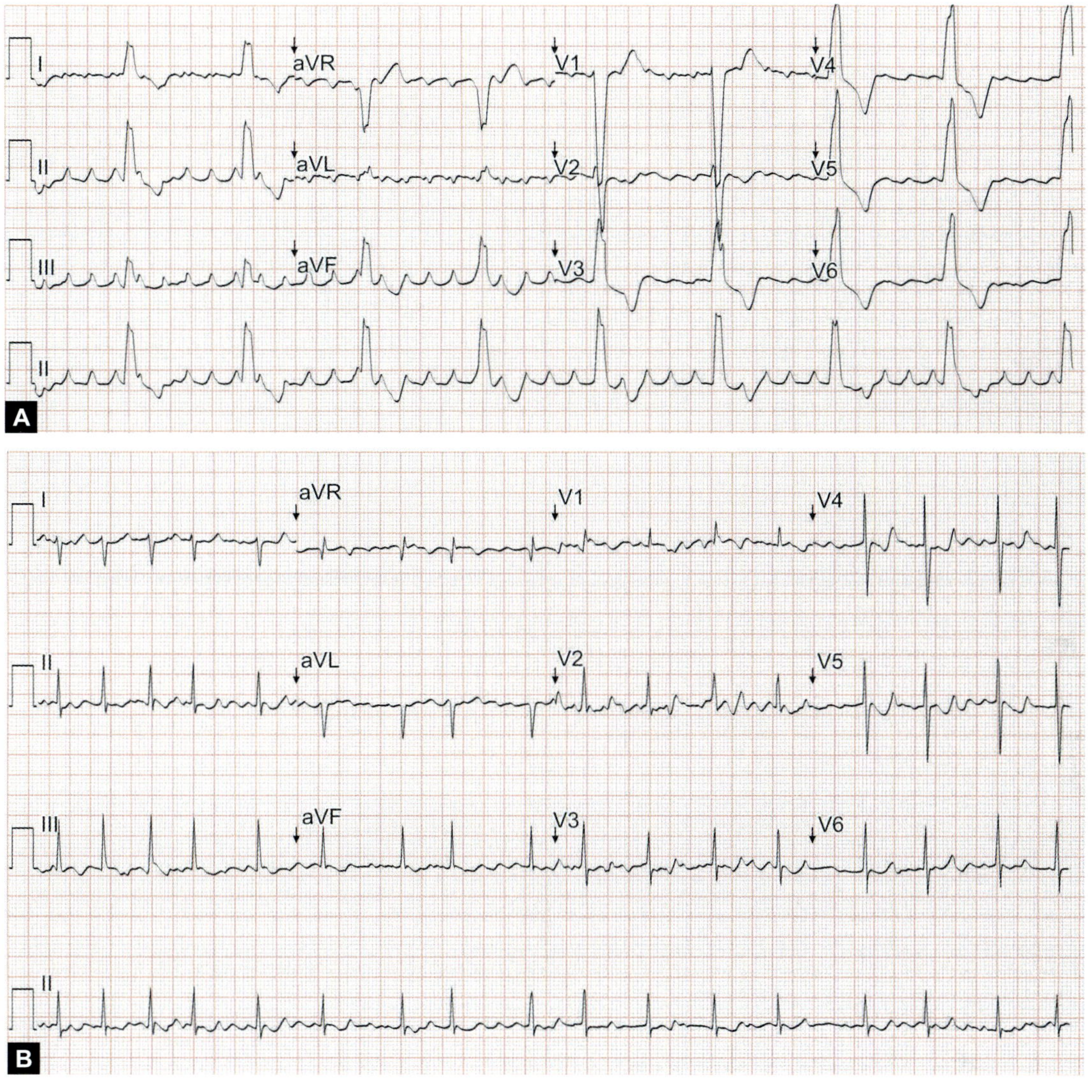

Figs. 6A and B: (A) A 12-lead electrocardiogram (ECG) showing the characteristic sawtooth pattern of P wave seen in atrial flutter; (B) A 12-lead ECG showing an irregularly irregular rhythm with no clear P wave seen. The features are suggestive of atrial fibrillation.

and from a vein close to the heart. The cubital vein should be the preferred site. However, in neonates and young infants, an upper limb cannula is preferable. A three-way stop valve should be used and the injection as well as flush should be connected before the injection is commenced (**Fig. 11**). The injections should be administered rapidly and should be followed by a rapid saline flush.

Adenosine can be safely administered in any regular monomorphic tachycardia. However, adenosine is contraindicated in irregular and polymorphic tachycardia. The major concern about administering adenosine is in a child with Wolff–Parkinson–White (WPW) syndrome who presents with atrial fibrillation. In such cases, blocking the AV node would paradoxically increase the heart rate and carry a risk of ventricular fibrillation. Atrial fibrillation is an irregular tachyarrhythmia and hence restricting adenosine use to regular and monomorphic tachycardia would avoid this potentially fatal complication. Adenosine is generally a safe drug. Its very short half-life ensures that any adverse event is also short-lasting. Transient chest pain has been reported after adenosine use in adults but rarely lasts more than a few minutes. The most concerning adverse effect due to adenosine is a propensity to cause atrial fibrillation. However, this is seldom seen in children.

Adenosine thus can be safely administered in any regular tachycardia with QRS complexes of the same morphology even if the pediatrician is not sure about the accurate diagnosis. However, it is important to ensure that the valuable diagnostic information available from the response of the tachyarrhythmia to adenosine is not lost. This is ensured by recording the response to adenosine on an ECG. As soon as the injection is ready, ECG recording should be commenced and the injection delivered. ECG recording should continue for a minimum of 20 seconds after administration. This will ensure that the adenosine response is recorded and any early recurrence of the arrhythmia is also documented.

The following case scenarios will help illustrate the utility of adenosine in tachyarrhythmias.

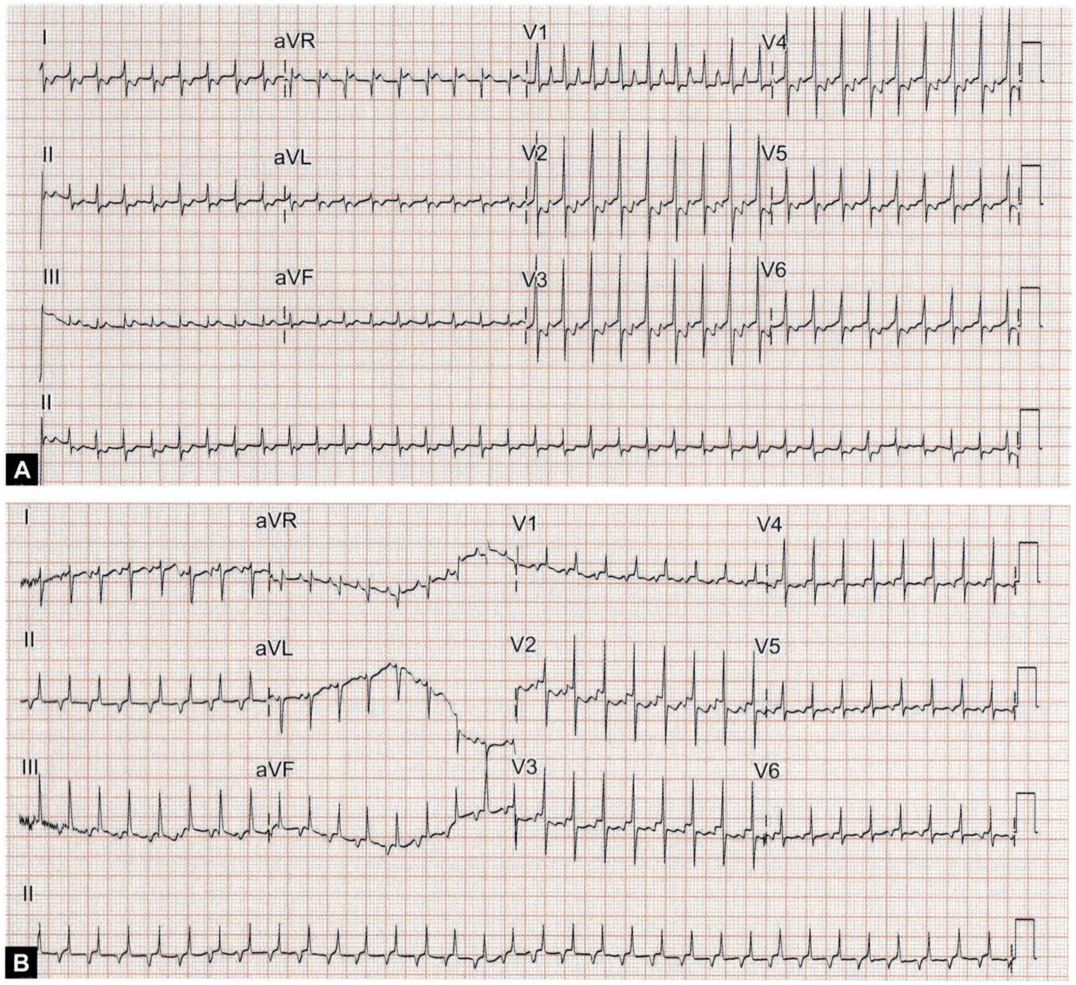

Figs. 7A and B: (A) A 12-lead electrocardiogram (ECG) showing a regular narrow complex tachycardia with a 1:1 relationship of P and QRS. The P wave is closer to the preceding QRS complex indicating a short R-P tachycardia; (B) A 12-lead ECG showing a regular narrow complex tachycardia with a 1:1 relationship of P:QRS. The P wave is closer to the following QRS complex indicating a long R-P tachycardia.

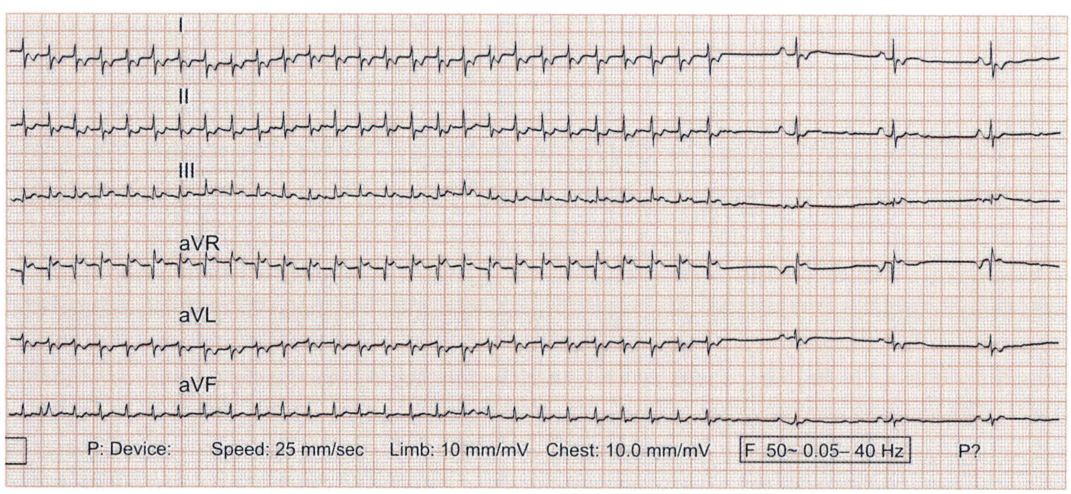

Fig. 8: A 6-lead electrocardiogram (ECG) showing a regular narrow complex tachycardia. On administration of adenosine, the tachyarrhythmia terminates abruptly resulting in the termination of the arrhythmia and return of sinus rhythm. This suggests the mechanism to be paroxysmal supraventricular tachycardia (PSVT).

Scenario 1

A 7-year-old boy presents to the outpatient clinic with palpitation. His heart rate is 250 per minute but there are no signs of hemodynamic instability. An ECG is obtained emergently (**Fig. 12A**). The stepwise evaluation of the ECG will be as follows:

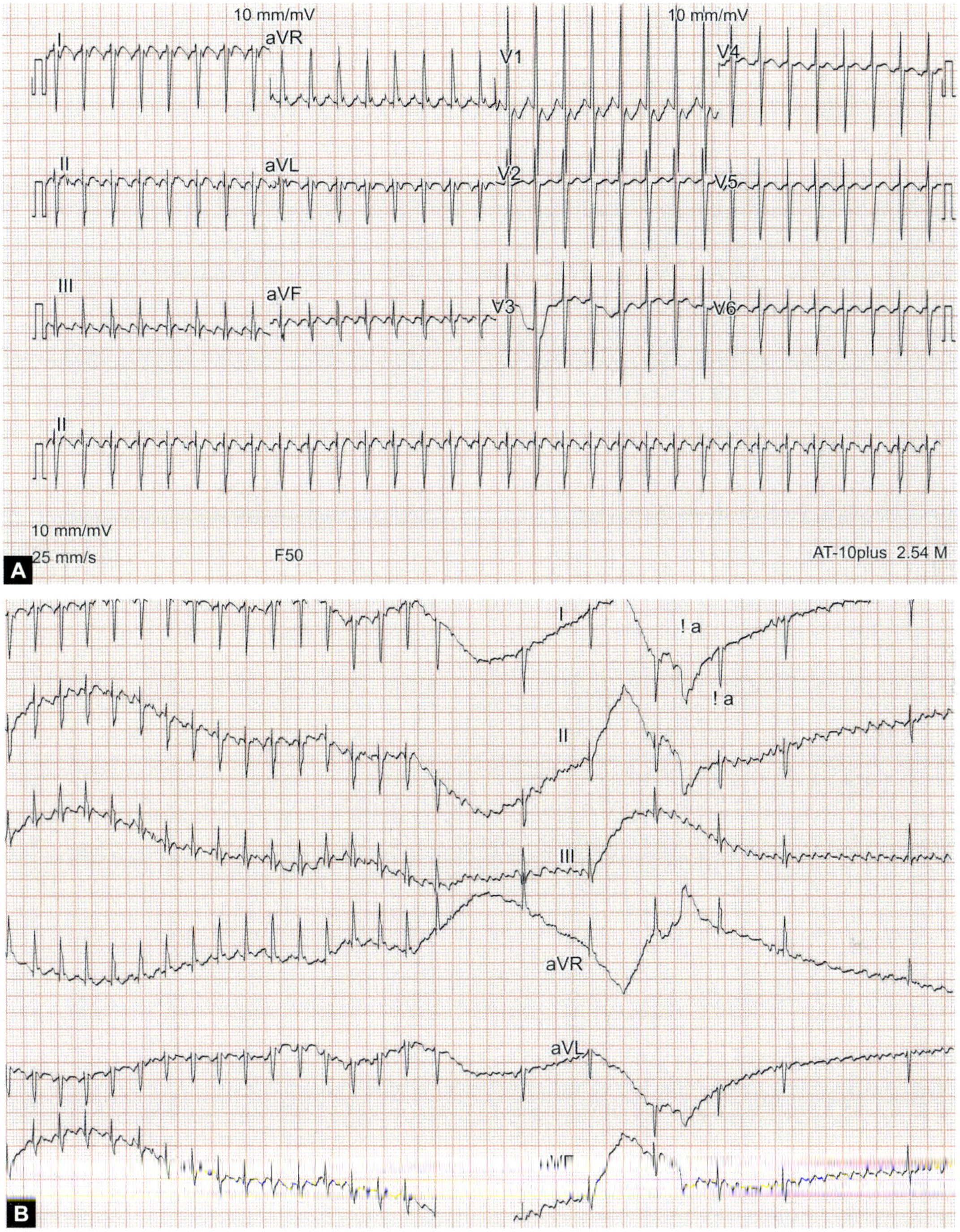

Figs. 9A and B: (A) A 12-lead electrocardiogram (ECG) demonstrating a regular narrow complex tachycardia. The P:QRS relationship is not readily apparent in this ECG; (B) Administration of adenosine blocks the atrioventricular (AV) node revealing the characteristic sawtooth pattern of P waves in atrial flutter.

Is the tachycardia regular? Yes.

How do the QRS complex appear? Narrow complex and monomorphic.

Are P waves visible? Yes.

What is the relationship of the P wave to the QRS complex? There is a 1:1 relationship with a short P-R interval.

Based on the assessment, the diagnosis is likely to be PSVT. However, if this is not apparent to the pediatrician, the next step would be:

Is it safe to administer adenosine? As this is a regular and monomorphic tachycardia, adenosine can be safely administered. The response to adenosine is demonstrated in **Figure 12B**.

Scenario 2

A 13-year-old boy presented to the outpatient clinic with palpitation. There were no signs of hemodynamic instability. An ECG was obtained and is shown in **Figure 13**.

Is the tachycardia regular? No.

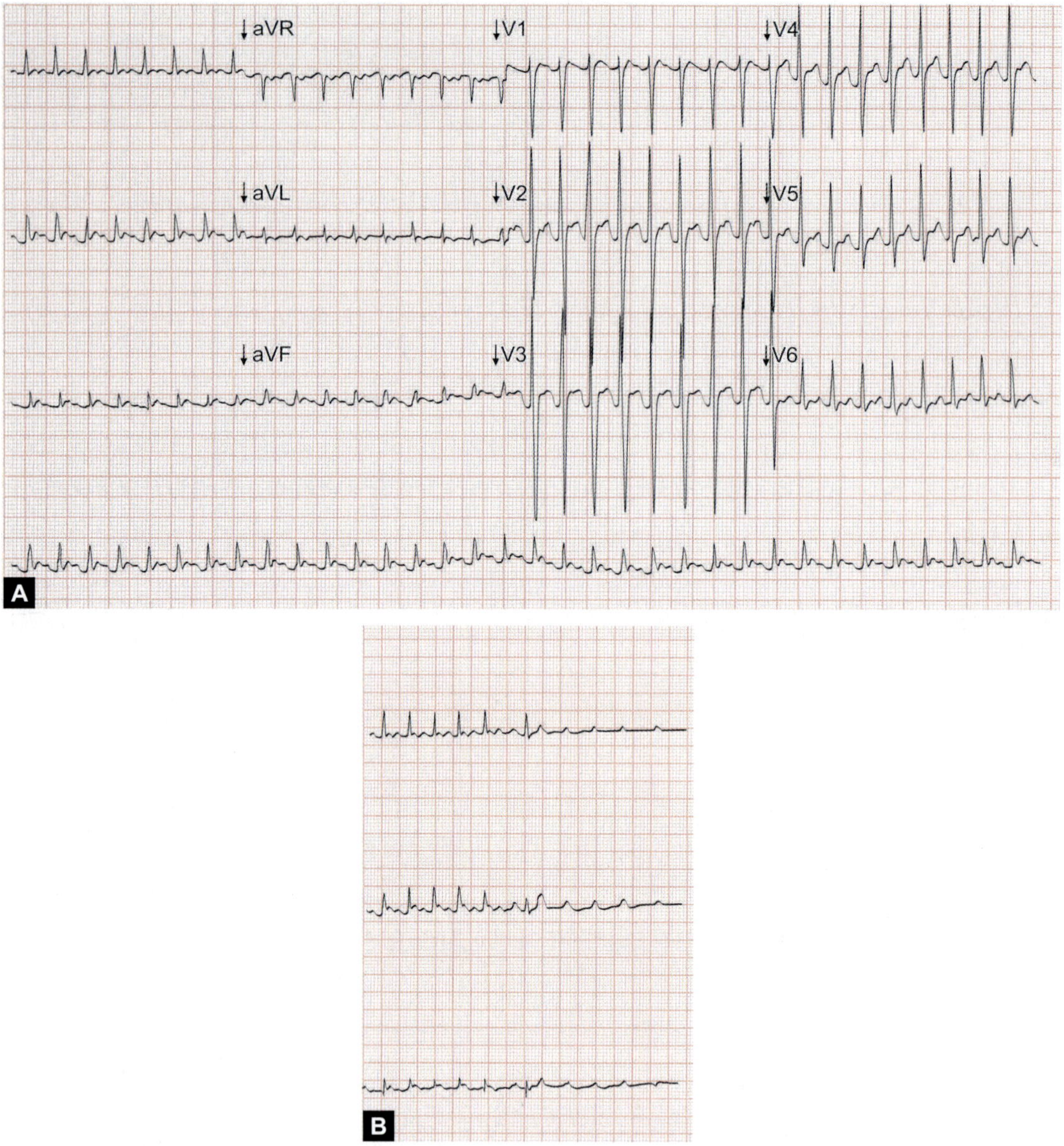

Figs. 10A and B: (A) A 12-lead electrocardiogram (ECG) showing a regular narrow complex tachycardia. The P waves are not readily apparent; (B) Administration of adenosine results in atrioventricular (AV) block and reveals the ectopic P waves of atrial tachycardia.

TABLE 1: Effect of adenosine administration on the various supraventricular tachyarrhythmias.

Arrhythmia	*Action of adenosine*
PSVT (re-entrant)	Terminates tachycardia
Atrial flutter	Unmasks flutter wave
Atrial tachycardia	Unmasks atrial rhythm
Adenosine sensitive atrial tachycardia	Terminates tachycardia (ends with P)
PJRT	Terminates transiently and returns (ends with QRS)
JET	No effect of adenosine

(JET: junctional ectopic tachycardia; PJRT: permanent junctional reciprocating tachycardia; PSVT: paroxysmal supraventricular tachycardia)

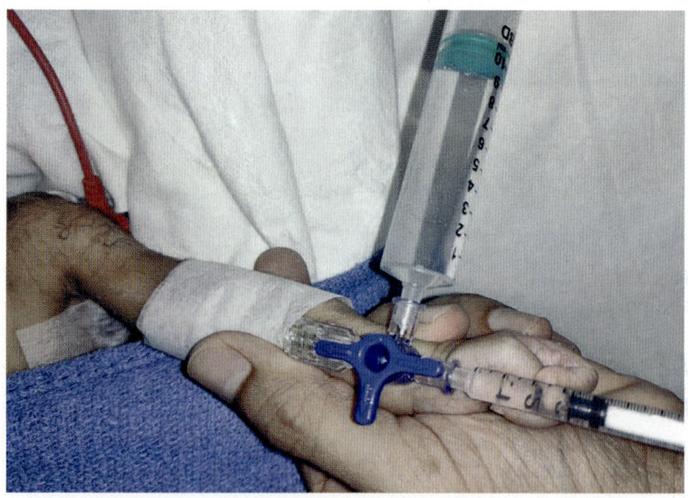

Fig. 11: The method of administering adenosine through an upper limb cannula with an attached three-way stop valve.

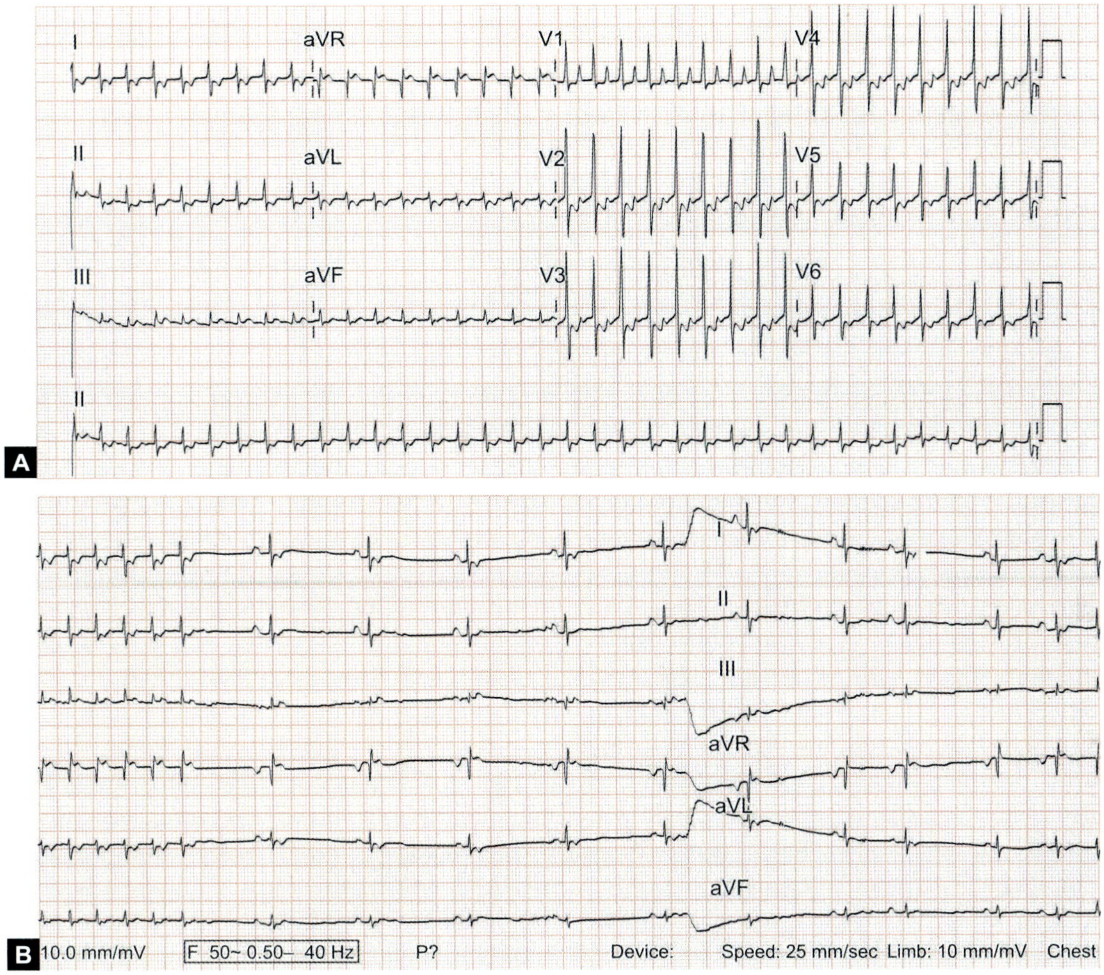

Figs. 12A and B: (A) A 12-lead electrocardiogram (ECG) of a regular monomorphic tachyarrhythmia; (B) Administration of adenosine results in the termination of tachyarrhythmia.

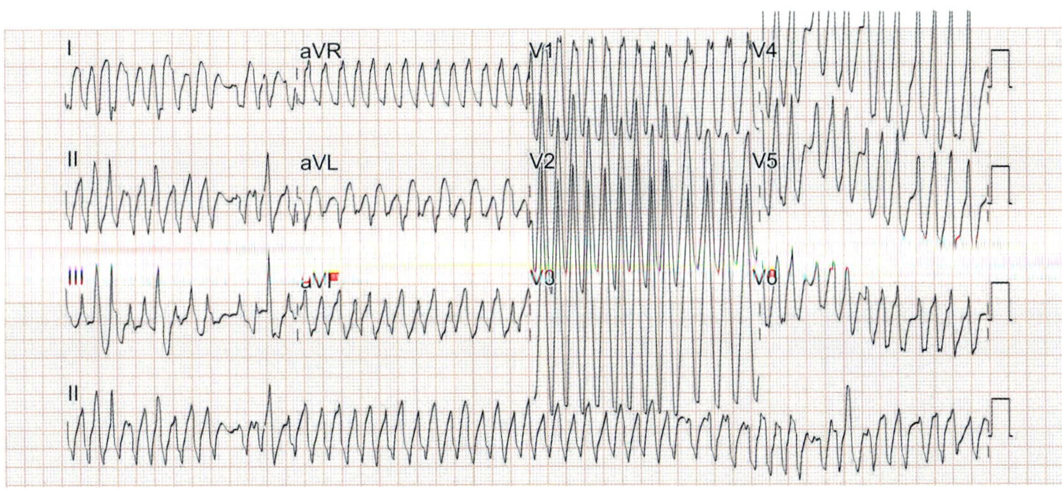

Fig. 13: A 12-lead electrocardiogram (ECG) of an irregular polymorphic tachyarrhythmia. Administration of adenosine is considered unsafe in this setting.

How do the QRS complexes appear? They are broad and polymorphic.

Are P waves seen? No.

Can adenosine be safely administered? No. As the tachycardia is irregular and polymorphic, adenosine should not be administered. This ECG shows atrial fibrillation with pre-excitation, an absolute contraindication for administration of adenosine.

Children frequently present to the pediatrician after the episode has subsided. In such cases, an ECG should be obtained. This is frequently normal. However, the presence of ventricular pre-excitation confirms WPW syndrome. All children with palpitation should be referred to a pediatric cardiologist for evaluation. An exercise stress test (EST) should be obtained if symptoms are triggered by exertion. A multiday ambulatory ECG, especially one available for >3 days, helps capture infrequent episodes.[8] An echocardiogram should be obtained to rule out coexistent CHD.

Treatment

Atrioventricular Node Blockage

Paroxysmal supraventricular tachycardia is AV node dependent and can be terminated by blocking the AV node. This can be achieved by vagal maneuvers or the administration of adenosine. Adenosine provides more reliable block of the AV node[9] and when available should be the preferred treatment of PSVT. In contrast, vagal maneuvers have a success rate of approximately 25%. The Valsalva maneuver is the most reliable of these but is impractical in children. The application of ice on the face is effective in neonates and young infants. A variety of vagal maneuvers are effective in older children. Older children with recurrent SVT can be taught vagal maneuvers to self-terminate the episode. Adenosine is administered at a dose of 0.1–0.3 mg/kg/dose. Adenosine has a half-life of only 6–8 seconds and is metabolized in the red blood cells. Hence, deactivation is initiated as soon as it is injected. It should hence be administered from an upper limb vein (preferably cubital vein) rapidly and followed by a saline flush. The adenosine should be administered first and the orientation of the stop valve changed to quickly flush saline. An experienced nurse or doctor should be able to administer both together. It results in termination of >90% of episodes of PSVT.[10] As discussed earlier, adenosine is both a diagnostic as well as a therapeutic tool. Hence, the ECG should be continuously recorded while administering adenosine and the recording should continue for 20 seconds after the administration of adenosine. Lack of response to adenosine in PSVT is almost always due to improper administration and hence many cardiologists prefer starting with a higher dose.[11]

Direct Current Cardioversion

Synchronized DC cardioversion can be utilized in all reentrant arrhythmias which present with hemodynamic instability. The dose used is usually 0.5–1 J/kg. In infants and toddlers, there may not be sufficient space to attach the paddles at the apex and the sternum. The paddles in this case can be placed anteroposteriorly (**Fig. 14**). Cardioversion could result in cutaneous burns in young children. This should be avoided by using a large amount of gel for lubrication. Cardioversion is a painful experience and the child should receive adequate analgesia/sedation. There are three important steps in cardioversion. After selection of the appropriate energy required, it is important to ensure synchronization to the QRS complex by pressing on the sync button on the defibrillator (**Fig. 15**). The paddles are then charged. Before the shock is delivered, it is important to ensure that oxygen supply is turned off. The PALS (Pediatric Advanced Life Support) algorithm encourages the operator to confirm "I am clear. You are clear. Everyone is clear. Oxygen is clear" before cardioversion. The paddles are then discharged. Most pediatricians do not routinely use defibrillators outside the intensive care unit and hence it is important that they become familiar with the model available in their hospital for use in an emergency.

Chronic Pharmacotherapy

Some form of pharmacological therapy will be required in most children with tachyarrhythmias and should be initiated in consultation with a pediatric cardiologist. The common drugs used, their dosage, and common adverse effects are

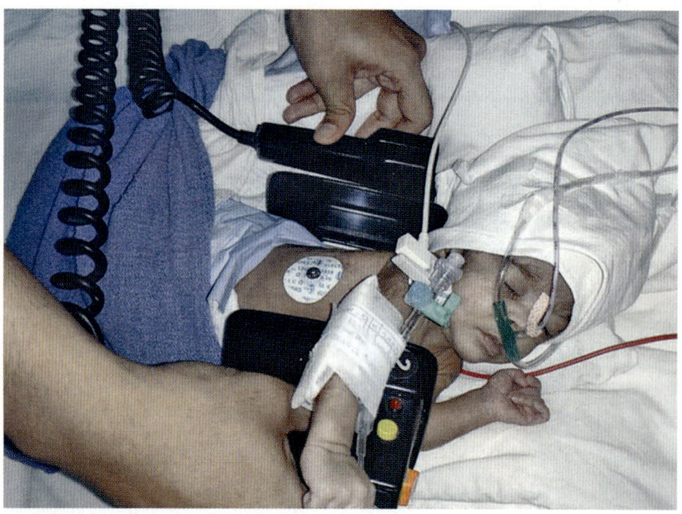

Fig. 14: Anteroposterior positioning of external defibrillator paddles for cardioversion in neonates and small infants.

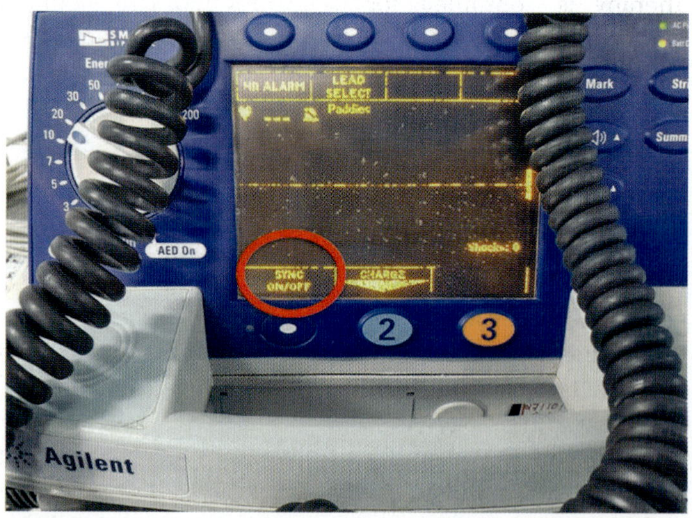

Fig. 15: External defibrillator demonstrating the SYNC button to ensure synchronized cardioversion.

TABLE 2: Common drugs used in chronic pharmacotherapy of tachyarrhythmias.

Drug	*Dose*	*Common indications*	*Adverse effects*
Propranolol	0.5–2 mg/kg/dose tds or qid	PSVT and atrial tachycardia	Fatigue and bronchospasm
Sotalol	1–2 mg/kg/dose tds	Refractory SVT and VT	Proarrhythmic effects (QTc to be monitored) and fatigue
Verapamil	1–2 mg/kg/dose tds	ILVT, PSVT (other than WPW)	Headache and constipation
Flecainide	1–2 mg/kg/dose bd or tds	Refractory PSVT	Proarrhythmic effects (QRSd to be monitored) and visual disturbances
Amiodarone	10 mg/kg/day for 1 week and then reduced to 5 mg/kg/day	Refractory arrhythmias	Proarrhythmic effects, hypotension, long-term effects on thyroid, liver, and lung
Digoxin	5 µg/kg/dose bd	PSVT (other than WPW)	Rare with correct dosing. Proarrhythmic effects on overdose, and GI intolerance

(ILVT: idiopathic left ventricular tachycardia; GI: gastrointestinal; PSVT: paroxysmal supraventricular tachycardia; SVT: supraventricular tachycardia; VT: ventricular tachycardia; WPW: Wolff–Parkinson–White syndrome)

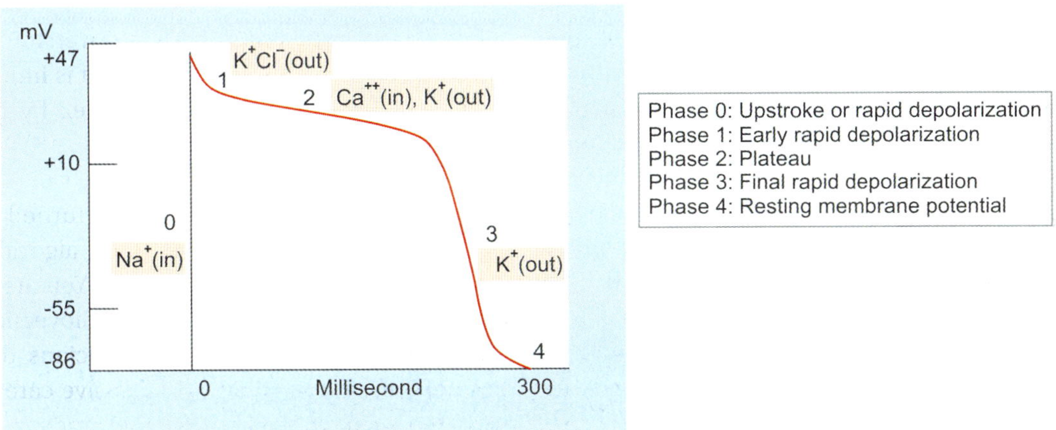

Fig. 16: Various phases of the cardiac action potential (AP) and the ions involved in each phase.

listed in **Table 2**. Beta-blockers are the drug of choice in PSVT and right ventricular outflow tract (RVOT) tachycardia. The calcium channel blockers, verapamil and diltiazem, are the drugs of choice in idiopathic left ventricular tachycardia (ILVT). In other conditions, the choice of drug is dictated by the availability and the choice of the treating cardiologist. Therapy is continued for 6–12 months with periodic monitoring before cessation can be considered in children with no further episodes.

Electrophysiological Study and Radiofrequency Ablation

An invasive study to identify the location of the AP or the automatic focus and ablate it using radiofrequency energy or cryotherapy should be considered in all recurrent tachycardia resistant to pharmacotherapy. Radiofrequency energy increases the local tissue temperature to >60°C and the resultant thermal injury causes destruction of tissue. An electrophysiology (EP) study should be offered to all children with WPW syndrome because of a small risk of sudden death in this condition. The procedure is safe in children weighing >15 kg. In children weighing <15 kg, it should be considered in children with recurrent episodes not responding adequately to medical management. The current recommendations list this as a Class IIb indication.[12] The most important adverse effect (albeit rare) is destruction of the AV node which results in heart block and the need of a pacemaker. The procedure has a success rate of above 90% in PSVT and atrial tachycardia.[12]

THE INHERITED ARRHYTHMIAS

The initiation and propagation of the heart beat as well as ventricular contraction involves a complex interplay of sodium, potassium, and calcium ions (**Fig. 16**). Changes in their relative intracellular and extracellular concentrations change the membrane potential and results in depolarization and repolarization. These ions are transported across the cell membrane through specialized ion channels. Mutations in these ion channels can alter the conduction of ions and the resultant abnormalities in membrane polarization could result in malignant ventricular arrhythmias and sudden unexpected death (SUD). The inherited arrhythmias include long QT syndrome (LQTS), catecholaminergic polymorphic ventricular tachycardia (CPVT), and Brugada syndrome (BrS). These disorders are mostly inherited in an autosomal dominant

(AD) fashion. However, the most severe of LQTS is Jervell-Lange-Nielsen syndrome which is autosomal recessive (AR). The clinical presentations of these disorders are varied and early recognition could facilitate appropriate management and reduce the risk of SUD. It is hence important that the pediatrician is aware of the heterogeneity of this disorder and recognizes it in time to facilitate early referral. These conditions are discussed together for ease of understanding of the pediatrician.

Etiopathogenesis

Long QT syndrome is the most prevalent of the channelopathies with an estimated incidence of 1 in 2,500.[13] Our understanding of this disorder has improved vastly since the times when it was classified into an AD Romano-Ward syndrome and AR JLNS. The genes implicated in the various channelopathies are listed in **Table 3**. The classical form of LQTS is caused by loss of function mutations in potassium channels or gain of function mutations in sodium channels. JLNS is due to homozygous mutations (both alleles affected) in the LQTS 1 gene and hence is the most severe form of the spectrum. These mutations result in prolonged repolarization as well as the time taken for repolarization to disperse in the myocardium. In the presence of an increased sympathetic tone, this triggers early after-depolarization potentials resulting in polymorphic ventricular arrhythmias and torsades de pointes (TdP). Tdp is the signature arrhythmia of LQTS characterized by rotation of the QRS axis around a point (**Fig. 17**). The triggers for arrhythmia in LQTS are physical exertion (LQTS 1 and 2), swimming (LQTS 1), auditory stimuli (LQTS 2), and bradycardia during deep sleep (LQTS 3).

TABLE 3: Genes implicated in the channelopathies.

Condition	*Genes implicated*
LQTS—genes deemed causative	KCNQ 1–LQTS 1 KCNH2–LQTS 2 SCN5A–LQTS 3 CALM 1,2,3—calmodulinopathy CACNA1C—Timothy syndrome KCNJ2—Andersen–Tawil syndrome TRDN—Triadin knockout syndrome
LQTS—genes with possible association	AKAP9 CAV3 KCNE1 KCNE2 KCNJ5 SCN4B SNTA1
CPVT	RyR2—ryanodine receptor 2 CASQ2—calsequestrin 2 CALM 1-3—calmodulinopathy
Brugada syndrome	SCN5A

(CPVT: catecholaminergic polymorphic ventricular tachycardia; LQTS: long QT syndrome)

Catecholaminergic polymorphic ventricular tachycardia is believed to have an incidence of 1 in 10,000.[14] It is caused by mutations in the calcium channel genes *RyR2*, *CASQ2*, and *CALM 1-3*. Of these, *CASQ2* has an AR inheritance. Calcium ions (Ca^{2+}) stored in the sarcolemma are released into the myocyte during systole and this binds to troponin resulting in muscle contraction. The Ca^{2+} are then returned to the sarcolemma during diastole. Mutations involved in CPVT result in diastolic accumulation of Ca^{2+} setting up delayed after depolarizations during sympathetic stimulation which result in ventricular ectopy and VT. The signature arrhythmia of CPVT is bidirectional ventricular ectopy or bidirectional VT (**Fig. 18**). The typical triggers in CPVT are physical activity and swimming.

Brugada syndrome is much less common in children than in adults. Studies in adults suggest a prevalence of 1 in 5,000.[15] However, symptomatic children are rare. The disease is characterized by right bundle branch block and typical "cove-type" ST elevation in the right side chest leads (**Fig. 19**). It is thought to be due to fibrosis in the RVOT causing delay in depolarization in this region. The late RVOT activation results in the typical ST elevation pattern of BrS. Unlike CPVT and LQTS, arrhythmias in BrS are not typically triggered by activity. However, fever is an important trigger for arrhythmias, especially in children, although the exact cause is not known.

Clinical Features

The clinical presentation of the channelopathies includes recurrent syncope, seizures, and a family history of sudden death. The most important clinical information in inherited arrhythmias is a detailed family history and it is worth investing time in a three-generation family history. In particular, the history should focus on SUD, drowning deaths, unexplained seizures in multiple family members, and alleged myocardial infarction without documented coronary angiogram in young family members (<45 years of age).

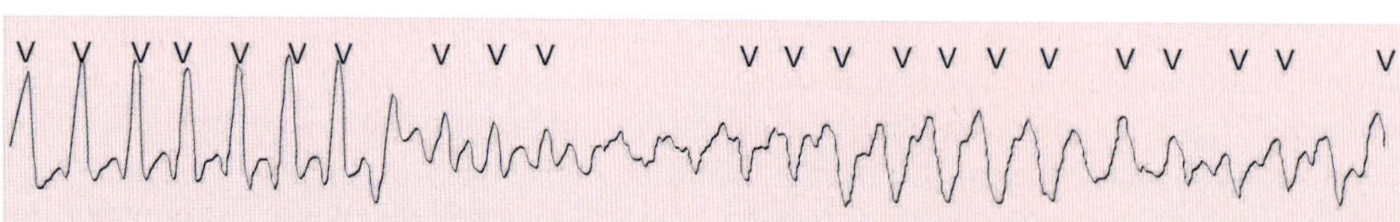

Fig. 17: An electrocardiogram (ECG) strip demonstrating a polymorphic broad complex tachyarrhythmia. The QRS axis in the middle portion appears to rotate around a point. This is termed torsades de pointes (TdP).

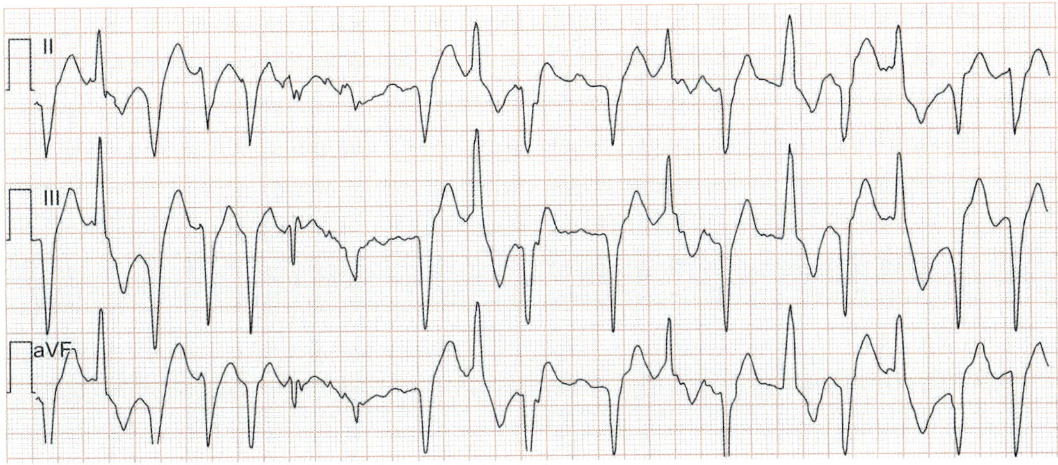

Fig. 18: An electrocardiogram (ECG) strip demonstrating a polymorphic tachycardia. The QRS axes in successive complexes are in opposite directions. This is termed bidirectional ventricular tachycardia.

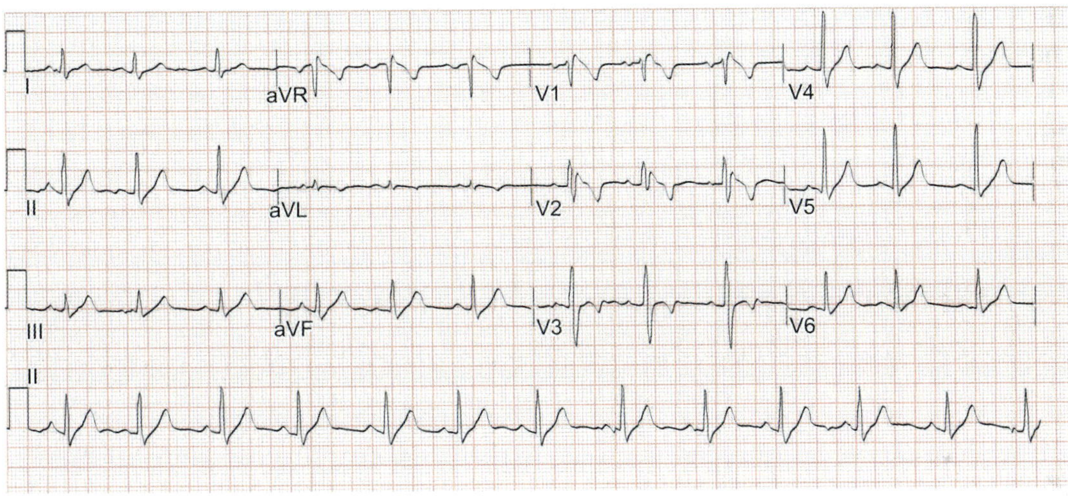

Fig. 19: A 12-lead electrocardiogram (ECG) in sinus rhythm. There is an incomplete right bundle branch block and a "cove-type" ST elevation in the right chest leads—typically seen in Brugada syndrome.

An important presentation of channelopathies is sudden infant death syndrome (SIDS). It is estimated that 20% of SIDS deaths can be attributed to channelopathies.[13] LQTS 1 and 3 contribute the biggest chunk of channelopathy associated SIDS and the incidence peaks at approximately 2 months of age. In the current era with good access to basic pediatric and neonatal care and low infant mortality, a family history of infant death with no clear diagnosis should be treated with suspicion of channelopathy and the family evaluated in these lines.

Both LQTS and CPVT can present as convulsive syncope or true seizures due to cerebral hypoperfusion. It is estimated that close to 50% of CPVT patients can be misdiagnosed and treated as drug-resistant epilepsy. Seizures not responding to standard treatment, seizures with repeated normal electroencephalograms (EEGs), seizures triggered by exertion or emotional trauma, and seizures with specific triggers (e.g., auditory stimuli) should raise the suspicion of a channelopathy.

A peculiar feature of BrS especially in children is the association of symptoms with fever.[15] The presenting feature may be recurrent syncope during febrile episodes as well as febrile seizures. Indeed some children may have normal ECG during the afebrile period with evidence of a Brugada pattern seen only with fever. Presentation as recurrent febrile seizures has also been reported in young children.

Evaluation

A 12-lead ECG should be obtained in all children suspected to have an inherited arrhythmia and the QTc interval should be calculated using the Bazett's formula. A prolonged QTc (**Fig. 20A**) along with an abnormal T wave morphology (asymmetric T wave in LQTS 1, bifid T wave in LQTS 2, and a long JT interval in LQTS 3) makes the diagnosis. Neonates and infants with LQTS may present with bradycardia due to a functional 2:1 AV block (**Fig. 20B**). The QTc is often significantly prolonged and hence only alternate P waves are conducted to the ventricle because of the prolonged

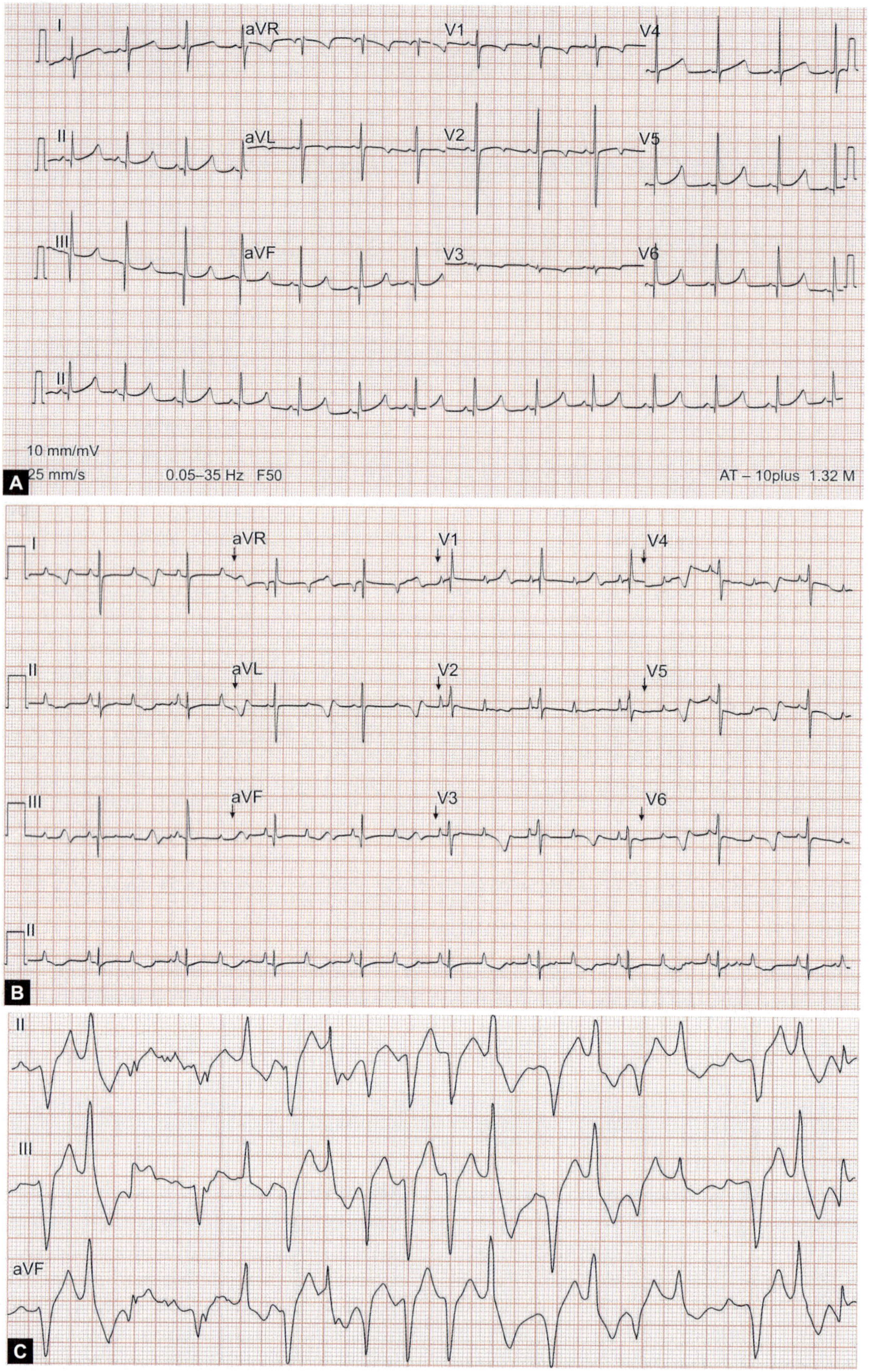

Figs. 20A to C: (A) A 12-lead electrocardiogram (ECG) in sinus rhythm with rightward axis. The corrected QT interval (QTc) is prolonged and the T wave has an abnormal asymmetric configuration; (B) A 12-lead ECG of a neonate with 2:1 atrioventricular (AV) block. Note that the QT interval is prolonged with the T wave only appearing after the next P wave. This is a functional AV block often seen in neonates with long QT syndrome; (C) ECG strip of a polymorphic ventricular tachycardia seen in catecholaminergic polymorphic ventricular tachycardia (CPVT).

refractory period. In BrS, there is a characteristic cove-shaped ST elevation >2 mm (*see* **Fig. 18**) in the right precordial leads (type 1) or a J point elevation of 2 mm with a saddleback ST elevation pattern (type 2). However, it is important to recognize that the interval ECG is frequently normal in channelopathies. Subtle clues could raise the suspicion and direct further evaluation. The heart rate in sinus rhythm is frequently lower than normal for age in children with LQTS and CPVT. The presence of a broad QRS complex (for age), especially with left axis deviation, may be seen in BrS. It is important to obtain ECG of all available family members whenever a channelopathy is suspected. This should be obtained in the very first clinical contact. A valuable opportunity may be lost especially in our country where it is often difficult to get family members to travel to a medical facility to obtain investigations.

If the ECG is normal, the next investigation would usually be an EST. It is logistically difficult to obtain an EST in children <8 years of age. In such cases, a reasonable alternative is to obtain ambulatory ECG recording (Holter). Young children are usually very active and capturing ECG recordings during activity can provide most of the information obtained from an EST. In LQTS 1, the QTc is prolonged during exercise with the longest QTc recorded during early recovery before normalizing. Children with CPVT would exhibit polymorphic ventricular ectopy during CPVT (**Fig. 20C**). If bidirectional ventricular ectopy or polymorphic VT is demonstrated, this is diagnostic. In children with suspected BrS but with normal ECG, obtaining ECG when the temperature is elevated may help unmask a typical Brugada pattern.

When first-line investigations are not contributory, it may be worthwhile considering provocation testing.[16] As the name implies, attempts are made to elicit ventricular arrhythmias. These tests are hence dangerous and should only be performed by a trained pediatric cardiologist in a center where all facilities for resuscitation are available and after a detailed discussion with the family about the potential dangers of this test. Provocation testing in LQTS and CPVT is performed with adrenaline. A number of different strategies and protocols for adrenaline challenge testing are described, each with its own advantages and risks and the choice of protocol depends on the individual center. In children with suspected BrS, ajmaline challenge testing is advocated. However, ajmaline is currently not available in our country. An alternative would be to perform a flecainide challenge test. This however carries a much higher risk than ajmaline and is not routinely used.

When the diagnosis is apparent on the above tests (and even in selected cases where there is a high index of clinical suspicion but with negative evaluation), genetic testing of the proband should be performed. This is done on peripheral blood by the technique of massive parallel sequencing [next generation sequencing (NGS)] which permits interrogation of a large number of genes simultaneously. Identification of a pathogenic mutation in a LQTS gene allows us to counsel the family about the prognosis of the condition, provide genotype specific treatment, and also perform cascade testing among family members to identify asymptomatic members at risk.[17]

Management

The general principles of management are broadly similar for the inherited arrhythmias. High levels of exertion as experienced in competitive sports should be avoided. However, leisure sports and low level physical activity should be encouraged as part of general fitness in these children. Swimming is prohibited for children with LQTS and CPVT. It is important to avoid drugs that could prolong the QTc in LQTS. Indeed avoidance of incriminatory drugs is the single most important intervention in LQTS. A number of common drugs used in pediatrics are contraindicated in LQTS and the pediatrician should consult the online database *www.crediblemeds.org* before prescribing any medication. The database is the most up-to-date reference available and is superior to any printed list which is usually provided to patients. A similar tool is also available for BrS (*www.brugadadrugs.org*). However, the incriminatory drugs in BrS are less frequently used in general practice. Children with BrS, especially those who have fever-related syndromes, should be advised hospitalization and ECG monitoring during febrile episodes. Efforts should be made to bring down temperature aggressively using paracetamol at standard doses.

The mainstay of treatment in LQTS and CPVT is beta-blocker therapy. The nonselective beta-blocker, propranolol, has been shown to be superior to other beta-blockers in channelopathies.[18] The dose required is usually higher (6–18 mg/kg/day in three to four divided doses). Another long-acting nonselective beta-blocker, nadolol, has shown superior efficacy in both CPVT and LQTS but is unfortunately not available in our country. Beta-blocker therapy is especially efficacious in LQTS 1 where it reduces the risk of SUD by close to 90% and CPVT. Mexiletine (a sodium channel blocker which targets the very channel affected in LQTS 3) is a specific agent in LQTS 3 and should be used whenever the diagnosis is confirmed.[19] Similarly, flecainide has been shown to be effective in children with CPVT in whom symptoms are not controlled by beta-blockers.

A proportion of children continue to experience symptoms despite adequate drug therapy. It is important to remember that no drug provides complete protection against ventricular arrhythmias and lifelong compliance to treatment is often challenging. Failure of medical treatment necessitates an implantable cardioverter defibrillator (ICD). This is a device placed inside the heart which constantly monitors the heart rhythm. Should a persistent ventricular arrhythmia be detected, the device provides a shock similar to the defibrillator and restores normal rhythm. This is often combined with a cervical sympathectomy in children with LQTS and CPVT. ICD implantation carries a higher risk of complications in children compared to adults and the decision should be made after detailed discussion with the family. It is also important to teach family members and caregivers basic life support (BLS). Should the child collapse suddenly, early institution of BLS can be life saving.

Prognosis

The most important prognostic feature in inherited arrhythmias is often establishing the correct diagnosis. Adherence to pharmacotherapy and lifestyle modifications can help reduce the risk of SUD to a significant extent. LQTS 3 with onset of symptoms in infancy and CALM mutations have been shown to carry a worse prognosis despite treatment.[20] When a genetic diagnosis is made, parents can be offered prenatal diagnostic testing. This allows us to start safety measures including drug therapy from the newborn period. The possibility of preimplantation genetic testing which allows the parents to choose a zygote which does not carry the mutation is also available.

BRADYARRHYTHMIAS

As the name implies, bradyarrhythmias are those where the heart rate is below the normal for age and level of activity. In adults, the cut-off for heart rate is universally 60 per minute. However, with the wide range of variability in heart rate between different ages, the same number cannot be used to define bradycardia in an infant as well as an 18-year old. The most popular definition is a heart rate below 100 per minute in infants and 60 per minute in older children. On a recent meta-analysis of published literature on heart rate range in children, the 1st centile for heart rate in neonates was 90 per minute increasing to 100 at 3 months of age before gradually dropping throughout childhood.[21]

Electrocardiographically, there are three major causes of bradycardia in children (**Fig. 21**)—(1) sinus bradycardia,

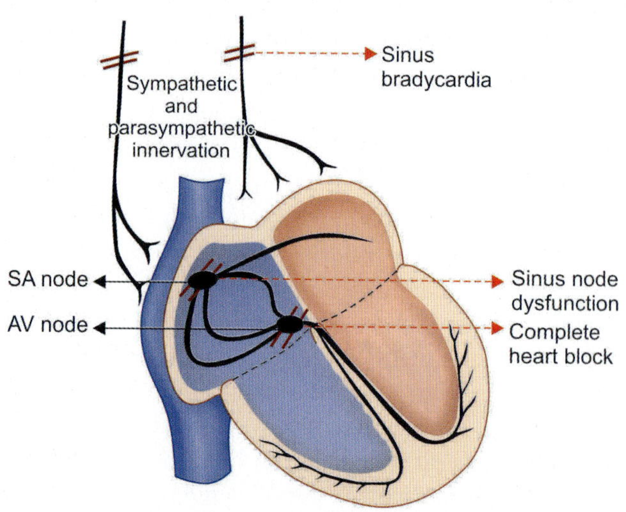

Fig. 21: A schematic diagram demonstrating the mechanisms of the common bradyarrhythmias seen in children.

(2) complete heart block (CHB), and (3) sinus node dysfunction (SND). The electrocardiographic features of each of this condition are depicted in **Table 4**. In this section, we will briefly discuss each of these conditions.

Sinus Bradycardia

Sinus bradycardia is the most common cause of bradycardia in children. The cause of sinus bradycardia may stem from any of the organ systems of the body from head to foot. Sinus bradycardia is unusual in younger children but a common feature in older children. In recent years, continuous hemodynamic monitoring by telemetry in hospitalized children, especially those requiring intensive care observation, has resulted in an increased recognition in children as well as referral for cardiological evaluation. During sleep, the heart rate can go below 60 per minute in normal children. An appropriate chronotropic response to awakening as well as a normal sinus rhythm on resting ECG is reassuring and should preclude further evaluation. Athletes who train regularly have a lower heart rate as a result of cardiac conditioning. The bradycardia response is lost within a few weeks of cessation of training. The various causes of sinus bradycardia are depicted in **Figure 22**. The clinical features may include symptoms related to the low heart rate as well as symptoms attributable to the underlying cause.[22] In most of these conditions, children present with symptoms of the disorder and bradycardia is picked up incidentally by the clinician. Symptoms attributable to bradycardia include feeding difficulty in infants and excessive fatigue, exercise intolerance, and syncope in older children. An ECG is warranted in all cases to ensure normal sinus rhythm. The bradycardia generally resolves with the treatment of the underlying condition.

Complete Heart Block

Atrioventricular block is classified into three types based on varying degrees of severity. First-degree AV block is characterized by a prolongation of the P-R interval beyond the normal range for age (**Fig. 23**). However, the P-R interval remains constant despite changes in the heart rate. It is usually associated with a small drop in the heart rate.

TABLE 4: Common bradyarrhythmias in children and their typical electrocardiographic findings.

Bradyarrhythmia	*ECG*
Sinus bradycardia	• Slow heart rate • P before every QRS • Regular PR interval
Sinus node dysfunction	• Slow heart rate • No P wave seen before QRS
Complete heart block	• Slow heart rate • P and QRS seen with no consistent relationship

(ECG: electrocardiogram)

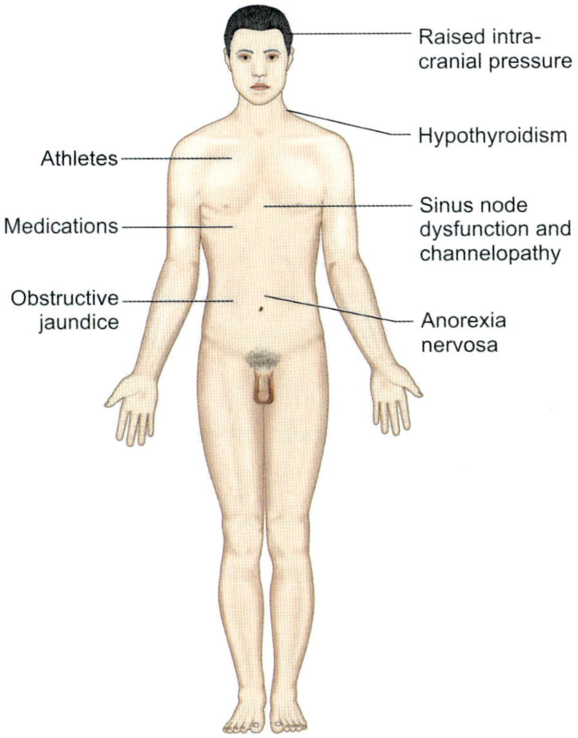

Fig. 22: A schematic diagram depicting the common causes of sinus bradycardia.

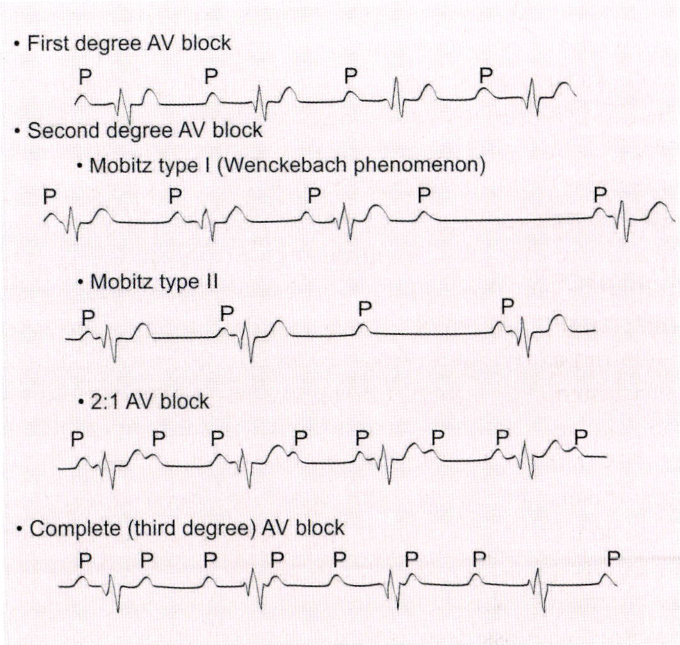

Fig. 23: Various degrees of atrioventricular (AV) block. The PR interval is above the normal limit for age in I degree AV block. In Mobitz type I AV block, there is progressive prolongation of PR interval until one P wave is not conducted. In Mobitz type II, the PR interval remains constant but one P wave is not conducted regularly. There is no consistent relationship between the P and QRS in III degree AV block.

Second-degree AV block is further divided into type 2A (Mobitz type I) and 2B (Mobitz type II). In Mobitz type I (**Fig. 23**), there is a progressive prolongation of the P-R interval until a P wave does not get conducted (dropped beat). This is also described as Wenckebach phenomenon after Karel Wenckebach who first described it in 1899. Interestingly, Wenckebach deduced the physiological basis of this condition even before ECG was invented by carefully timing the pulse and jugular venous pulsations of a female patient with irregular pulse and noticing the variation of the AV interval and that there is no drop beat in the jugular venous pulsations.[23] In Mobitz type II (**Fig. 23**), the PR interval remains constant but there is periodic nonconduction of the P wave (drop beat). Mobitz type II can be described as 2:1, 3:2, 4:3, etc., based on the number of conducted and nonconducted P waves.

Third-degree AV block is termed as CHB. There is no consistent relation between the atrial (P wave) and ventricular (QRS waves). The rhythm in CHB is characterized by the following (**Fig. 23**):

- Normal P wave rate and axis for age and level of activity
- Regular QRS complexes at a rate less than normal for age and lesser than the atrial rate
- No consistent relation between the P waves and the QRS complexes (AV disassociation).

Etiopathogenesis

Complete heart block in children may be congenital or acquired. Congenital CHB has an incidence of approximately 1 in 22,000 births.[24] Approximately 80% of these are associated with maternal autoimmune disorders. The antibodies implicated in CHB are the anti-Ro (SS-A) and anti-La (SS-B) antibodies. Fetal CHB occurs in approximately 3% of mothers with anti-Ro antibodies. The risk increases to as high as 17% in a subsequent pregnancy and 50% when more than one fetus has been affected. The immunoglobulin G (IgG) antibodies cross the placenta after 12–14 weeks of gestation and target specific cells of the cardiac conduction system. The resultant inflammatory process causes fibrosis of the conduction system fibers.

Complete heart block can also occur secondary to genetic causes. The most common single gene disorders associated with CHB are Holt–Oram syndrome and familial NKX 2.5 mutations. Holt–Oram syndrome is an autosomal disorder characterized by hand abnormalities, atrial septal defects (ASDs), and AV block of varying degrees. It is caused by a mutation in the TBX 5 gene. Familial mutations in the NKX 2.5 gene are also inherited in an AD fashion and causes familial ASD and CHB. Kearns–Sayre syndrome presents a classic triad of pigmentary retinal dystrophy, external ophthalmoplegia, and AV block. It is caused by a mitochondrial DNA deletion and is maternally transmitted.[25] Although a genetic condition, AV block frequently manifests only in late childhood.

Complete heart block can also occur in the setting of a CHD. Congenitally corrected transposition of the great arteries (ccTGA) and CHD in the setting of heterotaxy have a high association with CHB. The prognosis of CHB with coexistent CHB is usually worse and a greater proportion of such children will need definitive treatment for CHB.

In the current era, the most common cause of acquired CHB is postoperative after surgical repair of CHD. This is usually dealt with by the treating pediatric cardiac team before the child is discharged from hospital and usually does not fall under the purview of a pediatrician and hence is not covered in this chapter. Acquired CHB occurs frequently in the setting of myocarditis secondary to bacterial and viral infections. Recently, diphtheria has seen a reemergence in India despite adequate implementation of the immunization program. Approximately, 20% of children with faucial diphtheria can develop myocarditis and a half of these children develop conduction system abnormalities including CHB.[26] The diphtheria toxin has been shown to be cardiotoxic and can result in disruption of the fibers in the AV node.

Clinical Features

In the current era, congenital CHB secondary to maternal immune conditions is diagnosed prenatally. If the condition is not diagnosed prenatally, the presentation in infancy is usually bradycardia noticed by the pediatrician on examination. The other clinical features of neonatal lupus such as a characteristic skin rash may also bring the condition to attention. If there is a coexistent CHD, symptoms specific to the CHD such as cyanosis or heart failure may be the dominant presentation.

Older children with CHB may be asymptomatic and bradycardia may be noted during evaluation for some other illness. The inability to augment cardiac output by increasing heart rate may cause easy fatigability and breathlessness on exertion. Symptoms may be subtle in the form of preference for a sedentary lifestyle, poor school performance, or the need for a nap on returning from school. In more severe forms of CHB, bradycardia-related drop in cardiac output results in syncope (Stokes–Adams attacks). Rarely, SUD may be the presenting feature and a diagnosis may only be made postmortem. An unusual presenting feature in toddlers and young children is the presence of night terrors and disturbed sleep. This is attributed to an increased sympathetic tone as a result of the low heart rate although the exact cause is not known.[27]

Acquired CHB may occur in the setting of myocarditis and the clinical presentation is that of myocarditis with fever, tachypnea, and heart failure.

Evaluation

The cause of bradycardia should be confirmed on an ECG. Apart from the diagnosis of CHB, attention should be placed on the ventricular rate as well as the QRS morphology. The duration of the QRS complex (QRSd) provides an indication of the origin of the escape rhythm. A narrow complex QRS (typically <80–90 ms) indicates a supra-Hisian origin of the escape rhythm which is more stable (**Fig. 24A**). However, a wider QRSd suggests infra-Hisian escape rhythm (**Fig. 24B**) which is generally unreliable and needs immediate attention. All infants and children diagnosed with CHB on ECG should undergo Holter evaluation. The indications for urgent referral to a pediatric cardiologist include:

- CHB with symptoms
- CHB with a broad QRS complex
- CHB with a heart rate <50/minute (irrespective of age)
- Average heart rate <50/minute on Holter
- Pauses >3 seconds on Holter
- Presence of frequent ventricular ectopy on Holter.

All children with CHB should undergo an echocardiogram to rule out associated CHD and to ensure that the ventricular function is normal. In neonates with CHB and a structurally normal heart, it is important to evaluate the mother for presence of anti-Ro and anti-La antibodies even in the absence of other symptoms of an autoimmune disorder.

Treatment

Drug therapy in CHB is usually temporary in CHB. In neonates with CHB and a very low heart rate, the drug of choice is intravenous isoprenaline which is started as an infusion at the rate of 0.05 μg/kg/min which can be titrated to 10 μg/kg/min till an adequate heart rate is obtained. This is usually achieved by diluting 0.3 mg/kg in 50 mL of saline and starting an infusion of 0.5–10 mL per hour depending on the dose required. Oral orciprenaline has also been used as a maintenance therapy in selected cases although evidence for its efficacy is anecdotal. The usual dose of orciprenaline is 0.25–0.5 mg/kg every 6–8 hours.

Acquired CHB secondary to myocarditis frequently results in hemodynamic instability and will need to be urgently addressed by the insertion of a temporary pacemaker to improve the heart rate. In the vast majority, sinus rhythm is restored once the inflammatory process subsides and the temporary pacemaker can be removed after restoration of sinus rhythm.

The definitive treatment of CHB is insertion of a permanent pacemaker. Not all infants and children with CHB require a pacemaker. The indications for pacemaker insertion in congenital CHB include the following:[28]

- CHB associated with clinical symptoms
- CHB with a broad QRS escape rhythm or frequent ventricular ectopy
- CHB in an infant with a heart rate <55 per minute (if the heart is structurally normal) or 70 per minute (with associated critical CHD)
- CHB in an older child with an average heart rate <50 per minute or pauses >3 seconds on Holter.

In children weighing >15 kg, the pacemaker can safely be implanted endocardial through the subclavian vein. Endocardial pacing carries the advantage of more stable pacing and a longer battery life. However, the small size of

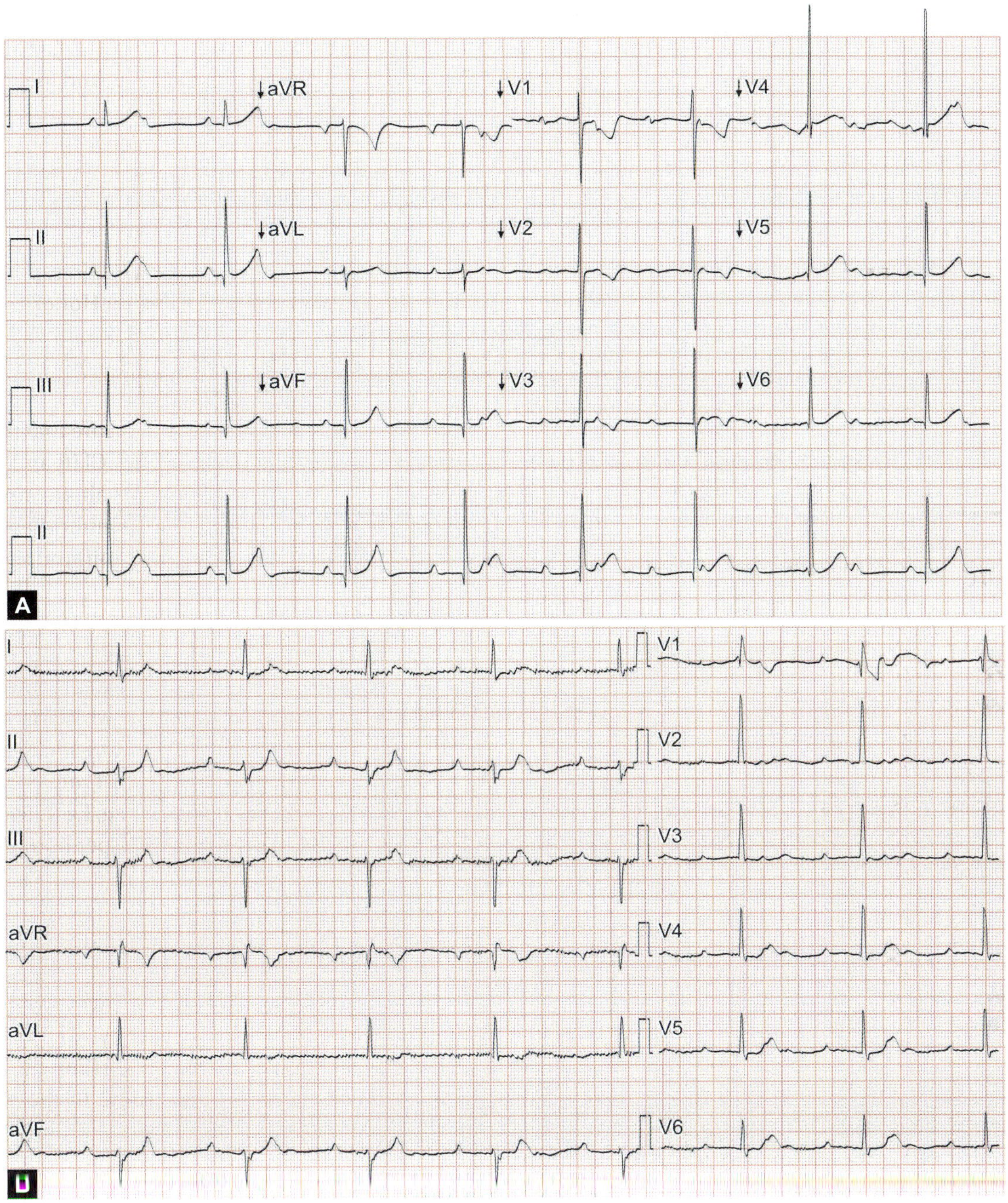

Figs. 24A and B: (A) A 12-lead electrocardiogram (ECG) of complete heart block. The QRS complexes are narrow with normal axis and this suggests a supra-Hisian escape rhythm; (B) A 12-lead ECG of complete heart block. The QRS complexes show a incomplete right bundle branch block with leftward axis suggesting a infra-Hisian escape rhythm.

the systemic veins precludes endocardial pacing in infants and the pacemaker hence has to be placed epicardial by a cardiothoracic surgeon. The long-term outcomes after pacemaker insertion are excellent although reinterventions are the rule due to lead malfunction and the need to replace the battery.

Sinus Node Dysfunction

Isolated SND is a very rare arrhythmia in children. It may be associated with structural heart disease particularly in the setting of left isomerism. However, it is more common in a postoperative setting, especially after complex surgeries involving the atrium. These include atrial switch operation after a late diagnosis of transposition of the great arteries (Senning or Mustard operation) or surgeries for children with a functional single ventricle (Fontan operation). The symptoms are usually those of a low heart rate and resultant drop in cardiac output. Some children with SND may present with palpitation due to episodic SVT—the so called tachybrady syndrome. Depending on the severity, the ECG may show a very slow sinus rhythm or a junctional escape rhythm with no visible P wave. In general, most children with SND will require treatment with a pacemaker.

REFERENCES

1. Hanash CR, Crosson JE. Emergency diagnosis and management of pediatric arrhythmias. J Emerg Trauma Shock. 2010;3(3): 251-60.
2. Ko JK, Deal BJ, Strasburger JF, Benson DW Jr. Supraventricular tachycardia mechanisms and their age distribution in pediatric patients. Am J Cardiol. 1992;69(12):1028-32.
3. Tse G. Mechanisms of cardiac arrhythmias. J Arrhythm. 2016;32(2):75-81.
4. Antzelevitch C, Burashnikov A. Overview of basic mechanisms of cardiac arrhythmia. Card Electrophysiol Clin. 2011;3(1):23-45.
5. KleinmanME,ChameidesL,SchexnayderSM,SamsonRA,Hazinski MF, Atkins DL, et al. Part 14: pediatric advanced life support: 2010 American Heart Association Guidelines for Cardiopulmonary Resuscitation and Emergency Cardiovascular Care. Circulation. 2010; 122(18 Suppl 3):S876-908.
6. Trappe HJ. Concept of the five 'A's for treating emergency arrhythmias. J Emerg Trauma Shock. 2010;3(2):129-36.
7. Pelleg A, Porter RS. The pharmacology of adenosine. Pharmacotherapy. 1990;10(3):157-74.
8. Bolourchi M, Batra AS. Diagnostic yield of patch ambulatory electrocardiogram monitoring in children (from a national registry). Am J Cardiol. 2015;115(5):630-4.
9. Sohinki D, Obel OA. Current trends in supraventricular tachycardia management. Ochsner J. 2014;14(4):586-95.
10. Blomstrom-Lundqvist C, Scheinman MM, Aliot EM, Alpert JS, Calkins H, Camm AJ, et al. ACC/AHA/ESC guidelines for the management of patients with supraventricular arrhythmias-executive summary. A report of the American college of cardiology/American heart association task force on practice guidelines and the European society of cardiology committee for practice guidelines (writing committee to develop guidelines for the management of patients with supraventricular arrhythmias) developed in collaboration with NASPE-Heart Rhythm Society. J Am CollCardiol. 2003; 42(8):1493-531.
11. Kothari DS, Skinner JR. Neonatal tachycardias: an update. Arch Dis Child Fetal Neonatal Ed. 2006;91(2):F136-44.
12. Philip Saul J, Kanter RJ, Writing C, Abrams D, Asirvatham S, Bar-Cohen Y, et al. PACES/HRS expert consensus statement on the use of catheter ablation in children and patients with congenital heart disease:developedinpartnershipwiththePediatricandCongenital Electrophysiology Society (PACES) and the Heart Rhythm Society (HRS). Endorsed by the governing bodies of PACES, HRS, the American Academy of Pediatrics (AAP), the American Heart Association (AHA), and the Association for European Pediatric and Congenital Cardiology (AEPC). Heart Rhythm. 2016; 13(6): e251-89.
13. Behere SP, Weindling SN. Inherited arrhythmias: the cardiac channelopathies. Ann Pediatr Cardiol. 2015;8(3):210-20.
14. Behere SP, Weindling SN. Catecholaminergic polymorphic ventricular tachycardia: an exciting new era. Ann Pediatr Cardiol. 2016;9(2): 137-46.
15. Behere SP, Weindling SN. Brugada syndrome in children—stepping into unchartered territory. Ann Pediatr Cardiol. 2017;10(3):248-58.
16. Obeyesekere MN, Klein GJ, Modi S, Leong-Sit P, Gula LJ, Yee R, et al. How to perform and interpret provocative testing for the diagnosis of Brugada syndrome, long-QT syndrome, and catecholaminergic polymorphic ventricular tachycardia. Circ Arrhythm Electrophysiol. 2011;4(6):958-64.
17. Sturm AC. Cardiovascular cascade genetic testing: exploring the role of direct contact and technology. Front Cardiovasc Med. 2016;3:11.
18. Chockalingam P, Crotti L, Girardengo G, Johnson JN, Harris KM, van der Heijden JF, et al. Not all beta-blockers are equal in the management of long QT syndrome types 1 and 2: higher recurrence of events under metoprolol. J Am Coll Cardiol. 2012;60(20):2092-9.
19. Mazzanti A, Maragna R, Faragli A, Monteforte N, Bloise R, Memmi M, et al. Gene-specific therapy with mexiletine reduces arrhythmic events in patients with long QT syndrome type 3. J Am Coll Cardiol. 2016;67(9):1053-8.
20. Crotti L, Spazzolini C, Tester DJ, Ghidoni A, Baruteau AE, Beckmann BM, et al. Calmodulin mutations and life-threatening cardiac arrhythmias: insights from the International Calmodulinopathy Registry. Eur Heart J. 2019; 40(35):2964-75.
21. Fleming S, Thompson M, Stevens R, Heneghan C, Pluddemann A, Maconochie I, et al. Normal ranges of heart rate and respiratory rate in children from birth to 18 years of age: a systematic review of observational studies. Lancet. 2011;377(9770):1011-8.
22. Baruteau AE, Perry JC, Sanatani S, Horie M, Dubin AM. Evaluation and management of bradycardia in neonates and children. Eur J Pediatr. 2016;175(2):151-61.
23. Fromell GJ, Root J, Barish R. The Wenckebach phenomenon. J Emerg Med. 1986;4(2):115-8.
24. Friedman D, Duncanson L, Glickstein J, Buyon J. A review of congenital heart block. Images Paediatr Cardiol. 2003;5(3):36-48.
25. Krishna MR. Kearns Sayre Syndrome: looking beyond A-V conduction. Indian Pacing Electrophysiol J. 2017;17(3):78-80.
26. Varghese MJ, Ramakrishnan S, Kothari SS, Parashar A, Juneja R, Saxena A. Complete heart block due to diphtheritic myocarditis in the present era. Ann Pediatr Cardiol. 2013;6(1):34-8.
27. Melles RB, Katz B. Night terrors and sudden unexplained nocturnal death. Med Hypotheses. 1988;26(2):149-54.
28. Epstein AE, DiMarco JP, Ellenbogen KA, Estes NA 3rd, Freedman RA, Gettes LS, et al. 2012 ACCF/AHA/HRS focused update incorporated into the ACCF/AHA/HRS 2008 guidelines for device-based therapy of cardiac rhythm abnormalities: a report of the American College of Cardiology Foundation/American Heart Association Task Force on Practice Guidelines and the Heart Rhythm Society. J Am Coll Cardiol. 2013;61(3):e6-75.

53
CHAPTER

Common Problems in Office Practice

Snehal Kulkarni, Tanuja Karande, Prashant Bobhate

INTRODUCTION

This chapter focuses on common situation that leads to a referral of children to a pediatric cardiology clinic. These conditions constitute the majority of outpatient practice. **Box 1** lists the conditions that constitute common reasons for referral of children to pediatric cardiology. Many of the conditions listed here are also discussed elsewhere in the book. In this chapter, we seek to provide a framework for addressing the common listed conditions.

THE CHILD WITH A MURMUR

Heart murmurs are common in healthy infants, children, and adolescents.[1] Most of them may not be pathologic, but murmur may be the sole manifestation of serious heart disease.[2] At the same time, murmur is mistakenly considered synonymous with heart disease also. It is very important to know that many significant heart diseases can present without murmur (especially true for neonates), and patients with significant murmurs can have minor heart defects or even no cardiac defects.[3] Clinically murmurs can raise the suspicion of heart defect. Isolated murmurs need to be evaluated carefully for clinical decision-making. Additional details on evaluation of heart murmurs are described in Chapter 5.

Examples of significant heart defects without murmur include the following conditions that are typically manifest in neonates or young infants include transposition of great arteries, pulmonary atresia with intact interventricular septum or associated with VSD and obstructed total anomalous pulmonary venous connections.

Similarly, there are examples of relatively benign heart defects with loud murmurs and they include restrictive ventricular septal defect or patent ductus arteriosus (PDA) and mild pulmonary stenosis.

It is quite common for a child to have a heart murmur at some point in their lives[4-6] and this is a very common reason for referral. The presence of a murmur could point to the presence of a significant heart disease. However, most children referred specifically for evaluation of a murmur usually have a relatively minor condition or no heart disease whatsoever.

Murmurs are considered "organic" when there is an underlying structural defect such as a valve obstruction or leak or a heart defect. They are labeled as functional when they occur as a result of excessive flow across the normal valves. While the vast majority of children are completely well and normal, some of these children may have a physiological basis such as anemia, fever, or thyrotoxicosis.

It is essential to recognize that the way the stethoscope is used impacts auscultation. The bell of the stethoscope enables listening to low frequency sounds while the diaphragm when pressed firmly selectively transmits the high frequency sounds. Apical mid-diastolic murmurs that are associated with large left-to-right shunts are best heard with the bell while high frequency murmurs of aortic regurgitation are best heard with the diaphragm firmly pressed.

Chapter 5 has an extensive description on cardiac murmurs. This section will focus on distinguishing between organic and functional murmurs.

BOX 1: Common reasons for referring a patient to pediatric cardiology outpatient clinic.

Condition

- Approach to a child with murmur (*see* Chapter 5 as well)
- Chest pain in a child
- Certification of fitness for sports
- Adolescent with heart disease
- Immunization of children with heart disease
- Follow-up after CHD surgery and intervention
- Cardiac assessment prior to anesthesia for noncardiac surgery
- Syncope (*see* Chapter 19)
- Cardiac involvement in other systems (*see* Chapter 55)
- Cardiac assessment in genetic conditions (*see* Chapter 54)

(CHD: congenital heart disease)

Functional Murmurs

They are very common in children especially in neonates.[7] The decision whether the murmur is organic and functional, does not just depend upon the location or intensity.

The decision should depend upon overall assessment of cardiovascular system. The most common reason for functional murmur in a child is a "hyperkinetic circulation".

The classic description of a still's murmur is that of a sound in the left second interspace that has characteristic vibratory nature. This is typically a mid-systolic murmur that tends to be louder during febrile illnesses. Often the murmur is identified by pediatricians during a fever and referred to the cardiologist for an evaluation. By the time the child is seen by the cardiologist, fever often subsides and so does the murmur.

Venous hum is a continuous murmur which originates in the jugular venous system where the diastolic component is louder than the systolic one. It is commonly audible in children between 3 and 6 years of age below infra- or supraclavicular area. It is only heard in sitting position as gravity exerts a stronger effect by pulling the blood toward the heart and is better heard after slight angulation of the neck. It is important to differentiate murmur of venous hum from the continuous murmur of PDA which is louder in systole and is best heard in the left 2nd intercostal space.

Common causes of benign murmurs in the newborns include the following:

- *Physiologic peripheral pulmonary stenosis*: This is particularly common in preterm neonate and results from flow acceleration in the proximal branch pulmonary arteries.
- *Small ventricular septal defects*: Small defects in the muscular septum are particularly common in neonates and they often close in a few months result in characteristically short- and high-pitched murmurs. Tricuspid regurgitation and PDA may also transiently result in a murmur.

It is very important to differentiate organic from functional murmurs. All diastolic murmurs are have an organic basis. Cardinal clinical signs of pathologic systolic murmurs include long and holosystolic murmurs, murmurs that are grade III or more, associated systolic clicks and abnormal second heart sound.[8]

The threshold for obtaining an echocardiogram for murmurs is considerably lowered these days because of the fear of missing a serious defect. However, in situations where echocardiogram is not easily obtained, children with suspected pathologic murmurs or those with associated cardiovascular symptoms, heart failure, cyanosis, and associated dysmorphic features should be evaluated further.[8,9]

CHEST PAIN IN CHILDREN

Chest pain is a relatively common presenting symptom in children that causes a great deal of anxiety in parents and healthcare professionals. A cardiac cause for chest pain is identifiable in a minority of children, in contrast to chest pain in adults with risk factors for coronary artery disease.

It is also important to recognize that children may label other symptoms as chest pain when they describe them. For example, children express that they have chest discomfort during episodes of tachyarrhythmia.

The initial evaluation should focus on exclusion of serious underlying cardiac pathologies and appropriate reassurance while acknowledging the fear that the parents have. Chest pain can be broadly classified into noncardiac and cardiac causes.

The purpose of history and physical examination should be to identfiy cardiac causes producing chest pain. Some of these conditions require urgent attention. These conditions are exceptionally rare.

The pointers to a possible cardiac basis include:

- Exertional retrosternal chest pain that is diffuse in nature, not limited to a specific location.
- Past history of Kawasaki disease, cardiac surgery sickle cell disease, hypercholesterolemia, and drug abuse (cocaine).
- *Association with other cardiac symptoms*: Palpitations, syncope or presyncope, breathlessness or in association with a positive family history of sudden death.
- Retrosternal and precordial pain associated with fever.

A comprehensive list of causes of chest pain is give in **Table 1**.

TABLE 1: Common causes of chest pain.

Category	*List of causes*
Chest wall (64%)	· Trauma · Costochondritis · Precordial muscle catch · Slipping rib · Infection · Mastalgia
Gastroesophageal (4%)	· Reflux · Foreign body · Gastritis
Pulmonary (13%)	· Asthma · Pneumonia · Pneumothorax · Pleuritis · Pulmonary embolus · Malignancy
Hematologic (<1%)	· Sickle cell disease · Thalassemia
Psychological (9%)	
Cardiac (5%)	· Angina · Congenital coronary abnormalities · Premature atherosclerosis · Post-Kawasaki disease · Hypercoagulable state · Cocaine · Outflow tract obstructions · Aortic regurgitation · Pericarditis · Arrhythmias · Myocarditis · Aortic dissection · Pulmonary hypertension · Pulmonary embolism

Source: Percentage distribution of causes from reference: Massin MM, Bourguignont A, Coremans C, Comté L, Lepage P, Gérard P. Chest pain in pediatric patients presenting to an emergency department or to a cardiac clinic. Clin Pediatr (Phila). 2004;43:231-8.

Apart from taking a careful history, it is essential to perform a complete general physical examination and cardiovascular examination. Dysmorphic features of Marfan syndrome or, Turner syndrome can lower the threshold for consideration of aortic dissection. Presence of xanthomas on extensors substantially increases the likelihood of atherosclerotic coronary artery disease as a cause of chest pain.

If concern about serious ethology is raised by history of physical examination or if pain is severe and disruptive to daily activities, further investigation is warranted. However, it is essential to note that the yield of these tests is low unless, there is a strong underlying reason to suspect a cardiac basis. The tests should be specifically targeted at the possible causes rather than just ordering them as a matter of "routine". The tests should look to refine the list of causes and arrive at an exact diagnosis. The electrocardiogram (ECG) and chest X-ray are considered as integral to initial cardiac evaluation. They must be obtained in all instances. Echocardiography has the advantage of being noninvasive, easily available, and low cost. However, it should be carefully targeted to rule out very specific causes. Structural heart diseases and cardiomyopathy are easily identified by echocardiography. It is relatively more challenging to be certain about the less common cardiac causes of chest pain. The list of these conditions include coronary abnormalities such as abnormal origin of coronary artery and post-Kawasaki coronary occlusion. Congenital coronary artery anomalies though rare (prevalence 0.21–5.79%) are potentially significant because of their association with myocardial ischemia and presentation of sudden death.[10]

Routine use of exercise testing for evaluation of chest pain in children and adolescents is not recommended. Exercise testing is appropriate for evaluation of the child having typical anginal chest pain which is consistently related to exercise, to uncover underlying ischemia, wherein no attributable causes are found on echocardiography.[11] Sometimes, however, it is useful to do the exercise test to reassure the family about the benign nature of the chest pain.

Computed tomography (CT) angiography forms the third line of investigation in evaluating a child with chest pain and is usually advised when cardiac or thoracic abnormality is suspected but not well delineated with other noninvasive diagnostic modes. It allows clear anatomical details of coronary abnormalities and is particularly useful to rule out aortic dissection and pulmonary thromboembolism.

CERTIFICATION FOR FITNESS FOR SPORTS: CARDIAC PERSPECTIVE

The overall rate of sudden death in athletes younger than 35 years is approximately 0.75 per 100,000 participants per year.[12] Congenital cardiac anomalies especially coronary anomalies and hypertrophic cardiomyopathy account for most sudden deaths in these patients.

The following outline can be used as a guideline by a pediatrician in his office practice while screening the general population.

The goal is to identify conditions that may put the athlete at higher risk of disability or life-threatening event. Considering that most of the fatalities in young athletes during sports participation occur as a consequence of cardiac pathology, it is important to identify the individuals at risk.

Children with known congenital heart defects, Marfan syndrome, hypertrophic cardiomyopathy, pulmonary and systemic hypertension, mitral valve propose, history of arrhythmogenic events, and family history of premature death require detailed cardiac evaluation and should be referred to a pediatric cardiologist for certification.

Particular attention should be given to the personal and family cardiac histories. Following questionnaire can be used as a checklist (**Box 2**). No scoring system is available based on screening history; however if answer to any of the below is "yes," it requires a cardiologists referral for ruling out serious underlying disorders (**Box 2**).

A thorough physical examination is mandatory. The general examination should include screening for physical stigmata of Marfan syndrome, measurement of height, arm-span, eye examination, and general evaluation of the skeletal system. Blood pressure (BP): Children with systolic or diastolic BP >90th percentile for height and age require further evaluation prior to fitness. Lower limb pulsations must be felt and lower limb BP should be recorded when there is concern about coarctation.

A careful cardiac examination is needed. Most patients with hypertrophic cardiomyopathy have a normal cardiac examination. A normal examination does not eliminate the chance of their being a substrate for sudden cardiac death.

The ECG enables identification of specific high-risk subsets. However, like physical examination, its specificity

BOX 2: Screening for participation in sports

- Do you cough, wheeze, or have difficulty breathing during or after exercise?
- Have you ever had discomfort, pain, tightness, or pressure in your chest during exercise?
- Do you get light-headed or feel shortness of breath sooner than your friends during exercise?
- Have you ever passed out or nearly passed out during or after exercise?
- Does your heart ever race, or skip beats (irregular beats) during exercise?
- Has a doctor ever told you that you have any heart problems?
- Has a doctor ever requested a test for your heart? For example, electrocardiography (ECG) or echocardiography.
- Has any family member or relative died of heart problems or had an unexpected or unexplained sudden death before the age of 35 years (including drowning or unexplained car crash)?
- Has anyone in your family had a pacemaker or an implanted defibrillator before the age of 35 years?
- Are you on any stimulants or performance-enhancing medications?

TABLE 2: Classification of sports based on contact.

Contact sports	*Limited contact*	*Non-contact*
· Basket ball	· Adventure racing	· Badminton
· Boxing	· Bicycling	· Body building
· Hockey	· Canoeing	· Bowling
· Football	· Fencing	· Canoeing
· Gymnastics	· High jump	· Kayaking
· Cricket	· Horseback riding	· Rowing
· Martial arts	· Pole vault	· Dance
· Water polo	· Racquet ball	· Golf
· Wrestling	· Ice skating	· Riflery
· Rugby	· Roller skating	· Rope jumping
· Race car driving	· Skiing	· Running
	· Squash	· Sailing
· Diving	· Volleyball	· Table tennis
· Lacrosse	· Weightlifting	· Tracks
· Rodeo	· Windsurfing	

is poor. Rare electrical disorders such as long QT syndrome, Wolff–Parkinson–White syndrome, catecholaminergic polymorphic ventricular tachycardia, Brugada syndrome, and short QT syndrome can potentially be identified on ECG. Presence of ST segment T wave abnormalities on resting ECG may give a clue toward hypertrophic cardiomyopathy. If a pediatric cardiologist suspects coronary anomalies, an exercise test may be prescribed to uncover underlying ischemia.

Currently there are no recommendations on the need for echocardiography prior to sports fitness, and the same can be reserved in case of any abnormality detected in history, physical examination, or ECG.[13]

During risk stratification of a particular athlete, one must consider the athlete's risk for harm, factoring in the type of sport he or she is playing, and the amount of contact or impact the athlete is likely to receive. Various classifications of different types of sports are available, based on intensity and level of bodily collision (**Table 2**). Those associated with higher incidence of impact have been known for higher risk of syncope and sudden death. Decisions have to be individualized taking into account the perceived risk status, expected level of physical activity, preferences of the affected individual and risk to others.

Once the history and examination parts are completed, one of the following decisions may be taken:

- Permitted all activities without restriction
- Permitted with recommendations for further evaluation or treatment
- Not permitted, or status to be reconsidered after further evaluation
- Not permitted for certain types of sports (contact) or for any sports.

The American College of Cardiology/American Heart Association (ACC/AHA) has published guidelines at the 36th Bethesda conference with regards to eligibility on the physical intensity of the sport and recommendations for competitive sport provide additional details for the interested reader.[13]

ADOLESCENT WITH HEART DISEASE

With the advances of practices in cardiology, many children born with congenital heart defects are expected to live up to adulthood with the expectation of living a near normal life. During the transition from childhood to adolescent period, these patients need to know their disease in relation to the health status, restriction for their physical activities, and future goals as well.[14-16] In addition, parents also need to be counseled regarding the need to take their children into confidence by sharing the magnitude of underlying heart disease. It is important to maintain a comprehensive cardiac record and share it with the family. It should include the details of cardiac problem, the intervention performed, stratification of the risk and complexity, and the specific issues that place the child at increased risk. The record also should mention possible future need for medical, transcatheter, or surgical intervention.

Adolescents who present with heart diseases can be categorized under following headings:

- *Simple heart defects*: Usually these are the types of heart defects, which might have been diagnosed in the childhood and are being followed over years or these are diagnosed first time during adolescent period. There are typically small atrial septal defects (ASDs), small ventricular septal defects (VSDs), mild pulmonary or aortic stenosis. Very rarely patients with mild cyanosis may present with underlying diagnosis of tetralogy of Fallot or univentricular heart lesions. They are exceptions and natural survivors.
- *Operated heart defects with no residual issues*: Some of the congenital heart defect which are diagnosed early in neonatal or infant life and corrected early may be completely repaired hearts. They need infrequent follow-ups after surgery and can be expected to lead a near normal life. Examples include closure of patent arterial duct, atrial and ventricular septal defects in infancy or early childhood.
- *Operated heart defects with residual issues*: This is the large subgroup of patients who are repaired in neonatal life or early infancy, but they need periodic follow-ups throughout their life. Examples include repair for tetralogy of Fallot, arterial switch repairs for transposition of great arteries, repair of atrioventricular septal defects, staged palliation of univentricular hearts, and repair involving the use of conduits.
- *Unoperated defects*: In India, unfortunately, a large number of adolescents with congenital heart disease (CHD) are survivors selected by natural history. These are patients with serious defects that were not corrected in infancy. Even today only a small minority of infants receive timely surgery. While many do not survive, some survive to reach adolescence and adulthood with significant residual issues that include activity

limitations, growth and developmental delay, hypoxia and cyanosis, learning disabilities, and heart failure. Examples include Eisenmenger syndrome resulting from development of pulmonary hypertension (PAH) in shunt lesions, unoperated tetralogy of Fallot, or partially palliated heart disease in whom corrective surgery has not been undertaken.

- *Acquired heart defects*: A number of acquired conditions such as rheumatic heart disease, idiopathic PAH, myocarditis, and aortoarteritis can present during adolescence.

Children with heart disease, either operated or unoperated, may face important medical problems. They require lifelong care and consultation with cardiologist for medical management. Following is the list of major cardiac issues that will need to be addressed on follow-up.

- *Heart failure*: Right heart failure is much more common especially with operated patients with tetralogy of Fallot. Left ventricular failure may be seen in few patients with aortic arch obstruction or after surgical repair of anomalous origin of left pulmonary artery from pulmonary artery or some univentricular heart repairs with significant atrioventricular valve regurgitation.
- *Persistent PAH*: Many patients with simple heart defects such as VSD or large PDA present late during life and they already have severe pulmonary artery hypertension with significantly elevated pulmonary vascular resistance. Even after surgical closures of the defect, they have elevated pulmonary artery pressures and vascular resistance. They may need treatment with pulmonary vasodilators and continued follow-up for long period of time.
- *Arrhythmias*: Many operated patients for complex univentricular hearts, develop arrhythmias on long-term follow-up. They need to be monitored and treated accordingly. Some of these children may need electrophysiology testing with radiofrequency ablation.
- Persistent cyanosis: In [illegible] hypoxia, and cyanosis will require to be managed carefully for the effects of erythrocytosis.
- *Pacemakers*: Few operated patients for heart defects or some patients with congenital complete heart blocks may have pacemakers and they have to be told to live with the pacemaker throughout their life. They need frequent pacemaker interrogation and change of the pacemaker battery every 8–10 years.

Some underlying issues may interfere with regular medical management. They are as follows:

- *Prophylaxis for infective endocarditis*: Recent guidelines by American College of Cardiology for prophylaxis for infective endocarditis need to be followed especially when there are residual cardiac problems.[17] Emphasis need to be given to have good dental hygiene and periodic visits to dental specialist.
- *Anticoagulation*: Patients who have metallic prosthesis for valve replacement or have undergone complex surgical procedures for univentricular repairs, may be on oral anticoagulation and their international normalized ratio (INR) need to be monitored periodically as per recommendations. Usually these patients are given a diet chart to be followed and a list of medications to be avoided while they are taking oral anticoagulants.
- *Imaging*: As these children get older, their echocardiographic windows become limited, and they may need other imaging techniques such as CT of magnetic resonance imaging (MRI) for better imaging. In addition guidelines for MRI imaging should be followed while imaging patients with prosthetic metallic valves or pacemakers.
- *Noncardiac surgeries*: Patients with defects with repaired/unrepaired heart defects may have increased risk for cardiac events. Preferably the surgeries should be planned in a tertiary care center. There needs to be careful planning of the procedure in consultation with primary cardiologist, anesthesiologist, and surgeon. The goal should be to identify the risk factors and try to modify them if possible.[18,19] These issues regarding antibiotics prophylaxis, anticoagulation monitoring, and arrhythmias need to be monitored strictly while planning noncardiac surgery.
- *Associated genetic defects*: Genetic evaluation for associated noncardiac defects or long-term prognosis may be required in select cases. This can be done with cytogenetic or molecular testing if required. It may be required regarding reproductive counseling.
- *Penicillin prophylaxis for rheumatic heart disease*: Patients with diagnosis of rheumatic valvular heart defects need to be on regular penicillin prophylaxis with injectable Benzathine penicillin every 3 weekly. The duration of prophylaxis needs to be decided by the treating cardiologist which recent guidelines (*see* Chapter [illegible]).[20]
- *Hematological abnormalities*: Many unrepaired cyanotic patients and patients with residual intracardiac shunts will have some degree of cyanosis. These patients with persistent cyanosis have hematological abnormalities and abnormal platelet functions. They need to be monitored periodically and they may have additional risk for undergoing noncardiac surgery.[21]

Adolescents with heart defects may face many noncardiac issues in daily life. They need to be addressed in consultation with the primary pediatrician, cardiologist, family members, and the patients themselves. The following are some important noncardiac issues which need to be addressed:

- *Career counseling*: Career and education issues should be discussed during early adolescence which depends upon their mental, physical, and social abilities. They need complete cardiac assessment prior to choosing carrier for fitness. This again will depend upon residual heart defects or underlying medical issues.

- *Contraception*: Barrier contraception, though relatively safe for these groups of patients, has a high failure rate. Contraception should be in consultation with a gynecologist and carefully individualized to each patient after taking into account their preferences, the underlying disease, and level of education.[22,23]
- *Pregnancy*: Pregnancy is considered high risk from psychological, medical, and sociological perspectives.[24,25] A carefully planned discussion on the potential risks of pregnancy should be arranged with a suitable councilor if possible for those who are at particular risk. They should also be counseled regarding the possible teratogenic effects of the medications.
- *Exercise and physical rehabilitation*: Exercise is an important component of maintenance of good health. Though exercise tolerance may not be normal for many patients, they may be able to perform some level of regular exercise.[26] Exercise capacity should be assessed by regular exercise testing, cardiopulmonary exercise testing, or 6-minute walk test. Many simple exercises such as walking, swimming, or cycling can be encouraged. But a word of caution—all patients need to be assessed individually. Patients with heart rhythm devices, dilated ascending aorta, heart failure, PAH, and coronary artery abnormalities need special attention. Guidelines on participation in sports are addressed previously in this chapter.
- *Insurance*: Patients with congenital heart defects either repaired or unrepaired may face problems for getting insurance cover for noncardiac procedures. Though some of the organizations are working for getting these patients insured, there are no clear guidelines at present.
- *Psychosocial aspects*: Many patients can have developmental delays, cognitive impairments, and learning difficulties. They lack the ability to manage their health care independently. They may need help from specialists from developmental pediatrics and their primary care pediatrician.
- *Disability guidelines*: Some of children with cardiac defect—either operated or unoperated may be eligible for disability benefits. A certificate can be issued after careful assessment of their status to help them cope with their challenges at work as well as to avail of specific benefits for which they may be eligible.

IMMUNIZATION IN CHILDREN WITH HEART DISEASE

Routine immunization is essential for prevention of several serious infections in children. Improvement in public health services has resulted in significant improvement in vaccine coverage both in urban and rural India.[27,28] Routine immunization and catch-up immunization schedule provided by the Indian Academy of Pediatrics and the World Health Organization should be followed for all patients with CHD.[29] In this section, we will discuss special issues related to CHD and immunization.

Congenital heart disease, the most common congenital malformation, poses increased risk to develop infections secondary to increase in the pulmonary blood flow and pressure as well as increased incidence of immunocompromised states such as DiGeorge syndrome and asplenia.[30] Children with CHD are more likely to miss routine vaccination schedule secondary to surgery as well as repeated hospital admissions and catch-up immunization might be required.

Prevention of Respiratory Illness and Influenza

Children with CHD, especially those with post-tricuspid shunts, are prone for increased respiratory tract infections secondary to increased pulmonary blood flow. Yearly global mortality due to acute respiratory illness in children <5 years of age is estimated at 28,000–150,000 and majority of these are secondary to vaccine-preventable diseases.[31]

Education of families regarding good hand hygiene and avoiding crowds reduces exposure. Nevertheless it is imperative to administer vaccine to prevent seasonal influenza as well as *Pneumococcus* and *Haemophilus influenzae* in children <5 years of age. Presence of certain comorbid factors such as PAH, systemic ventricular dysfunction, and single ventricular physiology would warrant for immunizations with the above vaccines even in older children.

Children with Reduced Immunocompetence

Of particular interest while discussing immunization in children with CHD is presence of DiGeorge syndrome and asplenia (functional or anatomical). In children with DiGeorge syndrome, an additional immunological consult and lymphocyte study might be warranted. Recent studies have demonstrated that live vaccines can be safely administered to patients with DiGeorge syndrome and mild-to-moderate immunosuppression.[32,33] Asplenia predisposes a patient to increased risk of infection by encapsulated organisms such as *Neisseria meningitides* and *Streptococcus pneumoniae*. Patients with asplenia have 200-fold greater risk of mortality than in patients with functional spleen.[34,35] Apart from antibiotic prophylaxis, children with asplenia should receive vaccine against *Pneumococcus, H. influenzae,* and *Meningococcus*. In susceptible children, it is recommended to administer 13-valent pneumococcal vaccine (PCV13) in between 2 and 59 months and an additional dose in between 60 and 71 months. Immunization against meningococcus with quadrivalent meningococcal vaccine (MCV4) is recommended between 2 and 10 years with an additional dose every 5 years.[36]

Children Receiving High-dose Intravenous Immunoglobulin (IVIg)

Patients with Kawasaki disease and some with myocarditis are administered high-dose intravenous immunoglobulin (IVIg) (2 g/kg) during acute phase of the disease. Live vaccines against measles, mumps, rubella, and varicella should be avoided for 11 months post-IVIg administration. In children with high endemicity or postexposure to a contact with measles, the vaccine may be administered earlier and a repeat vaccine should be given at least 11 months post-IVIg if the serological response is inadequate.[37]

Children on Low-dose Aspirin and Anticoagulation

Postcardiac surgery, some children might receive low-dose aspirin or anticoagulation such as warfarin. Children with systemic-to-pulmonary artery shunt [Blalock–Taussig (BT) shunt or PDA stent] or placement of a biological valve or conduit are given low-dose aspirin.[38] There is a concern of developing Reye syndrome in children administered aspirin following natural varicella infection or vaccine. However, the risk of developing Reye syndrome is significant in patients who are administered aspirin in anti-inflammatory doses and not with the ones on antiplatelet doses (low dose, 3–5 mg/kg).[39,40] Hence, children with heart disease should receive varicella vaccine at appropriate age and low-dose aspirin should be continued.

Immunization around Time of Surgery

Although, recent or upcoming surgeries are not a contraindication for immunization, routine immunization should preferably be avoided 1 week prior and until 4–6 weeks after a cardiac surgery. Exposure to cardiopulmonary bypass impairs the ability of children to mount an immune response.[41] Children also receive blood and blood products during the surgery hence it is recommended to avoid live vaccines such as measles, mumps, and rubella (MMR) and varicella for 3–6 months postcardiac surgery.[42]

Risk Stratification of Patients with Congenital Heart Disease and Monitoring Postvaccination

Some children with CHD before or after surgery are at increased risk of deterioration after immunization. It is important to identify and closely monitor these children to prevent life-threatening adverse events postvaccination. **Box 3** enlists the patients in high-risk category. Such patients should preferably be admitted for 24 hours postvaccination under cardiac monitoring (SpO_2, BP, and heart rate). Cyanotic children should be well hydrated before and after vaccination. Should the child develop hypotension postvaccination due to fever or vasodilatation, this should be managed with intravenous fluids and inotropes as deemed appropriate.

FOLLOW-UP AFTER CONGENITAL HEART DEFECT SURGERY AND INTERVENTION

With a birth prevalence of CHD of 8–9/1,000, the estimated number of children born with CHD in India is >200,000 per year.[43]

Advances in treatment and palliation of CHD have resulted in more patients being treated and discharged to be taken care of by their primary care providers (general pediatricians and internists). Primary care providers are

BOX 3: Risk stratification of children with congenital heart disease.

High-risk group:
- Uncorrected cyanotic congenital heart disease
  - [illegible]
  - Pulmonary atresia
  - Univentricular heart with pulmonary stenosis
  - Any other condition with significant cyanosis (SpO_2 <85%)
- Significant ventricular dysfunction (ejection fraction <40%): Children with dilated cardiomyopathy and ventricular dysfunction postcardiac surgery
- Moderate-to-severe atrioventricular valve regurgitation
- Significant ventricular outflow tract obstruction (peak gradient of > 60 mm Hg across right or left ventricular outflow tract)
- Moderate-to-severe pulmonary hypertension
- *Palliative procedures*: Blalock–Taussig shunt, pulmonary artery band, Norwood procedure, etc.
- Unrepaired defects with hemodynamically significant left-to-right shunt (large ventricular septal defect and patent arterial duct)
- Children with persistent or incessant arrhythmia

Moderate-risk group:
- Presence of postoperative residual lesions, e.g., severe pulmonary regurgitation, peak outflow tract gradient of 40–60 mm Hg
- Use of prosthetic valve/conduit
- Patients with single ventricular physiology status post-Glenn shunt or Fontan completion
- Children on anticoagulation/antiplatelet medications
- Children on antihypertensive or antiarrhythmic medications

Low-risk group:
- Completely repaired congenital heart disease with no/hemodynamically insignificant residual lesions
- Unrepaired CHD which are hemodynamically insignificant such as small left-to-right shunts, insignificant valve stenoses

being tasked with providing multiple health care needs of these children. A brief guide to managing postoperative and postinterventional patients in office practice is presented here:

- An early follow-up visit around 1 month postdischarge following a cardiac surgery is generally recommended. In some instances, earlier visits are recommended if there are special concerns.
  - *Wound care*: Usually all wounds are covered by a loose dry dressing, which can be removed after 14 days from surgery. No lotions or powder applications are needed. If there are any signs of inflammation or discharge, it would be best to get in touch with the surgical team and refer patient to the center where surgery was performed for further management to rule out underlying surgical wound infection and mediastinitis. Delayed surgical wound infections although relatively rare are well described and they require prompt and aggressive attention. Clues to a potentially serious major surgical wound infection with our without mediastinitis include, incessant crying in, extreme irritability, and fever. The surgical site may only show subtle features in the form of redness and tenderness. Discharge from the scar may not always be seen.
  - *Immunizations*: This is described above in the section on immunization. All live vaccines should be avoided for 4–6 weeks from the date of surgery. This does not hold true for cardiac catheterizations and interventions, for which immunization can be resumed immediately. All optional vaccines such as influenza and pneumococcal should be included in the schedule in all cardiac patients.
  - *Activities*: No restrictions required for infants and toddlers. Parents should be instructed to avoid picking up the child under the arms for first 2 weeks. For school-aged children, activity is restricted for 4–8 weeks to allow sternum to heal completely. It is important during this time to avoid jarring activities, twisting movements, jumping or using a single arm to strain, push or pull and lifting heavy weights (including backpacks).
  - *Cardiac*: It is essential to look for signs of cardiac failure such as tachypnea, tachycardia, facial or generalized edema. The saturations need to be interpreted in the context of the original operation. Some cyanosis will remain after palliative operations such as the Glenn Shunt or the BT shunt. Saturations that are much lower than the immediate predischarge saturations definitely merit concern and must be communicated to the team that performed the operation. Rhythm disturbances may be seen uncommonly during this period. Unexplained bradycardia or tachycardia warrants a 12-lead ECG to rule out late occurrence of complete heart block or tachyarrhythmia, respectively. A persistent murmur should not necessarily be a source of concern after a heart operation. Murmurs are always heard after palliative operations such as the BT shunt or pulmonary artery band. They are also common after certain corrective operations such as repair of tetralogy of Fallot or after a conduit repair of pulmonary atresia.
  - *Need to report early*: Parents should be instructed to follow early if fever (temperature over 100.5°F), increased tiredness, new onset of dry cough, change in appearance of incision or cloudy yellow drainage, increased pain, vomiting, diarrhea, or irritability.
  - *Medications*: Most corrective cardiac operations do not require cardiac medications on discharge. Occasionally diuretics are necessary. This is especially true for operations such as repair of tetralogy of Fallot with a transannular patch. It is essential to review the need for these medications on the first visit after discharge. If the patient has no residual lesions and no features of heart failure, cardiac medications such as diuretics, digoxin, angiotensin-converting enzyme (ACE) inhibitors can all be withdrawn. There are specific recommendations for antiplatelet and anticoagulant medications that need to continue as per standard recommendations. For majority of the patients, there are no dietary restrictions. Patients receiving warfarin are instructed to limit foods high in vitamin K such as green leafy vegetables. Target INR levels required are specific to each type of surgery and type of prosthetic material used. For example, metallic valve in mitral position would require INR levels between 2.5 and 3.5. It is imperative that these specifics are mentioned in the discharge summary. Drugs interfering with warfarin metabolism and its action tend to alter the INR levels. Concomitant use of drugs given in **Box 4** should be avoided.
- *Late follow-up*: (beyond 1 month postdischarge)
  - *Growth*: Children who have undergone complete repair of their cardiac lesion such as shunt closures (ASD, VSD, and PDA) or intracardiac repairs for tetralogy of Fallot should usually demonstrate good weight gain with improvement in appetite and activity comparable to their peers. Those with uncorrected lesions or staged repairs or children with syndromes may continue to remain below the standard growth curve. Early weaning and nutritional supplements may be required to meet the extracaloric demands. It is vital to carefully monitor growth, weight gain, and dietary intake during each visit. Suboptimal growth needs to be investigated.
  - *Neurodevelopmental milestones*: Children with CHD are at increased risk of neurodevelopmental disorders and learning disabilities and psychosocial limitations.

BOX 4: Drugs that interfere with the action of warfarin and INR levels.

- Acetaminophen
- Alcohol (binge)
- Amiodarone
- Aspirin
- Azithromycin
- Carbamazepine
- Chloral hydrate
- Ciprofloxacin
- Clarithromycin
- Diltiazem
- Disopyramide
- Doxycycline
- Erythromycin
- Fluconazole
- Isoniazid
- Levofloxacin
- Metronidazole
- Norfloxacin
- Propranolol
- Phenobarbital
- Phenytoin
- Rifampicin
- Sucralfate
- Sulfamethoxazole
- Voriconazole

These include cognitive, adaptive, motor, speech, behavioral, and executive functioning deficits, as well as autism spectrum disorder and psychiatric conditions. These patients would require long-term neurodevelopmental follow-up and rehabilitation. The neurodevelopmental status of all children should be monitored after cardiac surgery and early intervention should be recommended for those with abnormalities and for the high-risk groups such as Catch 22 and other chromosomal abnormalities and those with documented seizures in the perioperative phase.

- *Infective endocarditis prophylaxis*: All children undergoing cardiac surgeries involving the use of prosthetic material for correcting heart defects would require infective endocarditis prophylaxis for 6 months. Those with palliative operations such as the BT shunt are at high risk and require prophylaxis as long as the shunt is in place. There have been multiple modifications to the infective endocarditis (IE) prophylaxiswith the latest consensus of antibiotic prophylaxis should be provided to high-risk individuals (*see* Chapter 41).[44]
- *Cardiac*: It is important to stress to the parents regarding the need for regular cardiac follow-up as advised by the primary cardiac center as most children require long-term cardiac monitoring. Fitness for participation in sports would be based on current cardiac status and residual lesions, type of sport and grade of contact sport, and presence of any risk factors. Most of the children with completely corrected lesions can participate in school (leisure) sports. It is important to stress a healthy diet and lifestyle, especially for the adolescent group.

PREOPERATIVE ASSESSMENT FOR NONCARDIAC SURGERIES

Patients with CHD are at increased risk of developing complications during anesthesia.[45] While significant improvement in diagnostic and therapeutic strategies has significantly improved outcomes of patients with CHD, the complexity and heterogenicity of CHD along with various comorbid conditions make it essential to have an individualized approach for each child. For an uneventful anesthesia in these patients, it is important to understand the physiology and recognize the patients who are high-risk for noncardiac surgery.

Risk Stratification

Identification of high-risk patients during preoperative assessment is essential for adequate perioperative management. It is essential to refer high-risk patients to a cardiac facility to mitigate the risk by anticipating and preparing for specific events. Children with unrepaired CHD, those with single ventricular physiology, PAH, ventricular dysfunction, or those who have undergone palliative surgeries are at highest risk of morbidity as well as mortality (*see* **Box 3**). Along with the above, presence of genetic syndromes (Down, DiGeorge, Williams syndrome), presence of comorbid conditions such as airway, lung parenchymal, renal, hepatic, or neurological conditions increases the risk of the impending surgery.

Suggested Approach

Preoperative Clinical Assessment

A comprehensive and thorough preoperative assessment is the most important step to minimize the risk of the upcoming surgery. This should begin with a careful review of all clinical records including past operations, interventions, and other noncardiac surgery, if any. Clinical evaluation should include recording of anthropometric measurements, detailed cardiovascular and respiratory system examination. Signs and symptoms of compromised cardiovascular system include breathing and feeding difficulty, poor weight gain, diaphoresis, and easy fatigue. Increased respiratory rate, chest retraction, nasal flaring, use of accessory muscles of respiration, pedal edema, jugular venous distention, enlarged liver, and rales suggest cardiac failure. Palpation of all peripheral pulses, BP, and saturation measurement from all four limb are a part of detailed cardiovascular examination and should be performed in all patients. Presence of signs and symptoms of low cardiac output, SpO_2 <85% and BP >95% percentile will qualify as a high-risk group and further cardiac evaluation by pediatric cardiologist is necessary. Patients in the high-risk group should ideally be referred to a cardiac facility for management by a multidisciplinary team.

Cardiac Review

Preoperative cardiac assessment is essential in patient of the high-risk group as well as if the last review was >6 months prior to the scheduled surgery in moderate and low risk groups (*see* **Box 3**). Along with clinical examination, cardiac review should include a detailed echocardiogram (unless a recent one is available) and ECG.

Infective Endocarditis Prophylaxis (see Chapter 41)

Infective endocarditis is a rare infection affecting patients with CHD and is associated with high morbidity and mortality. In-hospital and 6-month mortality with IE is approximately 25–30%.[46] In 2007, American Heart Association revised its recommendation for administering IE prophylaxis to patients with high risk for developing IE.[44] Studies assessing the impact of these guidelines have shown conflicting results. Several studies have shown no increase in the annual incidence of IE.[47,48] In contrast, a study from United States (US) nationwide inpatient sample demonstrated a 2.4% increase in the age-adjusted annual incidence of IE.[49] A study from Germany also demonstrated a relative increase of 26% in annual incidence of IE.[50] A recent study by Garg et al. demonstrated an increase in IE in both high- and moderate-risk groups 3 years postchange in guidelines but demonstrated a relative decrease in proportion of streptococcal versus staphylococcal infections thus concluding that the increase in the incidence of IE was not secondary to the change in the guidelines.[51]

From a practical standpoint, it is very essential to stress on oral–dental hygiene among all patients with CHD and this is perhaps the most important preventive measure.

Anticoagulation and Antiplatelet Medications (see Chapter 12)

Patients undergoing palliative procedures such as BT shunt, PDA stent, Glenn shunt or Fontan surgery, and surgeries using biological prosthesis (conduits and bioprosthetic valves) are usually prescribed antiplatelet medications (aspirin and/or clopidogrel). Children with mechanical prosthetic valves or in selected patients with fenestrated Fontan surgery are prescribed vitamin K-dependent anticoagulants (VKA) such as warfarin. Children on these medications who are scheduled for noncardiac surgery are at higher risk for bleeding complications. However, in certain patients (BT shunt, PDA stent, and mechanical prosthesis), the risk of stopping these medications abruptly far outweighs the risk for bleeding during surgery. Such patients should preferably be referred to institutions with cardiac facility for noncardiac surgeries. In children who are on VKA, need to stop them at least 4 days prior and need to be administered unfractionated heparin (UFH) until 4 hours prior to surgery. These patients can then be restarted on UFH 12 hours postsurgery once adequate hemostasis is achieved. VKA can be restarted 24 hours postsurgery. UFH needs to be continued till the desired therapeutic range of VKA is achieved.

Antihypertensive, Antiarrhythmic, Pulmonary Vasodilators and Other Medications (see Chapter 12)

In certain conditions, children with CHD might have been prescribed medications to lower their BP, to control the heart rhythm and to decrease the pulmonary artery pressures. Such patients are usually high risk for any surgery and the medications need to be continued in the perioperative period in consultation with the pediatric cardiac team.

Multidisciplinary Team Approach

Children with high risk CHD or those with moderate-risk CHD and comorbid conditions need to be managed at institutions with a multidisciplinary team. Such multidisciplinary teams should include pediatrician, pediatric cardiologist, pediatric intensivist, pediatric surgeons, and pediatric cardiac anesthesia. In patients with very high risk, for example patients with systemic or suprasystemic PAH and severe ventricular dysfunction, an individualized comprehensive plan for perioperative management helps in mitigating the risk of surgery.

CONCLUSION

This chapter examines some of the common circumstances that lead to referral of a child or an adolescent with heart disease to a pediatric cardiologist and provides an outline to enable their optimal management. There is considerable overlap of the contents of this chapter with the rest of the book and the reader is encouraged to refer to specific sections if and when additional information is desired.

REFERENCES

1. Biancaniello T. Innocent murmurs. Circulation. 2005;111(3):e20-2.
2. Bansal M, Jain H. Cardiac murmur in neonates. Indian Pediatr. 2005;42(4):397-8.
3. Frommelt MA. Differential diagnosis and approach to a heart murmur in term infants. Pediatr Clin North Am. 2004;51(4):1023-32.
4. Poddar B, Basu S. Approach to a child with a heart murmur. Indian J Pediatr. 2004;71(1):63-6.
5. Advani N, Menahem S, Wilkinson JL. The diagnosis of innocent murmurs in childhood. Cardiol Young. 2000;10(4):340-2.
6. Pelech AN. Evaluation of the pediatric patient with a cardiac murmur. Pediatr Clin North Am. 1999;46(2):167-88.
7. McCrindle BW, Shaffer KM, Kan JS, Zahka KG, Rowe SA, Kidd L. Cardinal clinical signs in the differentiation of heart murmurs in children. Arch Pediatr Adolesc Med. 1996;150(2):169-74.

8. McConnell ME, Adkins SB, 3rd, Hannon DW. Heart murmurs in pediatric patients: when do you refer? Am Fam Physician. 1999; 60(2):558-65.
9. Yi MS, Kimball TR, Tsevat J, Mrus JM, Kotagal UR. Evaluation of heart murmurs in children: cost-effectiveness and practical implications. J Pediatr. 2002;141(4):504-11.
10. Pérez-Pomares JM, de la Pompa JL, Franco D, Henderson D, Ho SY, Houyel L, et al. Congenital coronary artery anomalies: a bridge from embryology to anatomy and pathophysiology-a position statement of the development, anatomy, and pathology ESC Working Group. Cardiovasc Res. 2016;109(2):204-16.
11. Gibbons RJ, Balady GJ, Bricker JT, Chaitman BR, Fletcher GF, Froelicher VF, et al. ACC/AHA 2002 guideline update for exercise testing: summary article: a report of the American College of Cardiology/American Heart Association Task Force on Practice Guidelines (Committee to Update the 1997 Exercise Testing Guidelines). Circulation. 2002;106(14):1883-92.
12. Van Camp SP, Bloor CM, Mueller FO, Cantu RC, Olson HG. Nontraumatic sports death in high school and college athletes. Med Sci Sports Exerc. 1995;27(5):641-7.
13. Maron BJ, Zipes DP. Introduction: eligibility recommendations for competitive athletes with cardiovascular abnormalities—general considerations. J Am Coll Cardiol. 2005;45(8): 1318-21.
14. Rosen DS, Blum RW, Britto M, Sawyer SM, Siegel DM. Transition to adult health care for adolescents and young adults with chronic conditions: position paper of the Society for Adolescent Medicine. J Adolesc Health. 2003;33(4):309-11.
15. Report of the British Cardiac Society Working Party Grown-up congenital heart (GUCH) disease: current needs and provision of service for adolescents and adults with congenital heart disease in the UK. Heart. 2002;88 Suppl 1(Suppl 1):i1-14.
16. American Academy of Pediatrics; American Academy of Family Physicians; American College of Physicians-American Society of Internal Medicine. A consensus statement on health care transitions for young adults with special health care needs. Pediatrics. 2002;110(6 Pt 2):1304-6.
17. Nishimura RA, Otto CM, Bonow RO, Carabello BA, Erwin JP, 3rd, Fleisher LA, et al. 2017 AHA/ACC Focused Update of the 2014 AHA/ACC guideline for the management of patients with valvular heart disease: a report of the American College of Cardiology/American Heart Association Task Force on Clinical Practice Guidelines. Circulation. 2017;135(25): e1159-e95.
18. Eagle KA, Brundage BH, Chaitman BR, Ewy GA, Fleisher LA, Hertzer NR, et al. Guidelines for perioperative cardiovascular evaluation for noncardiac surgery. Report of the American College of Cardiology/American Heart Association Task Force on Practice Guidelines (Committee on Perioperative Cardiovascular Evaluation for Noncardiac Surgery). J Am Coll Cardiol. 1996;27(4):910-48.
19. Galli KK, Myers LB, Nicolson SC. Anesthesia for adult patients with congenital heart disease undergoing noncardiac surgery. Int Anesthesiol Clin. 2001;39(4):43-71.
20. Gerber MA, Baltimore RS, Eaton CB, Gewitz M, Rowley AH, Shulman ST, et al. Prevention of rheumatic fever and diagnosis and treatment of acute Streptococcal pharyngitis: a scientific statement from the American Heart Association Rheumatic Fever, Endocarditis, and Kawasaki Disease Committee of the Council on Cardiovascular Disease in the Young, the Interdisciplinary Council on Functional Genomics and Translational Biology, and the Interdisciplinary Council on Quality of Care and Outcomes Research: endorsed by the American Academy of Pediatrics. Circulation. 2009;119(11):1541-51.
21. Territo MC, Rosove MH. Cyanotic congenital heart disease: hematologic management. J Am Coll Cardiol. 1991;18(2):320-2.
22. Silversides CK, Sermer M, Siu SC. Choosing the best contraceptive method for the adult with congenital heart disease. Curr Cardiol Rep. 2009;11(4):298-305.
23. Canobbio MM. Contraception for the adolescent and young adult with congenital heart disease. Nurs Clin North Am. 2004;39(4):769-85.
24. Canobbio MM. Health care issues facing adolescents with congenital heart disease. J Pediatr Nurs. 2001;16(5):363-70.
25. Klein JD. Adolescent pregnancy: current trends and issues. Pediatrics. 2005;116(1):281-6.
26. Swan L, Hillis WS. Exercise prescription in adults with congenital heart disease: a long way to go. Heart. 2000;83(6):685-7.
27. Francis MR, Nuorti JP, Kompithra RZ, Larson H, Balraj V, Kang G, et al. Vaccination coverage and factors associated with routine childhood vaccination uptake in rural Vellore, southern India, 2017. Vaccine. 2019;37(23):3078-87.
28. Singh S, Sahu D, Agrawal A, Jeyaseelan L, Nadaraj A, Vashi MD. Coverage, quality, and correlates of childhood immunization in slums under national immunization program of India: a cross-sectional study. Heliyon. 2019; 5(9):e02403.
29. Balasubramanian S, Shah A, Pemde HK, Chatterjee P, Shivananda S, Guduru VK, et al. Indian Academy of Pediatrics (IAP) Advisory Committee on Vaccines and Immunization Practices (ACVIP) Recommended Immunization Schedule (2018-19) and Update on Immunization for Children Aged 0 Through 18 Years. Indian Pediatr. 2018;55(12):1066-74.
30. Lantin-Hermoso MR, Berger S, Bhatt AB, Richerson JE, Morrow R, Freed MD, et al. The care of children with congenital heart disease in their primary medical home. Pediatrics. 2017;140(5).
31. Rudan I, Theodoratou E, Zgaga L, Nair H, Chan KY, Tomlinson M, et al. Setting priorities for development of emerging interventions against childhood pneumonia, meningitis and influenza. J Glob Health. 2012;2(1):010304.
32. Hofstetter AM, Jakob K, Klein NP, Dekker CL, Edwards KM, Halsey NA, et al. Live vaccine use and safety in DiGeorge syndrome. Pediatrics. 2014;133(4):e946-54.
33. Miranda M, Martins AT, Carvalho S, Serra-Caetano A, Esteves I, Marques JG. Live vaccine in children with DiGeorge/22q11.2 deletion syndrome. Acta Medica Portuguesa. 2019;32(7-8):514-9.
34. Ashorobi D, Fernandez R. Asplenia. StatPearls. Treasure Island (FL): StatPearls Publishing LLC.; 2020.
35. Theilacker C, Ludewig K, Serr A, Schimpf J, Held J, Bogelein M, et al. Overwhelming postsplenectomy infection: a prospective multicenter cohort study. Clinical Infect Dis. 2016;62(7):871-8.
36. Carrico RM, Goss L, Wojcik J, [illegible], Pentecost K, Frisbie M, et al. Postsplenectomy vaccination guideline adherence: opportunities for improvement. J Am Assoc Nurse Pract. 2017;29(10):612-7.
37. McCrindle BW, Rowley AH, Newburger JW, Burns JC, Bolger AF, Gewitz M, et al. Diagnosis, treatment, and long-term management of Kawasaki disease: a Scientific Statement for Health Professionals from the American Heart Association. Circulation. 2017;135(17): e927-e99.
38. Li JS, Yow E, Berezny KY, Rhodes JF, Bokesch PM, Charpie JR, et al. Clinical outcomes of palliative surgery including a systemic-to-pulmonary artery shunt in infants with cyanotic congenital heart disease: does aspirin make a difference? Circulation. 2007;116(3):293-7.
39. Dinakaran D, Sergi CM. Co-ingestion of aspirin and acetaminophen promoting fulminant liver failure: a critical review of Reye syndrome in the current perspective at the dawn of the 21st century. Clin Exp Pharmacol Physiol. 2018;45(2): 117-21.
40. Schror K. Aspirin and Reye syndrome: a review of the evidence. Paediatr Drugs. 2007;9(3):195-204.

41. Laudanski K, Zawadka M, Polosak J, Modi J, DiMeglio M, Gutsche J, et al. Acquired immunological imbalance after surgery with cardiopulmonary bypass due to epigenetic over-activation of PU.1/M-CSF. J Transl Med. 2018;16(1):143.
42. Shane AL. Red book: 2006 Report of the Committee on Infectious Diseases, 27th edition. Emerg Infect Dis. 2006;12(12):2003-4.
43. Saxena A. Congenital heart disease in India: a status report. Indian Pediatr. 2018;55(12):1075-82.
44. Wilson W, Taubert KA, Gewitz M, Lockhart PB, Baddour LM, Levison M, et al. Prevention of infective endocarditis: guidelines from the American Heart Association: a guideline from the American Heart Association Rheumatic Fever, Endocarditis, and Kawasaki Disease Committee, Council on Cardiovascular Disease in the Young, and the Council on Clinical Cardiology, Council on Cardiovascular Surgery and Anesthesia, and the Quality of Care and Outcomes Research Interdisciplinary Working Group. Circulation. 2007;116(15):1736-54.
45. Ramamoorthy C, Haberkern CM, Bhananker SM, Domino KB, Posner KL, Campos JS, et al. Anesthesia-related cardiac arrest in children with heart disease: data from the Pediatric Perioperative Cardiac Arrest (POCA) registry. Anesth Analg. 2010;110(5):1376-82.
46. Thornhill MH, Gibson TB, Cutler E, Dayer MJ, Chu VH, Lockhart PB, et al. Antibiotic prophylaxis and incidence of endocarditis before and after the 2007 AHA recommendations. J Am Coll Cardiol. 2018;72(20):2443-54.
47. Duval X, Delahaye F, Alla F, Tattevin P, Obadia JF, Le Moing V, et al. Temporal trends in infective endocarditis in the context of prophylaxis guideline modifications: three successive population-based surveys. J Am Coll Cardiol. 2012;59(22):1968-76.
48. Bikdeli B, Wang Y, Kim N, Desai MM, Quagliarello V, Krumholz HM. Trends in hospitalization rates and outcomes of endocarditis among Medicare beneficiaries. J Am Coll Cardiol. 2013;62(23):2217-26.
49. Bor DH, Woolhandler S, Nardin R, Brusch J, Himmelstein DU. Infective endocarditis in the U.S., 1998-2009: a nationwide study. PLoS One. 2013;8(3):e60033.
50. Keller K, von Bardeleben RS, Ostad MA, Hobohm L, Munzel T, Konstantinides S, et al. Temporal trends in the prevalence of infective endocarditis in Germany between 2005 and 2014. Am J Cardiol. 2017;119(2):317-22.
51. Garg P, Ko DT, Bray Jenkyn KM, Li L, Shariff SZ. Infective endocarditis hospitalizations and antibiotic prophylaxis rates before and after the 2007 American Heart Association Guideline Revision. Circulation. 2019;140(3):170-80.

54 CHAPTER

Genetic Disorders Associated with Congenital Heart Disease

Dhanya Yesodharan, Sheela Nampoothiri

INTRODUCTION

Congenital heart disease (CHD) is the most common birth defect, affecting 1% live births and 1 in 500 fetal ultrasound examinations. Around one-third of babies with potentially lethal CHD undergo surgical intervention in the first year of life.[1] An extensive population-based study over 26 years from France has identified the frequency of extracardiac structural malformations to be around 26% in patients presenting with CHD.[2] Anomalies of the urinary tract, musculoskeletal, digestive, central nervous system, ear, face, and eyes are the most common extracardiac anomalies associated with CHD. The presence of associated malformations has a significant impact on the quality of life in patients with CHD.

Congenital heart disease may be due to a chromosomal anomaly (aneuploidy or microdeletion disorder), a single gene defect, exposure to a teratogen, familial inheritance, or unknown causes. Population studies have identified that between 9 and 18% of patients with CHD have chromosomal anomalies detectable by karyotype (KT).[3] If trisomy 21, trisomy 13, trisomy 18, and Turner syndrome are excluded, the yield from KT analysis is as low as 1.6%. Approximately 30% of patients diagnosed with CHD have a syndromic phenotype with extracardiac manifestations. Here the focus is on three main aspects: (1) physical examination, (2) classification of the cardiac lesion, and (3) three generation pedigree. After initiating a universal genetic testing protocol, it has been estimated that nearly 36% of infants are diagnosed with an underlying genetic defect once trisomy 21 has been excluded. By seeking a genetic consultation, the diagnostic yield increases by an additional 7–13% which has a great impact for the overall management of the case and also for the counseling and prenatal diagnosis for the family. The exact cause of CHD is unknown in over half the cases.

INVESTIGATIONS

When to Investigate a Child with Congenital Heart Disease for Genetic Causes? (Flowcharts 1 and 2)

- The proband has syndromic features in addition to CHD.
- First or second-degree relative has been diagnosed with CHD.
- When there are associated extracardiac malformations (**Flowchart 2**).

Choosing the Right Test

*Approach to genetic testing for patients with CHD is illustrated in **Flowchart 1**.*

Karyotyping

This is the initial test to be performed when the patients have features suggestive of trisomy 21, 13, 18, or Turner syndrome.

Fluorescent In Situ Hybridization

This detects microdeletions, as in DiGeorge syndrome, William syndrome, 4p deletion syndrome, and 1p36 deletion syndrome.

Copy number variants (CNV) are areas of chromosomal deletions or duplications that are too small to be detected by karyotyping but can be identified by fluorescent in situ hybridization (FISH), multiple ligand probe amplification (MLPA), or chromosomal micro array (CMA). Owing to the high diagnostic yield, CMA is the first line evaluation for patients with CHD in association with multiple congenital anomalies and in those with major cardiovascular anomalies. CNV has been found to be causative in approximately 15% of cases of TOF.[4] In patients with single ventricle physiology, CNV >300 kb is a risk factor for poor neurodevelopmental outcome, independent of whether the CNV is known to cause CHD or not. Hence, before contemplating major surgical correction in patients with single ventricle physiology, it is advisable to do CMA.

Subtelomeric Fluorescent In Situ Hybridization

Congenital heart disease when associated with dysmorphic features and mental handicap.

Array Comparative Genome Hybridization

Probable chromosome syndrome with a normal KT result. This test detects CNV (deletion, duplication, unbalanced

Flowchart 1: Genetic testing approach for patients with congenital heart disease (CHD).

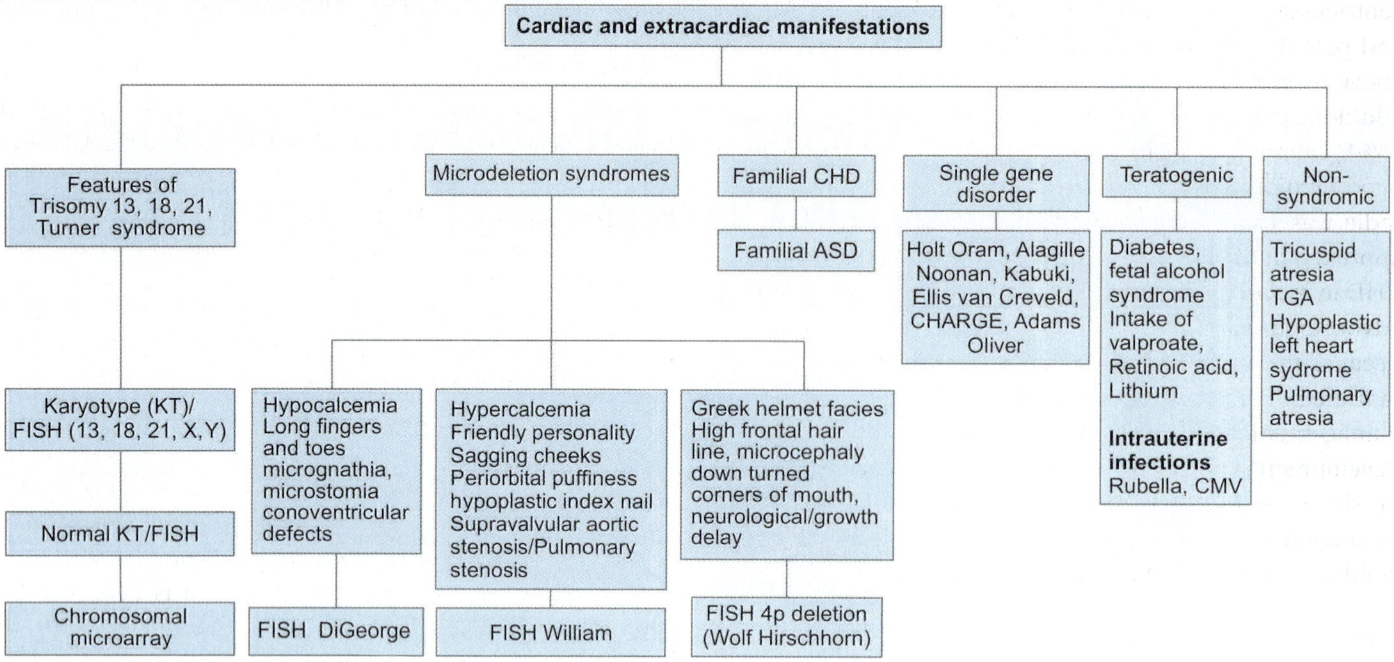

(ASD: atrial septal defect; FISH: fluorescent in situ hybridization; CMV: cytomegalovirus; TGA: transposition of the great arteries)

Flowchart 2: Approach to patients with congenital heart disease and extracardiac anomalies.

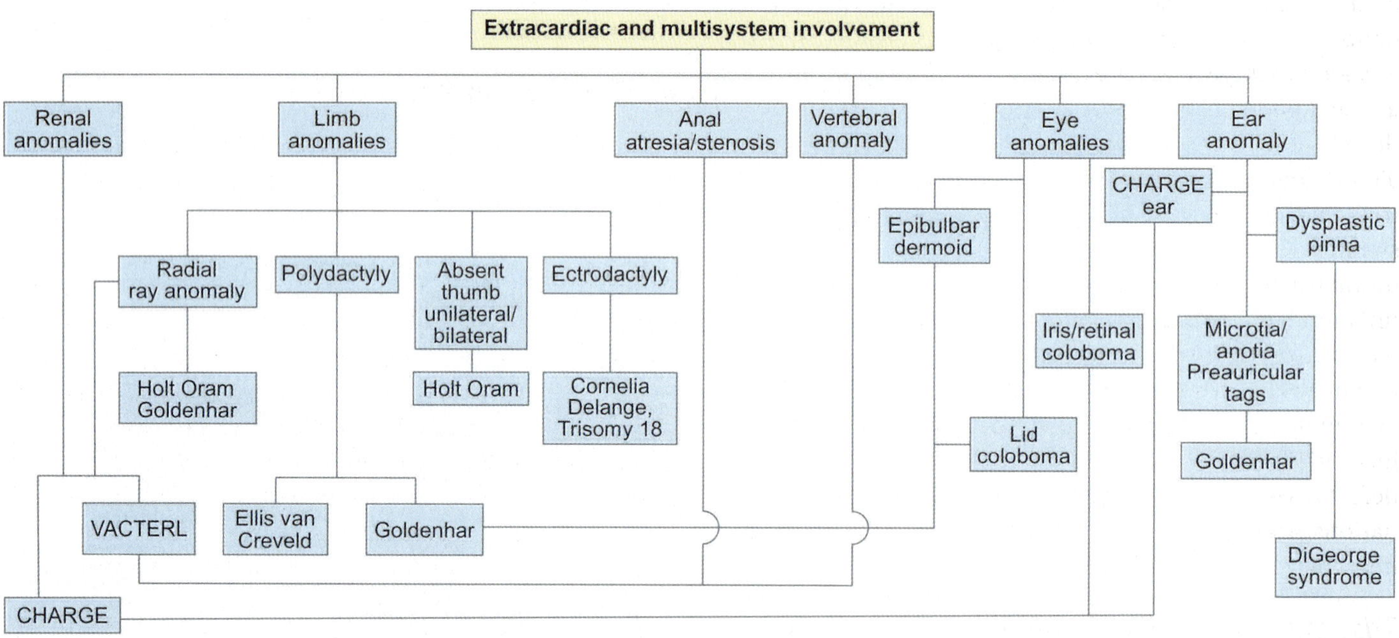

translocation, and aneuploidies). This has a potential to identify the underlying cause in 10–25% of cases.

Gene Sequencing

This is useful for single gene disorders. The family should be counseled in detail prior to testing regarding the possibility of having (1) a negative result, (2) a genetic variant for which the pathogenic potential is difficult to determine (VUS, i.e., variant of unknown significance), and (3) the possibility of picking up a variant that may have a familial recurrence risk.

CHROMOSOMAL ANOMALY

Aneuploidies

Aneuploidies refer to the presence of an abnormal number of chromosomes in a cell. The common aneuploidies associated with CHD include the trisomies (21, 18, and 13) and Turner syndrome.

Trisomy 21

Congenital heart disease is associated with up to 50% of the live born babies with trisomy 21. The most common heart diseases include atrioventricular septal defect (AVSD), ventricular septal defect (VSD), tetralogy of Fallot (TOF), and patent ductus arteriosus (PDA). Combinations of the above lesions (e.g., TOF with AVSD) may also be seen. In addition, they should be screened for hypothyroidism (4–18%), cataracts, and hearing disability. The prevalence of hypothyroidism in trisomy 21 in a recent study from South India was 13.6%.[5] There has been a significant shift in the approach in the management of babies with trisomy 21 and CHD in recent times. Most institutions across the world now advocate for early correction of the underlying heart defect because this markedly improves survival and quality of life in these patients.[5] While there are specific challenges in the management of CHD in these patients that include early development of pulmonary vascular obstructive disease in shunt lesions, an aggressive approach towards early correction often yields results that are no different from children without trisomy 21.

Trisomy 18 (Edward Syndrome)

This is the second most common multiple malformation syndrome. These babies present with prominent occiput, narrow palpebral fissure, low set malformed pinna, microstomia, and micrognathia (**Figs. 1A and C**). Clenched hands with overlapping fingers (**Fig. 1B**) and rocker-bottom feet are two important clues for trisomy 18. More than 75% of affected patients have cardiac anomalies; VSD, atrial septal defect (ASD), and PDA are the common cardiac anomalies. 95% of the babies expire within 1 year of age. Clues for trisomy 18 in the antenatal period include polyhydramnios, symmetric intrauterine growth restriction (IUGR), single umbilical artery, congenital diaphragmatic hernia, CHD, unilateral or bilateral choroid plexus cysts (30% association with trisomy 18). The diagnosis can be confirmed by karyotyping (*see* **Fig. 5B**) or with FISH. Because of the extremely poor long-term outcome in these patients, most institutions do not prefer to correct the underlying heart defects. However, in selected programs in high-income nations, attempts are being made to correct the underlying heart defect in selected cases.

Trisomy 13 (Patau Syndrome)

This condition should be suspected in patients presenting with cleft lip with or without cleft palate, microphthalmia, coloboma, hypotelorism, holoprosencephaly, and polydactyly of the hands or feet. Additional clues include capillary hemangioma and aplasia cutis congenita (**Fig. 1D**) over the scalp in the parieto-occipital area. 80% of babies have associated cardiac anomalies which include VSD, PDA, and ASD. In a few cases, they may have cyclopia (single-fused eye), anophthalmia, proboscis (**Fig. 1E**) and single nostril (**Fig. 1F**) due to abnormal development of the forebrain in association with holoprosencephaly. Like trisomy 18, the poor long-term outlook associated with trisomy 13 is a reason to avoid intervening on the heart defect.

Turner Syndrome

This condition can present in newborns with webbing of the neck (**Fig. 1G**), puffiness of the dorsum of hands and feet (**Fig. 1H**), and a broad chest with wide-spaced nipples. They also have narrow hyperconvex nails. Between 42 and 65% of cases of Turner present with hydrops, which is the most common chromosomal cause for nonimmune hydrops fetalis. Left ventricular outflow tract obstructive lesions predominate in Turner syndrome; 30% have bicuspid aortic valves and 10% present with coarctation of aorta. The growth rate is normal till around 3 years of age but height velocity then drops. The mean adult height in untreated patients is 140–143 cm. Families should be counseled regarding the need for hormone replacement therapy after 12 years of age and also about the option of growth hormone replacement therapy for augmentation of height, which is approved by US Food and Drug Administration (FDA). The diagnosis can be confirmed by karyotyping (*see* **Fig. 5C**) or with FISH. It is essential to remember that the coarctation associated with Turner syndrome may be challenging to manage in the catheterization laboratory. Balloon dilation can result in serious aortic injury because of the fragile aortic wall.

Microdeletion Syndromes

DiGeorge Syndrome (22q11.2 Deletion)

This is the most common microdeletion syndrome (1 in 4,000), with a deletion ranging from 0.7 to 3 Mbp. The phenotype arises from failure of development of derivatives of the 3rd and 4th branchial arches. The classical features include CHD in 75% of cases, which includes conotruncal anomalies especially TOF, truncus arteriosus, aortic arch anomalies, and right aortic arch. Other anomalies include cleft palate or palatal insufficiency, hypocalcemia in approximately 60% of cases due to hypoparathyroidism, immune deficiency, and development delay. The dysmorphic features include micrognathia, microstomia, a squared nasal tip (**Fig. 1I**) with a dysplastic pinna and long fingers and toes (**Figs. 1J and K**). Additional clues include asymmetric crying facies due to deficiency of depressor anguli oris muscle and extensive dental caries.

Diagnosis is confirmed by FISH (*see* **Fig. 5A**). 94% of deletions are de-novo (new) and 6% are inherited from either of the parents. This condition has marked intrafamilial variability of expression. DiGeorge syndrome is caused by a mutation in the transcription factor *TBX1* which has a major role in the development of the outflow tract and right ventricle and are also represented in the pharyngeal mesenchyme. In a resource-limited setting where FISH analysis is not available, analysis of mean platelet volume (MPV) is a bedside clue to the diagnosis of DiGeorge syndrome. In deletion versus

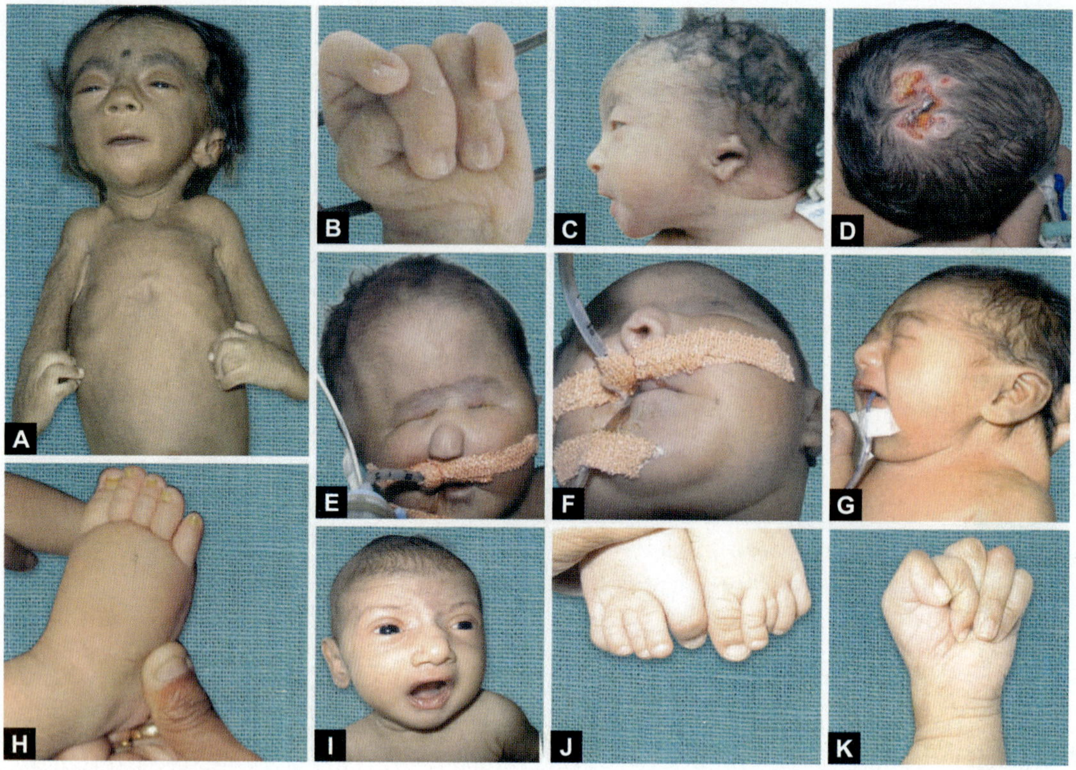

Figs. 1A to K: Trisomy 18 (A to C): (A) Hypertrichosis, low set ears, microstomia, micrognathia with bilateral radial ray anomaly; (B) Overlapping fingers classical of trisomy 18; (C) Low set malformed ears. Trisomy 13 (D to F): (D) Aplasia cutis congenita; (E) Bilateral anophthalmia, severe hypotelorism with proboscis; (F) Single nostril as part of holoprosencephaly spectrum. Turner syndrome (G and H): (G) Prominent webbing with short neck; (H) Puffiness of dorsum of feet which is a clue for Turner syndrome. DiGeorge syndrome (I to K): (I) Classical facies—narrow palpebral fissure, squared nasal tip, micrognathia; (J) Long toes; (K) Long-tapering fingers.

no deletion group, the MPV was 10.5 ± 2.5 versus 7.6 ± 1.5 fL with a sensitivity of 90.9% and specificity of 79.6%.[6] The diagnosis of DiGeorge syndrome is extremely important for a patient before planning a cardiac surgery. In view of the possible association of cell-mediated immune deficiency, they should be transfused only with irradiated blood products. Hypothyroidism should also be ruled out in all patients with DiGeorge syndrome. They should be on regular calcium supplementation and calcitriol should be started for those with associated hypoparathyroidism. Parents should be carefully evaluated for evidence of DiGeorge syndrome as variable penetrance is a well-recognized entity in this condition. If either of the parents is a carrier, the risk of having another affected child is 50% and the couple should be counseled regarding the option of prenatal diagnosis by FISH in subsequent pregnancies. There are additional specific long-term implications that include learning disabilities and a high incidence of neuropsychiatric conditions later in life.

William Syndrome

This microdeletion syndrome is caused by a deletion at 7q11.23 region affecting between 1:7,500 and 1:10,000 individuals. Cardiovascular anomalies have been seen in around 75–80% of the affected individuals. The most common CHDs are supravalvular aortic stenosis and branch pulmonary artery stenosis, and are due to haplo-insufficiency of the elastin gene that results in an abnormally thick vessel wall. The supravalvar aortic stenosis may extend along the entire length of the ascending aorta. Rarely, they have coarctation as well with involvement of a long segment of the descending thoracic aorta. 15% of the infants develop hypercalcemia but usually do not need any specific treatment. The facial gestalt include a long philtrum, wide mouth, everted full lips, full cheeks, periorbital puffiness, flat nasal bridge, medial eyebrow flare, hypochromic iris (**Fig. 2A**), hypoplastic index nails, and hoarse voice. They have an extremely sociable personality and have an increased tendency to have inguinal and umbilical hernia. Diagnosis is by FISH and the etiology is usually sporadic.

Wolf–Hirschhorn Syndrome (4p Deletion Syndrome)

This microdeletion syndrome is caused by loss of the distal portion of chromosome 4p with a breakpoint between 4p15 and 16. This is a rare microdeletion syndrome with a frequency of 1 in 50,000 live born babies. The phenotypic clues include Greek helmet facies, high frontal hairline, microcephaly, broad nose with prominent bridge, corners of mouth turned downward, hypertelorism (**Fig. 2B**), short philtrum, arched eyebrows, cleft palate/lip, neurological and growth delay, and seizures. CHD is associated in nearly 50% of cases which include ASD, VSD, and PDA. Ophthalmological clues include microphthalmia and coloboma and a few

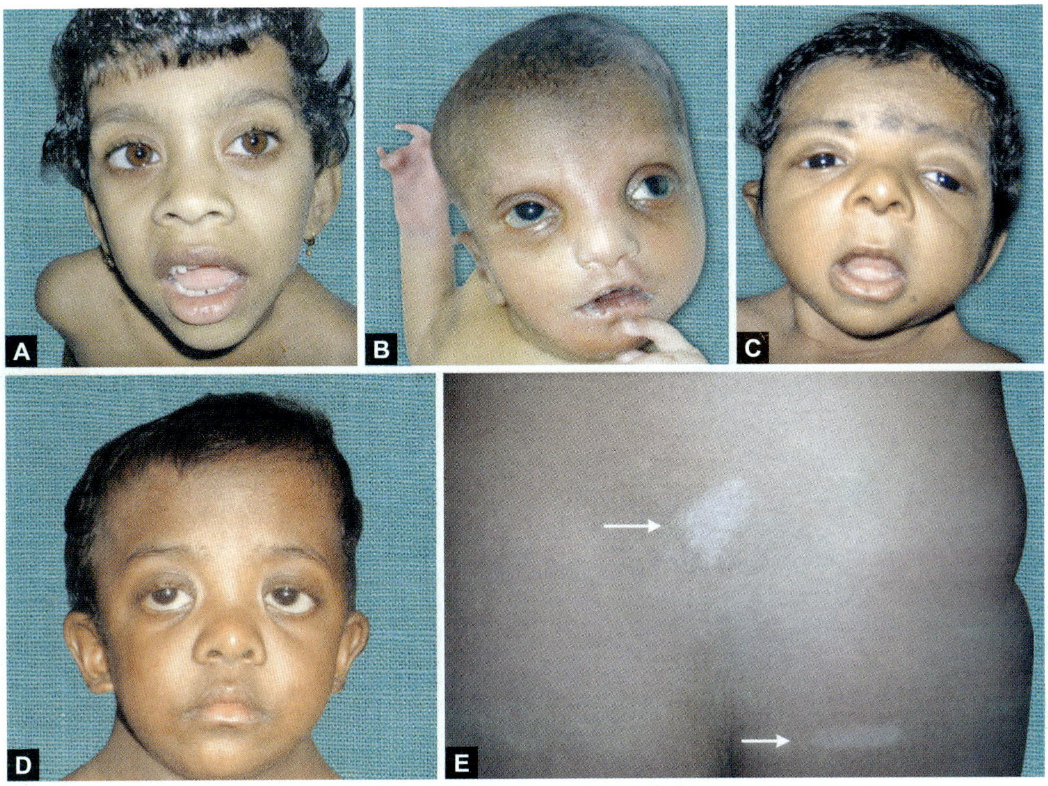

Figs. 2A to E: William syndrome (A). Typical facial gestalt with short nose, thick everted lips, medial eyebrow flare, and hypochromic iris. Wolf–Hirschhorn syndrome (B). Typical Greek helmet facies with high frontal hair line, prominent bridge of nose, hypertelorism, downturned corners of mouth. Noonan syndrome (C and D): (C) Bilateral downslanting eyes, short nose, long philtrum, bilateral ptosis in an infant; (D) Older child with ptosis, short neck with webbing, bilateral low set posteriorly rotated pinna, bilateral epicanthic folds, short nose, flat nasal bridge; (E) Ash leaf macules in tuberous sclerosis.

have associated renal anomalies including hydronephrosis and dysplastic kidneys. FISH is the ideal modality for the confirmation of the diagnosis.

1p36 Deletion Syndrome

This is the second most common microdeletion syndrome. These patients present with intellectual disability, epilepsy and dysmorphic features including microbrachycephaly, low anterior hairline, deep set eyes, hypertelorism, long philtrum, pointed chin, and straight eye brows. 50% of them have associated CHD especially cardiomyopathy and a high prevalence of left ventricular noncompaction.

SINGLE GENE DISORDERS

Noonan Syndrome

An RASopathy is a syndrome caused by a mutation in a gene of the Ras-MAPK pathway, e.g., Noonan syndrome, cardio-facio-cutaneous syndrome (CFC), Costello syndrome, and LEOPARD syndrome. Between 60 and 90% of patients with an RASopathy have a CHD, which include pulmonary valve stenosis, ASD, and hypertrophic cardiomyopathy (HCM).

Noonan syndrome is one of the most common single gene disorders associated with CHD, with a prevalence of 1 in 1,000 to 2,500 live births. It is an autosomal dominant disorder and the clinical clues include short stature, coarse face, low set posteriorly rotated ears, ptosis, antimongoloid slant of eyes, triangular face, deep philtrum, short neck, hypertelorism, cryptorchidism, and sparse scalp hair (**Figs. 2C and D**). 50% of cases of Noonan syndrome are associated with a mutation in the *PTPN11* gene, though 12 other genes may be causative, and they include *KRAS, SOS1, RAF1, NRAS, BRAF, SHOC2, PPP1CB, CBL, SOS2, RRAS, RIT1*, and *LZTR1*. Among these *SOS1, RIT1* and *RAF1* are the commonly mutated genes. The prevalence of HCM is very high in patients with *RIT1* gene mutation, and they also have an increased association with lymphatic problems. Owing to the autosomal dominant inheritance, the chance of transmission of this condition to the offspring from an affected parent is 50%. The unique feature of the pulmonic stenosis in Noonan syndrome is the fact that the valve is dysplastic and generally responds poorly to balloon dilation.

Tuberous Sclerosis

This is an autosomal dominant disorder with predilection to the development of hamartomatous lesions in multiple tissues especially in the skin and the brain. These patients have a high incidence of seizures, mental handicap, and behavioral problems. Skin lesions include adenoma sebaceum over the cheek and nasolabial folds, ash leaf macules (**Fig. 2E**), shagreen patches and small confetti macules, and fibromatous plaques. Other clues include subungual fibromas on fingers or toes, gingival fibroma, and dental pits with enamel defects. Angiomyolipomas are multiple benign cystic lesions in the kidneys and are seen in around 45–80% of patients. Subependymal tubers are classically seen in the periventricular region and retinal or optic nerve hamartoma can also develop in these patients. Cardiac rhabdomyomas (*see* **Fig. 5D**) are seen in 40–86% of fetuses and are identifiable with anomaly scan at 18–20 weeks. They are often multiple. Both parents should be carefully examined for adenoma sebaceum, ash leaf macules, shagreen patches, and subungual fibromas. Mutation in TSC1 or TSC2 can cause this disorder. Patients with rhabdomyoma which has been detected antenatally should be kept under close surveillance for the development of subependymal tubers in the brain and also for evaluation of angiomyolipoma of the kidneys. The interesting feature of these rhabdomyomas is that they tend to decrease in size after birth. The parents should be counseled regarding the possibility of seizure disorder in the proband, and mutation analysis should be offered for the confirmation of the diagnosis.

CHARGE Syndrome

This name is an acronym for Coloboma (retina or iris), Heart defects, choanal Atresia, Retarded growth and development, Genital hypoplasia (**Fig. 3C**), and Ear anomalies. There is a 70% association with CHD [TOF, double-outlet right ventricle (DORV), PDA, VSD, and ASD]. The typical "CHARGE" ears are cup-shaped wide ears with reduced vertical height (**Fig. 3B**). Ophthalmological clues include microphthalmia, microcornea, and coloboma of the retina and/or iris (**Fig. 3A**). Inner ear anomalies are associated in 90% of cases. Aplasia of the semi-circular canals and hypoplastic uncus are the most specific anomalies. The diagnostic criteria of Verloes (3C triad) include Coloboma, choanal atresia, and hypoplasia of semi-circular canals. If all the three features are present, then the patient has typical CHARGE syndrome. More than two-thirds cases are caused by mutations of *CHD 7* gene; *SMA3E* gene is less common.

Holt–Oram Syndrome

This syndrome has a combination of skeletal and cardiovascular abnormalities. The skeletal phenotype affects only the upper limbs. Thumbs may be absent, hypoplastic, triphalangeal, or bifid (**Figs. 4A and E**). Phocomelia may be seen in around 10% of cases. The limb anomaly is always asymmetric with more severe involvement of the left side. Sloping or narrow shoulders and hypoplastic pectorals are seen in mildly affected individuals (**Fig. 4D**). Cardiac association is seen in 85% of cases and the most common CHD is ostium secundum ASD and VSD. Hypoplastic or absent radius and absence or hypoplasia of the first metacarpal and phalanges and hypoplastic scaphoid are the radiological associations (**Fig. 4B and C**). This autosomal dominant disorder has marked intra- and interfamilial variation. It is caused by a mutation in the *TBX5* gene, which is expressed in the upper limbs and heart.[4] In view of the marked variability of expression, parents should be evaluated clinically for mild skeletal changes. Radiographs of the wrist and arms may reveal subtle radiological clues in the thumbs and carpal bones. An echocardiogram should also be suggested for the parents.

Kabuki Syndrome

This is a genetic disorder leading to short stature, microcephaly, and a typical facial gestalt reminiscent of the makeup worn by actors in Kabuki theater. The main diagnostic feature is the presence of an everted lateral one-third of the lower eyelid, long palpebral fissure, arched eyebrows, and ptosis. A break in the junction of the medial 2/3rd and lateral 1/3rd of the eyebrows is a good clue for the diagnosis. They also have a broad nasal tip, prominent ear lobes, and high arched or cleft palate. Persistence of fetal pads in fingers and brachydactyly of fingers are additional clues. Associated heart defects include coarctation and VSD. Three genes are implicated and the most common one is *MLL2* and others are *KMT2D* and *KDM6A*.

CONDITIONS WITHOUT IDENTIFIED CAUSES

The two examples in this category are Goldenhar syndrome and VACTERL association.

Goldenhar Syndrome

This sporadic syndrome is due to a defect in the morphogenesis of the first and second branchial arches, which in turn leads to a combination of vertebral, renal, and ocular abnormalities. Hemifacial microsomia is the classical feature and there is a right-sided predilection for this feature. Macrostomia with cleft-like extension of the corner of the mouth is common (**Fig. 3D**). Ear anomalies include microtia, and preauricular tags or pits which are common in the line joining the tragus to the corner of the mouth (**Fig. 3D**). Vertebral anomalies including hemivertebrae or hypoplastic vertebrae are most commonly seen in the cervical region. Epibulbar dermoid (**Fig. 3E**) with vertebral anomalies are an important association of this disorder. Cleft of the upper eyelid is yet another clue (**Fig. 3E**). CHDs are usually seen and include VSD, PDA, and TOF. Ultrasound evaluation for renal anomalies is advisable in view of associated anomalies such as ectopic or fused kidneys and renal agenesis. The cause of this disorder is unknown. Most of these patients have normal intelligence. They benefit from cosmetic corrective surgeries.

VACTERL Association

This is a malformation pattern with sporadic occurrence and unknown etiology. The acronym includes Vertebral anomaly, Anal atresia, Cardiac anomalies, Tracheoesophageal fistula,

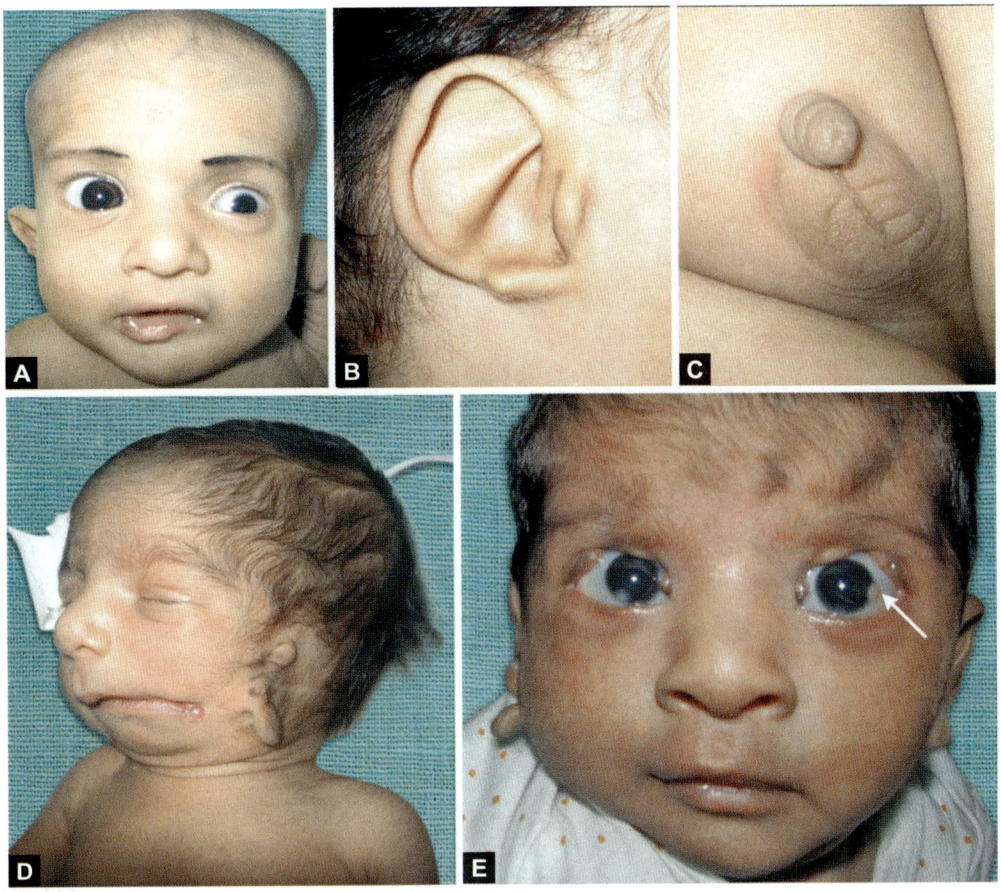

Figs. 3A to E: CHARGE syndrome (A to C): (A) Left microphthalmia, microcornea and left facial asymmetry, deficiency of left depressor anguli oris muscle; (B) Typical CHARGE ear with short vertical height and complete absence of ear lobule; (C) Micropenis with bilateral undescended testes. Goldenhar syndrome (D and E): (D) Severe microtia with preauricular tags on left with macrostomia with facial clefting; (E) Bilateral upper eyelid coloboma with classical limbal dermoid on left eye and corneal opacity in 7'o clock position in right eye. Also, note a skin tag in the line joining tragus and angle of mouth.

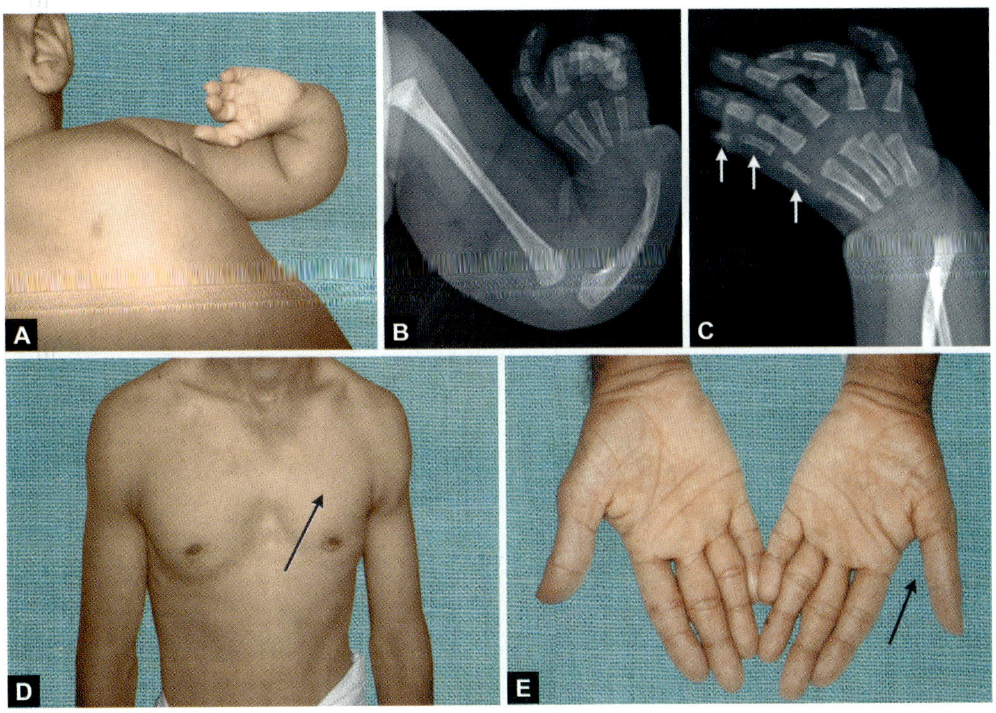

Figs. 4A to E: Holt–Oram syndrome: (A) Radial ray anomaly of left hand with absent thumb and preaxial remnant of thumb; (B) Radiograph showing complete absence of radius with curved ulna and complete absence of first metacarpal and phalanges; (C) Radiograph showing hypoplastic first metacarpal and triphalangeal thumb (arrows); (D) Parent of a child with Holt–Oram syndrome with reduced expressivity. Flat and asymmetric left chest with drooping of left shoulder (arrow); (E) Left hand showing triphalangeal thumb (arrow) and flat thenar eminence.

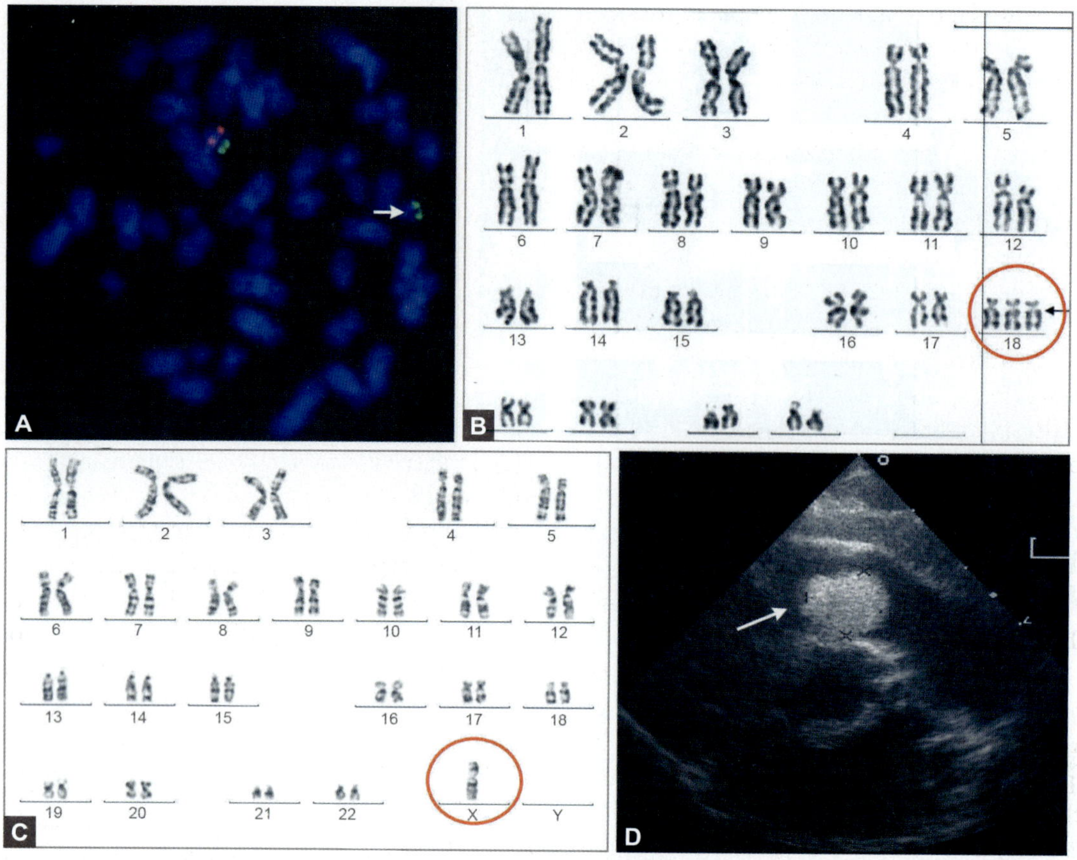

Figs. 5A to D: (A) Metaphase fluorescent in situ hybridization showing deletion of critical region for DiGeorge syndrome (22q11.2-orange) on one of the chromosome 22. Green signal shows the control probe (22q11.3); (B) Karyotype showing three copies of chromosome 18 in trisomy 18; (C) Karyotype showing single X in Turner syndrome; (D) Echocardiogram showing intracardiac rhabdomyoma in tuberous sclerosis.

Radial dysplasia with or without thumb anomalies, Renal anomaly, and Limb anomaly. Single umbilical artery is an association in approximately 35% of cases. Associated CHD is present in 75%. The common cardiac anomalies associated with this condition include VSD and TOF. Surgical management of these lesions is often challenging in the face of associated extracardiac malformations that are generally serious.

TERATOGENIC EXPOSURE

The known associations of exposure to teratogens and prenatal events with CHD include the following:

- *Rubella*: PDA and branch pulmonary stenosis
- *Gestational diabetes*: Transposition of great arteries (TGA) and tricuspid atresia
- *Sodium valproate*: Coarctation of aorta, ASD, VSD, and hypoplastic left heart syndrome (HLHS)
- *Isotretinoin (retinoic acid)*: TGA, HLHS, VSD, and TOF
- *Lithium*: Ebstein anomaly.

FAMILIAL INHERITANCE

Genetic assessment serves as a useful tool to predict the recurrence risk, define the pattern of inheritance within the family and assess the need for family screening, and to provide targeted follow-up and personalized medical care (**Table 1**).

TABLE 1: Genes linked to congenital heart disease.[7]

ASD	MYH6 and TBX20 (embryonic formation of atrial septum)
ASD, VSD, Ebstein anomaly, and TOF	NKX 2-5
ASD, VSD, and PS	GATA 4
AVSD	GATA-SMAD4
TOF and interrupted aortic arch	TBX 1
ASD, VSD, and valve defects	TBX 20

(ASD: atrial septal defect; AVSD: atrioventricular septal defect; PS: pulmonic stenosis; TOF: tetralogy of Fallot; VSD: ventricular septal defect)

NONSYNDROMIC CONGENITAL HEART DISEASE

Around 70% of CHD occur as isolated anomalies which include TGA, HLHS, tricuspid atresia, and pulmonary atresia. There are many unidentified genes, probably de-novo variants without clear Mendelian inheritance, responsible for CHD among this group. Between 5 and 10% of sporadic nonsyndromic CHD patients with normal KT and FISH analysis is due to a rare CNV (≤1% population frequency).[4] A "two hit" model has been considered for the causation for CHD wherein one CNV has been inherited from an unaffected parent and another de-novo CNV has originated in the affected child. This explanation could account for the very low recurrence risk rate for offspring of CHD patients when compared with other monogenic disorders.[4]

As most of the children with complex anomalies are subjected to corrective surgery, the recognition of specific genetic alteration underlying the heart disease not only helps for prognostication but also provides an opportunity for the family to choose the right reproductive option. This also gives an option for the first-degree relatives to identify the carrier status, which in turn would help them to be under surveillance for specific cardiac conditions such as progressive aortic dilatation and cardiomyopathy so that they have a provision for preventive therapy.

IMPLICATION OF IDENTIFYING THE VARIANTS IN SYNDROMIC AND NONSYNDROMIC CASES

- Patients who harbor NKX 2-5 mutation (transcription factor) are more likely to have atrioventricular block as NKX 2-5 has a major function in myocytes of conductive systems. A few of them have a tendency for dilated cardiomyopathy and progressive ventricular dysfunction and need close follow-up.
- Cardiac hypertrophy can evolve in patients with Noonan syndrome and other RASopathies. Hence, patients with Noonan syndrome should be counseled for cardiac evaluation every 5 years even if the initial echocardiogram is normal.
- Myosin Heavy Chain 6 (*MYH6*) gene sequencing is indicated in all patients with hypoplastic left heart. Patients with MYH6 mutation have reduced transplant-free survival and this evaluation helps to choose the right candidate for surgery.[1]
- MYH6 mutation is also associated with CHD and cardiomyopathy (dilated and HCM). Hence, a few carriers of MYH6 mutation can have CHD and others are at risk of cardiomyopathy necessitating the need for follow-up in first d[illegible]

As a general rule, the recurrence risk for siblings is between 1 and 6% if the parents are unaffected and increases to 10% if two siblings are affected (**Table 2**). Recurrence risk in the offspring is greater than in siblings, e.g., 10–14% for AVSD.

TABLE 2: Recurrence risk for CHD.[7]

Type of CHD	*First-degree relative*
AVSD	3.3%
TOF, DORV, TGV, TA	3.7%
ASD	3.2%
Coarctation of aorta, HLHS, AS	3.1%

(AS: aortic stenosis; ASD: atrial septal defect; AVSD: atrioventricular septal defect; CHD: congenital heart disease; DORV: double-outlet right ventricle; HLHS: hypoplastic left heart syndrome; TA: truncus arteriosus; TGV: transposition of the great vessels; TOF: tetralogy of Fallot; VSD: ventricular septal defect)

It is higher if the mother is the proband and more for left-sided obstructive lesions (8–10%).[7] This information is important as many women who have undergone corrective surgeries consider reproductive options and hence they should be counseled regarding the need for fetal echocardiogram at 18–20 weeks. Preimplantation genetic diagnosis is already in vogue for Holt-Oram syndrome and Marfan syndrome.[8]

REFERENCES

1. Geddes GC, Earing MG. Genetic evaluation of patients with congenital heart disease. Curr Opin Pediatr. 2018;30(6):707-13.
2. Stoll C, Dott B, Alembik Y, Roth MP. Associated noncardiac congenital anomalies among cases with congenital heart defects. Eur J Med Genet. 2015;58(2):75-85.
3. Saliba A, Figueiredo ACV, Baroneza JE, Afiune JY, Pic-Taylor A, Oliveira SF, et al. Genetic and genomics in congenital heart disease: a clinical review. J Pediatr (Rio J). 2019;96(3):279-88.
4. Fahed AC, Gelb BD, Seidman JG, Seidman CE. Genetics of congenital heart disease: the glass half empty. Circ Res. 2013;112(4):707-20.
5. Narayanan DL, Yesodharan D, Kappanayil M, Kuthiroly S, Thampi MV, Hamza Z, et al. Cardiac spectrum, cytogenetic analysis and thyroid profile of 418 children with Down syndrome from South India: a cross-sectional study. Indian J Pediatr. 2014;81(6):547-51.
6. Anilkumar A, Vasudevan DM, Kappanayil M, Sundaram KR, Krishna Kumar R, Nampoothiri S. Platelet parameters in children with chromosome 22q11 deletion and conotruncal heart defects. Congenit Heart Dis. 2018;13(3):[illegible]
[illegible] [illegible], [illegible] G, Khairy P. Genetic testing in congenital heart disease: a clinical approach. World J Cardiol. 2016;8(2):180-91.
8. He J, McDermott DA, Song Y, Gilbert F, Kligman I, Basson CT. Preimplantation genetic diagnosis of human congenital heart malformation and Holt-Oram syndrome. Am J Med Genet A. 2004;126A(1):93-8.

55
CHAPTER

Cardiac Manifestations in Systemic Conditions

Sumitra Venkatesh, Swati Garekar, Shakuntala S Prabhu

INTRODUCTION

Numerous primary systemic illnesses have cardiovascular manifestations as part of the disease process. The list of such illnesses is long, varied, and includes storage and metabolic disorders, collagen vascular diseases, endocrine diseases, neuromuscular disorders, and infections. Additionally, malnutrition is rampant in our country with micro- and macronutrient deficiencies, which also have significant effects on the heart.

The cardiac involvement by systemic diseases may be due to deposits in the myocardium/valves/coronary artery walls or genetic alteration of intracytoplasmic molecules or at times cause damage to the conduction system of the heart or inflammation of the vessel walls. The cause of mortality in many such systemic illnesses remains cardiac failure. With increasing survival of children with chronic systemic diseases, it is vital to diagnose cardiac involvement at a subclinical stage whenever possible. Advances in echocardiography like tissue Doppler imaging, strain calculation, and various Doppler indices have helped us to achieve this. Cardiac magnetic resonance (CMR) imaging also plays an important role in subclinical diagnosis of cardiac manifestations. This chapter briefly discusses the cardiovascular manifestations of the common systemic conditions that we come across in pediatric population in the Indian subcontinent.

STORAGE DISORDERS

Glycogen Storage Disorders

This is a group of inheritable disorders occurring due to quantitative or qualitative deficiency of one of the enzymes involved in glycogen metabolism.

Perhaps the most illustrative example of a glycogen storage disorder (GSD) with cardiac manifestation is GSD type II or Pompe disease (which accounts for roughly 15% of all GSDs). Cardiomyopathy has also been reported with GSD types III and IV.

Pompe Disease (Glycogen Storage Disorder Type II)

Pompe disease results from deficiency of the lysosomal enzyme acid alpha 1,4 glucosidase which is required for the degradation of lysosomal glycogen. The enzyme defect causes a progressive deposition of glycogen within lysosome-derived vacuoles in nearly all types of tissues with a predilection for myocardium, skeletal muscle, and liver.[1] Cellular injury leads to enlargement and dysfunction of the entire organ involved, manifesting as hypertrophic cardiomyopathy, weak bulky skeletal muscles, etc. The clinical manifestations depend on the severity of the enzyme deficiency. The more severe the deficiency, the earlier the presentation and more relentless the course. Thus, there are three major clinical phenotypes depending on age of onset; infantile, juvenile, or adult.

Infantile onset (classical Pompe) is the most severe variant, characterized by massive glycogen deposition in heart, liver, and skeletal muscles. These patients usually present within first 6 months of life with history of feeding difficulties, breathing difficulty, hypotonia, weak cry, enlarged protruding tongue, and features of congestive cardiac failure. Gross motor development, usually normal in the initial weeks or months of life, shows retardation as the disease (and the associated hypotonia) progresses. The disease relentlessly progresses to death, commonly from cardiac or respiratory failure, usually between 6 months and 2 years of life.

The cardiac manifestation of infantile Pompe disease is progressively worsening severe hypertrophic cardiomyopathy and resultant cardiac failure. Since glycogen also gets deposited in the conduction tissue, alteration in the form of short PR interval and conduction blocks may be seen on the electrocardiogram (ECG). Biochemical investigations may reveal elevated levels of creatine kinase (up to 2,000 IU/L), alanine aminotransaminase (ALT), aspartate transaminase (AST), lactate dehydrogenase (LDH), and alkaline and acid phosphatase. Juvenile and adult forms have less universal cardiac findings.

Investigations

Chest roentgenogram shows cardiomegaly and occasionally pulmonary congestion (**Fig. 1**). ECG may show characteristic tall QRS complexes and short PR interval as mentioned above. ST-T changes may also be seen. Atrioventricular (AV) block, bundle branch blocks, Wolff–Parkinson–White (WPW) syndrome, and atrial dysrhythmias have been reported (**Fig. 2**). Echocardiogram shows severe septal or concentric left ventricular hypertrophy (LVH), reduced left ventricular (LV) ejection fraction, and increased LV mass index (**Figs. 3A and B**). There is associated diastolic dysfunction as well. The LVH may occasionally cause obstruction of the LV outflow tract. The right ventricle may also be hypertrophied.

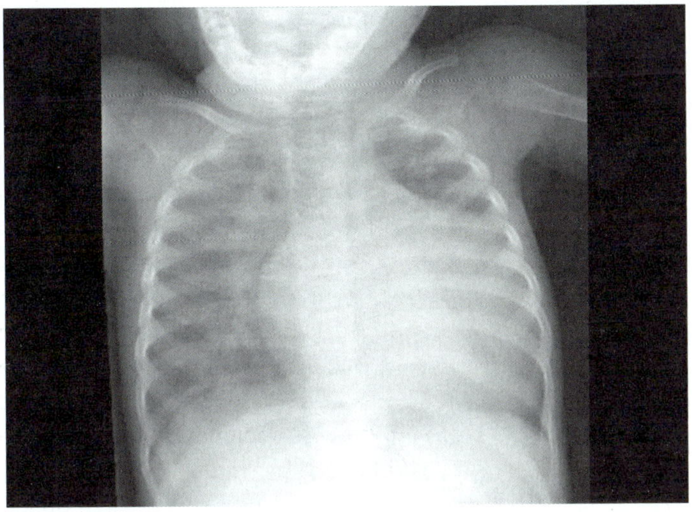

Fig. 1: Chest X-ray posteroanterior (PA) view showing massive cardiomegaly with computed tomography (CT) ratio of 70%.

CMR imaging allows for tissue definition and in a few instances myocardial fibrosis may be seen on late-gadolinium enhancement (LGE). Confirmation of diagnosis is by demonstration of absent or deficient enzyme (acid maltase) levels in muscle biopsy, cultured skin fibroblasts, or peripheral blood lymphocytes. Prenatal diagnosis is possible by determination of the enzyme levels in chorionic villus biopsy sampling or amniocentesis.

Management

It is principally symptomatic and supportive and includes medical therapy for cardiac and respiratory failure, ventilatory assistance, physiotherapy, and rehabilitative training. First-line anti-heart failure medications include diuretics, angiotensin-converting-enzyme (ACE) inhibitors, and angiotensin receptor blockers. There are anecdotal reports of benefits from dietary management (high protein, low carbohydrate diets, L-alanine supplementation, etc.) and exercise regimens. Advances in management include development of a recombinant human acid-alpha glucosidase enzyme (Myozyme™), designated enzyme replacement therapy (ERT). The sooner the ERT is begun, the better are the results. ERT is associated with a regression in cardiac hypertrophy, normalization of ECG changes, and reduction in cardiomegaly.[2,3]

Mucopolysaccharidosis

Mucopolysaccharidosis (MPS) are a group of rare inherited disorders that result from the deficiency of one or more of the lysosomal enzymes required for glycosaminoglycan (GAG) catabolism. GAGs are complex macromolecules that form a

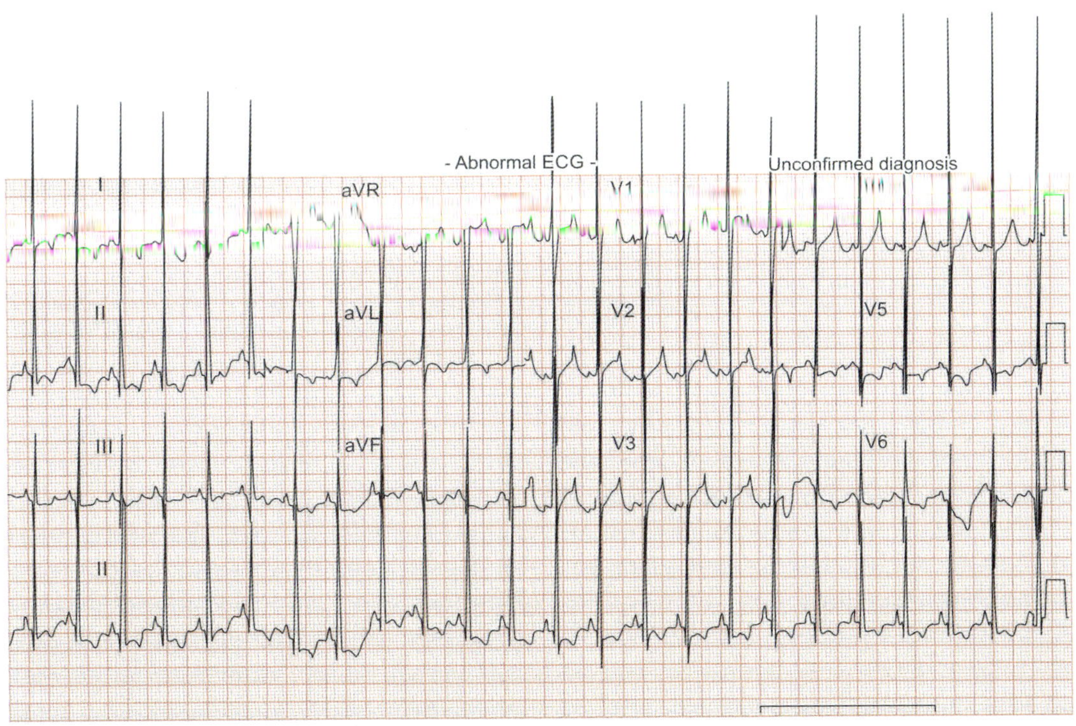

Fig. 2: Pompe disease: A 12-lead electrocardiogram (ECG) showing a short PR interval with very prominent QRS voltages in all leads.

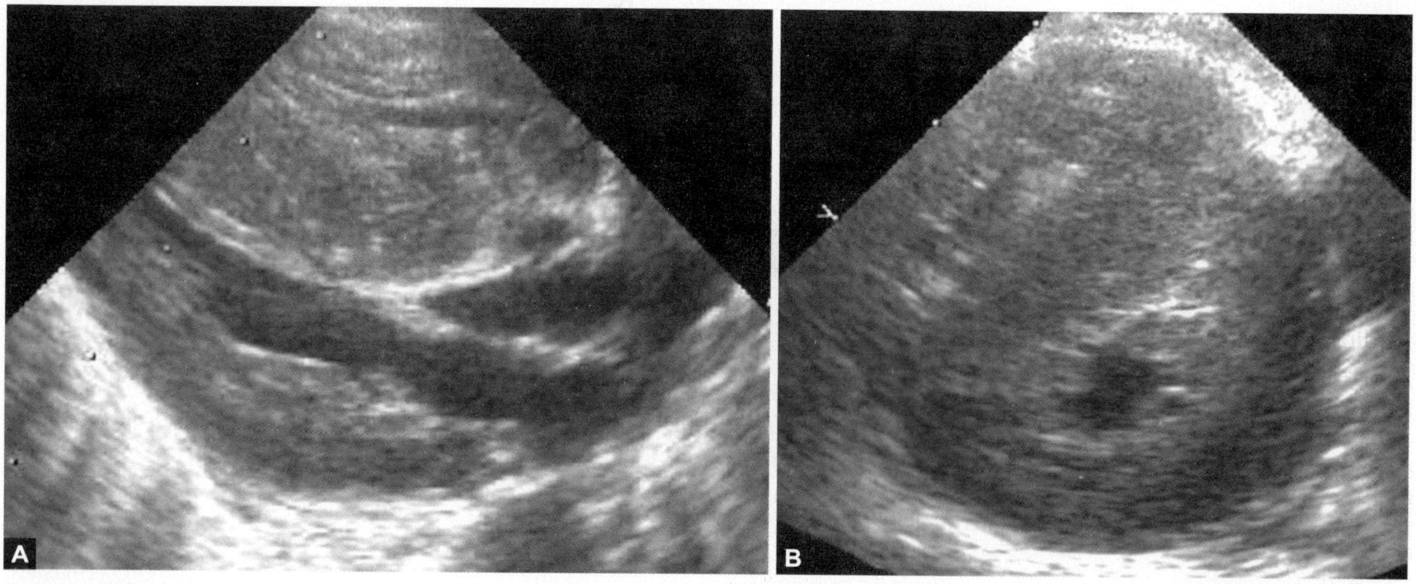

Figs. 3A and B: Echocardiographic images in parasternal long axis (A) and parasternal short axis (B) views showing massive left ventricular hypertrophy involving the entire left ventricle (LV).

major constituent of connective tissues. Enzyme deficiency therefore results in lysosomal accumulation of excessive amounts of GAGs at various sites including the skeleton, cardiac valves, myocardium, aorta, and coronaries. Since the inheritance is autosomal recessive, family history may be negative. Cardiovascular involvement is not an uncommon feature of this group of disorders and can be found in all types of MPS. MPS type I, II, and VI show the most severe and early cardiac involvement. Valve distortion due to GAG deposition with resultant stenosis or regurgitation of mitral, aortic, and tricuspid valves are the common cardiac manifestations. Cardiac failure associated with GAG myocardial deposits (cardiomyopathy) or endocardial fibroelastosis has also been reported to be a presenting feature, although rare.[3] Acute infantile cardiomyopathy has been reported with MPS type VI. Focal or diffuse deposits in the coronary arteries can lead to significant stenosis and sudden cardiac death. Depositions of mucopolysaccharides in the arterial walls produce lesions similar to atherosclerosis. At times, systemic hypertension is also seen. Conduction disturbances and complete heart block (CHB) have also been described. Typically, extracardiac clinical features include coarse facies, corneal clouding, skeletal abnormalities (joint stiffness, dysostosis multiplex), hernias, short stature, deafness, and mental subnormality (in certain types), depending upon the specific enzymatic deficiency and the resultant pattern of GAG degradation products. Cardiovascular findings may be a murmur or those of heart failure. Clinical examination has to be followed by an echocardiogram.

Investigations

Urine can be studied quantitatively and qualitatively for GAG excretion. Specific enzyme deficiency can be demonstrated in cultured fibroblasts or isolated leukocytes. Radiological, ophthalmological, and other specific systemic evaluations would elucidate the other manifestations of this disorder. B-type natriuretic peptide (BNP) or N-terminal pro B-type natriuretic peptide (NT-pro BNP) levels will help differentiate cause of dyspnea (heart failure versus worsening pulmonary function). Increasingly, an echocardiogram is being used to diagnose MPS early in the types with subtle clinical features and early screening should be recommended in such patients.[4] An ECG may show varying degrees of AV conduction block. Serial ECGs should be performed to detect worsening of blocks. Echocardiography shows valvar involvement manifesting as thickening and redundancy of the mitral valve with mitral regurgitation. Over time, calcification of the valve leaflets and the chordae will lead to stenosis. The aortic valve may also be involved. Deposit of GAG is not as common as other storage disorders. A detailed LV morphology/size/function quantification is essential. This will include indexed wall thickness, mass, and systolic function measurements. Aortic root measurements should also be made to detect aortopathy. The LV endocardium may be echogenic in certain types of MPS. Direct or indirect estimates of pulmonary pressure should also be obtained. A coronary angiography may be required to diagnose coronary stenosis in patients with high clinical suspicion of ischemia.

Management

The emphasis is on early diagnosis and early treatment. Cardiac evaluation and echocardiography are advisable as a screening tool and then at least annually. Management is guided by a multidisciplinary approach aimed at symptomatic and supportive care. Orthopedic and ophthalmological surgeries may be required. Standard heart failure therapies may be used for heart failure.

Infective endocarditis prophylaxis should be advised in all patients with valvular abnormalities. There are reports of surgical valve replacement in severely stenosed or regurgitant cardiac valves. Recombinant ERTs are now available for some types of MPS (e.g., Aldurazyme™ for MPS type I and Naglazyme™ for MPS type VI) which have been shown to improve physical capacity and respiratory functions. Hematopoietic stem cell transplant is also becoming an increasingly viable option. Patients with severe cardiomyopathy may benefit from ERT followed by the stem cell transplant. Cardiac function and ventricular hypertrophy resolve after treatment but valvular issues persist.

COLLAGEN VASCULAR DISEASES (CONNECTIVE TISSUE DISORDERS AND RHEUMATOID DISEASES)

The collagen vascular diseases are a group of diseases that result from abnormally regulated immune responses, leading to inflammation of target organs. They have varied pathogenetic mechanisms, and a wide spectrum of organ involvement and clinical presentation. Cardiac involvement is common, though there is no unified mechanism to explain its occurrence.

Systemic Lupus Erythematosus

Pediatric systemic lupus erythematosus (SLE) is a relatively uncommon disorder with a reported prevalence of 4–250/100,000. It is unusual before 8 years of age, though it has been reported as early as first year of life. There is an overwhelming predilection for female sex with an overall ratio of 6.3:1. The cardiac manifestations in SLE are seen in about 31% of the children, affecting all layers of the heart including myocardium, valves, coronaries, and the pulmonary arteries.[5] Children are more likely to have cardiac involvement within the first year of diagnosis. SLE is diagnosed by a combination of clinical criteria and laboratory manifestations. Clinical features include constitutional symptoms of fever, fatigue, malaise, weight loss with joint involvement (pain with/without swelling), skin rash (butterfly/malar rash), oral ulcers, photosensitivity, serositis, hematological derangements (thrombocytopenia, anemia, neutropenia), psychosis, chorea, and renal involvement in the form of hypertension. Any four of the above should raise a suspicion of SLE. Pericarditis is the most common cardiovascular manifestation of SLE, seen in about 25–30% of patients with active disease. It may be asymptomatic, or may present with fever, sharp chest pain that worsens with deep inspiration, and fever. Pericardial effusion is usually present in symptomatic patients, though tamponade is rare (in <1%). Patients may present with hepatomegaly and jugular venous distension from slowly accumulating fluid resulting in a large effusion. The pericardium may show fibrous adhesions obliterating the pericardial space.

Myocarditis is clinically diagnosed in up to 10% of patients; in another 40%, it may be subclinical. The myocardial abnormality may be in the form of myocardial cell atrophy, mild-to-moderate infiltrating foci scattered in the interstitium, or vascular lesions such as perivasculitis or necrotizing vasculitis of intramural arteries. Cardiomyopathy may develop due to accelerated atherosclerosis or platelet aggregation or due to fibrin accumulation causing myocardial ischemia. Myocardium may also be secondarily affected by hypertension or lupus valvulopathy. The child usually presents with chest pain, dyspnea, enlarged cardiac shadow on chest X-ray (CXR), and elevated ST-T wave segment with depressed QRS voltage on ECG. Echocardiography confirms the myocardial dysfunction. Valvar lesions are more common in adults compared to children. The characteristic valvular lesion in SLE is verrucous Libman–Sacks endocarditis. These lesions are 2–4 mm, pea-sized lesions consisting of proliferative or degenerating valve tissue with clumps of fibrin and platelet thrombi and are located on the ventricular side of the valve and along the chordae tendinae.[6] Libman–Sacks lesions are more common on the mitral valve. Embolization to coronary or cerebral artery is a rare complication. The other less typical valve afflictions include acute necrotizing valvulitis, valve thickening, and fibrosis with occasional calcification and distortion. Conduction system abnormality is seen especially in neonates. Maternal SLE is a well-established cause of fetal bradycardia and CHB leading to hydrops fetalis. AV block (I, II, III degree), bundle branch block, sick sinus syndrome, sinus tachycardia, atrial premature contractions, and atrial fibrillation have all been reported in patients with lupus. These may be secondary to vasculitis, focal myocarditis, or ischemic injury to the nodal vasculature due to thrombosis or atherosclerosis. Coronary involvement in the form of thrombosis, embolism, accelerated atherosclerosis, or combination of these may cause myocardial infarction. Aneurysms in coronaries have also been reported. Rarely, pulmonary arterial hypertension has been reported in patients with lupus and requires lifelong follow-up.[7]

Investigations

Antinuclear antibody (ANA) is usually positive (≥1:160), though not essential for diagnosis of SLE. Anti-double stranded-DNA, anti-smooth muscle antibody, and anti-RNP are more specific for SLE. Hypocomplementemia provides a measure of disease activity.[8] Supportive evidence is provided by complete blood count, platelet count, erythrocyte sedimentation rate (ESR), urinalysis, rheumatoid factor, blood urea nitrogen (BUN), creatinine, serum glutamic oxaloacetic transaminase (SGOT), serum glutamic pyruvate transaminase (SGPT), gamma-glutamyl transpeptidase (GGTP), amylase, lipase, venereal disease research laboratory (VDRL), Coombs test, and prothrombin time/partial thromboplastin time (kaolin) (PT/PTTK). Echocardiography forms the mainstay of diagnosis of cardiac involvement. Attention must be paid to the pericardial space, the myocardial function, the valves, and an estimate of the pulmonary artery pressure.

Management

Pericarditis producing pain and tachycardia may be treated with indomethacin or prednisone. Significant pericardial effusion rarely requires drainage; emergency pericardiocentesis has been described in a few cases. Control of disease (SLE) activity usually suffices. Myocarditis causing significant myocardial dysfunction will benefit from standard anti-heart failure therapy and a course of prednisone.

Neonatal Lupus

Neonatal lupus is characterized by CHB (50% of cases), a transient rash and mild hepatobiliary disease. This is associated with transplacental passage of maternal autoantibodies (16–28 weeks gestational age)—anti-SSA, anti-SSB, or both. Approximately 2% of women with such antibodies have fetuses with CHB. The damage becomes evident at 22–24 weeks of gestation by which time there is destruction of the AV nodal tissue and replacement of normal nodal tissue with fibrotic tissue. This causes fetal bradycardia, which is at times associated with congestive cardiac failure, hydrops fetalis, or pericarditis. Fluorinated glucocorticoids (dexamethasone and betamethasone) have been used in fetal CHB but multiple studies have failed to demonstrate its efficacy.[9] Maternal therapy with beta-agonists (salbutamol and terbutaline) is occasionally used, in the hope of elevating the fetal heart rate.[10]

About 65% of babies born with CHB due to neonatal lupus require pacemakers, often in the newborn period.[11] Mortality rate of 20% is usually due to congestive cardiac failure in infancy. 20% of children with neonatal lupus/complete congenital heart block (CCHB) develop dilated cardiomyopathy (DCM) despite receiving a pacemaker in a timely fashion. Aortic root dilatation has been reported in 13.5% cases of neonatal lupus.

Polyarteritis Nodosa

This is a necrotizing vasculitis affecting the small and medium-sized vessels (most commonly those of renal, gastrointestinal tract, muscles, and the nervous system). Thrombosis and microaneurysm formation may occur at the site of vessel injury with healing occurring by the proliferation of fibrous tissue (at times causing vessel occlusion). Cardiac involvement includes mitral or tricuspid regurgitation, depressed ventricular function, and pericardial thickening. Less frequently, pericardial effusion, coronary arteritis, myocardial infarction, and ventricular hypertrophy may be seen. These may manifest as arrhythmias in the form of supraventricular tachycardia (SVT), cardiomegaly, and congestive cardiac failure.[12]

Investigations

Definite diagnosis is difficult and requires either tissue biopsy (muscle, kidney, skin, or sural nerve) or angiography of medium/small-sized arteries. Echocardiography detects ventricular dysfunction or valvar regurgitation.

Management

Corticosteroid therapy—oral prednisolone 1–2 mg/kg/day for 4 weeks and subsequent tapering of the dose is the recommended therapy. Cyclophosphamide has also been used for nonresponders and also those developing steroid toxicity.

Takayasu Arteritis

This is a chronic inflammatory disease that involves the aorta, the proximal portions of the major branches, and the pulmonary arteries, resulting in varying degrees of stenosis, occlusion, or dilatation of the involved vessels. Predominantly, a disease of young adults in their second or third decade of life, it may occur in children, but rarely in infants. It is relatively more common in the Asian and Mexican population. Female:male ratio varies from 9:1 in Japanese population and 1.3:1 in India. Genetic predisposition to Takayasu arteritis has been extensively studied and has revealed association of the disease with HLA B-52 and DR-2 in Japanese population, HLA B-39 in the Mexican population, and HLA B-52 and B-5 in the Indian population.

Exact pathogenesis of this disease is unknown. Its relationship to tuberculosis (TB) has been long debated. Possibly, the pathogenetic mechanism may be related to genetically linked immune responses to an unidentified antigen inciting autoimmune damage by cell-mediated pathways resulting in the disease and its relapses.[13]

The clinical features have been characterized by two overlapping phases:

1. An acute, active inflammatory prepulseless phase
2. A chronic pulseless end-stage phase.

Based on angiographic morphology, Takayasu arteritis is divided into type I (involving aortic arch and its branches), type II (thoracoabdominal aorta and its branches), type III (involving lesions both type I and II), and type IV (involvement of pulmonary arteries in addition to any of the other types).

Clinical Presentation

The child may present with the usual constitutional symptoms in the acute phase with normally palpable peripheral pulses and blood pressure. As the disease progresses into the chronic, pulseless phase, the child may present with claudication, absent or decreased brachial and radial pulses, wide pulse pressure, aortic incompetence, hypertension, congestive cardiac failure, and syncope. Hypertension is usually a result of renal artery stenosis or aortic narrowing or aortic fibrosis. This may even be severe enough to cause hypertensive encephalopathy or heart failure. Heart failure (resulting from hypertension, coronary involvement, valvar involvement, or pulmonary artery involvement) is common in Takayasu arteritis in children and contributes significantly to mortality. Neurological symptoms such as headache, visual disturbances, amaurosis fugax, syncope, transient ischemic attacks, or cerebrovascular accidents can also be present.

Investigations

Diagnosis is made on the basis of clinical history and the angiographic morphology. Diagnostic criteria have been suggested by Ishikawa and the American College of Rheumatology (**Table 1**) which have incorporated clinical features (age of onset, blood pressure, peripheral pulses, and ESR) and angiographic morphology.[14,15] Though none of the diagnostic criteria are entirely satisfactory, they aid in arriving at an accurate diagnosis.

Takayasu arteritis is diagnosed if at least three of these six criteria are present.

Diagnosis is easier in the chronic phase by ultrasonography with color Doppler showing mural thickening and a turbulent flow in the aorta and branches. Echocardiography may detect aortic root dilation, aortic regurgitation, mitral regurgitation, or coronary artery involvement. Computed tomography (CT) angiography and magnetic resonance (MR) angiography can effectively reveal the thickening and calcification of the aorta and its branches and also the enhancement with inflammation with activity of the disease.

TABLE 1: 1990 criteria of American College of Rheumatology for the classification of Takayasu arteritis.

Criteria	*Definition*
Age at disease onset in year	Development of symptoms or findings related to Takayasu arteritis at age <40 years
Claudication of extremities	Development and worsening of fatigue and discomfort in muscles of one or more extremity while in use, especially the upper extremities
Decreased brachial artery	Decreased pulsation of one or both brachial arteries pulse
BP difference >10 mm Hg	Difference of >10 mm Hg in systolic blood pressure between arms
Bruit over subclavian arteries or aorta	Bruit audible on auscultation over one or both subclavian arteries or abdominal aorta
Arteriogram abnormality	Arteriographic narrowing or occlusion of the entire aorta, its primary branches, or large arteries in the proximal upper or lower extremities, not due to arteriosclerosis, fibromuscular dysplasia, or similar causes: changes usually focal or segmental

Assessment of Disease Activity

The presence of systemic symptoms, raised ESR (>20 mm/1st hour), and worsening vessel stenosis (claudication, disappearance of pulses, bruit, vascular pain, asymmetric blood pressures, angiographic features) are considered evidence of disease activity.

Management

During the pulseless phase, an elevated ESR or other signs of disease activity warrants oral steroids for 4 weeks (1 mg/kg/day) followed by slow tapering. Immunomodulation using cyclophosphamide (1–2 mg/kg/day), azathioprine (1–2 mg/kg/day), or methotrexate (0.15–0.35 mg/kg/week) may be tried in resistant cases or in order to facilitate reduction in steroid dose. Duration of treatment is guided by clinical assessment of disease activity. Control of hypertension with antihypertensives and management of cardiac failure is mainstay in therapy. Surgical intervention is required in case of severe arterial damage, when the arteritis is not active or has been adequately suppressed. Transcatheter balloon dilatation with or without stenting of the stenosed vessels has revolutionized the management of Takayasu arteritis though restenosis has also been well described.

Juvenile Idiopathic Arthritis

Juvenile idiopathic arthritis (JIA) or Still's disease is the most common form of chronic arthritis in the pediatric age group. Cardiac involvement is well-recognized and all layers of the heart may be affected. Cardiovascular complications form the second most common cause of mortality in JIA. According to the clinical presentation, JIA is classified into various forms, of which oligoarticular is the most common. However, cardiac involvement is most common in the systemic JIA.

Systemic Onset

Patients present with persistent fever (usually of [illegible] weeks duration) with an evanescent rash, hepatosplenomegaly, and generalized lymphadenopathy. Arthritis may or may not be present. Pericarditis and myocarditis are frequently seen along with pleuritis. Some patients with systemic JIA may develop cardiac tamponade or myocarditis during the acute phase; which may even cause death. Valvulitis is rare and manifests as aortic or mitral regurgitation. Other abnormalities seen are pulmonary hypertension (PH) and conduction system disturbances.[16] Due to better disease-modifying drugs being available, survival is enhanced, but effects of premature atherosclerosis are manifest. This causes myocardial infarction due to coronary atherosclerosis.

Investigations

Baseline investigations may reveal anemia, leukocytosis, and increased ESR. Rheumatoid factor and ANA are rarely seen. HLA-B27 histocompatibility is seen in 25% of the cases.

Cardiomegaly is noted on chest radiograph. ECG shows nonspecific ST-segment and T-wave changes. Echocardiography outlines the cardiac involvement in terms of pericardial, myocardial, or valvar involvement. Cardiac biomarkers will be elevated with myocardial inflammation. CMR imaging is increasingly being used to pick up subtle cardiac involvement. Tissue characterization with T1/T2 mapping indices and LGE protocol may help detect subclinical myocardial inflammation or fibrosis.

Management

Pericarditis is treated with high-dose salicylates or nonsteroidal anti-inflammatory drugs (NSAIDs) and steroids. Steroids are also useful in decreasing the risk of cardiac tamponade. Tamponade is managed with pericardiocentesis. Myocarditis warrants high-dose steroids and standard anti-heart failure regimen (ACE inhibitors or angiotensin receptor blockers along with beta-blockers and diuretics). Intravenous (IV) immunoglobulins (Igs) have also been used successfully in myocarditis related to JIA.

DISORDERS OF COLLAGEN SYNTHESIS

Marfan Syndrome

Marfan syndrome is autosomal dominant in inheritance with an incidence of 1/3,000–4,000 people. The phenotypic features of this condition are present from birth and the patients manifest with tall stature, arm span more than their height, long and thin fingers (arachnodactyly), high arched palate, chest deformity, kyphoscoliosis, ectopia lentis, and myopia. Ocular abnormalities are seen in almost 75% of the cases.

The cardiovascular manifestations of this disorder include mitral valve prolapse and mitral regurgitation along with aortic root dilatation. Mitral abnormalities are seen in almost two-thirds of the patients with annular dilation and occasional calcification. Aortic root dilation is seen in 50% of young children and progresses with age (**Fig. 4**). This leads to aortic valve noncoaptation and aortic regurgitation, valve rupture, and at times even dissection of the diseased aortic wall. Left ventricle and left atrium undergo progressive dilatation and LV dysfunction ensues.

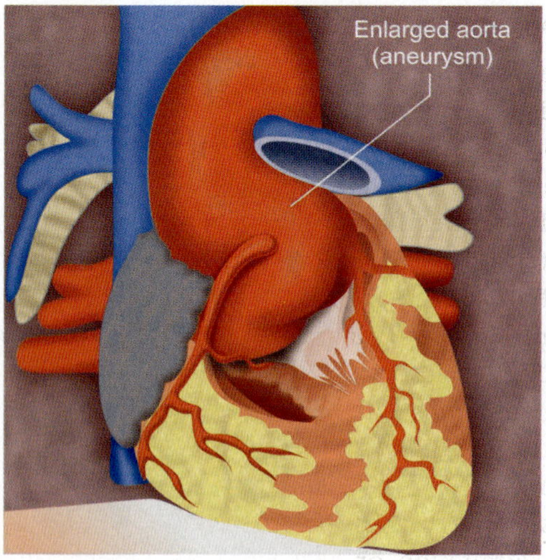

Fig. 4: Typical aortic root in Marfan syndrome.
(*Source*: Mayo Clinic: www.mayoclinic.org)

Diagnosis

The revised Ghent criteria gives weightage to systemic features, family history, lens dislocation, and aortic root dilatation as also mutation in fibrillin 1 (FBN1) gene.[17] In the absence of family history, aortic root dilation and ectopia lentis are sufficient to diagnose Marfan syndrome. As systemic features may manifest over time, a diagnosis of potential Marfan syndrome may be made. Other overlapping clinical syndromes such as Loeys–Dietz and Shprintzen-Goldberg have to be considered if the genetic tests do not support the diagnosis of Marfan syndrome. ECG shows signs of left ventricle and left atrial enlargement in the presence of significant valvar regurgitation. Arrhythmias viz. AV block (first degree), atrial flutter, fibrillation, and ventricular arrhythmias are also common. Screening with an echocardiogram is essential at the time of suspicion of Marfan/Marfan spectrum disorder. Careful and serial measurements of the aortic root dimensions (sinus of Valsalva diameter is vital) must be made. There are aortic root dimension calculators available online (*www.parameterz.com*). Mitral valve prolapse and regurgitation is also followed serially. Occasionally chordal rupture is seen. CMR in children with Marfan syndrome is sensitive in detection of aortic vascular disease along with accurate measurements of the aortic root.

Management

Beta-blockers (propranolol, atenolol, and metoprolol) are used to slow progression of aortic valve disease. Occasionally angiotensin receptor blockers are added. The guidelines for surgical intervention for elective root replacement/repair are based on a combination of aortic root dimensions and/or rate of growth of the aortic root and worsening of aortic regurgitation and positive family history of aortic dissection and death.

Ehlers–Danlos Syndrome

The features of this syndrome include flat nasal bridge; epicanthic folds with hyperextensibility of joints and increased skin elasticity, poor wound healing, and easy bruising. They may also have other ocular signs such as blue sclera, dislocated lens, and easy eversion of upper eyelid (Ménétrier's sign).

Cardiac manifestations in vascular Ehlers–Danlos syndrome include mitral valve prolapse or tricuspid valve prolapse. Rarely, death may also occur due to hemorrhage from arterial or aortic rupture, secondary to minor trauma. Premature death is also known in most severe forms.

Osteogenesis Imperfecta

Osteogenesis imperfecta or brittle bone disease is a generalized connective tissue disorder and the most common genetic cause of osteoporosis. It is autosomal dominant in inheritance with an incidence of 1 in 20,000 live births. Five types have been described of varying severity and all types are caused by structural or quantitative defects in type I procollagen genes.

Fragile/brittle bones is the hallmark of this condition with multiple, subperiosteal fractures. Skull usually consists of wormian bones with frontoparietal bossing. Sclera is blue in most types (except in type IV). Short stature and dental abnormalities are common associations. Cardiovascular manifestations include aortic root dilatation and mitral valve regurgitation or at times mitral valve prolapse due to ruptured chordae. Congenital heart diseases such as tetralogy of Fallot and atrial septal defect (ASD) have also been reported in association with osteogenesis imperfecta.

INFECTIONS

Diphtheria

Diphtheria is a vaccine-preventable disease that has become less prevalent in the developing world in the recent decades. However, India remains the country with a disproportionately larger number of cases as per current World Health Organization data. The causative organism is a gram-positive bacillus, *Corynebacterium diphtheriae*, and the toxicity is mediated through a toxin. The age group most affected is under 10 years population which is a change from the previously affected age profile of <5 years.[18] The common presenting symptoms and signs are fever, pseudomembrane in throat, sore throat, neck swelling, dysphagia, and cough. The heart is involved in 10–20% of cases and is the most common cause of death in genetically susceptible individuals.[19] The exotoxin causes myocardial inflammation and disruption of the conduction tissue leading to arrhythmias (tachycardias or heart block) and/or heart failure. This can appear at any time point in the illness, from early on to weeks later. The conduction block may be rapidly progressive and life-threatening.

Investigations

Diagnosis of diphtheria is by clinical presentation and demonstrating toxin production in isolated diphtheria bacillus from a throat swab. The ECG shows ventricular tachycardias or conduction block. The echocardiogram may show ventricular dilatation and dysfunction in patients with myocarditis.

Management

Isolation, antibiotics, and diphtheria antiserum are mainstay of therapy. A higher dose of the antiserum is required in the presence of cardiac disease. The control of ventricular tachycardia is via usual antiarrhythmics. A temporary or permanent pacemaker may be required for conduction block. The treatment of heart failure is with standard therapy.[20] Digoxin is avoided as it may worsen heart block or cause fatal arrhythmias in acute myocarditis.

Dengue Fever

Dengue is an important mosquito-borne viral disease endemic to the tropical and subtropical zones of the world. It is caused by any of the four dengue virus serotypes (DENV 1, 2, 3, 4). The clinical presentation usually varies from a milder flu-like symptoms to severe disease characterized by respiratory distress, arrhythmias, and cardiogenic shock.[21] Cardiac involvement is seen in 15–20% of cases with dengue infection requiring hospitalization and may manifest with only elevation of biomarkers at times to fulminant myocarditis and/or pericarditis leading to death. The pathophysiology for cardiac involvement is activation of the immune system leading to injury by proinflammatory cytokines and mediators, endothelial damage, and increased vascular permeability. This leads to myocardial edema, altered coronary microcirculation, and altered intracellular calcium metabolism. The viral load or severity of infection has shown no correlation to the severity of cardiac manifestations. Pericarditis and pericardial effusion rarely require intervention.

Investigations

Confirmation of dengue is by viral serology. The cardiac biomarkers creatine phosphokinase-MB (CPK-MB), NT-Pro-BNP, and troponin I or T are elevated in those with myocardial injury. ECG in myocardial involvement shows disproportionate sinus tachycardia, conduction abnormalities, tachycardias, and pattern of acute myocardial infarction. Targeted and functional echocardiography in pediatric intensive care settings is extremely useful in these cases to check the LV ejection fraction, wall motion abnormalities, and volume status.[22] Inappropriate tachycardia, unresponsive shock, and falling hematocrit despite fluid resuscitation are signs that there is cardiac dysfunction.

Management

Intravenous inotropes may be required. Standard anti-heart failure therapy can be used. IVIgs and steroid therapy may be tried in fulminant myocarditis.

COVID-19 Infection

The novel Coronavirus or SARS-CoV-2 is the latest addition to the long list of viruses that affect the heart. The cardiac manifestations of Covid-19 infection in children are believed to be due to a late immunological response (usually after 2–3 weeks of the acute infection) unlike the acute myocarditis as seen in adults. Children have a less severe viral prodrome and manifest with pediatric multisystem inflammatory syndrome, which shares overlapping features with conditions such as Kawasaki disease and toxic shock syndrome.[23] Clinical manifestations of this disease include fever with nonspecific abdominal pain, gastrointestinal symptoms, myocarditis, and shock.[24]

Investigations

Nasopharyngeal swab for viral RNA detection and also serum antibody (IgG and IgM) presence or absence is helpful. There have been cases where the antibody is positive but viral swab is negative. Neutrophilia with relative lymphopenia, elevated C-reactive protein and ESR, and a normal platelet count are generally seen. Serum ferritin, fibrinogen, AST, and triglycerides, d-dimers, and interleukin-6 (IL-6) are likely to be elevated. Elevated troponin I/T and CPK-MB indicate acute myocardial injury.[25] Chest radiograph shows cardiomegaly with pleural/pericardial effusion and pulmonary infiltrates. Echocardiography shows depressed myocardial function, pericardial effusion, and at times coronary dilation (as seen in Kawasaki disease).

Management

Most children have responded to inotropic drugs along with IV immunoglobulin and IV steroids (pulse methylprednisolone) with a better response when given early in the course of the illness. Though there is no conclusive data regarding the temporal relation between Covid-19 and Kawasaki disease, pediatricians should be aware of this atypical presentation and the need for early referral to a tertiary care center.

Human Immunodeficiency Virus

Cardiovascular involvement in human immunodeficiency virus (HIV)-infected children is very common and prevalence ranges from 75% to over 90% and is the cause of death in 10–25% of the cases.[26] The prevalence is higher in children lacking access to HAART (highly active antiretroviral treatment).[27] The pathogenesis of cardiac involvement in HIV infection is uncertain; but probable theories are autoimmunity, prolonged immunosuppression, cardiotoxicity from antiretroviral drugs (zidovudine), opportunistic infections, and coexisting nutritional deficiencies.[28] Cardiac lesions in HIV are often subclinical and progressive to include ventricular dilation, cardiomyopathy, myocarditis, valvulitis, pulmonary hypertension, and pericardial effusion.[29] Pericardial effusion has been noted in at least 11% of cases infected with HIV implying that HIV should be ruled out in all children presenting with unexplained pericardial effusion or tamponade. The rate of infective endocarditis due to the usual organisms and also opportunistic infections is high with at least 30% higher mortality than in non-HIV affected patients. HIV-related primary PH is a well-known entity, though the pathogenesis is still unclear and is considered to be multi-factorial. Affected children present with right ventricular failure for which therapy with anticoagulation and vasodilators is recommended. The antiretroviral therapy (HAART) may also cause cardiac side effects, thus warranting a regular or annual cardiac assessment to evaluate the progression of cardiac involvement in these children.

Investigations

Manifest or overt cardiac disease can be picked up on history, clinical examination, chest radiography, and ECG. The subclinical manifestations such as LV dilatation, dysfunction (systolic and diastolic), and hypertrophy need to be detected on echocardiography. Serial echocardiographic studies showing LV dilation may be a predictor for congestive cardiac failure in future. CMR with tissue characterization may help in diagnosing myocarditis.

Management

Few centers have reported use of IV immunoglobulin to normalize LV dysfunction in children with HIV-1 infection.[30]

Tuberculosis

Though TB leads the list of infectious diseases in India, cardiovascular manifestations in TB are seen only in 1–2% of the cases. Pericardium is the most commonly affected part of the heart, but myocardium and endocardium (valves) may also be rarely involved. The most common finding is that of pericardial effusion (acute or chronic) which may lead to a cardiac tamponade when compared to most other extrapulmonary TB. Constrictive pericarditis, which occurs due to the thickening of the visceral pericardium, is the late sequelae of the disease and accounts for more than two-thirds of the cases of constrictive pericarditis in India. TB pericarditis is always a secondary presentation to a focus elsewhere in the body, which spreads by direct extension from the tracheobronchial tree, spine, and hilar or mediastinal lymph nodes. Hematogenous spread from a pulmonary focus has also been noted in a few cases. Diagnosis of isolated myocarditis due to TB is very uncommon in children, though not unknown.[31] The mode of spread is through lymphatics, direct seeding from the pericardium, or hematogenous. It may present as acute, fulminant myocarditis with severe ventricular dysfunction and failure. The other features seen are conduction abnormalities such as AV blocks and ventricular arrhythmias which may lead to sudden cardiac death. Valvar (endocardial) involvement due to TB is more often a postmortem finding. A diffuse infiltrative form has also been reported.[32] Timely diagnosis and appropriate therapy is the key to managing these cases.

Investigations

Gastric aspiration is used to collect specimen for microscopic examination/culture of mycobacteria or gene amplification. Lymph node biopsy (maybe CT-guided) may also help. Pericardial fluid may also be examined. Cardiac catheterization is occasionally used to diagnose constrictive pericarditis where clinical or echocardiographical tools are insufficient to distinguish between constrictive pericarditis and restrictive cardiomyopathy.[33]

Management

The infection is treated with sensitive antitubercular drugs for an appropriate duration of 6 months along with a 4-week adjunctive therapy of oral corticosteroids. Pericardiocentesis is necessary in patients with massive pericardial effusion and those in cardiac tamponade. Pericardiectomy may be required in cases with constrictive pericarditis who are symptomatic with signs of right heart failure. Creating a pericardial window with insertion of pigtail catheter or drain is carried out for cases of pyopericardium (if facilities for pericardiectomy is unavailable).

Lyme Disease

Lyme disease is caused by the spirochete, *Borrelia burgdorferi*, which is transmitted by the bite of Ixodes tick. Most patients present with the classic rash of Lyme disease, erythema migrans, and arthritis. The disease is rare in the Indian subcontinent but must be kept as a possibility in children presenting with rash, arthritis, or cardiac involvement. Male-to-female ratio for Lyme carditis is 3:1. There is a 16% chance of carditis.[34] Older children who present with arthralgia are more likely to develop carditis. The cardiac manifestations generally present in stage 2 of the illness (early disseminated phase), which is 3–4 weeks after the onset of other symptoms. The cardiac involvement may range from first-degree AV block to CHB and myocarditis. There have been studies from Europe implicating Lyme disease as a cause of DCM on endomyocardial biopsy. The unique feature about the conduction abnormality in Lyme disease is that it can fluctuate to different degrees of AV block within minutes. Clinical manifestations of Lyme carditis vary widely ranging from being asymptomatic to pre-syncope/syncope, chest pain, palpitations, and dyspnea.

Investigations

Diagnosis is established by a history of exposure to ticks, travel, clinical symptoms, and serological evidence. Cardiac evaluation usually reveals varying degrees of AV block on ECG and ST segment depression, T-wave changes in case of myopericarditis. Echocardiography is diagnostic for systolic dysfunction and pericarditis. Electrophysiological studies have been reported with direct, diffuse involvement of the AV node conduction system with no increase in the vagal tone and hence no response to atropine. Fortunately, AV blocks are generally transient and the acquired AV block responds well to antibiotic therapy. In fact, early initiation of antibiotics has shown to decrease the incidence of cardiac involvement.

Management

Most cases respond to a 14-day course of oral doxycycline (older than 8 years) or amoxicillin or cefuroxime. Sick children may require parenteral ceftriaxone therapy. Temporary pacing is necessary in a small population of cases, but the need for permanent pacemaker implantation is extremely rare.

Malaria

Malaria has played a major role in human history, having caused more harm to people than any other infectious disease. Malaria is of overwhelming importance in the developing world today as most malarial deaths occur in infants and young children. In endemic countries such as India, children <5 years get repeated and often serious attacks of malaria. Cardiovascular manifestations are responsible for the major morbidity in malaria in children. The main aim of antimalarial treatment in children, which is also the basis of National Antimalarial Program, is to prevent early morbidity and death by early diagnosis and prompt treatment. Cardiac involvement in malaria used to be limited to *Plasmodium falciparum* monoinfection rather than mixed infections (with *Plasmodium vivax/malariae*) but *P. vivax* appears to be causing frequent systemic illnesses and cardiac involvement as well.[35] The cardiac manifestations include pericardial effusion, myocarditis, and conduction blocks.[36,37] Mortality due to cardiac cause alone is extremely rare.

Investigations

Cardiomegaly on X-ray and prolonged PR interval on ECG are seen in about 6–10% of the cases. Echocardiography may show pericardial effusion, LV dysfunction with AV valve regurgitation.

Management

Standard antimalarial medications are used in addition to anti-heart failure medications as required.

Chikungunya

Chikungunya is a mosquito borne illness caused by an RNA-type arbovirus species that belongs to the Togaviridae family. The word "Chikungunya" means "which contorts or bends up" in Makonde language from Tanzania, due to the classical symptom of severe bone involvement and difficulty in ambulation along with a self-limiting febrile illness in those affected. It has three phases spread over several weeks: acute, subacute, and chronic with 20% of affected people remaining asymptomatic. The cardiovascular system is the second most affected system after joints with gastrointestinal, dermatological, hepatic, and hematological manifestations also seen. Cardiovascular involvement is severe in children when associated with an underlying heart disease and presents with clinical features of heart failure, myocarditis, arrhythmias, and pericarditis.[38] The virus penetrates the myocytes causing direct damage to the muscle fibers. Additionally, the inflammatory response leads to secondary damage by hypersensitivity reaction and necrosis.[39] The initial phase has nonspecific symptoms. Arrhythmias in the form of atrial fibrillation progressing to severe ventricular arrhythmias and sudden cardiac death have been reported in the second phase of the illness. The third phase is that of heart failure with circulatory shock which requires intensive care with vasoactive medications.

Investigations

Epidemiological and clinical features are useful to make a diagnosis. Diagnosis is established by polymerase chain reaction (PCR) techniques in the acute phase and thereafter by serological/immunological testing for presence of CHIKV IgG. The initial investigations may show mild cardiomegaly on chest radiography with nonspecific T-wave changes on ECG. CMR may be needed in a few cases of myocarditis leading to DCM on follow-up.

Management

A specific management protocol is lacking. Standard anti-heart failure therapy is useful. There have been anecdotal reports of successful usage of levocarnitine, steroids in anti-inflammatory doses, and aspirin.

Parasitic Infections

Parasitic infections are very common in children in tropical countries and range from helminths to protozoa. *Ascaris lumbricoides* (roundworm), *Ancylostoma duodenale* (hookworms), *Enterobius vermicularis* (pinworm, threadworm), *Wuchereria bancrofti* (filarial worm), *Brugia malayi*, *Trichuris trichiura* (whip worm), *Taenia solium* (pig tapeworm), *Echinococcus granulosus* (dog tapeworm), dog heartworm, etc., are a few common helminths and they usually infest humans through the feco-oral route. Protozoan parasites include *Entamoeba histolytica*, *Trypanosoma cruzi*, *Toxoplasma gondii*, etc. These parasites produce toxic metabolites with eosinophilia causing direct cell-mediated damage to cardiac myocytes, microvasculature, and neurons. This leads to hyaline degeneration of the myocytes, pulmonary eosinophilia, and tropical endomyocardial fibrosis resulting in congestive cardiac failure, myocardial dysfunction, pulmonary arterial hypertension, and cardiac arrhythmias (tachyarrhythmias or heart block). The parasites and migratory larvae may also attack normal or prosthetic valves causing valvar regurgitation.

Many cases of primary PH have been diagnosed secondary to filariasis (*Wuchereria bancrofti*/*B. malayi*), and schistosomiasis (flatworms).[40] This occurs due to the tropical pulmonary eosinophilia (TPE) caused by type I hypersensitivity reaction to the filarial antigen leading to interstitial fibrosis and restrictive lung function. The eosinophils in the lungs degranulate to produce toxic free oxygen radicals that lead to a chronic pulmonary inflammatory process leading to PH. The circulating cytokines and immune complexes induced by schistosomula and egg depositions is the cause for PAH in schistosomiasis.

Filariasis is common in Uttar Pradesh, Bihar, Odisha, and some areas of South India. Diagnosis of PH secondary to TPE is made on clinical history of wheezy cough (predominantly nocturnal) with intermittent fever and progressive breathlessness with signs of right heart failure. Laboratory investigations show peripheral eosinophilia with increased IgE levels and presence of microfilaria on peripheral smear or antigen positivity for filariasis. CXR shows pulmonary infiltrates with prominent pulmonary artery and increased reticular shadows. ECG is suggestive of right axis deviation with right ventricular hypertrophy (RVH) and echocardiography shows evidence of right heart enlargement with tricuspid regurgitation. Treatment includes diuretics, diethylcarbamazine (DEC) @ 6 mg/kg/day for 3 weeks and steroids (low-dose for 6 weeks) with a good response on follow-up. Hence, exclusion of TPE as etiology for PH in tropical parts of the world is advisable. Conversely, all cases of eosinophilia should have PH ruled out.

Scorpion Sting Envenomation

Scorpion sting is an acute, life-threatening, rural emergency. The case fatality rates range from 3 to 22% in children hospitalized for scorpion sting in India, Saudi Arabia, and South Africa. There are over 80 species of scorpions in India, of which only two are of medical importance. Cardiovascular effects are particularly prominent following the stings by the species called *Mesobuthus tamulus* (Indian red scorpion). The venom contains various amino acids, serotonin, hyaluronidase, and other enzymes. The toxin acts by opening sodium channels and inhibiting calcium dependent potassium channels, thus causing an autonomic storm that presents as vomiting, excessive salivation, sweating, hypertension, tachycardia, cold extremities, myocardial dysfunction, and pulmonary edema.[41] Severe vasoconstriction occurs due to the catecholamine surge. Hypertensive stress leading to myocyte toxicity with LV failure and arrhythmias is common in children. Hypotension and bradycardia may be seen in the first 1–2 hours of sting due to cholinergic stimulation, but persistent bradycardia with hypotension beyond 4 hours of the sting suggests severe LV dysfunction. The level of toxicity depends on the species and the dosage of venom to weight ratio. Symptoms are most severe within 4–5 hours after the sting and subside within 1–2 days. Pulmonary edema may occur within half hour after the sting and can present as tachypnea and refractory cough in pale-looking children with respiratory distress. At times, this can occur even when the child seems to be recovering and hence a periodic, thorough clinical examination is important in such cases.

Investigations

Serial ECGs are recommended. CXR shows pulmonary vascular congestion with a normal cardiac silhouette and interlobar effusions. Echocardiography shows LV systolic dysfunction but LV dilation or regional wall motion abnormalities are rare. Cardiac markers such as CPK-MB and BNP may be elevated.

Management

Prazosin forms the mainstay of therapy and acts by suppressing sympathetic outflow and activating the venom-inhibited potassium channels.[42] It causes a decrease in the preload, afterload, and blood pressure. It is also a phosphodiesterase inhibitor and prevents myocardial injury. Pediatric dosage is 30 μg/kg/dose in all those with an autonomic storm, given as an emergency drug through nasogastric tube in cases of severe vomiting. Blood pressure, pulse rate, and respiration must be monitored every 30 minutes for 3 hours, every hour for next 6 hours and later every 4 hours till improvement. A repeat dose of prazosin can be given at the end of 3 hours according to clinical response and later every 6 hours till extremities are warm, dry, and peripheral veins are seen easily. Diazepam is often used to keep the child calm and some may require NSAIDs for pain management. In case of pulmonary edema, diuretics forms the mainstay of therapy to decrease the fluid load along with dobutamine and sodium nitroprusside or nitroglycerin. Scorpion antivenom if available should be given within 30 minutes of the sting for optimal effect.

ENDOCRINE AND METABOLIC CONDITIONS

Diabetes Mellitus

Diabetes mellitus increases the risk of cardiac, cerebral, and vascular diseases by two- to seven-fold. The annual incidence of juvenile diabetes is 8–10/100,000. Since the cardiac complications occur later in age, the pediatric cardiologist usually gets to manage the infants of diabetic mothers. There is an increased risk of ventricular septal defect (VSD) and transposition of great vessels in these babies. Even in the absence of these structural abnormalities, the infants of diabetic mothers have a host of other cardiac problems. Some infants have asymmetric septal hypertrophy. These infants are usually macrosomic due to increased body fat and have organomegaly due to increased fetal insulin and synthesis of glycogen, lipids, and proteins in response to hyperglycemia. After birth, they are jittery due to the hypoglycemia secondary to hyperinsulinemia, but some may be lethargic and hypotonic. Cardiomegaly is found in 30% and cardiac failure occurs in 5–10% of these infants. Echocardiography shows thickening of the right ventricular and LV free wall with septal hypertrophy. A spectrum of abnormalities ranging from mild ventricular hypertrophy to hypertrophic obstructive cardiomyopathy (HOCM) may occur in these infants. In case of HOCM, a harsh ejection systolic murmur may be heard due to the obstruction to the LV outflow.

There have been few studies in older children with type I DM, where there is an increase in the carotid intima media thickness (CIMT) and also LV dilation in almost 25% of the poorly controlled cases with a disease duration of over 6 months. Systemic hypertension with abnormal lipid profiles are also commonly associated features in these children.

Treatment

Children with diabetes-induced ventricular hypertrophy need only supportive care and the condition is usually reversible. Cardiac failure is treated with diuretics. Digitalis is avoided in the presence of obstruction. Subaortic obstruction improves with propranolol and may regress spontaneously within 1–2 months.

Pheochromocytoma

This is a catecholamine-secreting tumor, which causes hypertension as the major cardiovascular manifestation. 50% of the cases have myocardial evidence of focal necrosis with perivascular inflammation and inflammatory infiltration. Uncontrolled hypertension and direct involvement of the myocardium may lead to reversible DCM.[43] Surgery is the treatment of choice and use of alpha- and beta-adrenoreceptor blockers is essential for control of hypertension both pre- and post-surgery.

Thyroid Disorders

Thyroid hormone is essential for protein synthesis, growth and development, metabolism of carbohydrates, vitamins and minerals, and increases oxygen consumption by the tissues. It also accelerates the heart rate and myocardial contractility, partly due to the changes in the intracellular calcium levels and partly due to the action on the sympathetic nervous system.

Hypothyroidism

This occurs due to deficiency in the production of thyroid hormone or a defect in the thyroid hormone receptors, which may be congenital or acquired.

- *Congenital hypothyroidism*: Children with congenital hypothyroidism may have cardiomegaly mainly due to the thickening of the interventricular septum and LV free wall. 50% of the cases show presence of a slow-filling pericardial effusion due to increased systemic capillary permeability and electrolyte imbalance. Although it may be a large effusion, it usually does not cause cardiac tamponade. A few studies have reported dilated ventricles with dysfunction in a small population of children with severe hypothyroidism.

The infant may present with bradycardia, weak arterial pulses, distant heart sounds, hypotension and peripheral, non-pitting edema. ECG reveals low-voltage complexes, prolonged PR and QT intervals, with bradycardia. All these features revert on thyroid replacement, once the child achieves euthyroid state.[44]

- *Acquired hypothyroidism*: This condition most commonly occurs due to autoimmunity during childhood and adolescence and is also called juvenile hypothyroidism. Acquired hypothyroidism may also result from thyroid surgery, prolonged ingestion of goitrogens or iodides, and may also be seen after treatment with amiodarone (antiarrhythmic drug).

The cardiac features are similar to those seen with congenital hypothyroidism. Laboratory investigations may show hypercholesterolemia, which also reverts on correction of the hypothyroid state.

Hyperthyroidism

This occurs due to the excess of tri-iodothyronine (T3) or thyroxine (T4) or both and is most commonly accompanied by a diffuse goiter (Graves' disease).

- *Congenital hyperthyroidism*: This condition occurs in 1–2% of infants born to mothers with history of hyperthyroidism due to the transplacental passage of the thyroid-stimulating Ig. This condition usually remits spontaneously by 6–12 weeks of postnatal life.

The infant is usually premature with an anxious and alert look. He may present with tachycardia, tachypnea, bounding pulses, elevated temperature, and occasionally even with episodes of paroxysmal atrial tachycardia. Severe hypertension has also been reported in some.

Electrocardiogram shows evidence of peaked P-waves and chamber hypertrophy, which is reversible on treatment.

Therapy consists of Lugol's solution and propylthiouracil. Propranolol and corticosteroids are indicated in case of severe thyrotoxicity. Digitalis is added in case of congestive cardiac failure. The infant usually improves within the second and third month of life.

Graves' Disease

This is the most common cause of juvenile hyperthyroidism. Incidence is almost five times higher in females especially between 11 and 19 years of age. The patient may experience palpitations with tachycardia, cardiac hyperactivity, and dyspnea along with the other constitutional symptoms. Precordium is hyperactive with presence of mid-systolic murmur heard along the left sternal border, most likely due to presence of mitral valve incompetence. Mitral valve prolapse is seen in almost 30% of cases. 15–20% of the cases have evidence of atrial fibrillation. Tricuspid regurgitation is also a commonly reported feature of hyperthyroidism with myxomatous tricuspid valve with associated pulmonary hypertension.

Definitive therapy includes surgical removal of the gland or irradiation. Treatment of cardiovascular disease is difficult in patients with hyperthyroidism as arrhythmias and congestive cardiac failure may be resistant to the conventional doses of cardiac glycosides. Beta-blockers help in atrial fibrillation by slowing the heart rate, and can be administered orally or intravenously.

Nutritional Deficiencies and the Heart

Macronutrients and micronutrient deficiencies are very common in children of the Indian subcontinent due to poverty, malnutrition, cultural, and social reasons.[45] These deficiencies cause significant cardiac morbidity ranging from arrhythmias to cardiomyopathy and cardiac failure. Urban food fads of fat-laden junk food also increase the risk of heart disease as young adults. Specific nutrient deficiencies cause specific cardiac issues, a few of which will be covered in this discussion. These nutrients are either antioxidants or those that are known to affect myocardial energy production. Endogenous antioxidants include those like zinc in superoxide dismutase or selenium in glutathione peroxidase, free radical scavengers (e.g., vitamins A, C, or E), and metal chelators. Early recognition and optimization of many vitamin deficiencies help in prevention of cardiac damage.

Protein Energy Malnourishment

Protein energy malnourishment (PEM) remains a major health issue in the third world with a reported prevalence of >50% of children aged under 5 years in India. There is atrophy of various organs in PEM, inclusive of the heart muscle. Malnourishment has definitive effects on the myocardium.[46] Affected children have thinner walls and lower mass of the left ventricle. In severe PEM, there is depressed LV contractility expressed as reduced ejection fraction, global longitudinal strain, and tissue Doppler velocities. Troponin levels may be elevated in PEM associated with anemia, sepsis, and electrolyte disturbances, indicating myocardial damage. PEM produces hypotension, arrhythmias, cardiomyopathy, and sudden cardiac death.[47]

Magnesium

Magnesium is an important mineral that is vital for normal functioning of the body. It is a cofactor of over 300 enzymes involved in nerve conduction, muscle contraction, heart rhythmicity, protein synthesis, calcium and potassium homeostasis, blood pressure control, and blood sugar regulation. Magnesium is found in most foods that have a high fiber content, example green leafy vegetables. The recommended dietary allowance for a child for magnesium is 80–340 mg/day. In normal healthy states, magnesium deficiency is uncommon because the kidney regulates its excretion. Children with chronic diarrhea and fat malabsorption or those on chronic furosemide or lansoprazole therapy develop magnesium deficiency. Low magnesium levels in pediatric patients undergoing heart surgery are associated with an increased incidence of junctional ectopic tachycardia in the immediate postoperative period.[48] Magnesium may act through mechanisms of membrane stabilization (decreases potassium efflux from cell) and calcium channel blocking thereby reducing automaticity and AV node conduction speed. It homogenizes ventricular repolarization and this is thought to explain its role in torsades de pointes of long QT syndrome.[49]

Zinc

Zinc is a micronutrient that acts like a catalyst in over 100 enzymes involved in protein and DNA synthesis, wound healing, antioxidant activity, and immune function. Daily intake of zinc is essential. The recommended dietary allowance of zinc for a child is 3–10 mg daily. Zinc is found in meat, beans, nuts, and whole grains, but bioavailability of zinc is higher in meat as plants have phytates that inhibit intestinal zinc absorption. Zinc deficiency appears to be deleterious in adult patients with heart failure where there is increase in reactive oxygen and nitrogen molecules.[50] The postulated mechanism of action include increase in oxidative stress, disruption of the extracellular matrix (zinc is a component of matric metalloproteinases), and apoptosis of the cardiomyocytes. The cause of zinc deficiency in heart failure could be poor intake, reduced absorption, increased urinary loss, and increased uptake by stressed tissues. Standard anti-heart failure medications, ACE inhibitors, and ARBs also reduce serum zinc level.

Selenium

Selenium is a trace element found in small quantities in the soil. It is an essential component for DNA synthesis, thyroid hormone metabolism, reproduction, antioxidant activity, and immunity. Selenium reduces platelet aggregation, prevents oxidation of lipids and reduces inflammation, and is considered to have a role in heart failure management. However, multicenter studies are not unanimous in recommending selenium supplements in heart failure. The recommended dietary allowance for children is 15–55 µg daily. Selenium is consumed as food grains, meat, eggs, and fish. Food grown in certain parts of the world may have poor concentrations of selenium due to low content in soil. Selenium deficiency in developed nations is seen more often in the chronically ill, malnourished patients with malabsorption, and those on unsupplemented total parenteral nutrition. Selenium deficiency also is encountered when nutrient-limited diets are used for patients with phenylketonuria and refractory epilepsy (ketogenic diet).

- *Keshan disease*: This describes a cardiomyopathy associated with dietary selenium deficiency and a strain of coxsackievirus. Keshan is a county in China where children (and women of childbearing age) were on such a diet and developed DCM with a high mortality rate from 1930s to 1980s.[51] Glutathione peroxidase activity was found to be reduced in the affected children due to selenium deficiency and this resulted in free radical damage to cardiac myocytes manifesting histologically as multifocal necrosis and fibrotic replacement of cardiomyocytes.[52] Distribution of oral sodium selenite tablets resulted in a drop in the incidence of new cases of the cardiomyopathy.

Thiamine

Vitamin B1 (thiamine) is a vital water-soluble micronutrient important in carbohydrate and amino acid metabolism, synthesis of nucleic acids, neurotransmitters, and myelin along with roles in immunity, anti-inflammatory processes, and gene regulation. Its role as a coenzyme in aerobic metabolism of carbohydrates implies that a deficiency results in anaerobic metabolism and build-up of lactic acid. The recommended dietary allowance of thiamine for children is 0.2–1.2 mg daily.[53] It is widely available in meat, legumes, and vegetables. Daily intake of thiamine is essential. Pediatric cases of thiamine deficiency are most often found in breastfed infants of mothers on a staple diet of nonparboiled polished rice. Other scenarios where there is thiamine deficiency are malnourishment leading to poor intestinal absorption, complication of treatment of severe acute malnourishment, or chronic diarrhea. Deficiency of thiamine causes high-output cardiac failure due to poorly understood reasons. The causes include accumulation of lactate and pyruvate that causes severe vasodilation; myocardial edema and depressed ventricular function. PH as a sole feature has been described in an Indian case study.[54] This was a series of prospectively evaluated 66 infants from the southern state of Andhra Pradesh. They presented with features of lower respiratory tract infection, congestive heart failure, and PH as well on echocardiographic evaluation. The biventricular function was normal. The erythrocyte transketolase activity was depressed in these infants and their mothers. The response to thiamine therapy was rapid and complete with no residual damage to the heart. They stated that testing the erythrocyte transketolase activity was expensive and that a therapeutic challenge may be given to infants with a particular maternal dietary history and presentation with acute refractory heart failure.

Folic Acid, Vitamin B2 (Riboflavin), B6 and B12 (Cobalamin)

These are necessary for the conversion of homocysteine to methionine and hence a deficiency would lead to elevated plasma homocysteine levels. High homocysteine has been associated with increase in reactive-oxygen species (free radical damage), thrombogenicity, and endothelial dysfunction. However, in a large randomized double-blind trial of 5,000 adult patients with vascular disease or diabetes, a supplement of these vitamins did not reduce the risk of major cardiovascular events (coronary artery disease or stroke) after 5 years.[55] Additional studies are required to establish their role in preventive treatment of vascular disease.

Folate deficiency during pregnancy is casually associated with neural tube defects and congenital heart defects in fetuses. This association with CHD has been demonstrated in areas of the world where staple diet may be deficient in folate and not as much in other areas.[56]

Vitamin C

Association of vitamin C deficiency with heart disease is unknown. It has been linked to cardiovascular health especially atherosclerosis, due to its role as an antioxidant. It may help in hypertension due to its action on the cardiac vasculature in adults as shown by some studies.

Co-enzyme Q10

Co-enzyme Q10 is an endogenous fat-soluble quinolone and an antioxidant with membrane-stabilizing properties which is found in the mitochondria of organs with high energy requirements namely myocardium, liver, and kidney. It is an essential component of the mitochondrial electron transport chain. Co-enzyme Q10 may help by increasing adenosine triphosphate (ATP) production (heart failure is an energy-depleting state), anti-inflammatory action, and improving endothelial function.[57] It is produced by the body, but in a catabolic state such as heart failure, its availability is reduced. The suggested dosage for use in children with cardiomyopathy and heart failure is 4–15 mg/kg/day (up to 200 mg/day in older children). There is data to suggest that it may help in improving the exercise capacity in children with cardiac failure.

Carnitine

Carnitine plays an essential role in utilization of fatty acids by the cardiac muscle and a primary or secondary deficiency of carnitine can cause impaired energy production. It is believed to be a useful supplement in patients with cardiomyopathy, cardiac surgery, and even myocardial infarction. The dose is 50–75 mg/kg/day in children.

HEMATOLOGICAL CONDITIONS

Thalassemia Major

The hereditary, hemolytic anemia occurring due to deficient synthesis of beta-globin chain is known as beta-thalassemia major and is one of the most common forms of hemolytic anemias in India. Regular blood transfusions are necessary to prevent extramedullary erythropoiesis. Hemosiderosis is an obvious complication and leading cause of death, unless the patient is on optimal and timely chelation therapy. The major cardiac manifestations in patients with thalassemia (and other iron storage disorders) are due to iron overload. The iron deposits in children who have received multiple blood transfusions exceed the storage and detoxification capacity of ferritin. This causes the "free" iron (nontransferrin bound iron), which is oxidatively active to enter cardiac myocytes through nonspecific, poorly regulated cation channels leading to cardiac overload and damage. The other reasons for cardiac injury are anemia-induced ventricular dilatation, chronic hypoxia-induced myocardial dysfunction, and an increase in the amount of highly reactive iron radicals leading to oxidative damage to lipid cell membranes, nucleic acids, and proteins of cardiac myocytes.

There is restrictive cardiomyopathy with large quantities of iron deposited in the myocardium.[58,59] Unabated iron deposits then causes DCM. Pericarditis is seen in about 50% of the unchelated patients, which may appear as acute, self-limiting episodes lasting for 4–5 days. Congestive cardiac failure and cardiac arrhythmias may occur due to the myocardial siderosis and may be the cause of death that occurs usually in second or third decade of life. Patients present with easy fatigability and dyspnea on exertion in the initial stages which progresses to cardiac failure in advanced cases. Unusual presentations include syncope due to ventricular tachycardia or CHB.

Investigations

Echocardiography allows for serial follow-up of myocardial hypertrophy (linear dimensions of ventricular walls and cavity size) as well as detailed systolic and diastolic function analysis.[60] Restrictive cardiomyopathy causes diastolic dysfunction while end-state cardiomyopathy is the dilated form where there is systolic and diastolic dysfunction. Global longitudinal strain and tissue Doppler indices have been demonstrated to be a sensitive marker of LV dysfunction. Cardiac MR relaxation time with T2* assessment has proven to be a sensitive method to detect myocardial iron deposit as iron deposits shorten T2*.[61] This will permit early identification and hence early treatment of patients.

Management

Therapy includes an adequate and supervised transfusion program along with early initiation of chelation therapy, which will prevent the above complications. It has also been noted that the cardiac complications are significantly less when the hemoglobin is maintained steadily at about 10 g% with frequent, small transfusions. Digitalis, diuretics, and ACE inhibitors and beta-blockers are recommended for the treatment of the cardiac complications. Bone marrow/stem cell transplantation is the treatment of choice.

Sickle Cell Anemia

This is another relatively common type of hemolytic anemia occurring due to the replacement of fetal hemoglobin by hemoglobin-S. As a result, the erythrocytes become rigid and "sickle" during times of stress, which leads to occlusion of the capillaries. The cardiac manifestations of sickle cell anemia (SCA) include LV diastolic dysfunction and PH. The etiology of PH in SCA is believed to be multifactorial and includes chronic hypoxia, thromboembolism, hemoglobin reaction with nitric oxide (NO), and deactivating it and reduction in arginine availability for NO synthesis. PH has been reported in 25% of children in a recent study.[62] This study looked at echocardiographic parameters in children older than 10 years with SCA who underwent screening. All of them had normal biventricular function although LV dilatation was present in 25% of cases. The diastolic dysfunction described in adults may take time to develop and maybe a rare observation in the pediatric age group. There have been reports of myocardial ischemia occurring during the sickle crises in adult patients.

NEUROMUSCULAR DISEASES AND SPINAL MUSCULAR ATROPHY

Most of the neuromuscular diseases have cardiac manifestations. The common ones are Duchenne muscular dystrophy (DMD), Becker muscular dystrophy (BMD), Emery–Dreifuss dystrophy, Friedreich's ataxia, Barth syndrome, spinal muscular atrophy (SMA), and limb girdle muscle dystrophy. The involvement is usually in the form of myocardial dysfunction (cardiomyopathy) but other manifestations include conduction abnormalities. Cardiomyopathy is now considered the leading cause of death in these patients as they approach adulthood, as most are on home-based ventilation therapy to help in the respiratory failure component.[63]

Duchenne Muscular Dystrophy

This condition occurs due to the defect in the sarcolemmal membrane of the muscular cells causing cellular necrosis. It is X-linked recessive in inheritance and the incidence is one in 3,600 live male infants. Most patients are unable to walk by 10 years of age and few survive up to the second decade of life. Deterioration is a continuous process in these cases with the proximal muscles being involved early in the course of the disease. Cardiac involvement is very common mainly affecting the myocardium and is progressive in nature, causing skeletal muscle dysfunction.[64]

Investigations

Elevated levels of creatine kinase activity and biopsy of the muscle aid in diagnosis of this condition. Electromyography shows a decreased mean action potential voltage and duration with an increase in the number of polyphasic potentials. The gold standard would be the specific molecular genetic diagnosis by demonstration of deficient dystrophin by immunohistochemical staining of the tissue from muscle biopsy or by the DNA analysis of the peripheral blood. ECG may show presence of tall R-waves in the right precordial leads with narrow and deep Q-waves in the left precordial leads and limb leads. Conduction abnormalities are also commonly noted in these patients. Echocardiography shows systolic and diastolic dysfunction with an increase in the end-systolic and end-diastolic dimensions of the left ventricle. Global longitudinal strain (GLS) has been shown to detect subclinical ventricular dysfunction prior to a reduction in the LV ejection fraction. CMR is a sensitive test to detect myocardial fibrosis. It should be first performed when diagnosed with DMD and then periodically after age 10 years.

Management

Cardiac dysfunction is treated with ACE inhibitors, angiotensin receptor blockers, and also aldosterone antagonists (eplerenone). These medications appear to have a role by reverse myocardial remodeling. The overall disease progression may be also delayed by administration of oral corticosteroids, deflazacort. Antenatal screening for detection of carriers is necessary for genetic counseling.

Becker Muscular Dystrophy

This condition is very similar to DMD, though the onset and progression of the disease is delayed. The patient is unable to walk by the third decade and death occurs in the fifth decade (though the range may vary in individual cases). Management is similar to that of DMD.

Friedreich's Ataxia

This is a rare spinocerebellar neuromyelopathy, transmitted as an autosomal recessive condition with presentation at around 5–6 years of age. The neurological presentation includes ataxic gait, positive Romberg's test, absent tendon reflexes, lower limb weakness, loss of vibration and position sense, muscular atrophy, incoordination, and dysarthria.

Cardiac involvement occurs in many patients in the form of a concentric, symmetrical, progressive hypertrophic cardiomyopathy. Acute DCM and hypertrophic obstructed cardiomyopathy have also been rarely noted. These patients may present with dyspnea on exertion, palpitations, or angina. At times, soft systolic murmur is heard in the left sternal border and the apex with third and fourth heart sound.

Investigations

Diagnosis of this condition is based on the clinical manifestations with nerve conduction studies revealing gross reduction in the sensory conduction. ECG shows nonspecific ST-segment and T-wave changes with signs of ventricular hypertrophy with right or left axis deviation. Echocardiography is imperative in every case, since the clinical, radiographic, and electrocardiographical evaluation may be nonspecific in many cases. Echocardiogram shows impaired LV function with the systolic function of the posterior wall being more severely affected than the septum along with the other structural changes as described earlier. Delayed mitral valve opening is seen in almost all cases. Cardiac failure in 50% of the cases, cardiac arrhythmias, and respiratory complications are the major causes of death in Friedreich's ataxia.

Management

Symptomatic therapy with diuretics, judicious use of digoxin, and calcium antagonists is the mainstay of treatment in these children.

Spinal Muscular Atrophy

This is a degenerative disorder of the motor neurons causing programmed cell death or "apoptosis", beginning in the fetal life and progressing into infancy and childhood. It is autosomal recessive in inheritance.

Depending on the age of presentation, severity, and clinical course, SMA is divided into three types:

1. Type I (Werdnig–Hoffmann disease): Infantile age
2. Type II (Kugelberg-Welander disease): Juvenile SMA
3. Type III: More adult pattern

The children present with weakness, flaccidity, and atrophy of the proximal limbs initially and have difficulty in walking, climbing, and lifting. Fasciculation is present in about 50% of the cases.

Cardiac manifestations are more common in type II/III SMA and is usually in the form of arrhythmias viz. atrial fibrillation, premature beats, atrial flutter, or AV block, at times requiring pacemakers. Some cases are also associated with DCM.[65] Recent reports have found a higher incidence of structural heart defects such as ASDs and VSDs and complex ones such as hypoplastic left heart syndrome, indicating a defect in cardiogenesis.[66]

CONCLUSION

Cardiovascular manifestations are varied and may be seen in association with many systemic illnesses. Often, treatment of the primary disease is therapeutic for the cardiac pathology, though many conditions warrant only symptomatic or supportive cardiac therapy. However, increasingly, there is evidence that cardiac involvement may precede or progress along with the systemic illness and cardiac involvement may be diagnosed early thereby promoting early diagnosis and early treatment of the systemic illness. The adage goes "Fore warned is better armed" and hence it behooves the clinicians to be aware of the cardiac manifestations of systemic illnesses that children commonly present with, to ensure the best outcome for the patient.

REFERENCES

1. Hirschhorm R. Glycogen storage disease Type II. Acid alpha-glycosidase (acid maltase) deficiency. In: Scriber CR, Beaudet AL, Sly WS, et al. (Eds). The Metabolic and Molecular Bases of Inherited Disease, 7th edition. New York: McGraw-Hill; 1995. pp. 2443-64.
2. Forsha D, Li JS, Smith PB, van der Ploeg AT, Kishnani P, Pasquali SK, et al. Cardiovascular abnormalities in late-onset Pompe disease and response to enzyme replacement therapy. Genet Med. 2011;13(7):625-31.
3. Levine JC, Kishnani PS, Chen YT, Herlong JR, Li JS. Cardiac remodeling after enzyme replacement therapy with acid alpha-glucosidase for infants with Pompe disease. Pediatr Cardiol. 2008;29(6):1033-42.
4. Boffi L, Russo P, Limongelli G. Early diagnosis and management of cardiac manifestations in mucopolysaccharidoses: a practical guide for paediatric and adult cardiologists. Ital J Pediatr. 2018;44(Suppl 2):122.
5. Moder KG, Miller TD, Tazelaar HD. Cardiac involvement in systemic lupus erythematosus. Mayo Clin Proc. 1999;74(3):275-84.
6. Galve E, Candell-Riera J, Pigrau C, Permanyer-Miralda G, Garcia-Del-Castillo H, Soler-Soler J, et al. Prevalence, morphologic types and evolution of cardiac valvular disease in SLE. N Eng J Med. 1988;319(13):817-23.
7. Adrovic A, Dedeoglu R, Sahin S, Barut K, Koka A, Cengiz D, et al. Evaluation of pulmonary artery pressure in patients with juvenile systemic lupus erythematosus (jSLE). Bosn J Basic Med Sci. 2018;18(1):66-71.
8. Malleson PN, Sailor M, Mackinnon MJ. Usefulness of antinuclear antibody testing to screen for rheumatic diseases. Arch Dis Child. 1997;77(4):299-304.
9. Levesque K, Morel N, Maltret A, Baron G, Masseau A, Orquevaux P, et al. Description of 214 cases of autoimmune congenital heart block: results of the French neonatal lupus syndrome. Autoimmun Rev. 2015;14(12):1154-60.
10. Saxena A, Izmirly PM, Mendez B, Buyon JP, Friedman DM. Prevention and treatment in utero of autoimmune-associated congenital heart block. Cardiol Rev. 2014;22(6):263-7.
11. Buyon JP, Hiebert R, Copel J, Craft J, Friedman D, Katholi M, et al. Autoimmune associated congenital heart block. J Am Coll Cardiol. 1998;31(7):1658-66.
12. Gunal N, Kara N, Cakar N, Koçak H, Kahramanyol O, Cetinkaya E. Cardiac involvement in childhood poly arteritis nodosa. Int J Cardiol. 1997;60(3):257-62.
13. Kothari SS. Takayasu arteritis in children - a review. Images Paediatr Cardiol. 2001;3(4):4-23.
14. Ishikawa K. Diagnostic approach and proposed criteria for the clinical diagnosis of Takayasu arteriopathy. J Am Coll Cardiol. 1988;12(4):964-72.
15. Arend WP, Michel BA, Bloch DA, Hunder GG, Calobrese IH, Edworthy SM, et al. The American College of Rheumatology 1990 criteria for the classification of Takayasu arteritis. Arthritis Rheum. 1990;33(8):1129-32.
16. Bernstein B, Takahashi M, Hanson V. Cardiac involvement in juvenile rheumatoid arthritis. J Pediatrics. 1974;85(3):313-7.
17. Loeys BL, Dietz HC, Braverman AC, Callewaert BL, De Backer J, Devereux RB, et al. The revised Ghent nosology for the Marfan syndrome. J Med Genet. 2010;47(7):476-85.
18. Meshram RM, Patil A. Clinical profile and outcome of diphtheria in central India: a retrospective observational study. Int J Contemp Pediatr. 2018;5(4):1600-5.
19. Gundam BR, Sudarsi RK, Gundam A. Study of cardiac involvement in diphtheria. J Evid Based Med Healthc. 2016;3(61):3309-19.
20. Chokhandre M, Solomon R, Garekar S. Cardiac emergencies in countries with limited resources. In: Cardiac Emergencies in Children. New York: Springer International Publishing; 2018.
21. Pothapregada S, Kamalakannan B, Thulasingam M. Clinical profile of atypical manifestations of dengue fever. Indian J Pediatr. 2016;83(6):493-9.

22. Kirawittaya T, Yoon IK, Wichit S, Green S, Ennis F, Gibbons R, et al. Evaluation of cardiac involvement in children with dengue by serial echocardiographic studies. PLoS Negl Trop Dis. 2015;9(7):e0003943.
23. European Centre for Disease Prevention and Control. Paediatric inflammatory multisystem syndrome and SARS-CoV-2 infection in children – 15 May 2020. ECDC: Stockholm; 2020.
24. Wolfler A, Mannarino S, Giacomet V, Camporesi A, Zuccotti G. Acute myocardial injury: a novel clinical pattern in children with COVID-19. Lancet Child Adolesc Health. 2020;4(8):e26-7.
25. Verdoni L, Mazza A, Gervasoni A, Martelli L, Ruggeri M, Ciuffreda M, et al. An outbreak of severe Kawasaki-like disease at the Italian epicentre of the SARS-CoV-2 epidemic: an observational cohort study. Lancet. 2020; 395(10239):1771-8.
26. Shah I, Prabhu SS, V Sumitra, Shashikiran HS. Cardiac dysfunction in HIV infected children: a pilot study. Indian Pediatr. 2005;42(2):146-9.
27. Pugliese A, Isnardi D, Saini A, Raddino R, Torre D. Impact of highly active antiretroviral therapy in HIV positive patients with cardiac involvement. J Infect. 2000;40(3):282-4.
28. Feinstein M, Hsue P, Benjamin L, Bloomfield G, Currier J, Matthew S, et al. Characteristics, prevention, and management of cardiovascular disease in people living with HIV: a scientific statement from the American Heart Association. Circulation. 2019;140(2):e98-124.
29. Singh P, Hemal A, Agarwal S, Kumar D. Cardiac manifestations in HIV infected children. Indian J Pediatr. 2015;82(3):230-4.
30. Barbaro G. HIV-associated cardiomyopathy etiopathogenesis and clinical aspects. Herz. 2005;30(6):486-92.
31. Kumar P, Sharma S, Bisht D, Panwar R. Tuberculous dilated cardiomyopathy with myocarditis. Indian J Pediatr. 2020;87(2):161.
32. Gulati G, Kothari S. Diffuse infiltrative cardiac tuberculosis. Annals of Ped Card. 2011;4(1):87-9.
33. Doshi S, Ramakrishnan S, Gupta SK. Invasive hemodynamics of constrictive pericarditis. Indian Heart J. 2015;67(2):175-82.
34. Costello J, Alexander M, Greco K, Perez-Atayde A, Laussen P. Lyme carditis in children: presentation, predictive factors, and clinical course. Pediatrics. 2009;123(5):e835-41.
35. Mustafa S, Patra V, Sadat S Balaji P. Plasmodium vivax myocarditis in a child. Int Multidiscip Res J. 2011;1(7):45-6.
36. Khan FY. Imported Plasmodium vivax malaria complicated by reversible myocarditis. J Family Community Med. 2019;26(3): 232-4.
37. Arora A, Mudalgiri M, Sharma D, Porwal Y. Myocarditis with sinus exit block: a rare presentation of Plasmodium vivax malaria. 2019;10(1):39-41.
38. Alvarez MF, Bolívar-Mejía A, Rodriguez-Morales AJ, Ramirez-Vallejo E. Cardiovascular involvement and manifestations of systemic Chi[illegible] infection: a systematic review. F1000Res. 2017;[illegible].
39. Mirabel M, Vignaux O, Lebon P, Legmann P, Weber S, Meune C. Acute myocarditis due to Chikungunya virus assessed by contrast-enhanced MRI. Int J Cardiol. 2007;121(1):e7-8.
40. Mullerpattan JB, Udwadia ZF, Udwadia FE. Tropical pulmonary eosinophilia—a review. Indian J Med Res. 2013;138(3):295-302.
41. Agrawal A, Kumar A, Consul S, Yadav A. Scorpion bite, a sting to the heart!. Indian J Crit Care Med. 2015;19(4):233-6.
42. Shoreit AH, Eltayeb AA, Ali SS. Role of prazosin in management of scorpion sting in pediatrics: a comparative study. J Curr Med Res Pract. 2019;4(2):174-9.
43. Zhang R, Gupta D, Albert SG. Pheochromocytoma as a reversible cause of cardiomyopathy: analysis and review of the literature. Int J Cardiol. 2017;249:319-23.
44. DiGeorge AM, La Franchi S. Disorders of the thyroid gland. In: Kleigman RM, Arvin AM (Eds). Nelson Textbook of Pediatrics, Behrman E, 15th edition. Philadelphia: WB Saunders; 1996. pp. 1587-605.
45. Bharadva K, Mishra S, Tiwari S, Yadav B, Deshmukh U, Elizabeth KE, et al. Prevention of micronutrient deficiencies in young children: Consensus Statement from Infant and Young Child Feeding Chapter of Indian Academy of Pediatrics. Indian Pediatr. 2019;56(7):577-86.
46. Hassan Abu FN, Khalid Ibrahim ES, Hamdy S, Hosni B. Myocardial dysfunction in malnourished children. Annals of Ped Card. 2010; 3(2):113-8.
47. El Razaky O, Naeem A, Donia A, El Amrousy D, Elfeky N. Cardiac changes in moderately malnourished children and their correlations with anthropometric and electrolyte changes. Echocardiography. 2017;34(11):1674-9.
48. Dorman BH, Sade RM, Burnette JS, Wiles HB, Pinosky ML, Reeves ST, et al. Magnesium supplementation in the prevention of arrhythmias in paediatric patients undergoing surgery for congenital heart defects. Am Heart J. 2000;139(3):522-8.
49. Ho KM. Intravenous magnesium for cardiac arrhythmias: jack of all trades. Magnesium Research. 2008; 21(1):65-8.
50. Rosenblum H, Wessler JD, Gupta A, Maurer MS, Bikdeli B. Zinc deficiency and heart failure: a systematic review of the current literature. J Card Fail. 2020;26(2):180-9.
51. Chen J. An original discovery: selenium deficiency and Keshan disease (an endemic heart disease). Asia Pac J Clin Nutr. 2012; 21(3):320-6.
52. Burke MP, Opeskin K. Fulminant heart failure due to selenium deficiency cardiomyopathy (Keshan disease). Med Sci Law. 2002;42(1):10-3.
53. Hiffler L, Rakotoambinina B, Lafferty N, Martinez GD. Thiamine deficiency in tropical pediatrics: new insights into a neglected but vital metabolic challenge. Front Nutr. 2006:3:16.
54. Rao SN, Chandak GR. Cardiac beriberi: often a missed diagnosis. J Trop Pediatr. 2010;56(4):284-5.
55. Lonn E, Yusuf S, Arnold MJ, Sheridan P, Pogue J, Micks M, et al. Homocysteine lowering with folic acid and B vitamins in vascular disease. N Engl J Med. 2006;354(15):1567-77.
56. Øyen N, Olsen SF, Basit S, Leirgul E, Strøm M, Carstensen L, et al. Association between maternal folic acid supplementation and congenital heart defects in offspring in birth cohorts from Denmark and Norway. J Am Heart Assoc. 2019:8(6):e011615.
57. Bhagavan HN, Chopra RK. Potential role of ubiquinone (coenzyme Q10) in paediatric cardiomyopathy. Clin Nutr. 2005;24(3):331-8.
58. Shulman LN, Braunwald E, Rosenthal DS. Hematological-oncological disorders and heart disease. In: Braunwald E (Ed). Heart Disease: A Textbook of Cardiovascular Medicine, 5th edition. Philadelphia: WB Saunders; 1997. pp. 1786-805.
59. Murphy CJ, Oudit GY. Iron-overload cardiomyopathy: pathophysiology, diagnosis, and treatment. J Card Fail. 2010;16(11): 888-900.
60. Chanpura VR, Modi D. A study of echocardiographic changes in patients of thalassemia major. Int J [illegible] 2016; [illegible].
61. [illegible] Houghton M, Porter JB, Walker JM, Tanner MA, Patel J, et al. Cardiac T2* magnetic resonance for prediction of cardiac complications in thalassemia major. Circulation. 2009;120(20):1961-8.
62. Allen KY, Jones S, Jackson T, DeCost G, Stephens P, Hanna BD, et al. Echocardiographic screening of cardiovascular status in pediatric sickle cell disease. Pediatr Cardiol. 2009;40(8):1670-8.
63. Cheeran D, Khan S, Khera R, Bhatt A, Garg S, Grodin JL, et al. Predictors of death in adults with Duchenne muscular dystrophy-associated cardiomyopathy. J Am Heart Assoc. 2017;6(10): e006340.
64. Feingold B, Mahle WT, Auerbach S, Clemens P, Domenighetti A, Jeffries JL, et al. Management of cardiac involvement associated with neuromuscular diseases. A scientific statement from the American Heart Association. Circulation. 2017;136(13):e200-31.
65. Tanaka H, Uemeura N, Toyama Y, Kudo A, Ohkatsu Y, Kanehisa T. Cardiac involvement in the Kugel-Welander Syndrome. Am J Cardiol. 1976;38(4):528-32.
66. Wijngaarde CA, Blank AC, Stam M, Wadman RI, van den Berg LH, van der Pol WL. Cardiac pathology in spinal muscular atrophy: a systematic review. Orphanet J Rare Dis. 2017; 12(1):67.

Index

Page numbers followed by b refer to box, f refer to figure, fc refer to flowchart, and t refer to table.

A

B

C

D

E

F

G

H

I

Q

R

W

Y

Z